Child and Adolescent Drug and Substance Abuse

By offering unique analysis and synthesis of theory, empirical research, and clinical guidance in an up-to-date and unbiased context, this book assists health and social care professionals in understanding the use of drugs and substances of abuse by children and adolescents.

A comprehensive reference for health and social care professionals, the book identifies and corrects related false narratives and, with the use of the authors' combined experience of over 70 years of clinical and academic experience in drug and substance abuse, provides current pharmacotherapeutic and psychotherapeutic approaches for the treatment of alcohol or other dependence or use disorders among children and adolescents. The book also provides a useful reference for identifying brand/trade and street names of the drugs and substances of abuse commonly used by children and adolescents. Also included is a comprehensive, cross-referenced subject index.

Clear, comprehensive, accessible, and fully referenced, this book is an invaluable resource for professionals and students who aim to treat children and adolescents. *Child and Adolescent Drug and Substance Abuse* is the 19th clinical pharmacology and therapeutic text that the Pagliaros have written over the past 40 years and is the sixth that deals exclusively with drug and substance abuse.

Louis A. Pagliaro is Professor Emeritus, University of Alberta, and Co-Director of the Substance Abusology and Clinical Pharmacology Research Group. He was formerly a tenured, full professor in the Faculty of Education, Department of Educational Psychology, as well as in the Faculty of Pharmacy and Pharmaceutical Sciences, at the University of Alberta where he taught and supervised undergraduate and graduate students in the areas of drug and substance abuse and the biological basis of both clinical pharmacology and clinical psychology for over 30 years.

Ann Marie Pagliaro is Professor Emeritus, University of Alberta, and Co-Director of the Substance Abusology and Clinical Pharmacology Research Group. She was formerly a tenured, full professor in the Faculty of Nursing at the University of Alberta where she taught and supervised undergraduate and graduate students in the clinical treatment of drug and substance dependence or use disorders and the epistemology of drug and substance abuse.

Child and Adolescent Drug and Substance Abuse

A Comprehensive Reference Guide

Louis A. Pagliaro and Ann Marie Pagliaro

Routledge
Taylor & Francis Group
NEW YORK AND LONDON

First published 2020
by Routledge
52 Vanderbilt Avenue, New York, NY 10017

and by Routledge
2 Park Square, Milton Park, Abingdon, Oxon, OX14 4RN

Routledge is an imprint of the Taylor & Francis Group, an informa business

Library of Congress Cataloging-in-Publication Data
A catalog record for this title has been requested

ISBN: 978-1-138-54214-3 (hbk)
ISBN: 978-1-138-54215-0 (pbk)
ISBN: 978-1-351-00948-5 (ebk)

Typeset in Bembo
by Swales & Willis, Exeter, Devon, UK

To all children and adolescents, who have been harmed by their exposure to, or use of, the drugs and substances of abuse during the new millennium in the U.S. It is our hope that the information presented and discussed in this reference text will help to generate a greater awareness and deeper understanding of the nature and extent of this devastating epidemic. We trust that this increased awareness and understanding will significantly assist health and social care professionals, during the third decade of the new millennium, as they strive to stem the ever-growing tide of child and adolescent drug and substance abuse and lessen the associated pain and suffering experienced by these children and adolescents, as well as that of their families and communities.

LAP/AMP
2020

Contents

Illustrations

Figures

Tables

About the Authors

Louis A. Pagliaro is currently Professor Emeritus, University of Alberta, and Co-Director of the Substance Abusology and Clinical Pharmacology Research Group. He was formerly a tenured, full professor in the Faculty of Education, Department of Educational Psychology, as well as in the Faculty of Pharmacy and Pharmaceutical Sciences, at the University of Alberta where he taught and supervised undergraduate and graduate students in the areas of drug and substance abuse and the biological basis of both clinical pharmacology and clinical psychology for over 30 years. As a registered psychologist, he served a three-year elected term as president of the College of Alberta Psychologists. His area of specialty clinical psychology practice is the treatment of people across the lifespan who have refractory substance use disorders, including contemporaneous diagnoses.

Ann Marie Pagliaro is currently Professor Emeritus, University of Alberta, and Co-Director of the Substance Abusology and Clinical Pharmacology Research Group. She was formerly a tenured, full professor in the Faculty of Nursing at the University of Alberta where she taught and supervised undergraduate and graduate students, for over 30 years, in the areas of theory development and clinical practice with a primary focus on the prevention and treatment of alcohol and other dependence or use disorders across the lifespan—with particular attention to children and adolescents. Her specialty area of research continues to be the epistemological study of human drug and substance use and abuse.

The Pagliaros, full-time members of the academic staff at the University of Alberta from 1977 to 2008, taught thousands of students, published over 300 professional scientific articles, and extensively consulted for numerous governmental and professional organizations, locally, nationally, including the White House Office of Drug Abuse, and internationally. Six of their previous textbooks have focused explicitly on drug and substance abuse—two of which focused exclusively on children and adolescents and were published in 1996 and 2012 by John Wiley and Sons. Other books include: *Pagliaros' Comprehensive Guide to Drugs and Substances of Abuse* (1st and 2nd editions), which were published in 2004 and 2009, respectively, by the American Pharmacists Association; and *Women's Drug and Substance Abuse* (1st and 2nd editions), which were published by Brunner/Mazel and Routledge (Taylor & Francis) in 2000 and 2018, respectively. *Child and Adolescent Drug and Substance Abuse: A Comprehensive Reference Guide* is the 19th professional reference text, which the Pagliaros have co-edited or co-authored since 1979, with several having received prestigious publishing awards—including, in 2013, the "Choices Award" as an outstanding academic title, from the Association of College and Research Libraries. The Pagliaros have been married for 47 years.

Acknowledgments

First, we would like to share our appreciation and thank our many colleagues, students, and child, adolescent, and young adult patients (including, in numerous cases, their parents), who brought us to a better understanding of real-life experiences and the ramifications of drug and substance exposure or use. We have attempted to share this understanding with the readers of this text. The published clinical and other research cited in this reference text, and the lived experiences that have been shared with us over the past 40 years, have provided us with an appreciation of the truly devastating nature and extent of drug and substance abuse in the U.S. during the new millennium—as well as inspiration for the significant healing outcomes that can be achieved by children, adolescents, young adults, and their families and communities.

Second, we would like to share our appreciation to the dedicated staff at Routledge (Taylor & Francis), who directly contributed to the development and production of this reference text, particularly Amanda Devine, Emma Starr, Katherine Tsamparlis, Sonnie Wills, Abigail Stanley, and Ashley Thorpe.

Preface and Introduction

Children and adolescents[1] throughout the U.S., regardless of continental or other descent, culture, education, gender, religion, sexual orientation, or socioeconomic status, are exposed to, or actively use, various drugs and substances of abuse—abusable psychotropics (Figure P.1, Table P.1) These drugs and substances of abuse are used in a variety of ways that adversely affect their health, safety, and well-being. Their exposure to and use of these drugs and substances of abuse also adversely affect the health, safety, and well-being of their families, friends, schoolmates, and communities of which they are an integral part.

Consequently, a number of health and social care professionals who work to promote the optimal growth, development, and well-being of neonates/infants; children; adolescents; and young adults—including clinical or school psychologists; family counselors/therapists; family physicians; health psychologists; neurologists and neuropsychologists; nurses (e.g., community/public health; hospital; mental health; school nurses); obstetricians; pediatric nurse practitioners; pediatricians; pharmacists (both community and clinical or hospital/institutional pharmacists); and social workers (e.g., clinical social workers; medical or hospital social workers) require a specialized and unbiased reference source that provides up-to-date information on the statistics and trends concerning embryo/fetus, neonate/infant, child, adolescent, and young adult exposure to, or use of, the drugs and substances of abuse.

In addition, these health and social care professionals require critically reviewed, state of the art clinical strategies that directly assist them to:

1. Identify embryos/fetuses, neonates/infants, children, adolescents, and young adults a priori, who are at significant risk for exposure to, or use of, drugs and substances of abuse;
2. Assess and diagnose actual or potential exposure to, or use of, the drugs and substances of abuse with attention to the personal and social consequences of such use or exposure;
3. Provide efficacious treatment (i.e., empirically-based "best practices") for detected alcohol or other dependence or use disorder when encountered, including related contemporaneous diagnoses involving other dependence or use disorder(s), other mental disorders (e.g., anxiety disorders), and physical medical disorders (HIV/AIDS);
4. Monitor the efficacy of prevention and treatment approaches that have been implemented;
5. Appropriately modify or revise treatment approaches, as needed to prevent—or actively treat—recidivism (i.e., relapsed use).

1 "Childhood" is defined as the first decade of life, and, thus, includes boys and girls who are one to 10 years-of-age. Accordingly, "adolescence" is currently widely defined as the second decade of life, and, thus includes boys and girls who are 10 to 20 years-of-age. However, we also use, when necessary and appropriate, the more conventional related definitions, including: "neonate," covering the first 30 days of life; "infant," covering the first year of life; "toddler," covering one to three years-of-age; "preschooler," covering three to five years of age; "child," covering five to 12 years-of-age; "preadolescent," covering 12 to 13 years-of-age; "adolescent," covering 13 to 18 years-of-age, and "young, or emerging, adult," covering 18 to 25 years-of-age. In addition, to minimize any confusion regarding the research studies that we cite, we provide, whenever possible, the: (1) age ranges of research subjects or participants as specified by the authors of the study; and/or (2) reported primary and secondary school grade levels of subjects or participants, when provided.

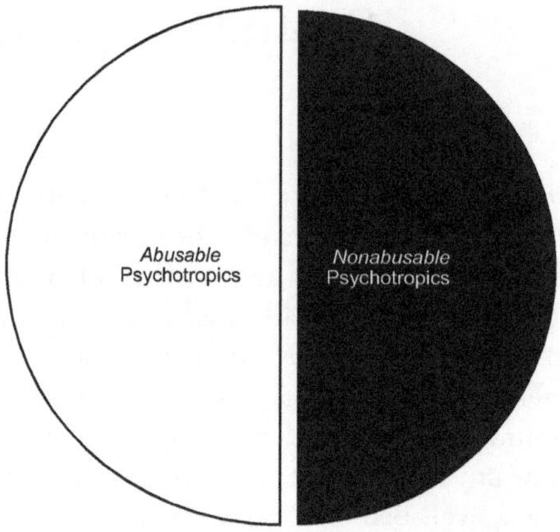

[a] The term, "psychotropics," refers to all exogenous substances (i.e., chemicals, including plant products, drugs, and xenobiotics) that: (1) elicit a direct effect on the CNS resulting in changes in cognition, learning, memory, behavior, perception, or affect; and (2) are used specifically for these major effects. The psychotropics can be further conveniently divided into either "abusable" or "nonabusable" psychotropics. The abusable psychotropics are represented by three classes of psychotropics—psychodepressants, psychostimulants, and psychodelics. (see Table P1.) The regular, long-term use of the abusable psychotropics is generally associated with the development of: (1) physical and/or psychological dependence characterized by (a) the need to use more and more of the drug or substance of abuse to achieve desired psychotropic actions (i.e., because of the development of tolerance); and (b) a withdrawal syndrome that occurs with the abrupt discontinuation of its regular, long-term use and that is immediately terminated when use is resumed.

The nonabusable psychotropics are represented by four classes of psychotropics—anticonvulsants, antidepressants, antiparkinsonians, and antipsychotics (see Table P.1). While used also for their major psychotropic actions, the nonabusable psychotropics have *not* been consistently associated with physical or psychological dependence and, thus, are *not* considered in this reference text. The proposed classification, presented here, has been found to be both accurate and parsimonious. However, because the term "abusable psychotropics" may be awkward for many readers, we consistently use the more common phrase, "drugs and substances of abuse" to denote this major class of chemicals, drugs, and xenobiotics.

Figure P.1 The Psychotropics

Obviously, an understanding of the unique nature of the use of drugs and substances of abuse—and their basic pharmacology and characteristics of use—is vital for the optimal professional practice of *all* health and social care professionals, who have an interest in, and/or provide direct care to, pregnant women, neonates/infants, children, adolescents, and young adults. However, a few specific examples are offered to help illustrate and support this claim. For example, this understanding will help to alert:

- All *Health and Social Care Professionals* to common patterns of adult violence and other criminal behavior perpetrated by parents, grandparents, and other family members (e.g., a mother's boyfriend or girlfriend; a step-parent; aunt or uncle), who are legally responsible for the protection of infants, children and adolescents in their care. These crimes typically involve exposure of children and adolescents to various: (1) drugs and substances of abuse; and (2) forms of physical, psychological, and sexual abuse. For example, in one such case, reported by Phillips (2016), a methamphetamine-abusing mother and her boyfriend drugged her young daughter with methamphetamine (just hours before the daughter's 10th birthday party), repeatedly sexually assaulted her, and then brutally stabbed her to death (see Chapter 2, "Amphetamine and Cocaine").

Table P.1 Major Psychotropic Classes and Subclasses[2]

Major Abusable Psychotropic Classes & Subclasses	
1. Psychodepressants	OPIATE ANALGESICS (e.g., codeine; fentanyl [Actiq®]; heroin; hydrocodone [Hysingla ER®]; meperidine [Demerol®]; morphine [MS Contin®]; oxycodone [OxyContin®]; oxymorphone [Numorphan®]; pentazocine [Talwin®])
	SEDATIVE-HYPNOTICS (e.g., barbiturates; benzodiazepines; z-drugs; miscellaneous sedative-hypnotics (e.g., alcohol [beer, wine, distilled liquor]; gamma-hydroxybutyrate [GHB]; suvorexant [Belsomra®])
	VOLATILE SOLVENTS & INHALANTS (e.g., gasoline; glue)
2. Psychostimulants	MISCELLANEOUS PSYCHOSTIMULANTS (e.g., amphetamines; caffeine; cocaine; nicotine [Tobacco])
3. Psychodelics	MISCELLANEOUS PSYCHODELICS (e.g., cannabis [i.e., marijuana, hashish, hash oil]; lysergic acid diethylamide [LSD]; mescaline [*peyote*]; methylenedioxymethamphetamine [MDMA]); phencyclidine [PCP]; psilocin, psilocybin ["magic mushrooms"]
Major Nonabusable Psychotropic Classes & Subclasses	
1. Anticonvulsants	MISCELLANEOUS ANTICONVULSANTS[3] (e.g., carbamazepine [Tegretol®]; phenytoin [Dilantin®]; primidone [Mysoline®]; valproic acid [Depakene®])
2. Antidepressants	MONOAMINE OXIDASE INHIBITORS (e.g., moclobemide [Manerix®]; phenelzine [Nardil®]; tranylcypromine [Parnate®])
	SELECTIVE SEROTONIN REUPTAKE INHIBITORS (e.g., Fluoxetine [Prozac®]; paroxetine [Paxil®]; sertraline [Zoloft®])[4]
	TRICYCLIC ANTIDEPRESSANTS (e.g., Amitriptyline [Elavil®]; desipramine [Norpramin®]; imipramine [Tofranil®]; Nortriptyline [Aventyl®])
	MISCELLANEOUS ANTIDEPRESSANTS (e.g., Amoxapine [Ascendin®]; Bupropion [Wellbutrin®]; maprotiline [Ludiomil®])
3. Antiparkinsonians	MISCELLANEOUS ANTIPARKINSONIANS (e.g., amantadine [Symmetrel®]; levodopa [Dopar®]; selegiline [Elderly®]; trihexyphenidyl [Artane®])
4. Antipsychotics	MISCELLANEOUS ANTIPSYCHOTICS (e.g., chlorpromazine [Thorazine®]; clozapine [Clozaril®]; Haloperidol [Haldol®]; olanzapine [Zyprexa®]; risperidone [Risperdal®])

2 Also see Figure P.1 "The Psychotropics."

3 Some abusable psychotropics (e.g., barbiturates; benzodiazepines) are clinically used as anticonvulsants. However, the listed anticonvulsants are not used as abusable psychotropics.

4 N.B. Generally, these antidepressants are considered to be, and are classified as, "nonabusable psychotropics." However, because of their mechanism of action, which is similar to the amphetamines and cocaine, they can be abused—although, rarely (Pagliaro & Pagliaro, 1993).

Also presented and discussed are patterns of criminal or violent behavior among adolescents—classmates, friends, siblings, and peers—that are associated with the use of the drugs and substances of abuse. For example, the use of:

1. Alcohol, gamma-hydroxybutyrate (GHB), or flunitrazepam ("Roofies") to perpetrate date-rape in the context of attending parties and raves. In addition, dating violence is both significant and increasing during the new millennium among U.S. high school students, particularly in the context of "episodic heavy drinking" (Black, Noonan, & Legg, 2006, p. 532) and the nonmedical use of prescription drugs (e.g., Clayton, Lowry, & Basile, 2017). (Also see Chapter 1, "Alcohol," Chapter 5, "Prescription Opiate Analgesics and Heroin," and Chapter 6, "Prescription-Sedative Hypnotics," for additional information and discussion.);
2. Amphetamines, cocaine, or phencyclidine (PCP),[5] which can cause, or exacerbate, violent behavior that can, and increasingly does, result in homicide (e.g., Pagliaro & Pagliaro, *Clinical Patient Data Files*; Salas-Wright, Vaughn, & Reingle Gonzalez, 2016). (Also see Chapter 2, "Amphetamines and Cocaine," and Chapter 4, "Cannabis and Other Psychodelics.")

In a related vein, it should be noted that adolescents are rarely criminally tried and sentenced as adults.[6] However, within the U.S. juvenile justice system, adolescents are increasingly being tried and sentenced to serve time in juvenile detention centers—often for drug trafficking-related crimes (e.g., selling crack cocaine on the street corner as a member of a criminal youth gang; transporting illicit drugs and substances of abuse from a drug dealer, who often is located in the "inner city," to users, who often are located in the "suburbs"). Sometimes, this transporting of drugs and substances of abuse occurs in the context of crossing international borders from, for example, Canada or Mexico to the U.S.—as noted, in a related article, by the Associated Press (2012):

> The U.S. Immigration and Customs Enforcement says that between 2008 and 2011, the number of youths aged 14 to 18 caught trying to cross the border between Tijuana and San Diego to sell drugs has grown tenfold … Most of them were high school students who carried drugs, usually methamphetamine or cocaine, hidden in their bodies or in their cars.
>
> (pp. 1-2)

In addition, adolescents, who are incarcerated in juvenile detention facilities, are at significantly higher risk for alcohol or other dependence or use disorder(s) (i.e., disorders that require active treatment) than are non-incarcerated youth (Sattler, 2017).

- *Health/Clinical/School Psychologists* to consider alcohol or other dependence or use disorder(s) as possible explanations for problem behavior (e.g., amotivational syndrome associated with cannabis use; decreased academic performance) or other dependence or use disorders that may be involved, or masked, such as:

5 For example, adolescent boys of Hispanic descent commonly use PCP deliberately to demonstrate to their peers—usually fellow criminal youth gang members—how "macho," or brave, they are (i.e., by being able to handle the often associated bizarre, unpredictable, and violent behavior associated with PCP use) (Pagliaro & Pagliaro, *Clinical Patient Data Files*). (Also see Chapter 4, "Cannabis and Other Psychodelics" for further related discussion.)

6 Trying an adolescent as an adult, is generally contingent on the nature, severity, and context of the crime committed—with most such cases involving a particularly violent or brutal offense (Pagliaro & Pagliaro, *Clinical Patient Data Files*; Rovner, 2017).

1. Anxiety disorders associated with excessive drinking of caffeinated beverages, including coffee, and, in particular, energy drinks;
2. Major depressive disorder associated with alcohol dependence or use disorder, which has been significantly related to suicide attempts and completions, particularly among Alaska Native and American Indian youth, who live on reservations (e.g., McGreal, 2015; Pagliaro & Pagliaro, *Clinical Patient Data Files*; Suicide Prevention Resource Center, 2013);
3. Psychotic disorders (e.g., cannabis-induced psychosis)—once rare in the U.S., but which now appear to be increasing among American adolescents in conjunction with the use of increasingly potent marijuana that now contains significantly higher tetrahydrocannabinol (THC) concentrations (Pagliaro & Pagliaro, 2012).

(See Chapter 1, "Alcohol;" Chapter 3, "Caffeine and Nicotine;" and Chapter 4, "Cannabis and Other Psychodelics.")

Health/Clinical/School psychologists also will be alerted to the fact that, while drugs and substances of abuse can cause, or exacerbate, mental disorders, they can also mask them. This clinical consideration becomes particularly significant in the context of the often-reported research finding that "approximately half of individuals with mental disorders have a comorbid drug and substance abuse diagnosis" (McClean, Anspikian, & Winters, 2014, p. 16).

- *Neurologists/Neuropsychologists* to child and adolescent exposure to, and use of, the drugs and substances of abuse (e.g., alcohol; methamphetamine; methylenedioxymethamphetamine [MDMA]) and the development of associated neurotoxicities. Depending on several factors—including the: (1) age of the child or adolescent—and related maturational brain development; (2) inherent neurotoxicity of the specific drug or substance of abuse; (3) extent of drug or substance use (i.e., dose; duration of use); and (4) risk factors, such as the concurrent exposure to, or use of, other neurotoxic drugs and substances of abuse—the drug or substance of abuse-related neurotoxicity can be either temporary (i.e., last for a few hours or days) or permanent (i.e., persist for long after the use of the drug or substance of abuse has been discontinued) (e.g., Bourgue, Baker, & Dagher, 2016; Pagliaro & Pagliaro, 2012; Shrot, Poretti, & Tucker, 2017).
- *Nurses* to the accidental injuries and adverse health consequences, including physical trauma and death, associated with child and adolescent use of the various drugs and substances of abuse. For example, to the prevention of contagious infections (e.g., hepatitis; HIV) that are commonly associated with: (1) the sharing of contaminated intravenous needles and syringes; (2) common use of a hookah mouthpiece during group cannabis smoking sessions; and (3) unprotected sex with multiple partners—as occurs, for example, in the context of both "sex-for-drug" exchanges and hazardous alcohol and other drug and substance use, particularly among high school students and "street-kids" (e.g., Fairbairn, Wood, & Dong, 2017; Lubman, Hides, & Yucel, 2007; Pagliaro & Pagliaro, 2012, 2018; Simmons & Suarez, 2016).[7]
- *Obstetricians* and *Nurse Midwives* to focus more attention on the prevention of teratogenic pathology related to maternal use of drugs and substances of abuse while pregnant (e.g., the FAS/FASD identified among neonates whose mothers drank

7 With this context in mind, we would encourage nurses to routinely screen all children and adolescents, who present with alcohol or other dependence or use disorders, for a history of violence, including physical and/or sexual abuse, as well as for sexually transmitted diseases (e.g., gonorrhea; hepatitis; human immunodeficiency virus [HIV] infection).

alcohol during their pregnancies). The signs and symptoms associated with FAS/FASD, as well as the clinical guidelines for its diagnosis (Hoyme, Kalberg, & Elliott, 2016), are presented and discussed. In addition, because of the significant escalation in opiate analgesic (e.g., oxycodone [Oxycontin®]) use (Pagliaro & Pagliaro, *Clinical Patient Data Files)*, among pregnant women in the U.S. during the new millennium, including adolescent girls, (e.g., Maguire, Taylor, & Armstrong, 2016; Pagliaro & Pagliaro, 2012, 2018), the American College of Obstetricians and Gynecologists recommended that "screening for substance use should be part of comprehensive obstetric care" (ACOG, 2017, p. 2). (See Chapter 1, "Alcohol," and Chapter 5, "Prescription Opiate Analgesics and Heroin").

- *Pharmacists* to be alert to adolescent or parent/caregiver "double doctoring," or "physician shopping," to obtain prescription drugs and substances of abuse (e.g., benzodiazepines; medical marijuana; prescription opiate analgesics) for personal use or for selling or trading for money, sexual favors, or other drugs and substances of abuse. For example, an adolescent selling his legitimate mixed amphetamines (Adderall®) prescription, which he received from his physician for the management of his attention-deficit/hyperactivity disorder (ADHD), to a friend at school to obtain money needed to purchase cannabis or methylenedioxymethamphetamine (MDMA) (i.e., "Ecstasy") for his own personal use at an upcoming rave. (See Chapter 2, "Amphetamines and Cocaine" and Chapter 4, "Cannabis and Other Psychodelics," for further information and discussion). Pharmacists also need to be aware of other related situations—such as a child, who has Type 1 diabetes mellitus, giving, selling, or trading her injection supplies (i.e., insulin needles and syringes) to her siblings, friends, or parents to inject heroin or prescription opiate analgesics (Pagliaro & Pagliaro, *Clinical Patient Data Files)*.

In addition, pharmacists need to be aware of potential and actual problems related to significant drug interactions, including the risk for fatal respiratory depression associated with using licit and illicit psychodepressant drugs—such as alcohol and prescription sedative-hypnotics (e.g., benzodiazepines) —together, and the risk for fatal overdosage. Related knowledge also is necessary to alert pharmacists, as well as other health care professionals, who work in drug information and/or poison control centers, to the rapidly increasing potential for the lethal exposure, both deliberate (i.e., suicide attempt) and unintentional (i.e., accidental poisoning), of children and adolescents to various drugs and substances of abuse (e.g., cocaine; heroin; methamphetamine) (e.g., Love, Davidson, & Valenti, 2014; McQuaid, 2017). For example, it has been noted that:

> Between 2000 and 2015, poison control centers in the United States received 188,468 calls about prescription opioid exposures in children and adolescents.
>
> (Reuters, 2017, p. 1)

- *Physicians* to *rule-out* the use of drugs and substances of abuse when diagnosing, prescribing, and monitoring medical problems among neonates/infants, child, adolescent, and young adult patients. It also alerts them to focus more carefully on the prevention of associated pathology (e.g., teratogenesis, such as the FAS/FASD; occurrence of the Neonatal Abstinence Syndrome [NAS]; sudden death; unexplained injuries) (e.g., Fischbach, 2017; Maguire, Taylor, & Armstrong, 2016). Related issues, such as the over-prescription of amphetamines to children and adolescents for the management of ADHD or opiate analgesics to adolescents for the management of chronic pain related to sports and other injuries, also are discussed. (See Chapter 2,

"Amphetamines and Cocaine," and Chapter 5, "Prescription Opiate Analgesics and Heroin," for additional related information and discussion.)
- *Social Workers* to investigate possible high-risk social dysfunction among children and adolescents, as well as their families. For example, the investigation of physical or sexual abuse of a child by a parent or the involvement of an adolescent in a criminal youth gang (e.g., Palmer, 2015; Walsh, MacMillan, & Jamieson, 2003). It also will help to facilitate their critical and accurate appraisal of social influences that may require attention and modification in order to decrease potential harm to children and adolescents and their families (e.g., living in a home that is used as either a marijuana "grow-op" or as a Mom and Pop "meth lab") (Butterfield, 2004; Pagliaro & Pagliaro, *Clinical Patient Data Files*.)

> Sandra Rupert, a counselor at an elementary school in this town tucked high up in the Blue Ridge Mountains, wondered last year about two sisters who were second and third graders. They had headaches, colds and coughs virtually every day. Sheriff Mark Shook found the explanation when he raided the children's home and discovered their mother and her boyfriend were cooking methamphetamine in the attic, next to where the girls slept.
>
> (Butterfield, 2004, p. 1)

In this context, it is informative to note that "the opioid crisis has caused more children than ever to be placed into the foster care system [in the U.S.]" (Cox, 2017, p. 3). In addition:

> Opioid overdoses have claimed more than 300,000 lives in the last 15 years, including some 33,000 in 2015 alone. But those numbers do not tell the full horror of this epidemic, which has devastated the lives of countless children whose parents have succumbed to addiction to prescription painkillers and other opiates. In one terrible case last month, a Pennsylvania couple died of apparent overdoses, and their baby perished from starvation a few days later.
>
> (The Editorial Board, 2017, p. 1)

Finally, as noted by Butchart and Poznyak (2006):

> Harmful alcohol use by parents and caregivers can impair their sense of responsibility and reduce the amount of time and money available to spend on the child. In such cases children's basic needs can be neglected.
>
> (p. 2)

As reported in a related news article:

> The youngest casualties of Florida's drug culture include Evan Longanecker, almost 2 months old when he was smothered by his drug-abusing mother, who passed out while breastfeeding him; 7-month-old Ella Moon Martin, whose mom stashed her pot in the baby's diaper bag; and Logan Suber, a 2-month-old who died in a barn surrounded by his mother's drugs and paraphernalia.
>
> (Marbin Miller & Burch, 2014, p. 1)

See Chapters 1, "Alcohol," 2, "Amphetamines and Cocaine," and 5, "Prescription Opiate Analgesics and Heroin," for additional related information and discussion.

Consequently, health and social care professionals desperately require, but, unfortunately, do not currently have, ready access to an objective and unbiased, reference—a scholarly reference that presents a deep depth and wide breadth of knowledge. The purpose of *Child and Adolescent Drug and Substance Abuse: A Comprehensive Reference Guide* is to fill this void of required knowledge (i.e., current and accurate information and informed, reflective interpretation).[8]

Thus, it is our intention that this text assists readers to understand the medical and nonmedical (i.e., "recreational") use of the drugs and substances of abuse by children and adolescents in a current and unbiased context reflecting a comprehensive interpretation of the published research literature and other related available information (e.g., clinical case reports; related U.S. government reports). Additionally, we have ensured that the data presented to the reader is fully supported with extensive reference documentation that has been carefully and critically reviewed by the authors.

Since we began work on our first textbook, *Problems in Pediatric Drug Therapy*, the 1st edition of which was published by Drug Intelligence in 1979, the needs of readers and our approach to preparing professional clinical pharmacology and therapeutics texts for publication have changed dramatically. For example, at that time there were no such things as a personal computer, smart cellular telephone, or the internet.

Consequently, at that time, the primary challenge for clinicians—our primary intended audience—was obtaining relevant published research findings that could be appropriately applied in their respective areas of clinical practice. This challenge motivated us in the early 1970s to begin work on our first text. At that time, because the necessary data were not yet "online," we had to go through printed volumes of the Index Medicus, by hand, to find needed published journal article citations and, then, physically, go into the medical library stacks (i.e., the storage area for bound copies of published journals from the mid-1800s to date) to access, extract and compile the necessary data for the users of our texts.

Today, the challenge for us, and our readers, has significantly changed from too "little" available data (i.e., a paucity of data) to too "much" available data (i.e., a surfeit of data). Consequently, the major challenge now is not so much the search for relevant available

8 On this point, it should be made explicit that we tend to view the use of the various drugs and substances of abuse as being neither good nor bad, neither moral nor immoral. As scientists rooted in several views of science (e.g., positivism; post-positivism; post-modernism) and as expert clinicians, our focus instead is on evaluating the results of these sciences based on their inherent assumptions, methods, and claims to fact (i.e., inherent truth). Most importantly as subscribers to the scientist-clinician model, we are concerned with the contribution of a study or research program regarding its ability to further knowledge that will lead to valuable outcomes for embryos/fetuses, children, adolescents, and young adults regarding their use of the drugs and substances of abuse. Thus, we are concerned with the result of the interaction of the use of a drug or substance of abuse by a child or adolescent in a certain context (i.e., did an opiate analgesic [e.g., morphine] provide relief from intractable pain or did it cause death because of an overdosage?). Thus, for us, it is not the use of a certain drug or substance of abuse by a certain child or adolescent that is "good" or "bad." Rather, it is the result, or outcome, of the use of the drug or substance of abuse by a certain child or adolescent in a certain specific context that is "good" or "bad."

To emphasize this point, we have often compared, in our related lectures and discussions, drugs and substances of abuse to a writing pen, which—as an inanimate object—is neither inherently "good" nor "bad". For example, if the pen is used to write a helpful textbook, it may be "good." However, if it is used to deliberately poke someone in the eye, it may be "bad." The pen, as an inanimate object is devoid of inherent goodness or badness. Thus, it is how the pen is used that can be interpreted as being "good" or "bad." We believe that the same is true for the drugs and substances of abuse.

N.B. Although, as professional mental health care professionals, we deliberately refrain from passing personal judgment regarding individual decisions to engage in various patterns of using drugs and substances of abuse, including "recreational use," these comments should not be interpreted, or construed in any manner, as an endorsement for this use.

Table P.2 Examples of "Common Misbeliefs" Discussed in the Text

Common Misbelief: Since the beginning of the new millennium, child and adolescent drug and substance abuse significantly decreased.
Common Misbelief: Children are not generally involved in the new millennial opioid epidemic in the U.S.
Common Misbelief: Regarding drug and substance abuse in the U.S., boys, overwhelmingly, outnumber girls.
Common Misbelief: Children and adolescents of certain continental or other descents are immune to drug and substance abuse.
Common Misbelief: Children and adolescents, who do become involved in drug and substance abuse, are primarily found in inner cities among families that are socioeconomically disadvantaged.
Common Misbelief: Effective drug and substance abuse prevention and treatment programs for children and adolescents are extremely limited in the U.S.
Common Misbelief: Most urban high school students who seek drugs and substances of abuse often find it hard to get them.

data of importance for the development of our ideas and texts, but, instead, it is the compilation, sorting, analysis, interpretation, reflection, synthesis, and assimilation from a virtual mountain of readily available data[9]—some relevant, much not; some accurate, much not; some useful, much not—into what is more valid, more reliable, more true, and most useful for clinical application before it is shared with the reader.

In addition to being of benefit to health and social care professionals, this text also should be of benefit to students who are assimilating knowledge in their respective fields of professional study. Last, but not least, we trust that *Child and Adolescent Drug and Substance Abuse: A Comprehensive Reference Guide* also may be of benefit to health and social policy makers (e.g., government officials, such as the Surgeon General; public health administrators, such as the members of boards of public health or health care authorities) who must increasingly address both the direct and indirect health and social consequences

9 For example, the input of a single "search term"–such as the name of a drug or substance of abuse–into a standard computer search engine will typically result in tens of thousands of apparently relevant "hits" (sometimes hundreds of thousands). How then does the reader select which citations (i.e., "hits") to use—particularly when the data presented in one citation contradict that which are found in another citation?

and costs[10] associated with the use of the various drugs and substances of abuse by children and adolescents; and then appropriately deal with the related significant adverse impact on all levels, and for all segments, of society in the U.S.

Also, the information presented in this text, which has been obtained from a wide variety of carefully selected sources and, subsequently, analyzed and/or synthesized, provides these health and social policy administrators with the status of child and adolescent drug and substance abuse in the U.S. during the new millennium—and identifies associated significant changes and trends that have occurred. One such change has been, for example, increasing use, particularly by adolescents, of drug and substance abuse-related sites on the "dark net" (e.g., "Silk Road;" "Valhalla;" and "Wall Street Market") (Gabler & Harris, 2017; Popper, 2019; Popper & Ruiz, 2017) from which they obtain information (often erroneous) concerning the production of the drugs and substances of abuse (e.g., hashish oil; methamphetamine) and/or directly purchase drugs—often utilizing "bitcoins."

Finally, throughout the text we have identified several "Common Misbeliefs" that have been widely promulgated and incorrectly accepted as "true"—by adolescents and other members of the lay public, as well as by many health and social care professionals. With current research findings and our own comprehensive analysis and reflective synthesis, we rectify these "common misbeliefs" for readers (see Table P.2 for several examples).

Also, as a pedagogical aid to facilitate application of knowledge directly to clinical practice, we have included throughout the text, "Related Professional Reminders." These represent a distillation and summary of approaches, reminders, and techniques—based both upon the published clinical literature and our own related clinical practice experiences—that are meant to assist clinicians to better understand and treat alcohol and other dependence or use disorder(s). In addition, we illustrate and make explicit (i.e., define), as related to the discussion in each chapter, the "secret language," or argot (e.g., "8-ball," "Molly," "pocket shot"), associated with the drugs and substances of abuse and their usage trends by children, adolescents, and young adults.

Data for this text have been purposely obtained from a variety of computerized database sources (e.g., CINAHL®; PubMed®; PsycINFO®) utilizing available internet search engines (e.g., BING®; Google®; YAHOO!®) to more accurately reflect the diverse scientific findings, theoretical orientations, and clinically relevant views that exist in our study of child and adolescent drug and substance abuse in the U.S. during the new millennium.

Organization

Child and Adolescent Drug and Substance Abuse: A Comprehensive Reference Guide, begins with a "Dedication" that presents the authors' commitment to the purpose and goals of the text. Following the dedication, is the Front Matter, which includes the: (1) Table of Contents; (2) About the Authors, which provides a synopsis of the relevant background of the authors; and (3) Preface and Introduction, which explains the nature, focus, and style of the text and provides an overview of, and glimpse into, the contents of each of the six chapters of this reference text. Each chapter focuses on specific drugs and substances of abuse and their use during the first and second decades of the new millennium, 2000 to 2020, in the U.S.:

10 These costs are: (1) biological (e.g., physical injuries to body systems, such as lung cancer related to tobacco smoking, which usually begins during adolescence); (2) psychological (e.g., emotional distress and mental disorders, such as amphetamine-related psychosis or cannabis-related memory impairment); and (3) sociological (e.g., child neglect and family violence related to the use of the drugs and substances of abuse, particularly alcohol, cocaine, or methamphetamine, by parents). In addition, a significant monetary cost is associated with drug and substance abuse in the U.S. As noted by the National Institute on Drug Abuse (NIDA, 2017):

> Abuse of tobacco, alcohol, and illicit drugs is costly to our Nation, exacting more than $740 billion annually in costs related to crime, lost work productivity and health care.
>
> (p.1)

Chapter 1, "Alcohol;" Chapter 2, "Amphetamines and Cocaine;" Chapter 3, "Caffeine and Nicotine;" Chapter 4, "Cannabis and Other Psychodelics;" Chapter 5, "Prescription Opiate Analgesics and Heroin;" and Chapter 6, "Prescription Sedative-Hypnotics."

Each of the chapters differs in length due to the variability of available and current relevant data. However, they follow the same general outline in relation to organization, levelling, depth, scope, and comprehensiveness. Additionally, Chapter 1, "Alcohol," is significantly longer than the other chapters. Being the first chapter in this reference text, it serves as the general model for needed information that applies to, and is further elaborated upon, in the later chapters, including the overview and discussion of the: (1) nine patterns of child and adolescent drug and substance abuse; (2) clinical approaches for assessing child and adolescent alcohol or other dependence or use disorders; (3) test statistics that can assist in the selection and use of available quick-screen psychometric tests for detecting adolescent and young adult alcohol or other dependence or use disorders; and (4) pharmacotherapy and psychotherapy/counseling approaches that have been found efficacious for treating children, adolescents, and young adults who have been diagnosed with alcohol or other dependence or use disorders.

Each of these chapters presents and discusses maternal exposure of embryos/fetuses during pregnancy and neonates/infants during breastfeeding. It also presents and discusses child, adolescent, and young adult exposure to—including overdosage/unintentional poisoning—and the medical and nonmedical (i.e. "recreational") use of these drugs and substances of abuse. As noted, for example, in relation to Chapter 1, "Alcohol:"

> These are soul-searching days in this Westchester County village, where teenage drinking has long been a fixture, as in other affluent suburbs. Last month's homecoming bacchanal here, which left scores of students falling-down drunk, 27 with three-day school suspensions and five hospitalized with acute alcohol poisoning, has Scarsdale shamefaced and reeling.
>
> (Gross, 2002, p. 1)

Remarks in a commentary by two physicians (Skolnik & Kiriakov, 2016) would tend to indicate that this pattern of alcohol use is not limited to Westchester County:

> Binge drinking is a common problem in adolescents as well as adults. In a 2013 survey, 60 million Americans, representing 22% of the population 12 years of age and older, engaged in binge drinking in the previous month. Among those 12–20 years of age, 14%, or one in seven, reported binge drinking ... Among young people who drink, a higher proportion drink heavily than among adult drinkers. For teenagers who drink, 28% to 60% report binge drinking [on at least one occasion]. Among high school seniors, 1 in 10 reports drinking more than 10 drinks in a row. The predominant liquor consumed by 13- to 20-year-olds is vodka (44%).
>
> (p. 1)

Each chapter begins with an introduction, including a brief history of the drugs and substances of abuse that are addressed in the chapter, followed by a thorough and current review of their general pharmacology, including: mechanisms of action; pharmacokinetics—absorption, distribution, metabolism, and excretion; drug-drug interactions; undesired, or harmful, effects and toxicities, including physical and psychological dependence; overdosage/unintentional poisoning; and effects of use during pregnancy and lactation.

New millennial trends in the use of the particular drugs and substances of abuse, which are addressed in the chapter, are then presented and discussed with particular attention to child and adolescent exposure and adolescent and young adult medical and nonmedical (i.e., "recreational") use. Attention is also given to genetic, psychological, and sociocultural factors that dissuade or conversely encourage use.

Each chapter also contains an in-depth, detailed section concerning the assessment and diagnosis of adolescent and young adult dependence or use disorders as related to the particular chapter. In addition, the use of DSM criteria and available quick-screen psychometric tests for detecting alcohol or other dependence or use disorders among adolescents and young adults are presented and discussed. A critical evaluation of the utility and limitations of DSM criteria and each of the psychometric-screening tests, including their appropriate use, administration, scoring, and associated statistics (i.e., measures of sensitivity, specificity, validity, and reliability) are included.

Attention also is given to the detection and occurrence of common contemporaneous diagnoses that, in addition to alcohol or other dependence or use disorders, concurrently involve: (1) other mental disorders, such as anxiety disorders, conduct disorder, eating disorders, major depressive disorder; and/or (2) physical medical disorders, such as direct or indirect, undesired, or harmful, effects and toxicities (e.g., accidental injury; HIV infection; STD) that can be acute or chronic. The occurrence of these disorders among children, adolescents, and young adults, as well as their interrelationship, are discussed with emphasis on the importance of accurate diagnoses, treatment selection, treatment implementation, and monitoring outcome. For example, as found by Weinberger, Platt, and Esan (2017):

> Continued smoking among smokers and smoking initiation among nonsmokers were associated with greater odds of SUD relapse.
>
> (p. e152)

This particular relationship between cigarette smoking (i.e., nicotine dependence or use disorder) and the occurrence of negative treatment outcomes for other SUDs also has been noted by others (e.g., Wilens, Biederman, & Martelon, 2016).

In another example involving of the relationship among alcohol or other dependence or use disorder and other mental disorders, Temcheff, Dery, and St. Pierre (2016) found an association between the diagnosis of conduct disorder in children and subsequent drug and substance abuse (e.g., alcohol and cannabis abuse). As reported by the researchers:

> These results suggest that conduct problems present in early elementary school can predict early initiation into potentially addictive behaviors among boys and girls.
>
> (p. 50)

The treatment section of each chapter focuses on the drugs and substances of abuse that are addressed in the chapter and age-appropriate secondary and tertiary prevention approaches for the pharmacotherapy and psychotherapy/counseling management of the diagnosed alcohol or other dependence or use disorder. Included in the treatment section of each chapter are established pharmacotherapeutic approaches for treating and managing adolescent alcohol or other dependence or use disorder(s) related to the drugs and substances of abuse addressed in the chapter, such as:

1. Assisted abstinence and replacement/substitution therapy (e.g., the use of nicotine products [Nicorette®; Nicotrol®] for tobacco smoking cessation programs);
2. Antidotes for acute overdosage (e.g., the use of naloxone [Narcan®] for opiate analgesic overdosage);
3. Treatment of withdrawal syndromes (e.g., the use of diazepam [Valium®] to prevent or manage sedative-hypnotic withdrawal syndrome).

Optimal current, evidence-based treatment protocols for specific dependence or use disorders associated with the drugs and substances of abuse that are addressed in the chapter, also are presented and discussed. For example, the use of buprenorphine versus morphine for the treatment of the neonatal abstinence syndrome (Kraft, Adenivi-Jones, & Chervoneva, 2017).

In addition, best practices also are presented and discussed regarding specific identified groups of children, adolescents, and young adults (e.g., boys of African continental descent [Flay, Graumlich, & Segawa, 2004][11]; LGBT youth [Aromin, 2016])—when these data are available.

The psychotherapy/counseling subsection presents and discusses behavioral approaches (e.g., cognitive-behavioral therapy), as well as family therapy; group therapy; social skills training; and short-term residential programs.

The text concludes with a comprehensive subject index. The index is extensively cross-referenced[12] and was carefully constructed by the authors to facilitate rapid and accurate retrieval of needed information by the readers. In addition to identifying the location of topics within the text, the index also contains: (1) abbreviations used in the text; and (2) common generic names, brand/trade names, and street names for both the illicit and licit drugs and substances of abuse discussed in this text.

Concluding Remarks

It is our hope that the information presented in this reference text will help health and social care professionals, students, and policy makers to better understand the:

1. Unique nature and extent of embryo/fetus, neonate/infant, child, adolescent, and young adult exposure to, and use of, the various drugs and substances of abuse in the U.S. during the new millennium;
2. Associated direct impact on the health, safety, and well-being, of this population group, as well as that of their families and communities.

By understanding the multitude of variables involved in child, adolescent, and young adult drug and substance abuse, and by applying the information presented in this text, it is our hope that health and social care professionals, students, and policy makers will be better able to provide appropriate and effective prevention and treatment services for children, adolescents, and young adults regarding their use of the various drugs and substances of abuse as the third decade of the new millennium begins.

It is our sincere desire that, by using the information presented in *Child and Adolescent Drug and Substance Abuse: A Comprehensive Reference Guide*—and working together, optimal health and well-being may be achieved by health and social care professionals for the countless numbers of embryos/fetuses, neonates/infants, children, adolescents, and young adults who, in various ways and to various degrees, have been, are, or will be adversely affected by the exposure to, or use of, the drugs and substances of abuse.

Louis A. Pagliaro
Ann Marie Pagliaro
2020

11 Interestingly, Flay, Graumlich, and Segawa (2004)—as have many others—demonstrated how specific treatment programs must be carefully selected and focused. As emphasized by the authors, while their program was quite successful for boys of African continental descent, "the lack of effects for girls [of African continental descent] deserves further research" (p. 377).

12 Extensive "cross-referencing" also has been used throughout the book—both within each chapter and, as appropriate, between chapters. This cross-referencing is generally denoted by the phrases, "See …" or "See also …"

References[13, 14, 15]

ACOG, American College of Obstetricians and Gynecologists, Committee Opinion No. 711. (2017). Opioid use and opioid disorder in pregnancy. *Obstetrics and Gynecology, 130*, e81–e94.

Aromin, R. A. (2016, December). Substance abuse prevention, assessment, and treatment for lesbian, gay, bisexual, and transgender youth. *Pediatric Clinics of North America, 63*(6), 1057–1077. doi:10.1016/j.pcl.2016.07.007

Associated Press. (2012, March 14). Mexico drug gangs using more children as "mules". *CBS News*, 1–4. Tijuana, Mexico. Retrieved August 2, 2017, from www.cbsnews.com/mexico-drug-gangs-using-more-children-as-mules/

Black, M. C., Noonan, R., & Legg, M. (2006, May 19). Physical dating violence among high school students– United States, 2003. *MMWR, Morbidity and Mortality Weekly Report, 55*(19), 532–535.

Bourgue, J., Baker, T. E., & Dagher, A. (2016, December 13). Effects of delaying binge drinking on adolescent brain development: A longitudinal neuroimaging study. *BMC Psychiatry, 16*(1), 445. doi:10.1186/s12888-016-1148-3

Butchart, A., & Poznyak, V. (2006). *Child Maltreatment and Alcohol.* Retrieved July 29, 2017, from WHO Facts on ... alcohol + violence: www/who.int/violence_injury_prevention/publications/violence/en/index.html

Butterfield, F. (2004, February 23). Home drug-making laboratories expose childen to toxic fallout. *The New York Times*, 1–5. Retrieved from www.nytimes.com/2004/02/232/us/home-drug-making-laboratories-expose-children-to-toxic-fallout.html

Clayton, H. B., Lowry, R., & Basile, K. C. (2017, December). Physical and sexual dating violence and nonmedical use of prescription drugs. *Pediatrics, 140*(6), e20172289. doi:10.1542/peds.2017-2289

Cox, E. (2017, June 22). The hidden victims of the opioid epidemic. *U. S. World and News Report.* Retrieved from www.usnews.com/topics/author/elaine-cox-md

Fairbairn, N., Wood, E., & Dong, H. (2017, April). Unsafe sexual behaviour associated with hazardous alcohol use among street-involved youth. *AIDS Care, 29*(4), 481–488. doi:10.1080/09540121.2016.1220480

Fischbach, P. (2017). The role of illicit drug use in sudden death in the young. *Cardiology in the Young, 27* (S1), S75-S79. doi:10.1017/S1047951116002274

Flay, B. R., Graumlich, S., & Segawa, R. (2004, April). Effects of 2 prevention programs on high-risk behaviors among African American youth: A randomized trial. *Archives of Pediatrics & Adolescent Medicine, 158*, 377–384.

Gabler, E., & Harris, R. (2017, July 20). On Reddit, intimate glimpses of addicts in thrall to opioids. *The New York Times*, 1–6. New York. Retrieved from www.nytimes.com/2017/07/20/us/opioid-reddit.html?rref=collection%2Ftimestopic%2FDrug%20Abuse%20Traffic&action=click&content.

Gross, J. (2002, October 8). Teenagers' binge leads Scarsdale to painful self-reflection. *The New York Times*, 1–5. Retrieved from www.nytimes.com/2002/10/08/nyregion/teenagers-binge-leads-to-painful-self-reflection.html

13 As per publisher style, only the first three authors are listed for each reference.

14 Several times the number of references listed were found, obtained, and analyzed by the authors during the preparation of this book. However, only the references that were cited at least once in the body of the text are included in the list. Major reasons for not citing other references, include that they: (1) did *not* provide any additional unique information or research findings; (2) were *not* well-researched or written (i.e., were evaluated as *not* being valid or reliable); (3) were based predominantly, or exclusively, on animal studies; (4) provided usage statistics from outside the U.S. or that focused exclusively on adults; and/or (5) were redundant with, or *not* as recent as, the already cited references.

15 The reference citation, "Pagliaro & Pagliaro, *Clinical Patient Data Files*," refers to unpublished data collected, with permission, over the last 50 years by the authors, in the formal course of their professional academic roles as clinician scientists and professors, from their patients, research subjects or participants, and students from the 1970s to date. Most of the related data previously have been made public (i.e., presented and discussed) in a wide and large number of formal academic presentations including: graduate seminars; grand rounds; guest lectures; and professional conference presentations.

Hoyme, H., Kalberg, W. O., & Elliott, A. J. (2016, August). Updated clinical guidelines for diagnosing fetal alcohol spectrum disorders. *Pediatrics*, *138*(2), e20154256. doi:10.1542/peds.2015-4256

Kraft, W. K., Adenivi-Jones, S. C., & Chervoneva, I. (2017, June 15). Buprenorphine for the treatment of the neonatal abstinence syndrome. *The New England Journal of Medicine*, *376*(24), 2341–2348. doi:10.1056/NEJMoa1614835

Love, C., Davidson, L., & Valenti, M. (2014, September 11). *Understanding the Connection between Suicide and Substance Abuse: What the Research Tells Us*. Rockville: SAMHSA.

Lubman, D. I., Hides, L., & Yucel, M. (2007, October). Intervening early to reduce developmentally harmful substance use among youth populations. *The Medical Journal of Australia*, *187*(7), S22-S25.

Maguire, D. J., Taylor, S., & Armstrong, K. (2016). Long-term outcomes of infants with neonatal abstinence syndrome. *Neonatal Network*, *35*(5), 277–286. doi:10.1891/0730-0832.35.5.277

Marbin Miller, C., & Burch, A. (2014, March 16). The littlest victims of Florida's drug binge. *Miami Herald*, 1–8. Retrieved July 30, 2017, from http://media.miamiherald.com/static/media/projects/2014/innocents-lost/stories/drugs/

McClean, J. M., Anspikian, A., & Winters, B. N. (2014). Factors that affect treatment initiation among individuals with serious mental illness and substance abuse disorder. *Addictive Diseases & Their Treatment*, *13*(1), 16–24.

McGreal, C. (2015, November 22). A reservation town fighting alcoholism, obesity and ghosts from the past. *The Guardian*, 1–15. Blackwater, Arizona. Retrieved July 30, 2017, from www.theguardian.com/us-news/2015/nov22/blackwater-arizona-native-americans-us-poorest-towns-

McQuaid, R. J. (2017, March 9). *Substance Use and Suicide Prevention among Youth: Prevention and Intervention Strategies*. Ottawa: Canadian Centre on Substance Abuse.

NIDA, National Institute on Drug and Substance Abuse. (2017, April). Costs of substance abuse. *Trends & Statistics*. National Institutes of Health. doi:www.drugabuse.gov/related-topics/trends-statistics

Pagliaro, A. M., & Pagliaro, L. A. (1996). *Substance Use among Children and Adolescents: Its Nature, Extent, and Effects from Conception to Adulthood* (1st ed.). New York, NY: John Wiley & Sons.

Pagliaro, A. M., & Pagliaro, L. A. (2000). *Substance Use among Women: A Reference and Resource Guide* (1st ed.). Philadelphia, PA: Brunner/Mazel (Taylor & Francis).

Pagliaro, A. M., & Pagliaro, L. A. (2018). *Women's Drug and Substance Abuse: A Comprehensive Assessment and Reflective Analysis* (2nd ed.). New York, NY: Routledge (Taylor & Francis).

Pagliaro, L. A., & Pagliaro, A. M. (1993). Fluoxetine abuse by an intravenous drug abuser. *The American Journal of Psychiatry*, *150*, 1898.

Pagliaro, L. A., & Pagliaro, A. M. (2004). *Pagliaros' Comprehensive Guide to Drugs and Substances of Abuse* (1st ed.). Washington, DC: American Pharmacists Association.

Pagliaro, L. A., & Pagliaro, A. M. (2009). *Pagliaros' Comprehensive Guide to Drugs and Substances of Abuse* (2nd ed.). Washington, DC: American Pharmacists Association.

Pagliaro, L. A., & Pagliaro, A. M. (2012). *Handbook of Child and Adolescent Drug and Substance Abuse: Pharmacological, Developmental, and Clinical Considerations* (2nd ed.). Hoboken, NJ: John Wiley & Sons.

Palmer, C. (2015, Spring). Drug trafficking, gang violence, and the U.S. immigration crisis. *Michigan Journal of Public Affairs*, *12*, 56–70.

Phillips, K. (2016, August 25). A girl was drugged with meth, abused and killed. One of the suspects: Her mother. *The Washington Post*, 1–3. Retrieved August 1, 2017.

Popper, N. (2019, June 11). Dark web drug sellers dodge police crackdowns. *The New York Times*, 1-4. Retrieved from https://www.nytimes.com/2019/06/11/technology/online-dark-web-drug-markets.html.

Popper, N., & Ruiz, R. R. (2017, July 20). 2 leading online black markets are shut down by authorities. *The New York Times*, 1–5. Retrieved from www.nytimes.com/2017/07/20/business/dealbook/alphabay-dark-web-opioids.html?rref=collection%2Ftimestopic%2FDrug%20Abuse%20and%.

Reuters. (2017, March 20). Studies shed light on opioid exposures among US children and young adults. Fox News. Retrieved from www.foxnews.com/health/2017/03/20/studies-shed-light-on-opioid-exposures-among-us-children-and-young-adults.html

Rovner, J. (2017). *Juvenile Life without Parole: An Overview*. Washington, DC: The Sentencing Project.

Salas-Wright, C. P., Vaughn, M. G., & Reingle Gonzalez, J. M. (2016). Attacks intended to seriously harm and co-occurring drug use among youth in the United States. *Substance Use & Misuse, 51*(13), 1681–1692.

Sattler, A. L. (2017, April). Treating youths in the juvenile justice system. *Pediatric Clinics of North America, 64*(2), 451–462. doi:10.1016/j.pcl.2016.11.012

Shrot, S., Poretti, A., & Tucker, E. W. (2017, April). Acute brain injury following illicit drug abuse in adolescent and young adult patients: Spectrum of neuroimaging findings. *The Neuroradiology Journal, 30*(2), 144–150. doi:10.1177/1971400917691994

Simmons, S., & Suarez, L. (2016, October). Substance abuse and trauma. *Child and Adolescent Psychiatric Clinics of North America, 25*(4), 723–734. doi:10.1016/j.chc.2016.05.006

Skolnik, N., & Kiriakov, D. O. (2016, February 16). *Binge Drinking in Adolescents*. Retrieved from Family Practice News: www.mdedge.com/familypracticenews/article/106533/mental-health/binge-drinking-adolescents?utm_source=TrendMD&utm_medium=TrendMD.

Suicide Prevention Research Center. (2013). *Suicide among Racial/Ethnic Populations in the U.S.: American Indians/Alaska Natives*. Waltham: Educational Development Center, Inc.

Temcheff, C. E., Dery, M., & St. Pierre, R. A. (2016, January). Precocious initiation into smoking, alcohol use, and gambling among children with conduct problems. *Canadian Journal of Psychiatry, 61*(1), 50–58. doi:10.1177/0706743715620402

The Editorial Board. (2017, January 16). Young victims of the opioid epidemic. *The New York Times*, 1–2. Retrieved from www.nytimes.com/2017/01/16/opinion/young-victims-of-the-opioid-epidemic.html

Walsh, C., MacMillan, H. L., & Jamieson, E. (2003). The relationship between parental substance abuse and child maltreatment: Findings from the Ontario Health Supplement. *Child Abuse & Neglect, 27* (12), 1409–1425.

Weinberger, A. H., Platt, J., & Esan, H. (2017, February). Cigarette smoking is associated with increased risk of substance use disorder relapse: A nationally representative, prospective longitudinal investigation. *Journal of Clinical Psychiatry, 78*(2), e152-e160. doi:10.4088/JCP.15m10062

Wilens, T. E., Biederman, J., & Martelon, M. (2016, October). Further evidence for smoking and substance use disorders in youth with bipolar disorder and comorbid conduct disorder. *Journal of Clinical Psychiatry*, 77(10), 1420–1427. doi:10.4088/JCP.14m09440

Epigraph[1]

For they have sown the wind, and they shall reap the whirlwind.
(Hosea 8:7)

1 This epigraph applies both to: (1) those who harmfully use the drugs and substances of abuse; and (2) those (e.g., family members; government agencies; health and social care professionals; teachers) who "turn a blind eye" to and, consequently, enable harmful drug and substance abuse.

1
Alcohol

Alcohol—whether provided by an older sibling, stolen from a parent's liquor supplies, purchased at a corner liquor store with a false I.D. or obtained by paying an adult standing outside of a liquor store, for a "six-pack" of beer—is widely used and abused by adolescents and young adults in the U.S. Whereas children often take a sip of a can of beer, while delivering it to a thirsty parent, "just to see what it tastes like," adolescents and young adults often drink large amounts of beer and other alcoholic beverages in small groups or at parties and celebrations to:

1. Achieve a desired dose-dependent disinhibition euphoria;
2. Attain a sense of well-being;
3. Be like "everyone else," whose "parents let them do it;"
4. Decrease social and sexual inhibitions;
5. Fit in with peers;
6. "Just have fun;"
7. Relieve anxiety, tension, or stress—to "cope" with "life's pains, disappointments, and impossible tasks."[1]

Unfortunately, the abuse of alcohol is associated with more harm than all of the other drugs and substances of abuse—combined.

In this chapter, we present and discuss alcohol with attention to its pharmacology—"pharmacodynamics" (i.e., mechanism of action); "pharmacokinetics" (i.e., absorption, distribution, metabolism, and excretion); and related undesired, or harmful, effects and toxicities. Also included in the pharmacology section are alcohol: drug–drug interactions; overdosage; and effects when used by adolescent girls and young women during pregnancy and lactation. We then present and discuss child alcohol exposure and patterns of adolescent and young adult alcohol use in the U.S., during the new millennium. The chapter concludes with a thorough discussion of the assessment, diagnosis, and treatment of alcohol dependence or use disorder (AUD) among children and adolescents.[2]

Pharmacologically, alcohol is classified as a psychodepressant that belongs to the "sedative-hypnotic" subclass, which also includes the prescription sedative-hypnotics (e.g., benzodiazepines;

1 The full quote from Sigmund Freud (1930/1989) is:

> Life as we find it, is too hard for us; it brings to many pains, disappointments and impossible tasks. In order to bear it we cannot dispense with palliative measures ... There are perhaps three such measures: powerful deflections, which cause us to make light of our misery; substitutive satisfaction, which diminish it; and intoxicating substances [e.g., alcohol], which make us insensible to it.

2 The terms (i.e., alcohol dependence or use disorder; AUD) subsume and replace the older established related term "alcoholism."

z-drugs).[3] However, we decided to separate alcohol from the prescription sedative-hypnotics and discuss it in its own chapter. There are several reasons for this decision, including the:

- Long history of medical and personal use of alcohol in the U.S.;
- Identification of alcohol as a neurotoxin in humans;
- Discontinued medical use of alcohol as a "psychostimulant" during the last century;
- Cultural inculcation of alcohol into social gatherings, parties, and celebrations in the U.S.;
- Potential for significant alcohol-related physical, mental, and social harm, including severe and irreversible teratogenic effects—Fetal Alcohol Syndrome/Spectrum Disorder (FAS/FASD)—when used by adolescent girls and young women during pregnancy;
- Use of alcohol, in the U.S., as a "rite of passage" from adolescence to adulthood;
- Current use of alcohol by more than 80% of adolescents and young adults in the U.S.

We begin with an overview and discussion of the pharmacology of alcohol.

Pharmacology

In this section we highlight the: basic chemistry; pharmacodynamics, or mechanism of action; pharmacokinetics; drug–drug interactions; and undesired, or harmful, effects and toxicities associated with alcohol use. Also discussed is alcohol overdosage and alcohol use during pregnancy and lactation.

Chemistry

In the scientific discipline of chemistry, "alcohol" is defined as any organic compound to which a hydroxyl (-OH) functional group is bound to a carbon atom. However, popularly it refers to beverage alcohol–ethyl alcohol or ethanol (Figure 1.1). Throughout this reference text, we use the word, "alcohol," to refer exclusively to beverage alcohol.

Beverage alcohol[4] is a colorless, flammable, and volatile liquid that is produced by fermenting various carbohydrate foodstuffs, including fruits, grains, and vegetables with the use of yeasts.[5, 6] Like other sedative-hypnotics, alcohol produces a progressive dose-related depression of the central nervous system (CNS) that ranges from mild sedation to deep sleep. Coma may rarely occur and can be fatal. These psychodepressant effects are generally predictable and depend on three major factors:

1. "Type" of the alcoholic beverage ingested (e.g., beer versus whiskey);
2. "Proof" (i.e., the equivalent to double the percentage concentration of the alcoholic beverage—for example, 40 proof indicates 20% alcoholic concentration);
3. "Amount" of the alcoholic beverage ingested (e.g., one can of beer or a six-pack of beer) per unit of time (e.g., hour, day, or week).

3 See the related discussion in Chapter 6, "Prescription Sedative-Hypnotics."

4 This form of alcohol is also used as: (1) a fuel; (2) an industrial solvent; and (3) a vehicle for various prescription and non-prescription drugs. These uses of alcohol are not further discussed in this chapter.

5 Yeasts are single cell fungi (genus, *Saccharomyces*) that are capable of fermenting (i.e., digesting or decomposing) carbohydrates (e.g., cellulose; starches; sugars) to ultimately produce alcohol, carbon dioxide, and water.

6 The concentration of the alcohol that is produced by fermentation is limited to approximately 16% because higher concentrations kill the yeast and, consequently, halt the fermentation process. To increase the alcohol concentration, for example, to 18%, as is done to produce sherry and other fortified wines, more alcohol is simply added to the already fermented product. Even higher concentrations of alcohol (e.g., concentrations of 30%, or higher) can be obtained by distilling the fermented product to obtain such distilled spirits as brandy and whiskey.

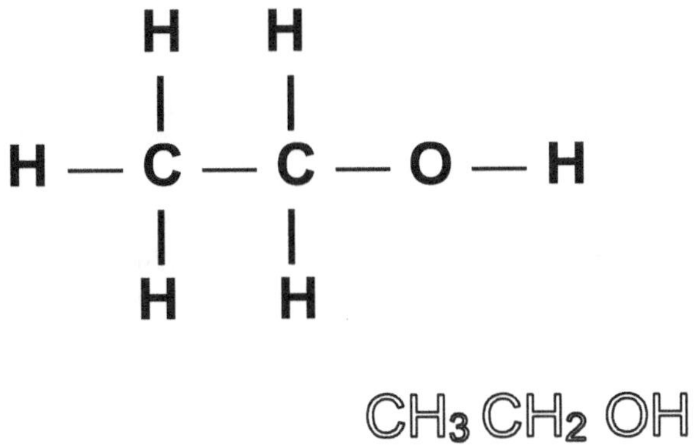

Figure 1.1 Chemical Structure of Alcohol

For further information regarding these factors, see the related discussion in the later section, "Blood Alcohol Concentrations."

Pharmacodynamics: Mechanism of Action and Blood Alcohol Concentrations

Common Misbelief: Alcohol is mostly used and abused for its psychostimulant actions.

Mechanism of Alcohol Actions

As recently as the last century, alcohol was considered to be a "psychostimulant" that was commonly used for such desired effects as to "have fun" and to "warm-up after coming in from the cold." It also was medically used for a variety of indications, including reviving someone who has fainted and treating the fatigue and weakness associated with cachexia. Although this belief was supported by lay and medical observations that drinking too much often resulted in such behaviors as taking off one's clothes and dancing naked on a table in a favorite bar or getting into a violent bar fight, alcohol possesses no psychostimulant actions (see the following subsection, "Blood Alcohol Concentrations").

Empirical findings in support of the psychodepressant actions of alcohol include the observation that as more alcohol is consumed during a drinking episode, drinkers do not become more wakeful, they become drowsier and, inevitably, uniformly fall asleep.

The exact mechanism of action by which alcohol depresses the entire CNS remains a mystery. However, research over the last several decades has resulted in two major plausible theories:

1. Alcohol readily crosses the blood-brain barrier disrupting the function of brain membrane lipids and glucose metabolism;
2. Alcohol acts at two specific receptor sites in the brain—gamma aminobutyric acid ($GABA_A$) receptor sites and N-methyl-D-aspartate (NMDA) receptor sites (e.g., Brower, 2001; Gonzales & Jaworski, 1997; Pagliaro & Pagliaro, 2009; Peoples, Li, & Weight, 1996).

While either theory may contribute to alcohol's actual mechanism of action, research in glucose metabolism supports the first theory, which also explains alcohol's effects on learning and memory. Research in support of the second theory suggests that alcohol acts to enhance GABAergic inhibition primarily by modifying the membrane environment of the $GABA_A$ receptor complex. This action significantly increases the affinity of the $GABA_A$ receptor complex for both endogenous (e.g., GABA) and exogenous sedative-hypnotics (e.g., barbiturates and benzodiazepines), thus, enhancing GABAergic inhibition.[7]

In addition, alcohol appears to inhibit the activity of glutamate, which is a naturally occurring excitatory neurotransmitter that functions largely at the NMDA receptors—as well as AMPA receptors and metabotropic glutamate receptors (mGluRs) (Gonzales & Jaworski, 1997). The regular, long-term use of alcohol results in "up-regulation of the NMDA receptors." The NMDA receptor has been posited, based on data obtained from laboratory animal studies, to play a significant role in both: (1) alcohol-induced neurotoxicity; and (2) the alcohol withdrawal syndrome, particularly the occurrence of withdrawal-related seizures (Chang-Mu, Jen-Kun, & Shing-Hwa, 2010; Charlton, Sweetnan, & Fitzgerald, 2002; Hoffman, 1995; Hoffman & Tabakoff, 1994). (For further related discussion of the $GABA_A$ receptor complex, see Chapter 6, "Prescription Sedative-Hypnotics.")

Additionally, other factors have been identified as contributing to both the pharmacological and toxicological effects related to alcohol use and withdrawal (Vezali Costardi, Teruaki Nampo, & Lourenco Silva, 2015). For example—regarding the serotonergic system:[8] (1) serotonin release and transmission are increased in the CNS by the acute administration of alcohol; (2) regular long-term, or chronic, use of alcohol leads to adaptive changes to the serotonin 5-HT_2 receptor (e.g., "up-regulation" or an increase in the number of 5-HT_2 receptors); and (3) serotonin levels are reduced during alcohol withdrawal (Lovinger, 1997; Tollefson, 1989).

Blood Alcohol Concentrations

Regardless of the actual mechanism of action, BACs that are associated with the amount of alcohol ingested during a drinking episode highly correlate with the direct and progressive depression of the CNS (Pagliaro & Pagliaro, 2009).[9] (See Table 1.1)

Lower BACs associated with the beginning of a drinking episode are often accompanied by excitement, happiness, and increased mental and physical activity. In fact, historically, these observed behaviors led researchers to commonly misclassify alcohol as a "psychostimulant" (see earlier related discussion). However, the stimulant-like behaviors were later found to be due to alcohol's general depression of the CNS—resulting in "disinhibition euphoria."

7 These posited actions of alcohol involving the $GABA_A$ receptor complex may also help to explain the: (1) development of tolerance to alcohol; and (2) cross-tolerance that is noted between alcohol and other sedative-hypnotics, specifically the barbiturates and the benzodiazepines—as well as the efficacy of these drugs in preventing/treating alcohol withdrawal (see related discussion in the later "Pharmacotherapy" sections—"Alcohol Tolerance" and "Alcohol Withdrawal Syndrome").

8 Serotonin has also been frequently associated with the positive pleasure and rewarding effects associated with alcohol use (Muller & Homberg, 2015; Schweighofer, Bertin, & Shishida, 2008).

9 The ingestion of a typical serving of alcohol (i.e., 12 fluid ounces of beer; five fluid ounces of wine; 1.5 fluid ounces of 80-proof distilled spirits) increases the BAC by approximately 0.02 gram% (i.e., 20 mg/100 ml of blood) in the average adolescent/young adult—traditionally calculated based on a 21-year-old male of European continental descent weighing 70 kg.

Table 1.1 Blood Alcohol Concentration (BAC) and Associated Physical and Mental Effects among Adolescents and Young Adults[10, 11]

BAC (gram % or grams per 100 ml)	*Physical Effects*	*Mental Effects*
0.01 to 0.03	Generally, *normal* appearance	Generally, *normal* behavior
0.03 to 0.06	Feel warm and relaxed with mild impairment of coordination and diminished ability to perform fine motor tasks	Mild euphoria (e.g., feelings of intense excitement and happiness) with decreased inhibitions and increased sociability and talkativeness Mild decreases in alertness and concentration
0.06 to 0.08	Increasing loss of coordination with a slight loss of both balance and speaking ability	Mild impairment of reasoning and memory with intensification of emotions Increased disinhibition euphoria with apparent "stimulant effect" on behavior and extroversion Lowered interest in sex
0.08 to 0.10	Mild impairment of hearing, speech, and vision	Mild impairment of both judgment and self-control with increased risk for and incidence of accidents
0.10 to 0.15	Continued loss of coordination with marked impairment of balance, slowed reaction time, and slightly slurred speech	Increased emotional instability with euphoria being increasingly replaced with the opposite feeling of dysphoria Significant impairment in judgment and ability to make good decisions with up to a 10-fold increase in the probability or incidence of accidents
0.15 to 0.20	Significant drowsiness, slurred speech, and prolonged reaction times Significant visual impairment with blurred vision, reduced glare recovery, and decreased peripheral vision	Significant impairment of perception Gross intoxication with further deterioration of judgment and up to a 30-fold increase in the probability or incidence of accidents

(*Continued*)

10 The BACs listed and their associated effects are meant to provide a general guideline. Variability from one adolescent or young adult to another does occur and can be significant, particularly in the context of genetics and acquired tolerance.

11 Because of a paucity of relevant available data for children and adolescents, this table was constructed from adult data. Given the known pharmacokinetics of alcohol, the extrapolation of these data to adolescents is expected to be quite valid and reliable. However, the data in this table should *not* be directly applied to children.

Table 1.1 (Cont.)

BAC (gram % or grams per 100 ml)	*Physical Effects*	*Mental Effects*
0.20 to 0.30	Severe motor and speech impairment with an appearance of a "sloppy drunk"—appears "smashed" May require assistance to stand upright or to walk Impaired gag reflex with risk of choking on food or own vomitus Risk of serious injury related to falls, walking into traffic, being attacked, robbed (i.e., being "rolled"), or raped	Significant mental confusion—may be dazed or disoriented Loss of normal understanding Significant pain tolerance ("feeling no pain") Memory loss and alcoholic blackouts May become stuporous, or achieve a state of near-unconsciousness ("a drunken stupor")
0.30 to 0.35	Total loss of motor control Significantly depressed or absent reflexes Incontinence, or loss of voluntary bladder control, "totally pissed" Significantly slowed heart and respiratory rates	Level of consciousness diminishes to a state of stupor, a complete lack of mental alertness or a condition of significantly impaired ability to respond to external environmental stimuli Level of consciousness diminishes to coma, or an extremely deep stupor—a condition in which the person cannot be aroused by external environmental stimuli (e.g., talking to the person, calling the person by name, or gentle shaking) Total lack of response to painful stimuli, such as pinching the skin or pricking the skin with a pin or needle (i.e., level of surgical anesthesia)
0.35 to 0.40+	Impaired circulation of the blood throughout the body Death, usually due to respiratory arrest LD_{50} = 0.4 grams %	Severe CNS depression and unconsciousness

Modified from: Pagliaro & Pagliaro (2012, p. 19–20).

The relatively low BACs achieved at the beginning of a drinking episode, diminish the control of the medulla oblongata over the higher cortical (i.e., executive functioning) centers of the brain impairing thinking and psychomotor performance. Social norms and related inhibitions, such as being polite or wearing clothes in public, also are impaired. There also is an incremental loss in discrimination, fine motor movement, concentration, memory performance, and conscious control over behavior.[12] Wide fluctuations in mood, with frequent emotional outbursts, also may occur.

As the BAC increases, the state of disinhibition euphoria is progressively impaired as the actions/control of the cerebral cortex are increasingly diminished.[13] As a consequence, "bar fights" and other aggressive behavior may occur. In this regard, women, when compared to men, are equally at risk for physically assaulting someone when they are drinking (Rothman, McNaughton Reyes, & Johnson, 2012; Timko, Moos, & Moos, 2009).

Instances of domestic violence, or intimate partner violence (IPV), often involve alcohol use—both acute intoxication and chronic drunkenness associated with regular, long-term use—and are often associated with alcohol dependence or use disorder (e.g., Pagliaro & Pagliaro, *Clinical Patient Data Files*; Stuart, Meehan, & Moore, 2006; Stuart, Moore, & Ramsey, 2004; Stuart, Temple, & Follansbee, 2008). This violence depends primarily upon the:

1. Pharmacological actions of alcohol;
2. Perpetrator's innate personality predisposition to engage in violent behavior;
3. Environmental circumstances.

Alcohol use–at any level—generally does not increase, or improve, cognitive or psychomotor performance.[14] With moderate to heavy alcohol ingestion: (1) visuospatial performance bias, which generally favors men, disappears; and (2) episodic memory performance bias, which generally favors women, is maintained. These observed actions may be mediated by the effects of alcohol on sex hormones (e.g., the facilitation of the conversion of testosterone to estrogen) (e.g., Yonker, Nilsson, & Herlitz, 2005).

When the BAC exceeds 0.1 gram %, usually within the first one to two hours after initiating a drinking episode (or approximately four drinks for women and five drinks for men),[15] further psychodepression occurs: judgment is impaired; coordination decreases; reaction time slows; and vision blurs. For this reason, the legal limit of intoxication in the U.S. is a BAC of 0.08 gram % (i.e., 0.08 gram of alcohol per 100 ml of blood). (For further related discussion, see later section, "Drinking and Driving.")

It is interesting to note that the psychodepressant actions associated with the ingestion of alcohol appear to be more marked when the BAC is increasing rather than when it is

12 The behavioral reaction to disinhibition, occurring at lower doses, is unpredictable and is determined by individual factors, including an adolescent's mental set and the setting in which the drinking occurs. Mental set and environmental setting become less important when increasing amounts of alcohol are consumed because sedation dominates and behavioral activity decreases. As alcohol ingestion increases, all drinkers experience progressive psychomotor incapacitation. Thus, for example, at low alcohol dosages/BACs, some drinkers—particularly women—may appear as "happy drunks," get on a table in a bar, take off their clothes, and dance naked without a care in the world. However, as alcohol BACs increase, all drinkers become "sleepy drunks" and soon fall asleep, or "pass-out."

13 The nature and extent of these psychodepressant actions depends upon such factors as gender, genetics, hepatic function, lean body weight, and tolerance to alcohol.

14 A noted exception is the case of an individual who is experiencing the alcohol withdrawal syndrome. In this case, "a bit of the hair of the dog that bit her" (i.e., an alcoholic drink) would increase BACs, relieve the signs and symptoms of the alcohol withdrawal syndrome, and, consequently, improve performance—at least temporarily. Thus, an experienced surgeon or pianist might perform better in this context "with a drink" rather than "without a drink," but not better than if sober—and free of withdrawal symptoms (Pagliaro & Pagliaro, *Clinical Patient Data Files*).

15 In the U.S., a standard drink is typically considered to be 0.5 ounces, or 15 grams, of absolute (i.e., 95% to 100%) alcohol. In relation to commonly consumed alcoholic beverages, this amount of alcohol is roughly equivalent to: 12 ounces (360 ml) of beer; 5 ounces (150 ml) of wine; or 1.5 ounces (45 ml) of 80-proof distilled spirits. Given these equivalencies, it is easy to see the truth in the adage, "a drink is a drink is a drink" (i.e., ultimately, it matters less what alcoholic beverage one drinks and more on how many drinks one has during a drinking episode).

decreasing.[16] As the ingestion of alcohol increases, the function of the CNS becomes increasingly impaired as a general anesthesia ultimately prevails. Several other body systems also are affected by acute alcohol ingestion, including: respiratory function; temperature regulation; sexual performance; and urinary output. See later pharmacology subsection, "Undesired, or Harmful, Effects and Toxicities."

Pharmacokinetics: Absorption, Distribution, Metabolism, and Excretion

Alcohol displays interesting and unique pharmacokinetics—from absorption to excretion. These processes are discussed in the following sections.

Absorption

Although only small amounts of alcohol (i.e., 10% to 20%) are directly absorbed from the stomach, overall, absorption is rapid, and virtually complete (i.e., 80% to 90%) from the small intestine. Any remaining amounts of alcohol are absorbed in the colon (i.e., in total, 90% to 100% of orally ingested alcohol is absorbed from the GI tract). The time from the last drink of alcohol to the maximal BAC usually ranges from 30 to 90 minutes, depending on gastric emptying time.

Gastric emptying time can be prolonged by the type and amount of food present in the stomach and, thus, slow both the rate by which alcohol is released into the small intestine and, in turn, the rate by which the BAC increases. The presence of food in the stomach also can slow the absorption of alcohol by diluting the alcohol and blocking absorption by covering some of the gastric mucosa through which alcohol is normally absorbed. In contrast, gastric emptying time can be shortened by ingesting an alcoholic beverage with a carbonated beverage (e.g., a "shot of whiskey" followed by a "beer chaser;" "gin and tonic;" or "rum and coke"). This conscious approach to drinking, allows drinkers to achieve higher BACs and associated desired effects more rapidly by:

1. Distending the stomach;
2. Relaxing the pyloric sphincter between the distal end of the stomach and the small intestine;
3. Promoting the rapid release of stomach contents into the small intestines—where alcohol is primarily absorbed.

However, regardless of the rate of absorption, any amount of alcohol that is ingested, under normal conditions, is virtually completely absorbed. This rule may be a deadly one regarding college/university students, who participate in "drinking games," or extremely risky methods of alcohol ingestion, such as "funneling" (i.e., pouring large amounts of alcohol through a funnel attached to a tube held in the mouth by a student or "pledge," who gulps it down as quickly as possible).[17]

These games are often associated with: high school proms and graduations; undergraduate university fraternity, or "frat," parties; and "Spring Break" celebrations. Another example is the heavy drinking that is frequently associated with school and university sport championship

16 This is probably due to the body's attempts to preserve homeostasis, or equilibrium, within the body (i.e., a state of dynamic equilibrium in response to both internal and external environmental changes). As such, it is more difficult to accommodate, or adapt to new changes (e.g., increasing BACs in the body) than those which occur after the body has adapted, or already made necessary changes (e.g., when BACs are decreasing).

17 "Funneling" large amounts of alcohol, rarely, may also be accomplished by inserting the funnel rectally (Pagliaro & Pagliaro, *Clinical Patient Data Files*).

celebrations or a favorite city team winning the "Orange Bowl" or the "Super Bowl." Unfortunately, these drinking games and sport celebrations can end in fatal alcohol overdosages. In many of these cases, the victim simply "passes out" (as a natural consequence of increasing alcohol concentrations), alone on the beach or in a hotel room (while friends continue to party). However, even while "passed-out," the alcohol continues to be absorbed, and, if a sufficient BAC is subsequently achieved, respiratory depression—and death—can occur (Pagliaro & Pagliaro, *Clinical Patient Data Files*). (See also the related discussion in the later pharmacology section—"Alcohol Overdosage" and the adolescent and young adult alcohol use section—"Pre-Partying and Drinking Games").

Distribution

Alcohol is a small molecule (see Figure 1.1) that is hydrophilic. In addition, alcohol is not protein-bound. Thus, it easily crosses biological membranes. For example, alcohol crosses from the GI tract into the bloodstream and from the bloodstream across the blood-brain barrier into the CNS. Crossing the "placental barrier" and "fetal blood-brain barrier," alcohol also is freely distributed to the fetus when ingested by women who are pregnant, and, consequently, easily achieves fetal BACs equivalent to those of the mother.

Figure 1.2 illustrates the: (1) basic principles of the transfer of free (i.e., "unbound") drugs across the human placenta and the fetal blood-brain barrier; and (2) effects of other factors, including protein binding—the binding of free drug to plasma protein [primarily albumin]—that prevents the cross-membrane transfer of "bound" drugs. These are important principles for health and social care professionals to understand because they help to explain the possible effects of the use of alcohol, or other drugs and substances of abuse, on developing embryos and fetuses when consumed by pregnant adolescent girls and young women (Also see the later discussion in the subsection, "Fetal Alcohol Syndrome [FAS]/Fetal Alcohol Spectrum Disorder [FASD]").

Although highly soluble in water, alcohol is not well-distributed into fatty (i.e., adipose) tissues. Thus, the distribution of alcohol is generally different for adolescent girls and young women when compared to adolescent boys and young men. On average, adolescent girls and young women, because of their significantly higher average percentage of body fat (10% to 13%), achieve higher BACs per drink ingested than adolescent boys and young men (2% to 5% essential body fat) of the same age, weight, and physical condition (Baraona, Abittan, & Dohmen, 2001). This difference accounts for the observations that:

1. Adolescent boys and young men, on average, can drink more than adolescent girls and young women before showing signs and symptoms of intoxication;
2. Binge drinking, on average for adolescent boys and young men, consists of consuming five drinks at one sitting, while for adolescent girls and young women, it consists of consuming four drinks at one sitting (see also the section, "Binge Drinking").

In general, for all body tissues, as emphasized by Cederbaum (2012):

> Equilibrium of alcohol within a tissue depends on the water content, rate of blood flow, and tissue mass.
>
> (p. 667)

Metabolism and Excretion

A relatively small amount of alcohol is metabolized by alcohol dehydrogenase (ADH) in the stomach, thus preventing its systemic absorption. The nature and extent of this effect is related to several factors, including the:

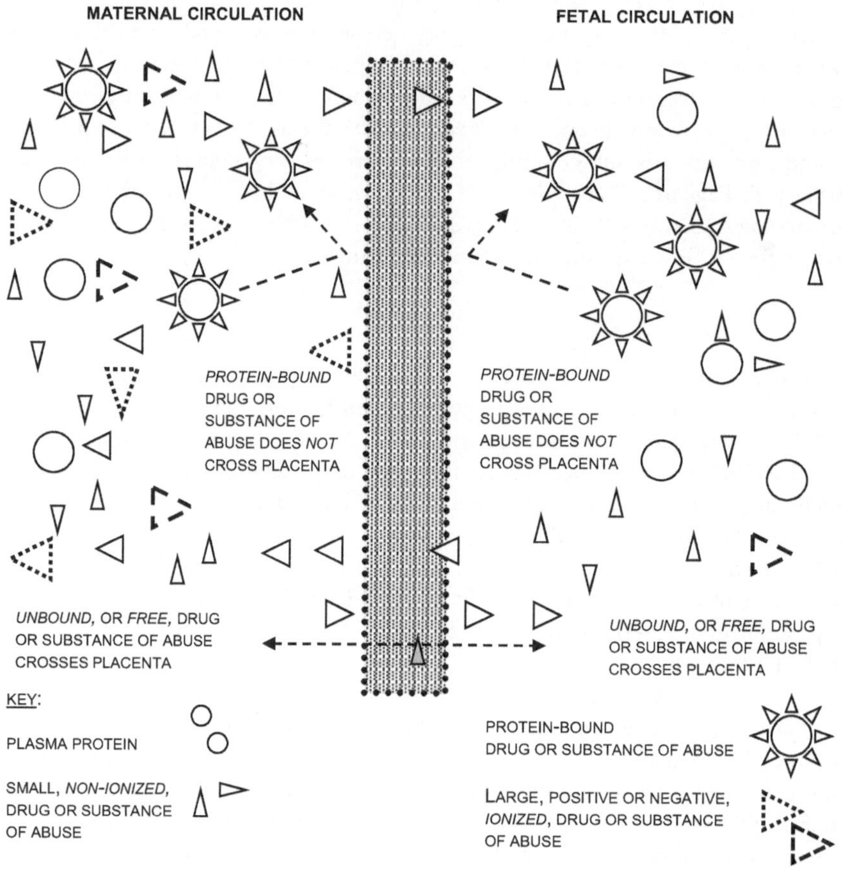

Figure 1.2 Drug Transfer across Biological Membranes

1. Length of time that the alcohol remains in the stomach, which itself depends on several factors including the presence of food (see the previous subsection, "Absorption");
2. Activity of ADH, which: (a) is influenced by genetics; and (b) is lower in alcoholics, particularly women (Cederbaum, 2012).[18]

Approximately 90% to 95% of ingested alcohol undergoes hepatic metabolism at a constant rate (Pagliaro & Benet, 1975) (see Figure 1.3). Ethanol's hepatic metabolism is mediated by ADH and cytochrome P450 CYP2E1 (Chan & Anderson, 2014; Lieber, 1999).[19] The remaining 5% to 10% of ingested alcohol, which is not metabolized in the liver, is excreted in unchanged form in the breath,[20] sweat, and urine. The energy released per gram of alcohol is approximately seven kilocalories (kcal). However, because alcohol

18 For example, Bosron and Li (1986) identified that the genetic polymorphism of the human alcohol dehydrogenase enzyme may contribute to an up to 3-fold variation in alcohol elimination rates.

19 CYP2E1 is also primarily responsible for the hepatic metabolism of fatty acids and xenobiotics (Chan & Anderson, 2014).

20 Thus, the physiological basis for the validity of the "alcohol breathalyzer test."

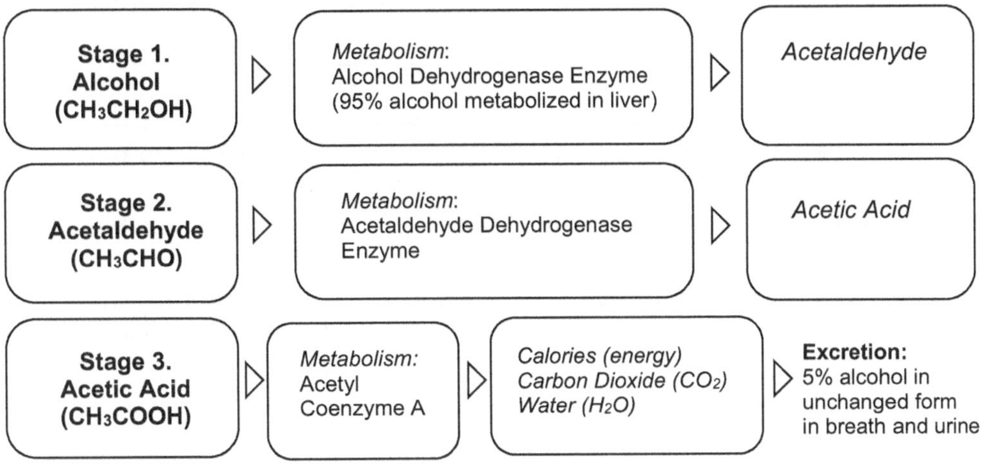

Figure 1.3 Alcohol Metabolism

has no nutritional value (e.g., vitamins and minerals) and is not "stored" in the body for later needed energy when required, it is considered to only provide "empty" calories when metabolized.

The rate of alcohol metabolism is linear with time and is minimally affected by variations in blood concentration.[21] For the average 21-year-old, 70 kg, male of European continental descent, the rate of metabolism is approximately 10 to 20 ml of 100% alcohol per hour. Thus, it takes approximately one hour to metabolize a "typical drink" (i.e., approximately 30 ml of whiskey or another distilled spirit; 150 ml of wine; or 360 ml of beer). If a larger amount of alcohol is ingested per hour than is capable of being metabolized, the BAC increases along with its corresponding psychodepressant actions, including desired and undesired, or harmful, effects and toxicities (see Table 1.2).

Common Misbelief: A drunk adolescent can quickly "sober up" by drinking several cups of strong coffee.

The process of "sobering up" is directly related to the half-life of elimination of alcohol (i.e., the equivalent number of drinks that is eliminated per hour). There are several factors (e.g., ingestion of fructose, or fruit sugar, and some vitamins) that may, theoretically, alter the rate of alcohol metabolism and, thus, increase its rate of elimination. However, none of these factors has proved clinically significant and, consequently, none have received FDA approval.[22] Thus, even though it is commonly thought that drinking

21 This form of metabolism is often referred to as "capacity limited," "dose-dependent," "zero order," or "Michaelis-Menten" kinetics (Holtzman, 1983; Pagliaro & Benet, 1975; Winek & Murphy, 1984).

22 In Europe, metadoxine (Metadoxil®), which is an ion pair of pyridoxines (i.e., vitamin B_6) and pyrrolidone-2-carboxylate, is used intravenously in cases of both acute and chronic alcohol intoxication. It has not yet received FDA approval.

Metadoxine appears to work by several mechanisms of action, including increasing the enzymatic activity of acetaldehyde dehydrogenase. Consequently, the metabolism of alcohol and acetaldehyde are increased and the half-life of elimination of alcohol is decreased (Addolorato, Ancona, & Capristo, 2003; Diaz Martinez, Diaz Martinez, & Villamil Salcedo, 2002; Shpilenya, Muzychenko, & Gasbarrini, 2002; Vonghia, Leggio, & Ferrulli, 2008).

Table 1.2 Acute and Chronic Toxicities Associated with Alcohol Use among Children, Adolescents, and Young Adults

Acute Toxicities	*Chronic Toxicities*	*Acute/chronic Toxicities*
Decreased social inhibitions	**Alcoholism**	**Absenteeism from school or work**
Diminished eye movements	**Alcohol withdrawal syndrome**	**Accidents (e.g., drownings; falls; MVCs)**
	Anemia	**Abusive and aggressive behavior, physical and psychological**
Hallucinations	**Cardiac dysrhythmias**	**Alcoholic "blackouts"**
Hangover	**Cardiovascular disease**	**Alcoholic ketoacidosis**
Homicide, perpetrator or victim	**Contemporaneous diagnosis**	**Amnesia**
Hypokalemia	**Decreased immune response**	**Boyfriend or girlfriend abuse, physical and psychological**
Hypothermia	**Diabetes mellitus**	**Child abuse, physical and psychological**
Peripheral vasodilation, or "flush"	**Dysmenorrhea**	**Cognitive dysfunction**
Psychomotor impairment	**FAS/FASD among off-spring of adolescent girls and young women**	**Coma**
Psychosis	**Hypertension**	**Criminal behavior**
Respiratory depression	**Hypertriglyceridemia**	**Dysfunctional parenting**
Risk-taking behavior, increased		**Gastritis**
Sexual activity, increased		**Guilt**
		Hypoglycemia
		Impaired relationships with parents and other family members, co-workers, employers, teachers, or others
Sexual assault (e.g., acquaintance rape, date rape, or IPV facilitation, perpetration, or participation)	**Malnutrition (e.g., thiamine deficiency)**	**Memory dysfunction**

Acute Toxicities	*Chronic Toxicities*	*Acute/chronic Toxicities*
Sexual dysfunction (adolescent boys and young men)	**Neuropathy**	**Mental depression**
Sexual inhibitions, decreased	**Peripheral neuropathy**	**Neurotoxicity**
Sexually transmitted diseases, increased	**Physical dependence**	**School work/academic performance, decreased**
Short-term memory impairment	**Psychological dependence**	**Self-neglect**
Slurred speech	**Sick days, increased**	**Social problems (e.g., absence from school or work; arguments with family members), increased**
Violent behavior, including homicide, physical assault, and rape		**Suicide, attempted or completed, increased**
Vomiting		**Victimization (e.g., physical and sexual assault), increased**
		Work productivity, decreased

"strong" coffee, taking a cold shower, or walking around can increase the elimination of alcohol and, thus, "speed-up" the process of "sobering-up" after a heavy drinking episode—they do not.

It also is commonly thought that caffeine in coffee (or energy drinks) can counteract drunkenness or prolong the desired effects of alcohol.[23] The only thing that these actions consistently accomplish is to change a drowsy adolescent, who is drunk, into a wide-awake adolescent, who is drunk. Of course, the more time that is devoted to these activities, the

23 Interestingly, McKetin, Coen, and Kaye (2015), in their comprehensive review of 62-related studies, reported that those who drank alcohol mixed with caffeinated energy drinks (AEDs) found that AEDs "increased stimulation and alertness, offset fatigue from drinking, and facilitated drinking" (p. 15). (See also related discussion in the later section, "Alcohol and Caffeinated Energy Drinks").

We would hasten to add that while these findings may help to account for a noted increase in the related consumption of alcohol/caffeine beverages among adolescents and young adults, it does not necessarily confirm the reported effects (i.e., believing these reports of behavior to be true while potentially reinforcing the related behavior among AED consumers does not make them "true" to the external objective observer). Several studies (e.g., Ferreira, de Mello, & Pompeia, 2006; Marczinski, 2014; Marczinski & Fillmore, 2006) support our observations and interpretations. See also the related discussion in the later section, "Alcohol Drug–Drug Interactions."

more time passes in which alcohol can be slowly, but steadily, eliminated and, thus, make these ineffective activities sometimes appear to be effective.

Presently, there is no practical way to increase the rate of alcohol metabolism. Once alcohol is ingested, absorbed, and distributed throughout the body, its ultimate elimination from the body primarily depends on its slow and steady rate of metabolism by the liver. This process may be impaired among adolescents who have liver disease (e.g., cirrhosis of the liver) or genetic polymorphism of both alcohol dehydrogenase and acetaldehyde dehydrogenase (i.e., enzymes involved in the hepatic metabolism of alcohol and in the occurrence of the "Asian Flush"). (See Figure 1.3.) Genetic polymorphism also may account, in part, for the variations in alcohol metabolism and elimination rates observed among adolescents of certain continental and other descents (e.g., Jewish adolescents versus American Indian and Alaska Native adolescents) (Pagliaro & Pagliaro, 1992) (See also the earlier related discussion in this subsection).

Alcohol Drug–Drug Interactions

Several clinically significant drug–drug interactions have been associated with the concurrent use of alcohol, involving:

- Other psychodepressants (e.g., opiate analgesics, prescription sedative-hypnotics, and volatile solvents and inhalants [e.g., gasoline; glue]);
- Other drugs that may be associated with depression (e.g., over-the-counter and prescription anticholinergics; antihistamines; tricyclic antidepressants);
- Psychostimulants (e.g., caffeine; nicotine);
- Alcohol abstinence maintenance drugs (e.g., disulfiram, Antabuse®; fomepizole, Antizol®).

These alcohol drug–drug interactions are presented and briefly discussed, in alphabetical order, in the following subsections.

Alcohol and Caffeine

See, in this subsection, "Alcohol and Psychostimulants."

Alcohol and Disulfiram

Disulfiram (Antabuse®) is an inhibitor of acetaldehyde dehydrogenase. Consequently, when used concurrently with alcohol, the metabolism of alcohol is blocked at the stage of acetaldehyde production (see earlier pharmacology subsection, "Pharmacokinetics—Metabolism and Excretion"). The resultant accumulation of acetaldehyde causes several unpleasant signs and symptoms including: facial flushing, hypotension, nausea, tachycardia, and vomiting—-collectively referred to as the "acetaldehyde syndrome" or "Antabuse® syndrome." The occurrence of this alcohol drug–drug interaction is therapeutically used for the management of alcohol abstinence maintenance (see the related discussion in the later subsection, "Alcohol Abstinence Maintenance—Disulfiram (Antabuse®) Pharmacotherapy").

Alcohol and Fomepizole

Fomepizole (Antizol®) is a potent inhibitor of the enzyme, alcohol dehydrogenase. It is therapeutically used for the treatment of ethylene glycol and methanol poisonings (see the related discussion in the later section, "Alcohol Overdosage/Poisoning"). Fomepizole, because of its mechanism of the action, can significantly increase the half-life of elimination of alcohol

(Kraut & Mullins, 2018). (See also the related discussion in the earlier pharmacology subsection, "Pharmacokinetics—Metabolism").

Alcohol and Nicotine

Alcohol and nicotine are often used together and each can influence the use of the other.[24] In summary:

1. Concurrent alcohol and nicotine use (i.e., e-cigarette vaping; tobacco smoking, or other nicotine use—chewing nicotine gum or using other nicotine replacement products):
   - Increases nicotine craving between nicotine use sessions;
   - Decreases the time between nicotine use sessions;
   - Increases the amount of nicotine vaped, tobacco smoked, or otherwise used per use session.

2. Concurrent nicotine and alcohol use (i.e., drinking beers, liqueurs, whiskey, wines, and other alcoholic beverages):
   - Increases craving for alcohol;
   - Decreases the subjective effects associated with alcohol use;
   - Increases the overall amount of alcohol ingested per drinking session.

(See also the later subsection, "Alcohol and Psychostimulants")

Alcohol and Other Psychodepressants

The concurrent use of alcohol and other psychodepressants (e.g., opiate analgesics; prescription sedative-hypnotics; volatile solvents and inhalants) results in additive effects. These additive effects can significantly increase both the incidence and severity of undesired, or harmful, effects and toxicities, including respiratory depression and death. (See the related discussion in Chapter 5, "Prescription Opiate Analgesics and Heroin," and Chapter 6, "Prescription Sedative-Hypnotics.")

Alcohol and Psychostimulants

The concurrent use of alcohol and psychostimulants (e.g., amphetamines; caffeine; cocaine) may reduce or ameliorate, respectively, the contributory psychodepressant and psychostimulant actions of both alcohol and the psychostimulant. However, in most of these cases, researchers found only negligible results, while others found mixed results. For example, Barkla, McArdle, and Newbury-Birch (2015) found "only a minimal increase in side-effects when ADHD medication (therapeutic doses) was taken with alcohol" (p. 270). More recently, McKetin, Coen, and Kaye (2015) found, "insufficient evidence" to conclude that mixing caffeinated energy drinks with alcohol "led to increased alcohol consumption or altered the nature of alcohol-related harm" (p. 15).

24 The contemporaneous occurrence of an AUD and nicotine use disorder (NUD) reinforces the operant, or cue mediated, use of both alcohol and nicotine. Although, not completely understood, the mechanism of these interactions appears to involve both "the stress hormone systems" and "adaptations" within the mesolimbic dopamine system (Little, Barron, & Prendergast, 2007; Ostroumov, Thomas, & Dani, 2015; Verplaetse & McKee, 2017).

However, others found significant results. For example, Striley and Khan (2014) found that:

> Harmful consequences, including involvement in risky driving, riding with an intoxicated driver, and being taken advantage of sexually, were reported significantly more often by adolescents and young adults who combined energy drinks with alcohol compared with those who did not.
>
> (p. 263)

(See also both the earlier subsection, "Alcohol and Nicotine" and the later subsection, "Alcohol and Caffeinated Energy Drinks").

***<u>Related Professional Reminder:</u> The clinical significance of drug–drug interactions involving the abusable psychotropics depends on several factors including the*:**

1. ***"Drug"—the drug or substance of abuse that is used, including dosage/amount and method of use;***
2. ***"Set"—personality characteristics and general mental and physical health of the user;***
3. ***"Setting"—the context of use*** [25]

Undesired, or Harmful, Effects and Toxicities

The myriad of adverse consequences, which are associated with alcohol use, should serve as a cautionary tale, particularly, for adolescents, who believe that "getting drunk" with friends while "partying" over the weekend is normal, "cool," something to brag about, or a "rite of passage." Unfortunately, most adolescents in the U.S. have not heeded this cautionary tale—as evidenced and discussed in the following subsections.

As identified by the USDHHS:

> Each year, approximately 5,000 young people under the age of 21 die as a result of underage drinking; this includes about 1,900 deaths from motor vehicle crashes, 1,600 as a result of homicides, 300 from suicide, as well as hundreds from other injuries such as falls, burns, and drownings.
>
> (NIAAA, 2006, p. 1)

Toward the end of the second decade of the new millennium, Delker, Brown, and Hasin (2016, p. 13)—based on their epidemiologic overview of alcohol consumption in the U.S.—concluded that:

> In the United States, AUD accounts for a high and potentially preventable proportion of overall disability and mortality.

As reported in the Global Burden of Disease (GBD, 2018) study:

> Alcohol use is a leading risk factor for death and disability . . . [and concluded] our results show that the safest level of drinking is none.
>
> (pp. 1, 12)

25 See also, Norman Zinberg (1986), for further related discussion of "drug," "set," and "setting."

Effects of Alcohol on Body Systems

With its desired psychotropic actions (e.g., disinhibition euphoria), and certain other positive qualities (e.g., legal availability; pleasant color, taste, bouquet; satisfying thirst), it is surprising to some—and often overlooked by many others—that alcohol use is associated with more harm than all of the other drugs or substances of abuse, combined (Pagliaro & Pagliaro, 2009).[26] The general effects of alcohol on many body functions are also not often recognized including its effects on: body temperature; executive processes; respiratory function; sexual behavior; sleep; and urination—all of which are directly affected by BAC (see also the earlier related discussion in the pharmacology subsection, "Blood Alcohol Concentrations").

Regarding "body temperature," alcohol ingestion generally causes peripheral vasodilation—along with a characteristic warm "flush"—and a decrease in body temperature.

Common Misbelief: When adolescents or young adults go inside from the winter cold, a "little sip" of brandy or whiskey can warm them up right away!

Unfortunately, they will only get a warm feeling in their stomachs. The vasodilation associated with alcohol ingestion, particularly that of blood vessels located near the skin surface, cools the body down in a manner similar to the automotive radiator cooling coils that cool the engine down. Thus, the fallacy of coming in from the cold and taking a drink of alcohol to "warm up."

Regarding "executive processes," Bickel, Moody, and Mueller (2013, p. 1), noted "significant executive dysfunction" among alcohol-dependent subjects. In a later study, Nguyen-Louie, Castro, and Matt (2015), recognizing that "adolescence is a period of neuromaturation concomitant with increased [drug or] substance involvement" (p. 738), examined the effects of adolescent emerging alcohol and marijuana use on neuropsychological functioning by conducting a four-year prospective study of 234 adolescents, 12- to 14-years-of-age. At baseline, the adolescents were administered a cognitive test battery that was re-administered approximately four years later, at which time, the researchers found that:

1. More alcohol use days predicted worse verbal memory;
2. More alcohol use days predicted worse visuospatial ability;
3. More alcohol use and more post-drinking effects predicted worse psychomotor speed;
4. Effects can occur independent of meeting established criteria for AUD.

Alcohol is a neurotoxin (NIAAA, 2005). Much research (e.g., Guerri & Pascual, 2010; Nguyen-Louie, Matt, & Jacobus, 2017; Squeglia & Gray, 2016) has demonstrated that regular (e.g., weekly) alcohol use/abuse during adolescence may result, as concluded by Nguyen-Louie, Tracas, and Squeglia (2016, p. 1895), in significant neurological impairment:

26 Consequently, alcohol consumption has been consistently cited as the third leading cause of death in the U.S. (CDC, 2004, 2012a). In addition to direct physical effects, these deaths are mediated, particularly among adolescents and young adults, by alcohol-related: accidents (e.g., MVCs); HIV infection; and suicides. See also the related discussion in the later "Undesired, or Harmful, Effects and Toxicities," subsections—"Mental Depression and Suicide;" "Risky Drinking and Driving;" and "Sexual Assault."

Drinking quantity during adolescence appears to affect verbal learning and memory in a dose-dependent manner.

These neurocognitive deficits appear to be accompanied, or be caused by, several noted changes in brain structure that include:

- Decreases in gray matter in the frontal and temporal cortexes;
- White matter deficits in the pons and corpus callosum;
- Decreased white matter integrity.

(e.g., Pfefferbaum, Kwon, & Brumback, 2017; Squeglia & Gray, 2016)

Regarding "respiratory function," moderate amounts of alcohol may stimulate or depress respiratory function.[27] In addition, the ingestion of large amounts of alcohol (e.g., BAC = 0.4 gram %, or higher), can be fatal due to associated severe respiratory depression and negative cardiac effects.

Regarding "sleep," the ingestion of alcohol slows the electroencephalogram (EEG) activity toward slow-wave sleep, depresses rapid eye movement (REM) sleep, and inhibits dreaming. The sleep induced by drinking alcohol is not always restful and peaceful—one reason, among others, why alcohol is not medically recommended as a sedative-hypnotic, even though it reduces sleep onset latency. In fact, large amounts of alcohol ingested at bedtime, as well as patterns of regular, long-term alcohol use that continues throughout the day, and which, is characterized by finally "falling down drunk," have been associated with several sleep-related problems including:

- Lower slow-wave sleep;
- Poor quality of sleep, particularly later in the night;
- Reduced REM sleep, particularly later in the first part of sleep;
- Sleep apnea;
- Urinary incontinence.

In addition, alcohol withdrawal is associated with: (1) decreased total sleep time; (2) problems falling asleep; and (3) REM rebound (Brower, 2001; Coltrain, Nicholas, & Baker, 2014; Ebrahim, Shapiro, & Williams, 2013).

Finally, regarding "urination," the use of alcohol exerts a diuretic effect by two principal mechanisms:

1. "Directly," by its suppressant action on the production and secretion of antidiuretic hormone by the hypothalamus and pituitary gland, respectively, which increases the reabsorption of water in the distal convoluted tubules of the kidneys;
2. "Indirectly," by the large quantity of liquid ordinarily ingested as alcoholic beverages, particularly beer.

27 However, health and social care professionals should be cognizant of the fact that both the: (1) "protective" effect of carbon dioxide on breathing—the increase in ventilation induced by the decreased availability of oxygen supply to the body tissues (i.e., hypoxic ventilatory response/drive); and (2) increase in ventilation induced by the increased levels of carbon dioxide in the blood (i.e., hypercapnic ventilator response/drive), are always depressed by alcohol intoxication (Roeggla, Roeggla, & Roeggla, 1995; Sahn, Lakshminarayan, & Pierson, 1975; White, Lindsey, & Vincente, 1981).

Although, these actions and effects may result in urinary incontinence, alcohol does not appear to directly cause permanent harm to the physical structure, or physiological function, of the kidneys.[28]

As identified in Table 1.2, there are many undesired, or harmful, effects and toxicities—both acute and chronic—that are "directly" and "indirectly" associated with alcohol use by adolescents and young adults. According to the National Institutes of Health (NIH):

> 28% of adults, aged 18 and older consume alcohol at levels that put them at risk for developing alcoholism, liver disease, and other medical and psychosocial problems.
>
> (Costin & Miles, 2014, p. 157)[29]

Several non-exclusive molecular mechanisms are suggested by Cederbaum (2012) as possible explanations for these alcohol-related undesired, or harmful, effects and toxicities, including:

- Acetaldehyde formation;
- Cytokine formation;
- Hypoxia;
- Immune actions;
- Kupffer cell activation;
- Membrane disruption;
- Mitochondrial damage;
- Oxidative stress;
- Redox state changes in the NAD/NADH ratio.

In the following subsections, four particularly serious harmful effects and toxicities, which are commonly associated with alcohol use by adolescents and young adults, are presented and discussed:

1. Mental depression and suicide;
2. Physical and psychological dependence;
3. Risky drinking and driving;
4. Sexual assault, acquaintance/date-rape, and intimate partner violence.[30]

28 The urinary incontinence that is often associated with heavy drinking episodes occurs primarily as a direct result of the psychodepressant actions of alcohol (i.e., drinkers fall into a deep sleep, or "pass out," and losing urinary bladder control, experience urinary incontinence—hence, the basis for the derivation, or origin, of the associated drinking phrase, "getting pissed") (Pagliaro & Pagliaro, *Clinical Patient Data Files*). These alcohol-related effects are most often noted among older adolescent drinkers who are living "on-the-street" (i.e., homeless) (Pagliaro & Pagliaro, *Clinical Patient Data Files*).

29 N.B. In a large study involving almost 600,000 adult current drinkers (without previous cardiovascular disease) from 19 high-income countries, Wood, Kaptoge, and Butterworth (2018) found that minimum all-cause mortality risk was associated with the consumption of 100 grams, or less, of alcohol (i.e., approximately seven standard drinks) per week.

30 N.B. Other serious health conditions related to alcohol use (e.g., alcoholic liver disease [e.g., Allampati & Mullen, 2016; Gutierez Garcia, Blasco-Algora, & Fernandez-Rodriguez, 2015]; alcohol-related dementia [e.g., Costin & Miles, 2014; Gupta & Warner, 2008]); cancers, such as esophageal squamous cell carcinoma and cancers of the oral cavity larynx, and pharynx [e.g., LoConte, Brewster, & Kaur, 2017; Matejcic, Gunter, & Ferrari, 2017; Tanaka, Yamamoto, & Suzuki, 2010]; cardiovascular disease [e.g., Rehm & Roerecke, 2017; Roerecke & Rehm, 2014]; and osteoporosis [e.g., Luo, Liu, & Liu, 2017; Maurel, Boisseau, & Benhamou, 2012]) quite often begin in adolescence with the adolescent's first drink—but do not become problematic or clinically significant until well into adulthood after many years of moderate to heavy drinking. Consequently, these alcohol-related disorders are not discussed in this text.

MENTAL DEPRESSION AND SUICIDE

In their critical systematic review of 30 related empirical studies, Galaif, Sussman, and Newcomb (2007), found that:

> Suicide is a serious health problem as it is currently the third leading cause of death for teenagers between the ages of 15 and 24 years. Depression, which is also a serious problem for adolescents, is the most significant biological and psychological risk factor for teen suicide. Alcohol use remains extremely widespread among today's teenagers and is related to both suicidality and depression.
>
> (p. 27)

DSM-5 diagnoses of alcohol use disorder and major depressive disorder frequently occur simultaneously among regular drinkers—including adolescents and young adults (e.g., Briere, Rohde, & Seeley, 2014; Sher, Stanley, & Harkavy-Friedman, 2008).

> Depression, alcohol abuse and suicidality each continue to threaten adolescent populations throughout the world. The comorbidity between these diseases has been found to be up to 73% with consistent positive correlations between adolescent drinking, depression and suicidality.
>
> (Ganz & Sher, 2009, p. 333)

This combination of disorders is highly correlated with the risk for suicide attempts and completions. As noted by Bailey, Patel, and Avenido (2011, p. 614), "Individuals with severe clinical depression and alcohol use disorder are at high risk [for suicide] if untreated." Whether depression precedes, or follows, alcohol abuse has not yet been fully determined. For example, Agrawal, Tillman, and Grucza (2017), in their prospective cohort study, the *Collaborative Study of the Genetics of Alcoholism*, found that "suicide attempts are associated with increased likelihood of substance [alcohol] dependence" (p. 96). However, in actuality, it is very likely, that the relationships among alcohol use/abuse, depression, and suicide differ among different adolescents—preceding for some, following for others, and co-occurring for still others (Pagliaro & Pagliaro, 2012). For example, as further identified by Ganz and Sher:

> Some studies suggest that depression encourages alcohol use as self-medication and then leads to suicidality, while others imply that the initial alcohol consumption is responsible for increasing depressive and suicidal symptoms in adolescents.
>
> (2009, p. 333)

Suicide attempts are typically five to 10 times higher for adolescents in association with alcohol use/abuse. In addition, as noted by several researchers (e.g., Pagliaro, 1995; Pagliaro & Pagliaro, *Clinical Patient Data Files*), suicide associated with alcohol use is significantly affected by other variables—in addition to depression, particularly gender and racial/ethnic affiliation. For example, as noted by Chartier, Vaeth, and Caetano (2013):

> Recent alcohol use was reported among suicides in 46 percent of Native Americans, 30 percent of Hispanics, 26 percent of Whites, 16 percent of Blacks, and 15 percent of Asians.
>
> (p. 231)

As significant as these statistics are, they are even higher among certain groups of adolescents in the U.S. For example, among Apache adolescents (mean 16 years-of-age), Cwik, Barlow, and Tingey (2015) found that 91% of suicide attempters used alcohol. In an earlier study of the relationship between suicide and substance use among Apache youth (15 to 24 years-of-age), Barlow, Tingey, and Cwik (2012) found that: 49% were "drunk or high" during suicide ideation; 76% were "drunk or high" at the time of suicide attempts; and 64% were "drunk or high" at the time of suicide.[31]

Dvorak, Lamis, and Malone (2013), in their cross-sectional, self-report study of undergraduate college/university students and the associations among alcohol use, depression, and suicide, found that two factors from their impulsivity model (i.e., "lack of perseverance" and "sensation seeking") significantly moderated the effect of alcohol use on suicidal behavior. It was also found that other intervening variables—being a "solitary binge drinker" compared to being a "social binge drinker" (Gonzalez, 2012) and "drinking to cope" (Gonzalez & Hewell, 2012)—play a significant role in affecting the relationships of alcohol use, depression, and suicide among college/university students. Regarding children and adolescents, "bullying" also has been clearly demonstrated to be a significant intervening variable in the context of alcohol use and suicide (e.g., Lardier, Barrios, & Garcia-Reid, 2016; Pagliaro & Pagliaro, *Clinical Patient Data Files*).

RISKY DRINKING AND DRIVING

One of the most significant examples of alcohol-related "preventable disability and mortality" among adolescents and young adults involves drinking and operating (or being a passenger in)[32] a motor vehicle—including all-terrain vehicles (ATVs), boats, cars, snow mobiles, and trucks (e.g., Denning, Harland, & Jennissen, 2014; Hadland, Xuan, & Sarda, 2017; Li, Brady, & Chen, 2013; Pagliaro & Pagliaro, 2003b, 2012, 2018).[33]

Consequently, adult drivers in all 50 states are currently prohibited from operating a motor vehicle if their BAC is 0.08% or higher. Several countries, including Austria, Denmark, and Japan, have lowered the BAC associated with impaired driving to 0.05% (e.g., Teutsch,

31 In the context of our forensic psychological practice we have consistently, over several decades, also noted a similar relationship between alcohol intoxication and charges of murder among native American male adolescents and young adults (Pagliaro & Pagliaro, *Clinical Patient Data Files*).

32 As noted by Williams and Tefft (2014):

> More than 40% of fatal crashes of 16- and 17-year-old drivers [in the U.S.] occur when transporting teenagers . . . Fatal crashes involving teen passengers, especially multiple passengers, are more likely to involve alcohol . . .
>
> (p. 37)

Unfortunately, these events—sometimes in unusual situations—commonly also occur among young adults as illustrated in the following example, as reported by Fox 46, 2018, p. 1:

> A UNC-Charlotte fraternity has suspended operations in connection to the death of a 20-year-old student and sorority member on Tuesday.

As followed-up by Lam (2018, p.1):

> A 20-year-old University of North Carolina at Charlotte student's blood alcohol level was more than double the legal limit when she was killed earlier this month after falling out of a party bus [and being run over by several cars], toxicology results revealed Tuesday.

33 In addition, a significant number of injuries and death incurred by bicycle riders and pedestrians is associated with alcohol impairment (e.g., Harada, Gangi, & Ko, 2015).

Baldwin & Degutis, 2018). The U.S. National Highway Traffic Safety Administration sponsored a study entitled, *Getting to Zero Alcohol-Impaired Driving Fatalities*, which was conducted by The National Academies of Sciences, Engineering, and Medicine. In January 2018, the Committee released its formal report that included a recommendation to modify the BAC associated with impaired driving in all 50 states from 0.08% to 0.05% (AP, 2018; Teutsch, Baldwin, & Degutis, 2018).

It is important to note that, since the legal minimal drinking age (MLDA) in all 50 states is 21 years-of-age, the previous discussion regarding BACs associated with impaired driving *should be only* of academic interest regarding adults (i.e., totally irrelevant for adolescents because the legally tolerated BAC for adolescents is zero).[34] Unfortunately, many adolescents in the U.S. do not appear to appreciate this "driving" distinction between themselves and adults. For example, countless adolescents have shared with us that "a drink or two" does not impair their ability to drive. In this context, the CDC noted that:

> Nearly one million high school teens drank alcohol and got behind the wheel in 2011.
>
> (NCIPC, 2012, p. 1)

According to the Office of Adolescent Health (2017), in the 30 days prior to the survey, approximately: (1) 10% of U.S. high school students reported driving a car or other vehicle when drinking alcohol; and (2) 20% of U.S. high school students reported that they had been a passenger in a car, or other vehicle, with a driver who had been drinking.

As noted earlier in this chapter, many of the undesired, or harmful, effects and toxicities (e.g., coronary artery disease; hepatic damage; various cancers), which are associated with regular, long-term alcohol use, begin during adolescence, but, typically, do not achieve clinical significance until later in life. However, the morbidity and mortality associated with "drinking and driving" is immediately (and all too often) tragically apparent among adolescents. Motor vehicle crashes (MVC) are a leading cause of death in the U.S. among all segments of the population, but particularly among adolescents.

As identified by Brady and Guohua (2013), in their review of data from the *Fatality Analysis Reporting System* for 2005–2009:

> Alcohol was the most commonly detected substance present in 40.2% of the fatally injured drivers [in the U.S.], followed by cannabinols (10.5%).
>
> (p. 104)

In this context, it should be noted that an even greater number of adolescents, who do not die, are seriously injured (e.g., experience/suffer brain damage; loss of a limb; quadriplegia) in alcohol-related motor vehicle accidents each year in the U.S. As found by Mattson, Cai, and Woodward (2015), utilizing emergency department (ED) data from 2004 to 2011, "alcohol is the prime source of MVC morbidity burden" (p. 45). Unfortunately, this number is increasing among adolescent drivers and is largely exacerbated due to "distracted driving" (e.g., texting while driving). As noted by Wilson, Stimpson, and Tibbits (2013), "Alcohol use is quickly increasing as an important factor behind distracted driving fatality."[35]

34 Many states have variously defined "zero tolerance" as BACs ranging from 0.00% to 0.02% (Voas, Tippetts, & Fell, 2003).

35 In this same context, we have also noted a significant and increasing trend—over the new millennium—of adolescents consuming both alcohol and cannabis prior to, and while, driving. This combination significantly increases their risk for involvement in serious MVCs (Pagliaro & Pagliaro, 2012; Pagliaro & Pagliaro, *Clinical Patient Data Files*). (For additional related discussion, see Chapter 4, "Cannabis and Other Psychodelics.")

> A teen accused of crashing a car carrying four of his Torrey Pines High School classmates, killing one of them as they left a party, will be held at Juvenile Hall until at least Oct 19, a judge ruled yesterday. The 17-year-old driver—who was not hurt in Sunday's crash—is charged with vehicular manslaughter with gross negligence while intoxicated and two counts of DUI causing great bodily injury.
>
> (CNS, 2009, p. 1)

> Five months after their friend was killed in a crash in Glastonbury, Conn, police have arrested three 17-year-old boys who are accused of letting her drive drunk. Police said the boys knew Jane Modlesky, 17, of Glastonbury, was "highly intoxicated" when she got behind the wheel of an [sic] SUV early on the morning of Sunday, July 14 and hit a tree on Woodhaven Road.
>
> (NBC News, 2013, p. 1)

> The teenager driver in an alcohol-related crash that claimed the life of a student from Sherwood High School and left another severely injured was sentenced to serve an 18-month jail term Thursday at an emotional hearing . . .
>
> (St. George, 2015, p. 1)

> A 17-year-old teenager has pleaded guilty to driving 119 miles per hour while drunk, causing a deadly crash that wreaked havoc on an entire community.
>
> (Lewis, 2015, p. 1)

> Police arrested a teenager suspected in a fatal drunk driving crash in Anaheim that left an expectant father dead, authorities said.
>
> (Tchekmedyian, 2017, p. 1)

> A 15-year-old boy died Sunday night after falling out of the window of a vehicle driven by an alleged [17-year-old] impaired driver, according to police.
>
> (The Bakersfield Californian, 2018, p. 1)

The relationship between drinking, driving, and consequent MVCs has been associated with various "pathways" for adolescents, including, as identified by McDonald, Sommers, and Fargo (2014, p. 365):

- Alcohol use disorder (AUD), or problem drinking, leading to drinking and driving;
- Major depressive disorder (MDD) leading to reckless driving;
- Conduct disorder (CD) leading to hostile driving.

As identified by Brown and Tapert (2004):

> Alcohol intoxication is associated with even greater risk of traffic accidents for youth as compared to adults, and adolescent drivers are more likely than adults to get into accidents at lower BACs.
>
> (p. 1)

Figure 1.4 illustrates the general related observation made by Brown and Tapert (2004), as well as others (e.g., Hingson, Heeren, & Levenson, 2002; Pagliaro & Pagliaro, 1996), that

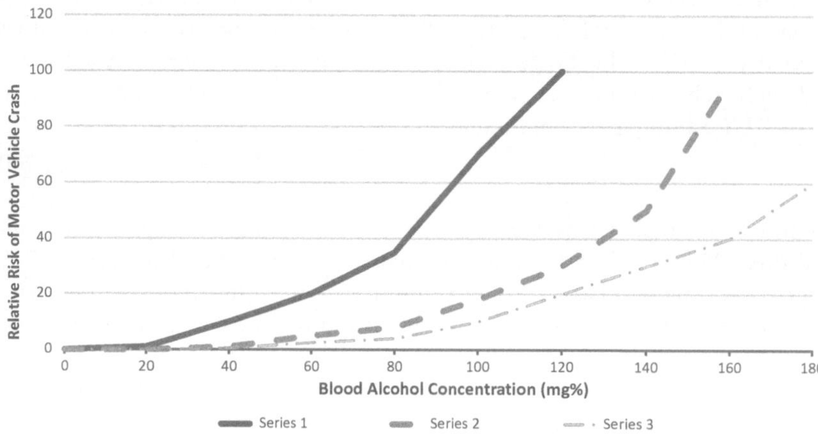

Figure 1.4 Adolescent Driving

relates the interacting variables of: BAC; driving experience; and MVCs. In this figure: Series 1 represents young, inexperienced drivers (i.e., younger drivers who are infrequent drinkers); Series 2 represents average drinkers; and Series 3 represents older, experienced drivers who are frequent drinkers.

SEXUAL ASSAULT

Sexual performance generally decreases as a direct response to increases in alcohol ingestion. However, of all the commonly used drugs and substances of abuse, alcohol is by far the one that is most often used for the perpetration of sexual assault, including acquaintance/date rape (A/DR) and intimate partner violence (IPV) (e.g., Anderson, Flynn, & Pilgrim, 2017; Madea & Musshoff, 2009; Slaughter, 2000; Young, Grey, & Abbey, 2008). In an attempt to better understand this behavior, Abbey, Buck, and Zawacki (2003) assessed the effects of alcohol use among college/university students on their perceptions of a potential date rape in a controlled laboratory setting. They found that:

> Participants' alcohol consumption during the study, self-reported alcohol expectancies, attitudes about casual sex, and usual drinking on dates had *significant* effects on their perceptions of the story. Participants' alcohol expectancy set and gender did *not* have significant effects on perceptions of the likelihood that the male character would force the female character to have sex . . . Intoxicated participants perceived the women in the vignette as being more sexually aroused and the man in the vignette as behaving more appropriately, and both of these variables were *negatively* related to ratings of how likely it was that forced sex would occur. These findings highlight the importance of mediating cues in intoxicated decision making.
>
> (p. 669)

Alcohol intoxication places adolescents, particularly adolescent girls, at increased risk for sexual assault (e.g., acquaintance/date rape) (e.g., McCauley, Calhoun, & Gidycz, 2010;

Parkhill, Norris, & Davi, 2014).[36] As identified by Young, Grey, and Abbey (2008), in their web-based survey of over 1,000 adolescents enrolled in the 7th through 12th grades:

> Findings from the study indicate that alcohol was involved in approximately 12%–20% of the assault cases, depending on age and gender of the respondent. For females, the presence of alcohol during assault differed significantly based on the location at which the assault occurred, ranging from 6% (at the survivor's home) to 29% (at parties or someone else's home). Furthermore, alcohol-related assault among females was more likely to involve physical force than non-alcohol-related assault.
>
> (p. 39)

Increased risk is also high among young women, including college/university students (e.g., Gilmore, Stappenbeck, & Lewis, 2015; Howard, Griffin, & Boekeloo, 2008; Mouilso, Fischer, & Calhoun, 2012). Testa and Livingston (2009), in their comprehensive review of the relationship between drinking alcohol and the sexual victimization of women, found that:

> At least half of sexual victimization incidents involve alcohol use and the majority of rapes of college women occur when the victim is too intoxicated to resist ("incapacitated rape").
>
> (p. 1349)

In addition, as noted in a related "Fact Sheet," from the Centers for Disease Control and Prevention (CDC, 2016):

> Binge drinking is a risk factor for sexual assault, especially among young women in college settings. Each year, about 1 in 20 college women are sexually assaulted. Research suggests that there is an increase in the risk of rape or sexual assault when both the attacker and victim have used alcohol prior to the attack.
>
> (p. 1)[37]

36 N.B. A medical/social history of IPV, and/or childhood sexual abuse, has been identified by several researchers (e.g., Hannan, Orcutt, & Miron, 2015; Hughes, Johnson, & Wilsnack, 2001; Skinner, Kristman-Valente, & Herrenkohl, 2016; Ullman & Sigurvinsdottir, 2015) as a significant risk factor for the development of harmful patterns of alcohol use later in life. Unfortunately, this pattern reflects a tragic cycle of alcohol use and harm (i.e., alcohol abuse leads to sexual abuse that leads to alcohol abuse, that leads to further sexual abuse, and so on—all of which also lead to increased risk for HIV). (See also the related discussion in the later sexual assault subsection, "Intimate Partner Violence.")

For over two decades, many researchers (e.g., Epstein, Saunders, & Kilpatrick, 1998; Felitti, Anda, & Nordenberg, 1998; Spatz-Widom & Hiller-Strumhofel, 2001) have suggested that post-traumatic stress disorder (PTSD) may be a mediator between childhood rape and/or physical abuse and later harmful patterns of alcohol use by adolescents and young adults. We, too, have, over the years, consistently noted this reported intercorrelation among these behaviors, particularly regarding: (1) adolescents and young women, who are lesbian; and (2) adolescents and young adults, who are homeless or living "on-the-street" (Pagliaro & Pagliaro, *Clinical Patient Data Files*).

This cyclic pattern of alcohol use and sexual abuse and/or unsafe/risky sexual behavior is most noteworthy among street-involved/homeless youth (e.g., Fairbairn, Wood, & Dong, 2017). Among this group, risk for this dangerous cycle of behavior is even more pronounced in "travelers"—"a subgroup of homeless youth . . . also known as 'gutter punks' and 'crusty punks' . . . who migrate from place to place, often following common travel routes across the Unites States" (Martino, Tucker, and Ryan, 2011, p. 1634).

> Travelers were almost twice as likely as non-travelers to exhibit heavy drinking in the past month . . . Travelers had more sex partners in the past three months than did non-travelers. They also were more likely to combine alcohol use with sex. (p. 1644)

37 Our own review and analysis of related behavior would indicate that the incidence during the new millennium is closer to one in 10 college/university women (Pagliaro & Pagliaro, *Clinical Patient Data Files*).

In the U.S., alcohol intoxication also promotes risky sexual behavior among adolescents of all continental or other descents (e.g., American Indian; Hawaiian Native; Hispanic) and sexual orientations, for which, bisexual and lesbian adolescents are at particular risk (e.g., George, Davis, & Masters, 2014; Hughes & Eliason, 2002; Hughes, Szalacha, & Johnson, 2010; Phillips, Turner, & Salamanca, 2017). For example, Sales, Brown, and Vissman (2012), in a review of 32 studies examining the association between alcohol use and sexual risk behaviors among adolescents of African continental descent found that: "increased use of alcohol is associated with increased sexual risk practices among African-American females" (p. 117) with associated increased risk of STDs, including HIV infection.[38] (See also the discussion in the related later section, "Binge Drinking.")

ACQUAINTANCE/DATE RAPE. Acquaintance rape is the perpetration of rape by a person who is known to the victim (e.g., classmate; co-worker; employer; family member; teacher). Although briefly discussed in the preceding section, date rape, as a form of acquaintance rape, generally involves some aspect of "romance." Both are frequently alcohol-related crimes that deserve additional specific attention by health and social care professionals. Alcohol, the original acquaintance/date rape drug, continues to be the most widely used drug for acquaintance/date rapes (see Chapter 6, "Prescription Sedative-Hypnotics," for additional related discussion of other drugs that are commonly used to facilitate acquaintance/date rape).

Alcohol use by either, or both, a perpetrator or victim, plays a significant role in facilitating this criminal behavior. A serious concern for researchers over the last three decades (e.g., Abbey, 1991; Pagliaro & Pagliaro, 1996, 2004, 2012, 2018), this abhorrent violence is neither rare nor restricted by population group, although statistics vary. For example, Rickert and Wiermann (1998) found that:

> Lifetime prevalence of date or acquaintance rape ranges from 13% to 27% among college-age women and 20% to a high of 68% among adolescents.
>
> (p. 167)

Alcohol use facilitates acquaintance/date rape by many of its direct actions, including:

- Decreasing social inhibitions;
- Impairing cognitive functioning, including judgment and risk assessment;
- Encouraging misinterpretation of friendly cues, both verbal and nonverbal, with "sexual invitations;"
- Reducing the ability to avoid, or ward-off, a potential or actual attack.

(e.g., Pagliaro & Pagliaro, 1996, 2004; Rickert & Wiermann, 1998)

A related context of this criminal behavior, which has become increasingly prominent during the new millennium, is the deliberate use of alcohol by teachers to facilitate sexual intercourse with their students. Typically, the teacher is married and female and the victim is one, or more, of her male junior or senior high school students:

> A 24-year-old high school teacher has been arrested for allegedly having sex with a male student and for providing him with alcohol.
>
> (Dailymail.com reporter, 2015, p. 1)

38 Interestingly, Thompson, McGee, and Mays (2012), utilizing data from the *Youth Risk Behavior Survey*, found that, although adolescents of European continental descent reported the highest incidence of binge drinking, "African Americans had the highest prevalence of having been forced to have sexual intercourse" (p. 283).

> A former Mount Clemens High School teacher has been charged with purchasing alcohol for a 17-year-old student and having sex with him, authorities said Wednesday.
>
> (Hotts, 2015, p. 1)

> Two female teachers who took male high school students on a camping trip to a San Clemente beach were charged Monday with supplying the students with alcohol and cocaine and having unlawful sexual intercourse, prosecutors said.
>
> (Hamilton, 2015, p. 1)

> California teen says he had booze-filled sex romps with married English teacher.
>
> (FoxNews.com, 2017, p. 1)

> Detectives say a Florida high school teacher has admitted she had sex with a student at least five times and also drank alcohol and used marijuana with the boy.
>
> (WFLA Staff, 2017, p. 1)

> West Fargo school documents show a Sheyenne High School English teacher recently resigned over concerns she had a sexual relationship with a student and gave alcohol to minors as well as having alcohol on school grounds.
>
> (Stanwood, 2017, p. 1)

Unfortunately, these cases of acquaintance/date rape are becoming increasingly common.[39] In response, many school districts have instituted specific programs concerning ethical behavior and "boundaries" for teachers. However, the outcome of these programs does not appear to have been particularly effective regarding the amelioration of the associated unethical and "out of bounds" criminal behavior—reported cases continue to increase (Pagliaro & Pagliaro, *Clinical Patient Data Files*).

Another context of acquaintance/date rape, which has also become increasingly prominent during the new millennium, is that which occurs on college/university campuses. As identified by Kerner, Kerner, and Herring (2017), in their systematic review of this issue:

> It is generally accepted that one in four women (25%) on college campuses report being sexually assaulted at some point in their lives, while nationally 17% of American women have been victims of sexual assault.
>
> (p. 41)

In this context, they also found that the following factors were most commonly related to the sexual assault of college coeds:

1. Alcohol use;
2. Living in residential college/university housing;
3. Sorority membership.

39 N.B. Although, in virtually all of these cases, the teachers claimed that the sex was consensual—with several further claims that it was the result of "true love"—it should be noted that, because all of the students, who were involved, were minors—at best, the cases may be considered to be cases of statutory rape involving the provision of alcohol to a minor. The position of "authority" that the teachers had, who in this capacity also were operating "in loco parentis," makes each of these cases even more egregious.

However, this behavior commonly is concealed and underreported by college and university administrators.[40, 41] Commenting on this phenomenon, Sharma (2007) emphasized that:

> Most rapes are unreported, perhaps giving campus administrators and police the false impression that current efforts are adequate. In addition, the police may be influenced by college administrators who fear that too strong an emphasis on the problem may lead potential students and their parents to believe that rape occurs more often at their school/college than at others.
>
> (p. 21)

It should also be noted that victims frequently choose not to report the incident of acquaintance/date rape for several reasons, including:

- Being labelled as an acquaintance/date rape victim or other undesired label;
- Concern that they will be unable to prove that the sexual act was nonconsensual;
- Being embarrassed or ashamed over the incident;
- Fear of retaliation by the perpetrator;
- Not wanting the perpetrator to be severely punished;
- Self-blame for drinking and/or placing themselves in a risky situation;
- Fear of social isolation from family and/or friends.

(Pagliaro & Pagliaro, *Clinical Patient Data Files*)

INTIMATE PARTNER VIOLENCE. Intimate partner violence (IPV)—economic, emotional, physical, sexual, and/or verbal abuse—usually occurs in the home. IPV is most often perpetrated by a current or former spouse or partner, who is in an intimate relationship with the victim and has been highly correlated with drug and substance abuse among adolescent girls and young women—and their intimate partners (e.g., Afifi, Henriksen, & Asmundson, 2012; Pagliaro & Pagliaro, 2018) (also see related discussion in Chapter 2, "Amphetamines and Cocaine"). Acute alcohol intoxication, or a history of AUD and/or SUDs, are strongly associated with IPV (Smith, Homish, & Leonard, 2012). As suggested by several studies (e.g., Devries, Child, & Bacchus, 2014), there is a distinct possibility of a bi-directional relationship involving these factors. For example, in some cases, adolescents and young adults, who experience IPV, are victims or, less often, are perpetrators, because of their own, or their partner's, use of alcohol. In other cases, adolescents and young adults may use alcohol to "self-medicate" (i.e., cope, or deal with) a traumatic experience associated with IPV.

40 We have found this observation to be true for many colleges/universities for which we have worked at, or consulted with, over our 40 years as academics. In addition, we have spoken widely to colleagues across the U.S. about this "hidden" problem and have discussed it specifically in undergraduate and graduate courses, as well as, formal academic presentations (Pagliaro & Pagliaro, *Clinical Patient Data Files*).

41 Of additional concern, Frinter and Rubinson (1993) noted that, in regard to acquaintance/date rape on college/university campuses, "fraternity members and members of sports teams were overrepresented among the accused." (p. 272). This observation appears to continue to be consonant with current media reports (e.g., Globe Newswire, 2017; Weikle, 2016; WVLT8, 2018). However, we would caution to add that other contributory factors (e.g., anabolic-androgenic steroid use; cocaine use; living independently, "away from home," for the first time) are likely involved as mediators.

Physical and Psychological Dependence.[42]

Alcohol has a high abuse potential and is associated with the development of both physical and psychological dependence. Physical dependence is characterized by the development of tolerance and the occurrence of an alcohol withdrawal syndrome, when regular, long-term and frequent use of increasing amounts of alcohol is abruptly discontinued, and is immediately relieved by resumed alcohol use. Physical dependence, previously identified as the medical disease, "alcoholism," has been more recently identified in the DSM-5, by the American Psychiatric Association (APA, 2013), as the "alcohol use disorder" (i.e., AUD). Psychological dependence accompanies physical dependence and is associated with intense "craving"—desire, longing, or "thirst"—for alcohol that contributes to the "loss of control" over its use.

Common Misbelief: The ability of adolescents and young adults to, "hold their liquor," indicates a developed "immunity," or resistance, to alcoholism, AUD, or physical and psychological dependence on alcohol.

The ability to "hold one's liquor" is, in fact, an indication of acquired tolerance—a characteristic sign of physical dependence on alcohol, or "alcoholism."

The extent to which physical and psychological dependence develop—as well as their associated physical, psychological, and social consequences—are directly related to the specific pattern and context of alcohol use. Infrequent use, or low to moderate "social use" of alcohol in small amounts—one or two drinks on holidays and special occasions or less than five drinks a week for adolescent girls and young women and seven drinks a week for adolescent boys and young men—is generally associated with few or no harmful effects.[43] However, for abusive and, finally, compulsive use, harmful effects and toxicities become more apparent and troublesome with the development of physical and psychological dependence, increasingly serious forms of dependence or use disorder—"alcoholism."[44]

Alcohol dependence or use disorder—alcoholism—is inherently complex in nature. It typically occurs insidiously with the regular, long-term moderate to heavy drinking of alcohol over months to years and is characterized by the development of tolerance to alcohol (i.e., adolescents and young adults find themselves drinking more frequently, and in

42 N.B. Over several decades—although not yet completely substantiated—several researchers (e.g., Deitrich, Zimatkin, & Pronko, 2006; Hipolito, Sanchez, & Polache, 2007) have posited that acetaldehyde, an intermediary product of alcohol metabolism (see related discussion in earlier pharmacology subsection, "Pharmacokinetics—Metabolism"), plays a significant role regarding several CNS actions that are associated with alcohol use—including increasing patterns of harmful use and physical and psychological dependence. In this context, it is commonly agreed that the acetaldehyde found in the brain is the result of the metabolism of alcohol—after the alcohol has crossed into the CNS—because acetaldehyde does not readily cross the blood-brain barrier. It has been further noted that acetaldehyde, in the CNS, contributes to the reinforcing effects of alcohol use—in contrast to acetaldehyde, in the peripheral circulation, which contributes to unpleasant, aversive effects (Quertemont, 2004).

43 Exceptions include, for example, adolescents who are: (1) alcohol dependent, but who are now abstinent (i.e., have achieved a pattern of resumed nonuse); (2) receiving disulfiram (Antabuse®) pharmacotherapy for alcohol abstinence maintenance (see the discussion in the later child, adolescent and young adult treatment subsection—"Pharmacotherapy"); and (3) pregnant (see related discussion in the later subsection, "Pregnancy and Lactation—Fetal Alcohol Syndrome/Fetal Alcohol Spectrum Disorder"). Additionally, ingesting all 5, or 7, drinks, respectively, during the same drinking episode would be considered to be harmful "binge drinking."

44 Genetics has been estimated to contribute to approximately 50% of the risk for developing alcohol dependence or use disorder. Polymorphisms in isoforms of alcohol dehydrogenase and acetaldehyde dehydrogenase (see related discussion in the earlier pharmacology subsection, "Pharmacokinetics—Metabolism") have been implicated in this risk, but specific loci of responsible genes have not yet been identified (e.g., Costin & Miles, 2014)

larger amounts, in an attempt to achieve the desired effects that they initially achieved with infrequent, low to moderate drinking). Severe alcohol dependence, or use disorder, is also characterized by the need to drink alcohol throughout the day to prevent, or ward off, the signs and symptoms associated with decreasing BACs, and the resultant alcohol withdrawal syndrome.

Consequently, we have, for a number of decades, considered alcohol dependence or use disorder to be more accurately considered as a syndrome characterized by many specific related signs and symptoms, as well as, varying levels of harm and/or associated risk. Most of these signs and symptoms are reflected in both the DSM-5 criteria for AUD and associated items/questions that have been constructed to detect alcohol dependence among adolescents and young adults (see the related discussion in the later assessment and diagnosis of alcohol dependence or use disorder subsection—"Selected Quick-Screen Psychometric Tests.") Traditionally, common characteristics include:

- Alcoholic "blackouts"—being unable to account for specific periods of time when drinking;[45]
- Drinking alone;
- Tolerance to alcohol—increasingly, drinking more alcohol, more frequently, to achieve initial desired effects;
- Drinking in the morning or "starting the day" with a drink;
- Experiencing signs and symptoms of withdrawal due to decreasing BACs when alcohol use is "cut-down" or suddenly discontinued;
- Feeling increasingly "guilty" about drinking behavior and/or associated effects;
- Gulping down drinks to rapidly increase BACs;
- Sneaking drinks;
- "Stashing" alcohol in the back of a computer desk drawer or other hiding place;
- Concealing alcohol in a Thermos® or water bottle in order to drink at school/work;
- Displaying negative affect or personality changes.[46]

Approximately one-third of adolescents and young adults in the U.S. are expected to develop patterns of abusive and, later, compulsive use of alcohol sometime during their lifetime (Hasin, Stinson, & Ogburn, 2007; Pagliaro & Pagliaro, 2012, 2018). These adolescents and young adults are usually characterized as belonging to one of two major groups:

1. "Bender" or "binge" drinkers—who drink heavily for a short period of time (e.g., weekends);
2. "Daily" drinkers—who drink heavily every day or whenever alcohol is available to them.

Approximately one-sixth of the adolescents and young adults, who meet the criteria for abusive or compulsive use of alcohol, manage to "cure themselves." Characteristic of the pattern of compulsive use, most of these adolescents and young adults have alternating periods of "complete abstinence," or resumed nonuse, followed by periods of "heavy drinking," or relapsed use—the

45 Blackouts, which were once primarily associated with alcoholism among older adults, who are regular, long-term drinkers, are now commonly reported by a significant percentage of high school and college/university students, who are regular, "long-term"—or acute, heavy—drinkers (Pagliaro & Pagliaro, *Clinical Patient Data Files*). For example, LaBrie, Hummer, and Kenney (2011), in their study of over 2,500 students from two universities who reported past month pre-partying (see the later section, "Pre-Partying and Drinking Games"), found that 25% reported experiencing at least one alcoholic blackout during the preceding month.

46 These "changes" are typically seen by others (e.g., classmate; coach; employer; minister; parent; teacher) as being annoying and/or problematic. Consequently, the adolescent or young adult is commonly urged to reduce or stop drinking alcohol (Pagliaro & Pagliaro, *Clinical Patient Data Files*).

return to compulsive use. Unfortunately, if they do not receive some form of external intervention, their alcohol use is likely to follow this typical pattern, which becomes increasingly harmful over time. The compulsive pattern of use has been described as beginning when the first major problems associated with alcohol use are recognized by those other than the drinker (e.g., coach; employer; friend; health or social care professional; parent; family physician; sibling; or teacher).

ALCOHOL WITHDRAWAL SYNDROME

> Depending on the amount of alcohol consumed and the duration of an individual's drinking habit, alcohol withdrawal syndrome can range from *minor* symptoms such as irritability, agitation, anxiety, headache, anorexia, diaphoresis, palpitations, insomnia, nausea and vomiting, and tremors; to *moderate* symptoms, including confusion and autonomic hyperactivity; to more *severe* symptoms, including muscle rigidity, seizures, and delirium tremens.
>
> (Costin & Miles, 2014, p. 8)

The alcohol withdrawal syndrome is characterized by a period of "rebound hyperexcitability," which may be quite severe—particularly for regular, long-term heavy drinkers, who abruptly discontinue alcohol use—and, consequently, may be fatal. As noted in the earlier pharmacology subsection, "Mechanism of Action," regular, long-term use of alcohol is associated with up-regulation of the NMDA glutamate receptors. Hence, during alcohol withdrawal, excess excitatory glutaminergic function is noted that significantly contributes to the signs and symptoms associated with the alcohol withdrawal syndrome (Gonzales & Jaworski, 1997; Hoffman, 1995)—including related seizure activity (Hoffman & Tabakoff, 1994).

Alcohol, like many other sedative-hypnotics, can suppress epileptic seizures. However, when regular, long-term alcohol use is abruptly discontinued, this anticonvulsant action may be followed by seizure-related hyperexcitability that lasts for several days. Whether adolescents or young adults, who are dependent on alcohol, have epilepsy or not, they commonly experience seizures (usually tonic-clonic, or grand mal, seizures, but may include partial seizures) when their regular, long-term, moderate to high use of alcohol is abruptly discontinued. During alcohol withdrawal, the associated seizures typically peak approximately eight to 12 hours after their last drink. The seizures associated with alcohol withdrawal are generally resistant to standard anticonvulsant pharmacotherapy (e.g., carbamazepine [Tegretol®] or phenytoin [Dilantin®]), but respond well —both in terms of prophylaxis and active treatment—to benzodiazepines (e.g., diazepam [Valium®]). (See the later discussion in the treating child and adolescent dependence and use disorder subsection, "Pharmacotherapy—Alcohol Withdrawal Syndrome.") As reported by Schmidt, Doshi, and Holzhausen (2016), "Approximately, 50% of patients with alcohol dependence experience alcohol withdrawal" (p. 389).[47]

HANGOVERS

Fortunately, for most adolescents who drink alcohol, a milder form of the alcohol withdrawal syndrome, commonly known as a "hangover," occurs. Hangovers are typically identified by the following characteristics that generally follow heavy drinking episodes: anxiety; cognitive deficits, particularly deficits in attention and memory; depressed mood; dry mouth; fatigue;

47 Interestingly, Dixit, Endicott, and Burry (2016) noted that:

> approximately 16–31% of patients in the intensive care unit (ICU) have an alcohol use disorder and are at risk for developing alcohol withdrawal syndrome.
>
> (p. 797)

general malaise; headache (often severe); hypersensitivity to light and sound; nausea; thirst; and vomiting.

In addition, as identified by several researchers (e.g., Ling, Stephens, & Heffernan, 2010; McKinney, 2010; Prat, Adan, & Perez-Pamies, 2008), hangovers also are associated with:

- Impaired job performance;
- Poor academic achievement;
- Potentially dangerous situations involving daily activities (e.g., child care, rearing, and supervision; driving a car; or operating heavy machinery);
- Reduced productivity;
- School or workplace absenteeism.

Many of these signs and symptoms are often self-managed by drinkers, themselves. For example, a commonly used remedy is to take "a little hair from the dog that bit me"[48]—have a "Bloody Mary" cocktail (tomato juice and vodka) for breakfast or a "Screwdriver" cocktail (orange juice and vodka)—to which vitamins, protein powder, and a raw egg may be added (Pagliaro & Pagliaro, *Clinical Patient Data Files*). These and other approaches that are used to self-manage hangovers are *not* recommended because they tend to promote, or reinforce, harmful drinking patterns that are likely to result in, or sustain, alcohol dependence or use disorder (Pagliaro & Pagliaro, 2012; Piasecki, Robertson, & Epler, 2010).

Alcohol Overdosage/Unintentional Poisoning

Alcohol overdosage[49] is generally self-limiting among adolescents and young adults, who are regular, long-term heavy drinkers, because they usually end their heavy drinking episodes by simply falling asleep (for related discussion, see also the earlier pharmacology subsection, "Pharmacokinetics—Absorption").[50]

A troubling trend, over the last two decades, is the increasing number of fatalities associated with the concurrent use of alcohol and other psychodepressants by adolescents and young adults. As reported by Jones, Paulozzi, and Mack (2014), working on behalf of the FDA and CDC, "alcohol was involved in 22.1% of opiate pain reliever and 21.4% of benzodiazepine drug-related deaths" (p. 881). The synergistic psychodepressant actions of alcohol—particularly respiratory depression—exacerbated by the concurrent use of other psychodepressants, such as, opiate analgesics (e.g., oxycodone) and prescription sedative-hypnotics (e.g.,

48 This common expression for treating a hangover originated from that associated with the ancient practice of treating rabid dog or other dog bites by placing some "hair from the dog that bit you" in the wound.

49 N.B. Unintentional poisonings also are noted among children and adolescents who have ingested "toxic alcohols" (i.e., diethylene glycol; ethylene glycol; isopropanol; methanol; propylene glycol) (Kraut & Mullins, 2018). Absorption of the toxic alcohols following ingestion is relatively complete and rapid achieving peak plasma concentrations within 30 minutes. Therefore, gastric lavage and the administration of activated charcoal generally are of limited clinical efficacy in cases of toxic alcohol poisonings (Ekka & Aggarwal, 2015; Kraut & Kurtz, 2008; Williams & Erickson, 1998). Because toxicities associated with the toxic alcohols is primarily a result of their metabolites—except in the case of isopropanol—treatment of poisonings involves, in addition to supportive medical care, inhibition of their metabolic conversion by alcohol dehydrogenase (see also the related discussion in the earlier pharmacology subsection, "Pharmacokinetics—Metabolism"). Although ethanol (i.e., alcohol) can be used, fomepizole (Antizol®, 4-methylpyrazole), a strong inhibitor of alcohol dehydrogenase, is the preferred antidote for these poisonings, particularly for ethylene glycol and methanol poisoning (Ekka & Aggarwal, 2015; Kraut & Kurtz, 2008).

50 Also, commonly associated with acute, non-fatal overdosages of alcohol are hangovers that occur during the post-drinking recovery phase. (See additional related discussion in the earlier alcohol pharmacology subsection, "Undesired, or Harmful, Effects and Toxicities—Hangovers.")

benzodiazepines), accounts for these increased mortality rates. (See also the related discussion in the earlier subsection, "Alcohol Drug–Drug Interactions").

Signs and symptoms of alcohol poisoning, in addition to those associated with alcohol intoxication (see earlier Table 1.2, "Blood Alcohol Concentrations"), include:

- Apnea;
- Bradycardia;
- Cyanosis;
- Delirium;
- Hypothermia;
- Seizures;
- Stupor;
- Unconsciousness;
- Vomiting.

***Related Professional Reminder:* Upon presentation to the ED—after the provision of urgent care, including respiratory support—it is highly recommended that the following laboratory analyses be obtained: (1) BAC in order to document the extent of the alcohol overdosage/unintentional poisoning; and (2) full toxicology screen in order to determine, or rule out, the use of other drugs and substances of abuse and/or the presence of other co-intoxicants.**

Although the incidence of mortality associated with alcohol overdosage/unintentional poisoning is relatively low in comparison to that associated with the toxic alcohols (see earlier related footnote #49), deaths do occur annually in the U.S.[51] As identified by the CDC (2015):

> An average of 6 people die of alcohol poisoning each day in the U.S.
>
> (p. 1)[52]

No specific antidote is available to treat alcohol poisoning. Treatment consists of symptomatic, supportive care. For example, in addition to maintaining respiratory function, those with alcoholic ketoacidosis require IV infusion of dextrose 5% in water (e.g., D_5W) and normal saline (NS) in order to restore volume deficits and prevent hypoglycemia (Kraut & Kurtz, 2008). Other common measures include: thiamine that may be required for correction of vitamin B_1 deficiency; and a urinary catheter to manage incontinence and monitor urinary function. Hemodialysis effectively removes alcohol from the blood and should be considered, particular in severe cases with BAC exceeding 400 mg/dl (see the related discussion in the earlier subsection, "Blood Alcohol Concentrations") (Atassi, Noghnogh, & Hariman, 1999; Quispe Gonzales, Gomez Giralda, & Ruiz-Zorrilla Lopez, 2011).[53]

Pregnancy, Breastfeeding, and Mothering

Among pregnant women, the prevalence of any alcohol use and binge drinking in the past 30 days were 10.2% and 3.1%, respectively. Among binge drinkers, pregnant women reported a

51 The lethal dose of alcohol for children is approximately 2–3 gm/kg and for adolescents and young adults, approximately 3–5 gm/kg (Hovda & Jacobsen, 2016).

52 Male college students of European descent residing in the midwestern or southwestern states are, as a group, particularly at risk for alcohol overdosage/unintentional poisoning.

53 Although not FDA approved, see also the discussion of metadoxine in the earlier pharmacology subsection, "Pharmacokinetics—Metabolism and Excretion."

significantly higher frequency of binge drinking than nonpregnant women (4.6 and 3.1 episodes, respectively); the largest amount consumed during binge drinking was also higher among pregnant women than nonpregnant women (7.5 versus 6.0 drinks). (Tan, Denny, & Cheal, 2015, p. 1042)

Consequently, biochemical testing of the newborn for exposure to alcohol and other drugs and substances of abuse is often required (see related discussion in the following subsection). General signs and systems that may indicate a need for this biochemical testing include:

- Abruptio placentae;
- Acknowledged maternal history of drug and substance abuse;
- Congenital abnormalities;
- Lack of prenatal maternal care;
- Maternal history of unexplained fetal death;
- Positive maternal toxicology screen;
- Preterm birth;
- Repeated spontaneous abortion;
- Signs and symptoms of neonatal abstinence syndrome;
- Unexplained CNS complications (e.g., intracranial hemorrhage; seizures);
- Uncharacteristic behavioral state of the newborn (e.g., jittery; lethargic);
- Unexplained intrauterine growth restriction.

(e.g., ACOG, 2015; Farst, Valentine, & Hall, 2011; Newman, 2016; Washington State Department of Health, 2015)

Fetal Alcohol Syndrome/Fetal Alcohol Spectrum Disorder

The term, "Fetal Alcohol Spectrum Disorder" (FASD), is now commonly used in lieu of the term, "Fetal Alcohol Effects" (FAEs), a term that was used to identify neonates, infants, and children who exhibit fewer of the characteristics deemed necessary, by definition or convention, to establish a diagnosis of FAS (Caruso & Ten Bensel, 1993; Ginsburg, Blacker, & Abel, 1991; Smitherman, 1994). Other diagnostic labels and definitions also have been used in this regard in the published clinical literature, including alcohol-related birth defects (ARBD) and alcohol-related neurodevelopment disorder (ARND) (Harris, Osborn, & Weinberg, 1993; Pagliaro & Levin, 1979; Sampson, Streissguth, & Bookstein, 1997; Sokol & Clarren, 1989). All such related terms are now generally subsumed by, or included within, the FASD.

Craniofacial characteristics that are commonly associated with FAS/FASD include:

1. Eyes
    a. Epicanthal folds;
    b. Microphthalmia;
    c. Ptosis;
    d. Shortened palpebral fissures;
    e. Strabismus.
2. Ears
    a. Abnormal (i.e., low-set, malformed, or smaller or larger than normal).
3. Nose
    a. Low or flattened nasal bridge;
    b. Short with high or upturned nasal tip.
4. Mouth
    a. Micrognathia or retrognathia;
    b. Philtrum: absent or underdeveloped;

   c. Teeth: absent enamel; malformed; or maloccluded;
   d. Thin vermillion border of upper lip;
   e. Wide mouth.
5. Head
   a. Abnormal shaped cranium;
   b. Microcephaly;
   c. Mid-face hypoplasia;
   d. Narrow receding forehead.

(Pagliaro & Levin, 1979; Pagliaro & Pagliaro, 1997, 2003a, 2018)

Alcohol, a known human teratogen, readily crosses the placental barrier from the maternal systemic circulation to the developing fetal systemic circulation and, consequently, results in exposure of the developing fetus to alcohol and its potential undesired, or harmful, effects and toxicities. As noted by Ross, Graham, and Money (2015), these adverse effects associated with alcohol exposure have been attributed to several diverse molecular mechanisms:

> Ethanol has diverse cellular targets, and produces wide-ranging effects depending on the dose, duration, and timing of exposure. Current evidence suggests that alcohol produces many of its damaging effects by exerting specific actions on molecules that regulate key developmental processes (e.g., L1 cell adhesion molecule, alcohol dehydrogenase catalase), interfering with trophic factors that regulate neurogenesis and cell revival, and/or inducing excessive cell death via oxidative stress or activation of caspase-3 proteases.
>
> (p. 75)

The most severe teratogenic effect associated with alcohol use during pregnancy is the FAS/FASD (Pagliaro & Pagliaro, 1987) (see Figure 1.5). In the U.S., the FAS/FASD:

- Is the leading cause of developmental disabilities (CDC, 2012b; Floyd, Weber, & Denny, 2009; Marchetta, Denny, & Floyd, 2012);
- Is the most common preventable cause of mental deficiency/intellectual deficit (Burd, Carlson, & Kerbeshian, 2007; Pagliaro & Pagliaro, 1995, 1997, 2000, 2012, 2018; Vaux, 2016);
- May be identified in up to 3% of live births (May, Baete, & Russo, 2014; May, Keaster, & Bozeman, 2015; Mengel, Searight, & Cook, 2006);[54]
- Is only caused by maternal alcohol use during pregnancy.

The detection of maternal alcohol use during pregnancy is an integral part of the diagnosis of FAS/FASD. However, retrospective self-report of alcohol use during pregnancy is not always reliable. As identified by Joya, Friguls, and Ortigosa (2012), "pregnant women tend to underreport alcohol drinking by questionnaires" (p. 209). Thus, to increase reliability, several researchers (e.g., Crunelle, Yegles, & van Nuijs, 2014; Pragst & Yegles, 2008) have recommended the analytical laboratory analysis of maternal hair

54 Significantly higher incidences have been reported for U.S. youth of various age groups and continental, or other descent—such as American Indians (see the related discussion later in this section).

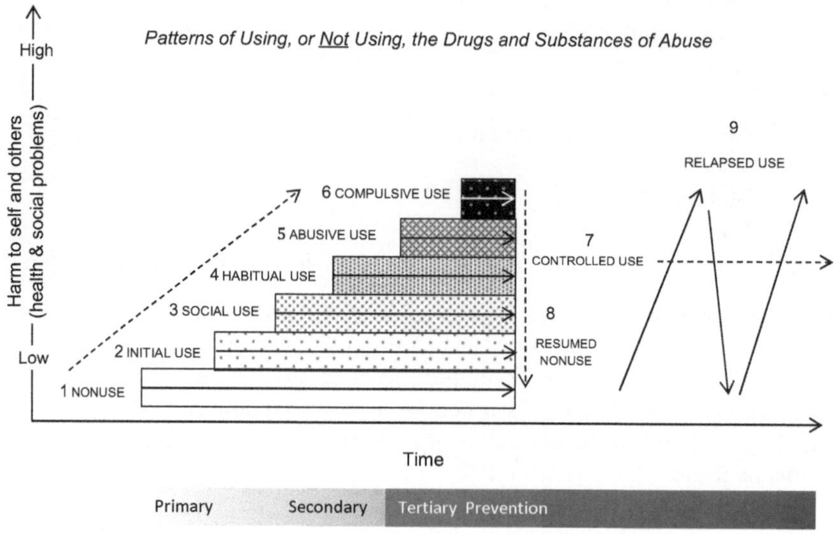

Figure 1.5 Nine Patterns of Abusable Psychotropic Use

samples—for the presence and level of fatty acid ethyl esters and/or ethyl glucuronide—in order to determine whether alcohol was used during pregnancy and, if so, the associated level of alcohol use (e.g., low, moderate, or heavy drinking).[55, 56, 57]

Serum microRNAs also have served as biomarkers of alcohol use during pregnancy (e.g., Gardiner, Gutierrez, & Luo, 2016). Some researchers also suggest the analysis of neonatal biological samples (e.g., hair; meconium), as well as placental and umbilical cord samples. Kvigne, Randall, and Simanton (2012) have suggested the analysis of neonatal BACs, positing that increased fetal alcohol dehydrogenase activity (as determined by increased alcohol elimination rates) is the result of, and thus, indicative of their mother's regular, long-term alcohol use during pregnancy.

The safety of alcohol ingestion during pregnancy (i.e., from conception to birth) has not been well-documented and appears to be highly variable. The ingestion of up to *two* drinks per

55 N.B. A wide variety of "biomarkers" have been identified and used to obtain better biological assessments of maternal alcohol use during the gestational period. These "indirect" measures of maternal BACs have been used in place of "direct" measures because alcohol has a relatively short and variable half-life of elimination (i.e., alcohol is subject to significant genetic effects) and, consequently, is only of value in terms of determining: (1) acute intoxication; or (2) relatively recent alcohol use. The biomarkers that have been used generally measure either maternal alcohol-induced pathology or derivatives of non-oxidative alcohol metabolism. They include: alanine aminotransferase; acetaldehyde-derived conjugates; aspartate aminotransferase; fatty acid ethyl esters; ethyl glucuronide; ethyl sulfate; gamma glutamyl transferase; mean corpuscular volume; and phosphatidylethanol (Joya, Friguls, & Ortigosa, 2012).

56 In addition, the "lack of candor" often noted during clinical interviews of pregnant women regarding self-reports of alcohol use, has resulted in the development and use of various related quick-screen psychometric tests (see discussion in the later section, "Selected Quick-Screen Psychometric Tests").

57 Obviously, consent must be obtained from the mother in order to test her, or her neonate, for exposure to drugs and substances of abuse. In addition, in most jurisdictions, cases involving neonates, who have been identified as being affected by maternal drug or substance abuse, including signs of neonatal withdrawal, must be reported by mental health care and other professionals to Child Protective Services.

day by pregnant adolescent girls and young women has been generally considered to be safe for the fetus. However, because of the serious, and irreversible, long-term/permanent physical and psychological effects associated with FAS/FASD, which may occur among offspring (e.g., behavioral problems; developmental deficits, including learning deficits), we have consistently recommended, over several decades, that adolescent girls and young women *completely avoid* the use of alcohol during pregnancy (e.g., Pagliaro & Pagliaro, 1987, 1996, 1997, 2000, 2002, 2003a, 2009, 2012, 2018).

> In 2005, the Surgeon General issued an advisory urging women, who are, or might be, pregnant, to abstain from alcohol consumption to eliminate the risk for FASD or other negative birth outcomes.
>
> (Tan, Denny, & Cheal, 2015, p. 1)

Despite these recommendations, a significant number of pregnant women in the U.S. continue to consume alcohol and many of these women knowingly engage in patterns of binge drinking while pregnant (Marchetta, Denny, & Floyd, 2012; Tan, Denny, & Cheal, 2015). In a large sample of "women with pregnancies that resulted in a live birth," 14% (i.e., approximately, one in seven) engaged in preconception binge drinking. These women tended to be single and of European continental descent. They also were found to be more likely to continue to both drink alcohol and smoke tobacco cigarettes during their pregnancies (Naimi, Lipscomb, & Brewer, 2003).

In addition, May, Keaster, and Bozeman (2015, p. 118), in their study of the mothers of 1278 children, found that the mothers of children with FAS/FASD were significantly more likely to have:

- Increased mental depression;
- Later recognition that they were pregnant;
- Lower educational achievement;
- Reported marijuana and methamphetamine use during pregnancy.

Montag (2016), in a review of published FAS/FASD studies, additionally identified significant correlations with other factors:

- Lower socioeconomic status;
- Older age;
- Single/Unmarried;
- Unemployed.

> Among pregnant women aged 15 to 44 in 2012–2013, an annual average of 9.4 percent reported current alcohol use, 2.3 percent reported binge drinking, and 0.4 percent reported heavy drinking.
>
> (SAMHSA, 2014, p. 37)

While published data since 1977 (e.g., Pagliaro & Levin, 1979; Pagliaro & Pagliaro, 1987) have implicated FAS with high maternal BACs during a critical time of embryonic or fetal development, the average daily alcohol consumption during pregnancy may not be as important as maximal concentrations obtained during binge drinking at critical periods. For example, alcohol consumption during pregnancy, particularly during the first trimester, has been associated with an increased risk for miscarriage (Avalos, Roberts, & Kaskutas, 2014). In addition, as noted by Riley and McGee (2005, p. 360), nonalcohol factors may contribute to the significance of the negative outcomes associated with FAS/FASD. These factors include:

- Genetic variation;
- Interaction with nutritional variables;
- Maternal characteristics;
- Socioeconomic status;
- Synergistic reactions with other drugs.

Available data suggest that neuronal apoptosis,[58] induced by maternal alcohol consumption during pregnancy, may be the primarily underlying pathophysiologic basis for the development of the FAS/FASD and its associated neurobehavioral deficits and impairments (Olney, Wozniak, & Jevtovic-Todorovic, 2002; Qi, Zhang, & Li, 2014). In this case, the third trimester of pregnancy—which correlates with the beginning of the brain growth spurt period—would appear to be the time of greatest vulnerability for the development of the FAS/FASD (Ikonomidou, Bittigau, & Koch, 2001; Pagliaro & Pagliaro, 1987).

Producers and marketers of alcohol have included warnings to women in their advertising that drinking alcohol during pregnancy should be avoided because of the possible risk for FAS/FASD. In addition, concerned groups have worked to encourage the display of signs—in bars and liquor stores—warning pregnant women *not* to drink during pregnancy because of the noted association between alcohol use and birth defects. During the new millennium, the use of alcohol has been identified as a form of child abuse and neglect and has resulted in legal action, in some jurisdictions, against women who excessively drink during pregnancy and, subsequently, give birth to infants with FAS/FASD. As noted by the *National Institutes on Alcohol Abuse and Alcoholism* (NIAAA), "State and Federal governments have established various policies in response to the risks associated with drinking during pregnancy" (*Pregnancy and alcohol*, 2015, p. 1). As further explained by Thomas, Cannon, and French (2015, p. 68):

> U.S. states have enacted a wide range of laws to address health challenges associated with alcohol use during pregnancy. Some have taken punitive approaches that restrain women's behavior, and some have taken supportive approaches aimed at improving women's health and supporting healthy pregnancies.[59]

Although these and other prevention efforts have been made, the incidence of the FAS/FASD in the U.S. remains at a significantly high level and, unfortunately, is increasing, particularly among women of American Indian descent (e.g., Eustace, Kang, & Coombs, 2003; Hanson, Winberg, & Elliott, 2012; Pagliaro & Pagliaro, 2009, 2012, 2018; Popova,

58 Neuronal apoptosis is the process by which brain cells disintegrate into particles that are consumed by other cells (e.g., leukocytes, macrophages). The process is, under normal circumstances, a physiologically important process that helps to regulate neurogenesis. However, when neuronal apoptosis is aberrant or premature, such as occurs with maternal alcohol use and with some neurological disorders (e.g., amyotrophic lateral sclerosis; Huntington's disease) the process of brain growth and development is abnormally prevented or slowed (e.g., Franklin-Tong & Gourlay, 2008; Mattson, 2000; Okouchi, Ekshyyan, & Maracine, 2007).

59 For further related discussion, see the *Alcohol Policy Information System* (Hilton, 2014), and Thomas, Cannon, and French (2015)

Lange, & Probst, 2017).[60, 61] In one of the most recently conducted related studies, May, Chambers, and Kalberg (2018) concluded that:

> Estimated prevalence of fetal alcohol spectrum disorders among more than 6,000 first-graders in 4 U.S. communities ranged from 1.1% to 5.0% using a conservative approach.
> (p. 474)

As identified in several studies and reports (e.g., Hanson, Winberg, & Elliott, 2012; Khan, Robinson, & Smith, 2013), including data from the Indian Health Services (IHS), in some Alaska Native and American Indian communities/reservations, women's use of alcohol during pregnancy has *exceeded* 50%, particularly during the first trimester (Pagliaro & Pagliaro, *Clinical Patient Data Files*).

Common Misbelief: Children with FAS/FASD will "outgrow" most of their associated mental and physical deficits during adolescence and young adulthood.

As noted by Riley and McGee (2005):

60 The significant variance noted in the reported incidence of FAS/FASD is primarily the result of five major factors: (1) genetics; (2) sociocultural drinking patterns; (3) year that the assessment was performed (i.e., drinking patterns change over time); (4) the criteria used to define FAS/FASD (e.g., all cases versus only clinically severe cases); and (5) experience and competence of researchers or research assistants—be they nurses, occupational speech therapists, physicians, psychologists, or others)—to note mild cases and be able to rule-out potentially overlapping conditions and syndromes that may affect appropriate diagnoses of FAS/FASD (e.g., Aarskog syndrome; Dubowitz syndrome; fetal anticonvulsant syndrome; toluene embryopathy; and Williams syndrome).

These factors are supported by several findings reported in the related published literature. For example, as identified by Chasnoff, Wells, and King (2015), "high rates of missed diagnoses and misdiagnosis" are commonly observed regarding FAS/FASD. In their study they found that:

> Among 156 children and adolescents who met criteria for a diagnosis within the fetal alcohol spectrum, 125 had never been diagnosed as affected by prenatal alcohol exposure, a missed diagnosis rate of 80.1%. Of the 31 who had been recognized before referral as affected by prenatal alcohol exposure, 10 children's FASD diagnoses were changed within the spectrum, representing a misdiagnosis rate of 6.4%. The remaining 21 (13.5%) children's diagnoses stayed the same.
> (p. 264)

Rojmahamongkol, Cheema-Hasan, and Weitzman (2015, p. 197) found that "pediatricians 'underrecognize' FASDs, lack confidence in making this diagnosis, and are unfamiliar with the diagnostic criteria." Finally, several researchers have provided additional insights into the reasons for these related observations. For example, Douzgou, Breen, and Crow (2012) found that "classification of FASD was difficult in children under a year old when data on growth and development were limited." Others (e.g., Cook, Green, & Lilley, 2016), subsequently provided revised guidelines to facilitate the diagnosis of FAS/FASD.

61 Significant variance in the incidence estimates of FASD has been identified in various countries. For example, Lange, Probst, and Gmel (2017, p. 948), utilizing WHO defined criteria, found that:

1. Overall global prevalence of FASD among children and youth in the general population was 7.7 per 1,000;
2. WHO European Region had the highest prevalence (i.e., 19.8 per 1,000);
3. WHO Eastern Mediterranean Region had the lowest prevalence (i.e., 0.1 per 1,000).

Of 187 counties for which data were available, the top three in terms of prevalence were: South Africa, 111.1 per 1,000; Croatia, 53.3 per 1,000; and Ireland, 47.5 per 1,000.

> Autopsy and brain imaging studies indicate reductions and abnormalities in overall brain size and shape, specifically in structures such as the cerebellum, basal ganglia, and corpus callosum. A wide range of neuropsychological deficits have been found in children prenatally exposed to alcohol, including deficits in visuospatial functioning, verbal and nonverbal learning, attention, and executive functioning. These children also exhibit a variety of behavioral problems that can further affect their daily functioning.
>
> (p. 357)

Consequently, the developmental deficits that are generally associated with FAS/FASD—both mental and physical—do not end in infancy, but persist into childhood, adolescence, and throughout adulthood (Pagliaro & Pagliaro, 1987, 2012, 2018; Smitherman, 1994; Spohr, Willms, & Steinhausen, 1993, 2007; Streissguth, Randels, & Smith, 1991).

As identified by Tan, Denny, and Cheal (2015):

> Community studies estimate that as many as 2% to 5% of first grade students in the United States might have an FASD.
>
> (p.1042)

Unfortunately, even with early identification and intervention, "the growth and neurological disabilities associated with alcohol consumption during pregnancy persist even when the child grows up in a good home" (Karp, Qazi, & Hittleman, 1993, p. 101). For example, common problems include: behavioral problems, such as a higher incidence of attention–deficit/hyperactivity disorder (ADHD), conduct disorder (CD), and externalizing behavior (e.g., acting out, aggressiveness, delinquency, and hostility) (Bada, Das, & Bauer, 2007; Pagliaro & Pagliaro, 2002, 2012; Sood, Delaney-Black, & Covington, 2001). These behavioral problems are not easily managed, even with appropriate pharmacotherapy or psychotherapy.

The lifelong effects of FAS/FASD require: (1) increased attention; (2) greater focus on prevention of the disorder; and, when it is identified, (3) appropriate and effective treatment. In this regard, we have long concurred with Streissguth, Randels, and Smith (1991) that, for infants and children affected with FAS/FASD—and their parents, teachers, and caregivers—less frustration and optimal behavioral outcomes during later adolescence and adulthood are most likely to be achieved with:

1. Realistic expectations for performance during childhood and adolescence;
2. Availability of more appropriate educational and health care services.

As noted over 25 years ago by Karp, Qazi, and Hittleman (1993), and many others (e.g., Spohr, Willms, & Steinhausen, 2007), FAS/FASD is a "permanent disease" in the literal sense (i.e., it cannot be reversed or cured).[62] Thus, it is essential that prevention and treatment programs be developed to assist women of reproductive age, including adolescent girls, to understand the: (1) risks

62 However, although FAS/FASD, as a teratogenic effect, is lifelong and incurable, it is treatable, and important advances have been made in this regard (Bertrand, 2009). As noted by Chudley, Conry, and Cook (2005), infants, children, and adolescents who have been diagnosed with FAS/FASD have an opportunity to achieve optimal outcomes with the help of specialized core teams of experts in the disorder, including: (1) nurses and social workers with expertise in case management and coordination of core team member activities; (2) physicians specially trained in the diagnosis and medical management of FAS/FASD; (3) clinical infant, child, and adolescent psychologists; (4) occupational therapists; and (5) speech language pathologists. These core team members, along with parents and caregivers, child care workers, family therapists, and teachers can help infants, children and adolescents, who are diagnosed with FAS/FASD, achieve optimal personal outcomes.

associated with alcohol use during pregnancy; and (2) need to discontinue alcohol use, particularly, if they are sexually active (and do not appropriately use available methods of birth control), or are pregnant. Attention also is needed regarding relapse prevention for women who have histories of abusive or compulsive use of alcohol, including binge drinking, and for whom abstinence during pregnancy, consequently, may be difficult to achieve or maintain.

Alcohol and Breastfeeding

Alcohol is excreted in significant amounts in breast milk (Pagliaro & Levin, 1979). As reported by Haastrup, Pottegard, and Damkier (2014):

> The amount of alcohol presented to nursing infants through breast milk is approximately 5-6% of the weight-adjusted maternal dose.
>
> (p. 168)

Gibson and Porter (2018, p. 1) suggest that maternal alcohol use may expose breastfed infants to BACs that result in "dose-dependent reductions in their cognitive abilities." However, the observed effects were not sustained beyond childhood and could have been due to a number of other intervening variables. The alcohol-related odor and taste of the breast milk produced by mothers, who have ingested alcohol, appear to significantly decrease the amount of breast milk ingested by nursing neonates and infants (Mennella, 2001a; Mennella & Beauchamp, 1999). In addition, as reported by Mennella (2001b), "maternal alcohol consumption may slightly reduce milk production" (p. 230).

Consequently, because of these reported effects, as well as the potential negative effects of alcohol use on mothering behaviors (see the next pharmacology subsection, "Alcohol and Mothering"), we recommend that adolescent girls and young women, who are breastfeeding, avoid drinking alcoholic beverages of any kind. The CDC (2018b, p. 1) generally concurs with this recommendation (i.e., "not drinking is the safest option for breastfeeding mothers") but notes that "one drink per day is not known to be harmful to the infant."

Alcohol and Mothering

An adolescent girl's or young woman's instinctive and protective care of her neonate, infant, toddler, preschooler, or child comprises natural[63] response—as well as uniquely learned physical, mental, and sociocultural behaviors. These behaviors involve concurrent behavioral responses from her offspring that lead to her offspring's healthy and optimal development. Unfortunately, for adolescent girls and young women, who abuse alcohol and other drugs and substances of abuse, mothering abilities can be significantly diminished—or destroyed, often with decidedly deleterious, and inter-generational, effects among offspring—particularly daughters (Pagliaro & Pagliaro, *Clinical Patient Data Files*).

A "special bulletin" for mental health and social care professionals, published by the U.S. Department of Health and Human Services, identified several deleterious effects associated with a parent's alcohol and other drug or substance use that can result in ineffective or inconsistent parenting:

63 Natural, or "innate," responses are generally associated with maternal instinct, as well as various ovarian and pituitary hormones (e.g., estradiol, oxytocin).

- Difficulties regulating emotions and controlling anger and impulsivity;
- Disruptions in healthy parent-child attachments;[64]
- Estrangement from family and other social supports;
- Incarceration, which can lead to separation from a child, inappropriate care, and lack of stability and supervision;
- Physical or mental impairment;
- Reduced capacity to respond to a child's cues and needs;
- Spending limited funds on alcohol and drugs rather than food and other household needs;
- Spending time seeking out, manufacturing, or using alcohol or other drugs and substances of abuse.

(Child Welfare Information Gateway, 2014, p. 3)[65]

As aptly noted by Connors, Bradley, and Whiteside Mansell (2003) in their longitudinal national study of women and their children from 50 publicly-funded residential substance abuse treatment programs:

> Findings from this study suggest that children whose mothers abuse alcohol or other drugs confront a high level of risk and are at increased vulnerability for physical, academic, and socioemotional problems. Children affected by maternal addiction are in need of long-term supportive services.
>
> (p. 744)

In a related "fact sheet" published by the WHO, "Child Maltreatment and Alcohol," identified that:

1. Numerous studies have established that alcohol is a significant contributory factor to child maltreatment;
2. In the U.S., 35% of offenders of parental child abuse had consumed either alcohol or drugs at the time of the incident.

(Butchart, Poznyak, & Bellis, 2006, p. 1, 3)

As illustrated in the following two vignettes:

64 As noted by Lander, Howsare, and Byrne (2013):

> It is estimated that more than eight million children younger than age 18 live with at least one adult who has a SUD that is a rate of more than one in 10 children. The majority of these children are younger than age five ... If the child experiences the primary caretaker as unresponsive or inconsistently responsive, an insecure attachment may form that can result in a variety of problems including anxiety, depression, and failure to thrive.
>
> (p. 194)

65 Others have noted similar findings. For example, Slesnick and Zhang (2016) reported that:

> Substance use is considered a stressor that negatively affects parenting of mothers ... Further, the parent-child relationship is often characterized by inconsistent care, unstable attachment and inadequate response to children's needs.
>
> (p. 619)

> A one-year-old baby covered in vomit and feces was discovered it the backseat of a car when officers in West Virginia pulled over a driver for a suspected DUI. . . . the driver of the vehicle—the child's mother—was too intoxicated to answer when she was asked for the child's name.
>
> (Sung, 2016, p. 1)

> Lehnardt told her Alcoholics Anonymous sponsor of a wild night in April that led to the mother losing custody of her children . . . she allowed the teens to smoke pot and drink booze in her home. The mother also joined the groups in a game of naked Twister. According to the police report, the mother left the game to have sex with an 18-year-old in the bathroom. The report said Lehnardt awoke around 3:30 am to find her daughter's 16-year-old boyfriend having sex with her [16 year-old-daughter].
>
> (Frisk, 2016, p. 1)

New Millennial Trends in Alcohol Use

Trends in alcohol use—including medical use and child, adolescent, and young adult exposure and use—are presented and discussed in the following subsections. Also included is a subsection, "Nine Patterns of Child, Adolescent, and Young Adult Alcohol Use." For a discussion of embryo/fetus, and neonate/infant exposure, see the earlier discussion in the pharmacotherapy subsections, "Pregnancy, Breastfeeding, and Mothering" and "Overdosage/ Unintentional Poisoning." We begin with the medical use of alcohol.

Medical Alcohol Use

Since its introduction in North America by European explorers and traders, alcohol was used to treat such varied conditions as the common cold and "rheumatism." Until approximately 80 years ago, alcohol was medically classified as a "psychostimulant" and was administered by nurses by the "syringeful" to their patients when "rapid stimulation" was required (Pagliaro, 1986, p. 10). It also was thought to possess nutritive and other benefits.

For the last 50 plus years, the only medical use for alcohol, other than its use as a topical antiseptic at injection sites, has been its use as a vehicle for the preparation of various pharmaceutical formulations (i.e., alcohol-containing solutions and elixirs). In response to both public and health care provider demands for alcohol-free liquid pharmaceutical products, particularly those formulated for children and older adults, the use of alcohol for the preparation of various pharmaceutical products has decreased significantly.[66] However, several pharmaceutical formulations—for prescription and non-prescription (i.e., over-the-counter) use—currently contain alcohol, including several:

- Liquid cough and cold formulations, such as Ambenyl®, Benylin®, Dilaudid Cough Syrup®, Novahistine®, Robitussin®, and Vicks®;
- Liquid vitamin drops, such as Ce-Vi-Sol®, Geritol®, and Nu-Iron®;
- Mouth washes, such as Cepacol® and Listerine®.

66 A commensurate reduction in the alcohol content of personal care products (e.g., aftershave; mouth wash) also occurred during the past 40 years. However, the reason for this reduction was to deter the use of these products by adolescents and young adults who were regular, long-term users of alcohol—generally homeless, "skid-row" alcoholics, primarily to avoid "getting sick" (i.e., to prevent, or self-manage, the alcohol withdrawal syndrome) at times when they were otherwise unable to obtain their usual wine, whiskey, or other alcoholic beverage (Pagliaro & Pagliaro, *Clinical Patient Data Files*). Because of the limited availability of personal care products that contain alcohol, a related concern is the drinking of household cleaning products that contain alcohol (e.g., "decanting" pressurized cans of Lysol® Disinfectant Spray for the same reasons) or other alcohol containing products (e.g., Chinese cooking wine; liquid shoe polish—usually "strained through a sock;" pure vanilla extract—which contains 35% alcohol) (Pagliaro & Pagliaro, *Clinical Patient Data Files*).

Health and social care professionals require a knowledge of the alcohol content of these and other pharmaceutical drug products, particularly when working in settings[67] where regular, long-term users of alcohol may substitute these products when beverage alcohol is unavailable to them. For example, when they are unable to purchase alcohol, obtain some from a friend, or are restricted from using it (e.g., when jailed or enrolled in drug treatment programs). In addition, it is particularly important for health and social care professionals to be aware of these alcohol-containing products if adolescents or young adults with AUD are initiating or being treated with disulfiram (Antabuse®) therapy, which requires a total restriction of the use of alcohol, because of the associated possibility of triggering an alcohol-induced "disulfiram reaction." (See also the related discussion of disulfiram [Antabuse®] in the earlier pharmacology subsection, "Alcohol Drug–Drug Interactions," and the later treating adolescent and young adult alcohol dependence or use disorder subsection, "Pharmacotherapy and Psychotherapy/Counseling—Pharmacotherapy").

Nine Patterns of Child, Adolescent, and Young Adult Alcohol Use

This section presents and discusses nine patterns of child, adolescent, and young adult alcohol use. It is followed by an overview of the trends identified in child, adolescent, and young adult alcohol use during the new millennium. For child exposure to alcohol, see also the earlier related-discussion in the "Pharmacology" subsections—"Alcohol Overdosage/Poisoning" and "Pregnancy, Breastfeeding, and Mothering."

The use of alcohol (and other abusable psychotropics) by children, adolescents, and young adults (as well as adults of all ages), is characterized by nine patterns of use from "nonuse" to "resumed nonuse" (see Figure 1.5).

Each of these patterns of use, which relate to the use of all abusable psychotropics, are presented and discussed in the following subsections, using alcohol as an example. We begin with "nonuse."

Nonuse

Nonuse, the first pattern of use, characterizes children, adolescents, and young adults who have never tasted, or tried, an alcoholic beverage.[68]

Initial Use

Initial use of alcohol during childhood may occur in association with religious ceremonies (i.e., Holy Communion) or because of curiosity (e.g., when a child takes a sip of beer—often provided by a parent)—to "see what it tastes like." For example, Jackson, Barnett, and Colby (2015), in their related study of initial alcohol use, found that: (1) approximately 30% of surveyed students "sipped" alcohol by the sixth grade; (2) in most cases the "sip" of alcohol occurred in their own homes; and (3) the primary supplier/source of the alcohol was a parent. Most significantly, they found that:

67 These settings include, for example: convenience stores; grocery stores; and pharmacies—particularly those located in, or near, alcohol-free Indian reservations and inner-city neighborhoods (Pagliaro & Pagliaro, *Clinical Patient Data Files*).

68 Of the 20% of people in the U.S. who do not drink alcohol, approximately one-half do not consume alcohol for religious reasons (e.g., Church of Jesus Christ of Latter-day Saints [Mormons]; Fundamentalist Moslems [Religion of Islam]; Seventh-Day Adventists) and the remaining one-half do not consume alcohol for medical reasons. Included in the latter group are those who are recovering from alcoholism and who subscribe to the principles of Alcoholics Anonymous (AA) or other similar 12-step programs.

> Youth who sipped alcohol by sixth grade had significantly greater odds of consuming a full drink, getting drunk, and drinking heavily by ninth grade than nonsippers.
>
> (p. 212)

Social Use

The most common form of alcohol use among adolescents and young adults is "social use," which involves the ingestion of alcohol, in the form of beer, wines, and distilled spirits (i.e., whiskey, vodka, liqueurs), at celebratory and other social situations with others (e.g., birthdays, holidays, and weddings; sport team victories; job promotions; graduation from high school or college/university). The social customs of various cultural/ethnic groups in the U.S. significantly affect adolescent and young adult drinking at this level. Other factors include:

- Age;
- Alcohol availability;
- Continental descent, including genetic predisposition for an ability to tolerate the use of alcohol (e.g., Jewish adolescents), or lack thereof (e.g., sensitivity of Asian adolescents and young adults to alcohol as characterized by the common occurrence of the "Asian Flush");[69]
- Family history of alcohol or other dependence or use disorder(s);
- Legal restrictions;
- Personal preferences;
- Religion;
- Sexual orientation.[70]

The *Office of Adolescent Health* for the SAMHSA (2014) reported that "Social Use" of alcohol (i.e., first "non-sip use") began prior to age 13 for approximately 20% of U.S. adolescents.

Habitual, Abusive, and Compulsive Use

Once the use of alcohol begins, it generally continues throughout an adolescent's or young adult's life and is characterized by habitual use (e.g., having a glass of wine with dinner; drinking a couple of cans of beer while watching a televised sporting event before going to bed) and is generally not associated with serious problems. However, for many adolescents, whose alcohol use is associated with characteristic patterns of abusive use (e.g., intermittent heavy drinking), increasingly suffer undesired, or harmful, effects and toxicities that, for some, may be fatal.

A history of childhood physical and/or psychological abuse, including sexual assault, has been highly correlated with the abusive pattern of alcohol use, which can spiral to compulsive

69 The "Asian Flush" also is known as the "Asian Flush Syndrome" or the "Oriental Flushing Syndrome." The characteristic "flushing," or "blushing," of the skin associated with drinking alcohol, usually involves the face, neck, and shoulders. This reaction is caused by the accumulation of acetaldehyde in the circulatory system associated with a deficiency of acetaldehyde dehydrogenase–the enzyme primarily responsible for the metabolism of acetaldehyde in the body. This genetically controlled, or inherited, deficiency is particularly common among adolescents and young adults (as well as adults) of Asian continental descent–thus, the name, "Asian Flush" (Crabb, Edenberg, & Bosron, 1989; Xiao, Weiner, & Crabb, 1996).

70 N.B. Formerly, males significantly outnumbered females in virtually every alcohol use category. However, male-female gender differences in the incidence of alcohol use by adolescents and young adults, in the U.S., have virtually been eliminated during the new millennium (Pagliaro & Pagliaro, 2012, 2018). In some cases, females now demonstrate superiority to males in various alcohol use categories—for example, "excess in newly incident drinking among 12–17 years" (Cheng & Anthony, 2017, p. 117).

use, particularly among bisexual, lesbian, and trans adolescents (Gilmore, Koo, & Nguyen, 2014; Pagliaro & Pagliaro, 2012, 2018).

It has been estimated that, annually, on college/university campuses across the U.S., alcohol use by young adults has been directly associated with: 1,400 student deaths; 500,000 unintentional injuries; and 600,000 physical assaults (including rape) (Hingson, Heeren, & Zakocs, 2002). In a later study of adolescents, 12 years-of-age to 18 years-of-age, Harland, Copelas, and Harris (2017) found that "trajectories of substance use" (i.e., the general "equivalent" of the progression through the nine patterns of use) revealed the following:

1. Adolescents, who abstained from drug and substance use, were most likely to have parents, who abstained from drug and substance use;
2. Adolescents, who increased their monthly use of drugs and substances of abuse, were more likely to have older siblings who abused drugs and substances of abuse;
3. Adolescents, who displayed the most frequent incidence of drug and substance abuse, were most likely to have siblings and peers who used drugs and substances of abuse.

Based on their analysis of data from a national survey study and their application of DSM criteria, Ahrnsbrak, Bose, and Hedden (2017, p. 25, 26) estimated that, in 2016, approximately:

- 488,000 adolescents, aged 12 to 17, had a past year alcohol use disorder;
- 3.7 million young adults, aged 18 to 25, had a past year alcohol use disorder.

Drinking Estimates[71]

The minimal legal drinking age across the entire U.S. (i.e., in all 50 states) is 21 years-of-age. As such, all alcohol use by children and adolescents in the U.S. (i.e., all "underage drinking") is "illicit." Once alcohol use begins, it generally continues throughout the life of a child, adolescent, or young adult —except for those, who are able to discontinue their alcohol use, primarily for health or religious reasons. This subsection focuses on estimates of new millennial statistics for alcohol use, particularly among adolescents and young adults with attention to recent trends in their drinking behavior, including: "binge drinking," "partying," and "drinking games." Also included is the more recent and growing trend among adolescents and young adults—drinking alcohol and caffeinated energy drinks.

Alcohol use, other than a "sip" or a "taste," generally increases with increasing age throughout late childhood and adolescence, from around eight years-of-age to around 20 years-of-age (Pagliaro & Pagliaro, 2009). As identified by Donovan (2007), in a review of children's alcohol use in the U.S., more than 6% of 9-year-old children and 15.5% of 12-year-old children reported having "more than a few sips of alcohol." This observation is also supported by Eaton, Kann, and Kinchen (2010), who found, in their analysis of data from the *Youth Risk Behavior Surveillance System* for 2009, that, nationwide, 21.1% of U.S. students, in grades nine through 12, reported having drunk alcohol (other than a few sips) for the first time before they were 13 years-of-age (a range of 11.5 % to 29.4 % across state surveys)—an age range reported by most adults as the time they ingested their first "non-sip" alcoholic drink (Alcohol Use USA, 2010; Office of Adolescent Health, 2017).[72]

71 Alcohol use estimates in the U.S. display significant variability for several reasons as discussed later in this chapter.

72 Similarly, Bracken, Rodolico, and Hill (2013), in their study of 939 adolescents admitted for drug or substance abuse treatment between 1995 and 2010, found that the reported age of "first alcohol use" was 13 years-of-age.

The NIDA-sponsored *Monitoring the Future (MTF)* survey for 2009, found that 14.9% of 8th grade students, 30.4% of 10th grade students, and 43.5% of 12th grade students reported past month use of alcohol (Johnston, O'Malley, & Bachman, 2010). In another study of over 3,000 adolescents in grades nine through 12, The Partnership for a Drug-Free America and the MetLife Foundation (2011), found that 39% of their adolescent participants reported having ingested alcohol during the past month. Regarding alcohol use, these findings—with a slight downward trend—have been relatively constant over the past several years.

Most studies indicate that approximately 80% of people in the U.S. regularly ingest alcoholic beverages. Regarding adolescents, Eaton, Kann, and Kinchen (2010), in their analysis of data from the *Youth Risk Behavior Surveillance System* for 2009, found that more than 72% of U.S. students, in grades nine through 12, reported alcohol use with a range of approximately 40% to 80% across state surveys. Over 25% of these students reported that they ingested alcohol on more than 100 days during the past year (Alcohol Use USA, 2010).

Interestingly, Eaton, Kann, and Kinchen (2010) also found that 4.5% of U.S. students nationwide, in grades nine through 12, ingested at least one alcoholic beverage while on school property during the previous 30 days (range, 2.7% to 8.0% across state surveys).[73] In addition, Johnston, O'Malley, and Bachman (2011) in their 2010 in-school survey, *Monitoring the Future*, found that 16.3% of 8th grade students, 36.9% of 10th grade students, and 54.1% of 12th grade students reported a lifetime prevalence of having been drunk.

As identified by Swendsen, Burstein, and Case (2012), in their analysis of data from the *National Comorbidity Survey—Adolescent Supplement*, which was based on a nationally representative face-to-face survey of over 10,000 adolescents, 13 to 18 years-of-age:

> By late adolescence, 78.2% of U.S. adolescents had consumed alcohol, 47.1% has reached regular drinking levels defined by at least 12 drinks within a given year, and 15.1% met criteria for lifetime abuse.
>
> (p. 390)

More recently, Lipari, Ahrnsbrak, and Pemberton (2017), based on the 2016 *National Survey on Drug Use and Health*, estimated that 2.3 million U.S. adolescents, 12 to 17 years-of-age began their use of alcohol in 2016.

Binge Drinking, Pre-Partying, and Drinking Games

This subsection describes and discusses the statistics, characteristics, and consequences of: (1) binge drinking; (2) pre-partying; and (3) drinking games.

Binge Drinking

"Binge drinking"—traditionally defined as the ingestion of 5, or more, alcoholic drinks per drinking episode for adolescent boys and young men, and 4, or more, alcoholic drinks per drinking episode for adolescent girls and young women—is highly correlated with acute CNS impairment and significant adverse health consequences (Pagliaro & Pagliaro, 2009, 2012).[74] In fact binge drinking significantly contributes to mortality in the U.S., as noted by the CDC:

73 The incidence was reportedly highest (i.e., 7.9%) for boys of Hispanic descent. (See also the related discussion of binge drinking among adolescents in the U.S. of Hispanic descent in the following section.)

74 Traditionally, the definition of binge drinking, for both adolescent boys and girls—as well as young women and men, was based on the amount of alcohol necessary to achieve a BAC of 0.08 gram% (i.e., 80 mg%; 80 mg/dL)—the legal level of alcohol intoxication in the U.S.

> Binge drinking was responsible for more than half of the estimated 79,000 deaths and two thirds of the estimated 2.3 million years of potential life lost as a result of excessive drinking each year in the United States during 2001–2005.
>
> (CDC, Centers for Disease Control and Prevention, 2010, p. 1274)

As identified by Chung, Creswell, and Bachrach (2018), "binge drinking . . . typically begins in adolescence" (p. 5). Of concern, the *Office of Adolescent Health* (2017, p. 3) found that ~45% of U.S. high school students reported having consumed "5 or more drinks of alcohol in a row within a couple of hours [during the 30 days before the survey]" (p. 3). They also found that when "compared to adults, adolescent drinkers tend to consume higher quantities of alcohol per occasion, but drink less frequently" (p. 5). Prior to, and throughout, the new millennium, binge drinking among adolescents and young adults has been repeatedly, and directly, associated with significantly increased incidence rates of:

- Academic problems;
- Acquaintance/date rape;
- Alcohol overdosage/poisoning;
- Alcohol-related blackouts;
- MVCs;
- Physical and/or sexual assault;
- Risky sexual behavior.

(e.g., Chung, Creswell, & Bachrach, 2018; Dunn, Bartee, & Perko, 2003; Pagliaro & Pagliaro, 1996, 2012)

These adverse consequences also contribute to many significant related adverse consequences for the families, peers, and communities of adolescent binge drinkers.

Using a modified version of the Widmark equation to calculate BACs for boys and girls, Donovan (2009) suggested a significant revision to the traditional definition of binge drinking. Specifically based on calculated estimates of the differences between children and adults in total body water (TBW) and alcohol elimination rates, Donovan (2009) recommended that "binge drinking" be more accurately defined as:

1. Three or more drinks per drinking episode for children and adolescents, nine to 13 years-of-age;
2. Three or more drinks per drinking episode for adolescent girls, 14 to 17 years-of-age;
3. Four or more drinks per drinking episode for adolescent boys, 14 and 15 years-of-age;
4. Five or more drinks per drinking episode for adolescent boys, 16 and 17 years-of-age.

While we would agree that the number of drinks required to detect binge drinking should be lowered for children and adolescents, we would also caution that: (1) there are, as of yet, no empirical data to support Donovan's recommendations; and (2) alcohol metabolism and elimination may significantly vary among children and adolescents in the U.S. Major contributing factors to this variance include differences in: body weight; gender; and genetics.

Regarding "body weight," it should be noted that alcohol is predominantly water soluble. As such, doses of alcohol based on body weight will yield a significantly higher BAC among obese children and adolescents when compared to children and adolescents of normal body weight for their height and age. Regarding "gender differences," for post-pubescent adolescents, on average, girls have significantly more body fat than boys (see related discussion in the earlier pharmacology subsection, "Pharmacokinetics—Volume of Distribution"). Regarding "genetic differences," for example, whereas American Indians and Asians, generally, are genetically more sensitive to the effects of alcohol, Jews, generally, are genetically more tolerant. Thus, we expect a significant amount of related variance regarding general definitions of binge drinking and the detection criteria for children and adolescents.

Regardless of this variance, the incidence of the occurrence of binge drinking episodes has increased significantly over the past two decades and appears to be continuing to increase across the U.S. (Naimi, Lipscomb, & Brewer, 2003; Pagliaro & Pagliaro, 2009, 2018). As noted by the U.S. Surgeon General:

> In 2015... over 66 million people (nearly a quarter of the adult and adolescent population) reported binge drinking in the past month.
>
> (USDHHS, 2016, p. ES-1)[75]

As further noted by Chung, Creswell, & Bachrach (2018):

> Most of the alcohol consumption of underage drinkers occurs during "binge" episodes.
>
> (p. 5)

The highest rates of binge drinking, in the U.S., are reported for the Northern states along the Canadian border—with the exception of Washington state—and the states of Alaska and Hawaii (Sacks, Gonzales, & Bouchery, 2015, p. e73). In addition, approximately 80% of these binge drinkers are males (Kanny, Naimi, & Liu, 2018). In comparison, adolescent rural high school seniors, living in the Midwest, have the highest incidence of binge drinking (Chung, Creswell, & Bachrach, 2018).[76]

Utilizing a sample of 8,110 adolescents, 12 to 17 years-of-age, who reported alcohol consumption during the past 30 days, Rossheim, Stephenson, and Thombs (2017) examined factors associated with binge drinking, "heavy episodic drinking"—defined as the consumption of five or more drinks for adolescent boys and four, or more, drinks for adolescent girls. The researchers found several factors that were characteristic for adolescent binge drinkers:

- Being given alcohol by a non-parental social source;
- Being older in age;
- Buying alcohol from liquor stores or from another person;
- Drinking at multiple locations;
- Drinking at someone else's house and not their own;
- Initiating alcohol use at a younger age.

Grucza, Norberg, and Bierut (2009) analyzed available data from the *National Survey on Drug Use and Health*—a pooled sample of more than 500,000 adolescent and young adult subjects. Overall, from 1979 to 2006, they found that the incidence of binge drinking decreased significantly for boys (i.e., by approximately 15%), but increased significantly for girls (i.e., by approximately 50%). Adolescent findings, classified according to gender and age cohorts, are presented in Table 1.3.

75 Similarly, Ahrnsbrak, Bose, and Hedden (2017) estimated that 65.3 million people in the U.S., 12 years-of-age and older, were current binge drinkers. In addition, they estimated that, of these binge drinkers, 4.5 million were adolescents between 12 and 20 years-of-age.

76 McKinnon, O'rourke, and Thompson (2004) examined the rates of binge drinking among high school students in the 9th through the 12th grades, who were sampled from 16 U.S. high schools along the U.S.-Mexico border. Most students, who participated in the study, were of Hispanic descent. Of these students, 45% reported binge drinking, 19% reported high risk driving behaviors (e.g., drinking and driving), and 46% reported riding with a driver who had been drinking. These percentages were found to be: (1) significantly higher than the U.S. national averages; and (2) highly correlated with reported "alcohol-related problems" and "lower academic grades." Equally significant and disturbing, the students who participated in the study reported even higher rates of binge drinking (i.e., OR = 6.44), risky driving (OR = 5.39), and riding with a driver who had been drinking (OR = 5.39) "when visiting Mexico."

Table 1.3 Incidence of Binge Drinking among Adolescent Girls and Boys in the U.S.[77]

Gender	*Age (Years)*	*% Binge drinkers (2009)*	*% Binge drinkers (2012)*
Girls	12 to 14	3.5	6.1
	15 to 17	15.1	12.7
	18 to 20	30.1	17.6
Boys	12 to 14	2.7	6.5
	15 to 17	18.1	16.5
	18 to 20	41.0	25.5

Source: Grucza, Norberg, and Bierut (2009); Patrick and Schulenberg (2012).

As illustrated in Table 1.3, the incidence of binge drinking among adolescents:

1. Increases with increasing age;
2. Is significantly higher among boys, although girls are in the same "ball park;"
3. Appears to be affected by an interaction effect between age and gender.

Similarly, Miller, Naimi, and Brewer (2007), in a study of approximately 14,000 high school students, found that 27.5% of boys and 23.5% of girls had engaged in binge drinking during the 30 days preceding their survey. Although the results indicate a higher incidence of binge drinking among boys, 18 to 20 years-of-age, this finding may be due to the use of "5, or more, drinks in a row on one, or more, of the 30 days preceding the survey"—instead of the standard measurement of binge drinking for girls as "4, or more, drinks" (see earlier discussion in this subsection).

Regarding the interaction effect between age and gender, Grucza, Norberg, and Bierut (2009) also noted that, in regard to the incidence of binge drinking:

4. For adolescents 12 to 14 years-of-age, girls had a significantly higher incidence of binge drinking than boys;
5. For adolescents 15 to 17 years-of-age, the incidence of binge drinking was essentially the same;
6. For adolescents 18 to 20 years-of-age, boys had a significantly higher incidence of binge drinking.

Bisexual and lesbian adolescent girls comprise another group that has relatively high rates of binge drinking and alcohol dependence or use disorder—regardless of continental or other descent (Pagliaro & Pagliaro, *Clinical Patient Data Files*). This group, when compared to heterosexual adolescent girls who drink, has been identified (e.g., Pagliaro & Pagliaro, 2012) as sharing the following characteristics:

77 The variance identified in this table may be confounded by the differences in the: (1) 8th, 10th, and 12th grade samples used in each of the source studies (e.g., differences in location—urban versus rural; differences in race/ethnicity—Hispanic versus Native American Indian); (2) definitions of binge drinking (e.g., five drinks versus four drinks); and (3) time frame for binge drinking (e.g., past two weeks versus past year).

- Higher incidence of binge-drinking;
- Higher incidence of heavy drinking;
- Higher incidence of problem drinking behaviors (e.g., driving while intoxicated; getting into fights);
- Higher rates of alcohol-related problems (e.g., accidents; physical assault);
- Higher rates of attendance at bars, clubs, and house parties for drinking purposes;
- Higher risk for alcohol dependence or use disorder;
- Higher risk for other dependence or use disorders;
- Lower rates of decline in binge-drinking, heavy drinking, and other problem drinking in relation to increasing age;
- Higher likeliness to seek formal treatment for alcohol dependence or use disorder.

Although, it has long been recognized that binge drinking is significantly higher among adolescent girls and young women, who are bisexual or lesbian (Pagliaro & Pagliaro, 1995, 2018), it also is significantly higher among trans-females (i.e., MTFs) (e.g., Drabble, Midanik, & Trocki, 2005; Hughes & Wilsnack, 1997; Hyde, Comfort, & McManus, 2009; Rowe, Santos, & McFarland, 2015). For example, Rowe, Santos, and McFarland (2015), in their study of MTF youth, found that:

> Most (81%) drank alcohol in the last six months whereas half (51%) engaged in binge drinking. (p. 162)

Pre-Partying and Playing Drinking Games

Pre-partying and playing drinking games can be considered to be "special cases" of binge drinking. In this context, Patrick, Terry-McElrath, and Miech (2017) identified that binge drinking and intoxication are higher among college students than non-college peers. For example, binge drinking within the past two weeks was reported by 32.4% of college students and 28.7% of non-college peers. In addition, alcohol intoxication within the past month was reported by 40.8% of college students and 30.4% of non-college peers.[78]

PRE-PARTYING

Pre-partying has also been referred to as "front-loading," "pre-drinking," and "pre-gaming"—terms that refer to "the consumption of alcohol prior to attending a planned event or activity (e.g., [meeting friends at a] bar, concert, dance, party, or sporting event), at which, more alcohol may or may not be consumed" (Pedersen & LaBrie, 2007, p. 238). In these contexts, alcohol is used to "loosen up," "get into the mood," "decrease sexual inhibitions," and engender "courage in a bottle," primarily by adolescents and young adults in their last two years of high school and first two years of college/university, respectively (Pagliaro & Pagliaro, *Clinical Patient Data Files*).[79] Researchers have consistently found that pre-partying is associated with significant increases in overall alcohol consumption (up to 50% greater) and resultant experiences of adverse alcohol-related consequences (e.g., Earleywine, LaBrie, & Pedersen, 2008; LaBrie, Earle, & Hummer, 2016; Paves, Pedersen, & Hummer, 2012; Pedersen & LaBrie, 2007).

LaBrie and Pedersen (2008) found that college women "drank significantly more drinks and reached higher BACs [than college men] on the pre-partying drinking day" (p. 955). In an

78 Interestingly, for undergraduate college/university students of European continental descent in the U.S., the rate of binge drinking has been significantly correlated with the use of volatile solvents and inhalants (e.g., gasoline; glue; nitrogen oxide) during childhood or adolescence (Bennett, Walters, & Miller, 2000; Pagliaro & Pagliaro, *Clinical Patient Data Files*).

79 Pre-partying is commonly observed among youth who deliberately intend to become intoxicated (i.e., "wasted").

earlier study, Pedersen and LaBrie (2007) found that, in comparison to college men, college women "were 1.75 times more likely to engage in heavy episodic drinking on pre-partying days" and that this behavior was "1.33 times more likely" to occur (p. 7).[80] These findings were subsequently duplicated by Paves, Pedersen, and Hummer (2012).

PLAYING DRINKING GAMES

Playing "drinking games" is a closely related behavior that is primarily used for the "same reasons" as pre-partying. As explained by Kenney, Hummer, and LaBrie (2010):

> An estimated 500 types of drinking games, including *Kings, Power Hour*, and *Quarters*, test players' drinking endurance and speed as they consume large amounts of alcohol in relatively short spans of time. Self-reports have revealed that students most commonly play drinking games for social enhancement, for instance to act as a social lubricant or to intoxicate themselves or others.
>
> (p. 999)

Several researchers (e.g., Borsari, 2004; Borsari, Bergen-Cico, & Carey, 2003; Kenney, Hummer, & LaBrie, 2010; Pedersen & LaBrie, 2007) have reported that participation in this risky drinking behavior is common among college students (i.e., over 50% self-report participation) and that most of those college students reported beginning this behavior while in high school. Two of these popular drinking games are described below by Kenney, Hummer, and LaBrie (2010, p. 1006):

> *Kings*. This game is typically played by four or more players. The dealer shuffles the cards and begins dealing one card at a time, face-up, to each player. The first person to be dealt a king picks a type of liquor. The second person to be dealt a king picks the mixer (if any). The third person makes the actual drink according to his/her discretion. And the fourth person who receives the final king consumes the drink that has been made.
>
> *Beer Pong*. This is one of the most popular drinking games. Beer Pong (also known as "Beirut") is a game in which players throw a ping-pong ball across a table with the intent of landing the ball in a cup of beer on the other end. The game typically consists of two, two-player teams. Six to 10 cups are set up on each side in triangle formation. The goal of the game is to eliminate the other teams' cups before one's own cups are eliminated. When a ball lands in a cup, which is generally filled with two–three oz. of beer, that cup is eliminated and the defending team must consume all the beer inside that cup. Once a team has eliminated all of the opposing cups (with the opponents having consumed all the beer in the cups), the losing team must also consume all the beer remaining in the winning team's cups.

In their narrative literature review of drinking games, Zamboanga, Tomaso, and Cloutier (2016, 24-E1) identified that: "Late adolescence (i.e., 17 to 19 years-of-age, which encompasses older high school students and younger college students) appears to be a period of peak risk for drinking games." These observations appear to be consistent with the "developmental" aspects of this period of life (i.e., late adolescence). A period during which individuals, as they move to young adulthood and increasing freedom from parental guidance/supervision (e.g., moving away from home to attend college), generally engage in more risky behavior than at earlier periods of life (in the absence of

80 Interestingly, Pedersen and LaBrie (2007) also found that, during pre-partying, college women were significantly more likely to drink "shots of liquor" or "wine" while college men were significantly more likely to drink "beer" (p. 14).

mental disorders, such as conduct disorder or risk-taking personality). They also found that adolescent girls were equally as likely as adolescent boys to participate in drinking games.[81]

Alcohol and Caffeinated Energy Drinks[82]

Energy drinks are non-alcoholic beverages (e.g., Red Bull®, RevItUp®, and Rock Star®) that are heavily laden with caffeine (see related discussion in Chapter 3, "Caffeine and Nicotine"). Throughout the first two decades of the new millennium, these beverages have become increasingly attractive to adolescents and young adults, including college/university students, who drink them to: stay awake; increase energy to "party all night and have fun;" "cram" for final examinations; or finish term papers (Nordt, Vilke, & Clark, 2012; Pagliaro & Pagliaro, 2009, 2012, 2018).

Malinauskas, Aeby, and Overton (2007) found that over 50% of U.S. college/university students reported regularly consuming energy drinks. They also found that almost half of these young adults reported commonly consuming three or more energy drinks, together with alcoholic drinks, while "partying." Miller (2008) found that, in the U.S., the association between the ingestion of energy drinks and aggression, insomnia, and other related problems among undergraduate college/university students was particularly significant for those of European continental descent, although not for those of African continental descent.[83] The use of "alcohol mixed with energy drinks" (AmED) has now become a well inculcated new millennial social phenomenon among adolescents and young adults.

Many adolescents and young adults assume that the psychostimulant actions of caffeine can "balance out" the psychodepressant actions of alcohol and, consequently, they can drink as much alcohol as they want without becoming drunk. However, the cognitive and psychomotor impairment associated with increasing BACs (see Table 1.1) are not significantly reduced by the caffeine consumed in energy drinks (Ferreira, de Mello, & Pompeia, 2006; Ferreira, de Mello, & Rossi, 2004)—even though these young adults generally incorrectly perceive themselves as being significantly "less intoxicated" than they are (Marczinski & Fillmore, 2006).

Undergraduate college/university students also use energy drinks to increase the amount of alcohol they can ingest during a drinking episode—without becoming "overly intoxicated." As identified by Marczinski (2011), "to get drunk and reduce sedation compared to alcohol alone" (p. 3232). However, as we have previously noted, what is achieved with a "caffeinated drunk" is simply a "wide-awake drunk." Instead of falling asleep, or "passing out," with a BAC of 0.25 to 0.30, these young adults remain awake and, consequently, often engage in hazardous behaviors that may result in harm to self and others (e.g., accidental falls; drunk driving; physical assault) (Pagliaro & Pagliaro, *Clinical Patient Data Files*). For example, Williams, Housman, and Woolsey (2018, p. 137) found that:

> 12th grade AmED users were significantly more likely to be in a motor vehicle accident ($p < .001$) and receive a ticket for a traffic violation ($p < .05$). Additionally, 12th grade AmED users were significantly less likely to wear a seatbelt as a driver or passenger ($p < .001$).

81 We believe that these observations are a function of changes in drug and substance use behaviors, including drinking, during the new millennium (i.e., previously, in most U.S. cultural contexts, adolescent boys would be expected to engage in this risky drinking behavior to a significantly greater degree than adolescent girls) (Pagliaro & Pagliaro, *Clinical Patient Data Files*).

82 See also the related discussion in the earlier pharmacology subsection, "Alcohol Drug–-Drug Interactions—Alcohol and Psychostimulants."

83 These continental and other descent biases, whether genetic or sociocultural, appear to contribute to the variability observed in the results of studies examining the drug interactions that involve alcohol and caffeine. For related discussion, see the earlier pharmacology subsection, "Alcohol Drug–-Drug Interactions."

(See Table 1.3 and previous related discussion in the pharmacology section, "Undesired, or Harmful, Effects and Toxicities.") Interestingly, Snipes, Green, and Javier (2014), in their study of the use of alcohol mixed with energy drinks and experiences of sexual victimization, found that the concurrent ingestion of alcohol and energy drinks was significantly associated with being "sexually victimized" for male college students, but not for female college students.

Diagnosis and Treatment of Adolescent and Young Adult Alcohol Dependence or Use Disorder[84]

The initiation of alcohol use, and the development of increasingly harmful alcohol-related problems, is beginning at younger ages. Those at particular risk for alcohol dependence or use disorder, are adolescents and young adults, who:

- Are in their late teens or early twenties;
- Are of Alaska Native or American Indian descent;
- Are poor, particularly those who are homeless or living on-the-street;
- Have been diagnosed with a conduct disorder during childhood;
- Have PTSD, including that associated with sexual assault (e.g., childhood sexual abuse; acquaintance/date rape; IPV);
- Have a genetic predisposition for alcohol dependence or use disorder (i.e., positive family history of alcoholism);
- Have a history of child neglect, physical abuse and/or mental abuse;
- Identify as bisexual, gay, lesbian, or trans.

(Forcehimes, Venner, & Bogenschutz, 2011; Green & Feinstein, 2012; Pagliaro & Pagliaro, 2000, 2012, 2018; Temcheff, Dery, & St-Pierre, 2016)

It is important to note that several physiological differences, as previously discussed (e.g., increased body fat among adolescent girls and young women; decreased alcohol metabolism among adolescent girls and young women), make adolescent girls and young women more physiologically vulnerable, than adolescent boys and young men, to both the acute and chronic effects associated with alcohol use, including the development of dependence or use disorder (see earlier related discussion in the pharmacology subsection, "Undesired, or Harmful, Effects and Toxicities—"Physical and Psychological Dependence")—despite drinking less alcohol and drinking for a shorter period of time. This accelerated progression to alcohol dependence among adolescent girls and young women, when compared to adolescent boys and young men, has been identified as the "telescoping effect" (Clarke, Kim, & White, 2013; Diehl, Croissant, & Batra, 2007; Keyes, Martins, & Blanco, 2010; Pagliaro & Pagliaro, 2018; Stewart, 2009). (See the *Index* for additional citations related to "telescoping.") (See also the related discussion in the earlier subsection, "Alcohol Dependence or Use Disorder.")

84 Alcohol dependence or use disorder occurs rarely among children younger than 10 years-of-age in the U.S. We have encountered this situation only in the most unusual circumstances that involved mutually contributory factors of severe poverty, social isolation, and parental alcoholism (Pagliaro & Pagliaro, *Clinical Patient Data Files*). Other researchers/clinicians (e.g., Temcheff, Dery, & St-Pierre, 2016) identified that the occurrence of conduct disorder in children is also an associated contributory factor to the early development of alcohol dependence or use disorder in this age group. Unfortunately, we are unable to present an empirically informed overview of this topic because, as noted by Donovan (2014, p. 1), "the study of alcohol use by children ages 12 and younger has been very limited." Additionally, Donovan, on behalf of the National Institute on Alcohol Abuse and Alcoholism (NIAAA), stated that:

> Chief among the factors inhibiting the estimation of alcohol burden in children and preadolescents is the absence of ongoing national surveillance data (p. 2).

Assessment and Diagnosis of Alcohol Dependence or Use Disorder

The use of alcohol, as well as other drugs and substances of abuse, among children, adolescents, and young adults, in the U.S., has reached significant and alarming proportions during the new millennium. However, only a small proportion of pediatricians and adolescent family physicians include the adequate assessment of AUD or SUDs during routine annual physical examinations or other office visits (Aspy, Mold, & Thompson, 2008; Habis, Tall, & Smith, 2007; Marcell, Halpern-Felsher, & Coriell, 2002; O'Brien, 2008a).

***Related Professional Reminder:* The assessment of alcohol dependence or use disorder includes a thorough history—both past and present—for the use of alcohol and its patterns of use, including concurrent use with other drugs and substances of abuse. If use is reported, then specific questions should be asked for alcohol, as well as for each of the other identified substances of abuse, including:**

- ***Age of initial use;***
- ***Circumstances associated with initial use, including involvement of boyfriends/girlfriends, parents, peers, siblings, or others;***
- ***Desire to address current alcohol or other dependence or use disorder (i.e., "readiness to change");***
- ***Duration;***
- ***Experience of adverse consequences including signs and symptoms of withdrawal;***
- ***Frequency of use;***
- ***Methods of use;***
- ***Positive experiences/benefits reportedly (believed to be) associated with use;***
- ***Previous related intervention or treatment and outcomes;***
- ***Quantity of use;***
- ***Severity of alcohol and other dependence or use disorder(s).***

Lack of attention to screening youth for alcohol or other drugs and substances of use is also true for other health and social care professionals (e.g., nurse practitioners; pediatricians; psychiatrists; school counselors/psychologists; social workers) who are involved in the promotion of child, adolescent, and young adult health and well-being. Thus, for many children, adolescents, and young adults, alcohol dependence or use disorder, as well as that for other drugs and substances of abuse, are left unidentified and remain untreated until associated personal and social problems escalate (see Table 1.4).

For example, Delaney-Black, Chiodo, and Hannigan (2010), in their longitudinal cohort study of over 400 urban, high-risk adolescents of African continental descent in the U.S., found that, "Teen specimens (hair) were 52 times more likely to identify cocaine use compared with self-report" (p. 887). In addition, none of the adolescent participants admitted to using opiate analgesics—even with the assurance that their responses would remain confidential. However, approximately 7% tested positive on laboratory analysis for opiate analgesic use. In a similar context, Bone, Gelberg, and Vahidi (2016), using drug analysis of urine samples to determine the accuracy of self-reported drug or substance abuse, found that:

> Under reporting of drug use is prevalent even among self-reported drug users in primary care patients of Federally Qualified Health Centers (22%).
>
> (p. 387)

Table 1.4 Alcohol or Other Dependence or Use Disorders: Missed Physician Diagnoses and Patient Responses

Percentage and type of physician respondents	*Physician diagnostic behavior in managing AUD and SUDs*
94% Primary Care Physicians	**Fail** to diagnose alcohol abuse when presented with early signs and symptoms in an adolescent or young adult patient
58% Physicians	**Fail** to discuss the use of drugs and substances of abuse with their patients because they believe their patients lie about it[85]
41% Pediatricians	**Fail** to diagnose illicit use of the drugs and substances of abuse when presented with a classic description of a drug-abusing teenage patient
35% Physicians	**Fail** to treat a patient who abuses the drugs and substances of abuse because of time constraints
30% Physicians	Identify they are prepared to diagnose drug abuse
20% Physicians	Identify they are prepared to diagnose alcoholism
17% Physicians	Identify they are prepared to diagnose illicit drug and substance abuse
11% Physicians	**Fail** to treat a patient who abuses drugs and substances of abuse because they are concerned that they won't be reimbursed for the time necessary to screen and treat the patient
Percentage of patient respondents	*Patient reports of physician behaviors in managing aud and suds*[86]
75%	Say their primary care physician was *not* involved in their decision to seek treatment for an AUD or SUDs
54%	Say their primary care physician did *nothing* about their addiction

Sources: Aspy, Mold, & Thompson, 2008; Habis, Tall, & Smith, 2007; Pagliaro & Pagliaro, 2012; Thompson, 2018.

Adolescent and young adult assessment and diagnosis of alcohol dependence or use disorder (i.e., Alcoholism; AUD) can be facilitated with the use of: DSM-5 criteria; screening, brief intervention, and referral to treatment (SBIRT) model; or specific quick-screen psychometric tests for alcohol dependence.[87]

Importance of Screening

It has long been established that delayed intervention or treatment can result in increasingly harmful consequences that are largely preventable. Selected quick-screen psychometric

85 Approximately, 58% of patients agree that they lie about their drug and substance abuse.

86 The typical patient had a substance use problem for 10 years before receiving treatment.

87 Tests for detecting other drugs and substances of abuse (i.e., amphetamines; caffeine; cannabis; cocaine; nicotine; opiate analgesics; psychodelics; sedative-hypnotics) are presented, respectively, in each of the following chapters.

tests offer health and social care professionals an accurate, economic, and efficient means for identifying adolescents and young adults for immediate necessary intervention (Eberhard, Nordstrom, & Hoglund, 2009), including referral to other appropriate health and social care providers (Searight, 2009), as needed (see Figure 1.6). Indeed, as we and others (e.g., Crome, Bloor, & Thom, 2006) have long noted, alcohol or other drug and substance of abuse dependence or use disorder—particularly when left unidentified or undiagnosed—can exacerbate, predispose, mask, or otherwise interfere with the diagnosis and management of other mental and physical disorders (see the later section in this chapter, "Child, Adolescent, and Young Adult Contemporaneous Diagnoses").

Related Professional Reminder:

- ***Obtain consent from parent or legal guardian and ascent/consent from child/adolescent—as appropriate;***
- ***Conduct a comprehensive assessment prior to planning and initiating treatment;***
- ***Maintain an appropriate level of confidentiality for the child or adolescent during all aspects of the assessment and treatment processes;***
- ***Recognize that different types of treatment may be required (i.e., the type of treatment that works best for one child or adolescent may not necessarily work best for another);***

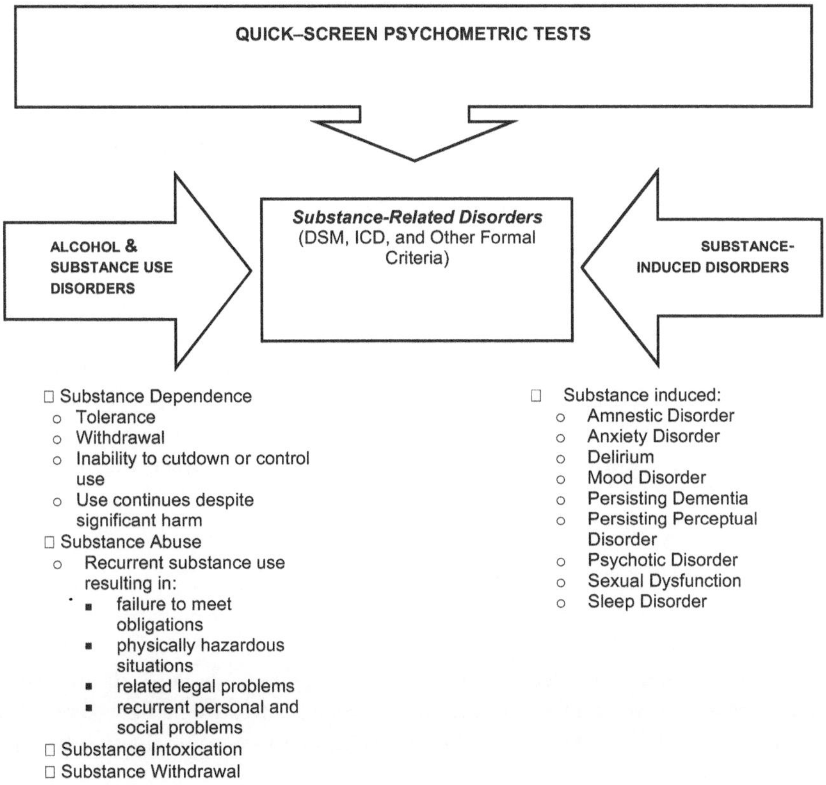

Figure 1.6 Diagnosing Alcohol or Other Dependence or Use Disorders

- ***Assess children and adolescents for any accompanying mental disorders (i.e., contemporaneous diagnoses) and refer or treat appropriately (see later section in this chapter, "Contemporaneous Diagnoses").***

Several professional organizations/societies (e.g., *American Academy of Pediatrics; American Society of Addiction Medicine; American College of Obstetricians and Gynecologists; U.S. Preventative Services Task Force*) have endorsed the use of screening tests to detect alcohol and/or other drug and substance of abuse dependence or use disorders (ACOG, 2011, 2015; ASAM, 1997, 2005; Levy & Williams, 2016; Moyer, 2013).

We recommend that, minimally, the following groups of adolescents and young adults be screened for alcohol, or other dependence or use disorder(s), because of the: (1) associated high incidence of drug and substance abuse among these groups of adolescents and young adults; and (2) significant potential and opportunity for preventing the development of associated increasingly undesired, or harmful, patterns of use:

- Adolescents and young adults, who are being assessed for, or who are already being treated for, any mental disorder, including any specific learning disorder;
- Adolescents and young adults, who are in the process of being committed, or have already been committed, to a youth detention or correctional facility;
- Adolescent girls and young women, who may become pregnant, or who are pregnant, because of the serious and lifelong teratogenic effects and related sequelae associated with the maternal use of alcohol and resultant FAS/FASD;
- Adolescents and young adults, who are being assessed, or who are being treated for, a sexually transmitted disease (STD);
- Adolescents and young adults, who are accessing ED services for: acute injuries associated with MVCs; violent assaults, including rape; or acute mental disorders (e.g., psychosis);
- Adolescents and young adults, who are suicidal or who have attempted suicide;
- Adolescents and young adults, who are homeless and living on-the-street;
- Adolescents and young adults who have positive family histories of drug or substance abuse, particularly among parents and/or siblings.

Additionally, as identified by Jones, Paulozzi, and Mack (2014)—in the context of the millennial opiate analgesic epidemic in the U.S.—alcohol was involved in 22% of deaths and 18% of ED visits associated with opiate analgesic use in 2010. Consequently, the CDC (2018a) recommended the use of alcohol screening and brief intervention (ASBI) for *all* patients who consume alcohol and use opiate analgesics (i.e., a focused special application of the widely known concept of, "Screening, Brief Intervention, and Referral to Treatment" [SBIRT]).

Screening, Brief Intervention, and Referral to Treatment (SBIRT)

In an effort to assist health and social care professionals, including pediatricians, psychiatrists, psychologists, and other health and social care providers, to assure the accurate and timely diagnosis and management of alcohol or other dependence or use disorder(s), several approaches for screening, brief intervention, and referral to treatment have been developed and implemented (e.g., Babor, McRee, & Kassebaum, 2007; Levy, Vaughan, & Knight, 2002; Madras, Compton, & Avula, 2009; Searight, 2009).

In 2011, the American Academy of Pediatrics (AAP) issued a policy statement endorsing the use of SBIRT. Specifically, pediatricians were encouraged to screen adolescents for drug and substance use at every: (1) "well" examination; and (2) acute care visit (when possible). In this context, the utilization of a validated quick-screen psychometric test was recommended (Beaton, Shubkin, & Chapman, 2016). However, in their analysis of the impact of the AAP recommendations among program directors and clinicians—in school-based health centers that served middle and high school students in New York state—Harris, Shaw, and Sherman (2016) found that:

1. Only 22% reported following the AAP SBIRT recommendations;
2. Less than 30% believed that they could effectively help students to reduce drug and substance use/abuse;
3. 63% did not believe that it was their professional role to utilize related quick-screen psychometric tests;
4. 30% did not feel competent to perform SBIRT.

In an attempt to: (1) positively address these issues; and (2) provide health and social care professionals with the data and tools necessary to perform SBIRT, we have included the following sections that present a detailed overview of the quick-screen psychometric tests that have been found to be particularly effective for detecting alcohol dependence or use disorder among adolescents. It should be kept in mind, that a positive screening test result does not, in and of itself, establish a related diagnosis of alcohol or other dependence or use disorder. While indicative of a related diagnosis, the actual diagnosis of an alcohol dependence or use disorder—for a specific adolescent—must be confirmed by an additional focused clinical assessment by the primary health or social care professional responsible for planning and delivering the adolescent's treatment. This assessment includes a:

1. Detailed history of the adolescent's use of alcohol and other drugs and substances of abuse;
2. Related personal data from any prior referrals to specific adolescent treatment programs, including information regarding completion and outcomes.

"Screening, brief intervention, and referral to treatment" is a treatment model that was developed early in the new millennium. It represents a major shift in the focus of the assessment and treatment of alcohol or other dependence or use disorder, from a focus on patients experiencing patterns of "abuse" or "compulsive use," to include a focus on "initial," "social," and "habitual use" of alcohol and other drugs and substances of abuse (i.e., it targets those, who have not yet developed significant related problems). As explained by SAMHSA:

> One of the strengths of the SAMHSA SBIRT model is that it screens all patients regardless of an identified disorder, allowing healthcare professionals in a variety of settings to address the spectrum of such behavioral health problems even when the patient is not actively seeking an intervention or treatment for his or her problems.
>
> (2013, p. 1)

The SBIRT model functions, in general, at the intersection between "prevention" and "treatment." (see Figure 1.7 The SBIRT Model)

The SAMHSA SBIRT model has six major characteristics:

1. Brevity. The initial screening is accomplished quickly (modal time about 5–10 minutes), and the intervention and treatment components indicated by the screening results are completed in significantly less time than traditional specialty alcohol or other dependence or use disorder(s);
2. Universality. All patients, clients, students, or other target populations are screened as part of other standard intake processes;

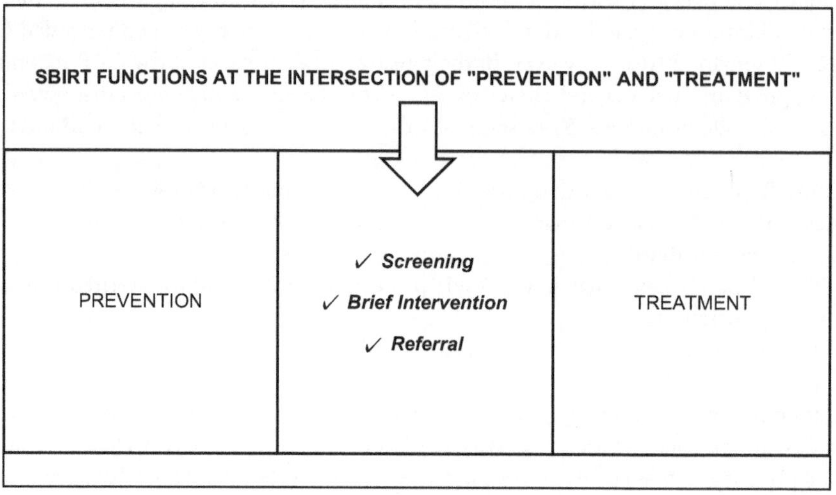

Figure 1.7 The SBIRT Model

3. Targets one or more specific behaviors. The screening tool addresses specific problematic behaviors or behaviors that are preconditional to alcohol or other dependence or use disorder(s);
4. Services occur in a public health, medical, or other non-alcohol or other dependence or use disorder treatment setting. The settings include, for example: EDs; primary care physicians' offices; and schools;
5. Comprehensive. The program includes a seamless transition between brief universal screening, a brief intervention (BI) and/or brief treatment (BT), and referral to specialty care for alcohol or other dependence or use disorder(s);
6. Strong research or substantial experimental evidence supports the model. At a minimum, programmatic outcomes demonstrate a successful approach.

(SAMHSA, 2013, p. 2)

The universal "screening" component of SBIRT is used to identify if a particular adolescent or young adult has a problem related to alcohol or other dependence or use disorder. "Brief intervention," or BI, provide behavioral intervention—generally motivational—over a single or several sessions as deemed necessary for adolescents and young adults who are at a minimal to moderate risk for alcohol or other drug- or substance of abuse-related problems. "Referral to Treatment," or "RT" is used for adolescents and young adults, who are deemed to be at moderate to high risk for alcohol or other drug- or substance of abuse-related problems and, consequently, involves more intensive and prolonged treatment than is provided by "BI."

In this context, health and social care or other professionals, who are conducting SBIRT determine, for example, whether an adolescent requires referral. They also determine whether he or she is at significant risk for self-harm and/or harm to others—in which cases, additional measures are warranted. In this regard, Levy and Williams (2016, p. e9), on behalf of the *Committee on Substance Use and Prevention of the American Academy of Pediatrics*, recommended the following:

- Break confidentiality and notify parents of risk;
- Make a verbal contract with patients not to use substances while awaiting treatment entry;
- Ask parents to monitor the adolescent closely while awaiting treatment entry;

- If parents know the adolescent is talking about self-harm, seek an emergency evaluation. Call 911, if the adolescent refuses;
- If parents note that the adolescent has an altered mental status, seek emergency evaluation;
- If the adolescent is unwilling to accept a parent's rules or becomes violent or threatening, advise the parent to call the local police station and request emergency assistance.

However, many clinicians have argued that screening adolescents and young adults for the use of drugs and substances of abuse, particularly when performed as a part of an annual physical examination, or as part of a routine office visit, is both: (1) time consuming; and (2) an inefficient use of valuable clinical resources (see Table 1.5). Other clinicians have argued that screening adolescents for their use of drugs and substances of abuse can result in both: (1) misdiagnoses; and (2) missed diagnoses (see the following section, "Type 1 and Type 2 Diagnostic Errors"). Thus, for screening to become more highly valued by clinicians, it is essential that it can be administered quickly and can contribute to the development of an accurate diagnosis.

To meet these needs, several quick-screen psychometric tests have been developed for use in clinical practice settings—both institutional and office settings—that are capable of: (1) being quickly administered (i.e., efficient); and, (2) providing high levels of accuracy (i.e., valid and reliable) regarding the specific detection of drug and substance abuse among male and female members of a particular group (e.g., adolescents; young adults). These quick-screen psychometric tests are presented and discussed in this chapter, with particular attention to their application, associated statistical strength, efficacy, and practicality regarding the diagnosis of alcohol or other dependence or use disorder, particularly among adolescent boys and girls.

Type 1 and Type 2 Diagnostic Errors

The accurate diagnosis of alcohol or other dependence or use disorder is the cornerstone for designing and implementing appropriate treatment plans for achieving optimal therapeutic outcomes. In this regard, the best designed treatment program in the world would be unsuccessful if an adolescent diagnosed with alcohol or other dependence or use disorder did not have the dependence or use disorder. As well, the best designed treatment program in the world for an adolescent, who does have an active alcohol or other dependence or use disorder, would have essentially no effect if the dependence or use disorder was not diagnosed (i.e., was "missed"). These two types of misdiagnosis are commonly conceptualized as "Type 1" and "Type 2" diagnostic errors (see Figure 1.8).[88] Type 1 diagnostic error represents the false "positive" diagnosis of an individual with alcohol or other dependence or use disorder—when, in fact, he or she does not have alcohol or other dependence or use disorder. Type 2 diagnostic error represents the false

88 The statistics discussed in this chapter are population statistics. That is, they are meant to represent the true state of affairs in a population (e.g., all adolescents in the U.S. with alcohol or other dependence or use disorder). The population is sampled to test various related assumptions or premises. Depending on the precision of the sampling procedures (e.g., random versus convenience sampling), the size of the sample used (e.g., 10 subjects versus 1,000 subjects), research design utilized (e.g., experimental versus quasi-experimental), the statistical results can be generalized, with more or less accuracy (i.e., validity) to the population under study (e.g., all adolescents with alcohol or other dependence or use disorder).

However, these statistics are not always applicable to the individual adolescent that a psychiatrist, psychologist, or other health or social care professional may be screening (e.g., he or she may be the exception to the rule because, in this statistical context, he or she is an outlier in the population. That is, he or she is one of the members of the population that resides at one extreme or the other of the normal distribution population curve—the normal, or bell-shaped, Gaussian curve). Therefore, when establishing a diagnosis of alcohol or other dependence or use disorder, health and social care providers should recognize the statistical limitations of these psychometric screening tests. With this in mind, the results always should be interpreted with due clinical caution and should be used in conjunction with other data sources (e.g., clinical interview).

Table 1.5 Major Constraints Affecting Appropriate Use of Quick-Screen Psychometric Tests Used for Adolescents

Major constraints	*Descriptions and examples*
Personal AND Professional Constraints	• Beliefs regarding professional role and responsibilities that do *not* include: ○ Testing for drug and substance abuse; ○ Treating drug and substance abuse; ○ Referring patients for needed help for drug and substance abuse. • Negative attitudes toward adolescents, particularly adolescents, who use drugs and substances of abuse. • Inadequate education/training or self-confidence regarding delivering optimal adolescent care concerning the use of the drugs and substances of abuse: ○ Poor interpersonal skills (e.g., uncomfortable with test administration procedures); ○ Poor social skills (e.g., unable to comfortably discuss alcohol or other dependence or use disorders with adolescents and their parents or legal guardians); ○ Poor technical skills (e.g., unable to answer related questions from adolescent test-taker); ○ Unable to effectively administer structured interviews; ○ Unable to discuss positive results with adolescent test-taker and parents or legal guardians.
Environmental Constraints	• Lack of time (already overbooked and overburdened); • Difficulties scheduling and conducting necessary follow-up appointments; • Lack of space; • Limited resources, including staff turnover of those who would administer quick-screen psychometric tests; • Inflexible electronic medical records; • Lack of standardized, validated quick-screen psychometric tests for adolescents.

Sources: Aspy, Mold, and Thompson (2008); Crome, Bloor, and Thom (2006); Habis, Tall, and Smith (2007); Searight (2009).

"negative" diagnosis of an individual (i.e., failure to detect alcohol or other dependence or use disorder when, in fact, he or she does have alcohol or other dependence or use disorder).

Unfortunately, in clinical practice, psychiatrists, psychologists, and other health and social care professionals are often faced with Type 1 and Type 2 diagnostic errors. This situation occurs because the science (i.e., Addictionology or Drug and Substance Abusology) guiding the understanding and treatment of alcohol or other dependence or use disorders, is not as precise a science as would be desired. As such, it suffers many limitations and is not devoid of human error (e.g., error of measurement)—as hard as clinicians strive to minimize error, they are not always as successful as they strive to be. Fortunately, selection criteria can be determined and set to adjust the

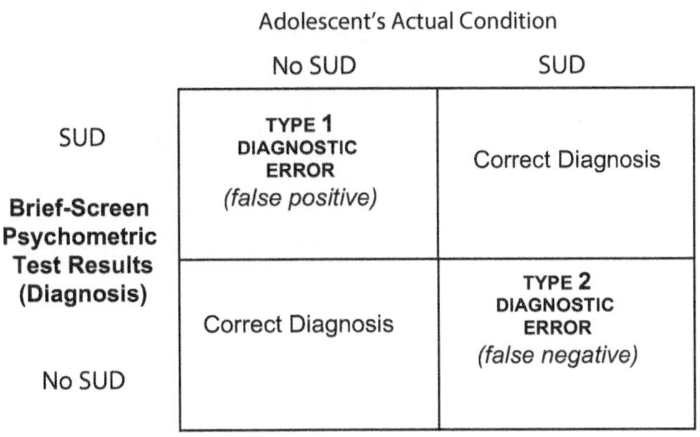

Figure 1.8 Type 1 and Type 2 Diagnostic Errors

"probability" of the occurrence of either Type 1 or Type 2 diagnostic errors. In general, when using standardized psychometric tests to screen for a possible alcohol or other dependence or use disorder among adolescents, test scores can be cutoff at various levels to provide better statistical discrimination and fewer false positives, or Type 1 diagnostic errors.

For example, increasing the cutoff score, or criterion value, reduces the number of false positive results (i.e., reduces Type 1 diagnostic error). However, it also increases the number of false negative results (i.e., increases Type 2 diagnostic error). Correctly diagnosing alcohol or other dependence or use disorder (i.e., minimizing Type 1 and Type 2 diagnostic errors) involves careful clinical assessment with both subjective data (e.g., data obtained from structured interviews, such as a medical or patient history or other assessment instruments; clinical observation) and objective data (e.g., data obtained from laboratory[89] and psychometric tests) along with professional clinical judgment and analysis, including the determination of potential diagnoses (i.e., multiple working hypotheses) and, subsequently, ruling out these diagnoses until the final and most probable diagnosis is determined.

In an effort to prevent or decrease diagnostic errors, and to also increase and expedite the delivery of needed clinical services, several quick-screen psychometric tests have been developed.[90] The goal

89 Laboratory tests (i.e., biological markers), such as those that are used to help to detect alcoholism (e.g., elevated bilirubin, gamma-glutamyl transpeptidase [GGT; GGTP; GTP], mean corpuscular volume [MCV], and carbohydrate-deficient transferrin [CDT]) generally have excellent reliability, but their validity is problematic (e.g., Bianchi, Ivaldi, & Raspagni, 2010; Golka & Wiese, 2004) (see, the later "Test Validity" and "Test Reliability" subsections for further discussion). For example, the GGT may be elevated by: alcoholic hepatic disease; pharmacotherapy (e.g., phenytoin [Dilantin®]); congestive heart failure; nonalcoholic hepatic disease; or various carcinomas—potentially resulting in many false positive results for alcoholism.

Laboratory tests also can be used to detect the actual physical presence of drugs and substances of abuse, including their concentrations and active or inactive metabolites. However, the accuracy of these tests, including their validity and reliability, as well as their sensitivity (see related discussion of these concepts later in this chapter), depend upon: (1) the method of analysis, such as the instruments used (e.g., immunoassay versus GC/MS); and (2) the drug or substance of abuse being detected (e.g., cocaine, which has a mean half-life of elimination of 1.25 hours, can be detected for less than half a day following last use, versus tetrahydrocannabinol, which has a mean half-life of elimination of 3.5 days, can be detected for over a week following last use or exposure) (Pagliaro & Pagliaro, 2009).

90 These quick-screen psychometric tests also are generally referred to, in the clinical literature, as "psychometric instruments," "psychometric questionnaires," "psychometric screening tests," or "psychometric tools." However, we generally use the term, "quick-screen psychometric tests," in this chapter. Although we may use the term that is used in the title of a particular screening test (e.g., "Maternal Substance Use Screening Questionnaire;" or "Michigan Alcoholism Screening Test") when discussing the test, we generally prefer and use the term quick-screen psychometric

of these tests is to quickly and accurately screen adolescents for alcohol or other dependence or use disorder so that further assessment and diagnosis can be completed (i.e., in an effort to provide optimal therapy as soon as possible and to reduce the unnecessary expenditure of human and other resources). Several brief, or quickly administered, psychometric screening tests have been commonly used to assess adolescents (and adults) for possible alcohol, or other dependence or use disorder, including, for example, cannabis use disorder, nicotine use disorder, or opiate analgesic (i.e., opioid) use disorder. Prior to discussing the specific quick-screen psychometric tests, basic test statistics—test specificity, sensitivity, validity, and reliability—are briefly reviewed.

Basic Test Statistics

For optimal selection and use of quick-screen psychometric tests, attention must be given to their basic test statistics: (1) specificity and sensitivity; (2) negative and positive predictive values; (3) test validity; and (4) test reliability. These and other related test statistics are reviewed in this section. Attention also is given to both the person administering the test, the "tester," and the adolescent who is completing the test, the "test-taker," regarding their roles in assuring accurate testing outcomes.

TEST SPECIFICITY, SENSITIVITY, AND POSITIVE AND NEGATIVE PREDICTIVE VALUES

Two closely related test statistics are test "specificity" and test "sensitivity." Test specificity is the term used to identify the probability that a subject, who does not have alcohol or other dependence or use disorder is correctly identified by a quick-screen psychometric test as not having an alcohol or other dependence or use disorder. For example, if the selected psychometric test only detects a total of five out of 10 people who actually do not have the disorder, how "specific" is the test, or what is its "specificity"? In this case, its specificity would be 50% (see Table 1.6 for related calculation formulae).

Conversely, test sensitivity is the probability that a subject, who actually has alcohol dependence, or use disorder, is correctly detected by a selected quick-screen psychometric test. For example, if the selected psychometric test only detects alcohol or other dependence or use disorder in a total of seven out of 10 people who actually have the disorder, how "sensitive" is it? In this case, its sensitivity would be 70% (see Table 1.6). While these test statistics are closely related, preferentially, we generally recommend using the sensitivity statistic when selecting quick-screen psychometric tests for clinical use based on their statistics for specificity or sensitivity—so as to err on the inclusive side of detecting an alcohol or other dependence or use disorder.

Two other related test statistics are "positive predictive value" and "negative predictive value." Positive predictive value is the probability that a subject, who actually has an alcohol or other dependence or use disorder, will be detected by the selected quick-screen psychometric test as having the disorder. For example, if the psychometric test detected that all 10 subjects in a sample were "positive" for the specific dependence or use disorder being screened for and only two subjects actually had the dependence or use disorder, then the "positive predictive value" would be 20% (see Table 1.6). Similarly, negative predictive value is the probability that a subject who actually does not have alcohol or other dependence or use disorder will be detected by the selected quick-screen psychometric test as not having the disorder (see Table 1.6).

test because each of the tests selected for discussion in this chapter was developed to expediently, and accurately, measure, or detect, patterns of behavior denoting problem use of the drugs and substances of abuse.

In this regard, basic statistical procedures were used to help to assure that each test, which often comprises a list of questions, expediently measures, by means of an objective score that was set a priori, the construct of concern every time it is administered to a member of the particular population for which it was designed and evaluated. As such, these quick-screen psychometric tests strive to provide desired levels of statistical robustness in test specificity, sensitivity, validity, and reliability that help to assure both accuracy and expediency in clinical diagnosis.

Table 1.6 Quick-Screen Psychometric Test Criterion Variables: Efficacy, Positive Predictive Value, Negative Predictive Value, Specificity, and Sensitivity

Quick-Screen Psychometric Test Results	*Actual Condition of Adolescent*		*Quick-Screen Psychometric Test Totals and Equations*
	Positive	*Negative*	
Positive	a[91]	b[92]	a + b
Negative	c[93]	d[94]	c + d
Totals	a + c	b + d	a + b + c + d
Where ***efficacy*** = $\frac{a+d}{a+b+c+d}$ = Overall percentage of correctly *categorized* subjects.			**Equation 1**
Where ***positive predictive value*** = $\frac{a}{a+b}$ = probability that a subject with a *positive* screening score has the SUD.[95]			**Equation 2**
Where ***negative predictive value*** = $\frac{d}{c+d}$ = probability that a subject with a *negative* screening score does *not* have the SUD.[96]			**Equation 3**
Where ***specificity*** = $\frac{d}{b+d}$ = probability that a subject, who actually does *not* have the SUD, is correctly detected as *not* having it.			**Equation 4**
Where ***sensitivity*** probability that a subject, who actually has the SUD, is correctly detected as having it.			**Equation 5**
Where the ***false positive rate*** = $\frac{b}{b+d}$ = 1 minus the specificity of the test.			**Equation 6**
Where the ***false negative rate*** = $\frac{c}{a+c}$ = 1 minus the sensitivity of the test.			**Equation 7**

TEST VALIDITY

The "validity" of a psychometric screening test is simply a test statistic that indicates whether the test measures what it purports to measure[97] (e.g., that an IQ test measures IQ or that an alcoholism screening test detects alcoholism). In this context, validity is determined by both empirical data and theoretical support. Validity, as a construct, is extremely important to psychometric tests because it provides evidence that the test measures what it

91 n for *true positives*.

92 n for *false positives*.

93 n for *false negatives*.

94 n for *true negatives*.

95 This value may be influenced by the characteristics of the sample population. Thus, if the attribute being screened for is common (e.g., screening is done in a clinical population), then a positive test will be more likely to detect drug or substance use (i.e., high positive predictive value). Conversely, a negative test will be less likely to detect the *absence* of drug or substance use (i.e., low negative predictive value).

96 This value may be influenced by the characteristics of the sample population. Thus, if the attribute being screened for is *rare* (e.g., screening is done in the general population), then a negative test will be more likely to detect *no* drug or substance use (i.e., high negative predictive value). Conversely, a positive test will be less likely to detect drug or substance use (i.e., low positive predictive value).

97 Most often, when tests do not measure what they purport to measure it is because of their poor design, particularly that related to the inadvertent incorporation of bias. A particular good review of this topic, which goes beyond the purview of this chapter and text, was prepared by Choi and Pak (2005) for the Centers of Disease Control and Prevention.

purports to measure. There are several types of related validity, including: "construct," "content," "concurrent," "criterion-related," "face," and "predictive validity."[98] These types of validity are defined and briefly reviewed with attention to their use and value regarding selecting quick-screen psychometric tests for detecting alcohol dependence or use disorder, or other drug and substance of abuse dependence or use disorder.

CONTENT VALIDITY. Content validity refers to how well the items that are included in a psychometric test measure the entire domain that the test purports to measure. As such, it is a measure of the comprehensiveness of a test. For example, if a test includes items that relate to only one form, or aspect, of adolescent alcoholism, then the other forms, or aspects, of alcoholism would be missed. In this regard, it is important to ask the question, if the test purports to measure adolescent alcoholism, does it measure all aspects of this disorder, including, for example, binge drinking or early onset versus late onset alcoholism? Thus, a test with high content validity would include as many measures of constructs, or factors, of the domain as possible–while excluding other constructs, or factors, which were not related to the domain of interest.

Content validity is commonly validated, by the degree of agreement (i.e., kappa scores—see the later subsection, "The Tester") among experts in the domain of interest. Content validity is often conceptualized as being subsumed within the concept of construct validity, which is validated by the statistical procedure of confirmatory factor analysis (CFA). Content validity is generally considered to be a requisite first step in determining test validity. (See also the following subsection, "Construct Validity.")

CONSTRUCT VALIDITY. Construct validity refers to the extent to which a test measures what it intended to measure—a quick-screen psychometric test that purports to measure, or detect, "harmful alcohol use," actually measures, or detects, "harmful alcohol use." Two statistics are generally used to demonstrate construct validity: (1) "convergent validity;" and (2) "divergent validity." Both statistics can be thought of in practical terms as measures of Type 1 and Type 2 error as applied to a specific construct (see the earlier discussion in the section, "Type 1 and Type 2 Diagnostic Errors").

CONVERGENT, OR CONCURRENT, VALIDITY Convergent validity is essentially the same as concurrent validity (see following discussion).

DIVERGENT, OR DISCRIMINANT, VALIDITY Divergent, or discriminant, validity is used primarily to help to establish construct validity. It is used to establish, for example, that a quick-screen psychometric test does not measure what it is not supposed to measure (i.e., divergent validity is the "flip-side" of convergent validity). Thus, as a measure of divergent validity, we would expect that a quick-screen psychometric test for detecting alcohol dependence or use disorder (i.e., AUD) would not have a high correlation with a test that detects being a devout Muslim (i.e., it would be incongruent to be both a devout Muslim and a heavy drinker of alcohol).

98 The different types of validity are not mutually exclusive and are presented here to assist readers to identify the similarities and differences of the terms used for this statistic by various authors in the related published clinical and research literature. Indeed, they can be conceptualized as all providing information regarding a particular aspect of the larger construct of validity by providing statistical information about, for example, test content, response process, internal structure, relationship to other constructs (or test items), and the consequences of testing (i.e., the application of test results) (Campbell & Fiske, 1959; Cronbach & Meehl, 1955; Kendell & Jablensky, 2003; Messick, 1995).

CONCURRENT VALIDITY. Concurrent validity is simply a measure of a test's similarity in results when compared to similar tests—generally with similar subjects, at the same point in time. It is commonly measured or validated by using Spearman's rank correlation coefficient (i.e., "Spearman's rho").[99] Convergent validity measures how similar, or convergent, a test is to other theoretically similar tests (also see, "Construct Validity"). For example, we would expect that one quick-screen psychometric test that detects alcohol dependence or use disorder would correlate well with a different quick-screen psychometric test that detects alcohol dependence or use disorder. For all practical purposes, "convergent" validity is one and the same as "concurrent" validity.

CRITERION-RELATED VALIDITY. Criterion-related validity is a measure of the extent to which the results of a quick-screen psychometric test agree with an independent indicator (i.e., most often a benchmark or "gold standard") for detecting a particular criterion. For example, finding agreement between a quick-screen psychometric test and a clinical interview or other established criteria (e.g., DSM or ICD criteria) when detecting "harmful drinking." Criterion-related validity is most often measured statistically by the correlation between the test (i.e., "predictor") and the criterion (e.g., "harmful drinking"). This correlation is generally referred to as the "criterion-related validity coefficient." Concurrent validity can be considered to be a type of criterion-related validity.

FACE VALIDITY. Face validity is simply an indicator that the items on a quick-screen psychometric test appear to be appropriate. For example, if a screening test claims that it measures cannabis use, it should include items that reflect a wide range of typical cannabis use behaviors. Face validity and content validity are generally closely related, but are not always statistically equivalent. In this context, content validity is considered to be the more important statistic. For example, the "MacAndrew Alcoholism Scale," a successful psychometric test for diagnosing alcoholism among adults, does not appear to have good face validity. However, it does include many questions that have good content validity. Thus, face validity is generally considered to be a good starting point in the development of quick-screen psychometric tests. However, it should be kept in mind that, because face validity is readily apparent, even to the test-taker, it makes "faking bad" (i.e., malingering) easier to accomplish.

PREDICTIVE VALIDITY. Predictive validity is concerned with a test's ability to predict a future outcome (e.g., future harm associated with regular, long-term heavy drinking). Most quick-screen psychometric tests for detecting alcohol or other dependence or use disorder, are concerned with detecting current behavior. Thus, concurrent predictive validity would be the more useful statistic (i.e., in terms of clinical performance) for measuring the ability of a test to detect current outcomes. Predictive validity can be considered to be a type of criterion-related validity.

99 Spearman's rho is a nonparametric statistic that is commonly used to determine the relationship between different rankings (as provided by different tests) on the same set of items (e.g., test-taker characteristics or responses to related questions). It is essentially the equivalent of the Pearson correlation coefficient (i.e., "r"), which is the statistic used for parametric data. Spearman Rho values range from +1, perfect positive correlation, to 0, absolutely no correlation, to -1, perfect correlation in the exact opposite direction (Spearman, 1904). The Kendall rank correlation coefficient (Kendall's tau [τ]) (Kendall, 1938) is a very closely related statistic that also is used in this context.

TEST RELIABILITY

In terms of quick-screen psychometric "tests," "test reliability" is simply an indicator that the test consistently provides the same results. Statistical synonyms for reliability in this context are "consistency," "repeatability," "replicability," "reproducibility," and "stability." Test reliability allows for both the comparison and generalization of the test with reliability estimates that have been obtained from various researchers. However, it should be noted that, some significant degree of variance can be expected to occur in measures of reliability for a specific quick-screen psychometric test because reliability, unlike validity (see the "Test Validity" section), is a property of the scores obtained from the test as opposed to the test, itself, and are, consequently, much more sample dependent.

The concept of test reliability is a necessary co-requisite, together with test validity, for determining the quality, or usefulness, of all quick-screen psychometric tests for alcohol use disorder or use, or other drug and substances of abuse dependence or use disorders. The two principle measures of reliability involve: (1) test-retest reliability; and (2) internal test consistency—the reliability of the items that comprise a test. It also has been noted that the "tester," "test-taker," and "drug or substance of abuse" (e.g., alcohol; heroin; tobacco),[100] can affect test reliability. These concepts are discussed in the following sections.

TEST-RETEST RELIABILITY. Test-retest reliability is concerned with the "temporal stability" of a test. That is, does the psychometric screening test, when re-administered in the same manner, to the same group of subjects, at a later date, provide the same results as originally obtained? Test-retest reliability is determined by: (1) administering a specific psychometric test to a group of subjects (TIME 1); (2) re-administering the same test, to the same group of subjects, in the same manner, at a later date (TIME 2); and (3) correlating the scores obtained from testing at both TIME 1 and TIME 2. This correlation between the two sets of scores (i.e., Pearson correlation coefficient [r]) is commonly known as the "reliability" or "stability" coefficient. The higher the correlation between the scores obtained for TIME 1 and TIME 2, the higher the test-retest reliability.

However, the time interval between initial testing (TIME 1) and retesting (TIME 2) can be a critical factor in assuring test reliability. For example, if the time interval is too short, correlations may be confounded by the subject's memory of his or her responses when initially tested (i.e., at TIME 1). If the interval is too long, correlations may be confounded by real changes in the characteristic being measured. For example, a subject when retested (TIME 2) may have since started to use the drug or substance of abuse in question and, consequently, report a much higher "current" use of a drug or substance of abuse than what was reported at initial testing (TIME 1)—when he or she was not using the drug or substance of abuse. In addition, other factors, including maturational and situational factors (e.g., the test-taker being older, hungrier, or more tired at pretest) and testing factors (e.g., effect of previously having taken the test), can confound the interpretation of the test-retest results. Typically, for research purposes, a test-retest time interval of at least one week is used in related reliability studies.

INTERNAL CONSISTENCY OR ITEM RELIABILITY. The reliability of test items, or components, is based on an average of the correlations of all the individual test items comprising a quick-screen psychometric test. Internal consistency, reliability, or inter-item consistency is typically indicated by Cronbach's alpha coefficient[101] or the Kuder-Richardson coefficient (of

100 The drug or substance of abuse can significantly affect the validity of self-reported use. For example, among adolescents being tested in a youth detention center, reporting the "current use" of heroin may have a pejorative connotation among staff members, whereas, admitting to current tobacco use would not.

101 The generally accepted criterion value for satisfactory item reliability is a Cronbach's alpha coefficient ≥ 0.70 (Cronbach, 1951).

equivalence—KR20). The calculation of KR20 is appropriate for use with dichotomously-scored items (e.g., True or False; Yes or No) while the Cronbach alpha is appropriate for use with non-dichotomously-scored items (e.g., multiple choice items). As such, it is a measure of the "internal consistency," or "homogeneity" of the test (i.e., a measure of if, and to what extent, all the items of a test measure the same latent variable). As the inter-correlations among the various test items increase, Cronbach's alpha will increase to a maximal statistic value of 1.0.

An important related corollary, based on classical test theory (CTT), is that adding additional items of equal reliability to the test will increase the test's reliability. While the addition of these items will increase the overall item reliability of the test, it also may impose several practical clinical limitations. For example, adding additional items may significantly increase testing time, which may result in increased subject fatigue or boredom and, consequently, increase the number of inaccurate or untruthful responses.

THE TESTER AND TEST-TAKER

The value and usefulness of a psychometric test depend on its validity and reliability. It also depends on the knowledge and experience, or ability, of the tester and the personal characteristics (e.g., "truthfulness") of the test taker.

The Tester. The tester should be able to select the appropriate test for detecting alcohol or other dependence or use disorder of concern for a particular adolescent or young adult. In this regard, testers and interpreters must be aware of the:

1. Basic principles, assumptions, and concepts that govern the test and its use;
2. Inherent strengths and limitations of the selected test;
3. Testing conditions under which the test should be administered;
4. Scoring procedures and interpretation of the test results;
5. Inherent ethical considerations and limitations of professional practice as related to his or her professional license as a tester or test interpreter;
6. Appropriate use of test results.

Inter-rater reliability (also referred to as: "inter-rater agreement;" "consensus;" or "concordance") is an important related construct. It is the correlation of test scores obtained when the same test is administered to the same subjects (or cohorts) at the same time (i.e., on the same day) by different raters, or testers (e.g., male testers of female subjects versus female testers; counselor versus psychologist). Low inter-rater reliability indicates that either one, or both, of the following are occurring:

1. The test is defective, or lacking in statistical robustness, and requires modification or replacement with a more robust test;
2. The tester is inadequately trained in testing skills and requires training or retraining.

Inter-rater reliability also has been used to verify the reliability of self-administered test results with the results obtained by structured interview. Either Pearson's correlation (for a rating scale that uses continuous data) or Spearman's rho (for a rating scale that uses ordinal data) can be used to measure the pairwise correlation among testers. A specific statistic developed to measure inter-rater reliability is "kappa"—Cohen's kappa to compare two raters and Fleiss' kappa for any number of raters (Shrout & Fleiss, 1979).

THE TEST-TAKER. The value and usefulness of a quick-screen psychometric test depend on its validity and reliability for detecting the potentially harmful use of drugs and substances of abuse by adolescents and young adults. It also depends on the truthfulness of the adolescent or young adult who is being tested (i.e., the "test-taker").[102] Thus, when psychometric tests are administered, testers, who are involved directly or indirectly in administering the test and in interpreting the results, must carefully consider the answers to each of the following 17 questions. Careful consideration of these questions and their answers will help to assure that truthful responses are obtained (i.e., increase the validity of self-report) and, consequently, increase the validity of the test results.[103]

1. Does the adolescent or young adult have a sufficient IQ to properly understand and follow the test-taking procedures?
2. Does the adolescent or young adult comprehend the items or questions comprising the test?
3. Is the adolescent or young adult aware of, and does he or she understand the possible consequences of, testing?
4. Is the adolescent or young adult sufficiently literate in English to understand and respond truthfully to the questions being asked?[104]
5. Does the adolescent or young adult have an adequate reading level for self-administered tests?
6. Does the adolescent or young adult have adequate vision for reading instructions and responding to test items?
7. Does the adolescent or young adult have adequate hearing for completing tester-administered tests?
8. Was the adolescent referred for psychometric testing primarily because of: a general parental concern; a driving while impaired (DWI/DUI) charge; parole sentencing; a threat of expulsion from school; the possible loss of a job; or a child custody proceeding?
9. Is the adolescent or young adult aware that self-report data will be corroborated with a clinical interview and other assessment procedures (e.g., interviews with a parent, parole officer, social worker, or teacher)?
10. Does the adolescent or young adult display characteristics indicative of such mental disorders as conduct disorder/antisocial personality disorder, major depressive disorder, or psychotic disorder?
11. Does the adolescent or young adult demonstrate inadequate test-taking behavior (e.g., leaves numerous items blank; answers "true" for all items)?

102 Deliberate conscious deviation from truthful responses in order to meet a personal agenda, such as to avoid incarceration or to continue unwarranted disability payments, is referred to as "faking good" and "faking bad," respectively.

103 When administering quick-screen psychometric tests or when supervising adolescents and young adults as they self-administer a particular related test, we conscientiously consider the 17 questions. In addition, we typically, while an adolescent is completing the next test, quickly look-over the previous completed self-administered test in order to identify items that may have been skipped or that may require further clarification. For example:

- Have some questions remained unanswered?
- Do some written responses require further exploration or elaboration?
- Has a response set bias been noted (i.e., the adolescent simply responds "true" to all items)?

104 If so, then a pencil and paper or computerized questionnaire may provide superior results in terms of both compliance and honesty of response in comparison to a structured diagnostic interview by a health or social care provider.

12. Is the adolescent or young adult currently receiving any pharmacotherapy (e.g., a psychotropic drug for the management of: attention deficit hyperactivity disorder [ADHD]; mental depression; insomnia or other sleep disorder; pain disorder; psychotic disorder [e.g., schizophrenia]; or seizure disorder) that may affect his or her test performance?[105]
13. Is the adolescent or young adult currently using alcohol or another drug or substance of abuse that may affect his or her test performance?
14. Is the adolescent or young adult currently intoxicated or "high"?
15. Is the adolescent or young adult currently in pain or in any other physical or emotional distress?
16. Does the adolescent or young adult have any current medical disorder (Type 1 diabetes mellitus) or condition (e.g., recent head injury) that may affect his or her test performance?
17. Is the adolescent or young adult accompanied by a parent or other legal guardian?[106]

In addition, building rapport with the test-taker and providing appropriate assurance of confidentiality (i.e., being truthful regarding who will have, or who will not have, access to self-report information) will help to increase the validity of self-reports regarding sensitive information, including the use of alcohol or other drugs and substances of abuse. In this regard, it has been long recognized (e.g., Williams, Perry, & Dudovitz, 1995) that adolescents, including young adolescents, should be expected to, and can provide, honest responses to sensitive questions about their use of alcohol and other drugs and substances of abuse. Attention to both the previous recommendations and the 17 questions presented earlier will help to ensure optimal performance for adolescent and young adult test-takers.

Selected Quick-Screen Psychometric Tests

Several quick-screen psychometric tests are commonly used to quickly and accurately detect possible alcohol or other dependence or use disorder among adolescents and young adults.[107] These tests include the tests designed specifically for adolescents and several general tests that can be used for both adolescents and adults (see Table 1.7).[108] This section presents an overview of these screening tests with attention to their development and scoring. To facilitate their selection and use, attention also is given to their basic test statistics—their sensitivity, specificity, validity, and reliability. Recommendations and limitations for the use of these tests for adolescents and young adults are also included at the conclusion of each test section.

105 For additional related information, see Pagliaro & Pagliaro, 1999, 2000, 2009, 2012.

106 Non-truthful reporting on sensitive items, such as the use of drugs and substances of abuse, is most frequently a motivated process deliberately engaged in by the test-taker to: (1) avoid embarrassment in the presence of the interviewer or others; (2) keep personal or family information private; and (3) avoid negative repercussions from a third party (e.g., legal system; parent; teacher or school principal) (McAllister & Makkai, 1991; Pagliaro & Pagliaro, *Clinical Patient Data Files*; Tourangeau & Yan, 2007).

107 This chapter focuses on the selection and use of the various quick-screen psychometric tests that are available for use with adolescents and young adults in order to detect alcohol use disorder. To date, no comparable statistically appropriate tests have been made available for detecting alcohol or other dependence or use disorders among children. Thus, mental health professionals and other clinicians must depend on other assessment methods (e.g., clinical observation and interview) to assist with this formidable task.

108 Other quick-screen psychometric tests, which have been specifically designed or recommended for detecting specific drug and substance abuse dependence or use disorder (e.g., cannabis use disorder), among adolescents or young adults. These are discussed, respectively, in the following chapters of this text.

Table 1.7 Selected Quick-Screen Psychometric Tests for Detecting Alcohol Dependence or Use Disorder among Adolescents.[109]

Identification Test	*Acronym or Abbreviation*	*Administration*	*Number of Items*	*Average Completion Time (Minutes)*
Alcohol Use Disorders Identification Test	AUDIT	Self-administered *or* structured interview	10	3
Alcohol Use Disorders Identification Test—Consumption	AUDIT-C	Self-administered *or* structured interview	3	1
Brief Michigan Alcoholism Screening Test	B-MAST	Self-administered *or* structured interview	10	3
The CAGE	CAGE	Self-administered *or* structured interview	4	1
Michigan Alcoholism Screening Test	MAST	Self-administered *or* structured interview	24	5
Michigan Alcoholism Screening Test- Adolescent	MAST-A	Self-administered *or* structured interview	24	5
Michigan Alcoholism Screening Test-Revised	MAST-R	Self-administered	22	5
Rapid Alcohol Problem Screen (Version 4)	RAPS4	Structured interview	4	2
Rutgers Alcohol Problem Index	RAPI	Self-administered *or* structured interview	23	5
Short Michigan Alcoholism Screening Test	Short MAST	Self-administered	13	3
T-ACE	T-ACE	Self-Administered *or* structured interview	4	2
TWEAK	TWEAK	Self-Administered *or* structured interview	5	2

Other related quick-screen psychometric tests also have been developed and clinically used (e.g., "Alcohol Beliefs Scale;" "Spouse Sobriety Influence Inventory"). However, these tests generally focus more on the severity of an already confirmed diagnosis of alcohol dependence or use disorder (i.e., alcoholism; AUD) and the identification of factors that may be of assistance in treatment. Thus, these quick-screen psychometric tests are not addressed in this chapter. Additionally, quick-screen psychometric tests that are not discussed in this chapter include those that are:

1. Specifically developed for, and primarily limited to, detecting drug and substance of abuse, other than alcohol, among adults (e.g., "Substance Abuse Questionnaire," or SAQ);

109 For additional discussion, see the section in this chapter, "Selection of Quick-Screen Psychometric Screening Tests."

2. Only, or primarily, used by the developer of the test (e.g., "Substances and Choices Scale," or SACS [Christie, Marsh, & Sheridan, 2007]; RAFFT [Bastiaens, Francis, & Lewis, 2000; Bastiaens, Riccardi, & Sakhrani, 2002]; Revised Mãlmo modification of the "Michigan Alcoholism Screening Test," or Mm-MAST [Osterling, Berglund, & Nilsson, 1993]);
3. Severely limited, or weak, in regard to statistical testing;
4. Long and/or difficult to administer or score (e.g., "Adolescent Drinking Index," or ADI, which recommends a minimum of a bachelor's degree in psychology to score the test and requires that the results be converted to "T-scores" and plotted on a profile sheet prior to interpretation).

We begin with the "Alcohol Use Disorders Identification Test," or AUDIT.

Alcohol Use Disorders Identification Test (AUDIT)

The AUDIT is a 10-item quick-screen psychometric test (Table 1.8) that was specifically designed for international use. It was developed from a six-country WHO collaborative project to detect "excessive drinking," or AUD (i.e., alcohol dependence; alcoholism) and to be administered in primary health care settings (Saunders, Aasland, & Babor, 1993). The 10-item core questionnaire for adolescents and adults, which requires a 7th grade reading level for completion (Hays, Merz, & Nicholas, 1995), appears to be particularly useful for the early detection of hazardous or harmful drinking (i.e., "risky drinking"). It measures the domains of: "alcohol consumption;" "alcohol dependence-related drinking behavior;" and "harmful alcohol use" (Babor, Higgins-Biddle, & Saunders, 2001; Saunders, Aasland, & Babor, 1993).[110]

The AUDIT was originally normed using a large representative sample of subjects who accessed services at several primary health care facilities. It has since been widely used with diverse populations of alcohol and other drug and substance of abuse users, such as inpatients, university students, and others in a variety of settings. The AUDIT has continuously been demonstrated to be a valuable and reliable psychometric screening test for detecting AUD (e.g., McCusker, Basquille, & Khwaja, 2002; Reinert & Allen, 2007). For example, the AUDIT was found to perform significantly better than either the CAGE or the TWEAK for detecting AUD among under-aged drinkers, 12 to 20 years-of-age, who were being treated in emergency departments (Kelly, Donovan, & Kinnane, 2002). (Also see the "AUDIT-C.")

SCORING THE AUDIT

Responses to each item of the AUDIT are scored from 0 to 4, except for items #9 and #10, which are scored 0, 2, or 4 (see Table 1.8 for scoring criteria). Summing all the scores provides a possible maximal score of 40. A total score of 2, or more, indicates some level of harmful alcohol use. A total score of 8, or higher, generally indicates an AUD (i.e., alcohol dependence, or alcoholism) (Conigrave, Saunders, & Reznik, 1995; MacKenzie, Langa, & Brown, 1996; Saunders, Aasland, & Babor, 1993).

Total scores of 12, or higher, provide increased discrimination, or specificity, for predicting alcohol-related social problems. However, this increased discrimination is at the cost of reduced test sensitivity (Conigrave, Hall, & Saunders, 1995). Approximately

110 N.B. All of the various screening tests used to detect alcohol use disorder (AUD) do not measure the same construct of alcohol use. See Table 1.9 for related definitions and descriptions of these constructs.

Table 1.8 The AUDIT

Item/Question	*Scoring Criteria [Point Allocation]*
1. How often did you have a drink containing alcohol in the past year?	Never, [0]; Monthly or less, [1]; Two to four times a month, [2]; Two to three times a week, [3]; Four or more times a week, [4]
2. How many drinks containing alcohol did you have on a typical day when you were drinking in the past year?	One or two drinks, [0]; three or four drinks, [1]; five or six drinks, [2]; seven to nine drinks, [3]; ten or more drinks, [4]
3. How often did you have six or more drinks on one occasion in the past year?	Never, [0]; Monthly or less, [1]; Two to four times a month, [2]; Two to three times a week, [3]; Four or more times a week, [4]
4. How often during the last year have you found that you were not able to stop drinking once you had started?	Never, [0]; Monthly or less, [1]; Two to four times a month, [2]; Two to three times a week, [3]; Four or more times a week, [4]
5. How often during the last year have you failed to do what was normally expected from you because of drinking?	Never, [0]; Monthly or less, [1]; Two to four times a month, [2]; Two to three times a week, [3]; Four or more times a week, [4]
6. How often during the last year have you needed a first drink in the morning to get yourself going after a heavy drinking session?	Never, [0]; Monthly or less, [1]; Two to four times a month, [2]; Two to three times a week, [3]; Four or more times a week, [4]
7. How often during the last year have you had a feeling of guilt or remorse after drinking?	Never, [0]; Monthly or less, [1]; Two to four times a month, [2]; Two to three times a week, [3]; Four or more times a week, [4]
8. How often during the last year have you been injured as a result of your drinking?	Never, [0]; Monthly or less, [1]; Two to four times a month, [2]; Two to three times a week, [3]; Four or more times a week, [4]
9. Have you or someone else been injured as a result of your drinking?	No/Never, [0]; Yes, but not in the last year, [2]; Yes, during the last year, [4]
10. Has a relative or friend or doctor or other health care worker been concerned about your drinking or suggested you cut down?	No/Never, [0]; Yes, but not in the last year, [2]; Yes, during the last year, [4]

Source: Saunders, Aasland, & Babor (1993).

97% of respondents with a score of 12, or higher, have a significant AUD. However, of all respondents with a significant AUD, approximately 72% have a lower AUDIT score (see previous discussion of "Type 1 and Type 2 Diagnostic Errors"). For adolescents and women, several authors (e.g., Reinert & Allen, 2007) have suggested a lower cutoff score (i.e., 4 or 5).

AVAILABLE TEST STATISTICS AND RECOMMENDATIONS

Test specificity, sensitivity, validity, and reliability for the AUDIT are presented and discussed in the following subsections, followed by our recommendations for its use with adolescents.

Table 1.9 Terms, Definitions, and Criteria for Various Forms of Alcohol Abuse

Type of Drinking and Definition	*Clinical Diagnosis*	*Diagnostic Criteria*
	Alcohol Use Disorder (AUD)	Meets criteria for: • Alcohol dependence; • Alcohol abuse; • Harmful drinking.
	Dependence (Alcoholism)	Meets criteria for at least three of the following: • Tolerance or the need to use increasing amounts alcohol to achieve desired effects; • Alcohol withdrawal with discontinuation of regular use; • Drinking to relieve alcohol withdrawal symptoms; • Impaired control (e.g., drinking more or longer than intended or planned); • Preoccupation with obtaining and/or using alcohol; • Increased time spent drinking or recovery from drinking episodes; • Persistent desire to use alcohol or unsuccessful effort to discontinue or quit alcohol use; • Sustains social, occupational, or recreational disability; • Alcohol use continues despite adverse consequences associated with its use.
	Abuse	Meets criteria for at least one of the following: • Fails to fulfill occupational or social obligations (at home, school, or work) due to drinking; • Use occurs in physically hazardous situations (e.g., drinking and driving a car or operating other hazardous machinery) or leads to recurrent legal problems; • Use continues despite persistent social or interpersonal problems.

(*Continued*)

Table 1.9 (Cont.)

Type of Drinking and Definition	*Clinical Diagnosis*	*Diagnostic Criteria*
	Harmful Drinking	• Clear evidence that alcohol is causing physical or psychological harm; • Nature of the harm is clearly identifiable; • Alcohol use has persisted at least one month or has occurred repeatedly over the past 12-month period; • Subject does not meet criteria for alcohol dependence.
Men: • 21 or more drinks per week or • Seven or more drinks per occasion at least three times per week **Women:** • 14 or more drinks per week or • Five or more drinks per occasion at least three times per week	Hazardous Drinking	• Quantity or pattern of use that places patients at risk for adverse consequences.
Men: • 14 or more drinks per week or • Five or more drinks per occasion **Women:** • Seven or more drinks per week or • Four or more drinks per occasion	Heavy Drinking, or Heavy Episodic Drinking	• Quantity or pattern of use that exceeds a defined threshold; • Does *not* meet criteria for harmful drinking.
Men/Women:	Risky Drinking	• Subject meets the criteria for either hazardous or heavy drinking.

Modified from: APA (2000); Bradley, DeBenedetti, & Volk (2007); Carrington Reid, Fiellin, & O'Connor (1999); Hasin (2003); Kriston, Holzel, & Weiser (2008); Seale, Boltri, & Shellenberger (2006).

SPECIFICITY AND SENSITIVITY. Specificity and sensitivity for the AUDIT range from 66% to 100% and approximately 38% to 96%, respectively, for identifying "at risk," "hazardous," or "harmful drinking" behavior (Fiellin, Reid, & O'Connor, 2000; Hill & Chang, 2007; McQuade, Levy, & Yanek, 2000). Much of this variability is related to the type of alcohol behavior being screened (Bradley, Bush, & McDonell, 1998). For example, when Saunders and Aasland (1987) first formally tested the AUDIT, they found that "harmful drinking" had a specificity of 81% and a sensitivity of 87%, while "hazardous drinking" had a specificity of 98% and a sensitivity of 96%. Similarly, Kriston, Holzel, and Weiser (2008) found that the mean AUDIT specificity results varied from 0.79 (for AUDs) to 0.88 (for risky/hazardous drinking) and the mean AUDIT sensitivity results varied from 0.84 (for AUD) to 0.81 (for risky/hazardous drinking) among patients in primary care settings.

The selected cutoff score also significantly affects, as expected, the observed specificity and sensitivity of the AUDIT (i.e., as the cutoff score of 6 is raised to a cutoff score of 12, the specificity increases, but the sensitivity decreases). For example, using a criterion value, or cutoff score, of 8 resulted in a specificity of 94% and a sensitivity of 92% (Saunders, Aasland, & Babor, 1993). A cutoff score of 10, for a clinical sample of participants with "first-episode psychosis," resulted in a specificity of 91% and a sensitivity of 85% (Cassidy, Schmitz, & Malla, 2008). Although variable, the generally high specificity and sensitivity statistics make the AUDIT a clinically acceptable quick-screen psychometric test for detecting alcohol abuse, AUD, or hazardous drinking behavior among adolescents (Cook, Chung, & Kelly, 2005; Gomez, Conde, & Santana, 2005; Kelly, Donovan, & Chung, 2009; Knight, Sherritt, & Harris, 2003).

VALIDITY AND RELIABILITY. The AUDIT has good construct validity. Criterion-related validity is demonstrated by the moderate to high correlations obtained between the AUDIT and, for example, the CAGE, which was 0.78 (Hays, Merz, & Nicholas, 1995) and the MAST, which was 0.88 (Bohn, Babor, & Kranzler, 1995). Concurrent criterion-related validity also has been demonstrated by excellent agreement between scores on the AUDIT and DSM-validated diagnoses of AUDs (Barry & Fleming, 1993; Fleming, Barry, & MacDonald, 1991; Isaacson, Butler, & Zacharek, 1994).

Good test-retest reliability (i.e., 0.88) has been reported for the AUDIT (Daeppen, Yersin, & Landry, 2000). The AUDIT also has very good internal consistency (reliability) with Cronbach's alpha coefficients reported in the 0.80 to 0.94 range (Kelly, Donovan, & Kinnane, 2002; Selin, 2003; Shields & Caruso, 2003). However, the average inter-item correlation among the 10 items comprising the AUDIT were found to be relatively low (i.e., 0.42) (Kelly, Donovan, & Kinnane, 2002).

RECOMMENDATIONS. The test appears to be quite robust. For example, comparisons of paper and pencil versus computerized administration of the AUDIT reported no significant differences (Chan-Pensley, 1999). In addition, the AUDIT appears to be more sensitive than the B-MAST, CAGE, Mm-MAST, and RAPS (Bradley, Bush, & McDonell, 1998; Cherpitel, 1997a; Cook, Chung, & Kelly, 2005). It also does not appear to be significantly affected by age, gender, or ethnic biases (Adewuya, 2005; Aertgeerts, Buntinx, & Ansoms, 2001; Giang, Spak, & Dzung, 2005; Nevitt, Lundak, & Codr, 2007). For example, when compared to the CAGE, POSIT, or TWEAK, the AUDIT was found to be an equally, or more, valid test for detecting excessive drinking or alcohol use disorders among adolescents (Chung, Colby, & Barnett, 2000; Knight, Sherritt, & Harris, 2003). However, some caution is advised when the test is administered to adolescents who are deaf because deaf subjects have found some of the wording of questions, or the phrases used, as being generally unfamiliar to members of the deaf culture because they are not widely or commonly used (Alexander, DiNitto, & Tidblom, 2005).

Shortened versions of the AUDIT (e.g., AUDIT-C; AUDIT-PC; AUDIT-3) generally appear to have lower sensitivity than the full AUDIT (Gomez, Conde, & Santana, 2005; McCambridge & Thomas, 2009). In addition, several researchers (e.g., Rist, Glockner-Rist, & Demmel, 2009), have suggested that the shorter versions of the AUDIT do not measure all the factors associated with AUD, and, therefore, assume that the assessment of alcohol use is equivalent to the assessment of alcohol-induced adverse consequences. Although we recommend the use of the AUDIT, we do not generally recommend the use of the shortened versions of the AUDIT, other than the AUDIT-C (see following discussion) because of their:

1. Reported lower sensitivity;
2. Incomplete measurement of all factors;
3. Significantly less available published data on validity and reliability;
4. Minimal savings related to testing time for both testers and test-takers when compared to the original AUDIT.

Alcohol Use Disorders Identification Test-Consumption (AUDIT-C)

The AUDIT-C is a three-question quick-screen psychometric test that was developed by Bush, Kivlahan, and McDonell (1998) to detect "heavy drinking." [111, 112] As a shortened version of the standard 10-question AUDIT, it contains the first three questions that deal explicitly and exclusively with patterns of alcohol consumption (Table 1.10). Also see the AUDIT.

SCORING THE AUDIT-C

Each response to the AUDIT-C questions is given a score of 1 to 4 for a possible maximal score of 12 (see Table 1.10 for scoring criteria). A total score of 4 or higher is considered to be indicative of heavy, or hazardous, drinking. The AUDIT-C was originally tested and normed using a sample of men who were general medical patients in several VA Medical Centers (Bush, Kivlahan, & McDonell, 1998). The subsequent findings of several studies (e.g., Bradley, DeBenedetti, & Volk, 2007; Caviness, Hatgis, & Anderson, 2009) supported this cutoff score of 4, or higher, for men and an optional cutoff score of 3, or higher, for women.

The scoring of the AUDIT-C is slightly more involved than that for other quick-screen psychometric tests. Consequently, the AUDIT-C has been criticized, by several health and

Table 1.10 The AUDIT-C

ITEM #	*QUESTION*	*SCORING CRITERIA* *[Point Allocation]*
1.	How often do you have a drink containing alcohol?	Never [0]; Monthly or less [1]; Two to four times a month [2]; Two to three times a week [3]; Four or more times a week [4]
2.	How many drinks containing alcohol do you have on a typical day when you are drinking?	One or two [0]; Three or four [1]; Five or six [2]; Seven to nine [3]; 10 or more [4]
3.	How often do you have six or more drinks on one occasion?	Never [0]; Less than monthly [1]; Monthly [2]; Weekly [3]; Daily or almost daily [4]

Source: Bush, Kivlahan, & McDonell (1998).

111 "Heavy drinking" was defined as 14 or more drinks per week, or five or more drinks per drinking episode, or occasion. (See also the earlier related discussion in the section, "New Millennial Trends in Child, Adolescent, and Young Adult Alcohol Use"—"Binge Drinking").

112 This pattern of alcohol use also has been referred to by some clinicians, who use the AUDIT-C, as "hazardous drinking." That is, 16 or more drinks per week for men, and 12 or more drinks per week for women (Gordon, Maisto, & McNeil, 2001).

social care professionals, particularly those who are practicing in emergency departments and other busy clinical settings (Kelly, Donovan, & Chung, 2009).

AVAILABLE TEST STATISTICS AND RECOMMENDATIONS

Published data have been found regarding the specificity and sensitivity of the AUDIT-C. Gender effects also have been observed and are discussed together with published data regarding the AUDIT-C's validity and reliability.

SPECIFICITY AND SENSITIVITY. The AUDIT-C was found to have a specificity of 72% and a sensitivity of 86% using a sample of men and a criterion value, or cutoff score, of 4.[113] Bradley, DeBenedetti, and Volk (2007) obtained similar results (i.e., specificity 89% and sensitivity 86%) with the same cutoff score using a similar sample. Bradley, McDonell, and Bush (1998) also reported similar results (i.e., sensitivity of 87%). Using collapsed data from four extant studies involving over 2,500 patients in primary care settings, both men and women, Kriston, Holzel, and Weiser (2008) determined that the mean specificity of the AUDIT-C varied from 0.68, when used to detect risky/hazardous drinking, to 0.78, when used to detect AUD. Similarly, they determined that the mean sensitivity of the AUDIT-C varied from 0.97, when used to detect risky/hazardous drinking, to 0.82, when used to detect AUD.

Since its development and initial use, the AUDIT-C, overall, appears to perform slightly better for women than for men in regard to detecting alcohol dependence (Dawson, Grant, & Stinson, 2005). Using a sample of women, Bradley, DeBenedetti, and Volk, (2007) found a specificity of 91% and a sensitivity of 73% using a cutoff score of 3. Again, with a cutoff score of 3, a moderate specificity of 71% and a high sensitivity of 98% were obtained using a sample of women who were pregnant (Burns, Gray, & Smith, 2010).

Also using a cutoff score of 3, Caviness, Hatgis, and Anderson (2009) reported excellent test statistics for a large sample of incarcerated women (i.e., efficacy 91.5%; specificity, 91.5%; sensitivity, 91.6%; positive predictive value, 93%; and negative predictive value, 90%). In addition, the AUDIT-C appears to display greater, although variable, sensitivity when used for women of different continental or other descent. For example, in their large cross-sectional validation study using a sample of women from their academic family practice clinic, Frank, DeBenedetti, and Volk (2008) reported a significantly higher sensitivity for women of Hispanic descent (i.e., 85%) than for women of European continental descent (i.e., 70%) or African continental descent (i.e., 67%).[114] In general, the AUDIT-C performs well for respondents from various continental and other descents (Frank, DeBenedetti, & Volk, 2008). However, sensitivity can vary within this high and acceptable range as noted in their study.

As with other quick-screen psychometric tests, increasing the criterion value (i.e., cutoff score) results in increased specificity, but reduced sensitivity (Aalto, Alho, & Halme, 2009; Dawson, Grant, & Stinson, 2005).

VALIDITY AND RELIABILITY. The questions of the AUDIT-C have good face validity. In addition, the results of the AUDIT-C correlate well with the results of the full AUDIT (Bush, Kivlahan, & McDonell, 1998; Reinert & Allen, 2007). When using a standard cutoff score of 4, the AUDIT-C did not appear to be significantly affected by the method of administration (i.e.,

113 A cutoff score of 3 was first proposed for men and then changed to a cutoff score of 4.

114 They also found variable sensitivity among men in the U.S. of different continental and other descents with a sensitivity of 95% for men of European continental descent, 85% for men of Hispanic descent, and 76% for men of African continental descent.

electronic delivery by computer; oral interview; self-administered paper and pencil test) (Graham, Goss, & Xu, 2007). In addition, it should also be noted that the AUDIT-C was originally tested by sending a hardcopy (a paper and pencil copy) of the test to sample respondents by mail (Bush, Kivlahan, & McDonell, 1998). Test-retest reliability, after a period of three months, ranged from 0.65 to 0.85 (Bradley, McDonell, & Bush, 1998).

RECOMMENDATIONS. The AUDIT-C has demonstrated acceptable test statistics for diverse groups of subjects. We recommend the use of the AUDIT-C for the detection of AUD among adolescents and young adults.

Brief MAST (B-MAST)

The B-MAST is a 10-item quick-screen psychometric test that was derived from the Michigan Alcoholism Screening Test (MAST) by Pokorny, Miller, and Kaplan (1972) to detect alcoholism, or alcohol dependence (see Table 1.11). Also see the MAST and the Short-MAST.

SCORING OF THE B-MAST

Each question in the B-MAST is assigned a weight of 0 to 5 (see Table 1.11, for scoring criteria). Items 1 and 2 are scored in reverse. A total score of 6, or higher, provides presumptive evidence of alcoholism.

Table 1.11 The B-MAST

Question	*Scoring Criteria [Point Allocation]*
1. Do you feel you are a normal drinker?	No [2] Yes [0]
2. Do friends or relatives think you are a normal drinker?	No [2] Yes [0]
3. Have you ever attended a meeting of Alcoholics Anonymous (AA)?	No [0] Yes [5]
4. Have you ever lost friends or girlfriends/boyfriends because of your drinking?	No [0] Yes [2]
5. Have you ever gotten into trouble at work because of drinking?	No [0] Yes [2]
6. Have you ever neglected your obligations, your family, or your work for two or more days in a row because you were drinking?	No [0] Yes [2]
7. Have you had delirium tremens (DTs), severe shaking, heard voices, or seen things that weren't there after heavy drinking?	No [0] Yes [2]
8. Have you ever gone to anyone for help about your drinking?	No [0] Yes [5]
9. Have you ever been in a hospital because of your drinking?	No [0] Yes [5]
10. Have you ever been arrested for drunk driving after drinking?	No [0] Yes [2]

Source: Pokorny, Miller, & Kaplan (1972).

AVAILABLE TEST STATISTICS AND RECOMMENDATIONS

Limited published data are available regarding the specificity, sensitivity, validity, and reliability for the B-MAST. These statistics are discussed in the following sections.

SPECIFICITY AND SENSITIVITY. The B-MAST has been found to be significantly less sensitive than the AUDIT, CAGE, or RAPS (Cherpitel, 1997b, 1998; MacKenzie, Langa, & Brown, 1996). The sensitivity of the B-MAST in detecting moderate alcohol problems in the general population is low (approximately 30%), presumably because the items deal primarily with severe alcohol problems (Chan, Pristach, & Welte, 1994). Overall, the reported specificity ranges from 80% to 99% and sensitivity ranges from 30% to 78% (Cherpitel, 1997b).

VALIDITY AND RELIABILITY. The B-MAST has good face validity. In addition, concurrent validity has been demonstrated in relation to both clinical assessment and the AUDIT (Connor, Grier, & Feeney, 2007).

RECOMMENDATIONS. Given the limited availability of published statistics for the B-MAST, we generally do not recommend its use, particularly for adolescents.

CAGE

The CAGE is a four-question quick-screen psychometric test (Table 1.12), which was developed by Ewing in 1968 as part of a clinical study to detect alcoholism (Ewing, 1984). A noted criticism of the CAGE is that it fails to detect "heavy drinkers," who may lack insight or who may be in "denial." Another concern is its focus on "alcoholism" and the expectation that, for this reason, the CAGE will miss a significant number of people who may display less harmful or hazardous patterns of alcohol use, but have significant related problems. Specifically, regarding this latter concern, the AUDIT has demonstrated clinical superiority to the CAGE (McCusker, Basquille, & Khwaja, 2002). Overall, the CAGE performs significantly better for men, when compared to women, in regard to detecting alcoholism (Dhalla & Kopec, 2007).

Although a version of the CAGE (i.e., CAGE-AA) was constructed with questions specifically adapted for adolescent use, its psychometric properties, specifically its internal consistency, or inter-item reliability, were found to be lacking (Knight, Goodman, & Pulerwitz, 2000).

Table 1.12 The CAGE

Question *{Alternate Phrasing}*	*Scoring Criteria* *[Point Allocation]*
1. Have you ever felt you ought to **C**utdown on your drinking? {have you ever felt the need to cutdown your drinking?}	No [0] Yes [1]
2. Have people **A**nnoyed you by criticizing your drinking? {have you ever felt annoyed by criticism of your drinking?}	No [0] Yes [1]
3. Have you ever felt bad or **G**uilty about your drinking? {have you ever had guilty feelings about drinking?}	No [0] Yes [1]
4. Have you ever had a drink first thing in the morning to steady your nerves or to get rid of a hangover (i.e., as an **E**ye-opener)? {have you ever taken a morning eye-opener?}	No [0] Yes [1]

Sources: Ewing (1984); Mayfield, McLeod, & Hall (1974).

SCORING OF THE CAGE

Each affirmative answer is given a score of 1 (see Table 1.12 for scoring criteria). A total score of 2, or higher, is indicative of "alcoholism" (Buchsbaum, Buchanan, & Centor, 1991; Kitchens, 1994; NIAAA, 1995). However, several researchers (e.g., Aertgeerts, Buntinx, & Kester, 2004) have found the CAGE to be of limited screening value at this cutoff score. O'Brien (2008b) recommends that a score of 2 or 3 is highly indicative of alcoholism and that a score of 4 is diagnostic of alcoholism. (See following related discussion.)

AVAILABLE TEST STATISTICS AND RECOMMENDATIONS

This section discusses the specificity, sensitivity, positive and negative predictive values, and reliability and validity of the CAGE. It concludes with our recommendations regarding its use.

SPECIFICITY, SENSITIVITY, POSITIVE PREDICTIVE VALUE, AND NEGATIVE PREDICTIVE VALUE. The CAGE has generally demonstrated both a high specificity (77% to 96%) and high sensitivity (61% to 100%) for alcoholism screening (i.e., alcohol dependence) with a general population of adults (Do Amaral & Malbergier, 2008; Fiellin, Reid, & O'Connor, 2000; McQuade, Levy, & Yanek, 2000). Similar values were reported (i.e., sensitivity, 68%, and specificity, 93%) for a sample of men, in the U.S., of American-Indian descent (Saremi, Hanson, & Williams, 2001). However, the CAGE was found to be relatively insensitive when used with a population of pregnant women of European continental descent (Bradley, Boyd-Wickizer, & Powell, 1998). In the U.S., it also demonstrated a low sensitivity for women of Hispanic (Steinbauer, Cantor, & Holzer, 1998) and American Indian descents (i.e., 62%) (Saremi, Hanson, & Williams, 2001).

With adolescent populations, the sensitivity of the CAGE was found to be only 37% (Knight, Sherritt, & Harris, 2003). This percentage is much lower than that reported for the AUDIT and the Mm-MAST, both of which also appear to have superior clinical application for this age group (Cook, Chung, & Kelly, 2005; Kelly, Donovan, & Chung, 2004). However, Knight, Sherritt, and Harris (2003) used a criterion value, or cutoff score, of 1 rather than the recommended cutoff score of 2.

Several other researchers (e.g., Aertgeerts, Buntinx, & Bande-Knops, 2000; Chung, Colby, & Barnett, 2000; Kelly, Donovan, & Kinnane, 2002) have reported poor performance of the CAGE with younger subjects. In this context, Dawe, Loxton, and Hides (2002) suggested that quick-screen psychometric tests, such as the AUDIT or TWEAK, which focus more on "psychological symptomatology," may be better suited for adolescents and young adults than other tests, such as the CAGE and MAST, which focus more on long-term alcohol related problems.

Aertgeerts, Buntinx, and Ansoms (2001), also using a cutoff score of 1, with a large sample of adults attending general medical practices in Belgium, found a specificity of 81% and a sensitivity of 62% for men. They also found that the CAGE had a high negative predictive value (i.e., 93%) and a low positive predictive value (i.e., 34%). Aertgeerts, Buntinx, and Ansoms (2001) also found that sensitivity (i.e., 54%) and positive predictive value (i.e., 24%) were significantly lower for women.

Similarly, Aertgeerts, Buntinx, and Bande-Knops (2000), using a cutoff score of 1, with a large sample of college freshmen in Belgium, obtained a specificity of 87%, a sensitivity of 42%, a negative predictive value of 90%, and a positive predictive value of 36%. As with other quick-screen psychometric tests, modifying the criterion variable set for the CAGE to increase its specificity, also decreases its sensitivity (Ewing, 1984)—regardless of what type of alcohol use behavior (e.g., "heavy or hazardous drinking;" "alcohol dependence") is screened (Bradley, Bush, & McDonell, 1998), as can be seen in Table 1.13.

Table 1.13 Specificity and Sensitivity of the CAGE

Number of Positive "yes" Responses Per Subject (Selected Criterion Level)	*Approximate* Specificity *for the General Population*	*Approximate* Sensitivity *for the General Population*
1	80%	98%
2	90%	81%
3	99%	66%
4	100%	37%

Source: Knight, Sherritt, & Harris (2003).

VALIDITY AND RELIABILITY. The CAGE has excellent "face," or content, validity. However, its strong face validity makes "faking" quite easy. In terms of performance, the CAGE has been found to be comparable to the S-MAST (Maisto, Connors, & Allen, 1995). Correlation with the S-MAST is 0.70 (Hays, Merz, & Nicholas, 1995) and 0.48 to 0.62 with the AUDIT (Hays, Merz, & Nicholas, 1995; Hodgson, Abbasi, & Hodgson, 2003). Criterion-related validity, as demonstrated by the correlation, or agreement, of the CAGE with DSM criteria, is high (Liskow, Campbell, & Nickel, 1995).

It also has an acceptable measure of test-retest reliability of 0.80 to 0.95 (Dhalla & Kopec, 2007; Teitelbaum & Mullen, 2000). However, the internal consistency (reliability) of the CAGE is lower and its standard error of measurement is higher (Hays, Merz, & Nicholas, 1995). In addition, the CAGE has a reported median internal consistency of 0.74 (range of 0.52 to 0.90) and its score reliability appears to vary with the median age of the sample being tested (Shields & Caruso, 2003).

Among adolescents seeking emergency department services, the internal consistency of the CAGE (i.e., Cronbach's alpha) was determined to be 0.66 (Kelly, Donovan, & Kinnane, 2002). Although an alpha of 0.70, or higher, is generally desired, an alpha of 0.66 is an acceptable indicator of internal consistency, particularly for a four-item test.

RECOMMENDATIONS. The CAGE is more quickly administered than the AUDIT or S-MAST (i.e., one minute versus three minutes). No significant differences were found when comparing results for the CAGE when administered by written paper-and-pencil format or by structured interview (Aertgeerts, Buntinx, & Fevery, 2000). Additionally, as with the AUDIT, caution is indicated when the CAGE is used for adolescents, who are hearing impaired or deaf, because some of the wording or phrases used in the questions have been found to be generally unfamiliar to members of the deaf community (Alexander, DiNitto, & Tidblom, 2005). Due to these limitations, we do not generally recommend the use of the CAGE for adolescents.

CRAFFT

The CRAFFT (**C**ar, **R**elax, **A**lone, **F**orget, **F**riends, **T**rouble) is a six-item, quick-screen psychometric test (Table 1.14) that was developed by Knight, Shrier, and Bravender (1999) specifically for adolescent medical patients, 14 to 18 years-of-age. This psychometric test screens for alcohol "use," "abuse," and "dependence." It also can be used to detect these patterns of use for other drugs and substances of abuse. Interestingly, the CRAFFT is the only quick-screen psychometric test that includes a question on "drinking and driving."

Table 1.14 The CRAFFT

Acronym	*Question*	*Scoring Criteria [Point Allocation]*
C	Have you ever ridden in a **C**ar driven by someone (including yourself) who was "high" or had been using alcohol or drugs?	No [0] Yes [1]
R	Do you ever use alcohol or drugs to **R**elax, feel better about yourself, or fit in?	No [0] Yes [1]
A	Do you ever use alcohol or drugs while you are by yourself (**A**lone)?	No [0] Yes [1]
F	Do you ever **F**orget things you did while using alcohol or drugs?	No [0] Yes [1]
F	Do your **F**amily or friends ever tell you that you should cutdown on your drinking or drug use?	No [0] Yes [1]
T	Have you ever gotten into **T**rouble while you were using alcohol or drugs?	No [0] Yes [1]

Source: Knight, Shrier, & Bravender (1999).

SCORING OF THE CRAFFT

Each affirmative response is given a score of 1 (see Table 1.14 for scoring criteria). A total score of 2, or higher, is indicative of problematic patterns of alcohol or other drug and substance use needing treatment, including "problem use," "abuse," and "dependence" (Knight, Sherritt, & Shrier, 2002; Knight, Shrier, & Bravender, 1999). At a cutoff score of 2, the CRAFFT demonstrates excellent correlation with related DSM-5 criteria (Mitchell, Kelly, & Gryczynski, 2014; Oesterle, Hitschfeld, & Lineberry, 2015).

AVAILABLE TEST STATISTICS AND RECOMMENDATIONS

Specificity, sensitivity, and positive and negative predictive values are discussed along with validity and reliability. The section concludes with our own recommendations.

SPECIFICITY, SENSITIVITY, POSITIVE PREDICTIVE VALUE, AND NEGATIVE PREDICTIVE VALUE. The optimal psychometrics obtained at the established criterion discrimination, or cutoff score of 2, are: specificity, 82% to 94%; sensitivity, 76% to 92%; positive predictive value, 67% to 83%; and negative predictive value, 91% to 97% (Knight, Sherritt, & Shrier, 2002; Knight, Shrier, & Bravender, 1999; Mitchell, Kelly, & Gryczynski, 2014). Lowering the cutoff score to 1, increased the sensitivity to 100%, but decreased the specificity to 58% (Knight, Shrier, & Bravender, 1999). In addition, when the CRAFFT was used with a cutoff score of 2 for adolescents of American Indian descent, the following statistics were obtained: specificities of 72% for "frequent alcohol use" and 86% for "high alcohol-related problems;" and sensitivities of 100% for "frequent alcohol use" and 95% for "high alcohol-related problems" (Cummins, Chan, & Burns, 2003).

VALIDITY AND RELIABILITY. The validity of the CRAFFT does not appear to be significantly affected by the age, continental descent, ethnicity, or gender of respondents. In addition, the score obtained from the CRAFFT highly correlates with related diagnostic classifications (i.e., Spearman rho = 0.72).

The CRAFFT also has acceptable reliability. The standardized item alpha is 0.68 (Knight, Shrier, & Bravender, 1999). Although an alpha of 0.70, or higher, is generally desired (see previous discussion in the earlier section, "item reliability"), an alpha of 0.68 is an acceptable indicator of internal consistency, particularly for a relatively short, six-item test (Knight, Sherritt, & Shrier, 2002). The use of the CRAFFT with a sample of adolescents of American Indian descent yielded an alpha of 0.81 (Cummins, Chan, & Burns, 2003). In a later study, test-retest reliability yielded kappa values in the range of 0.71 to 0.84 (Levy, Sherritt, & Harris, 2004). In addition, test-retest reliability for the CRAFFT was found to be high (i.e., approximately 0.91) (Levy, Sherritt, & Harris, 2004).

RECOMMENDATIONS. The CRAFFT is a valid quick-screen test for detecting adolescent drug and substance abuse and has acceptable reliability. Although, we recommend its use to detect AUD among adolescents, prior to administration, we specifically delete all test references to "drugs" (i.e., "alcohol or drugs," is changed to "alcohol").

Michigan Alcoholism Screening Test (MAST)

The MAST is a 24-item quick-screen psychometric test[115] (Table 1.15, The MAST) that was designed by Selzer (1971) to detect "harmful or hazardous drinking" or "alcoholism" among adults while accommodating for an expected lack of candor among respondents. It was normed, for use in the U.S., with samples that were primarily comprised of men of European continental descent, who were 25 to 44 years-of-age. An adolescent version, the MAST-A, also was developed and is used for screening adolescents. The MAST-A, having only

Table 1.15 The MAST[116]

Scoring Criteria [Point Allocation]	*Question*
Yes [0], No [2]	1. Do you feel you are a normal drinker?
Yes [1], No [0]	2. Have you ever awakened the morning after some drinking the night before and found that you could not remember a part of the evening before?
Yes [1], No [0]	3. Does your wife, husband, a parent, or other near relative ever worry or complain about your drinking?
Yes [0], No [2]	4. Can you stop drinking without a struggle after one or two drinks?
Yes [1], No [0]	5. Do you ever feel guilty about your drinking?
Yes [0], No [2]	6. Do friends or relatives think you are a normal drinker?
Yes [0], No [2]	7. Are you able to stop drinking when you want to?
Yes [5], No [0]	8. Have you ever attended a meeting of Alcoholics Anonymous (AA)?
Yes [1], No [0]	9. Have you ever gotten into physical fights when drinking?

(Continued)

115 Since its initial development, several different versions of the full MAST have become available. These different versions can include from 22 to 25 items. For example, the question, "Do you enjoy a drink now and then?" is sometimes included as Question #0. In addition, the question, "Do you ever try to limit your drinking to certain times of the day or to certain places?" has been included as the last question and is scored, "No, 0; Yes, 1."

116 In the original version, a "pre-question" was included as Question #0, "Do you enjoy a drink now and then?"

Table 1.15 (Cont.)

Scoring Criteria [Point Allocation]	*Question*
Yes [2], No [0]	10. Has drinking ever created problems between you and your wife, husband, a parent, or other near relative?
Yes [2], No [0]	11. Has your wife, husband, a parent, or other near relative ever gone to anyone for help about your drinking?
Yes [2], No [0]	12. Have you ever lost friends or girlfriends/boyfriends because of your drinking?
Yes [2], No [0]	13. Have you ever gotten into trouble at work because of drinking? [The MAST-A replaces "work" with "school"]
Yes [2], No [0]	14. Have you ever lost a job because of drinking?
Yes [2], No [0]	15. Have you ever neglected your obligations, your family, or your work for two or more days in a row because you were drinking? [The MAST-A replaces "work" with "school"]
Yes [1], No [0]	16. Do you drink before noon fairly often? [The MAST-A does not include, "fairly often"]
Yes [2], No [0]	17. Have you ever been told you have liver trouble? Cirrhosis?
Yes [5], No [0]	18. After heavy drinking, have you ever had delirium tremens (DTs) or severe shaking, or heard voices, or seen things that weren't really there?
Yes [5], No [0]	19. Have you ever gone to anyone for help about your drinking?
Yes [5], No [0]	20. Have you ever been in a hospital because of drinking?
Yes [2], No [0]	21. Have you ever been a patient in a psychiatric hospital or on a psychiatric ward of a general hospital where drinking was part of the problem that resulted in hospitalization?
Yes [2], No [0]	22. Have you ever been seen at a psychiatric or mental health clinic, or gone to a doctor, social worker, or clergyman for help with any emotional problem where drinking was part of the problem?
Yes [2], No [0]	23. Have you ever been arrested for drunken driving while intoxicate or driving under the influence of alcoholic beverages?
Yes [2], No [0]	24. Have you ever been arrested, even for a few hours, because of other drunken behavior?

Source: Selzer (1971).

minor rewording of three questions, is essentially the same as the full MAST (see Table 1.15).

The MAST was originally designed to be verbally administered to the test-taker by a tester (e.g., health or social care professional). However, it is frequently used in paper-and-pencil format as a self-administered quick-screen psychometric test. The MAST is one of the most widely used quick-screen psychometric tests for detecting alcoholism and harmful or hazardous drinking (i.e., AUD; alcohol physical dependence) and, for these indications, is often considered to be one of the benchmarks, or standards, to which other quick-screen psychometric tests are compared. However, a noted short-coming of the MAST is its inability to distinguish between present alcohol problems and past alcohol problems. Also see the B-MAST and the SMAST.

SCORING OF THE MAST

Each item comprising the MAST is assigned a weight of 0 to 5 as specified in the left-hand column of the test (see Table 1.15 for scoring criteria). Items #1, #4, #6, and #7 are scored in reverse. The scores are summed for a possible maximal score of 55. Selzer (1971) originally recommended a cutoff score of 5, or higher, to identify harmful or hazardous drinking. Ross, Gavin, and Skinner (1990) later recommended a total score of 13, or higher, to detect alcoholism. The overall accuracy, or efficacy, of the MAST is 88% (Ross, Gavin & Skinner, 1990).

AVAILABLE TEST STATISTICS AND RECOMMENDATIONS

Available test statistics for the MAST include specificity, sensitivity, validity and reliability, which are discussed in the following section, followed by our recommendations.

SPECIFICITY AND SENSITIVITY. Overall, the MAST has good specificity (i.e., up to 95%) and sensitivity (i.e., up to 98%). However, poor results also have been reported, including a specificity of 50% and an overall efficacy of 58% (Zung, 1982). Using a cutoff score of 13, Ross, Gavin, and Skinner (1990) obtained a specificity of 76% and a sensitivity of 91%.

VALIDITY AND RELIABILITY. The MAST has excellent validity correctly identifying over 90% of men who have alcoholism. However, a significant variance in measures of criterion-related validity has been reported that appears to be primarily related to the: (1) correlation of the diagnostic test or other criterion against which the MAST is validated; and (2) population group that is sampled and tested (Storgaard, Nielsen, & Gluud, 1994).

For example, in a sample of patients with psychiatric or mental disorders, which was primarily comprised of women, validity estimates were found to be higher than for samples comprised of lower proportions of women (Teitelbaum & Mullen, 2000). Interestingly, for adolescents, MAST scores demonstrate no gender differences (Nevitt, Lundak, & Galardi, 2006). Construct-validity for the MAST has been demonstrated by the: (1) moderate correlation between the MAST and AUDIT; and (2) high correlation between the MAST and DSM criteria (Conley, 2001).

Regarding reliability, the MAST has been generally found to have excellent internal consistency with a reported Cronbach's alpha coefficient of 0.95 (Selzer, Vinokur, & Van Rooijen, 1975). Later studies (e.g., Conley, 2001) have found a lower, but still a strong, measure of internal consistency (i.e., 0.86). The MAST's test-retest measures of reliability range from 0.83 to 0.95 for samples of psychiatric patients when test-retest intervals ranged from one day to approximately five months (Skinner & Sheu, 1982; Zung, 1982).

RECOMMENDATIONS. In general, we have found the MAST and the MAST-A to be valid and reliable quick-screen psychometric tests and recommend their use for adolescents. However, some caution is advised regarding their use for Muslim adolescents because the MAST and MAST-A were not developed for this group, or other groups for which religious restrictions forbid the use of alcohol (Luczak, 2003).

Rapid Alcohol Problems Screen—Version 4 (RAPS4)

The RAPS4 is a 4-item, quick-screen psychometric test (Table 1.16) that was developed by Cherpitel (2000) to detect alcohol dependence, or alcoholism. The original Rapid Alcohol Problems Screen (RAPS), which was developed by Cherpitel in 1995, received its name from

Table 1.16 The RAPS4

Question	*Scoring Criteria [Point Allocation]*
1. DURING THE PAST YEAR, HAVE YOU HAD A FEELING OF GUILT OR REMORSE AFTER DRINKING?	No [0] Yes [1]
2. DURING THE PAST YEAR, HAS A FRIEND OR FAMILY MEMBER EVER TOLD YOU ABOUT THINGS YOU SAID OR DID WHILE YOU WERE DRINKING THAT YOU COULD NOT REMEMBER?	No [0] Yes [1]
3. DURING THE PAST YEAR, HAVE YOU FAILED TO DO WHAT WAS NORMALLY EXPECTED OF YOU BECAUSE OF DRINKING?	No [0] Yes [1]
4. DURING THE PAST YEAR, DO YOU SOMETIMES TAKE A DRINK WHEN YOU FIRST GET UP IN THE MORNING?	No [0] Yes [1]

Source: Cherpitel (2000).

the acronyms obtained for each of these four items, or questions, about drinking: **R** for "remorse;" **A** for "amnesia;" **P** for "performance;" and **S** for "starter"—the need to ingest alcohol upon awakening in the morning (Cherpitel, 1995) (See Table 1.16.) As its name implies, the RAPS4 is the fourth revision of the original RAPS. The items, or questions, about drinking that comprise the RAPS4 were taken from other quick-screen psychometric tests that were used for detecting "harmful, or hazardous, drinking" (i.e., AUD; alcohol dependence; or alcoholism). A Spanish language version also is available (Borges & Cherpitel, 2001; Cherpitel & Borges, 2000)

SCORING OF THE RAPS4

A positive response to any one of the four questions on the RAPS4 is considered a positive test for harmful, or hazardous, drinking (i.e., alcohol dependence), or alcoholism (see Table 1.16 for scoring criteria for the RAPS4).

AVAILABLE TEST STATISTICS AND RECOMMENDATIONS

RAPS4 test statistics include those for specificity and sensitivity. These data are discussed in the following section, followed by our recommendations regarding the use of the RAPS4.

SPECIFICITY AND SENSITIVITY. Like the original RAPS, the RAPS4 reportedly performs better than most similar quick-screen psychometric tests in terms of specificity and sensitivity for men and women in the U.S. of African or European continental or Hispanic descents (Cherpitel, 1997a, 1998, 2000, 2002; Cherpitel & Bazargan, 2003).[117] Using a cutoff total score of 1, with a large

117 The RAPS, RAPS4, and RAPS4-QF have been used in several foreign countries (e.g., Argentina, India, Poland). However, their reported test statistics have been disappointing (Cremonte & Cherpitel, 2008; Cherpitel, Ye, & Bond, 2005; Cherpitel, Ye, & Moskalewicz, 2005; Nayak, Bond, & Cherpital, 2009). These findings do not support the use of the RAPS, or its derivatives, in this context.

sample of patients accessing emergency department services, Cherpitel (2000) reported a specificity of 87% and a sensitivity of 93% for alcohol dependence. However, for harmful, or hazardous, drinking, a significantly lower specificity of 79% and a sensitivity of 55% were found.[118]

VALIDITY AND RELIABILITY. Published data concerning the validity and reliability of the RAPS4 are not available.

RECOMMENDATIONS. We do not recommend the use of the RAPS4 for adolescents because of its: (1) generally limited published statistics; and (2) total lack of test statistics for adolescents in the U.S.

Rutgers Alcohol Problem Index (RAPI)

The RAPI is a 23-item,[119] self-administered quick-screen psychometric test (Table 1.17) that was developed by White and Labouvie (1989) to detect problem drinking among adolescents. Factor analysis of the RAPI indicates that it is composed of three factors: (1) abuse/dependence symptoms; (2) personal consequences of alcohol use; and (3) social consequences of alcohol use (Martens, Neighbors, & Dams-O'Connor, 2007). It was normed on a non-clinical sample of adolescent girls and boys, 12 years-of-age to 21 years-of-age. The RAPI requires a 7th grade reading level.

Several brief versions of the RAPI have been proposed to reduce gender bias (Earleywine, LaBrie, & Pedersen, 2008)[120] and to facilitate clinical utility (Neal, Corbin, & Fromme, 2006). However, related test statistics are not generally available for these versions of the RAPI.

SCORING OF THE RAPI

Each item of the RAPI is scored from 0 to 3 (see Table 1.17) and is summed for a possible maximal score of 69. The RAPI was developed for use with "normed samples" and, thus, it can be administered with any sample. For example, for the initial clinical sample (age range, 14 to 18 years-of-age), the mean scores ranged from 21 to 25, depending on age and gender. Similarly, for a non-clinical sample (age range, 15 to 18 years-of-age), mean scores ranged from 4 to 8, depending on age and gender.

AVAILABLE TEST STATISTICS AND RECOMMENDATIONS

Available statistical data for the RAPI's specificity, sensitivity, variability, and reliability are discussed. Our recommendations, regarding the use of the RAPI as a quick-screen psychometric test for adolescents, follow.

118 The low sensitivity has been significantly increased to 90% with the addition of two quantity–frequency questions: (1) "During the past year, have you consumed five or more drinks on at least one occasion?" and (2) "During the past year, have you consumed alcohol at least once per month?" (Cherpitel, 2002). The modified RAPS4 is referred to as the "RAPS4-QF."

119 An 18-item version was developed by White and Labouvie (2000) to replace the original 23-item RAPI. The two tests are exactly alike, except for the deletion of items #14, #17, #18, #20, and #22. Although there are very little psychometric data available for the 18-item version of the RAPI, the correlation between the two versions is reported to be 0.99.

120 The S-RAPI was developed to address concerns regarding men's and women's significantly different biological responses to drinking alcohol. Statistical analyses revealed 7 items (#3, #4, #11, #16, #17, #18, and #19) that displayed bias, which were subsequently removed from the test. According to the authors "dropping these items created a shorter scale with almost identical psychometric properties but less potential for bias" (p. 1249). Unfortunately, detailed, related psychometric analysis of their data were not provided.

Table 1.17 The RAPI

Question Number and Behavior Affected *How many times has this happened to you while you were drinking or because of your drinking during the last year?*	*Scoring Criteria* *[Point Allocation]*
1. NOT ABLE TO DO YOUR HOMEWORK OR STUDY FOR A TEST	None [0]; One to two times [1]; Three to five times [2]; More than five times [3]
2. GOT INTO FIGHTS WITH OTHER PEOPLE (FRIEND, RELATIVE, STRANGER)	None [0]; One to two times [1]; Three to five times [2]; More than five times [3]
3. MISSED OUT ON OTHER THINGS BECAUSE YOU SPENT TOO MUCH MONEY ON ALCOHOL	None [0]; One to two times [1]; Three to five times [2]; More than five times [3]
4. WENT TO WORK OR SCHOOL "HIGH" OR DRUNK	None [0]; One to two times [1]; Three to five times [2]; More than five times [3]
5. CAUSED SHAME OR EMBARRASSMENT TO SOMEONE	None [0]; One to two times [1]; Three to five times [2]; More than five times [3]
6. NEGLECTED YOUR RESPONSIBILITIES	None [0]; One to two times [1]; Three to five times [2]; More than five times [3]
7. RELATIVES AVOIDED YOU	None [0]; One to two times [1]; Three to five times [2]; More than five times [3]
8. FELT THAT YOU NEEDED MORE ALCOHOL THAN YOU USED TO IN ORDER TO GET THE SAME EFFECT	None [0]; One to two times [1]; Three to five times [2]; More than five times [3]
9. TRIED TO CONTROL YOUR DRINKING (TRIED TO DRINK ONLY AT CERTAIN TIMES OF THE DAY OR IN CERTAIN PLACES, THAT IS, TRIED TO CHANGE YOUR PATTERN OF DRINKING)	None [0]; One to two times [1]; Three to five times [2]; More than five times [3]
10. HAD WITHDRAWAL SYMPTOMS, THAT IS, FELT SICK BECAUSE YOU STOPPED OR CUT DOWN ON DRINKING	None [0]; One to two times [1]; Three to five times [2]; More than five times [3]
11. NOTICED A CHANGE IN YOUR PERSONALITY	None [0]; One to two times [1]; Three to five times [2]; More than five times [3]
12. FELT THAT YOU HAD A PROBLEM WITH ALCOHOL	None [0]; One to two times [1]; Three to five times [2]; More than five times [3]
13. MISSED A DAY (OR PART OF A DAY) OF SCHOOL OR WORK	None [0]; One to two times [1]; Three to five times [2]; More than five times [3]
14. WANTED TO STOP DRINKING BUT COULDN'T	None [0]; One to two times [1]; Three to five times [2]; More than five times [3]
15. SUDDENLY FOUND YOURSELF IN A PLACE THAT YOU COULD NOT REMEMBER GETTING TO	None [0]; One to two times [1]; Three to five times [2]; More than five times [3]
16. PASSED OUT OR FAINTED SUDDENLY	None [0]; One to two times [1]; Three to five times [2]; More than five times [3]

(*Continued*)

Table 1.17 (Cont.)

Question Number and Behavior Affected *How many times has this happened to you while you were drinking or because of your drinking during the last year?*	*Scoring Criteria* *[Point Allocation]*
17. HAD A FIGHT, ARGUMENT OR BAD FEELING WITH A FRIEND	None [0]; One to two times [1]; Three to five times [2]; More than five times [3]
18. HAD A FIGHT, ARGUMENT OR BAD FEELING WITH A FAMILY MEMBER	None [0]; One to two times [1]; Three to five times [2]; More than five times [3]
19. KEPT DRINKING WHEN YOU PROMISED YOURSELF NOT TO	None [0]; One to two times [1]; Three to five times [2]; More than five times [3]
20. FELT YOU WERE GOING CRAZY	None [0]; One to two times [1]; Three to five times [2]; More than five times [3]
21. HAD A BAD TIME	None [0]; One to two times [1]; Three to five times [2]; More than five times [3]
22. FELT PHYSICALLY OR PSYCHOLOGICALLY DEPENDENT ON ALCOHOL	None [0]; One to two times [1]; Three to five times [2]; More than five times [3]
23. WAS TOLD BY A FRIEND, NEIGHBOR OR RELATIVE TO STOP OR CUTDOWN ON DRINKING	None [0]; One to two times [1]; Three to five times [2]; More than five times [3]

Source: White & Labouvie (1989).

SPECIFICITY AND SENSITIVITY. A specificity of approximately 76% was obtained for adolescents of American Indian descent (i.e., 76.2%, cutoff score of 21) and, for adolescents not of American Indian descent, a specificity of approximately 75% (i.e., 74.6%, cutoff score of 27). Corresponding sensitivities were 80.0% and 53.3%, respectively (Noel, O'Connor, & Boudreau, 2010). In other studies, the specificity of the RAPI increased for both groups of adolescents as the cutoff score was increased (i.e., at a cutoff score of 38, specificity increased to 90.5% for adolescents of American Indian descent and increased to 85.7% for adolescents not of American Indian descent). However, the sensitivity decreased (i.e., at a cutoff score of 38, the sensitivity for adolescents of American Indian descent decreased to 40.0% and to 46.7% for adolescents not of American Indian descent (Noel, O'Connor, & Boudreau, 2010).

VALIDITY AND RELIABILITY. The items selected for inclusion in the RAPI were selected from other similar quick-screen psychometric tests that had good face validity. Therefore, the RAPI tends to have good face validity, as well. Good convergent validity has been established for the RAPI when compared with DSM-IV criteria for harmful, or hazardous, drinking and alcohol dependence (Ginzler, Garrett, & Baer, 2007). The internal consistency of the RAPI also is good as demonstrated by a Cronbach's alpha coefficient of 0.88 (Earleywine, LaBrie, & Pedersen, 2008) and 0.92 (White & Labouvie, 1989).

RECOMMENDATIONS. The RAPI contains more items than the other quick-screen psychometric tests used to detect an AUD among adolescents. These additional items increase the time required to complete the test, but also increase its validity. We recommend the use of the RAPI for the detection of AUD among adolescents with the caution that testers pay particular attention to the selected cutoff score.

Short Michigan Alcoholism Screening Test (SMAST)

The Short Michigan Alcoholism Screening Test, "Short Mast" or "SMAST," is a 13-item psychometric screening test (Table 1.18) that was developed by Selzer, Vinokur, and Van Rooijen (1975) to detect "alcoholism" (i.e., AUD; alcohol dependence). Also see the B-MAST (Table 1.11) and MAST (Table 1.15).

SCORING OF THE SMAST

Each of the items of the SMAST is scored, 0 or 1—with the exception of #1, #4, and #5, which are scored in reverse (see Table 1.18). All scores are summed to provide a possible maximal score of 13. It is recommended that the total scores achieved by respondents be interpreted as: 0 or 1, "non-alcoholic;" 2, "possible alcoholic;" and 3, or higher, "alcoholic."

Table 1.18 The SMAST

Scoring Criteria	*Item #/Question*
PLEASE CIRCLE EITHER YES *OR* NO *FOR EACH ITEM AS IT APPLIES TO YOU*	
YES [0] NO [1]	1. Do you feel you are a normal drinker?
YES [1] NO [0]	2. Does your wife, husband, a parent, or other near relative ever worry or complain about your drinking?
YES [1] NO [0]	3. Do you ever feel guilty about your drinking?
YES [0] NO [1]	4. Do friends or relatives think you are a normal drinker?
YES [0] NO [1]	5. Are you able to stop drinking when you want to?
YES [1] NO [0]	6. Have you ever attended a meeting of Alcoholics Anonymous (AA)?
YES [1] NO [0]	7. Has drinking ever created problems between you and your wife, husband, a parent, or other near relative?
YES [1] NO [0]	8. Have you ever gotten into trouble at work because of drinking?
YES [1] NO [0]	9. Have you ever neglected your obligations, your family, or your work for two or more days in a row because you were drinking?
YES [1] NO [0]	10. Have you ever gone to anyone for help about your drinking?
YES [1] NO [0]	11. Have you ever been in a hospital because of drinking?
YES [1] NO [0]	12. Have you ever been arrested for drunken driving while intoxicated or driving under the influence of alcoholic beverages?
YES [1] NO [0]	13. Have you ever been arrested, even for a few hours, because of drinking?

Source: Selzer, Vinokur, & Van Rooijen (1975).

AVAILABLE TEST STATISTICS AND RECOMMENDATIONS

The specificity and sensitivity of the SMAST, as well as its validity and reliability, are discussed in the following sections. We conclude with our recommendations.

SPECIFICITY AND SENSITIVITY. The SMAST was used to discriminate between social drinkers (i.e., "non-alcoholics") and heavier drinkers (i.e., "possible alcoholics and alcoholics") with a sample of traditional Muslim men living in Kuwait. The SMAST demonstrated a good specificity of 82.5% and an excellent sensitivity of 100% (al-Ansari & Negrete, 1990). In contrast, samples of American Southwestern and Plains Indians—both men and women—demonstrated an unacceptable specificity range of 23% to 47% using the recommended cutoff score of 3, although a very good sensitivity (range, 86% to 95%) was obtained. Using a cutoff score of 2 to detect lifetime alcohol abuse/dependence for samples of primary care patients, specificities ranged from 88% to 97% and sensitivities ranged from 38% to 82% (Brown & Rounds, 1995; Cleary, Miller, & Bush, 1988; Fleming & Barry, 1991).

VALIDITY AND RELIABILITY. As a quick-screen psychometric test, the SMAST is comparable to the CAGE in regard to detecting alcoholism (Maisto, Connors, & Allen, 1995). Internal reliability has been reported as 0.85 (Barry & Fleming, 1993). However, the variability in internal consistency estimates, particularly among women and nonclinical respondents, have been found to adversely affect the overall reliability of the SMAST (Shields, Howell, & Potter, 2007).

RECOMMENDATIONS. The lack of sufficient published adolescent test statistics and the amount of variability in the internal consistency estimates affecting overall test reliability, prevent us from recommending the clinical use of the SMAST for adolescents.

T-ACE

The T-ACE is a four-item psychometric screening test (see Table 1.19) that was developed by Sokol, Martier, and Ager (1989) to detect alcoholism. Based on the CAGE (see earlier discussion), it was originally used in obstetric settings to detect alcoholism or "risk drinking" and associated potential danger for the development of FAS/FASD among pregnant women. Although initially designed to be administered by structured interview, the T-ACE is frequently self-administered.

Table 1.19 The T-ACE

Scoring Criteria [Point Allocation]	*Item Number and Question*
NO [0] YES [1]	1. Does it take more than it used to for you to get "high?" (**T**olerance)
NO [0] YES [1]	2. Have you become **A**ngry or Annoyed when others express concern about your alcohol use? (**A**ngry)
NO [0] YES [1]	3. Have you tried to **C**utdown or quit? (**C**utdown)
NO [0] YES [1]	4. Have you had an **E**ye opener? (**E**ye opener)

Source: Sokol, Martier, & Ager (1989).

SCORING OF THE T-ACE

Each affirmative response to the questions on the T-ACE is given a score of 1 (see Table 1.19 for scoring criteria). The scores are summed for a possible maximal score of 4. A total score of 2, or higher, is considered to be indicative of alcoholism, or "risk drinking."

AVAILABLE TEST STATISTICS AND RECOMMENDATIONS

Statistical data regarding the specificity and sensitivity of the T-ACE are discussed in the following sections, which conclude with our recommendations. Published data regarding the validity and reliability of the T-ACE, and other test statistics, are not available.

SPECIFICITY AND SENSITIVITY. The reported specificity of the T-ACE for a cohort of pregnant women was 79% (Russell, Martier, & Sokol, 1994, 1996). Among the male partners of a similar cohort of pregnant women, the T-ACE had a specificity of approximately 50% and a sensitivity of approximately 84% (Chang, McNamara, & Orav, 2006). In comparison, the specificity of the T-ACE was found to be 59% and the sensitivity to be 88% for a formal structured clinical interview conducted with patients in a psychiatric clinic (Hill & Chang, 2007).

In another study, poor specificity (19% to 34%) was reported with a sample of pregnant women using recommended cutoff scores (Sarkar, Einarson, & Koren, 2010). Increasing the criterion value (i.e., cutoff point) to a score of 3 for a similar sample of women of both European and African continental descents, significantly increased the specificity of the T-ACE (Chiodo, Delaney-Black, & Sokol, 2014).

The sensitivity of the T-ACE is reportedly higher than that for the CAGE (Russell, Martier, & Sokol, 1994), particularly for pregnant women of African continental descent (Bradley, Boyd-Wickizer, & Powell, 1998). The T-ACE also has been reported to be more sensitive than obstetric staff assessment for detecting alcoholism or risk drinking by pregnant women (Chang, Wilkins-Haug, & Berman, 1998). The overall sensitivity of the T-ACE with samples of pregnant women ranges from 85% to 100% (Chang, Goetz, & Wilkins-Haug, 1999; Russell, Martier, & Sokol, 1996; Sarkar, Einarson, & Koren, 2010). For a randomly selected sample of outpatients, 18 years-of-age and older, McQuade, Levy, and Yanek (2000) found the overall sensitivity to be 74%. The sensitivity performance results that were obtained were: (1) superior to both the AUDIT (i.e., 68%) and the CAGE (i.e., 68%); and (2) significantly higher for men (i.e., 81%) than for women (i.e., 70%). McQuade, Levy, and Yanek (2000) also found that the T-ACE outperformed both the AUDIT and the CAGE.

RECOMMENDATIONS. Test statistics for the T-ACE are limited. In addition, data regarding its use with adolescents, other than that reported by McQuade, Levy, and Yanek (2000) for a random sample of participants, 18 years-of-age and older, is generally lacking. Thus, we do not recommend the use of the T-ACE for adolescents.

TWEAK

The TWEAK is a five-item psychometric screening test (Table 1.20) that was designed by Russell, Martier, and Sokol (1994). It was adapted from the CAGE in order to better detect "heavy drinking" or alcoholism among women during pregnancy and was initially tested in the U.S. with pregnant women of African continental descent. Although initially designed to be administered by structured interview, the TWEAK is frequently self-administered. A computerized version also is available.

SCORING OF THE TWEAK

The TWEAK is comprised of five questions (see Table 1.20 for scoring criteria). Positive responses for questions #1 and #2 are each given a score of 2. Positive responses for questions

Table 1.20 The TWEAK

Scoring Criteria [Point Allocation]	*Item #, Acronym, and Question*
Five or more drinks [2]	**1. T**OLERANCE: How many drinks can you hold?[121]
No [0] Yes [2]	**2. W**ORRIED: Have close friends or relatives worried or complained about your drinking in the past year?
No [0] Yes [1]	**3. E**YE OPENER: Do you sometimes take a drink in the morning when you first get up?
No [0] Yes [1]	**4. A**MNESIA: Has a friend or family member ever told you about things you said or did while you were drinking that you could not remember?
No [0] Yes [1]	**5.** C**[K]**UTDOWN: Do you sometimes feel the need to c[k]utdown on your drinking?

Source: Russell, Martier, & Sokol (1996).

#3, # 4, and #5 are each given a score of 1. The scores are then summed for a possible maximal score of 7. A final total score of 2, or higher, for women (Cherpitel, 1995; Russell, Martier, & Sokol, 1996) and a final total score of 3, or higher, for men (Cherpitel, 1998, 1999) suggests harmful or hazardous alcohol use.

AVAILABLE TEST STATISTICS AND RECOMMENDATIONS

Specificity, sensitivity, reliability, and other available test statistics for the TWEAK are discussed in the following sections, along with our recommendations. Published data regarding the validity of the TWEAK are not available.

SPECIFICITY AND SENSITIVITY. The TWEAK has a reportedly higher specificity and sensitivity than the CAGE or B-MAST regarding the detection of heavy drinking or alcoholism (Chan, Pristach, & Welte, 1993) among pregnant women (Chang, Wilkins-Haug, & Berman, 1998; Russell, Martier, & Sokol, 1996). The TWEAK—although, overall, more sensitive for men than for women—has been reported to out-perform both the CAGE and the MAST in detecting "heavy drinking" or alcoholism (i.e. alcohol dependence; AUD) among women (Bradley, Boyd-Wickizer, & Powell, 1998; Cherpitel, 1997b). Overall, the TWEAK has a demonstrated specificity of approximately 90% and a sensitivity of approximately 74% (O'Connor & Whaley, 2003; Russell, Martier, & Sokol, 1994).

These statistics vary, as previously noted in the discussion of other quick-screen psychometric tests in this chapter, with both the population sampled and the cutoff score selected. For example, using a cutoff score of 2, or higher, for detecting "alcohol problems" among women, the TWEAK was found to have a specificity range of 77% to 87% and a sensitivity range of 89% to 91 % (Cherpitel, 1995, 1997b; Russell, Martier, & Sokol, 1996). For adolescents accessing emergency room services, Chung, Colby, and Barnett (2000), using a cutoff score of 1, found the TWEAK to have a specificity of 80% and a sensitivity of 84%.

However, overall, the TWEAK is generally considered to be inferior to the AUDIT, particularly when used to detect alcohol problems among women (Bush, Kivlahan, & Davis,

121 "Version 2," an alternative version of the TWEAK (Chan, Pristach, & Welte, 1993), replaces this question and point allocation for scoring with, "How many drinks does it take you to get high?" *Three or more drinks* [2].

2003; Chung, Colby, and Barnett 2000). The TWEAK also appears to be equally sensitive (approximately 90%) when used for men and women of either African or European continental descents (Cherpitel, 1997a).

RELIABILITY AND OTHER AVAILABLE TEST STATISTICS. Published data regarding the TWEAK that are available regarding its reliability are cause for concern. A comparison of the AUDIT, RAPS4, and TWEAK found the TWEAK to have the lowest reliability of the three tests (Cremonte, Ledesma, & Cherpitel, 2010). In addition, as found in an earlier study by Kelly, Donovan, and Kinnane (2002), the internal consistency of the TWEAK is low (i.e., Cronbach's alpha of 0.50) and the average inter-item correlation is low (i.e., 0.17).

RECOMMENDATIONS. Based on the available statistics indicating poor reliability, and other poor test statistics, we generally do not recommend the use of the TWEAK for detecting AUD among pregnant adolescents or young women.

***Related Professional Reminder:* Always keep in mind that quick-screen psychometric tests, no matter how valid and reliable, are by definition, "screening tests." Thus, they require carefully administered psychiatric/psychological interview and other objective data (laboratory test results; consideration of parent and teacher reports; other professional reports) as needed to develop and substantiate a "correct" diagnosis.**[122]

Before moving to an overview of treatment approaches for AUD—both pharmacotherapy and psychotherapy/counseling—we discuss contemporaneous diagnoses, which may commonly occur among adolescents and young adults, that involve an AUD and/or one, or more: (1) SUDs; (2) other mental disorders (OMDs); and (3) physical medical disorders (PMDs).

Child, Adolescent, and Young Adult Contemporaneous Diagnoses

A "contemporaneous diagnosis" occurring in a child, adolescent, or young adult (or adult) is defined as a diagnosis of alcohol (AUD) and/or one or more other dependence or use disorders (i.e., substance use disorders, or SUDs), together with one or more other mental disorders (OMDs), and/or one or more physical medical disorders (PMDs) (Pagliaro & Pagliaro, 2018). Over the years, several other closely related terms have been commonly used to denote this diagnosis, such as:

- "Dual addiction"—concomitant alcoholism and drug abuse (Kreek & Stimmel, 1984);
- "Dual disorder"—concurrent diagnosis of alcoholism plus a psychiatric diagnosis (Daley, Moss, & Campbell, 1987);
- "Dual diagnosis"—the identification of an adolescent (or young adult) as having two, or more, mental disorders at the same time (Pagliaro, 1990);
- "Comorbidity"—cases of two diagnosable entities in the realm of substance abuse and mental illness (Belfer, 1993);

122 In this regard, we tend to find ourselves, as clinician-scientists, particularly favoring a positive empiricist stance. Consequently, we are very comfortable with the use of fully structured interviews. However, given our academic appreciation of other views of many sciences, we also value the arguments offered by others (e.g., Nordgaard, Sass, & Parnas, 2013), who have noted the limitations of quantitative, or fully structured interviews and present arguments for a more phenomenologically informed, semi-structured conversation approach. We also appreciate other approaches, which include, for example, the consideration of gestalt-based approaches that we have found to be particularly helpful in understanding the nature of physical and psychological dependence with a particular patient. This understanding generally exceeds a "collection" of specific signs and symptoms—as used by DSM.

- "Dual diagnosis"—the concurrence of another disorder (psychiatric or medical) existing independent of an addictive disorder (Miller, Leukefeld, & Jefferson, 1994);
- "Dual diagnosis"—the concurrence of substance abuse and severe mental illness (i.e., long-term psychiatric disorders) (Drake, Essock, & Shaner, 2001);
- "Multiple diagnosis"—two or more mental health diagnoses in addition to a substance use diagnosis (Slesnick & Prestopnik, 2005).

The diversity of these terms and definitions has contributed to much semantic confusion in the published literature and in clinical settings. Thus, for clarity, the term, "contemporaneous diagnosis," is used in this reference text and is defined as:

> The detection—in a child, adolescent, or young adult—of an AUD and/or one or more SUDs, and/or one or more OMDs,[123] and/or one or more PMDs[124] that may, or may not, be directly related.

Contemporaneous Diagnoses Involving OMDs

As originally recognized by Keller, Lavori, and Beardslee (1992), the presence of more than one OMD with an AUD, and/or SUD, is more common than once thought. In fact, among the adolescents they studied, who had been diagnosed with an AUD and/or a SUD, almost three-quarters (74%) had two to four OMDs (see Table 1.21).

In cases in which an AUD and/or SUD and OMD are "directly" related, the AUD and/or SUD most commonly occur as an antecedent to, or as a consequence of, the OMD (e.g., Lehman, Myers, & Corty, 1994; Pagliaro, 1995)[125] An example of the former is an 18-year-old adolescent boy, who, over a few weeks of heavy drinking and cannabis use, developed cannabis-induced paranoid psychosis.[126] An example of the latter is a young man, who began regular cocaine use to self-medicate his undiagnosed mental depression and, consequently, developed cocaine-induced psychosis.[127] An "indirect" relationship also may occur.

123 For the sake of parsimony, and to further reduce semantic confusion, we use the term, "other mental disorder" (OMD), to include all related disorders, diseases, and conditions that are typically diagnosed and treated by psychiatrists and psychologists (i.e., all psychiatric disorders and all psychological disorders).

124 In addition, for the sake of parsimony, and to further reduce semantic confusion, we use the term, "physical medical disorder" (PMD), to include all related disorders, diseases, and health conditions that are typically diagnosed and treated by physicians (i.e., all physical medical disorders, including neurological disorders).

125 Usually, the distinction, as to whether, or not, a co-occurring mental disorder is an "antecedent" or a "consequence" to an AUD/SUD, is not particularly relevant in many clinical contexts. However, in cases where the co-occurring mental disorder is an "antecedent" to the AUD/SUD, intervention aimed at ameliorating the co-occurring mental disorder (e.g., major depressive disorder) will also ameliorate the related AUD/SUD (Deas & Brown, 2006).

126 He was living in the basement of his parents' home. One evening after heavy drinking and cannabis use, he threatened his parents and punched his father, thinking that they were strangers who had invaded the house to kill his parents. In fear, the father subsequently called 911 for assistance. The police arrived in full tactical gear because the adolescent was known to them from previous encounters. The adolescent boy did not believe that they were police officers and a violent struggle ensued as he "tried to protect his family." The adolescent was finally restrained by the police, handcuffed, and placed in leg restraints. However, he continued to violently resist arrest—he was quite strong and muscular, being a body-builder, around six feet tall, and weighed approximately 200 pounds. He finally succumbed when the paramedics arrived and injected him with an antipsychotic tranquilizer. The adolescent boy was formally charged, as an adult, with resisting arrest (one charge) and assault (five charges) on the five different police officers who were directly involved in his arrest. All charges were dismissed at trial subsequent to our expert forensic testimony that explained his uncharacteristic alcohol and cannabis-induced behavior (Pagliaro & Pagliaro, *Clinical Patient Data Files*).

127 Sadly, the cocaine-induced psychosis, which developed from his heavy cocaine use, resulted in a "high-speed" police chase and tragic motor vehicle crash that killed a recently married couple (Pagliaro, Jaglalsingh, & Pagliaro, 1992).

Table 1.21 Eleven Mental Disorders Commonly Involved in Adolescent and Young Adult Contemporaneous Diagnoses

Mental Disorders
1. Attention-Deficit/Hyperactivity Disorder (ADHD)
2. Bipolar Disorder (BD)
3. Borderline Personality Disorder (BPD)
4. Conduct Disorder (CD)
5. Gender Dysphoria
6. Major Depressive Disorder (MDD)
7. Oppositional Defiant Disorder (ODD)
8. Panic Disorder (PD)
9. Post-Traumatic Stress Disorder (PTSD)
10. Psychotic Disorder (Schizophrenia)
11. Sleep Disorders: Insomnia

For example, a SUD may be an antecedent to the development of an OMD as occurs, for example, when an adolescent with latent schizophrenia (a co-factor) uses LSD and develops LSD-induced psychotic disorder—schizophrenia. Figure 1.9 illustrates the components of contemporaneous diagnoses. These relationships can often be complicated when adolescents and young adults are involved because, as noted by Deas (2006), while adolescents and young adults may be actively developing a SUD, and have one or more diagnostic signs and symptoms, they may not yet have developed sufficient signs and symptoms to meet established diagnostic criteria (e.g., from DSM-5; or the cutoff score required for a related quick-screen psychometric test), which are required to satisfy a formal diagnosis of the SUD.

As previously noted, a significant percentage of adolescents and young adults, who present with a primary diagnosis of an AUD, an SUD, or an OMD, can be expected to have a contemporaneous diagnosis.[128] Although several studies and reports have suggested that a diagnosis of an AUD or SUD can be generally expected in approximately 10% to 20% of patients, who have an OMD, our own clinical experiences, and the published literature (e.g., Drake, Essock, & Shaner, 2001; Kaminer, Goldberg, & Connor, 2010), suggest that the actual incidence of contemporaneous diagnoses is significantly higher (i.e., more than 50% and often closer to 100%) among patients whose primary disorder is a clinically significant AUD or SUD (i.e., involving physical and psychological dependence on alcohol or another drug or substance of abuse) (Pagliaro & Pagliaro, *Clinical Patient Data Files*).

As identified by several researchers and clinicians (e.g., Deas, 2006; Pagliaro & Pagliaro, *Clinical Patient Data Files*), when compared to adolescents and young adults, who have a single AUD, SUD, or OMD, adolescents and young adults, who concurrently have an AUD, SUD, and OMD, generally have:

128 In our clinical practice, which specializes in the treatment of patients who have contemporaneous diagnoses, we have noted that the vast majority of patients, themselves, are generally unaware that they have a contemporaneous diagnosis that has not been previously identified or diagnosed. Generally, these patients are only consciously aware that they are "depressed" or that they have a "drinking problem" (i.e., the reason for their referral), or smoke cigarettes "more than they should." They are not aware that they have two, or generally more, active OMDs—all of which are generally highly interrelated (Pagliaro & Pagliaro, *Clinical Patient Data Files*).

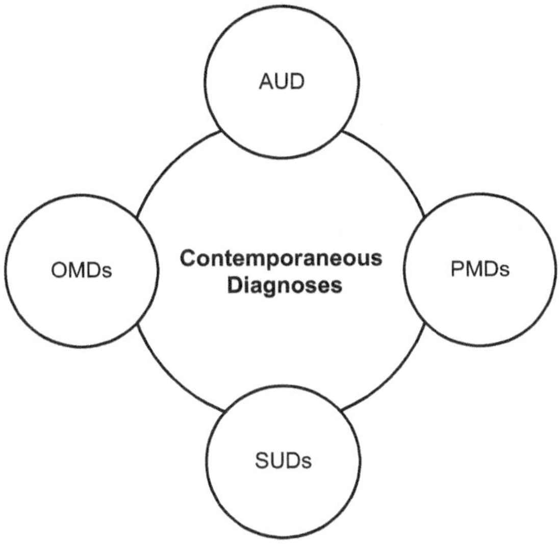

Figure 1.9 Components of Contemporaneous Diagnoses

1. A significantly more severe form of the related disorders;
2. A poorer prognosis regarding therapeutic outcomes;
3. Additional major PMDs often associated with significant related health and social care requirements (e.g., hepatitis; HIV; pregnancy among adolescent girls; tuberculosis).

In addition, these adolescents and young adults are more likely to present with increased rates of:

- Academic difficulties (e.g., absenteeism; dropping out of, or not completing, high school; low academic performance);
- Arrest and incarceration;
- Homelessness and reliance on social assistance;
- Hospitalization or institutionalization;
- Job loss and unemployment;
- Poor compliance with prescribed pharmacotherapy, psychotherapy (e.g., family; group; individual), and other treatment interventions;
- Poor interpersonal relationships (i.e., difficulty making friends);
- Little or no response to treatment interventions;
- Recidivism or relapse;
- Suicide, attempted or completed.[129]

As identified, almost three decades ago, by Stowell (1991): "dual diagnosis patients are [generally] heterogeneous as to their psychiatric diagnoses, as well as the various substances they abuse" (p. 98). However, a review of the published literature suggests that the majority of cases of contemporaneous diagnoses detected among adolescents and young adults involve: (1) one or more SUDs—related to the use of alcohol, amphetamines,

129 See the related discussion in the earlier pharmacology section, "Undesired, or Harmful, Effects and Toxicities—Depression and Suicide."

cannabis, cocaine, nicotine, or opiate analgesics—and (2) one, or more, OMDs from the following eight categories:[130]

1. Disorders usually first diagnosed in infancy, childhood, or adolescence (e.g., attention-deficit/hyperactivity disorder [ADHD]; conduct disorder [CD]; oppositional defiant disorder [ODD]);
2. Anxiety disorders (e.g., panic disorder [PD]; post-traumatic stress disorder [PTSD]);
3. Eating disorders (e.g., anorexia nervosa; bulimia nervosa);
4. Gender dysphoria;
5. Mood disorders (e.g., bipolar disorder [BD]; major depressive disorder [MDD]);
6. Personality disorders (e.g., borderline personality disorder [BPD]);
7. Psychotic disorders (e.g., schizophrenia);
8. Sleep disorders.

(Pagliaro & Pagliaro, 2012, 2018)

Of these mental disorders, those that are most frequently implicated with a contemporaneous diagnosis are:

1. Attention-deficit/hyperactivity disorder (ADHD);
2. Conduct disorder (CD);
3. Oppositional defiant disorder (ODD);
4. Major depressive disorder (MDD).

Interestingly, ADHD, CD, and ODD involve marked externalizing behaviors and are generally diagnosed during childhood and "prior" to the development of an AUD or a SUD, which usually tends to be diagnosed during late adolescence or early adulthood. Each of these disorders are also discussed in more detail in the later, respective chapters (e.g., Chapter 2, "Amphetamines and Cocaine;" Chapter 4, "Cannabis and Other Psychodelics;" Chapter 5, "Prescription Opiate Analgesics and Heroin")

AUD/SUDs & ADHD

Worldwide, including the U.S., the incidence of ADHD is approximately 8%, or one in 13 children (Dopheide & Pliszka, 2009; Mayes, Bagwell, & Erkulwater, 2008). Several researchers (e.g., Bukstein, 2008; Shrier, Harris, & Kurland, 2003) have found that the co-occurrence of SUDs among adolescents and young adults with ADHD is several times higher than that among matched cohorts, or the general population.

ADHD also has been implicated in the development of an AUD and/or SUD among adolescents and young adults. For example, both the incidence of adolescent drunkenness and binge drinking (see the earlier subsection, "New Millennial Trends—Binge Drinking") are significantly higher for adolescents and young adults who have ADHD (Molina & Pelham, 2001; Molina, Pelham, & Gnagy, 2007). It has also been found that the association of ADHD with an AUD and/or SUD is particularly significant among boys—which is not surprising given the approximately 10-fold over-representation of boys in comparison to girls with ADHD. In these and other cases, the ADHD is noted to "precede" the development of the AUD or SUD (Bukstein, 2008).

130 For example, over 90% of individuals with an AUD also have a nicotine use disorder (e.g., Van Skike, Maggio, & Reynolds, 2015; Verplaetse & McKee, 2017).

Marshal and Molina (2006) suggested that children with ADHD and either CD or ODD (i.e., comorbid antisocial behavior—see following section),[131] are at significant risk for developing a "peer-mediated" AUD and/or SUDs during adolescence. Arias, Gelernter, and Chan (2008) suggested that the impulsivity associated with ADHD underlies its correlation with AUD and/or SUDs and their increased severity and associated sequelae (e.g., hospitalizations; suicide attempts).[132] In addition, the significant association between ADHD and AUD/SUDs has increased concern regarding the diversion and illicit use, particularly among adolescent boys, of the psychostimulants that are medically prescribed to adolescents and young adults for the medical management of ADHD, including methylphenidate (Ritalin®) and mixed amphetamines (Adderall®) (Bukstein, 2008; Pagliaro & Pagliaro, 2009; Upadhyaya, 2008; Wilens, Adler, & Adams, 2008). (Also see related discussion in Chapter 2, "Amphetamines and Cocaine.") Contemporaneous diagnoses detected among adolescents with ADHD also have been related to CD and ODD, as well. See following discussion.

AUD/SUDs & Conduct Disorder (CD)

Conduct disorder appears to be more commonly associated with an AUD and/or SUD among adolescents than are OMDs, including MDD (Armstrong & Costello, 2002; Slesnick & Prestopnik, 2005). A positive parental history of an AUD and/or SUD is significantly correlated with a childhood diagnosis of CD—most likely because of both genetic and environmental factors (e.g., learned parenting styles) (Button, Rhee, & Hewitt, 2007; Haber, Bucholz, & Jacob, 2010; Haber, Jacob, & Heath, 2005; Kramer, Han, & Leukefeld, 2009). Conduct disorder also is significantly more common among boys than girls (Kramer, Han, & Leukefeld, 2009; Shrier, Harris, & Kurland, 2003).

Quite often, children who are diagnosed with CD also have been diagnosed with ADHD "prior" to the subsequent development and diagnosis of an AUD and/or SUD during adolescence or early adulthood (e.g., Burke, Loeber, & Lahey, 2001; Molina, Pelham, & Gnagy, 2007). Marshal and Molina (2006) suggested that a contemporaneous diagnosis involving CD may be mediated among adolescents, who have been identified as having childhood ADHD, by the factor of deviant peer affiliation (i.e., children and adolescents, with ADHD and co-morbid CD or ODD, are at significantly increased risk for developing a peer-mediated AUD and/or SUD during adolescence).

In an earlier study of "runaway" youth living in youth shelters, Slesnick and Prestopnik (2005) found that a CD-related contemporaneous diagnosis usually accompanied an AUD and two, or more, SUDs—15% of research participants had AUD and one SUD; 27% had AUD and two SUDs; and 38% had AUD and three SUDs. A diagnosis of CD made during childhood often "precedes" a diagnosis of AUD and/or SUD during adolescence with the resultant AUD/SUD tending to be more severe than usual (Fergusson, Horwood, & Ridder, 2005, 2007; Nock, Kazdin, & Hiripi, 2006). In these cases, during late adolescence or early adulthood, these adolescents may be also diagnosed with "antisocial personality disorder" (APD).

131 Several researchers (e.g., Masi, Manfredi, & Nieri, 2017; Sinzig, Dopfner, & Lehmkuhl, 2007) have reported an increased risk for both aggressive and antisocial behavior among adolescents with ADHD.

132 Several clinicians and researchers (e.g., Furman, 2005, 2008; Pagliaro & Pagliaro, *Clinical Patient Data Files*) view ADHD as a "grouping" of neurobehavioral signs and symptoms (e.g., hyperactivity; impulsivity; inattentiveness) that have diverse etiologies related to several different mental or neurological conditions, rather than a single mental disorder (i.e., as a multivariate as opposed to a univariate disorder). In addition, we have, for some time, viewed ADHD as a "spectrum" disorder (i.e., not a simple, single, quantitatively invariant disorder, but rather as a complex, variant disorder) with significant variance in presenting signs and symptoms, particularly in regard to "intensity" and associated clinical consequences (Pagliaro & Pagliaro, *Clinical Patient Data Files*).

AUD/SUDs & ODD

The combination of AUD and/or SUD with ODD is another common contemporaneous diagnosis identified among adolescents (Armstrong & Costello, 2002). Many of the adolescents, in this category, also have a diagnosis of co-morbid ADHD, which, according to Marshal and Molina (2006), may be mediated through deviant peer affiliation. Not surprisingly, a contemporaneous diagnosis involving an AUD and/or SUD and ODD among boys during middle childhood has been highly correlated with delinquent behavior.

Contemporaneous Diagnoses Involving PMDs

Adolescents and young adults can present with any of a number of possible contemporaneous diagnoses involving one or more PMDs. In fact, there seems to be an unending number of combinations and permutations of diagnoses involving an AUD, SUDs, and PMDs.

AUD/SUDs/OMDs & PMDs

AUD and/or SUDs, and OMDs are often associated with increasingly high-risk behaviors among adolescents and young adults that often result in serious injuries (i.e., PMDs), including, for example, alcohol-related: bar fights; falling down stairs; and MVCs. They also are associated with behaviors that place them at increased risk for HIV infection and AIDS due to unprotected sex with multiple partners (e.g., Pagliaro & Pagliaro, 2012, 2018). These injuries and infections, as well as other medical concerns, demonstrate the need for the designation of contemporaneous diagnoses that include the diagnosis of PMDs such as serious injury and HIV infection and AIDS, which has become increasingly recognized, particularly in regard to bisexual and gay adolescent boys and young adult men, and "run-away" and homeless adolescents, who often live "on-the-streets" (e.g., Slesnick & Prestopnik, 2005).

In fact, generally "heavy drinkers" and "concurrent-users" of drugs and substances of abuse, these adolescents and young adults have an extremely high incidence of AUD, SUDs, and OMDs that are reported to be between 60% (Slesnick & Prestopnik, 2005) and 90% (Pagliaro & Pagliaro, *Clinical Patient Data Files*).

Appropriate pharmacotherapy and psychotherapy are a common and integral component of the management of the "quad" contemporaneous diagnoses commonly presented by adolescents and young adults. As identified by several researchers (e.g., McCarthy, Tomlinson, & Anderson, 2005), the symptomatic management of AUD, various SUDs, OMDs, and PMDs may be adversely affected by the inadequate treatment of one or more of these disorders. The complexity of diagnosing, planning therapeutic intervention, and delivering appropriate pharmacotherapy, together with optimal psychotherapy/counseling and needed medical treatment, requires multidisciplinary expertise, communication, and coordination. We now turn to the approaches for treating alcohol dependence or use disorder.

Treating Child, Adolescent, and Young Adult Alcohol Dependence or Use Disorder

Reus, Fochtmann, and Bukstein (2018b), in an AUD practice guideline for the American Psychiatric Association (APA), noted that:

> Despite its high prevalence and numerous negative consequences, AUD remains undertreated.
>
> (p. 4)

The treatment[133] of alcohol dependence or use disorder involves both pharmacotherapy and psychotherapy/counseling, including 12-step programs and other approaches. In fact, more research is available on the treatment of alcohol dependence or use disorder than for all of the other drugs and substances of abuse, combined. We have consistently found that a combination of both efficacious pharmacotherapy and psychotherapy/counseling provide optimal results in terms of achieving and maintaining abstinence (i.e., "resumed nonuse"),[134] by: (1) dealing with the alcohol withdrawal syndrome; and (2) preventing "relapsed use," or "resumed compulsive use." Each of these approaches are discussed separately in the following sections, "Pharmacotherapy" and "Psychotherapy/Counseling."

Pharmacotherapy

There is no pharmacotherapy available for preventing the development of alcohol dependence or use disorder among adolescents or young adults. However, pharmacotherapeutic approaches have been developed and found to be efficacious in the management of adolescent and young adult: (1) "alcohol withdrawal syndrome;" and (2) abstinence maintenance. In the following subsections, we present and discuss these pharmacotherapeutic approaches.[135]

***Related Professional Reminder:* As with all pharmacotherapy, before initiating the selected pharmacotherapeutic approach, assure that the adolescent or young adult:**

- ***Does not have any contraindications to the use of the selected pharmacotherapy;***
- ***Is not at risk for any clinically significant drug–drug interactions (i.e., risk has been identified and has been appropriately dealt with);***
- ***Has been identified as having appropriate renal and hepatic function and that any other necessary related adjustments to the dosage or dosing interval of the associated pharmacotherapy has been carefully addressed.***

Alcohol Withdrawal Syndrome[136]

Acute alcohol withdrawal is often managed quite successfully with a long-acting benzodiazepine—usually chlordiazepoxide (Librium®) or diazepam (Valium®). Benzodiazepine pharmacotherapy for

133 Treatment can also be conceptualized as involving "primary prevention," which is generally directed at preventing initial drug use. Obviously considering the current nature and extent of adolescent and young adult drug and substance use in the U.S., primary prevention has generally been a dismal failure. For a discussion of the factors that contribute to this failure, see Pagliaro and Pagliaro (2018).

In this context, it is interesting to consider Lipari's (2017, p. 1) findings, from an analysis of data concerning adolescent exposure to drug and substance abuse prevention messages from the 2002 to 2015 *National Survey on Drug Use and Health*, that in 2015:

- 75% of adolescents, 12 to 17 years-of-age were "exposed to substance use prevention messages in the media or at school;"
- 50% of adolescents, 12 to 17 years-of-age, "talked with their parents about substance use;"
- Exposure of adolescents to drug and substance abuse prevention messages was lower than in the years 2002 to 2015.

134 Although controlled use has been found to be successful in some cases, complete abstinence is the preferred goal for adolescents and young adults who are diagnosed with AUD.

135 The approaches discussed in this section, particularly those related to "psychotherapy/counseling," often may be applied in the context of other SUDs, which are discussed in the following chapters.

136 See also the related discussion in the earlier pharmacology subsection, "Alcohol Withdrawal Syndrome."

the management of alcohol withdrawal requires a gradual reduction of dosage over a one to two-week period. When appropriately used, benzodiazepine therapy can make the alcohol withdrawal syndrome virtually "symptomless" (Pagliaro & Pagliaro, 1999). In their literature review of treatment for the alcohol withdrawal syndrome among hospitalized patients, Muzyk, Leung, and Nelson (2013) found that, "diazepam loading"[137] provided rapid symptom relief as well as reduced the incidence of seizures and the duration of delirium tremens, or "DTs" (p. 113). Currently, the benzodiazepines are considered to be the cornerstone for the treatment of the alcohol withdrawal syndrome (e.g., Long, Long, & Koyfman, 2017; Ricks, Replogle, & Cook, 2010).

For the treatment of cases that are resistant to benzodiazepine pharmacotherapy, the barbiturate, phenobarbital (Luminal®), and the general anesthetic, propofol (Diprivan®; "Milk of Amnesia"), have been recommended alone, or in combination with a benzodiazepine (e.g., Brotherton, Hamilton, & Kloss, 2016; Long, Long, & Koyfman, 2017; Mo, Thomas, & Karras, 2016; Schmidt, Doshi, & Holzhausen, 2016).

Although pharmacologically not as efficacious as other pharmacotherapeutic approaches, the alpha-adrenergic agonist, clonidine (Catapres®), which is generally clinically used for its antihypertensive effects, has been used as an adjunct for the management of moderate to severe alcohol withdrawal syndrome (Bayard, McIntyre, & Hill, 2004; Stanley, Worrall, & Lunsford, 2005). In this context, the signs and symptoms of withdrawal are generally managed by gradually decreasing the clonidine dosage over a one- to two-week period.

The use of other pharmacological approaches for treating the alcohol withdrawal syndrome, such as the: (1) muscle relaxant, baclofen (Lioresal®); and (2) anticonvulsant, topiramate (Topamax®), are limited and inconclusive (e.g., Guglielmo, Martinotti, & Quatrale, 2015). However, gabapentin (Neurontin®), another anticonvulsant, also has been utilized—"off-label"—to treat alcohol withdrawal.[138] Results, particularly at higher dosages, appear both promising and significantly superior to placebo (Hammond, Niciu, & Drew, 2015; Leung, Hall-Flavin, & Nelson, 2015; Mason, Quello, & Goodell, 2014).[139] Regardless, for adolescents and young adults, particularly those who also have a positive history of drug and substance abuse, we do not recommend the use of gabapentin for the treatment of the alcohol withdrawal syndrome because of the significant potential for gabapentin: (1) abuse; (2) physical dependence; and (3) withdrawal syndrome.

Alcohol Abstinence Maintenance

Pharmacotherapy for alcohol abstinence maintenance helps to assure continued "resumed nonuse" of alcohol, by means of either:

137 Diazepam loading (i.e., administration of fixed 20 mg oral doses every two hours) has long been demonstrated to be a generally safe and effective treatment for alcohol withdrawal. Use is predicated on the pharmacology of diazepam, as well as its pharmacokinetics—rapid achievement of peak concentrations following oral use and a relatively long half-life of elimination (Heinala, Piepponen, & Heikkinen, 1990; Muzyk, Leung, & Nelson, 2013; Sellers, Naranjo, & Harrison, 1983; Weintraub, 2017). See Chapter 6, "Prescription Sedative-Hypnotics," for additional related discussion concerning diazepam (Valium®).

138 Although the APA has recommended the use of gabapentin for the treatment of alcohol dependence or use disorder (Reus, Fochtmann, & Bukstein, 2018a, 2018b), until significantly more data are available supporting its therapeutic efficacy, we cannot recommend gabapentin pharmacotherapy for the management of the alcohol withdrawal syndrome, particularly for adolescents and young adults.

139 It should be noted that, because gabapentin is predominantly excreted in unchanged form in the urine, dosage reduction is required in the presence of mild to severe renal impairment (Raouf, Atkinson, & Crumb, 2017).

1. Aversive stimulation (i.e., pairing unpleasant effects with the use of alcohol);
2. Prevention of rewarding effects (i.e., "blocking" the desired effects associated with alcohol use).[140]

Three drugs have been developed, and have received FDA approval, to help to assure continued resumed nonuse of alcohol among people who have discontinued their regular, long-term abusive and compulsive use of alcohol:

1. Acamprosate (Campral®);
2. Disulfiram (Antabuse®);
3. Naltrexone (ReVia®).

(Garbutt, 2009, 2010; Oural, Paris, & Sullivan, 2008; Swift, 2007)

In addition, topiramate (Topamax®), an anticonvulsant, has been clinically used, "off-label," for this indication and has demonstrated some noted clinical efficacy. Each of these drugs are presented and discussed in the following sections.

ACAMPROSATE (CAMPRAL®) PHARMACOTHERAPY

The use of acamprosate (Campral®), approved for use by the FDA in 2004, has been demonstrated to be both safe and effective for the prevention of relapsed alcohol use among abstinent drinkers (e.g., Jung & Namkoong, 2006; Kennedy, Leloux, & Kutscher, 2010; Rosner, Hackl-Herrwerth, & Leucht, 2010). Its use is generally well-tolerated (Mason & Heyser, 2010b; Yahn, Watterson, & Olive, 2013) with diarrhea being the most commonly reported adverse effect (Boothby & Doering, 2005; Crowley, 2015; Diehl, Ulmer, & Mutschler, 2010). Overall, clinical efficacy has been found to be acceptable and similar to that obtained with naltrexone. Additionally, some researchers (e.g., Crowley, 2015; Plosker, 2015) have noted that acamprosate pharmacotherapy has a generally superior efficacy in comparison to that obtained with other pharmacotherapy approaches.

The exact neurochemical mechanism of action for the success of acamprosate pharmacotherapy has not yet been determined (Kiefer & Mann, 2010; Yahn, Watterson, & Olive, 2013). However, it has been identified that the regular long-term use of alcohol (i.e., alcohol dependence or use disorder) is associated with an increase of N-methyl-D-aspartate (NMDA) receptors. Consequently, during alcohol withdrawal, the NMDA receptors are stimulated by a surge in the release of neurotransmitters, such as glutamate. Given these observations, it has been suggested that acamprosate may work as a neuromodulator by reducing the glutamate surge (i.e., glutamatergic neurotransmission is restored to normal) (De Witte, Littleton, & Parot, 2005; Mennella & Heyser, 2010a; Swift, 2007). Thus, acamprosate may have a dual role as a neuromodulator (i.e., as a GABA agonist and as an NMDA glutamate antagonist).

Available from the manufacturer as a 333 mg, delayed-release, enteric coated oral tablet, acamprosate is ingested daily in three divided dosages (i.e., two tablets three times daily). To increase GI absorption due to its low oral bioavailability (i.e., ~ 11%), it has been suggested that acamprosate should be ingested on an empty stomach. However, because the associated increase is only approximately 20%, acamprosate is generally ingested without regard to meals (Mason & Heyser, 2010b; Wright & Myrick, 2006).

Acamprosate does not undergo hepatic metabolism and is primarily eliminated in unchanged form in the urine (Mason & Heyser, 2010b; Saivin, Hulot, & Chabac, 1998).

140 Abstinence, in this context, is actually a form of relapse prevention (see the "Relapse Prevention" section later in this chapter).

Consequently, the use of acamprosate is contraindicated for patients, who have severe renal impairment (i.e., creatinine clearance less than 30 ml/minute).[141] Although not generally recommended as the "drug of first choice" for patients who have moderate renal impairment, acamprosate can be used with an appropriate reduction in dosage (i.e., one 333-mg tablet, three times daily) (Plosker, 2015; Reus, Fochtmann, & Bukstein, 2018a; Wright & Myrick, 2006). The half-life of elimination of acamprosate is 24 to 32 hours (Kalk & Lingford-Hughes, 2014; Wright & Myrick, 2006).

Acamprosate combination pharmacotherapy for alcohol abstinence maintenance (e.g., acamprosate and naltrexone), along with adjunctive psychotherapy (e.g., acamprosate and cognitive-behavioral therapy), have been found to significantly increase positive therapeutic outcomes (Boothby & Doering, 2005; Kennedy, Leloux, & Kutscher, 2010; Mason, 2001, 2003).

DISULFIRAM (ANTABUSE®) PHARMACOTHERAPY

In 1951, disulfiram (Antabuse®) became the first drug that was approved by the FDA for the management of alcoholism (Soghoian, Wiener, & Diaz-Alcala, 2016). It is well-absorbed following oral ingestion and is highly protein bound. Disulfiram is extensively metabolized in the liver to both toxic and nontoxic metabolites with 10% to 20% of disulfiram being excreted in unchanged form in the feces (Soghoian, Wiener, & Diaz-Alcala, 2016).

Disulfiram blocks the metabolism of alcohol at the "acetaldehyde stage" by means of inhibition of the enzyme, acetaldehyde dehydrogenase (See Figure 1.3, "Alcohol Metabolism," and the related discussion in the earlier pharmacology subsection, "Pharmacokinetics—Metabolism"). Consequently, when alcohol is ingested, even in small amounts, acetaldehyde accumulates in the circulatory system and elicits many undesired, or harmful, effects and toxicities throughout the body, including:

- Blurred vision;
- Chest pain;
- Confusion;
- Copious vomiting;
- Dyspnea;
- Facial flushing;
- Hyperventilation;
- Hypotension;
- Nausea;
- Respiratory distress;
- Syncope;
- Tachycardia;
- Throbbing headache;
- Vertigo;
- Weakness.

The intensity of this reaction, which is known as the "disulfiram-alcohol (-ethanol) reaction" (or more commonly, "Antabuse® reaction" or "disulfiram flush"), is generally proportional to both the amount of:

141 Acamprosate is also contraindicated for: (1) patients who are hypersensitive to acamprosate; and (2) mothers who are breastfeeding.

1. Disulfiram used as a component of the alcohol abstinence maintenance program;
2. Alcohol ingested during a drinking session.

(Pagliaro & Pagliaro, 1999)

Disulfiram pharmacotherapy is initiated following at least one day of abstinence from alcohol use to avoid inadvertently precipitating the disulfiram reaction. Subsequently, disulfiram is orally ingested in doses of 500 mg, on a daily basis each morning, for a period of months to years until abstinence can be maintained without the aid of the drug.[142] Daytime drowsiness/tiredness and night-time sleep disturbances are the most commonly reported adverse effects (Diehl, Ulmer, & Mutschler, 2010). Several contraindications to the use of disulfiram have been identified including: breastfeeding; coronary occlusion; hypersensitivity; metronidazole pharmacotherapy; myocardial disease (severe); pregnancy; and psychosis (Pagliaro & Pagliaro, 1999; Rundio, 2010).

***Related Professional Reminder:* Adolescent and young adult disulfiram pharmacotherapy for alcohol abstinence maintenance, requires health and social care professionals to clearly explain and discuss:**

1. ***Before the initiation of disulfiram pharmacotherapy, the mechanism of disulfiram action as a means for maintaining alcohol abstinence.***
2. ***When receiving disulfiram pharmacotherapy, the need to avoid alcohol and alcohol-containing items that may precipitate a disulfiram reaction, including:***
   - ***Alcohol-containing cough syrups;***
   - ***Alcohol-containing after-shave products;***
   - ***Alcohol-containing mouthwashes;***
   - ***Candies that contain liqueurs;***
   - ***Chinese cooking wine;***
   - ***Cosmetics that contain alcohol.***
3. ***When discontinuing disulfiram pharmacotherapy, because of its long-lasting effects related to its half-life of elimination, the need to avoid the use of alcohol for two weeks following the last dose of disulfiram in order to prevent the precipitation of a disulfiram reaction.***

NALTREXONE (REVIA®) PHARMACOTHERAPY

Another approach for promoting alcohol abstinence maintenance is naltrexone (ReVia®) pharmacotherapy, which received FDA approval in 1994. Naltrexone is a long-acting oral opiate analgesic antagonist (see Chapter 5, "Prescription Opiate Analgesics and Heroin") that was originally developed and marketed under the brand name, "Trexan®," for the treatment

142 Systematic reviews (e.g., Skinner, Lahmek, & Pham, 2014) generally have not supported significant efficacy for disulfiram pharmacotherapy when used alone—particularly in the context of double-blind controlled studies. However, we have found disulfiram pharmacotherapy to be effective for highly motivated, compliant young adults in their early twenties when used as an initial adjunct to Alcoholics Anonymous, or other 12-Step programs, and weekly psychotherapy. However, we do *not* recommend disulfiram pharmacotherapy for promoting alcohol abstinence maintenance for adolescents—although case reports of such use have appeared in the clinical literature with mixed results over the past 30 years (e.g., Myers, Donahue, & Goldstein, 1994). Both acamprosate and naltrexone are safer to use and more efficacious in this clinical context (see related discussion in this chapter).

of opiate analgesic dependence or use disorder (Kirchmayer, Davoli, & Verster, 2000). However—by serendipity—naltrexone was also found to block the disinhibitory euphoria associated with alcohol use.[143] Naltrexone is usually ingested on a daily basis (i.e., 50 mg/day) without regard to meals. Overall, the clinical efficacy of naltrexone is acceptable and similar to that obtained for acamprosate. Naltrexone combination therapy with appropriate psychotherapy/counseling increases efficacious outcomes.

An injectable form of naltrexone (Vivitrol®) also is available and is considered a major pharmaceutical advancement regarding alcohol abstinence maintenance (Garbutt, Kranzier, & O'Malley, 2005). The naltrexone injectable form is an extended-release, microsphere injectable suspension formulation (380 mg). It is injected IM, generally once a month, in a major gluteal muscle by a health care provider or trained family member. The IM injection of naltrexone significantly increases compliance with alcohol abstinence pharmacotherapy (Naltrexone injection, 2010; Swift, 2007).

The endogenous opiate system plays a significant role in the mediation of the disinhibitory euphoria and other desired effects associated with alcohol use, particularly those related to the modulation of dopaminergic neurotransmission in the mesolimbic area of the brain (Jung & Namkoong, 2006; Soyka & Rosner, 2010).[144] Consequently, when the receptors are blocked by naltrexone, the associated "urge" to drink is reduced, thus, strengthening the ability to abstain from drinking. Although additional research is required, it appears that carriers of a variant of the mu-opiate receptor gene may be particularly receptive to the efficacious effects of naltrexone abstinence pharmacotherapy for promoting self-restraint among regular, continuous long-term users of alcohol—including, for example, those who are identified as: addicted to alcohol; physically and psychologically dependent on alcohol; having alcoholism; or having been diagnosed with AUD (Mann & Hermann, 2010; Pagliaro & Pagliaro, 2012, 2018). As a result of these actions, the use of naltrexone can be of particular benefit for those adolescents and young adults who have a contemporaneous diagnosis involving both alcohol and opiate analgesics.

As an adjunct to effective psychotherapy, naltrexone pharmacotherapy demonstrates:

1. A significant clinical utility with reports of less craving for alcohol;
2. A lower rate of relapse;
3. When drinking, the ingestion of fewer drinks per drinking episode.

(Liang & Olsen, 2014; Naltrexone, 2009; Volpicelli, Clay, & Watson, 1995)

Nausea is the most common adverse effect associated with naltrexone pharmacotherapy. However, its long-term safety and efficacy have not yet been clearly established. Additionally, the FDA has added a "boxed warning" to its official monograph stating that: "Naltrexone may cause liver damage when taken in large doses" (Naltrexone, 2009, p. 1).

As a potent opiate analgesic antagonist, naltrexone can precipitate the opiate analgesic withdrawal syndrome among regular, long-term users of the opiate analgesics, including those who are being medically managed for pain (e.g., acute, severe pain; chronic cancer, or other malignant, pain). Thus, caution must be exercised when naltrexone pharmacotherapy is

143 The CNS depressant effects, including alcohol-related effects on cognition, do not appear to be significantly affected by naltrexone. Thus, it is not a "sobriety pill."

144 This current theory is based upon the observation originally expressed in the Walsh-Davis hypothesis. The Walsh-Davis hypothesis, first posited in the 1970s, proposed that a common molecular biochemical mechanism may be responsible for, or at least contribute to, addiction to both alcohol and the opiate analgesics (Davis & Walsh, 1970a, 1970b).

implemented for these users, who also would require alternative pain relief measures until the effects of naltrexone have dissipated (Pagliaro & Pagliaro, 1999; Volpicelli, Clay, & Watson, 1995).[145] Of note, because of both naltrexone's primary hepatic metabolism and its propensity for hepatotoxicity, the use of naltrexone pharmacotherapy is contraindicated for adolescents and young adults, who have acute hepatitis or hepatic failure.

TOPIRAMATE (TOPAMAX®) PHARMACOTHERAPY

Topiramate (Topamax®) is an anticonvulsant that has been used to symptomatically manage various seizure disorders among children and adolescents, as well as adults in the U.S., for well over 30 years (Maryanoff, Nortey, & Gardocki, 1987). While not FDA approved for alcohol abstinence maintenance, its "off-label" use for this indication has been reported for well over a decade (Johnson, Ait-Daoud, & Bowden, 2003; Johnson, Rosenthal, & Capece, 2007). Several published studies and reviews (e.g., De Sousa, 2010; Florez, Saiz, & Garcia-Portilla, 2010; Johnson & Ait-Daoud, 2010; Kenna, Lomastro, & Schiesl, 2009) have indicated that, when compared to either placebo or naltrexone pharmacotherapy for alcohol abstinence maintenance, topiramate pharmacotherapy resulted in:

1. Fewer drinks per day;
2. Fewer drinks per drinking day;
3. Fewer heavy drinking days;
4. Greater reduction in reports of craving;
5. More days abstinent.

The mechanism of action for topiramate, in regard to alcohol abstinence maintenance, has not yet been determined. However, topiramate appears to modulate dopaminergic neurotransmission in the mesolimbic area of the brain by decreasing the changes in NMDA receptor activity associated with the damage caused by regular, continuous long-term alcohol use—or "heavy drinking." Consequently, dopamine release is inhibited, and GABA function is enhanced (Johnson, Ait-Daoud, & Bowden, 2003; Olmsted & Kockler, 2008).

Topiramate is ingested orally in dosages of 200 to 300 mg daily. It is rapidly and well-absorbed from the GI tract with approximately 70% excreted in unchanged form in the urine. Consequently, dosage adjustment may be required for patients with renal impairment. The most common reported undesired effects associated with the use of topiramate, include: cognitive impairment (e.g., short-term memory impairment); dizziness; GI distress; paresthesia; psychomotor slowing; sedation; and weight loss. These undesired effects may significantly limit its use for alcohol abstinence maintenance (Arbaizar, Diersen-Sotos, & Gomez-Acebo, 2010; Shinn & Greenfield, 2010).

Psychotherapy/Counseling

Whereas, children generally respond best to individual psychotherapy and counseling for the management of AUD, as well as SUDs and OMDs, both individual and group psychotherapeutic and counseling approaches can be used for adolescents and young adults, alone, or as an adjunct to pharmacotherapy (e.g., Azorin, Bowden, & Garay, 2010; Miller & Roache, 2009; Pagliaro & Pagliaro, *Clinical Patient Data Files*). These approaches include:

145 Alternatively, if the use of opiate analgesic pharmacotherapy for the treatment of severe pain is clinically indicated, the naltrexone should be discontinued and appropriately replaced with alternative pharmacotherapy (e.g., acamprosate; topiramate).

1. Cognitive therapy and cognitive behavioral therapy;
2. Family therapy;
3. Social skills training;
4. Group therapy;
5. Therapeutic communities;
6. Short-term residential treatment programs;
7. Ethnic-specific programs for adolescents and young adults of various continental (e.g., African; Asian; European) or other descents (e.g., American Indian; Hispanic) in the U.S.;
8. Gay-, lesbian-, or trans-specific adolescent and young adult programs.

Each of these eight approaches is briefly discussed in the following sections.[146]

Related Professional Reminder: ***The success of psychotherapy/counseling depends on many factors—the most important of which are the professional commitment, capabilities, and experiences of the individual psychotherapist/counselor in relation to the specific form of psychotherapy/counseling individually selected for a specific child or adolescent or group of children or adolescents.***

Cognitive Therapy & Cognitive Behavioral Therapy

"Cognitive therapy" (CT) is explicitly based on the original cognitive model of depression proposed by Aaron T. Beck (1961, 1967) for the treatment of mental depression. Breaking from his initial psychoanalytical focus, Beck proposed that behavior change could be best accomplished by altering three levels of cognition:

1. "Core Beliefs," which are learned early in life and are deeply held;
2. "Dysfunctional Assumptions," which are rules for living that are generally maladaptive;
3. "Negative Automatic Thoughts," which are irrational, but accepted as plausible by the patient.

Cognitive therapy is often referred to, in the broader context, as "cognitive-behavioral therapy" (CBT). CBT is "problem focused" and emphasizes the present-day with specific attention to:

- Identifying problem behaviors or relationships, including those associated with alcohol or other drug or substance of abuse dependence or use disorder and/or OMD(s);
- Developing—in both individual and group treatment settings—"action-oriented" or "personal coping" strategies that can later be used by children, adolescents, and young adults to effectively deal with, or manage, their problem behavior(s).

In essence, CBT guides therapists to teach children, adolescents, and young adults to "be their own therapist."

146 Although pharmacotherapy and psychotherapy/counseling approaches are discussed separately, optimal therapeutic outcomes for adolescents—as clearly and consistently demonstrated by many researchers (e.g., Hudmon, Corelli, & Prokhorov, 2010; McCaul & Petry, 2003; Swift, 2007)—generally involve various combinations of these approaches.

Cognitive behavioral therapy (CBT) is a "psychosocial" intervention that empirically has clearly and consistently demonstrated significant efficacy (e.g., Carroll, 2014; Kaminer, 2002; McHugh, Hearon, & Otto, 2010; Waldron & Kaminer, 2004). Although originally used for the treatment of MDD, CBT has been used to treat AUD and virtually every other type of SUD (e.g., cannabis, cocaine, nicotine, and opiate analgesic use disorders). It also has been used for the treatment of several OMDs that are commonly identified among children, adolescents, or young adults (e.g., ADHD; CD; eating disorders; GAD; gender dysphoria; MDD; OCD; PTSD). In addition, it has been used to successfully treat several PMDs including obesity and premenstrual syndrome. As well, CBT has been used with children, adolescents, and young adults in the context of both individual and group therapy, as well as couples and family therapy (see the later discussion in the following section, "Family Therapy").

CBT, often the first choice in terms of the form of psychotherapy/counseling selected for children, adolescents, and young adults, generally follows 10 specific steps:

1. Establishing and maintaining rapport with the patient/family/group;
2. Assessing:
    - Presenting "problems"
    - Problem-related behavior
    - Behavior "deficits"
    - Incidence and severity of related behaviors, or lack thereof;
3. Re-conceptualizing the "problem(s)"
    - Helping the child or adolescent to recognize the problem, including its duration and extent;
4. Teaching and developing needed skills, including skills to cope with "craving" and to assertively resist offers for drugs;
5. Applying needed skills and monitoring results;
6. Re-assessing and adjusting the therapy plan, as needed;
7. Generalizing and continuing the maintenance of needed skills;
8. Assessing or evaluating post-treatment outcomes;
9. Following-up, as deemed necessary and appropriate for the child, adolescent, or young adult, in terms of both form and duration of treatment;
10. Terminating therapy, which actually begins during the first session with a child, adolescent, or young adult, with clarification of treatment approach, goals, objectives, and expected general time frame for needed CBT.[147]

Cognitive behavioral therapy assumes that harmful patterns of using alcohol, and other drugs and substances of abuse, are indicative of maladaptive coping in which "learning processes" play a major role (i.e., the child, adolescent, or young adult has not learned effective ways to cope with problems or to meet certain individual needs, particularly

147 In the context of CBT for children, adolescents, and young adults with alcohol or other drug and substance abuse dependence or use disorder, intervention terminates at the end of the formal scheduled treatment as the child, adolescent, or young adult successfully meets his or her goals and expectations. However, this involves the realization that reinforcement may be needed during the long-term because of the general nature and characteristics of alcohol or other drug and substance abuse dependence or use disorder that may result in a need for help to maintain nonuse and prevent the occurrence of relapsed use.

developmental needs).[148] Integral to this theory, is the acceptance that "feelings/emotions," "thoughts," and "behaviors" all influence each other (see Figure 1.10). As illustrated in the Figure 1.10, the triangle in the center represents the CBT tenet that the "core beliefs" of all humans can be divided into three categories: (1) "view of self;" (2) "view of others/world;" and (3) "view of future."

Consequently, successful intervention is predicated upon helping a child, adolescent, or young adult to both: (1) recognize or admit specific problems; and (2) learn to correct these problems by applying a range of different effective strategies including:

- Changing maladaptive/dysfunctional core beliefs (e.g., "no one likes me;" "people can't be trusted");[149]
- Learning and developing new and effective coping mechanisms (e.g., distraction; imagery; minimizing negative thoughts; motivational self-talk) to deal with related anticipated problems;
- Learning and developing better information processing skills.

Thus, CBT is directed at the correction, or modification, of:

1. Faulty thinking patterns or styles;
2. Irrational belief systems;
3. Maladaptive or deficient coping skills.

Sharing of thoughts and feelings/emotions with a therapist is attempted as part of the training process of CBT. This training in self-observation involves the systematic analysis of the validity of negative and irrational self-statements, and the gradual substitution of positive, logical thinking patterns based on rational belief systems.[150] Through this training process, children, adolescents, and young adults are gradually made more aware of their problems associated with their use of alcohol or other drugs and substances of abuse, which may have been denied or avoided. Through CBT, they are helped to develop the coping strategies, skills, and abilities that they need to effectively deal with these problems.

The development, or strengthening, of specific intrapersonal and interpersonal skills, including anger control, leisure time management, problem solving, and resistance training, is an integral component of cognitive therapy. Cognitive behavioral therapy is often used, in the context of alcohol dependence or use disorder, to help children, adolescents, and young adults to both achieve resumed nonuse of alcohol and prevent the occurrence of relapsed use. Thus, attention is focused on the positive gains achieved during early abstinence and how these gains can be maintained in order to prevent relapse. A central component in the achievement of this goal involves teaching children, adolescents, and young adults to: (1)

148 In comparison to, for example, treatment using traditional psychoanalysis, during which the therapist utilizing observed/reported behaviors, dreams, or memories, looks for "unconscious" meaning, which, subsequently results in the formulation of a diagnosis.

149 These dysfunctional core beliefs, or identified "errors" in patient thinking, can often be non-exclusively categorized as: catastrophizing; dichotomous reasoning; emotional reasoning; magnification; minimization; mind reading; overgeneralizing; personalization; and selective abstraction.

150 For example, the health and social care professional, or other clinician, can help patients to self-identify irrational "automatic" thoughts (also referred to as: "cognitive distortions;" or "negative automatic thoughts") by asking questions such as, "What was going through your mind at that time?" or "What are you thinking right now?" These irrational thoughts generally occur spontaneously and, thus, are not immediately self-evident to the patient, who, consequently, generally accepts them as plausible.

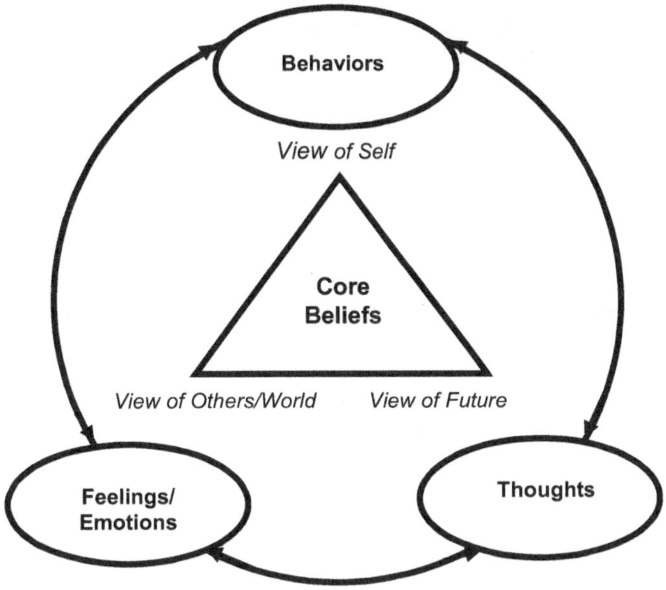

Figure 1.10 Basic Tenets of CBT

identify and anticipate high-risk situations that may lead to relapsed use; and (2) apply previously learned and rehearsed techniques to effectively avoid or deal with them.[151]

Finally, although often ignored or given insufficient attention, the process of "termination" in CBT is of clinical significance. In this regard, Vidair, Feyijinmi, and Feindler (2017, p. 20), based on their review of theories and research related to the termination of CBT with children and parents, developed a seven-point model that focuses on specific aspects aimed at successfully completing the process of termination that may also be of value for adolescents and young adults:

1. Teach children to become their own therapists from the start of treatment, clarifying expectations and eliciting parental assistance as developmentally appropriate;
2. Foster a therapeutic alliance early on to engage children and parents in the process of skills acquisition;
3. Facilitate skills generalization and maintenance to prepare families for termination;
4. Consolidate treatment gains and a final therapy "product" in the final sessions;
5. Plan for relapse prevention and booster sessions;
6. Celebrate child and parent progress;
7. Facilitate a "good goodbye" by modeling, eliciting, and validating positive and negative feelings while reinforcing the idea that the child is ready to be her or his own therapist.

151 Although a relatively simple strategy, with efficacy that has been questioned, the "Just Say No Campaign" is an example of the application of cognitive rehearsal techniques that may be used to prevent initial use of alcohol or other drugs and substances of abuse. Interestingly, this particular program has demonstrated particular success when used for children rather than adolescents (or adults) (Pagliaro & Pagliaro, *Clinical Patient Data Files*).

***Related Professional Reminder:* When a behavior changes, the new behavior does not completely erase the old behavior. Consequently, appropriate follow-up strategies must be planned and implemented in order to maintain/sustain the therapeutic gains/successes associated with behavior change.**

Unfortunately, behavior change—even when successfully achieved with CBT or other forms of psychotherapy—is often temporary. As explained by Bouton (2014), many factors contribute to this situation:

> The research suggests that methods used to create behavior change (including extinction, counterconditioning, punishment, reinforcement of alternative behavior, and abstinence reinforcement) tend to inhibit, rather than erase, the original behavior.
>
> (p. 29)

Hence, children, adolescents, and young adults, who have developed patterns of "compulsive use" of alcohol or other drugs and substances of abuse (see the earlier related discussion, "Nine Patterns of Using Drugs and Substances of Abuse") may require periodic reinforcement following successful intervention. This periodic reinforcement, in many cases, may be required over their lifetime.

CBT, primarily delivered by direct face-to-face interaction between the child, adolescent, or young adult and the therapist, also can be effectively delivered to small groups of similarly-aged children, adolescents and young adults. In addition, CBT can be delivered with the use of a (1) computerized, or internet-based delivery system;[152] or (2) a self-help guide. We generally recommend that the latter be used only in conjunction with direct face-to-face interaction with the therapist.

***Related Professional Reminder:* Indirect methods of CBT delivery generally are associated with lower rates of compliance to, and completion of, planned psychotherapy. They also are associated with a higher incidence of negative effects associated with uncorrected self-rumination.**

Family Therapy

> Alcohol isn't a spectator sport. Eventually, the whole family has to play.
>
> Anonymous

As denoted in this chapter, and the other chapters of this reference text, the family often plays a significant role in the etiology and maintenance of harmful patterns of alcohol and other drug and substance use among children, adolescents, and young adults. Some general guidelines that can assist family therapists and other health and social care professionals, regardless of their specific theoretical orientations, are presented in Table 1.22. As identified by Bukstein and Van Hasselt (1993), almost 30 years ago regarding adolescents:

152 Several researchers (e.g., Kiluk, Nich, & Buck, 2018) have found computer-delivered CBT to be equally efficacious as clinician-delivered CBT. Sarlin (2018), in a report for the NIDA, noted that:

> - Patients, who self-administer cognitive behavioral therapy (CBT) using computerized training modules reduced their drug use as much as patients who received clinician-delivered CBT, and they maintained this advantage through a 6-month follow-up;
> - By reducing the time that clinicians need to spend with individual patients, computer-based CBT training may enable treatment programs to accommodate larger caseloads and increase access to treatment.
>
> (p. 1)

Table 1.22 General Guidelines for Family Therapists

	General Guidelines
1.	Respect the hierarchal structure of the family, if appropriate. If not, try to help the family re-establish a functional hierarchy.
2.	Listen to what is being said and not said, asking relevant questions for both.
3.	Don't interrupt a family member while he or she is speaking to ask for clarification. Wait until they have finished.
4.	Observe nonverbal behavior closely, as a basis for understanding family relationships and for possible intervention.
5.	Give equal attention to each family member.
6.	Do not attempt to minimize problems to the family. Be honest and open.
7.	Empathize with the stated family issues.
8.	Be nonjudgmental so that the family feels free to discuss problems without fear of censure.
9.	Establish open communication patterns early in therapy.
10.	Be aware of your own biases (and countertransference tendencies).
11.	Be flexible enough to shift your approach if you find that it is not working.
12.	Do not give advice, only suggestions as they fit the therapeutic plan.
13.	Do not allow yourself to be triangulated or manipulated. *You* are the therapist.
14.	Evaluate each individual in terms of depression, guilt, self-esteem, etc.
15.	When you sense the family feels it has failed, attempt to bring up past successful experiences as reinforcement.
16.	Become a role model to the family.
17.	Allow the family to see you as a person who can make mistakes and own up to these mistakes.
18.	Allow them to see you as a person with feelings.
19.	Try to have a purpose and reason for all of your actions or lack of action.
20.	Do not copy another therapist's style. Be yourself. Act in a manner that is comfortable for you and fits your personality.
21.	Your role is to provide options for the family to select and pursue. You plant a seed for positive growth that will enable the therapeutic process to bring about change.

Modified from: Frankel & Piercy (1990).

> Intervention with substance-abusing adolescents that fails to proactively involve the family in treatment is unlikely to yield significant short- or long-term improvements.
>
> (p. 465)[153]

Cognizant of these associations, family therapy attempts to correct the dysfunctional behavior of family members, both individually and as a group (e.g., Lewis, Piercy, & Sprenkle, 1990; Szapocznik & Williams, 2000).

Family Therapy, in its various forms, is largely based on "Family Systems Theory" (FST), which was developed from "General Systems Theory," and examines the relationships among

153 In addition, several studies have validated the efficacy of family therapy for the treatment of both: (1) children and adolescents with FASD (e.g., Peadon, Rhys-Jones, & Bower, 2009); and (2) adolescent mothers who use the drugs and substances of abuse and neglect or physically abuse their children (e.g., Donohue, 2004; Slesnick & Zhang, 2016).

the members of a family and the family unit itself. Three major concepts associated with the FST are: (1) "boundaries;" (2) "feedback;" and (3) "homeostasis."

"Boundaries" define the internal and external limits of the family system. Healthy families define roles that are intended to support optimal functioning and provide protection of the family unit. In unhealthy families, for example, in which a child, adolescent, or young adult—or a parent—has alcohol or other dependence or use disorder, the boundary between parents and their children becomes "permeable." Consequently, family roles can become confused (e.g., sometimes "reversed") and the family is unable to perform optimally as a cohesive unit.

"Feedback" refers to the reciprocal/circular manner by which members of the family communicate with each other. In this context, the behavior of one family member becomes feedback which facilitates and reinforces the behavior of another family member. See for example, the concept of "maternal-infant attachment" discussed in the earlier section, "Mothering."

"Homeostasis" is the inherent tendency of the family system to maintain equilibrium—even if this equilibrium is not in the overall best interest of individual members of the family or the family unit itself. For example, a parent may routinely report that his/her son is "sick with the flu" when in fact he is drunk or too "hung-over" to go to school or to his part-time job. This behavior may help to promote equilibrium by protecting the son from: being expelled from school (and potentially not meeting the criteria for graduation from high school or losing his job); social services (potential removal from the home); and a possible "fight" with the father when he comes home from work (for "drinking again"). However, the parent's protective behavior also may serve as an enabling behavior that helps to maintain the son's AUD and/or SUDs.

Applying family therapy to treat "drug-abusing adolescents," Lewis, Piercy, and Sprenkle (1990, p. 88) described the "Purdue Brief Family Therapy Model," a "mixed" family therapy model, noting its seven major goals, which we believe are applicable to many types of family therapy:

1. To decrease a family's resistance to treatment;
2. To redefine substance use as a family problem;
3. To re-establish appropriate parental influence;
4. To interrupt dysfunctional family sequences of behavior;
5. To assess the interpersonal function of the substance use;
6. To implement change strategies consistent with the family's interpersonal functioning;
7. To provide assertion training skills for child and adolescent family members to resist peer pressures to engage in substance use.

Family therapy[154] attempts to correct the dysfunctional behavior of family members, both individually and as a group. Behavioral and strategic-structural family therapies are the most commonly used forms of family therapy, excluding mixed therapies. These systemic

154 When the concept of circular or reciprocal causality is applied, this approach also is commonly referred to as a systemic (i.e., family systems oriented) approach or model (Lewis, Piercy, & Sprenkle, 1990). This approach or model should not be confused with "systemic family therapy," a particular model of family therapy that uses a cybernetic process. Systemic intervention or treatment differs from psychologic and pharmacologic approaches because of the inherent focus of these intervention strategies. Whereas the focus of the latter is on the child or adolescent as an individual, the focus of the former is on the entire family as a group that includes a member(s) (i.e., the adolescent) who displays harmful patterns of using the drugs and substances of abuse. In this regard, the drug and substance using adolescent member is often identified as the "thermostat" of family health and functioning. Thus, therapists attempt (optimally) to assess and treat all the members of the family, including nuclear and extended family members, or significant others, as a group.

approaches are briefly discussed in the context of their application to the treatment of AUD and SUDs among children, adolescents, and young adults.

BEHAVIORAL FAMILY THERAPY (BFT)

Behavioral family therapy for children and adolescents, who have been diagnosed with alcohol or other dependence or use disorder, and their families predominantly consists of techniques that were: (1) developed and validated by empirical studies of children and adolescents who were identified as delinquent; and (2) applied in child welfare and criminal justice contexts (e.g., Donovan, Azrin, & Allen, 2009; Donovan, Azrin, & Bradshaw, 2014). These techniques typically include "contingency management" and "behavioral contracting."

Contingency management and behavioral contracting involve identifying, operationally defining, and agreeing to a set of desired child or adolescent target behaviors. These behaviors include, for example: (1) completing household chores (e.g., taking out the garbage; cleaning one's room; getting homework done well, and on time); and (2) complying with time schedules (e.g., specified times for coming home after school or returning from an evening date).

Consequences, or punishments, for breaking agreed upon contracts (e.g., being "grounded," or restricted to the home premises for a period of time; taking away computer or cell phone privileges; or restricting use of the family car) are upheld and immediately implemented. Explicitly defined rewards for complying to the agreed-upon contracts (e.g., an allowance; access to the child's or adolescent's cell phone; or permission to drive the family car) are used as reinforcements to positively modify the child's or adolescent's behavior.

Over the new millennium, contingency management has been widely empirically validated for the management of AUD and various SUDs among adolescents (e.g., Corby, Roll, & Ledgerwood, 2000; Henggeler, Chapman, & Rowland, 2008; Stranger, Lansing, & Budney, 2016; Walter & Petry, 2016). As found by Petry, Alessi, and Olmstead (2017):

> Contingency management (CM) interventions consistently improve substance abuse treatment outcomes.
>
> (p. 1)

The contingency management interventions were derived from the operant behavioral psychology of B. F. Skinner (1938) and are based on, "the belief that behavior is learned and reinforced by interaction with environmental contingencies" (Bigelow & Silverman, 1999, p. 16). As explained by Higgins and Petry (1999, p. 5), contingency management interventions almost always involve one or more of the following generic contingencies to motivate increases and decreases in the frequency of a "therapeutically desirable" and "undesirable" behavior, respectively:

- "Positive reinforcement" that delivers a desired consequence (e.g., a voucher exchangeable for retail items), contingent on the individual meeting a therapeutic goal (e.g., negative urinalysis test results);
- "Negative reinforcement" that removes an aversive or confining circumstance (e.g., living at home under parent or legal guardian supervision with a judicial requirement for ankle bracelet monitoring), contingent on meeting a target therapeutic goal (e.g., attending counseling sessions);
- "Positive punishment" that delivers a punishing consequence (e.g., a professional reprimand), contingent on evidence of undesirable behavior (e.g., positive urine test results);

- "Negative punishment" that removes a positive condition (e.g., reducing the monetary value of a voucher to be earned), contingent on evidence of the occurrence of an undesirable behavior (e.g., missing a scheduled counseling session).

Although first used in the U.S. in the context of methadone maintenance programs (Carroll, 2014), contingency management techniques (e.g., Stranger, Lansing, & Budney, 2016) have, quite often, been applied in closed youth detention and treatment facilities and other settings amenable to the use of a token economy system (e.g., Godley, Godley, & Dennis, 2014; Rohsenow, Tidey, & Kahler, 2015), including juvenile drug courts (e.g., Chapman, McCart, & Letourneau, 2013). As identified by Petry (2000), seven core factors need to be adequately identified and addressed in order to maximize the potential for success:

1. Target behavior, which must be both observable and measurable;
2. Target population (e.g., adolescents who are users of a particular drug or substance of abuse, or who have a contemporaneous diagnosis, or who have a high recidivism rate);
3. Type of incentive (e.g., youth detention center privileges; on-site prize distribution; token economy voucher);
4. Amount or value of the incentive (i.e., generally, the greater the incentive, the greater the response);
5. Frequency of incentive distribution (i.e., generally, the response will be greater if the incentive is presented soon after the target behavior is achieved or demonstrated);
6. Timing of incentive distribution (i.e., generally the more rapidly the incentive is distributed in relation to the target behavior, the more effective it will be);
7. Duration of the reinforcement intervention (i.e., the longer the duration, the greater the success)—it appears that a minimal duration of six months is generally required for individuals to internalize the desired behavior.[155]

The training component of behavioral family therapy is often directed toward assertiveness, parent management, and problem-solving skills training. "Assertiveness training" assists children and adolescents to learn and rehearse techniques that can help them to resist peer pressure to use drugs and substances of abuse. "Parent management training" helps parents to improve their communication with their children, establish common goals, and re-establish their appropriate influence within the family structure. Parent training focuses on: (1) altering inappropriate parental behavior(s); and (2) teaching parents using role playing and practicing new skills for managing positive and negative behaviors identified in their children or adolescents.

"Problem-solving skills training" is aimed at assisting all family members to learn to become less dogmatic and more accepting of applying alternative strategies for solving family problems. The problem-solving approach has four principal components:

155 Interestingly, advances in technology (e.g., cell phones; internet) have been utilized to facilitate and extend the delivery and duration of contingency management in the treatment of alcohol dependence or use disorder and other drug and substance of abuse dependence or use disorders. As identified by Kurti, Davis, and Redner (2016):

> The use of technology to facilitate the remote implementation of incentive-based interventions to improve health is a burgeoning area of research, especially interventions targeting substance use . . .
>
> (p. 145)

1. Defining the problem;[156]
2. Generating a number of alternative solutions for the defined problem;[157]
3. Evaluating the positive and negative aspects of each solution;
4. Selecting the best available (practical and doable) solution for that particular family unit.

Stormshak and Dishion (2009) describe "The Family Check-Up" intervention that integrates aspects of BFT into schools (i.e., establishing a family resource center in schools). Twenty years of related research (e.g., Stormshak, Fosco, & Dishion, 2010) have demonstrated efficacy in reducing the long-term risk for adolescent use of drugs and substances of abuse. However, caregiver participation and adolescent results are extremely variable.

STRATEGIC-STRUCTURAL FAMILY THERAPY (SFT)

Strategic-structural family therapy, or simply structural family therapy, attempts to "restructure" maladaptive family boundaries that separate family members from each other in destructive ways (Szapocznik & Williams, 2000). For example, a mother and son may form a close, protective alliance that excludes the father from the knowledge that his son is a homosexual and that he also abuses several drugs and substances of abuse because of his frequent participation in both local and distant "circuit parties." In reaction to this exclusion, the father may feel alienated from his once close family and becomes increasingly indifferent to his wife and distant and unsupportive of, or openly hostile toward, his son.

In another example, a young adolescent mother may be involved in constant, bitter conflicts with her fiancé over her cannabis use and involve their young children in the conflict by making them "take her side." In this situation, the mother may also physically or verbally abuse one of her children, using him or her as a "scapegoat" for the displacement of her own anger, frustration, and sense of blame (i.e., responsibility for the situation).

The general strategies incorporated with strategic-structural family therapy include:

1. Reframing;
2. Validation;
3. Facilitated Communication.

"Reframing," a method also used in cognitive psychotherapy, simply refers to the process of conceptualizing a problem in a new and different way. The purpose of reframing is generally to first place a problem in proper (generally smaller) perspective, and second, to lessen the negative views that the family members have regarding their perceived notion of the cause of the problem. For example, a mother may identify her daughter's alcohol use as an act of defiance. Whereas, the therapist may reframe the adolescent daughter's alcohol use as an expression of insecurity, low self-esteem, or a need to establish autonomy. This reframing of the reasons related to the daughter's alcohol use may then facilitate shifting the treatment approach from one of punishment to one of understanding and support.

"Validation" refers to the process by which the therapist, in acting as a role model for family members, acknowledges and expresses an understanding of each family member's concerns, feelings, and desires. This approach encourages each family member to listen to or "hear out" the concerns, feelings, and desires of other family members before reacting to them or judging them.

156 This component of the problem-solving approach is conceptually equivalent to what has been referred to in a scientific or medical context as the generation of "multiple working hypotheses."

157 This component of the problem-solving approach is often referred to as "brainstorming."

For "facilitated communication," various techniques are taught and used during family therapy sessions to facilitate communication among family members. For example, individual family members may be taught to use the expression "I feel" as opposed to "you feel." This communication technique helps to avoid casting blame based on "mind-reading" and allows other family members to clarify their own feelings. It also allows them to state for themselves what they feel—as opposed to responding to what a family member "thinks" they feel. As such, the "I feel" communications tend to engender more empathetic responses than do "you feel" communications, which tend to elicit decidedly more defensive responses.

Social Skills Training

Social skills training attempts to help children and adolescents, who have insufficient social skills, to interact more effectively with their friends, peers, teachers, parents, and employers.[158] Social skills training involves detailed, focused training sessions that deal with common child and adolescent problems related to their poor social skills (Oei & Jackson, 1980) and, thus, include:

- Nonverbal expression;
- Refusing unreasonable requests;
- Making difficult requests;
- Expressing and receiving positive emotions;
- Replying appropriately to criticism;
- Initiating social conversations.

The training approach also has been successfully applied in juvenile closed-custody correctional settings (Pagliaro & Pagliaro, *Clinical Patient Data Files*).[159]

Children and adolescents, who engage in harmful patterns of using alcohol and other drugs and substances of abuse, have been commonly identified as having interpersonal, family, school, and vocational problems that appear to be related to deficits in social skills. In response to this observation, several social skills, school-based programs and other individual and group training programs have been initiated. These programs generally rely on therapist role modeling, role playing, and homework assignments, to help children and adolescents to:

- Deal with anger and frustration;
- Reduce high levels of social anxiety;
- Communicate more effectively with others;
- Become more assertive;
- Avoid being pressured by peers to do things they do *not* really want to do.

Group Therapy

It has been well established for over 30 years that peer group psychotherapy for adolescents and young adults can be extremely effective. For example, Stead and Lancaster (2005), in their meta-analysis of group behavioral therapy programs for smoking cessation, found that group participants were able to:

158 Social skills training also has been demonstrated to be of potential benefit for the treatment of children with FAS/FASD (e.g., Peadon, Rhys-Jones, & Bower, 2009).

159 The "targeted" behavior among youth for these social skills, school-based programs has not been limited to reducing the use of alcohol or other drugs and substances of abuse, but also has included reducing problems with bullying and violence (e.g., Mytton, DiGuiseppi, & Gough, 2002, 2006; Vreeman & Carroll, 2007).

1. Learn behavioral techniques for smoking cessation;
2. Provide each other with mutual support.

In terms of smoking cessation, they also found that outcomes were:

1. Superior to those achieved with self-help;
2. Similar to those achieved with individual counseling.

However, not all psychotherapists are equally adept at effectively practicing group psychotherapy. Bratter (1989) observed that "those psychotherapists who can work with addicted adolescents effectively in a group setting possess a quintessential quality that the theologian, Paul Tillich, has defined as caritas, which connotes a non-compromising and non-possessive form of caring" (p. 167).[160]

For additional details and discussion of group therapy, see also the Psychotherapy/Counseling subsections: "Family Therapy;" "Social Skills Training;" "Therapeutic Communities;" and "Short-Term Residential Treatment Programs."

Therapeutic Communities (TCs)

Therapeutic communities assume that problematic, or harmful, patterns of using the drugs and substances of abuse are primarily symptomatic of psychosocial maladaptation to society, often as a result of incompetence in dealing with alienation, social privation, and stress. Reflective of the growing egalitarian, anti-establishment movements of the 1960s, TCs were developed to operate more democratically and less rigidly than were the more traditional and authoritarian mental health and psychiatric residential facilities at the time. Residents were viewed as active and equal co-participants with staff in dealing with their own, and each other's, issues regarding the use of drugs and substances of abuse (i.e., providing both self-help and mutual self-help, respectively). As noted by O'Brien and Biase (1984, p.16), the goals of TC programs are:

1. To eliminate the resident's drug-taking behavior;
2. To assist the resident to learn to respond to personal and environmental distress in a healthier manner;
3. To assist residents to readjust and return to the outside community as a functioning, independent person.

These goals are achieved by providing "24/7" therapeutic community care for adolescents and young adults, who display patterns of abusive or compulsive use of alcohol or other drugs and substances of abuse. The residential care is usually provided for three to 12 months, giving adolescents and young adults the opportunity, often mandated in the context of the juvenile criminal justice system, to live with others, who have similar problems, in a highly structured home-like environment. As such, the TC provides a setting where everyone shares in the work and responsibility of minimizing community problems. Ideally, during their residential treatment, adolescents and young adults are able to increasingly assume skills and responsibilities that are needed to successfully transfer to the larger community upon their completion of the program.

TC also requires that regular meetings be held throughout the day in "informal" settings (e.g., sitting around the kitchen table). These meetings serve to facilitate the operation of the

160 Caritas has also been variably defined as "Christian love of humankind."

TC (e.g., division of work; provision of feedback on the quality of resident work performance) and provide a format for decision making processes. A significant amount of TC therapy also occurs informally throughout the day during which residents learn to take responsibility for, and perform, required tasks while interacting with the other residents. Recreational and leisure activities also provide a means for socializing and learning to interact more positively with others.

Most TCs practice a form of egalitarianism. For example, in regard to deciding how to handle a resident, who is having difficulty "getting on the program" or dealing with setting a program policy, all residents have an equal opportunity to share input and have an equal vote with the staff members.[161] Generally, all TCs require total abstinence from the use of alcohol, cocaine, heroin, LSD, and marijuana, but may allow caffeine (i.e., coffee) and nicotine (i.e., tobacco) use.

Although TC programs have been widely used across the U.S. for the last 60-plus years, research studies demonstrating their superior efficacy over other treatment approaches are lacking. As found by Smith, Gates, and Foxcroft (2006), in their review of randomized controlled studies of the use of TC programs for the Cochrane Database:

> There is little evidence that TCs offer significant benefits in comparison with other residential treatment, or that one type of TC is better than another.
>
> (p. 1)

However, several researchers (e.g., Dye, Ducharme, & Johnson, 2009) have conversely demonstrated that some modifications to traditional TCs (e.g., outpatient TCs; short-term residential TCs) have resulted in significant reductions in efficacy outcomes.

Adolescents and young adults, who complete TC programs, have been found to show a success rate of more than 75%. However, most adolescents (i.e., approximately 75%) do not complete the entire TC treatment program. For these adolescents, outcome results indicate that the reduction of illicit drug use, involvement in crime, and unemployment corresponded to: (1) the length of time they participated in the TC (Coombs, 1981); and (2) during post-treatment, not associating with deviant peers. In an effort to increase adolescent and young adult attendance and participation in TCs, several authors (e.g., Hanson, 2002) have suggested several specific changes aimed at making TCs more responsive to the needs of adolescents and young adults. These changes include:

1. Reducing the waiting time between initial contact with the program and entry into the program;
2. Employing more staff members who are older adolescents or young adults;
3. Developing and using gender- and sociocultural-specific therapy groups;
4. Using onsite school teachers;
5. Including addressing mothering or parenting issues;

161 The primary clinical and custodial staff members, who are employed by TCs, are generally paraprofessionals, who, with the assistance of a TC program, have successfully rehabilitated themselves from previous patterns of abusive or compulsive use of alcohol and/or other drugs and substances of abuse. Ancillary staff members include professionals from various disciplines (e.g., law; medicine; psychology), who are generally used on a contractual basis (Pagliaro & Pagliaro, *Clinical Patient Data Files*). Although this staffing pattern is beginning to change with the use of more certified addictions counselors and social workers, the utilization of clinical psychologists and other university educated mental health care and social care professionals generally remains low in these programs (e.g., De Leon, Hawke, & Jainchill, 2000; Dye, Ducharme, & Johnson, 2009).

6. Incorporating childcare programs;
7. Integrating visiting family therapy.[162]

Short-Term Residential Treatment Programs

In comparison to TCs, short-term residential treatment programs (e.g., Hazelden) began to be developed during the early 1970s (Laundergan & Williams, 1993) in response to several identified issues, including the:

- Lack of adequate treatment services, particularly for adolescents and young adults, who had problems related to cocaine use;
- Desire for treatment services other than those that "institutionalize" for months;
- Limitations placed by third party insurance carriers for the reimbursement of fees paid for provided treatment services (i.e., often with a 30-day limit).

For an overview of the program objectives and elements employed by a "typical" short-term residential treatment program, see Table 1.23.

The major problem with residential treatment programs is the risk for resumed use of alcohol or other drugs and substances of abuse following discharge. Recidivism is extremely high and begins to significantly increase as soon as the adolescent is released in

Table 1.23 Short-Term Residential Treatment Program Objectives and Key Elements

PROGRAM OBJECTIVES AND KEY ELEMENTS
PROGRAM OBJECTIVES
1. Maintain "sobriety," or nonuse
2. Learn about alcohol or other dependence or use disorder and the process of recovery
3. Recognize the effects of alcohol or other dependence or use disorder on self and others (e.g., family; friends; co-workers)
4. Develop strategies to "maintain sobriety" or nonuse
5. Share thoughts and feelings with others (e.g., in group therapy sessions)
6. Utilize the basics of the AA program
PROGRAM KEY ELEMENTS
1. Personal inventory and plan
2. Daily schedule of program activities
3. Educational component
4. Group therapy sessions
5. Provision of a safe and supportive environment

Modified from: Laundergan & Williams (1993), Pagliaro & Pagliaro (2012).

162 We would add, "# 8"—Increasing the use of competent, academically prepared, health and social care professionals.

a "clean and sober" condition from supervised residential treatment. As identified by Godley, Godley, and Dennis (2014):

> Most adolescents relapse within 90 days of discharge from residential substance treatment. (p. 40)

Ethnic-Specific Treatment Programs

In the U.S., children, adolescents, and young adults of African continental descent generally have significantly lower rates of using alcohol and other drugs and substances of abuse than do those of other continental, or other, descents. As noted by O'Malley, Johnston, and Bachman (2006), schools that have predominantly students of African continental descent typically have lower rates of using the drugs and substances of abuse "at all grades" (p. 409). However, perhaps surprisingly—given the support over the last five decades by the federal government for ethnic minority programs (e.g., McBride, Terry-Elrath, & VanderWaal, 2008)—there is a paucity of data to support ethnic-specific treatment programs.

For example, Huey and Polo (2008), from their review of evidence-based psychosocial treatments for youth of African, Asian, or other continental descent in the U.S., as well as youth of Alaska Native, American Indian, and Hispanic descent, reported that "no well-established treatments were identified" (p. 262). Part of the reason for this paucity of associated published data appears to be related to the under-representation of minority youth in treatment studies concerned with patterns of adolescent use and treatment of alcohol and other drugs and substances of abuse—which, in turn, is at least partially due to the significantly higher than expected drop-out rates of youth in the U.S. of African descent who have been involved in these studies (Magruder, Bichun Ouyang, & Miller, 2009). Interventions that provided evidence for possible or probable efficacious tertiary prevention among ethnic minority youth, who used drugs and substances of abuse, all involved a central component involving family therapy. Based on self-report responses at post-treatment—directed by professional family therapists in community clinics—Multidimensional Family Therapy (MDFT) appears to be efficacious in regard to decreasing alcohol use among minority ethnic youth (Liddle, Dakof, & Parker, 2001; Liddle, Jackson-Gilfort, & Marvel, 2006). (See the related discussion in the earlier subsection, "Family Therapy.")

Bisexual-, Gay-, Lesbian-, and Trans-Oriented Treatment Programs

As noted by several researchers (e.g., Corliss, Rosario, & Wypij, 2010; Ott, Wypij, & Corliss, 2013; Rosario, Reisner, & Corliss, 2014), adolescents and young adults, who have bisexual, gay, or lesbian sexual orientations, are significantly more likely to display harmful patterns of using alcohol and other various drugs and substances of abuse than are their heterosexual peers. Consequently, research studies and findings concerning efficacious treatment approaches aimed at better meeting the needs of bisexual, gay, lesbian, and trans adolescents are urgently needed. Unfortunately, such research is not available. Until it becomes available, other treatment programs, which have demonstrated success with heterosexual adolescents, should be used with appropriate therapeutic modifications.[163]

163 In this regard, we have, when possible—and with good results, used group therapy approaches for small groups of gay or lesbian adolescents in order to focus therapy more specifically on the: (1) alcohol and other drugs and substances of abuse that are commonly used by bisexual, gay, lesbian, or trans- adolescents; and (2) life-style issues that contribute to the use of alcohol and/or other drugs and substances of abuse by bisexual, gay, lesbian, or trans adolescents. Although we do not practice family therapy—when deemed beneficial, we do make referrals to qualified family therapists who specialize in providing family therapy for bisexual, gay, lesbian, or trans-adolescents.

Alcoholics Anonymous[164]

Alcoholics Anonymous (AA) was started in 1935 in Akron, Ohio by Bill W. (a stockbroker) and Bob S. (a physician), who were its first two members. Alcoholics Anonymous has since spread across North America and now holds meetings worldwide. AA has become, particularly in North America, the most frequently used form of alcohol treatment with over one-million recovering members. According to several researchers and therapists (e.g., Room & Greenfield, 1993; Weisner, Greenfield, & Room, 1995), the popularity of AA is due in large part to its American themes of individualism, equality, and spirituality, which are embodied in the 12-steps (see later in this subsection).[165] The organizational structure of AA also supports these themes in that: there is no central authority or hierarchy, the only officer in AA groups is a secretary; and members avoid the use of last names.

The key distinguishing principles of AA include that:

1. There is no cure for alcoholism;
2. Abstinence is the only viable goal;
3. Peer support is vital to maintain recovery;
4. Recidivism, or resumed use (i.e., "slips" or "falling off the wagon"), is less important than what one does in response;
5. Progress is more important than perfection.

These principles are actualized by active participation in the 12-step program that includes:

- Avoiding the first drink;

164 Alcoholics Anonymous (AA) is considered to be the prototypical 12-step program for many other programs, including:

- Cocaine Anonymous (CA);
- Emotions Anonymous (EA);
- Gamblers Anonymous (GA);
- Men's Way through the 12-Steps;
- Narcotics Anonymous (NA);
- Overeaters Anonymous (OA);
- Sixteen Steps to Empowerment;
- Women for Sobriety;
- Women's Way through the 12-Steps.

165 The same themes that account for much of the success attributed to AA, also make it an inappropriate treatment approach for some adolescents. The spiritual characteristics of AA are reflected by the wording in the 12-Steps, and also in both the generally accepted moto, "Let Go and Let God," and the "Serenity Prayer," which is often used to conclude group meetings:

> God grant me the serenity to accept the things I cannot change, the courage to change the things I can, and the wisdom to know the difference.
>
> (Reinhold Niebuhr, 1892–1971)

Our clinical experience indicates that regardless of gender, ethnicity, or sexual orientation, most adolescents who have alcoholism and other problems related to using the drugs and substances of abuse, can generally derive significant benefit from AA as a component of their psychotherapy. However, we also have found over the last two decades that an increasing number of adolescents, who identify themselves as agnostic, generally reject AA as a component of their therapy because they generally find the tenets of AA philosophically incompatible with their own personal views of the world (i.e., lack of a strong belief in God) (Pagliaro & Pagliaro, *Clinical Patient Data Files*).

- Focusing on each day;
- Actively dealing with "slips."

Alcoholics Anonymous is regarded as neither a medical nor a psychological approach for the treatment of alcoholism (Borkman, 2008). As such, the organization maintains that alcoholism is a disease without cure and that treatment is social or spiritual (McGee, 2000).[166] Consequently, a number of slogans have been adopted and are frequently used by AA members, including:

- Be part of the solution, not the problem;
- But for the grace of God;
- Don't quit before the miracle happens;
- Easy does it;
- Faith without works is dead;
- Feelings are not facts;
- First things first;
- I am an alcoholic;
- Keep it simple, stupid;
- Let go and let God;
- Nothing changes, if nothing changes;
- One day at a time;
- Progress, not perfection;
- Sick and tired of being sick and tired;
- Sobriety is a journey . . . not a destination;
- When all else fails, follow instructions.

As identified by Valliant (2005):

> The suggested mechanism of action of AA is that it employs four factors widely shown to be effective in relapse prevention in addictions: (1) external supervision; (2) substitute dependency; (3) new caring relationships; and (4) increased spirituality.
>
> (p. 431)

Alcoholics Anonymous relies on a rather informal form of "group" therapy and social support (i.e., frequent meetings with other fellow recovering members who attempt total abstinence from alcohol use) and a "buddy" system (i.e., the use of sponsors who have remained sober for a period of time by "working" the 12-steps and who can, thus, show "newcomers" the way to sobriety) as guided by the following 12-steps:

1. We admitted we were powerless over alcohol—that our lives had become unmanageable;
2. Came to believe that a Power greater than ourselves could restore us to sanity;
3. Made a decision to turn our will and our lives over to the care of our God as we understood Him;
4. Made a searching and fearless moral inventory of ourselves;
5. Admitted to God, to ourselves, and to another human being the exact nature of our wrongs;
6. Were entirely ready to have God remove all these defects of character;
7. Humbly asked Him to remove our shortcomings;
8. Made a list of all person we had harmed, and became willing to make amends to them all;

166 For this reason, AA has often been labeled as a "social" form of treatment.

9. Made direct amends to such people wherever possible, except when to do so would injure them or others;
10. Continued to take personal inventory and when we were wrong promptly admitted it;
11. Sought through prayer and meditation to improve our conscious contact with God, as we understood Him, praying only for knowledge of His will for us and the power to carry that out;
12. Having had a spiritual awakening as the result of these steps, we tried to carry this message to alcoholics, and to practice these principles in all our affairs.

(AA, 1939)

As part of the "group therapy," members hear from other members that they are not alone and that they share common, painful experiences in relation to their alcohol use. In addition, in conjunction with Step 1, members learn to overcome their strong denial of their own drinking problem. The confrontation of denial is both clearly and directly reflected in the members' introductions of themselves at AA group meetings, "Hello, my name is ____ and I'm an alcoholic."

"Denial," which is typically characterized by such statements as, "I don't have a drinking (or other drug or substance of abuse) problem," or "I can stop drinking (or using another drug or substance of abuse) whenever I want to," is a hallmark of the development of compulsive use of alcohol (or other drugs or substances of abuse). Compulsive use of alcohol (or other drugs or substances of abuse), which follows the earlier patterns of habitual and abusive use: (1) prevents early therapeutic intervention; (2) after achieving "resumed nonuse," contributes to "relapsed use;" and (3) encourages the progressive development of increasingly undesired, or harmful, effects and toxicities (see Figure 1.5). (Also see, respectively, the section in each chapter, "Undesired, or Harmful, Effects and Toxicities.")

Consequently, to optimize assessment and subsequent treatment approaches, a major primary goal is to breakdown the defensive wall of denial. Commonly identified as simply a "weakness in character," traditionally, denial was also largely viewed psychoanalytically as a means to protect the ego. More recently, denial is considered to be a psychological construct that can best be dealt with by using other psychological approaches (e.g., CBT).

<u>Related Professional Reminder</u>: Regardless of selected therapeutic intervention, denial, as a prominent characteristic feature of harmful patterns of alcohol, as well as other drug and substance abuse behavior, must be effectively addressed for all adolescents and young adults.

> Kristin, now 17, started using meth when she was 15: Her mother had asked her if she was doing meth but, until she was in rehab, Kristin never admitted it.
>
> (Irvine, 2005, p. 1)

Nowinski, Baker, and Carroll (1992/1999, pp. 39–40) identified several common forms of "denial:"

- Refusing to face facts: refusing to do a serious alcohol history, refusing to acknowledge negative consequences of use, rejecting clear evidence of tolerance, refusing to go to AA meetings;
- Minimizing the facts: Understating negative consequences, tolerance, and so forth;
- Avoiding: Sleeping a lot, becoming socially isolated, or becoming compulsive (addictive) in some other way, such as work or eating;
- Exaggerating others' use in an effort to "normalize" one's own use;
- Blaming someone/something else for alcohol use (a "bad" marriage; family conflicts; feeling depressed) as opposed to accepting the fact that cravings for alcohol are responsible for use;

- Bargaining: Trying to limit or control either the amount or type of alcohol used or when it is used;
- Rationalizing: Making up "good" reasons (usually ones that will get sympathy) for drinking.

Members are encouraged to "work through" and "practice" the 12-steps on a daily basis. This encouragement is particularly important given that, the AA model is based on the premise that there is no cure for alcoholism[167] and that the maintenance of lifelong abstinence is achieved by continued membership in the "fellowship" (i.e., AA) with regular attendance at meetings.

<u>Related Professional Reminder</u>: In the context of the philosophical underpinnings of AA, it is important for both health and social care professionals and members to keep in mind that while alcoholics are* not *responsible for their illness, they* are *responsible for their recovery.

The number of AA meetings that an active member attends generally ranges from one daily to one weekly. The number of meetings attended on a regular basis is dictated, in large part, by such factors as the:

- Amount of time that a member has been sober (e.g., one day versus one year);
- Personality of the member (e.g., avoidant, dependent, or compulsive);
- Accessibility of scheduled meetings for a member (e.g., meetings are nearby or transportation, both to and from meetings, is readily available);
- Style of the meeting is compatible with the member's needs.

For many alcoholics, AA provides both the social support necessary to maintain abstinence and an effective surrogate for their previously patterned "drinking time" or "familiar bar scene" (i.e., AA meetings serve as a place to go on evenings, weekends, and holidays for socializing with "friends" who, in addition to other benefits, provide understanding and help to alleviate social isolation and loneliness).[168]

The overall effectiveness of AA is difficult to ascertain because:

- AA does not maintain formal records;
- Very few scientific studies have been conducted to formally measure the efficacy of AA;
- Available data are primarily observational;
- There is a lack of sufficient theory to explain the inherent mechanisms of AA;
- Research is not an AA mandate;
- The amount of time that members remain active in AA is extremely variable;
- Drop-out rates are high.

167 This AA belief would be consonant with what we describe as "compulsive use" (see Figure 1.5). In this regard, we would concur with the AA philosophy that, once compulsive use has been achieved, treatment, in order to have optimal opportunity for success, must include a lifetime of "total" abstinence.

168 In some cases, however, an individual member will develop a "cult-like" relationship with AA (i.e., will become obsessive and compulsive regarding AA doctrine; will limit social interaction to AA meetings and members; will increasingly become estranged from other social groups such as family and colleagues) (Pagliaro & Pagliaro, *Clinical Patient Data Files*). These situations, although relatively infrequently encountered, should be appropriately monitored for and dealt with as part of the patient's program of psychotherapy.

Obviously, the approach used by AA will *not* be suitable for all adolescents or young adults and we would not recommend it as the sole approach to therapy. However, for patients who are willing to attend the AA meetings, we have found AA to be an effective and useful adjunct to individual psychotherapy—as have others (e.g., Ferri, Amato, & Davoli, 2006; Hoeppner, Hoeppner, & Kelly, 2014; Kelly, Dow, & Yeterian, 2010; Sussman, 2010)—and can highly recommend it in this context.,[169, 170] In addition, the efficacy of AA programs appears to be substantiated de facto by the: (1) large number of members who speak positively about it; and (2) use of the AA approach by groups that have been based on, or extended from, it (e.g., Cocaine Anonymous [CA], Crystal Meth Anonymous [CMA], Gamblers Anonymous [GA], and Narcotics Anonymous (NA]). It also has been extended to other 12-Step self-help groups for families who have parents or members, respectively, who have harmful patterns of using drugs and substances of abuse (e.g., Al-ATEEN; Al-ANON; Families of Alcoholics [FA]) (Laudet, 2008). (See also the related discussion in the following section, "12-Step Facilitation.") In addition, AA has generally been rated highly by health and social care professionals.

12-Step Facilitation

12-step facilitation, as opposed to AA (or the "12-Steps"), is a specific method of therapeutic intervention for adolescent and young adults, who have contemporaneous diagnoses involving alcohol and other dependence or use disorder, and/or other related mental disorder(s) (e.g., eating disorders). Also referred to as "Twelve Step Facilitation" (TSF), these programs are generally: (1) brief in duration (i.e., 12 to 15 sessions); (2) structured; and (3) manual-driven or guided. As explained by Nowinski, Baker, and Carroll (1992/1999, pp. 1–4), it is a process guided by a written manual and delivered by a drug counselor or therapist. Usually, 12 sessions are used to accomplish three major goals:

1. To facilitate acceptance—acceptance by patients that they suffer from the chronic and progressive illness of alcoholism, that they have lost the ability to control their drinking, and since there is no effective cure for alcoholism, the only viable alternative is complete abstinence from the use of alcohol;
2. To facilitate surrender—acknowledgment on the part of the patient that there is hope for recovery (sustained sobriety) but only through accepting the reality of loss of control and by having faith that some Higher Power can help the individual whose own willpower has been defeated by alcoholism. Acknowledgment by the patient that the fellowship of AA has helped millions of alcoholics to sustain their sobriety and that the patient's best chances for success are to follow the AA path;

169 Although adolescents and young adults have been reported to attend adolescent AA meetings, mixed adolescent-young adult meetings, and primarily adult AA meetings (Kelly, Myers, & Brown, 2002), we recommend that adolescent boys and girls *only* attend AA meetings that are comprised of other adolescent members (e.g., those AA programs that meet in youth correctional treatment centers). Due to their age and the possible psychopathology related to their use of alcohol and/or other drugs and substances of abuse (e.g., active contemporaneous diagnoses), adolescents comprise a population group that is particularly "vulnerable." Thus, attention to this consideration is required when identifying and selecting appropriate AA groups for adolescents (as has been noted in the same context for young adults [Labbe, Greene, & Bergman, 2013]). In addition, consideration should be given to gender-specific (e.g., all female; all male) and sexual orientation-specific (e.g., lesbian) groups.

170 As with most forms of psychotherapy or counseling, the efficacy of AA for adolescents is highly correlated with the frequency (Kelly, Dow, & Yeterian, 2010; Kelly, Myers, & Brown, 2002) and duration of their attendance at meetings (Chi, Kaskutas, & Sterling, 2009).

3. To facilitate active involvement or participation in 12-step meetings and related activities—maintenance of a personal journal that is reviewed with the therapist[171] at the beginning of each session; attendance at AA (or other 12-step) meetings; and bibliotherapy usually involving readings from the "AA Service Manual" or "Big Book."

As identified by Nowinski, Baker, and Carroll (1992/1999) in the introduction to the original "AA Service Manual" that they prepared on behalf of the National Institute on Alcohol Abuse and Alcoholism (NIAAA):

> The [12-Step] facilitation program described in this manual is intended for use in brief individual outpatient treatment for persons who satisfy the criteria for a diagnosis of alcohol dependence and abuse.
>
> (p. 1)

Relapse Prevention

The rate of relapsed use, or recidivism, following the "successful" treatment of alcohol or other dependence use disorder(s) among children, adolescents, and young adults is quite high (see Figure 1.11). Although much research has examined treatment factors (e.g., family involvement in treatment; provision of special services; staff characteristics; and time in treatment), these factors have not been able to account for the majority of variance in post-treatment return to harmful patterns of alcohol and other drug and substance use. Obviously, much more research is required in this area.

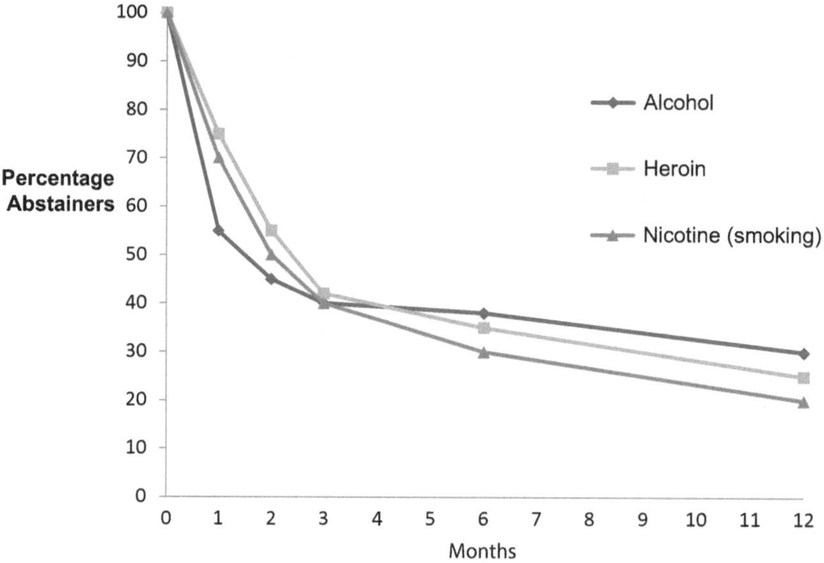

Figure 1.11 Typical Relapse Rates

171 N.B. In the context of 12-step facilitation, the major agent of change (i.e., the active therapeutic modality) is the fellowship of AA and not the individual therapist, who is seen more as a facilitator or coach.

Factors that have been implicated as contributory to relapse include:

- Cognitive factors ("stinking-thinking");
- Increased desire for alcohol or other drugs and substances of abuse ("craving");
- Interpersonal problems;
- Lack of, or poor, coping abilities;
- Negative affective states.

(McKay 1999, p. 566)

In addition, it has been noted that a complicated and dynamic interplay of "proximal" and "distal" factors plays a major role in the relapse process (e.g., Feingold, Capaldi, & Owen, 2015; McKay, Franklin, & Patapis, 2006). Examples of "proximal factors," include current drinking behavior, and social influences. Examples of "distal factors," include genetic predisposition, and inappropriate parenting (Pagliaro & Pagliaro, *Clinical Patient Data Files*).

Our own clinical experience and the currently available published research data suggest that the use of the following three recommendations would, at least, minimize the potential for the relapsed use of alcohol, or other drugs and substances of abuse:

1. Individualize treatment to the specific needs and characteristics of the child, adolescent, or young adult (i.e., "cut the shoe to fit the foot").[172]
2. Employ specific indicators or performance goals to objectively evaluate the success of treatment outcomes and, subsequently, the degree of relapse or efficacy of relapse prevention.
3. Periodically, as individually indicated, prophylactically re-assess children, adolescents, and young adults and proactively intervene to prevent the occurrence of relapsed use.

Some of this periodic monitoring is addressed, for example, in "aftercare" programs and in continued attendance at AA meetings, which have both been positively correlated with significantly higher rates and duration of post-treatment abstinence, or "resumed nonuse" (Chi, Kaskutas, & Sterling, 2009; Pagliaro & Pagliaro, *Clinical Patient Data Files*). We would suggest, particularly for children and adolescents, who have engaged in abusive or compulsive use of alcohol or other drugs or substances of abuse, that the propensity for relapsed use and, thus, the return to compulsive use, be considered a "life-long" concern (i.e., we do not subscribe to, nor do we endorse, the often noted belief among many addiction counselors, health, social, and other care professionals, parents, and therapists that the harmful use of drugs and substances of abuse—at the compulsive level of use—is "just a phase" or something that the adolescent or young adult "addict" will simply "grow out of" [i.e., "mature out of"]).

Whenever possible, once children, adolescents, and young adults are abstinent, we gradually decrease the frequency and length of their psychotherapy sessions (e.g., from biweekly, to weekly, to every other week, to monthly, to every other month, to phone contact every six months). This strategy helps to maintain a communication link and "help-line" or "safety line," for each patient. This strategy also demonstrates continued concern and support, while providing an opportunity for the early detection of problems by the health or social care

172 The use of "patient-treatment matching" has been known and used for almost three decades (e.g., Kaminer & Francis, 1991; Mattson & Allen, 1991; Mattson, Allen, & Longabaugh, 1994; Project MATCH, 1993). However, usually due to economic and/or time constraints, patient-treatment matching now remains the "exception to the rule."

professional and for patients to request needed assistance before problems get "out of control." In our practice, this strategy (i.e., if we can maintain patient contact), has resulted in a long-term (i.e., generally longer than five years) relapse rate of less than 20% (Pagliaro & Pagliaro, *Clinical Patient Data Files*).

As succinctly concluded by Godley, Godley, & Dennis (2014):

> Providing continuing care following addiction treatment can improve clinical outcomes. (p. 40)

<u>Related Professional Reminder</u>:

- ***Be willing to consider available and appropriate treatment approaches and strategies (e.g., AA; cognitive therapy; pharmacotherapy) that may be efficacious for a particular child, adolescent, or young adult.***
- ***Individualize treatment approaches.***
- ***Remember that reasons for using drugs and substances of abuse may differ from one child, adolescent, or young adult to another child, adolescent, or young adult and may also differ for the same child, adolescent, or young adult over time.***
- ***Be nonjudgmental in approaching treatment.***
- ***Break the denial of problems associated with the use of the drugs and substances of abuse.***
- ***Respect children, adolescents, and young adults, who have problems with drugs and substances of abuse, including those with contemporaneous diagnoses (i.e., AUD and/ or SUDS and/or OMDs; do not treat them in a condescending manner.***
- ***Provide education in a straightforward, nonbiased manner that is appropriately tailored to the child, adolescent, or young adult and his or her cognitive abilities, developmental level, and learning and social needs.***
- ***Work toward realistic and achievable goals that have been mutually agreed upon.***
- ***Appropriately address underlying problems (e.g., low self-esteem; poor coping skills; history of sexual assault).***
- ***Involve family, friends, and others, as appropriate, in confrontation, treatment planning, and program implementation.***
- ***Group children, adolescents, and young adults according to their specific age; continental or other descent; culture or ethnicity; gender; primary language; socioeconomic level; sexual orientation; or other specific grouping as deemed appropriate and beneficial for the child, adolescent or young adult and his or her optimal treatment and recovery.***
- ***Use community social agencies designed for children, adolescents, and young adults, as appropriate.***
- ***Provide appropriate childcare services for adolescent and young adult parents in treatment.***
- ***Assure that pregnant adolescent girls and young women have access to, or are provided with referral services, as appropriate, for birthing and mothering programs and classes.***
- ***Make referrals to other appropriate health and social care professionals and agencies.***
- ***Develop and use procedures and techniques that help to: (1) minimize treatment attrition, or drop-out; and (2) maximize treatment compliance and completion of treatment programs.***
- ***Anticipate, and provide, effective cognitive rehearsal strategies for high-risk situations that may be associated with relapse.***
- ***Provide appropriate follow-up, or aftercare, services.***
- ***Remember that success or failure is ultimately the child's, adolescent's, and young adult's responsibility (i.e., do not become co-dependent or over-responsible).***

- ***If for any reason, and at any time, you feel that you cannot provide optimal treatment for a specific child, adolescent, or young adult, then discuss your concerns with the child, adolescent, or young adult (and their parent(s) or legal guardian, as necessary and appropriate) and, following this discussion, and with their concurrence and permission:***
  - ***make an appropriate referral to another therapist/program that you feel would be better able to provide optimal treatment;***
  - ***ensure that contact is made, and that the child, adolescent, or young adult is accepted by the therapist/program that you referred him or her to;***
  - ***provide "bridge" treatment/support services until the child, adolescent, or young adult begins his/her new program.***

References

AA, Alcoholics Anonymous. (1939). *Alcoholics Anonymous* (1st ed.). New York: Works Publishing Company.

Aalto, M., Alho, H., & Halme, J. T. (2009). AUDIT and its abbreviated versions in detecting heavy and binge drinking in a general population survey. *Drug and Alcohol Dependence, 103*(1–2), 25–29.

Abbey, A. (1991). Acquaintance rape and alcohol consumption on college campuses: How are they linked? *Journal of American College Health, 39*(4), 165–169.

Abbey, A., Buck, P. O., & Zawacki, T. (2003). Alcohol's effects on perceptions of a potential date rape. *Journal of Studies on Alcohol, 64*(5), 669–677.

ACOG, American College of Obstetricians and Gynecologists. (2011). Committee on Health Care for Underserved Women. Committee opinion no. 496: At-risk drinking and alcohol dependence: Obstetric and gynecologic implications. *Obstetrics and Gynecology, 118*, 383–388.

ACOG, American College of Obstetricians and Gynecologists. (2015, June). Alcohol abuse and other substance use disorders: Ethical issues in obstetric and gynecologic practice. *Committee Opinion Number 633*. American College of Obstetricians and Gynecologists.

Addolorato, G., Ancona, C., & Capristo, E. (2003, September–December). Metadoxine in the treatment of acute and chronic alcoholism: A review. *International Journal of Immunopathology and Pharmacology, 16*(3), 207–214.

Adewuya, A. O. (2005, November–December). Validation of the alcohol use disorders itentification test (audit) as a screening tool for alcohol-related problems among Nigerian university students. *Alcohol and Alcoholism, 40*(6), 575–577. doi:10.1093/alcalc/agh197

Aertgeerts, B., Buntinx, F., & Ansoms, S. (2001). Screening properties of questionnaires and laboratory tests for the detection of alcohol abuse or dependence in general practice population. *British Journal of General Practice, 51*, 206–217.

Aertgeerts, B., Buntinx, F., & Bande-Knops, J. (2000). The value of CAGE, CUGE, and AUDIT in screening for alcohol abuse. *Alcoholism: Clinical and Experimental Research, 24*(1), 53–57.

Aertgeerts, B., Buntinx, F., & Fevery, J. (2000). Is there a difference between CAGE interviews and written CAGE questionnaires? *Alcoholism: Clinical and Experimental Research, 24*(5), 733–736.

Aertgeerts, B., Buntinx, F., & Kester, A. (2004). The value of the CAGE in screening for alcohol abuse and alcohol dependence in general clinical populations: A diagnostic meta-analysis. *Journal of Clinical Epidemiology, 57*(1), 30–39. doi:10.1016/S0895-4356(03)00254-3

Afifi, T. O., Henriksen, C. A., & Asmundson, G. J. (2012). Victimization and perpetration of intimate partner violence and substance use disorders in a nationally representative sample. *Journal of Nervous and Mental Disease, 200*(8), 684–691. doi:10.1097/NMD.0b013e3182613f64

Agrawal, A., Tillman, R., & Grucza, R. A. (2017, April 15). Reciprocal relationships between substance use and disorders and suicidal ideation and suicide atempts in the Collaborative Study of the Genetics of Alcoholism. *Journal of Affective Disorders, 213*, 96–104. doi:10.1016/j.jad.2016.12.060.

Ahrnsbrak, R., Bose, J., & Hedden, S. L. (2017, September). *Key Substance Use and Mental Health Indicators in the United States: Results from the 2016 National Survey on Drug Use and Health. SAMHSA*. Rockville, MD: Center for Behavioral Health Statistics and Quality.

al-Ansari, E. A., & Negrete, J. C. (1990). Screening for alcoholism among alcohol users in a traditional Arab Muslim society. *Acta Psychiatrica Scandinavica, 81*(3), 284–288.

Alcohol Use USA. (2010, January 6). *Alcohol Use USA*. Retrieved from Alcohol and Drug Guide: www.alcohol-and-drug-guide.com/alcohol-use-usa.html

Alexander, T., DiNitto, D. M., & Tidblom, I. (2005). Screening for alcohol and other drug use problems among the deaf. *Alcoholism Treatment Quarterly, 23*(1), 63–78.

Allampati, S., & Mullen, K. D. (2016, August). Long-term management of alcoholic liver disease. *Clinical Liver Disease, 20*(3), 551–562. doi:10.1016/j.cid.2016.02.011.

Anderson, L. J., Flynn, A., & Pilgrim, J. L. (2017, April). A global epidemiological perspective on the toxicology of drug-facilitated sexual assault: A systematic review. *Journal of Forensic and Legal Medicine, 47*, 46–54. doi:10.1016/j.jflm.2017.02.005.

AP, Associated Press. (2018, January 17). Science panel recommends lowering blood-alcohol threshold for drunken driving. *U.S. World & News Report*, 1–7. Washington, DC. Retrieved from http:///ww.syracuse.com/us-news/index.ssf/2018/01/science_panel_recommends_lowingh_blood-alcohol_threshold_for_drunken_driving.html

APA, American Psychiatric Association. (2000). *Diagnostic and Statistical Manual of Mental Disorders* (4th ed., TR). Arlington, VA: American Psychiatric Association.

APA, American Psychiatric Association. (2013). *Diagnostic and Statistical Manual of Mental Disorders* (5th ed.). Arlington, VA: American Psychiatric Association.

Arbaizar, B., Diersen-Sotos, T., & Gomez-Acebo, I. (2010). Topiramate in the treatment of alcohol dependence: A meta-analysis. *Actas Espanolas De Psiquiatria, 38*(1), 8–12.

Arias, A. J., Gelernter, J., & Chan, G. (2008). Correlates of co-occurring ADHD in drug-dependent subjects: Prevalence and features of substance dependence and psychiatric disorders. *Addictive Behaviors, 33*(9), 199–1207. doi:10.1016/j.addbeh.20078.05.003

Armstrong, T. D., & Costello, E. J. (2002, December). Community studies on adolescent substance use, abuse, or dependence and psychiatric comorbidity. *Journal of Consulting and Clinical Psychology, 70*(6), 1224–1239.

ASAM, American Society of Addiction Medicine. (1997). Screening for addiction in primary care settings. *Public Policy Statement.* Chevy Chase, MD: American Society of Addiction Medicine.

ASAM, American Society of Addiction Medicine. (2005). Public Policy Statement. *Screening for Addiction in Primary Care Settings.* Chevy Chase, MD: American Society of Addiction Medicine. Retrieved July 1, 2018.

Aspy, C. B., Mold, J. W., & Thompson, D. M. (2008). Integrating screening and interventions for unhealthy behaviors into primary care practices. *American Journal of Preventive Medicine, 53*(Supplement 5), S373–S380.

Atassi, W. A., Noghnogh, A. A., & Hariman, R. (1999). Hemodialysis as a treatment of severe ethanol poisoning. *The International Journal of Artificial Organs, 22*(1), 18–20.

Avalos, L. A., Roberts, S. C., & Kaskutas, L. A. (2014). Volume and type of alcohol during early pregnancy and the risk of miscarriage. *Substance Use & Misuse, 49*(11), 1437–1445. doi:10.3109/10826084

Azorin, J. M., Bowden, C. L., & Garay, R. P. (2010). Possible new ways in the pharmacological treatment of bipolar disorder and comorbid alcoholism. *Neuropsychiatric Disease and Treatment, 6*, 37–46.

Babor, T. F., Higgins-Biddle, J. C., & Saunders, J. B. (2001). *AUDIT: The Alcohol Use Disorders Identification Test: Guidelines for Use in Primary Care* (2nded.). Geneva, Switzerland: World Health Organization (WHO).

Babor, T. F., McRee, B. G., & Kassebaum, P. A. (2007). Screeing, brief intervention, and referral to treatment (SBIRT): Toward a public health approach to the management of substance abuse. *Substance Abuse, 28*(3), 7–30. doi:10.1300/J465v28n03_03

Bada, H. S., Das, A., & Bauer, C. R. (2007). Impact of prenatal cocaine exposure on child behavior problems through school age. *Pediatrics, 119*, e348–e359.

Bailey, R. K., Patel, T. C., & Avenido, J. (2011). Suicide: Current trends. *Journal of the National Medical Association, 103* (7), 614–617.

Baraona, E., Abittan, C. S., & Dohmen, K. (2001). Gender differences in pharmacokinetics of alcohol. *Alcoholism: Clinical and Experimental Research, 25*(4), 502–507.

Barkla, X. M., McArdle, P. A., & Newbury-Birch, D. (2015, October 30). Are there any potentially dangerous pharmacological effects of combining ADHD medication with alcohol and drugs of abuse? A systematic review of the literature. *BMC Psychiatry, 125*, 270. doi:10.1186/sd12888-015-0657-9.

Barlow, A., Tingey, L., & Cwik, M. (2012). Understanding the relationship between substance use and self-injury in American Indian youth. *The Journal of Drug and Alcohol Abuse, 38*(5), 403–408. doi:10.3109/00952990.2012.696757

Barry, K. L., & Fleming, M. F. (1993). The Alcohol Use Disorders Identification Test (AUDIT) and the SMAST-13: Predictive validity in a rural primary care sample. *Alcohol and Alcoholism, 28*(1), 33–42.

Bastiaens, L., Francis, G., & Lewis, K. (2000). The RAFFT as a screening tool for adolescent substance use disorders. *The American Journal on Addictions, 9*(1), 10–16.

Bastiaens, L., Riccardi, K., & Sakhrani, D. (2002). The RAFFT as a screening tool for adult substance use disorders. *American Journal of Drug and Alcohol Abuse, 28*(4), 681–691.

Bayard, M., McIntyre, J., & Hill, K. R. (2004, March 15). Alcohol withdrawal syndrome. *American Family Physician, 69* (5), 1443–1450.

Beaton, A., Shubkin, C. D., & Chapman, S. (2016, April). Addressing substance misuse in adolescents: A review of the literature on the screening, brief intervention, and referral to treatment model. *Current Opinion in Pediatrics, 28* (2), 258–265. doi:10.1097/MOP.0000000000000333.

Beck, A. T. (1961). A systematic investigation of depression. *Comprehensive Psychiatry, 2*, 163–170.

Beck, A. T. (1967). *Depression: Clinical, Experimental and Theoretical Aspects.* New York: Harper & Row.

Belfer, M. L. (1993). Substance abuse with psychiatric illness in children and adolescents: Definitions and terminology. *American Journal of Orthopsychiatry, 63*(1), 70–79.

Bennett, M. E., Walters, S. T., & Miller, J. H. (2000). Relationship of early inhalant use to substance use in college students. *Journal of Substance Abuse, 12*(3), 227–240.

Bertrand, J. (2009). Interventions for children with fetal alcohol spectrum disorders (FASDs): Overview of findings for five innovative research projects. *Research in Developmental Disabilities, 30*(5), 986–1006.

Bianchi, V., Ivaldi, A., & Raspagni, A. (2010). Use of carbohydrate-deficient transferrin (CDT) and a combination of GGT and CDT (GGT-CDT) to assess heavy alcohol consumption in traffic medicine. *Alcohol and Alcoholism, 45* (3), 247–251.

Bickel, W. K., Moody, L., & Mueller, E. T. (2013). Executive dysfunction among alcohol- and cocaine-dependent women. *American Psychological Association 2013 Convention Presentation.*

Bigelow, G. E., & Silverman, K. (1999). Theoretical and empirical foundations of contingency management treatments for drug abuse. In S. T. Higgins & K. Silverman, *Motivating Change among Illicit-drug Abusers: Research on Contingency Management Interventions* (pp. 125–131). Washington, DC: American Psychological Association.

Bohn, M. J., Babor, T. F., & Kranzler, H. R. (1995). The Alcohol Use Disorders Identification Test (AUDIT): A screening instrument for use in medical settings. *Journal of Studies on Alcohol, 56*(4), 423–432.

Bone, C., Gelberg, L., & Vahidi, M. (2016). Under-reporting of risky drug use among primary care patients in federally qualified health centers. *Journal of Addiction Medicine, 10*(6), 387–394. doi:10.1097/ADM.0000000000000246

Boothby, L. A., & Doering, P. L. (2005). Acamprosate for the treatment of alcohol dependence. *Clinical Therapeutics, 27* (6), 695–714.

Borges, A., & Cherpitel, C. J. (2001). Selection of screening items for alcohol abuse and alcohol dependence among Mexicans and Mexican Americans in the emergency department. *Journal of Studies on Alcohol, 62*, 277–285.

Borkman, T. (2008). The twelve-step recovery model of AA: A voluntary mutual help association. *Recent Developments in Alcoholism, 18*, 9–35.

Borsari, B. (2004). Drinking games in the college environment: A review. *Journal of Alcohol & Drug Education, 48*(2), 29–51.

Borsari, B., Bergen-Cico, D., & Carey, K. B. (2003). Self-reported drinking-game participation of incoming college students. *Journal of American College Health, 51*(4), 149–154.

Bosron, W. F., & Li, T. (1986, May-June). Genetic polymorphism of human liver alcohol and aldehyde dehydrogenases, and their relationship to alcohol metabolism and alcoholism. *Hepatology*. doi: 10.1002/hep.1840060330.

Bouton, M. E. (2014, November). Why behavior change is difficult to sustain. *Preventive Medicine*, 29–36. doi:10.1016/j.ypmed.2014.06.010.

Bracken, B. K., Rodolico, J., & Hill, K. P. (2013). Sex, age, and progression of drug use in adolescents admitted for substance use disorder treatment in the northeastern United States: Comparison with a national survey. *Substance Abuse, 34*(3), 263–272. doi:10.1080/08897077.2013.770424

Bradley, K. A., Boyd-Wickizer, J., & Powell, S. H. (1998). Alcohol screening questionnaires in women: A critical review. *JAMA: the Journal of the American Medical Association, 280*(2), 166–171.

Bradley, K. A., Bush, K. R., & McDonell, M. B. (1998). Screening for problem drinking: Comparison of CAGE and AUDIT. *Journal of General Internal Medicine, 13*(6), 379–389.

Bradley, K. A., DeBenedetti, A. F., & Volk, R. J. (2007). AUDIT-C as a brief screen for alcohol misuse in primary care. *Alcoholism: Clinical and Experimental Research, 31*(7), 1208–1217. doi:10.111/j.1530-0277.2007.00403.x

Bradley, K. A., McDonell, M. B., & Bush, K. (1998). The AUDIT alcohol consumption questions: Reliability, validity, and responsiveness to change in older male primary care patients. *Alcoholism: Clinical and Experimental Research, 22* (8), 1842–1849.

Brady, J. E., & Guohua, L. (2013). Prevalence of alcohol and other drugs in fatally injured drivers. *Addiction, 108*(1), 104–114. doi:10.1111/j.1360-0443.2012.03993.x

Bratter, T. E. (1989). Group psychotherapy with alcohol and drug addicted adolescents: Special clinical concerns and challenges. In F. J. Azina & L. H. Richmond, *Adolescent Group Psychotherapy* (pp. 163–189). Madison, CT: International Universities.

Briere, F. N., Rohde, P., & Seeley, J. R. (2014). Comorbidity between major depression and alcohol use disorder from adolescence to adulthood. *Comprehensive Psychiatry, 55*(3), 526–533. doi:10.1016/j.comppsych.2013.10.007

Brotherton, A. L., Hamilton, E. P., & Kloss, H. G. (2016). Propofol for treatment of refractory alcohol withdrawal syndrome: A review of the literature. *Pharmacotherapy, 36*(4), 433–442. doi:10.1002/phar.1726

Brower, K. J. (2001). Alcohol's effects on sleep in alcoholics. *Alcohol Research & Health, 25*(2), 110–125.

Brown, R. L., & Rounds, L. A. (1995). Conjoint screening questionnaires for alcohol and other drug abuse: Criterion validity in a primary care practice. *Wisconsin Medical Journal, 94*, 135–140.

Brown, S. A., & Tapert, S. F. (2004). Health consequences of adolescent alcohol involvement. In R. J. Bonnie & M. E. O'Connell (Eds.), *Reducing Underage Drinking: A Collective Responsibility.* (pp. 383–401) Washington D.C.: National Academies Press.

Buchsbaum, D., Buchanan, R., & Centor, R. (1991). Screening for alcohol abuse using CAGE scores and likelihood ratios. *Annals of Internal Medicine, 15*, 774–777.

Bukstein, O. (2008, August). Substance use disorders in adolescents with attention-deficit/hyperactivity disorder. *Adolescent Medicine: State of the Art Reviews, 19*(2), 242–253.

Bukstein, O. G., & Van Hasselt, V. B. (1993). Alcohol and drug abuse. In A. S. Bellack & M. Hersen, *Handbook of Behavior Therapy in the Psychiatric Setting* (pp. 453–475). New York: Springer Science. doi:10.1007/978-1-4899-2430-8.

Burd, L., Carlson, C., & Kerbeshian, J. (2007). Fetal alcohol spectrum disorders and mental illness. *International Journal on Disability and Human Development, 6*(4), 383–396. doi:10.1515/IJDHD.2007.6.4.383

Burke, J. D., Loeber, R., & Lahey, B. B. (2001, May). Which aspects of ADHD are associated with tobacco use in early adolescence? *The Journal of Child Psychology and Psychiatry, 42*(4), 493–502.

Burns, E., Gray, R., & Smith, L. A. (2010). Brief screening questionnaires to identify problem drinking during pregnancy: A systematic review. *Addiction, 105*(4), 601–614. doi:10.111/j.1360-0443.2009.02842.x

Bush, K. R., Kivlahan, D. R., & Davis, T. M. (2003). The TWEAK is weak for alcohol screening among female Veterans Affairs outpatients. *Alcoholism: Clinical and Experimental Research, 27*(12), 1971–1978. doi:10.1097/01.ALC.0000099262,50094.98

Bush, K. R., Kivlahan, D. R., & McDonell, M. B. (1998). The AUDIT acohol consumption questions (AUDIT-C): An effective brief screening test for problem drinking. Ambulatory Care Quality Improvement Project (ACQUIP). Alcohol Use Disorders Identification Test. *Archives of Internal Medicine, 158*(16), 1789–1795.

Butchart, A., Poznyak, V., & Bellis, M. (2006). Child maltreatment and alcohol. *WHO Facts On.*, 1–11. Geneva, Switzerland: World Health Organization. Retrieved October 10, 2016, from www.who.int/violence_injury_prevention/publications/violence/en/index/html

Button, T. M., Rhee, S. H., & Hewitt, J. K. (2007, February 23). The role of conduct disorder in explaining the comorbidity between alcohol and illicit drug dependence in adolescence. *Drug and Alcohol Dependence, 87*(1), 46–53. doi:10.1016/j.drugalcodep.2006.07.012.

Campbell, D. T., & Fiske, D. W. (1959). Convergent and discriminant validation by the multitrait-multimethod matrix. *Psychological Bulletin, 56*(2), 81–105.

Carrington Reid, M., Fiellin, D. A., & O'Connor, P. G. (1999). Hazardous and harmful alcohol consumption in primary care. *Archives of Internal Medicine, 159*(15), 1681–1689.

Carroll, K. M. (2014, October). Lost in translation? Moving contingency management and cognitive behavioral therapy into clinical practice. *Annals of the New York Academy of Sciences, 1327*(1), 94–111. doi:10.1111/nyas.12501.

Caruso, K., & Ten Bensel, R. (1993). Fetal alcohol syndrome and fetal alcohol effects. The University of Minnesota experience. *Minnesota Medicine, 76*(4), 25–29.

Cassidy, C. M., Schmitz, N., & Malla, A. (2008). Validation of the alcohol use disorders identification test and the drug abuse screening test in first episode psychosis. *Canadian Journal of Psychiatry, 53*(1), 26–33.

Caviness, C. M., Hatgis, C., & Anderson, B. J. (2009). Three brief alcohol screens for detecting hazardous drinking in incarcerated women. *Journal of Studies on Alcohol and Drugs, 70*(1), 50–54.

CDC, Centers for Disease Control and Prevention. (2010). Vital signs: Binge drinking among high school students and adults–United States 2009. *MMWR, Morbidity and Mortality Weekly Report, 59*(39), 1274–1279.

CDC, Centers for Disease Control and Prevention. (2004). Alcohol-attributable deaths and years of potential life lost–United States, 2001. *MMWR, Morbidity and Mortality Weekly Report, 53*(37), 866–870. Retrieved from MMWR, Morbidity and Mortality Weekly Report.

CDC, Centers for Disease Control and Prevention. (2012a). *Underlying cause of death, 1999-2008 results form*, pp. 1–9. Retrieved from CDC.gov: http://wonder.cdc.gov/controller/datarequest/D67;jsessionid=B09E7BE6825E31EB884.

CDC, Centers for Disease Control and Prevention. (2012b, July 20). Alcohol use and binge drinking among women of childbearing age–United States, 2006-2010. *MMWR, Morbidity and Mortality Weekly Report, 61*(28), 534–538.

CDC, Centers for Disease Control and Prevention. (2015, January). Alcohol poisoning deaths: A deadly consequence of binge drinking. *CDC Vital Signs*, 1–4. Atlanta, GA: CDC.

CDC, Centers for Disease Control and Prevention. (2016, March 7). *Fact Sheets - Excessive alcohol use and risks to women's health.* Retrieved from CDC, Centers for Disease Control and Prevention: Division of Population Health: www.cdc.gov/NCCDPHP/dph/

CDC, Centers for Disease Control and Prevention. (2018a, February). Prescribing guideline. *Alcohol screening and brief intervention for people who consume alcohol and use opioids.* Atlanta, GA: U.S. Department of Health & Human Services.

CDC, Centers for Disease Control and Prevention. (2018b, March 21). Breastfeeding. *Alcohol.* Atlanta, GA: U.S. Department of Health & Human Services.

Cederbaum, A. I. (2012). Alcohol metabolism. *Clinical Liver Disease, 16*(4), 667–685. doi:10.1016/j.cld.2012.08.002

Chan, A. W., Pristach, E. A., & Welte, J. W. (1993). Use of TWEAK test in screening for alcoholism/heavy drinking in three populations. *Alcoholism: Clinical and Experimental Research, 17*(6), 1188–1192.

Chan, A. W., Pristach, E. A., & Welte, J. W. (1994). Detection by the CAGE of alcoholism or heavy drinking in primary care outpatients and the general population. *Journal of Substance Abuse, 6*(2), 123–135.

Chan, L. N., & Anderson, G. D. (2014). Pharmacokinetics and pharmacodynamic drug interactions with ethanol (alcohol). *Clinical Pharmacokinetics, 53*(12), 1115–1136. doi:10.1007/s40262-014-0190-x

Chang, G., Goetz, M. A., & Wilkins-Haug, L. (1999). Identifying prenatal alcohol use: Screening instruments versus clinical predictors. *American Journal on Addictions, 8*(2), 87–93.

Chang, G., McNamara, T., & Orav, E. J. (2006). Identifying risk drinking in expectant fathers. *Birth Issues in Perinatal Care, 33*(2), 110–116.

Chang, G., Wilkins-Haug, L., & Berman, S. (1998). Alcohol use and pregnancy: Improving identification. *Obstretrics & Gynecology, 91*(6), 892–898.

Chang-Mu, C., Jen-Kun, L., & Shing-Hwa, L. (2010). Characterization of neurotoxic effects of NMDA and the novel neuroprotection by phytopolyphenols in mice. *Behavioral Neuroscience, 124*(4), 541–553.

Chapman, J. E., McCart, M. R., & Letourneau, E. J. (2013). Comparison of youth, caregiver, therapist, trained, and treatment expert raters of therapist adherence to a substance abuse treatment protocol. *Journal of Consulting and Clinical Psychology, 81*(4), 674–680. doi:10.1037/a0033021

Charlton, M. E., Sweetnan, P. M., & Fitzgerald, L. W. (2002). Chronic ethanol administration regulates the expression of GABBA receptor alpha1 and alpha5 subunit in the ventral tegmental area and hippocampus. *Journal of Neurochemistry, 68*(1), 121–127.

Chartier, K. G., Vaeth, P. A., & Caetano, R. (2013). Focus on: Ethnicity and the social and health harms from drinking. *Alcoholism Research: Current Reviews, 35*(2), 229–237.

Chasnoff, I. J., Wells, A. M., & King, L. (2015). Misdiagnosis and missed diagnoses in foster and adopted children with prenatal alcohol exposure. *Pediatrics, 135*(2), 264–270.

Cheng, H. G., & Anthony, J. C. (2017). A new era for drinking? Epidemiological evidence on adolescent male-female diferences in drinking incidence in the United States and Europe. *Social Psychiatry and Psychiatric Epidemiology, 52* (1), 117–126. doi:10.1007/s00127-016-1318-0

Cherpitel, C. J. (1995). Analysis of cut points for screening instruments for alcohol problems in the emergency room. *Journal of Studies on Alcohol, 56*(6), 695–700.

Cherpitel, C. J. (1997a, November). Comparison of screening instruments for alcohol problems between black and white emergency room patients from two regions of the country. *Alcoholism: Clinical and Experimental Research, 21*(8), 1391–1397.

Cherpitel, C. J. (1997b). Brief screening instruments for alcoholism. *Alcohol Health & Research World, 21*(4), 348–351.

Cherpitel, C. J. (1998). Differences in performance of screening instruments for problem drinking among blacks, whites and Hispanics in an emergency room population. *Journal of Studies on Alcohol, 59*(4), 420–426.

Cherpitel, C. J. (1999). Screening for alcohol problems in the U. S. general population: A comparison of the CAGE and TWEAK by gender, ethnicity, and services utilization. *Journal of Studies on Alcohol, 60*, 705–711.

Cherpitel, C. J. (2000). A brief screening instrument for problem drinking in the emergency room: The RAPS4. Rapid Alcohol Problems Screen. *Journal of Studies on Alcohol, 61*(3), 447–449.

Cherpitel, C. J. (2002). Screening for alcohol problems in the US general population: Comparison of the CAGE, RAPS4, and RAPS4-QF by gender, ethnicity, and service utilization. Rapid Alcohol Problems Screen. *Alcoholism: Clinical and Experimental Research, 26*(11), 1686–1691. doi:10.1097/01.ALC.0000036300.26619.78

Cherpitel, C. J., & Bazargan, S. (2003). Screening for alcohol problems: Comparison of the AUDIT, RAPS4 and RAPS4-QF among African American and Hispanic patients in an inner city emergency department. *Drug and Alcohol Dependence, 71*(3), 275–280.

Cherpitel, C. J., & Borges, A. (2000, November). Performance of screening instruments for alcohol problems in the ER: A comparison of Mexican-Americans and Mexicans in Mexico. *American Journal of Drug and Alcohol Abuse, 26*(4), 683–702.

Cherpitel, C. J., Ye, Y., & Bond, J. (2005). Cross-national performance of the RAPS4/RAPS4-QF for tolerance and heavy drinking: Data from 13 countries. *Journal of Studies on Alcoholism, 66*(3), 428–432.

Cherpitel, C. J., Ye, Y., & Moskalewicz, J. (2005). Screening for alcohol problems in two emergency service samples in Poland. Comparison of the RAPS4, CAGE, and AUDIT. *Drug and Alcohol Dependence, 80*(2), 201–207.

Chi, F. W., Kaskutas, L. A., & Sterling, S. (2009). Twelve-Step affiliation and 3-year substance use outcomes among adolescents: Social support and religious service attendance as potential mediators. *Addiction, 104*(6), 927–939. doi:10.111/j.1360-0443.2009.02524.x

Child Welfare Information Gateway. (2014). *Parental Substance Use and the Child Welfare System* (pp. *1–13*). Washington, DC: U.S. Department of Health and Human Services, Children's Bureau.

Chiodo, L. M., Delaney-Black, V., & Sokol, R. J. (2014). Increased cut-point of the TACER-3 screen reduces false positives without losing sensitivity in predicting risk alcohol drinking in pregnancy. *Alcoholism: Clinical and Experimental Research, 38*(5), 1401–1408. doi:10.1111/acer.12368

Choi, B. C., & Pak, A. W. (2005). A catalog of biases in questionnaires. *Preventing Chronic Disease: Public Health Research, Practice and Policy, 2*(1), 1–13.

Christie, G., Marsh, R., & Sheridan, J. (2007). The Substances and Choices Scale (SACS)–The development and testing of a new alcohol and other drug screening and outcome measurement instrument for young people. *Addiction, 102*(9), 1390–1398.

Chudley, A. E., Conry, J., & Cook, J. L. (2005). Fetal alcohol spectrum disorder: Canadian guidelines for diagnosis. *CMAJ, Canadian Medical Association Journal, 172*(5 Supplement), S1–S21.

Chung, T., Colby, S. M., & Barnett, N. P. (2000). Screening adolescents for problem drinking: Performance of brief screens against DSM-IV alcohol diagnoses. *Journal of Studies on Alcohol, 61*(4), 579–587.

Chung, T., Creswell, K. G., & Bachrach, R. (2018). Adolescent binge drinking: Developmental context and opportunities for prevention. *Alcohol Research Current Reviews, 39*(1), 5–15.

Clarke, N., Kim, S.-Y., & White, H. R. (2013). Associations between alcohol use and alcohol-related negative consequences among black and white college men and women. *Journal of Studies on Alcohol and Drugs, 74*, 521–531.

Cleary, P. D., Miller, M., & Bush, B. T. (1988). Prevalence and recognition of alcohol abuse in a primary care population. *The American Journal of Medicine, 85*, 466–471.

CNS, California News Service. (2009, October 8). Teen driver charged in fatal drunk driving crash. *Worldnow*.

Coltrain, I. M., Nicholas, C. L., & Baker, F. C. (2014). Alcohol and the sleeping brain. *Handbook of Clinical Neurology, 125*, 415–431. doi:10.1016/B978-0-444-62619-6.00024-0

Conigrave, K. M., Hall, W. D., & Saunders, J. B. (1995). The AUDIT questionnaire: Choosing a cut-off score. Alcohol Use Disorder Identification Test. *Addiction, 90*(10), 1349–1356.

Conigrave, K. M., Saunders, J. B., & Reznik, R. B. (1995). Predictive capacity of the AUDIT questionnnaire for alcohol-related harm. *Addiction, 90*, 1479–1485.

Conley, T. B. (2001, July). Construct validity of the MAST and AUDIT with multiple offender drunk drivers. *Journal of Substance Abuse, 20*(4), 287–295. doi:10.1016/s0740-5472(01)00159-3.

Connor, J. P., Grier, M., & Feeney, G. F. (2007). The validity of the Brief Michigan Alcohol Screening Test (B-MAST). *Journal of Studies on Alcohol and Drugs, 68*(5), 771–779.

Connors, N. A., Bradley, R. H., & Whiteside Mansell, L. (2003). Children of mothers with serious substance abuse problems: An accumulation of risks. *The American Journal of Drug and Alcohol Abuse, 29*(4), 743–758. doi:10.1081/ADA-120026258

Cook, J. L., Green, C. R., & Lilley, C. M. (2016, February 16). Fetal alcohol spectrum disorder: A guideline for diagnosis across the lifespan. *CMAJ, Canadian Medical Association Journal, 188*(3), 191–197. doi:10.1503/cmaj.141593.

Cook, R. L., Chung, T., & Kelly, T. M. (2005). Alcohol screening in young persons attending a sexually transmitted disease clinic. Comparison of AUDIT, CRAFFT, and CAGE instruments. *Journal of General Internal Medicine, 20* (1), 1–6. doi:10.1111/j.1525-1497.2005.40052.x

Coombs, R. H. (1981). Back on the streets: Therapeutic communities' impact upon drug users. *American Journal of Drug and Alcohol Abuse, 8*(2), 185–201.

Corby, E. A., Roll, J. M., & Ledgerwood, D. M. (2000). Contingency management interventions for treating the substance abuse of adolescents: A feasibility study. *Experimental and Clinical Psychopharmacology, 8*(3), 371–376. doi:10.1037/1064-1297.8.3.371

Corliss, H. L., Rosario, M., & Wypij, D. (2010). Sexual orientation and drug use in a longitudinal cohort study of US adolescents. *Addictive Behaviors, 35*(5), 517–521. doi:10.1016/j.addbeh.2009.12.019

Costin, B. N., & Miles, M. F. (2014). Molecular and neurologic responses to chronic alcohol use. *Handbook of Clinical Neurology (on-line Version, ScienceDirect.com), 125*, 157–171. doi:10.1016/B978-0-444-62619-6.00010-0

Crabb, D. W., Edenberg, H. J., & Bosron, W. F. (1989). Genotypes for aldehyde dehydrogenase deficiency and alcohol sensitivity. The inactive ALDH2(2) allele is dominant. *Journal of Clinical Investigation, 83*(1), 314–316.

Cremonte, M., & Cherpitel, C. J. (2008). Performance of screening instruments for alcohol use disorders in emergency department patients in Argentina. *Substance Use & Misuse, 43*(1), 125–138.

Cremonte, M., Ledesma, R. D., & Cherpitel, C. J. (2010). Psychometric properties of alcohol screening tests in the emergency department in Argentina, Mexico, and the United States. *Addictive Behaviors, 35*(9), 818–825.

Crome, I. B., Bloor, R., & Thom, B. (2006). Screening for illicit drug use in psychiatric hospitals: Whose job is it? *Advances in Psychiatric Treatment, 12*, 375–383.

Cronbach, L. J. (1951). Coefficient alpha and the internal structure of tests. *Psychometrika, 16*(3), 297–334.

Cronbach, L. J., & Meehl, P. E. (1955). Construct validity in psychological tests. *Psychological Bulletin, 52*, 281–302.

Crowley, P. (2015). Long-term drug treatment of patients with alcohol dependence. *Australian Prescriber, 38*, 41–43. doi:10.18773/austprescr.2015.015

Crunelle, C. L., Yegles, M., & van Nuijs, A. L. (2014, January 1). Hair ethyl glucuronide levels as a marker for alcohol use and abuse: A review of the current state of the art. *Drug and Alcohol Dependence, 134*, 1–11. doi:10.1016/j.drugalcdep.2013.10.008.

Cummins, L. H., Chan, K. K., & Burns, K. M. (2003, September). Validity of the CRAFFT in American-Indian and Alaska-Native adolescents: Screening for drug and alcohol risk. *Journal of Studies on Alcohol, 64*(5), 727–732.

Cwik, M., Barlow, A., & Tingey, L. (2015). Exploring risk and protective factors with a community sample of American Indian adolescents who attempted suicide. *Archives of Suicide Research, 19*(2), 172–189. doi:10.1080/13811118.2015.1004472

Daeppen, J. B., Yersin, B., & Landry, U. (2000). Reliability and validity of the Alcohol Use Disorders Identification Test (AUDIT) imbedded within a general health risk screening questionnaire: Results of a survey in 332 primary care patients. *Alcoholism: Clinical and Experimental Research, 24*(5), 659–665.

DAILYMAIL.COM.REPORTER. (2015, April 1). *Teacher Kayla Mooney gave student alcohol and had sex wtih him.* Retrieved December 31, 2017, from Daily Mail Online: www.dailymail.co.uk/news/article-3021813/Science-teacher-24-gave-male-student-alcohol-sex-him.html

Daley, D. C., Moss, H., & Campbell, F. (1987). *Dual Disorders: Counseling Clients with Chemical Dependency and Mental Illness.* Center City, MA: Hazelden.

Davis, V. E., & Walsh, M. J. (1970a, February 13). Alcohol, amines, and alkaloids: A possible biochemical basis for alcohol addiction. *Science, 167*(3920), 1005–1007.

Davis, V. E., & Walsh, M. J. (1970b, September 11). Alcohol addiction and tetrahydropapaveroline. *Science, 169*(3950), 1105–1106.

Dawe, S., Loxton, N. J., & Hides, L. (2002). *Review of Diagnostic Screening Instruments for Alcohol and Other Drug Use and Other Psychiatric Disorders* (2nd ed.). Canberra, Australia: Commonwealth Department of Health and Ageing Care.

Dawson, D. A., Grant, B. F., & Stinson, F. S. (2005). The AUDIT-C: Screening for alcohol use disorders and risk drinking in the presence of other psychiatric disorders. *Comprehensive Psychiatry, 46*(6), 405–416.

De Leon, G., Hawke, J., & Jainchill, N. (2000, December). Therapeutc communities. Enhancing retention in treatment using "senior professor" staff. *Journal of Substance Abuse Treatment, 19*(4), 375–382.

De Sousa, A. (2010). The role of topiramate and other anticonvulsants in the treatment of alcohol dependence: A clinical review. *CNS Neurological Disorders – Drug Targets, 9*(1), 45–49.

De Witte, P., Littleton, J., & Parot, P. (2005). Neuroprotective and abstinence-promoting effects of acamprosate: Elucidating the mechanism of action. *CNS Drugs, 19*(6), 517–537.

Deas, D. (2006). Adolescent substance abuse and psychiatric comorbidities. *The Journal of Clinical Psychiatry, 67* (Supplement 7), 18–23.

Deas, D., & Brown, E. S. (2006). Adolescent substance abuse and psychiatric comorbidities. *The Journal of Clinical Psychiatry, 67*(7), e02.

Deitrich, R., Zimatkin, S., & Pronko, S. (2006). Oxidation of ethanol in the brain and its consequences. *Alcohol Research & Health, 29*(4), 266–273.

Delaney-Black, V., Chiodo, L. M., & Hannigan, J. H. (2010, November). Just say "I don't": Lack of concordance between teen report and biological measures of drug use. *Pediatrics, 126*(5), 887–893. doi:10.1542/peds.2009-3059.

Delker, E., Brown, Q., & Hasin, D. S. (2016). Alcohol consumption in demographic subpopulations: An epidemiologic overview. *Alcohol Research: Current Reviews, 38*(1), 7–15.

Denning, G. M., Harland, K. K., & Jennissen, C. A. (2014, December). Age-based risk factors for pediatric ATV-related fatalities. *Pediatrics, 134*(6), 1094–1102. doi:10.1542/peds.2014-1993.

Devries, K. M., Child, J. C., & Bacchus, L. J. (2014). Intimate partner violence victimization and alcohol consumption in women: A systematic review and meta-analysis. *Addiction, 109*(3), 379–391. doi:10.1111/add.12393

Dhalla, S., & Kopec, J. A. (2007). The CAGE questionnaire for alcohol misuse: A review of reliability and validity studies. *Clinical and Investigative Medicine, 30*(1), 33–41.

Diaz Martinez, M. C., Diaz Martinez, A., & Villamil Salcedo, V. (2002, January-February). Efficicacy of metadoxine in the management of acute alcohol intoxication. *The Journal of International Medical Research, 30*(1), 44–51.

Diehl, A., Croissant, B., & Batra, A. (2007). Alcoholism in women: Is it different in onset and outcome compared to men? *European Archives of Psychiatry and Clinical Neuroscience, 257*(6), 344–351. doi:10.1007/s00406-007-0737-z

Diehl, A., Ulmer, L., & Mutschler, J. (2010). Why is disulfiram superior to acamprosate in the routine clinical setting? A retrospective long-term study in 353 alcohol-dependent patients. *Alcohol and Addiction, 45*(3), 271–277.

Dixit, D., Endicott, J., & Burry, L. (2016). Managemnt of acute alcohol withdrawal syndrome in critically ill patients. *Pharmacotherapy, 36*(7), 797–822. doi:10.1002/phar.1770

Do Amaral, R. A., & Malbergier, A. (2008). Effectiveness of the CAGE questionnaire, gamma-glutamyltransferase and mean corpuscular volume of red blood cells as markers for alcohol-related problems in the workplace. *Addictive Behaviors, 33*(6), 772–781. doi:10.1016/j.addbeh.2007.12.006

Donohue, B. (2004, March). Coexisting child neglect and drug abuse in young mothers: Specific recommendations for treatment based on a review of the outcome literature. *Behavior Modification, 28*(2), 206–233. doi:10.1177/0145445503259486.

Donovan, B., Azrin, N. H., & Bradshaw, K. (2014, August). A conrolled evalutation of family behavior therapy in concurrent child neglect and drug abuse. *Journal of Consulting and Clinical Psychology, 82*(4), 706–720. doi:10.1037/a0036920.

Donovan, B., Azrin, N., & Allen, D. N. (2009, September). Family behavior therapy for substance abuse and other associated problems: A review of its intervention components and applicability. *Behavior Modification, 33*(5), 495–519. doi:10.1177/0145445509340019.

Donovan, J. E. (2007, September). Really underage drinkers: The epidemiology of children's alcohol use in the United States. *Prevention Science, 8*(3), 192–205.

Donovan, J. E. (2009). Estimated blood alcohol concentrations for child and adolescent drinking and their implications for screening instruments. *Pediatrics, 123*(6), e975–e981. doi:10.1542/peds.2008-0027

Donovan, J. E. (2014). The burden of alcohol use: Focus on children and preadolescents. *Alcohol Research: Current Reviews, 35*(2), 1–7.

Dopheide, J. A., & Pliszka, S. R. (2009). Attention-deficit-hyperactivity disorder: An update. *Pharmacotherapy, 239*(6), 656–679. doi:10.1592/phco.29.6.656

Douzgou, S., Breen, C., & Crow, Y. J. (2012). Diagnosing fetal alcohol syndrome: New insights from newer genetic technologies. *Archives of Disease in Childhood, 97*(9), 812–817.

Drabble, L., Midanik, L. T., & Trocki, K. (2005). Reports of alcohol consumption and alcohol-related problems among homosexual, bisexual and heterosexual respondents: Results from the 2000 National Alcohol Survey. *Journal of Studies on Alcohol, 66*(1), 111–120.

Drake, R. E., Essock, S. M., & Shaner, A. (2001). Implementing dual diagnosis services for clients with severe mental illness. *Psychiatric Services, 52*(4), 469–476.

Dunn, M. S., Bartee, R. T., & Perko, M. A. (2003). Self-reported alcohol use and sexual behaviors of adolescents'. *Psychological Reports, 92*, 339–348.

Dvorak, R. D., Lamis, D. A., & Malone, P. S. (2013). Alcohol use, depressive symptoms, and impulsivity as risk factors for suicide proneness among college students. *Journal of Affective Disorders, 149*(1–3), 326–334. doi:10.1016/j.jad.2013.01.046

Dye, M. H., Ducharme, L. J., & Johnson, J. A. (2009). Modified therapeutic communities and adherence to traditional elements. *Journal of Psychoactive Drugs, 41*(3), 275–283.

Earleywine, M., LaBrie, J. W., & Pedersen, E. R. (2008). A Brief Rutgers Alcohol Problem Index with less potential for bias. *Addictive Behaviors, 33*(9), 1249–1253.

Eaton, D. K., Kann, L., & Kinchen, S. (2010, June 4). Youth risk behavior surveillance — United States, 2009. *Morbidity and Mortality Weekly Report, 59*(SS-5), 1–9.

Eberhard, S., Nordstrom, G., & Hoglund, P. (2009). Secondary prevention of hazardous alcohol consumption in psychiatric out-patients: A randomized controlled study. *Social Psychiatry and Psychiatric Epidemiology, 44*(12), 1013–1021. doi:10.1007/s00127-009-0023-7

Ebrahim, I. O., Shapiro, C. M., & Williams, A. J. (2013). Alcohol and sleep I: Effects on normal sleep. *Alcoholism: Clinical & Experimental Research, 37*(4), 539–549. doi:10.1111/acer.12006

Ekka, M., & Aggarwal, P. (2015, March). Toxic alcohols. *Journal of Mahatma Gandhi Institute of Medical Sciences, 20*(1), 38–45.

Epstein, J. N., Saunders, B. E., & Kilpatrick, D. G. (1998). PTSD as a mediator between childhood rape and alcohol use in adult women. *Child Abuse & Neglect, 22*(3), 223–234.

Eustace, L. W., Kang, D. H., & Coombs, D. (2003). Fetal alcohol syndrome: A growing concern for health care professionals. *Journal of Obstetric, Gynecologic, & Neonatal Nursing, 32*(2), 215–221.

Ewing, J. A. (1984, October 12). Detecting alcoholism: The CAGE questionnaire. *JAMA, Journal of the American Medical Association, 252*(14), 1905–1907.

Fairbairn, N., Wood, E., & Dong, H. (2017). Unsafe sexual behaviour associated with hazardous alcohol use among street-involved youth. *The Journal of the Association of Nurses in AIDS Care, 29*(4), 481–488. doi:10.1080/09540121.2016.1220480

Farst, K. J., Valentine, J. L., & Hall, R. W. (2011, July 11). Drug testing for newborn exposure to illicit substances in pregnancy: Pitfalls and pearls. *International Journal of Pediatrics*, 951616. doi:10.1155/2011/951616.

Feingold, A., Capaldi, D. M., & Owen, L. D. (2015, August). Proximal vs. distal predictors of alcohol use disorders and treatment utilization in at-risk men in early middle age. *Comprehensive Psychiatry, 61*, 54–71. doi:10.1016/j.comppsych.2015.05.010.

Felitti, V. J., Anda, R. F., & Nordenberg, D. (1998). Relationship of childhood abuse and household dysfunction to many of the leading causes of death in adults: The Adverse Childhood Experiences (ACE) Study. *American Journal of Preventive Medicine, 14*(4), 245–258.

Fergusson, D. M., Horwood, L. J., & Ridder, E. M. (2005). Show me the child at seven: The consequences of conduct problems in childhood for psychological functioning in adulthood. *Journal of Child Psychology and Psychiatry, 46*(8), 837–849. doi:10.1111/j.1469-7610.2004.00387.x

Fergusson, D. M., Horwood, L. J., & Ridder, E. M. (2007, April). Conduct and attentional problems in childhood and adolescence and later substance use, abuse and dependence: Results of a 25-year longitudinal study. *Drug and Alcohol Dependence, 88*(Supplement 1), S14–S26. doi:10.1016/j.drugalcdep.2006.12.011.

Ferreira, S. E., de Mello, M. T., & Pompeia, S. (2006). Effects of energy drink ingestion on alcohol intoxication. *Alcoholism: Clinical and Experimental Research, 30*(4), 598–605.

Ferreira, S. E., de Mello, M. T., & Rossi, M. V. (2004). Does an energy drink modify the effects of alcohol in a maximal effort test? *Alcoholism: Clinical and Experimental Research, 28*(9), 1408–1412.

Ferri, M., Amato, L., & Davoli, M. (2006, July 19). Alcoholics Anonymous and other 12-step programmes for alcohol dependence. *Cochrane Database of Systematic Reviews, 3,* CD005032.

Fiellin, D. A., Reid, M. C., & O'Connor, P. G. (2000). Screening for alcohol problems in primary care: A systematic review. *Archives of Internal Medicine, 160*(13), 1977–1989.

Fleming, M. F., & Barry, K. L. (1991). The effectiveness of alcoholism screening in an ambulatory care setting. *Journal of Studies on Alcohol, 52*(1), 33–36.

Fleming, M. F., Barry, K. L., & MacDonald, R. (1991). The Alcohol Use Disorders Identification Test (AUDIT) in a college sample. *International Journal of Addictions, 26,* 1173–1185.

Florez, G., Saiz, P. A., & Garcia-Portilla, P. (2010). Topiramate for the treatment of alcohol dependence: Comparison with naltrexone. *European Addiction Research, 17*(1), 29–36.

Floyd, R. L., Weber, M. K., & Denny, C. (2009). Prevention of fetal alcohol spectrum disorders. *Developmental Disabilities Research Reviews, 15*(3), 193–199. doi:10.1002/ddrr.75

Forcehimes, A. A., Venner, K. L., & Bogenschutz, M. P. (2011). American Indian methamphetamine and other drug use in the southwestern United States. *Cultural Diversity & Ethnic Minority Psychology, 17*(4), 366–376. doi:10.1037/a0025431

Fox 46 web staff. (2018, May 7). Party bus owner cited after UNC-Charlotte student falls to her death. *Fox 46 WJZY.* Charlotte, NC: Fox News.

FoxNews.com. (2017, December 20). *California teen says he had booze-filled sex romps with married English teacher, cops say.* FoxNews.com. Retrieved from www.foxnews.com/us/2017/12/20/california-teen-says-had-booze-filled-sex-romps-with-married-english-teacher-cops-say.html

Frank, D., DeBenedetti, A. F., & Volk, R. J. (2008). Effectiveness of the AUDIT-C as a screening test for alcohol misuse in three race/ethnic groups. *Journal of General Internal Medicine, 23*(6), 781–787. doi:10.1007/s11606-008-0594-0

Frankel, B. R., & Piercy, F. P. (1990). The relationship among selected supervisor, therapist, and client behaviors. *Journal of Marital and Family Therapy,* 16(4), 407–421.

Franklin-Tong, V. E., & Gourlay, C. W. (2008, August 1). A role for actin in regulating apoptosis/programmed cell death: Evidence spanning yeast, plants and animals. *Biochemical Journal, 413*(3), 389–404. doi:10.1042/BJ0080320.

Freud, S. (1930/1989). *Civilization and Its Discontents.* New York, NY: Norton.

Frinter, M. P., & Rubinson, L. (1993). Acquaintance rape: The influence of alcohol, fraternity membership, and sports team membership. *Journal of Sex Education and Therapy, 19*(4), 272–284.

Frisk, A. (2016, July 7). *Alcoholic mother who hosted naked twister party with teen daughter won't face jail.* Retrieved July 11, 2016, from Globalnews.ca, p. 1: http://globalnews.ca/news/2809582/alcoholic-mother-who-hosted-naked-twister-party-with-teen-daughter-wont-face-jail/

Furman, L. (2005). What is attention-deficit hyperactivity disorder (ADHD)? *Journal of Child Neurology, 20*(12), 994–1002. doi:10.1177/08830738050200121301

Furman, L. M. (2008). Attention-deficit hyperactivity disorder (ADHD): Does new research support old concepts? *Journal of Child Neurology, 23*(7), 775–784. doi:10.1177/0883073808318059

Galaif, E. R., Sussman, S., & Newcomb, M. D. (2007). Suicidality, depression, and alcohol use among adolescents: A review of empirical findings. *International Journal of Adolescent Medicine and Health, 19*(1), 27–35.

Ganz, D., & Sher, L. (2009). Suicidal behavior in adolescents with comorbid depression and alcohol abuse. *Minerva Pediatrica, 61*(3), 333–347.

Garbutt, J. C. (2009). The state of pharmacotherapy for the treatment of alcohol dependence. *Journal of Substance Abuse Treatment, 36*(1), S15–S23.

Garbutt, J. C. (2010). Efficacy and tolerability of naltrexone in the management of alcohol dependence. *Current Pharmaceutical Design, 16*(19), 2091–2097.

Garbutt, J. C., Kranzier, H. R., & O'Malley, S. S. (2005). Efficacy and tolerability of long-acting injectable naltrexone for alcohol dependence: A randomized controlled study. *JAMA, the Journal of the American Medical Association, 293,* 1617–1625.

Gardiner, A. S., Gutierrez, H. L., & Luo, L. (2016). Alcohol use during pregnancy is associated with specific alterations in microRNA levels in maternal serum. *Alcoholism: Clinical and Experimental Research, 40*(4), 826–837. doi:10.1111/acer.13026

GBD, Global Burden of Diseases. (2018). Alcohol use and burden for 195 countries and territories, 1990-2016: A systematic analysis for the global Burden of Disease Study 2016. *The Lancet,* 1–21. doi:10.1016/S0140-6736(18)31310-2

George, W. H., Davis, K. C., & Masters, N. T. (2014). Sexual victimization, alcohol intoxication, sexual-emotional responding, and sexual risk in heavy episodic drinking. *Archives of Sexual Behavior, 43*(4), 645–658. doi:10.1007/s10508-013-0143-8

Giang, K. B., Spak, F., & Dzung, T. (2005, August 23). The use of AUDIT to assess level of alcohol problems in rural Vietnam. *Alcohol and Alcoholism, 40*(6), 578–583.

Gibson, L., & Porter, M. (2018, August). Drinking or smoking while breastfeeding and later cognition in children. *Pediatrics, 142*(2), 1–11. doi:10.1542/peds.2017-4266.

Gilmore, A. K., Koo, K. H., & Nguyen, H. V. (2014). Sexual assault, drinking norms, and drinking behavior among a national sample of lesbian and bisexual women. *Addictive Behaviors, 39*(3), 630–636. doi:10.1016/j.addbeh.2013.11.015

Gilmore, A. K., Stappenbeck, C. A., & Lewis, M. A. (2015). Sexual assault history and its association with the use of drinking protective behavioral strategies among college women. *Journal of Studies on Alcohol and Drugs, 76*(3), 459–464.

Ginsburg, K. A., Blacker, C. M., & Abel, E. L. (1991). Fetal alcohol exposure and adverse pregnancy outcomes. *Contributions to Gynecology and Obstetrics, 18*, 115–129.

Ginzler, J. A., Garrett, S. B., & Baer, J. S. (2007). Measurement of negative consequences of substance use in street youth: An expanded use of the Rutgers Alcohol Problem Index. *Addictive Behaviors, 32*(7), 1519–1525.

Globe Newswire. (2017, September 28). *New Survey Finds that Adults are Most Likely to Believe Stricter Campus Policies are Most Effective Approach to Decrease Campus Sexual Assault.* Harrisburg, PA: *National Sexual Violence Resource Center.*

Godley, M. D., Godley, S. H., & Dennis, M. L. (2014, February). A randomized trial of assertive contining care and contingency management for adolescents with substance use disorders. *Journal of Consulting and Clinical Psychology, 82*(1), 40–51. doi:10.1037/a0035264.

Golka, K., & Wiese, A. (2004). Carbohydrate-deficient transferrin (CDT)–A biomarker for long-term alcohol consumption. *Journal of Toxicology and Environmental Health, Part B: Critical Reviews*, 7(4), 319–337.

Gomez, A., Conde, A., & Santana, J. M. (2005). Diagnostic usefulness of brief versions of Alcohol Use Disorders Identification Test (AUDIT) for detecting hazardous drinkers in primary care settings. *Journal of Studies on Alcohol, 66*(2), 305–308.

Gonzales, R. A., & Jaworski, J. N. (1997). Alcohol and glutamate. *Alcohol Health & Research World, 21*(2), 120–127.

Gonzalez, V. M. (2012). Association of solitary binge drinking and suicidal behavior among emerging adult college students. *Psychology of Addictive Behavior, 26*(3), 609–614. doi:10.1037/a0026916

Gonzalez, V. M., & Hewell, V. M. (2012). Suicidal ideation and drinking to cope among college binge drinkers. *Addictive Behaviors, 37*(8), 994–997. doi:10.1016/j.addbeh.2012.03.027

Gordon, A. J., Maisto, S. A., & McNeil, M. (2001). Three questions can detect hazardous drinkers. *Journal of Family Practice, 50*(4), 313–320.

Graham, A., Goss, C., & Xu, S. (2007). Effect of using different modes to administer the AUDIT-C on identification of hazardous drinking and acquiescence to trial participation among injured patients. *Alcohol and Alcoholism, 42*(5), 423–429.

Green, K. E., & Feinstein, B. A. (2012). Substance use in lesbian, gay, and bisexual populations: An update on empirical research and implications for treatment. *Psychology of Addictive Behaviors, 26*(2), 265–278. doi:10.1037/a0025424

Grucza, R. A., Norberg, K. E., & Bierut, L. J. (2009). Binge drinking among youth and young adults in the United States: 1979-2006. *Journal of the American Academy of Child & Adolescent Psychiatry, 48*(7), 692–702.

Guerri, C., & Pascual, M. (2010, February). Mechanisms involved in the neurotoxic, cognitive, and neurobehavioral effects of alcohol consumption during adolescence. *Alcohol, 44*(1), 15–26. doi:10.1016/j.alcohol.2009.10.003.

Guglielmo, R., Martinotti, G., & Quatrale, M. (2015). Topiramate in alcohol use disorders: Review and update. *CNS Drugs, 29*(5), 383–395. doi:10.1007/s40263-015-0244-0

Gupta, S., & Warner, J. (2008). Alcohol-related dementia: A 21st-century silent epidemic? *The British Journal of Psychiatry, 193*, 351–353. doi:10.1192/bjp.bp.108.051425

Gutierez Garcia, M. L., Blasco-Algora, S., & Fernandez-Rodriguez, C. M. (2015, July 28). Alcohol liver disease: A review of current therapeutic approaches to achieve long-term abstinence. *World Journal of Gastroenterology, 21* (28), 8516–8526. doi:10.3748/wjg.v21.i28.8516.

Haastrup, M. B., Pottegard, A., & Damkier, P. (2014). Alcohol and breast feeding. *Basic & Clinical Pharmacology & Toxicology, 114*(2), 168–173. doi:10.1111/bcpt.12149

Haber, J. R., Bucholz, K. K., & Jacob, T. (2010, September). Effect of paternal alcohol and drug dependence on offspring conduct disorder: Gene-environment interplay. *Journal of Studies on Alcohol and Drugs, 71*(5), 652–663.

Haber, J. R., Jacob, T., & Heath, A. C. (2005, April). Paternal alcoholism and offspring conduct disorder: Evidence for the 'common genes' hyposthesis. *Twin Research and Human Genetics, 8*(2), 120–131. doi:10.1375/1832427053738782.

Habis, A., Tall, L., & Smith, J. (2007). Pediatric emergency medicine physicians' current practices and beliefs regarding mental health screening. *Pediatric Emergency Care, 23*(6), 387–393.

Hadland, S. E., Copelas, S. H., & Harris, S. K. (2017, May). Trajectories of substance use frequency among adolescents seen in primary care: Implications for screening. *The Journal of Pediatrics, 184*, 178–185. doi:10.1016/j.jpeds.2017.01.033.

Hadland, S. E., Xuan, Z., & Sarda, V. (2017). Alcohol policies and alcohol-related motor vehicle crash fatalities among young people in the US. *Pediatrics, 139*(3), e20163037. doi:10.1542/peds.20126-3037

Hamilton, M. (2015, March 2). *Teachers charged with having sex with students, giving them cocaine.* Retrieved December 31, 2018, from LA Times: www.latimes.com/local/lanow/la-me-in-teachers-charged-sex-cocaine-camping-trip-20150302-story.html

Hammond, C. J., Niciu, M. J., & Drew, S. (2015). Anticonvulsants for the treatment of alcohol withdrawal syndrome and alcohol use disorders. *CNS Drugs, 29*(4), 293–311. doi:10.1007/s40263-015-0240-4

Hannan, S. M., Orcutt, H. K., & Miron, L. R. (2015, June 30). Childhood sexual abuse and later alcohol-related problems: Investigating the roles of revictimization, PTSD, and drinking motivations among college women. *Journal of Interpersonal Violence*, [Epub ahead of print]. Retrieved March 6, 2016, from www.ncbi.nlm.nih.gov/pubmed

Hanson, G. R. (2002). Therapeutic Community. *National Institute on Drug Abuse Research Report Series*. Rockville, MD: National Institute on Drug Abuse.

Hanson, J. D., Winberg, A., & Elliott, A. (2012). Development of a media campaign on fetal alcohol disorders for Northern Plains American Indian communities. *Health Promotion Practice, 13*(6), 842–847. doi:10.1177/1524839911404232

Harada, M. Y., Gangi, A., & Ko, A. (2015, December). Bicycle trauma and alcohol intoxication. *International Journal of Surgery, 24*(Part A), 14–19. doi:10.1016/j.ijsu.2015.10.013.

Harris, B. R., Shaw, B. A., & Sherman, B. R. (2016). Screening, brief intervention, and referral to treatment for adolescents: Attitudes, perceptions, and practice of New York school-based health center providers. *Substance Abuse, 37*(1), 161–167. doi:10.1080/08897077.2015.1015703

Harris, S. R., Osborn, J. A., & Weinberg, J. (1993). Effects of prenatal alcohol exposure on neuromotor and cognitive development during early childhood: A series of case reports. *Physical Therapy, 73*(9), 608–617.

Hasin, D. (2003). Classification of alcohol use disorders. *Alcohol Research & Health, 27*(1), 5–17.

Hasin, D. S., Stinson, F. S., & Ogburn, E. (2007). Prevalence, correlates, disability, and comorbidity of DSM-IV alcohol abuse and dependence in the United States: Results from the National Epidemiologic Survey on Alcohol and Related Conditions. *Archives of General Psychiatry, 64*(7), 830–842.

Hays, R. D., Merz, J. F., & Nicholas, R. (1995). Response burden, reliability, and validity of the CAGE, Short MAST, and AUDIT alcohol screening measures. *Behavioral Research Methods, Instruments, & Computers, 27*, 277–280.

Heinala, P., Piepponen, T., & Heikkinen, H. (1990). Diazepam loading in alcohol withdrawal: Clinical pharmacokinetics. *International Journal of Clinical Pharmacology, Therapy and Toxicology, 28*(5), 211–217.

Henggeler, S. W., Chapman, J. E., & Rowland, M. D. (2008). Statewide adoption and initial implementation of contingency management for substance-abusing adolescents. *Journal of Consulting and Clinical Psychology, 76*(4), 556–567. doi:10.1037/0022-006X.76.4.556

Higgins, S. T., & Petry, N. M. (1999). Contingency management. Incentives for sobriety. *Alcohol Research & Health, 23* (2), 122–127.

Hill, K. P., & Chang, G. (2007). Brief screening instruments for risky drinking in the outpatient psychiatry clinic. *The American Journal on Addictions, 16*(3), 222–226.

Hilton, M. (2014). APIS: The NIAAA alcohol policy information system. *Alcohol Research: Current Reviews, 35*(2), 184–185.

Hingson, R. W., Heeren, T., & Zakocs, R. C. (2002). Magnitude of alcohol-related mortality and morbidity among U. S. college students ages 18-24. *Journal of Studies on Alcohol, 63*(2), 136–144.

Hingson, R., Heeren, T., & Levenson, S. (2002). Age of drinking onset, driving after drinking, and involvement in alcohol related motor-vehicle crashes. *Accidents; Analysis and Prevention, 34*, 85–92.

Hipolito, L., Sanchez, M. J., & Polache, A. (2007, October). Brain metabolism of ethanol and alcoholism: An update. *Current Drug Metabolism, 8*(7), 716–727.

Hodgson, R. J., Abbasi, J. B., & Hodgson, R. C. (2003, October). Fast screening for alcohol misuse. *Addictive Behaviors, 28*(8), 1453–1463.

Hoeppner, B. B., Hoeppner, S. S., & Kelly, J. F. (2014, October 1). Do young people benefit from AA as much, and in the same ways, as adult aged 30+? A moderated multiple mediation analysis. *Drug and Alcohol Dependence, 143*, 181–188. doi:10.1016/j.drugalcdep.2014.07.023.

Hoffman, P. L. (1995, March). Glutamate receptors in alcohol withdrawal-induced neurotoxicity. *Metabolic Brain Disease, 10*(1), 73–79.

Hoffman, P. L., & Tabakoff, B. (1994). The role of the NMDA receptor in ethanol withdrawal. *EXS, 71*, 61–70.

Holtzman, J. L. (1983). Definition and implications of dose-dependent kinetics in clinical medicine. *Drug Metabolism Reviews, 14*(6), 1103–1117.

Hotts, M. (2015, June 17). *Ex-Mount Clemens teacher charged with sex with student*. Retrieved 31 2018, from The Macomb Daily: www.macombdaily.com/article/MD/20150617/NEWS/150619675

Hovda, K. E., & Jacobsen, D. (2016). Management of alcohol poisoning. In A. Webb, D. Angus, & S. Finfer (Eds.), *Oxford Textbook of Critical Care* (2nd ed., pp. 1–11). Oxford: Oxford University Press.

Howard, D. E., Griffin, M. A., & Boekeloo, B. O. (2008). Prevalence and psychosocial correlates of alcohol-related sexual assault among university students. *Adolescence, 43*(172), 733–750.

Hudmon, K. S., Corelli, R. L., & Prokhorov, A. V. (2010, February). Current approaches to pharmacotherapy for smoking cessation. *Therapeutic Advanvces in Repiratory Disease, 4*(1), 35–47. doi:10.1177/1753465809353768.

Huey, S. J., & Polo, A. J. (2008). Evidence-based psychological treatments for ethnic minority youth. *Journal of Clinical Child & Adolescent Psychology, 37*(1), 262–301. doi:10.1080/15374410701820174

Hughes, T. L., & Eliason, M. (2002, Spring). Substance use and abuse in lesbian, gay, bisexual and transgender populations. *The Journal of Primary Prevention, 22*(3), 263–298. doi:0278-095X/02/0300-0263/0

Hughes, T. L., & Wilsnack, S. C. (1997). Use of alcohol among lesbians: Research and clinical implications. *American Journal of Orthopsychiatry, 67*(1), 20–36.

Hughes, T. L., Johnson, T., & Wilsnack, S. C. (2001). Sexual assault and alcohol abuse: A comparison of lesbians and heterosexual women. *Journal of Substance Abuse, 13*(4), 515–532.

Hughes, T. L., Szalacha, L. A., & Johnson, T. P. (2010). Sexual victimization and hazardous drinking among heterosexual and sexual minority women. *Addictive Behaviors, 35*(12), 1152–1156. doi:10.1016/j.addbeh.2010.07.004

Hyde, Z., Comfort, J., & McManus, A. (2009, September). Alcohol, tobacco and illicit drug use amongst same-sex attracted women: Results from the Western Australian Lesbian and Bisexual Women's Health and Well-Being Survey. *BMC Public Health - BioMed Central, 9*, 317.

Ikonomidou, C., Bittigau, P., & Koch, C. (2001). Neurotransmitters and apoptosis in the developing brain. *Biochemical Pharmacology, 62*(4), 401–405.

Irvine, M. (2005, July 24). Teenagers lured into meth's net. *The Washington Post*, 1–2.

Isaacson, J. H., Butler, R., & Zacharek, M. (1994). Screening with the Alcohol Use Disorders Identification Test (AUDIT) in an inner city population. *Journal of General Internal Medicine, 9*, 550–553.

Jackson, K. M., Barnett, N. P., & Colby, S. M. (2015, March). The prospective association between sipping alcohol by the sixth grade and later substance use. *Journal of Studies on Alcohol and Drugs, 76*(2), 212–221. Retrieved from www.jsad.com/doi/pdf/10.15288/jsad.20125.76.212

Johnson, B. A., & Ait-Daoud, N. (2010). Topiramate in the new generation of drugs: Efficacy in the treatment of alcoholic patients. *Current Pharmaceutical Design, 16*(19), 2103–2112.

Johnson, B. A., Ait-Daoud, N., & Bowden, C. L. (2003). Oral topiramate for treatment of alcohol dependence: A randomized controlled study. *The Lancet, 361*(9370), 1677–1685.

Johnson, B. A., Rosenthal, N., & Capece, J. A. (2007). Topiramate for treating alcohol dependence: A randomized controlled study. *JAMA, the Journal of the American Medical Association, 298*(14), 1641–1685.

Johnston, L. D., O'Malley, P. M., & Bachman, J. G. (2010, May). Monitoring the future national results on adolescent drug use: Overview of key findings, 2009. *NIH Publication No. 10-7583*. Bethesda, MD: National Institute on Drug Abuse.

Johnston, L. D., O'Malley, P. M., & Bachman, J. G. (2011, February). *Monitoring the Future, National Results on Adolescent Drug Use: Overview of Key Findings, 2010*. Ann Arbor: Institute for Social Research, The University of Michigan.

Jones, C. M., Paulozzi, L. J., & Mack, K. A. (2014). Alcohol involvement in opioid pain reliever and benzodiazepine drug abuse-related emergency department visits and drug-related deaths – United States, 2010. *MMWR, Morbidity and Mortality Weekly Report, 63*(40), 881–885.

Joya, X., Friguls, B., & Ortigosa, S. (2012). Determination of maternal-fetal biomarkers of prenatal exposure to ethanol: A review. *Journal of Pharmaceutical and Biomedical Analysis, 69*, 209–222. doi:10.1016/j.jpba.2012.01.006

Jung, Y. C., & Namkoong, K. (2006). Pharmacotherapy for alcohol dependence: Anticraving medications for relapse prevention. *Yonsei Medical Journal, 47*(2), 167–178.

Kalk, N. J., & Lingford-Hughes, A. R. (2014). The clinical pharmacology of acamprosate. *British Journal of Clinical Pharmacology*, 77(2), 315–323. doi:10.1111/bcp.12070

Kaminer, Y. (2002, October). Adolescent substance abuse treatment: Evidence-based practice in outpatient services. *Current Psychiatry Reports, 4*(5), 397–401.

Kaminer, Y., & Francis, R. J. (1991). Inpatient treatment of adolescents with psychiatric and substance abuse disorders. *Hospital & Community Psychiatry, 42*(9), 894–896.

Kaminer, Y., Goldberg, P., & Connor, D. F. (2010). Psychotropic medications and substances of abuse interactions in youth. *Substance Abuse, 31*(1), 53–57. doi:10.1080/08897070903442665

Kanny, D., Naimi, T. S., & Liu, Y. (2018). Annual total binge drinks consumed by U.S. adults, 2015. *American Journal of Preventive Medicine, 54*(4), 486–496.

Karp, R. J., Qazi, Q., & Hittleman, J. (1993). Fetal alcohol syndrome. In R. J. Karp (Ed.), *Malnourished Children in the United States: Caught in the Cycle of Poverty* (pp. 101–108). New York: Springer.

Keller, M. B., Lavori, P. W., & Beardslee, W. R. (1992). The disruptive behavioral disorder in children and adolescents: Comorbidity and clinical course. *Journal of the American Academy of Child & Adolescent Psychiatry, 31*(2), 204–209. doi:10.1097/00004583-199203000-00005

Kelly, J. F., Dow, S. J., & Yeterian, J. D. (2010, July 1). Can 12-step group participation strengthen and extend the benefits of adolescent addiction treatment? A prospective analysis. *Drug and Alcohol Dependence, 110*(1–2), 117–125. doi:10.1016/j.drugalcdep.2010.02.019.

Kelly, J. F., Myers, M. G., & Brown, S. A. (2002). Do adolescents affiliate with 12-step groups? A multivariate process model of effects. *Journal of Studies on Alcohol and Drugs, 63*(3), 293–304.

Kelly, T. M., Donovan, J. E., & Chung, T. (2004). Alcohol use disorders among emergency department-treated older adolescents: A new brief screen (RUFT-Cut) using the AUDIT, CAGE, CRAFFT, and RAPS-QF. *Alcoholism: Clinical and Experimental Research, 28*(5), 746–753.

Kelly, T. M., Donovan, J. E., & Chung, T. (2009). Brief screens for detecting alcohol use disorder among 18-20 year old young adults in emergency departments: Comparing AUDIT-C, RAPS4-QF, FAST, RUFT-Cut, and DSM-IV 2-Item Scale. *Addictive Behaviors, 34*(8), 668–674.

Kelly, T. M., Donovan, J. E., & Kinnane, J. M. (2002, September–October). A comparison of alcohol screening instruments among under-aged drinkers treated in emergency departments. *Alcohol and Alcoholism, 37*(5), 444–450.

Kendall, M. (1938). A new measure of rank correlation. *Biometrika, 30*(1–2), 81–89.

Kendell, R., & Jablensky, A. (2003). Distinguishing between validity and utility of psychiatric diagnoses. *The American Journal of Psychiatry, 160*(1), 4–12.

Kenna, G. A., Lomastro, T. L., & Schiesl, A. (2009). Review of topiramate: An antiepileptic for the treatment of alcohol dependence. *Current Drug Abuse Reviews, 2*(2), 135–142.

Kennedy, W. K., Leloux, M., & Kutscher, E. C. (2010). Acamprosate. *Expert Opinion on Drug Metabolism & Toxicology, 6* (3), 363–380.

Kenney, S. R., Hummer, J. F., & LaBrie, J. W. (2010). An examination of prepartying and drinking games playing during high-school and their impact on alcohol-related risk upon entrance into college. *Journal of Youth and Adolescence, 39*(9), 999–1011. doi:10.1007/s10964-009-9473-1

Kerner, L. L., Kerner, J., & Herring, S. D. (2017, Fall). Sexual assaults on college campuses. *Journal of Academic Administration in Higher Education, 13*(2), 41–45.

Keyes, K. M., Martins, S. S., & Blanco, C. (2010). Telescoping and gender differences in alcohol dependence: New evidence from two national surveys. *The American Journal of Psychiatry, 167*(8), 969–976. doi:10.1176/appi.ajp.2009.09081161

Khan, B. A., Robinson, R. F., & Smith, J. J. (2013, August 5). Prenatal alcohol exposure among Alaska Native/American Indian infants. *International Journal of Circumpolar Health*, 72. doi:10.3402/ijch.v72i0.20973.

Kiefer, F., & Mann, K. (2010). Acamprosate: How, when, and for whom does it work? Mechanisms of action, treatment targets, and individualized therapy. *Current Pharmaceutical Design, 16*(19), 2098–2102.

Kiluk, B. D., Nich, C., & Buck, M. B. (2018, May 24). Randomized clinical trial of computerized and clinician-delivered CBT in comparison with standard outpatient treatment for substance use disorders: Primary within-treatment and follow-up outcomes. *The American Journal of Psychiatry*. doi: 10.1176/appi.ajp.2018.17090978.

Kirchmayer, U., Davoli, M., & Verster, A. (2000). Naltrexone maintenance treatment for opioid dependence. *The Cochrane Database of Systematic Reviews, 2*, CD0013333. doi:10.1002/14651858.CD001333

Kitchens, J. M. (1994, December 14). Does this patient have an alcohol problem? *JAMA, 272*(22), 1782–1787.

Knight, J. R., Goodman, E., & Pulerwitz, T. (2000). Reliabilities of short substance abuse screening tests among adolescent medical patients. *Pediatrics, 105*(4, part 2), 948–953.

Knight, J. R., Sherritt, L., & Harris, S. K. (2003). Validity of brief alcohol screening tests among adolescents: A comparison of the AUDIT, POSIT, CAGE, and CRAFFT. *Alcoholism: Clinical and Experimental Research, 27*(1), 67–73. doi:10.1097/01.ALC.0000046598.59317.3A

Knight, J. R., Sherritt, L., & Shrier, L. A. (2002). Validity of the CRAFFT substance abuse screening test among adolescent clinic patients. *Archives of Pediatric & Adolescent Medicine, 156*(6), 607–614.

Knight, J. R., Shrier, L. A., & Bravender, T. D. (1999). A new brief screen for adolescent substance abuse. *Archives of Pediatric & Adolescent Medicine, 153*(6), 591–596.

Kramer, T. L., Han, X., & Leukefeld, C. (2009, Winter). Childhood conduct problems and other early risk factors in rural adult stimulant users. *The Journal of Rural Health, 25*(1), 50–57. doi:10.1111/j.1748-0361.2009.00198.x

Kraut, J. A., & Kurtz, I. (2008). Toxic alcohol ingestion: Clinical features, diagnosis, and management. *Clinical Journal of the American Society of Nephrology, 3*, 208–225. doi:10.2215/CJN.03220807

Kraut, J. A., & Mullins, M. E. (2018, January 18). Toxic alcohols. *The New England Journal of Medicine, 378*(3), 270–280. doi:10.1056/NEJMra1615295.

Kreek, M. J., & Stimmel, B. (Eds.). (1984). *Dual Addiction: Pharmacological Issues in the Treatment of Concomitant Alcoholism and Drug Abuse*. Binghamton, NY: Haworth.

Kriston, L., Holzel, L., & Weiser, A. (2008). Meta-analysis: Are 3 questions enough to detect unhealthy alcohol use? *Annals of Internal Medicine, 149*(12), 879–888.

Kurti, A. N., Davis, D., & Redner, R. (2016). A review of the literature on remote monitoring technology in incentive-based interventions for health-related behavior change. *Translational Issues in Psychological Science, 2*(2), 128–152. doi:10.1037/tps0000067

Kvigne, V. L., Randall, B., & Simanton, E. G. (2012). Blood alcohol levels for American Indian mothers and newborns. *Pediatrics, 130*(4), e1015–e1018. doi:10.1542/peds.2011-1400

Labbe, A. K., Greene, C., & Bergman, B. G. (2013, December 1). The importance of age composition of 12-step meetings as a moderating factor in the relation between young adults' 12-step participation and abstinence. *Drug and Alcohol Dependence, 133*(2), 541–547. doi:10.1016/j.drugalcdep.2013.07.021.

LaBrie, J. W., & Pedersen, E. R. (2008). Prepartying promotes heightened risk in the college environment: An event-level report. *Addictive Behaviors, 33*(7), 955–959. doi:10.1016/j.addbeh.2008.02.011

LaBrie, J. W., Earle, A. M., & Hummer, J. F. (2016, July 2). Is prepartying a cause of heavy drinking and consequences rather than just a correlate? A longitudinal look at the relationship between prepartying, alcohol approval, and subsequent drinking and consequences. *Substance Use & Misuse, 51*(8), 1013–1023. doi:10.3109/10826084.2016.1152493.

LaBrie, J. W., Hummer, J., & Kenney, S. (2011). Identifying factors that increase the likelihood for alcohol-induced blackouts in the prepartying context. *Substance Use & Misuse, 46*(8), 992–1002. doi:10.3109/10826084.2010.542229

Lam, K. (2018, May 29). UNCC student killed after falling out of party bus was extremely intoxicated, report says. *Fox News*, 1–2.

Lander, L., Howsare, J., & Byrne, M. (2013). The impact of substance use disorders on families and children: From theory to practice. *Social Work in Public Health, 28*, 194–205. doi:10.1080/19371918.2013.759005

Lange, S., Probst, C., & Gmel, G. (2017). Global prevalence of fetal alcohol spectrum disorder among children and youth: A systematic review and meta-analysis. *JAMA Pediatrics, 171*(10), 948–956. doi:10.1001/jamapediatrics.2017.1919

Lardier, D. T., Barrios, V. R., & Garcia-Reid, P. (2016). Suicidal ideation among suburban adolescents: The influence of school bullying and other mediating risk factors. *Journal of Child and Adolescent Mental Health, 28*(3), 213–231. doi:10.2989/17280583.2016.1262381

Laudet, A. B. (2008). The impact of alcoholics anonymous on other substance abuse-related twelve-step programs. *Recent Developments in Alcoholism, 18*, 71–89.

Laundergan, J. C., & Williams, T. (1993). The Hazelden Residential Family Program: A combined systems and disease model approach. In T. J. O'Farrell (Ed.), *Treating Alcohol Problems: Marital and Family Interventions* (pp. 145–169). New York: Guilford.

Lehman, A. F., Myers, C. P., & Corty, E. (1994, March-April). Prevalence and patterns of "dual diagnosis" among psychiatric inpatients. *Comprehensive Psychiatry, 35*(2), 106–112.

Leung, J. G., Hall-Flavin, D., & Nelson, S. (2015). The role of gabapentin in the management of alcohol withdrawal and dependence. *The Annals of Pharmacotherapy, 49*(8), 897–906. doi:10.1177/1060028015585849

Levy, S. J., & Williams, J. F. (2016). Substance use screening, brief intervention, and referral to treatment. *Pediatrics, 138*, e1–e15. doi:10.1542/peds.2016-1211

Levy, S., Sherritt, L., & Harris, S. K. (2004). Test-retest reliability of adolescents' self-report of substance use. *Alcoholism: Clinical & Experimental Research, 28*(8), 1236–1241.

Levy, S., Vaughan, B. L., & Knight, J. R. (2002, April). Office-based intervention for adolescent substance abuse. *Pediatric Clinics of North America, 49*(2), 329–343.

Lewis, K. (2015, July 17). Police: Car cruising at 119 mph before fatal crash, teen driver drunk. *ABC 7 News*. Washington, DC: WJLA.

Lewis, R. A., Piercy, F. P., & Sprenkle, D. H. (1990). Family-based interventions for helping drug-abusing adolescents. *Journal of Adolescent Research, 5*(1), 82–95.

Li, G., Brady, J. E., & Chen, Q. (2013, November). Drug use and fatal motor vehicle crashes: A case-control study. *Accident Analysis & Prevention, 60*, 205–210. doi:10.1016/j.aap.2013.09.001.

Liang, J., & Olsen, R. W. (2014). Alcohol use disorders and current pharmacological therapies: The role of GABA(A) receptors. *Acta Pharmacologica Sinica, 35*(8), 981–993. doi:10.1038/aps.2014.50

Liddle, H. A., Dakof, G. A., & Parker, K. (2001, November). Multidimensional family therapy for adolescent drug abuse: Results of a randomized clinical trial. *The American Journal of Drug and Alcohol Abuse, 27*(4), 651–688.

Liddle, H. A., Jackson-Gilfort, A., & Marvel, F. A. (2006, April). An empirically supported and culturally specific engagement and intervention strategy for African American adolescent males. *American Journal of Orthopsychiatry, 76*(2), 215–225. doi:10.1037/0002-9432.75.2.215.

Lieber, C. S. (1999). Microsomal ethanol-oxidizing system (MEOS): The first 30 years (1968-1998) – A review. *Alcoholism: Clinical & Experimental Research, 23*(6), 991–1007.

Ling, J., Stephens, R., & Heffernan, T. M. (2010). Cognitive and psychomotor performance during alcohol hangover. *Current Drug Abuse Reviews, 3*(2), 80–87.

Lipari, R. N. (2017, October 3). Exposure to substance use prevention messages among adolescents. *SAMHSA: The CBHSQ Report*, pp. 1–7. Retrieved from www.samhsa.gov/data/sites/default/files/report_3380/ShortReport-3380.html

Lipari, R. N., Ahrnsbrak, R. D., & Pemberton, M. R. (2017). *Risk and Protective Factors and Estimates of Substance Use Initiation: Results from the 2016 National Survey on Drug Use and Health.* Rockville: Substance Abuse and Mental Health Services Administration.

Liskow, B., Campbell, J., & Nickel, E. J. (1995, May). Validity of the CAGE questionnaire in screening for alcohol dependence in a walk-in (triage) clinic. *Journal of Studies on Alcohol, 56*(3), 277–281.

Little, J., Barron, S., & Prendergast, M. (2007, May-June). Smoking kills (alcoholics)! Shouldn't we do something about it? *Alcohol and Alcoholism, 42*(3), 167–173. doi:10.1093/alcalc/agm019

LoConte, N. K., Brewster, A. M., & Kaur, J. S. (2017). Alcohol and cancer: A statement of the American Society of Clinical Oncology. *Journal of Clinical Oncology, 36*(1), 83–93. doi:10.1200/JCO.2017.76.1155

Long, D., Long, B., & Koyfman, A. (2017). The emergency medicine management of severe alcohol withdrawal. *The American Journal of Emergency Medicine, 35*(7), 1005–1011. doi:10.1016/j.ajem.2017.02.002

Lovinger, D. M. (1997). Serotonin's role in alcohol's effects on the brain. *Alcohol Health & Research World, 21*(2), 114–120.

Luczak, S. E. (2003). Construct of alcohol problems: Invariance across religions. *Dissertation Abstracts International, 63*(9), 4377B.

Luo, Z., Liu, Y., & Liu, Y. (2017, December). Cellular and molecular mechanisms of alcohol-induced osteopenia. *Cellular and Molecular Life Sciences, 74*(24), 4443–4453. doi:10.1007/s00018-017-2585-y.

MacKenzie, D., Langa, A., & Brown, T. M. (1996). Identifying hazardous or harmful alcohol use in medical admissions: A comparison of audit, cage and brief mast. *Acohol and Alcoholism, 31*(6), 591–599.

Madea, B., & Musshoff, F. (2009, May). Knock-out drugs: Their prevalence, modes of action, and means of detection. *Deutsches Arzteblatt International, 106*(20), 341–347. doi:10.3238/arztebl.2009.0341.

Madras, B. K., Compton, W. M., & Avula, D. (2009, January). Screening, brief interventions, referral to treatment (SBIRT) for illicit drug and alcohol use at multiple sites: Comparison at intake and 6 months later. *Drug and Alcohol Dependence, 99*(1–3), 280–295. doi:10.1016/j.drugalcdep.23008.08.003.

Magruder, K. M., Bichun Ouyang, B., & Miller, S. (2009, June). Retention of under-represented minorities in drug abuse treatment studies. *Clinical Trials, 6*(3), 252–260. doi:10.1177/1740774509105224.

Maisto, S. A., Connors, G. J., & Allen, J. P. (1995). Contrasting self-report screens for alcohol problems: A review. *Alcoholism: Clinical & Experimental Research, 19*(6), 1510–1516.

Malinauskas, B. M., Aeby, V. G., & Overton, R. F. (2007). A survey of energy drink consumption patterns among college students. *Nutrition Journal, 6*, 35.

Mann, K., & Hermann, D. (2010). Individualised treatment in alcohol-dependent patients. *European Archives of Psychiatry & Clinical Neuroscience, 260*(Supplement 2), S116–S120.

Marcell, A. V., Halpern-Felsher, B., & Coriell, M. (2002). Physicians' attitudes and beliefs concerning alcohol abuse prevention in adolescents. *American Journal of Preventive Medicine, 22*(1), 49–55.

Marchetta, C. M., Denny, C. H., & Floyd, R. L. (2012, July 20). Alcohol use and binge drinking among women of childbearing age–United States, 2006-2010. *MMWR, Morbidity and Mortality Weekly Report, 61*(28), pp. 534–538. Retrieved July 7, 2014.

Marczinski, C. A. (2011). Alcohol mixed with energy drinks: Consumption patterns and motivations for use in U. S. college students. *International Journal of Environmental Research and Public Health, 8*(8), 3232–3245.

Marczinski, C. A. (2014). Combined alcohol and energy drink use: Hedonistic motives, adenosine, and alcohol dependence. *Alcoholism: Clinical and Experimental Research, 38*(7), 1822–1825. doi:10.1111/acer.12493

Marczinski, C. A., & Fillmore, M. T. (2006). Clubgoers and their trendy cocktails: Implications of mixing caffeine into alcohol on information processing and subjective reports of intoxication. *Experimental and Clinical Psychopharmacology, 14*(4), 450–458.

Marshal, M. P., & Molina, B. S. (2006, June). Antisocial behaviors moderate the deviant peer pathway to substance use in children with ADHD. *Journal of Clinical Child & Adolescent Psychology, 35*(2), 216–226. doi:10.1207/s15374424jccp3502_5.

Martens, M. P., Neighbors, C., & Dams-O'Connor, K. (2007). The factor structure of a dichotomously scored Rutgers Alcohol Problem Index. *Journal of Studies on Alcohol and Drugs, 68*(4), 597–606.

Martino, S. C., Tucker, J. S., & Ryan, G. (2011). Increased substance use and risky sexual behavior among migratory homeless youth: Exploring the role of social network composition. *Journal of Youth and Adolescence, 40*(12), 1634–1648. doi:10.1007/s10964-011-9646-6

Maryanoff, B., Nortey, O., & Gardocki, J. (1987). Anticonvulsant O-alkyl sulfamates. 2, 3:4,5-Bis-O-(1-methyethylidene)-beta-D-fructopyranosesulfamate and related compounds. *Journal of Medicinal Chemistry, 30*(5), 880–887.

Masi, G., Manfredi, A., & Nieri, G. (2017, October). A naturalistic comparison of methylphenidate and risperidone monotherapy in drug-naive youth with attention-deficit/hyperactivity disorder comorbid with oppositional defiant disorder and aggression. *Journal of Clinical Psychopharmacology, 37*(5), 590–594. doi:10.10976/JCP.0000000000000747.

Mason, B. J. (2001). Treatment of alcohol-dependent outpatients with acamprosate: A clinical review. *The Journal of Clinical Psychiatry, 62*(Supplement 20), 42–48.

Mason, B. J. (2003). Acamprosate. *Recent Developments in Alcoholism, 16*, 203–215.

Mason, B. J., & Heyser, C. J. (2010a). The neurobiology, clinical efficacy and safety of acamprosate in the treatment of alcohol dependence. *Expert Opinion on Drug Safety, 9*(1), 177–188.

Mason, B. J., & Heyser, C. J. (2010b, March). Acamprosate: A prototypic neuromodulator in the treatment of alcohol dependence. *CNS & Neurological Disorders Drug Targets, 9*(1), 23–32.

Mason, B. J., Quello, S., & Goodell, V. (2014). Gabapentin treatment for alcohol dependence: A randomized clinical trial. *JAMA Internal Medicine, 174*(1), 70–77. doi:10.1001/jamainternmed.2013.11950

Matejcic, M., Gunter, M. J., & Ferrari, P. (2017). Alcohol metabolism and oesephageal cancer: A systematic review of the evidence. *Carcinogenesis, 38*(9), 859–872. doi:10.1093/carcin/bgx067

Mattson, M. E., & Allen, J. P. (1991). Research on matching alcoholic patients to treatments: Findings, issues, and implications. *Journal of Addictive Diseases, 11*(2), 33–49.

Mattson, M. E., Allen, J. P., & Longabaugh, R. (1994, December). A chronological review of empirical studies matching alcoholic clients to treatment. *Journal of Studies on Alcohol Supplement, 12*, 16–29.

Mattson, M. E., Cai, R., & Woodward, A. (2015, June). Emergency department visits vs. fatalities among substance-impaired underage youths involved in motor vehicle crashes. *Journal of Safety Research, 53*, 45–51. doi:10.1016/j.jsr.20125.03.007.

Mattson, M. P. (2000, November 1). Apoptosis in neurodegenerative disorders. *Nature Reviews Molecular Cell Biology, 1*, 120–130.

Maurel, D. B., Boisseau, N., & Benhamou, C. L. (2012). Alcohol and bone: Review of dose effects and mechanisms. *Osteoporosis International, 23*(1), 1–16. doi:10.1007/s00198-011-1787-7

May, P. A., Baete, A., & Russo, J. (2014). Prevalence and characteristics of fetal alcohol spectrum disorders. *Pediatrics, 134*(5), 855–866. doi:10.1542/peds.20123-3319

May, P. A., Chambers, C. D., & Kalberg, W. O. (2018). Prevalence of fetal alcohol spectrum disorders in 4 US communities. *Journal of the American Medical Association, 319*(5), 474–482. doi:10.1001/jama.2017.21896

May, P. A., Keaster, C., & Bozeman, R. (2015, October 1). Prevalence and characteristics of fetal alcohol syndrome and partial fetal alcohol syndrome in a Rocky Mountain Region City. *Drug and Alcohol Dependence, 155*, 118–127. doi:10.1016/j.drugalcdep.20125.08.006.

Mayes, R., Bagwell, C., & Erkulwater, J. (2008). ADHD and the rise in stimulant use among children. *Harvard Review of Psychiatry, 16*(3), 151–166. doi:10.1080/10673220802167782

Mayfield, D., McLeod, G., & Hall, P. (1974). The CAGE questionnaire: Validation of a new alcoholism screening instrument. *American Journal of Psychiatry, 131*(10), 1121–1123.

McAllister, I., & Makkai, T. (1991). Correcting for the underreporting of drug use in opinion surveys. *The International Journal of the Addictions, 26*(9), 945–961.

McBride, D. C., Terry-Elrath, Y. M., & VanderWaal, C. J. (2008). US Public Health Agency involvement in youth-focused illicit drug policy, planning, and prevention at the local level, 1999-2003. *APHA, American Journal of Public Health, 98*(2), 270–277. doi:10.2105/AJPH.2007.112524

McCambridge, J., & Thomas, B. A. (2009). Short forms of the AUDIT in a Web-based study of young drinkers. *Drug and Alcohol Reviews, 28*(1), 18–24. doi:10.1111/j.1465-3362.2008.00010.x

McCarthy, D. M., Tomlinson, K. L., & Anderson, K. G. (2005, March). Relapse in alcohol- and drug-disordered aldolescents with comorbid psychopathology: Changes in psychiatric symptoms. *Psychology of Addictive Behaviors, 19*(1), 28–34. doi:10.1037/0893-164X.19.1.28.

McCaul, M. E., & Petry, N. M. (2003). The role of psychosocial treatments in pharmacotherapy for alcoholism. *The American Journal on Addictions, 12*(Supplement 1), S41-S52.

McCauley, J. L., Calhoun, K. S., & Gidycz, C. A. (2010). Binge drinking and rape: A prospective examination of college women with a history of previous sexual victimization. *Journal of Interpersonal Violence, 25*(9), 1655–1668. doi:10.1177/0886260509354580

McCusker, M. T., Basquille, J., & Khwaja, M. (2002). Hazardous and harmful drinking: A comparison of the AUDIT and CAGE screening questionnaires. *The Quarterly Journal of Medicine, 95*, 591–595.

McDonald, C. C., Sommers, M. S., & Fargo, J. D. (2014, December). Risky driving, mental health, and health-compromising behaviors: Risk clustering in late adolescents and adults. *Injury Prevention, 20*(6), 365–372. doi:10.1136/injurypre-2014-041150.

McGee, E. M. (2000). Alcoholics Anonymous and nursing: Lessons in holism and spiritual care. *Journal of Holistic Nursing, 18*(1), 11–26.

McHugh, R. K., Hearon, B. A., & Otto, M. W. (2010). Cognitive behavioral therapy for substance use disorders. *Psychiatric Clinics of North America, 33*(3), 511–525.

McKay, J. R. (1999). Studies of factors in relapse to alcohol, drug and nicotine use: A critical review of methodologies and findings. *Journal of Studies on Alcohol, 60*(4), 566–576.

McKay, J. R., Franklin, T. R., & Patapis, N. (2006). Conceptual, methodological, and analytical issues in the study of relapse. *Clinical Psychology Reviews, 26*(2), 109–127.

McKetin, R., Coen, A., & Kaye, S. (2015, June 1). A comprehensive review of the effects of mixing caffeinated energy drinks with alcohol. *Drug and Alcohol Dependence, 151*, 15–30. doi:10.1016/j.drugalcdep.20125.01.047.

McKinney, A. (2010). A review of the next day effects of alcohol on subjective mood ratings. *Current Drug Abuse Reviews, 3*(2), 88–91.

McKinnon, S. A., O'rourke, K. M., & Thompson, S. E. (2004). Alcohol use and abuse by adolescents: The impact of living in a border community. *Journal of Adolescent Health, 34*(1), 88–93.

McQuade, W. H., Levy, S. M., & Yanek, L. R. (2000). Detecting symptoms of alcohol abuse in primary care settings. *Archives of Family Medicine, 9*, 814–821.

Mengel, M. B., Searight, H. R., & Cook, K. (2006). Preventing alcohol-exposed pregnancies. *The Journal of the American Board of Family Medicine, 19*(5), 494–505.

Mennella, J. (2001a). Alcohol's effect on lactation. *Alcohol Research & Health, 25*(3), 230–234.

Mennella, J. A. (2001b). Regulation of milk intake after exposure to alcohol in mothers' milk. *Alcoholism, Clinical & Experimental Research, 25*(4), 590–593.

Mennella, J. A., & Beauchamp, G. K. (1999, November). Experience with flavor in mother's milk modifies the infant's acceptance of flavored cereal. *Developmental Psychobiology, 35*(3), 197–203.

Messick, S. (1995). Validity of psychological assessment: Validation of inferences from persons' responses and performances as scientific inquiry into score meaning. *American Psychologist, 50*, 741–749.

Miller, J. W., Naimi, T. S., & Brewer, R. D. (2007). Binge drinking and associated health risk behaviors among high school students. *Pediatrics, 119*(1), 76–85.

Miller, J., & Roache, J. (2009). Benefits of topiramate treatment in a dual-diagnosis patient. *Psychosomatics, 50*(4), 426–427.

Miller, K. E. (2008). Energy drinks, race, and problem behaviors among college students. *Journal of Adolescent Health, 43* (5), 490–497.

Miller, T. W., Leukefeld, C., & Jefferson, B. (1994, September). Dual diagnosis: Clinical issues in substance abuse treatment. *Journal of Contemporary Psychotherapy, 24*(3), 169–177.

Mitchell, S. G., Kelly, S. M., & Gryczynski, J. (2014). The CRAFFT cut-off points and DSM-5 criteria for alcohol and other drugs: A reevaluation and reexamination. *Substance Abuse, 35*(4), 376–380. doi:10.1080/08897077.2014.936992

Mo, Y., Thomas, M. C., & Karras, G. E. (2016, April). Barbiturates for the treatment of alcohol withdrawal syndrome: A systematic review of clinical trials. *Journal of Critical Care, 32*, 101–107. doi:10.1016/j.jcrc.2015.11.022.

Molina, B. S., & Pelham, W. E. (2001, July-August). Substance use, substance abuse, and LD among adolescents with a childhood history of ADHD. *Journal of Learning Disabilities, 34*(4), 333–342. doi:10.1177/002221940103400408.

Molina, B. S., Pelham, W. E., & Gnagy, E. M. (2007). Attention-deficit/hyperactivity disorder risk for heavy drinking and alcohol use disorder is age specific. *Alcoholism: Clinical & Experimental Research, 31*(4), 643–654. doi:10.1111/j.1530-0277.20076.00349.x

Montag, A. (2016). Fetal alcohol-spectrum disorders: Identifying at-risk mothers. *International Journal of Women's Health, 8*, 311–323.

Mouilso, E. R., Fischer, S., & Calhoun, K. S. (2012). A prospective study of sexual assault and alcohol use among first-year college women. *Violence and Victims, 27*(1), 78–94.

Moyer, V. A. (2013). Screening and behavioral counseling interventions in primary care to reduce alcohol misuse: U.S. Preventive Services Task Force recommendations statement. *Annals of Internal Medicine, 159*(3), 210–218. doi:10.7326/0003-4819-159-3-201308060-00652

Muller, C. P., & Homberg, J. R. (2015, January). The role of serotonin in drug use and addiction. *Behavioural Brain Research, 277*, 146–192.

Muzyk, A. J., Leung, J. G., & Nelson, S. (2013, March-April). The role of diazepam loading for the treatment of alcohol withdrawal syndrome in hospitalized patients. *The American Journal on Addictions, 22*(2), 113–118. doi:10.1111/j.1521-0391.2013.00307.x.

Myers, W. C., Donahue, J. E., & Goldstein, M. R. (1994, May). Disulfiram for alcohol use disorders in adolescents. *Journal of the American Academy of Child and Adolescent Psychiatry, 33*(4), 484–489.

Mytton, J. A., DiGuiseppi, C., & Gough, D. A. (2002). School-based violence prevention programs: Systematic review of secondary prevention trials. *Archives of Pediatrics & Adolescent Medicine, 156*(8), 752–762.

Naimi, T. S., Lipscomb, L. E., & Brewer, R. D. (2003). Binge drinking in the preconception period and the risk of unintended pregnancy: Implications for women and their children. *Pediatrics, 111*(5, Part 2), 1136–1141.

Naltrexone. (2009, February 1). *Medline Plus*, 1–4. Retrieved from www.nlm.nih.gov/medlineplus/druginfo/meds/a685041.html

Naltrexone injection. (2010, May 1). *Medline Plus*, 1–4. Retrieved from www.nlm.nih.gov/medlineplus/druginfo/meds/a609007.html

Nayak, M. B., Bond, J. C., & Cherpital, C. J. (2009). Detecting alcohol-related problems in developing countries: A comparison of 2 screening measures in India. *Alcoholism: Clinical & Experimental Research, 33*(12), 2057–2066.

NBC News. (2013, December 6). Teens arrested for letting friend drive drunk before fatal crash. *NBC News*.

NCIPC, National Center for Injury Prevention and Control. (2012, October). Teen drinking and driving: A dangerous mix. *CDC Vitalsigns*. Atlanta, GA: Centers for Disease Control and Prevention.

Neal, D. J., Corbin, W. R., & Fromme, K. (2006). Measurement of alcohol-related consequences among high school and college students: Application of item response models to the Rutgers Alcohol Problem Index. *Psychological Assessment, 18*(4), 402–414.

Nevitt, J. R., Lundak, J., & Codr, J. (2007). An analysis of AUDIT scores of adolescent offenders in two Midwestern counties. *Psychological Reports, 100*(3, part 1), 700–706.

Nevitt, J. R., Lundak, J., & Galardi, G. (2006, April). A profile of adolescent alcohol offenders in two rural Midwestern counties. *Psychological Reports, 98*(2), 379–384. doi:10.2466/pr0.98.2.379-384.

Newman, L. (2016, March 1). As substance abuse rises, hospitals drug test mothers, newborns. *Applied Laboratory Medicine*, 1–5.

Nguyen-Louie, T. T., Castro, N., & Matt, G. E. (2015). Effects of emerging alcohol and marijuana use behaviors on adolescents' neuropsychological functioning over four years. *Journal of Studies on Alcohol and Drugs*, *76*, 738–748.

Nguyen-Louie, T. T., Matt, G. E., & Jacobus, J. (2017). Earlier alcohol use onset predicts poorer neuropsychological functioning in young adults. *Alcoholism: Clinical & Experimental Research*, *41*(12), 2082–2092. doi:10.1111/acer.13503

Nguyen-Louie, T. T., Tracas, A., & Squeglia, L. M. (2016). Learning and memory in adolescent moderate, binge, and extreme-binge drinkers. *Alcoholism: Clinical & Experimental Research*, *40*(9), 1895–1904. doi:10.1111/acer.13160

NIAAA, National Institute on Alcohol Abuse and Alcoholism. (1995). *The Physician's Guide to Helping Patients with Alcohol Problems*. Washington, DC: Government Printing Office.

NIAAA, National Institute on Alcohol Abuse and Alcoholism. (2005, April). The neurotoxicity of alcohol. *Alcohol and the Brain: Neuroscience and Neurobehavior*, 134–146. Bethesda, MD: National Institutes of Health.

NIAAA, National Institute on Alcohol Abuse and Alcoholism. (2006, January). Underage drinking. *Alcohol Alert(67)*. Rockville, MD: U.S. Department of Health and Human Services.

Nock, M. K., Kazdin, A. E., & Hiripi, E. (2006). Prevalece, subtypes, and correlates of DSM-IV conduct disorder in the National Comorbidity Survey Replication. *Psychological Medicine*, *36*(5), 699–710. doi:10.1017/S0033291706007082

Noel, M., O'Connor, R. M., & Boudreau, B. (2010). The Rutgers Alcohol Problem Index (RAPI): A comparison of cut-points in First Nations Mi'Kmaq and Non-Aboriginal adolescents in rural Nova Scotia. *International Journal of Mental Health and Addiction*, *8*, 336–350.

Nordgaard, J., Sass, L. A., & Parnas, J. (2013). The psychiatric interview: Validity, structure, and subjectivity. *European Archives of Psychiatry and Clinical Neurosciences*, *263*, 353–364.

Nordt, S. P., Vilke, G. M., & Clark, R. F. (2012). Energy drink use and adverse effects among emergency department patients. *Journal of Community Health*, *37*(5), 976–981. doi:10.1007/s10900-012-9549-9

Nowinski, J., Baker, S., & Carroll, K. (1992/1999). *Twelve Step Facilitation Therapy Manual: A Clinical Research Guide for Therapists Treating Individuals with Alcohol Abuse and Dependence*. Rockville, MD: National Institute on Alcohol Abuse and Alcoholism.

O'Brien, C. P. (2008a, November). The CAGE questionnaire for detection of alcoholism: A remarkably useful but simple tool. *JAMA, Journal of the American Medical Association*, *300*(17), 2054–2056. doi:10.1001/jama.2008.570.

O'Brien, M. P. (2008b, June). *Epidemiologic Trends in Drug Abuse, Proceedings of the Community Epidemiology Work Group*. National Institutes of Health, National Institute on Drug Abuse. Washington, DC: US Department of Health and Human Services.

O'Brien, W., & Biase, D. V. (1984). The therapeutic community: A current perspective. *Journal of Psychoactive Drugs*, *16*, 9–21.

O'Connor, M. J., & Whaley, S. E. (2003). Alcohol use in prenant low-income women. *Journal of Studies on Alcohol*, *64* (6), 773–783.

Oei, T., & Jackson, P. (1980). Long-term effects of group and individual social skills training with alcoholics. *Addictive Behaviors*, *5*, 129–136.

Oesterle, T. S., Hitschfeld, M. J., & Lineberry, T. W. (2015). CRAFFT as a substance use screening instrument for adolescent psychiatry admissions. *Journal of Psychiatry Practice*, *21*(4), 259–266. doi:10.1097/PRA.0000000000000083

Office of Adolescent Health. (2017, January 25). *United States Adolescent Substance Abuse Facts*. Washington, DC: U.S. Department of Health & Human Services.

Okouchi, M., Ekshyyan, O., & Maracine, M. (2007, August). Neuronal apoptosis in neurodegeneration. *Antioxidants & Redox Signaling*, *9*(8), 1059–1096.

Olmsted, C. L., & Kockler, D. R. (2008). Topiramate for alcohol dependence. *Annals of Pharmacotherapy*, *42*(10), 1475–1480.

Olney, J. W., Wozniak, D. F., & Jevtovic-Todorovic, V. (2002). Drug-induced apoptotic neurodegeneration in the developing brain. *Brain Pathology*, *12*(4), 488–498.

O'Malley, P. M., Johnston, J. L., & Bachman, J. G. (2006, December). How substance use differs among American secondary schools. *Prevention Science*, 7(4), 409–420. doi:10.1007/s11121-006-0050-5.

Osterling, A., Berglund, M., & Nilsson, L. H. (1993). Sex differences in response style to two self-report screening tests on alcoholism. *Scandinavian Journal of Social Medicine*, *21*(2), 83–89.

Ostroumov, A., Thomas, A. M., & Dani, J. A. (2015, October 15). Cigarettes and alcohol: The influence of nicotine on operant alcohol self-administration and the mesolimbic dopamine system. *Biochemical Pharmacology*, *97*(4), 550–557. doi:10.1016/j.bcp.2015.07.038.

Ott, M. Q., Wypij, D., & Corliss, H. L. (2013). Repeated changes in reported sexual orientation identity linked to substance use behaviors in youth. *Journal of Adolescent Health*, *52*(4), 465–472. doi:10.1016/j.jadohealth.2012.08.004

Oural, L., Paris, M. V., & Sullivan, O. (2008, January-February). Pharmacological review of alcoholic dependence treatment. *Vertex, 19*(77), 512–521.

Pagliaro, A. M. (1986). Pharmacologic aspects of nursing: A historical overview. In A. M. Pagliaro & L. A. Pagliaro (Eds.), *Pharmacologic Aspects of Nursing* (pp. 3–29). St. Louis, MI: C. V. Mosby.

Pagliaro, A. M., & Pagliaro, L. A. (1995). Abusable psychotropic use among children and adolescents. In L. A. Pagliaro & A. M. Pagliaro (Eds.), *Problems in Pediatric Drug Therapy* (3rd ed., pp. 507–540). Hamilton, IL: Drug Intelligence.

Pagliaro, A. M., & Pagliaro, L. A. (1996). *Substance Use among Children and Adolescents.* New York: John Wiley & Sons.

Pagliaro, A. M., & Pagliaro, L. A. (1997). Teratogenic effects of in utero exposure to alcohol and other abusable psychotropics. In P. Budetti & M. Haack (Eds.), *Drug-Dependent Mothers and Their Children: Issues in Public Policy and Public Health* (pp. 31–63). New York: Springer.

Pagliaro, A. M., & Pagliaro, L. A. (2000). *Substance Use among Women: A Reference and Research Guide.* Philadelphia, PA: Brunner/Mazel.

Pagliaro, A. M., & Pagliaro, L. A. (2003a). Alcohol and other drug use during pregnancy: Effects on the developing fetus, neonate, and infant. In R. Saitz (Ed.), *Principles of Addiction Medicine* (3rd ed.). Washington, DC: American Society of Addiction Medicine.

Pagliaro, A. M., & Pagliaro, L. A. (2003b). An addictionologist's perspective on catastrophic injury. In K. N. Anchor, J. Shmerling, & J. M. Anchor (Eds.), *The Catastrophic Injury Handbook* (pp. 213–0227). Dubuque, IA: Kendall/Hunt.

Pagliaro, A. M., & Pagliaro, L. A. (2018). *Women's Drug and Substance Abuse: A Comprehensive Analysis and Reflective Synthesis.* New York: Routledge.

Pagliaro, L. A. (1990). Dual diagnosis. *Alberta Psychology, 19*(5), 23–24.

Pagliaro, L. A. (1995). Adolescent depression and suicide. *Canadian Journal of School Psychology, 11*, 191–201.

Pagliaro, L. A. (1995a). The straight dope: A consideration of substance-induced disorders. *Psynopsis, 17*(Spring), 14.

Pagliaro, L. A., & Benet, L. Z. (1975). Critical compilation of terminal half-lives, percent excreted unchanged, and changes of half-life in renal and hepatic dysfunction for studies in humans with references. *Journal of Pharmacokinetics and Biopharmaceutics, 3*, 333–383.

Pagliaro, L. A., & Levin, R. (Eds.). (1979). *Problems in Pediatric Drug Therapy.* Bethesda, MD: Drug Intelligence Publications.

Pagliaro, L. A., & Pagliaro, A. M. (Eds.). (1987). *Problems in Pediatric Drug Therapy* (2nd ed.). Hamilton, IL: Drug Intelligence Publications.

Pagliaro, L. A., & Pagliaro, A. M. (1992). Alcohol metabolism. *CMAJ: Canadian Medical Association Journal, 146*(12), 2141.

Pagliaro, L. A., & Pagliaro, A. M. (1999). *PNDR: Psychologists' Neuropsychotropic Drug Reference.* Philadelphia, PA: Brunner/Mazel.

Pagliaro, L. A., & Pagliaro, A. M. (Eds.). (2002). *Problems in Pediatric Drug Therapy* (4th ed.). Washington, DC: American Pharmaceutical Association.

Pagliaro, L. A., & Pagliaro, A. M. (2004). *Pagliaros' Comprehensive Guide to Drugs and Substances of Abuse* (1st ed.). Washington, DC: American Pharmacists Association.

Pagliaro, L. A., & Pagliaro, A. M. (2009). *Pagliaros' Comprehensive Guide to Drugs and Substances of Abuse* (2nd ed.). Washington, DC: American Pharmacists Association.

Pagliaro, L. A., & Pagliaro, A. M. (2012). *Handbook of Child and Adolescent Drug and Substance Abuse.* Hoboken, NJ: Wiley & Sons.

Pagliaro, L. A., Jaglalsingh, L. H., & Pagliaro, A. M. (1992). Cocaine use and depression. *Canadian Medical Association Journal, 147*, 1636–1637.

Parkhill, M. R., Norris, J., & Davi, K. C. (2014). The role of alcohol use during sexual situations in the relationship between sexual revictimization and women's intentions to engage in unprotected sex. *Violence and Victims, 29*(3), 492–505.

Patrick, M. E., & Schulenberg, J. E. (2012). Prevalence and predictors of adolescent alcohol use and binge drinking in the United States. *Alcohol Research: Current Reviews, 35*(2), 193–200.

Patrick, M. E., Terry-McElrath, Y. M., & Miech, R. A. (2017). Age-specific prevalence of binge and high-intensity drinking among U.S. young adults: Changes from 2005 to 2015. *Alcoholism, Clinical and Experimental Research, 41* (7), 1319–1328. doi:10.1111/acer.13413

Paves, A. P., Pedersen, E. R., & Hummer, J. F. (2012). Prevalence, social contexts, and risks for prepartying among ethnically diverse college students. *Addictive Behaviors, 37*(7), 803–810. doi:10.1016/j.addbeh.2012.02.003

Peadon, E., Rhys-Jones, B., & Bower, C. (2009, May 25). Systematic review of interventions for children with Fetal Alcohol Spectrum Disorders. *BMC Pediatrics, 9*(35), 35. doi:10.1186/1471-2431-9-35.

Pedersen, E. R., & LaBrie, J. (2007). Partying before the party: Examining pepartying behavior among college students. *Journal of American College Health, 56*(3), 237–245. doi:10.3200/JACH.56.3.237-246

Peoples, R. W., Li, C., & Weight, F. F. (1996). Lipid versus protein theories of alcohol action in the nervous system. *Annual Review of Pharmacology and Toxicology, 36*, 185–201.

Petry, N. M. (2000, February 1). A comprehensive guide to the application of contingency management procedures in clinical settings. *Drug and Alcohol Dependence, 58*(1-2), 9–25.

Petry, N. M., Alessi, S. M., & Olmstead, T. A. (2017, June 22). Contingency management treatment for substance use disorders: How far has it come, and where does it need to go? *Psychology of Addictive Behaviors*, 1–10. doi:10.1037/adb0000287.

Pfefferbaum, A., Kwon, D., & Brumback, T. (2017, October 31). Altered brain developmental trajectories in adolescents after initiating drinking. *The American Journal of Psychiatry*. doi: 10.1176/appi.ajp.2017.17040469.

Phillips, G., Turner, B., & Salamanca, P. (2017, September 1). Victimization as a mediator of alcohol use disparities between sexual minority subgroups and sexual majority youth using the 2015 National Youth Risk Behavior Survey. *Drug and Alcohol Dependence, 178*, 355–362. doi:10.1016/j.drugalcdep.2017.05.040.

Piasecki, T. M., Robertson, B. M., & Epler, A. (2010). Hangover and risk for alcohol use disorders: Existing evidence and potential mechanisms. *Current Drug Abuse Reviews, 3*(2), 92–102.

Plosker, G. L. (2015, July). Acamprosate: A review of its use in alcohol dependence. *Drugs, 75*(11), 1255–1268. doi:10.1007/s40265-015-0423-9.

Pokorny, A. D., Miller, B. A., & Kaplan, H. B. (1972). The Brief MAST: A shortened version of the Michigan Alcoholism Screening Test. *The American Journal of Psychiatry, 129*(3), 342–345.

Popova, S., Lange, S., & Probst, C. (2017). Prevalence of alcohol consumption during pregnancy and fetal alcohol spectrum disorders among the general and Aboriginal populations in Canada and the United States. *European Journal of Medical Genetics, 60*(1), 32–48. doi:10.1016/j.ejmg.2016.09.010

Pragst, F., & Yegles, M. (2008). Determination of fatty acid ethyl esters (FAEE) and ethyl glucuronide (EtG) in hair: A promising way for retrospective detection of alcohol abuse during pregnancy? *Therapeutic Drug Monitoring, 30*(2), 255–263. doi:10.1097/FTD.0b013e318167d602

Prat, G., Adan, A., & Perez-Pamies, M. (2008). Neurocognitive effects of alcohol hangover. *Addictive Behaviors, 33*(1), 15–23. doi:10.1016/jaddbeh.2007.05.002

Pregnancy and alcohol: Limitations on criminal prosecution. (2015, January 1). Retrieved March 3, 2016, from APIS- Alcohol Policy Information System, pp. 1–4: http://alcoholpolicy.niaaa.nih.gov/alcohol_and_pregnancy_limitations_on_criminal_prosecution.html

Project MATCH. (1993, December). Project MATCH (Matching Alcoholism Treatment to Client Heterogeneity): Rationale and methods for a multisite clinical trial matching patients to alcoholism treatment. *Alcoholism: Clinical & Experimental Research, 17*(6), 1130–1145.

Qi, Y., Zhang, M., & Li, H. (2014). MicroRNA-29b regulates ethanol-induced neuronal apoptosis in the developing cerebellum throuh SP1/RAX/PKR cascade. *The Journal of Biological Chemistry, 289*(14), 10201–10210.

Quertemont, E. (2004). Genetic polymorphism in ethanol metabolism: Acetaldehyde contribution to alcohol abuse and alcoholism. *Molecular Psychiatry, 9*, 570–581. doi:10.1038/sj.mp.4001497

Quispe Gonzales, J. O., Gomez Giralda, B., & Ruiz-Zorrilla Lopez, C. (2011). Severe ethanol poisoning treated by haemodialysis. *Nefrologia, 31*(2), 226–227.

Raouf, M., Atkinson, T. J., & Crumb, M. W. (2017). Rational dosing of gabapentin and pregabalin in chronic kidney disease. *Journal of Pain Research, 10*, 275–278. doi:10.2147/JPR.S130942

Rehm, J., & Roerecke, M. (2017, November). Cardiovascular effects of alcohol consumption. *Trends in Cardiovascular Medicine, 27*(8), 534–538. doi:10.1016/j.tcm.2017.06.002.

Reinert, D. F., & Allen, J. P. (2007). The alcohol use disorders identification test: An update of research findings. *Alcoholism: Clinical and Experimental Research, 31*(2), 185–199.

Reus, V. I., Fochtmann, L. J., & Bukstein, O. (2018a). The American Psychiatric Association practice guidelines for the pharmacological treatment of patients with alcohol use disorder. *American Journal of Psychiatry, 175*(1), 86–90.

Reus, V. I., Fochtmann, L. J., & Bukstein, O. (2018b). *The American Psychiatric Association Practice Guidelines for the Pharmacological Treatment of Patients with Alcohol Use Disorder*. Washington, DC: American Psychiatric Association.

Rickert, V. I., & Wiermann, C. M. (1998, November). Date rape among adolescents and young adults. *Journal of Pediatric and Adolescent Gynecology, 11*(4), 167–175.

Ricks, J., Replogle, W. H., & Cook, N. J. (2010, August 15). FPIN's clinical inquiries. Management of alcohol withdrawal syndrome. *American Family Physician, 82*(4), 344–347.

Riley, E. P., & McGee, C. L. (2005). Fetal alcohol spectrum disorders: An overview with emphasis on changes in brain and behavior. *Experimental Biology and Medicine, 230*, 357–365.

Rist, F., Glockner-Rist, A., & Demmel, R. (2009). The Alcohiol Use Disorders Identification Test revised: Establishing its structure using nonlinear factor analysis and identifying subgroups of respondents using latent class factor analysis. *Drug and Alcohol Dependence, 100*(1–2), 71–82.

Roeggla, G., Roeggla, H., & Roeggla, M. (1995). Effect of alcohol on acute ventilatory adaptation to mild hypoxia at moderate altitude. *Annals of Internal Medicine, 122*(12), 925–927.

Roerecke, M., & Rehm, J. (2014, October 21). Alcohol consumption, drinking patterns, and ischemic heart disease: A narrative review of meta-analyses and a systematic review and meta-analysis of the impact of heavy drinking occasions on risk for moderate drinkers. *BMC Medicine, 12*, 182. doi:10.1186/s12916-014-0182-6.

Rohsenow, D. J., Tidey, J. W., & Kahler, C. W. (2015, April). Intolerance for withdrawal discomfort and motivation predict voucher-based smoking treatment outcomes for smokers with substance use disorders. *Addictive Behaviors, 43*, 18–24. doi:10.1016/j.addbeh.2014.12.003.

Rojmahamongkol, P., Cheema-Hasan, A., & Weitzman, C. (2015, April). Do pediatricians recognize fetal alcohol spectrum disorders in children with developmental and behavioral problems? *Journal of Developmental & Behavioral Pediatrics, 36*(3), 197–202.

Room, R., & Greenfield, T. (1993). Alcoholics Anonymous, other 12-step movements and psychotherapy in the US population, 1990. *Addiction, 88*, 555–562.

Rosario, M., Reisner, S. L., & Corliss, H. L. (2014, September). Sexual-orientation disparities in substance use in emerging adults: A function of stress and attachment paradigms. *Psychology of Addictive Behaviors, 28*(3), 790–804. doi:10.1037/a0035499.

Rosner, S., Hackl-Herrwerth, A., & Leucht, S. (2010). Acamprosate for alcohol dependence. *Cochrane Database of Systematic Reviews, 9*, CD004332.

Ross, E. J., Graham, D. L., & Money, K. M. (2015). Developmental consequences of fetal exposure to drugs: What we know and what we still must learn. *Neuropsychopharmacology, 40*(1), 61–87. doi:10.1038/np.2014.147

Ross, H. E., Gavin, D. R., & Skinner, H. A. (1990). Diagnostic validity of the MAST and the alcohol dependence scale in the assessment of DSM-III alcohol disorders. *Journal of Studies on Alcoholism, 51*(6), 506–513.

Rossheim, M. E., Stephenson, C. J., & Thombs, D. L. (2017). Characteristics of drinking events associated with heavy episodic drinking among adolescents in the United States. *Drug and Alcohol Dependence, 181*, 50–57. doi:10.1016/j.drugalcdep.2017.09.018

Rothman, E. F., McNaughton Reyes, R. L., & Johnson, R. M. (2012). Does the alcohol make them do it? Dating violence perpetration and drinking among youth. *Epidemiologic Reviews, 34*(1), 103–119.

Rowe, C., Santos, G. M., & McFarland, W. (2015, February 1). Prevalance and correlates of substance use among trans female youth ages 16-24 years in the San Francisco Bay Area. *Drug and Alcohol Dependence, 147*, 160–166. doi:10.1016/j.drugalcdep.2014.11.023.

Rundio, A. (2010, March). Disulfiram (Antabuse). *Journal of Addictions Nursing, 21*(1), 54–55.

Russell, M., Martier, S. S., & Sokol, R. J. (1994, October). Screening for pregnancy risk-driving. *Alcoholism, Clinical and Experimental Research, 18*(5), 1156–1161.

Russell, M., Martier, S. S., & Sokol, R. J. (1996). Detecting risk drinking during pregnancy: A comparison of four screening questionnaires. *American Journal of Public Health, 86*(10), 1435–1439. doi:10.2105/AJPH.86.10.1435

Sacks, J. J., Gonzales, K. R., & Bouchery, E. E. (2015). 2010 National and state costs of excessive alcohol consumption. *AJPM, American Journal of Preventive Medicine, 49*(5), e73–e79.

Sahn, S. A., Lakshminarayan, S., & Pierson, D. J. (1975). Effect of ethanol on the ventilatory responses to oxygen and carbon dioxide in man. *Clinical Science and Molecular Medicine, 49*(1), 33–38.

Saivin, S., Hulot, T., & Chabac, S. (1998, November). Clinical pharmacokinetics of acamprosate. *Clinical Pharmacokinetics, 35*(5), 331–345.

Sales, J. M., Brown, J. L., & Vissman, A. T. (2012). The association between alcohol use and sexual risk behaviors among African American women across three developmental periods: A review. *Current Drug Abuse Reviews, 5*(2), 117–128.

SAMHSA, Substance Abuse and Mental Health Services Administration. (2013). Systems-Level Implementation of Screening, Brief Intervention, and Referral to Treatment. *Technical Assistance Publication (TAP) Series 33*. Rockville, MD: Substances Abuse and Mental Health Services Administration.

SAMHSA, Substance Abuse and Mental Health Services Administration. (2014). Results from the 2013 National Survey on Drug Use and Health: Summary of National Findings. *NSDUH Series H-48*, 1–170. Rockville, MD: SAMHSA.

Sampson, P. D., Streissguth, A. P., & Bookstein, F. L. (1997). Incidence of fetal alcohol syndrome and prevalence of alcohol-related neurodevelopmental disorder. *Teratology, 56*(5), 317–326. doi:10.1002/%28SICI%291096-9926(199711)56:5<317::AID-TERA5>3.0XO:2-U

Saremi, A., Hanson, R. L., & Williams, D. E. (2001). Validity of the CAGE questionnaire in an American Indian population. *Journal of Studies on Alcoholism, 62*(3), 294–300.

Sarkar, M., Einarson, T., & Koren, G. (2010). Comparing the effectiveness of TWEAK and T-ACE in determining problem drinkers in pregnancy. *Alcohol and Alcoholism, 45*(4), 356–360. doi:10.1093/alcalc/agq022

Sarlin, E. (2018, June 25). Outcomes of computerized CBT rival those of clinician-delivered CBT. *NIDA Notes*, 1–2. National Institute on Drug Abuse.

Saunders, J. B., & Aasland, O. G. (1987). *WHO Collabortative Project on Identification and Treament of Persons with Harmful Alcohol Consumption. Report on Phase I. Development of a Screening Instrument*. Geneva, Switzerland: World Health Organization.

Saunders, J. B., Aasland, O. G., & Babor, T. F. (1993). Development of the Alcohol Use Disorders Identification Test (AUDIT): WHO Collaborative Project on Early Detection of Persons with Harmful Alcohol Consumption – II. *Addiction, 88*(6), 791–804.

Schmidt, K. J., Doshi, M. R., & Holzhausen, J. M. (2016). Treatment of severe alcohol withdrawal. *The Annals of Pharmacotherapy*, *50*(5), 389–401. doi:10.117/1060028016629161

Schweighofer, N., Bertin, M., & Shishida, K. (2008). Low-serotonin levels increase delayed reward discounting in humans. *The Journal of Neuroscience*, *28*(17), 4528–4532.

Seale, J. P., Boltri, J. M., & Shellenberger, S. (2006). Primary care validation of a single screening question for drinkers. *Journal of Studies on Alcohol*, *67*(5), 778–784.

Searight, R. (2009). Realistic approaches to counseling in the office setting. *American Family Physician*, *79*(4), 277–284.

Selin, K. H. (2003). Test-retest reliability of the Alcohol Use Disorder Identification Test in a general population sample. *Alcoholism: Clinical & Experimental Research*, *27*(9), 1428–1435.

Sellers, E. M., Naranjo, C. A., & Harrison, M. (1983, December). Diazepam loading: Simplified treatment of alcohol withdrawal. *Clinical Pharmacology and Therapeutics*, *34*(6), 822–826.

Selzer, M. L. (1971). The Michigan Alcoholism Screening Test: The quest for a new diagnostic instrument. *The American Journal of Psychiatry*, *127*(12), 1653–1658. doi:10.1176/ajp.127.12.1653

Selzer, M. L., Vinokur, A., & Van Rooijen, L. J. (1975). A self-administered Short Michigan Alcohol Screening Test (SMAST). *Journal of Studies on Alcohol*, *36*(1), 117–126.

Sharma, B. R. (2007). Acquaintance rape among adolescents and the youth: A fast emerging public health problem. *Trends in Medical Research*, *2*(1), 21–26.

Sher, L., Stanley, B. H., & Harkavy-Friedman, J. M. (2008). Depressed patients with co-occurring alcohol use disorders: A unique patient population. *The Journal of Clinical Psychiatry*, *69*(6), 907–915.

Shields, A. L., & Caruso, J. C. (2003). Reliability generalization of the Alcohol Use Disorders Identification Test. *Educational and Psychological Measurement*, *63*(3), 404–413.

Shields, A. L., Howell, R. T., & Potter, J. S. (2007). The Michigan Alcoholism Screening Test and its shortened form: A meta-analytic inquiry into score reliability. *Substance Use & Misuse*, *42*(11), 1783–1800.

Shinn, A. K., & Greenfield, S. F. (2010). Topiramate in the treatment of substance-related disorders: A critical review of the literature. *The Journal of Clinical Psychiatry*, *71*(5), 634–648.

Shpilenya, L. S., Muzychenko, A. P., & Gasbarrini, G. (2002). Metadoxine in acute alcohol intoxication: A double-blind, randomized, placebo-controlled study. *Alcoholism, Clinical and Experimental Research*, *26*(3), 340–346.

Shrier, L. A., Harris, S. K., & Kurland, M. (2003, June). Substance use problems and associated psychiatric symptoms among adolescents in primary care. *Pediatrics*, *111*(6 Part 1), e699–e705.

Shrout, P., & Fleiss, J. L. (1979). Intraclass correlation: Uses in assessing rater reliability. *Psychological Bulletin*, *86*(2), 420–428.

Sinzig, J., Dopfner, M., & Lehmkuhl, G. (2007, August). Long-acting methylphenidate has an effect on aggressive behavior in children with attention-deficit/hyperactivity disorder. *Journal of Child and Adolescent Psychopharmacology*, *17*(4), 421–432. doi:10.1089/cap.2007.0011.

Skinner, B. F. (1938). *The Behavior of Organisms: An Experimental Analysis*. Englewood Cliffs, NJ: Prentice-Hall.

Skinner, H. A., & Sheu, W. J. (1982). Reliability of alcohol use indices: The Lifetime Drinking History and the MAST. *Journal of Studies on Alcohol*, *43*, 1157–1170.

Skinner, M. D., Lahmek, P., & Pham, H. (2014). Disulfiram efficacy in the treatment of alcohol dependence: A meta-analysis. *PLoS One*, *9*(2), e87366. doi:10.1371/journal.pone.0087366

Skinner, M. L., Kristman-Valente, A. N., & Herrenkohl, T. I. (2016, March 1). Adult binge drinking: Childhood sexual abuse, gender and the role of adolescent alcohol-related experiences. *Alcohol and Alcoholism*, *51*(2), 136–141.

Slaughter, L. (2000). Involvement of drugs in sexual assault. *Journal of Reproductive Medicine*, *45*(5), 425–430.

Slesnick, N., & Prestopnik, J. (2005). Dual and multiple diagnosis among substance using runaway youth. *The American Journal of Drug and Alcohol Abuse*, *31*(1), 179–201.

Slesnick, N., & Zhang, J. (2016, September). Family systems therapy for substance-using mothers and their 8- to 16-year old children. *Psychology of Addictive Behaviors*, *30*(6), 619–629. doi:10.1037/adb0000199.

Smith, L. A., Gates, S., & Foxcroft, D. (2006, January 25). Therapeutic communities for substance related disorder. *Cochrane Database of Systematic Reviews*, *1*, CD005338.

Smith, P. H., Homish, G. G., & Leonard, K. E. (2012). Intimate partner violence and specific substance use disorders: Findings from the National Epidemiologic Survey on Alcohol and Related Conditions. *Psychology of Addictive Behaviors*, *26*(2), 236–245. doi:10.1037/a0024855

Smitherman, C. H. (1994). The lasting impact of fetal alcohol syndrome and fetal alcohol effect on children and adolescents. *Journal of Pediatric Health Care*, *8*, 121–126.

Snipes, D. J., Green, B. A., & Javier, S. J. (2014). The use of alcohol mixed with energy drinks and experiences of sexual victimization among male and female college students. *Addictive Behaviors*, *39*(1), 259–264. doi:10.1016/j.addbeh.2013.10.005

Soghoian, S., Wiener, S. W., & Diaz-Alcala, J. E. (2016, January 6). Disulfiram toxicity. *Medscape*.

Sokol, R. J., & Clarren, S. K. (1989). Guidelines for use of terminology describing the impact of prenatal alcohol on the offspring. *Alcoholism: Clinical and Experimental Research*, *13*(4), 597–598.

Sokol, R. J., Martier, S. S., & Ager, J. W. (1989). The T-ACE questions: Practical prenatal detection of risk-drinking. *AJOG, American Journal of Obstetrics & Gynecology*, *160*(4), 863–868.

Sood, B., Delaney-Black, V., & Covington, C. (2001). Prenatal alcohol exposure and childhood behavior at age 6 and 7 years: I. dose-response effect. *Pediatrics, 108*, E34.

Soyka, M., & Rosner, S. (2010). Nalmefene for treatment of alcohol dependence. *Expert Opinion on Investigational Drugs, 19*(11), 1451–1459.

Spatz-Widom, C., & Hiller-Strumhofel, S. (2001). Alcohol abuse as a risk factor for and consequence of child abuse. *Alcohol Research & Health, 25*(1), 52–57.

Spearman, C. (1904). The proof and measurement of association between two things. *The American Journal of Psychology, 15*, 72–101.

Spohr, H. L., Willms, J., & Steinhausen, H. C. (1993). Prenatal alcohol exposure and long-term developmental consequences. *The Lancet, 341*(8850), 907–910.

Spohr, H. L., Willms, J., & Steinhausen, H. C. (2007). Fetal Alcohol Spectrum Disorders in young adulthood. *The Journal of Pediatrics, 150*(2), 175–179.

Squeglia, L. M., & Gray, K. M. (2016). Alcohol and drug use and the developing brain. *Current Psychiatry Reports, 18*(5), 46. doi:10.1007/s11920-016-0689-y

St. George, D. (2015, September 10). Teen driver in fatal alcohol-related crash is sentenced to 18 months in jail. *The Washington Post.*

Stanley, K. M., Worrall, C. L., & Lunsford, S. L. (2005). Experience with an adult alcohol withdrawal syndrome practice guideline in internal medicine patients. *Pharmacotherapy, 25*(8), 1073–1083. doi:10.1592/phco.2005.25.8.1073

Stanwood, C. (2017, September 14). *Reports show WF teacher allegedly had sexual relationship with student, gave alcohol to minors.* Retrieved from West Fargo, N. D. (Valley News Live): www.valleynewslive.com/content/news/Reports-show-WF-teacher-allegedly-had-sexual-relationship-with-student-gave-alcohol-to-minors-444530

Stead, L. F., & Lancaster, T. (2005, April 18). Group behavior therapy programmes for smoking cessation. *Cochrane Database of Systematic Reviews, 2*, CD001007.

Steinbauer, J. R., Cantor, S. B., & Holzer, C. E. (1998). Ethnic and sex bias in primary care screening tests for alcohol use disorders. *Annals of Internal Medicine, 129*(5), 353–362.

Stewart, S. H. (2009). Women, girls, and alcohol. In K. T. Brady (Ed.), *Women and Addiction: A Comprehensive Handbook* (pp. 341–359). New York, NY: Guilford.

Storgaard, H., Nielsen, S. D., & Gluud, C. (1994, September). The validity of the Michigan Alcoholism Screening Test (MAST). *Alcohol and Alcoholism, 29*(5), 493–503.

Stormshak, E. A., & Dishion, T. J. (2009). A school-based, family-centered intervention to prevent substance use: The family check-up. *The American Journal of Drug and Alcohol Abuse, 35*(4), 227–232. doi:10.1080/00952990903005908

Stormshak, E. A., Fosco, G. M., & Dishion, T. J. (2010, June). Implementing interventions with families in schools to increase youth school engagement: The Family Check-Up model. *School Mental Health, 2*(2), 82–92. doi:10.1007/s12310-009-9025-6.

Stowell, R. J. (1991). Dual diagnosis issues. *Psychiatric Annals, 21*(2), 98–104. doi:10.3928/0048-5713-19910201-09

Stranger, C., Lansing, A. H., & Budney, A. J. (2016, October). Advances in research on contingency management for adolescent substance use. *Child & Adolescent Psychiatric Clinics of North America, 25*(4), 645–659. doi:10.1016/j.chc.2016.05.002.

Streissguth, A. P., Randels, S. P., & Smith, D. F. (1991). A test-retest study of intelligence in patients with fetal alcohol syndrome: Implications for care. *Journal of the American Academy of Child & Adolescent Psychiatry, 30*(4), 584–587. doi:10.1097/00004583-199107000-00009

Striley, C. W., & Khan, S. R. (2014, July). Review of the energy drink literature from 2013: Findings continue to support most risk from mixing with alcohol. *Current Opinion in Psychiatry, 27*(4), 263–268. doi:10.1097/YCO.0000000000000070.

Stuart, G. L., Meehan, J. C., & Moore, T. M. (2006). Examining a conceptual framework of intimate partner violence in men and women arrested for domestic violence. *Journal of Studies on Alcohol, 67*(1), 102–112.

Stuart, G. L., Moore, T. M., & Ramsey, S. E. (2004). Hazardous drinking and relationship violence perpetration and victimization in women arrested for domestic violence. *Journal of Studies on Alcohol, 65*(1), 46–53.

Stuart, G. L., Temple, J. R., & Follansbee, K. W. (2008). The role of drug use in a conceptual model of intimate partner violence in men and women arrested for domestic violence. *Psychology of Addictive Behaviors, 22*(1), 12–24. doi:10.1037/0893-164X.22.1.12

Sung, J. (2016, August 26). *Baby covered in vomit bathed by cops after being found in backseat of drunk driver.* Retrieved August 26, 2016, from http://globalnews.ca/news/2905718/baby-covered-in-vomit-bathed-by-cops-after-being-found-in-backseat-of-drunk-driver/?utm_source=Article&utm_m.

Sussman, S. (2010, March). A review of Alcoholics Anonymous/Narcotics Anonymous programs for teens. *Evaluation & the Health Professions, 33*(1), 26–55. doi:10.1177/0163278709356186.

Swendsen, J., Burstein, M., & Case, B. (2012). Use and abuse of alcohol and illicit drugs in US adolescents. *Archives of General Psychiatry, 69*(4), 390–398. doi:10.1001/archgenpsychiatry.2011.1503

Swift, R. (2007). Emerging approaches to managing alcohol dependence. *AJHP, American Journal of Health-System Pharmacy*, *64*(5, Supplement 3), S12–S22.

Szapocznik, J., & Williams, R. A. (2000). Brief Strategic Family Therapy: Twenty-five years of interplay among theory, resaearch and practice in adolescent behavior problems and drug abuse. *Clinical Child and Family Psychological Review*, *3*(2), 117–134.

Tan, C. H., Denny, C. H., & Cheal, N. E. (2015, September 25). Alcohol use and binge drinking among women of childbearing age – United States, 2011-2013. *Morbidity and Mortality Weekly Report (MMWR)*, *64*(37), 1042–1046.

Tanaka, F., Yamamoto, K., & Suzuki, S. (2010). Strong interaction between the effects of alcohol consumption and smoking on oesophageal squamous cell carcinoma among individuals with ADH1B and/or ALDH2 risk alleles. *Gut*, *59*(11), 1457–1464. doi:10.1136/gut.2009.205724

Tchekmedyian, A. (2017, July 30). Teen arrested in drunk driving crash that left expectant father dead, police say. *Los Angeles Times*.

Teitelbaum, L., & Mullen, B. (2000). The validity of the MAST in psychiatric settings: A meta-analytic integration. *Journal of Studies on Alcoholism*, *61*(2), 254–261.

Temcheff, C. E., Dery, M., & St-Pierre, R. A. (2016). Precocious initiation into smoking, alcohol use, and gambling among children with conduct disorder. *The Canadian Journal of Psychiatry*, *61*(1), 50–58. doi:10.1177/0706743715620402

Testa, M., & Livingston, J. A. (2009). Alcohol consumption and women's vulnerability to sexual victimization: Can reducing women's drinking prevent rape? *Substance Use & Misuse*, *44*(9–10), 1349–1376. doi:10.1080/1086080902961468

Teutsch, S. M., Baldwin, J. A., & Degutis, L. C. (2018, January 17). New report calls for lowering blood alcohol concentration levels for driving, increasing federal and state alcohol taxes, increasing enforcement, among other recommendations. *News, The National Academies of Sciences, Engineering, and Medicine*, 1–6. Washington, DC.

The Bakersfield Californian. (2018, January 15). Teen dies after falling out of car window, driver arrested on suspicion of DUI. *The Bakersfield Californian*. Retrieved from www.bakersfield.com/news/breaking/teen-dies-after-falling-out-of-car-window-driver-arrested/article_c9a3c4ce-fa02-11e7-b892-ff17cfa94be2.html

The Partnership at Drugfree.org; MetLife Foundation. (2011, April 6). *2010 partnership attitude tracking study: Teens and parents*. MetLife Foundation. Retrieved November 23, 2017, from www.drugfree.org

Thomas, S., Cannon, C., & French, J. (2015). The effects of state alcohol and pregnancy policies on women's health and healthy pregnancies. *Journal of Women, Politics & Policy*, *36*, 68–94.

Thompson, N. J., McGee, R. E., & Mays, D. (2012). Race, ethnicity, substance use, and unwanted sexual intercourse among adolescent females in the United States. *Western Journal of Emergency Medicine*, *13*(3), 283–303. doi:10.5811/westjem.2012.3.11774

Thompson, W. (2018, November 27). Which factors lead to misdiagnosis of alcohol-related problems? *Medscape*, 1–2.

Timko, C., Moos, B. S., & Moos, R. H. (2009). Gender differences in 16-year trends in assault- and police-related problems due to drinking. *Addictive Behaviors*, *34*(9), 744–750. doi:10.1016/j.addbeh.2009.04.013

Tollefson, G. D. (1989). Serotonin and alcohol: Interrelationships. *Psychophathology*, *22*(Supplement 1), 37–48.

Tourangeau, R., & Yan, T. (2007). Sensitive questions in surveys. *Psychological Bulletin*, *133*(5), 859–883.

Ullman, S. E., & Sigurvinsdottir, R. (2015). Intimate partner violence and drinking among victims of adult sexual assault. *Journal of Agression, Maltreatment, & Trauma*, *24*(2), 117–130. doi:10.1080/10926771.2015.996312

Upadhyaya, H. P. (2008). Substance use disorders in children and adolescents with attention-deficit/hyperactivity disorder: Implications for treatment and the role of the primary care physician. *Primary Care Companion to the Journal of Clinical Psychiatry*, *10*(3), 211–221.

USDHHS, U.S. Department of Health and Human Services, Office of the Surgeon General. (2016). *Facing Addiction in America: The Surgeon General's Report on Alcohol, Drugs, and Health, Executive Summary*. Washington, DC: Health and Human Services. Retrieved December 14, 2016.

Valliant, G. E. (2005). Alcoholics Anonymous: Cult or cure? *Australian & New Zealand Journal of Psychiatry*, *39*(6), 431–436. doi:10.1080/j.1440-1614.2005.01600.x

Van Skike, C. E., Maggio, S. E., & Reynolds, A. R. (2015, February 4). Critical needs in drug discovery for cessation of alcohol and nicotine polysubstance abuse. *Progress in Neuropsychopharmacology & Biological Psychiatry*, *65*, 269–287. doi:10.1016/j.pnpbp.2015.11.004.

Vaux, K. K. (2016, October 22). Fetal alcohol syndrome. *Medscape*, 1–2.

Verplaetse, T. L., & McKee, S. A. (2017, March). An overview of alcohol and tobacco/nicotine interactions in the human laboratory. *The American Journal of Drug and Alcohol Abuse*, *43*(2), 186–196. doi:10.1080/00952990.2016.1189927.

Vezali Costardi, J. V., Teruaki Nampo, R. A., & Lourenco Silva, G. (2015). A review on alcohol: From the central action mechanism to chemical dependency. *Revista Da Associacao Medica Brasileira*, *61*(4), 381–387.

Vidair, H. B., Feyijinmi, G. O., & Feindler, E. L. (2017, March). Termination in cognitive-behavioral therapy with children, adolescents, and parents. *Psychotherapy, 54*(1), 15–21. doi:10.1037/pst0000086.

Voas, R. B., Tippetts, A. S., & Fell, J. C. (2003). Assessing the effectiveness of minimum legal drnking age and zero tolerance laws in the United States. *Accident Analysis and Prevention, 35*, 579–587.

Volpicelli, J. R., Clay, K. L., & Watson, N. T. (1995). Naltrexone in the treatment of alcoholism: Predicting response to naltrexone. *The Journal of Clinical Psychiatry, 56*(Supplement 7), 39–44.

Vonghia, L., Leggio, L., & Ferrulli, A. (2008). Acute alcohol intoxication. *European Journal of Internal Medicine, 19*, 561–567. doi:10.1016/j.ejim.2007.06.033

Vreeman, R. C., & Carroll, A. E. (2007). A systematic review of school-based interventions to prevent bullying. *Archives of Pediatric and Adolescent Medicine, 161*(1), 78–88. doi:10.1001/archpedi.161.1.78

Waldron, H. B., & Kaminer, Y. (2004). On the learning curve: The emerging evidence supporting cognitive-behavioral therapies for adolescent substance abuse. *Addiction, 99*(Supplement 2), 93–105.

Walter, K. N., & Petry, N. M. (2016). Motivation and contingency management treatments for substance use disorders. *Current Topics in Behavioral Neurosciences, 27*, 569–581. doi:10.1007/7854_2015_374

Washington State Department of Health. (2015, July) *Gudelines for Testing and Reporting Drug Exposed Newborns in Washington State*. Olympia, Washington: Author.

Weikle, B. (2016, September 13). Universities face increasing pressure to address campus sexual assault. *CBC News*. CBC News.

Weintraub, S. J. (2017). Diazepam in the treatment of moderate to severe alcohol withdrawal. *CNS Drugs, 31*(2), 87–92. doi:10.1007/s40263-016-0403-y

Weisner, C., Greenfield, T., & Room, R. (1995). Trends in the treatment of alcohol problems in the US general population: 1979 through 1990. *AJPH, American Journal of Public Health, 85*, 55–60.

WFLA Staff (2017, March 23). *Deputies: Teacher and student had sex, drank alcohol, used drugs*. Retrieved from NBC4i.com: http://nbc4i.com/2017/03/23/deputies-teacher-and-student-had-sex-drank-alcohol-used-drugs/

White, C., Lindsey, S., & Vincente, C. (1981). Alcohol increases sleep apnea and oxygen desaturation in asymptomatic men. *The American Journal of Medicine, 71*(2), 240–245.

White, H. R., & Labouvie, E. W. (1989). Toward the assessment of adolescent problem drinking. *Journal of Studies on Alcohol, 50*(1), 30–37.

White, H. R., & Labouvie, E. W. (2000). Longitudinal trends in problem drinking as measured by the Rutgers Alcohol Problem Index. *Alcoholism: Clinical & Experimental Research, 24*(5, Supplement 1), 76A.

Wilens, T. E., Adler, L. A., & Adams, J. (2008). Misuse and diversion of stimulants prescribed for ADHD: A systematic review of the literature. *Journal of the American Academy of Child & Adolescent Psychiatry, 47*(1), 21–31. doi:10.1097/chi.0b013e31815a56f1

Williams, A. F., & Tefft, B. C. (2014, February). Characteristics of teens-with-teens fatal crashes in the United States, 2005-2010. *Journal of Safety Research, 48*, 37–42. doi:10.1016/j.jsr.2013.11.001.

Williams, C. L., Perry, C. L., & Dudovitz, B. (1995, December). A home-based prevention program for sixth-grade alcohol use: Results from project Northland. *The Journal of Primary Prevention, 16*(2), 125–147. doi:10.1007/BF02407336.

Williams, R. D., Housman, J. M., & Woolsey, C. L. (2018). High-risk driving behaviors among 12th grade students: Differences between alcohol-only and alcohol mixed with energy drink users. *Substance Use & Misuse, 53*(1), 137–142. doi:10.1080/10826084.2017.1327973

Williams, R. H., & Erickson, T. (1998). Evaluating toxic alcohol poisoning in the emergency setting. *Laboratory Medicine, 29*(2), 102–108.

Wilson, F. A., Stimpson, J. P., & Tibbits, M. K. (2013, November). The role of alcohol use on recent trends in distracted driving. *Accident Analysis & Prevention, 60*, 189–192. doi:10.1016/j.aap.2013.08.025.

Winek, C. L., & Murphy, K. L. (1984, July). The rate and kinetic order of ethanol elimination. *Forensic Science International, 25*(3), 159–166.

Wood, A. M., Kaptoge, S., & Butterworth, A. S. (2018, April 14). Risk thresholds for alcohol consumption: Combined analysis of individual-participant data for 599,912 current drinkers in 83 prospective studies. *The Lancet, 391*, 1513–1523.

Wright, T. M., & Myrick, H. (2006, December). Acamprosate: A new tool in the battle against alcohol dependence. *Neuropsychiatric Disease and Management, 2*(4), 445–453.

WVLT8. (2018, May 31). Rape reported at UT campus fraternity. *WVLT*. Knoxville, TN: WVLT.

Xiao, Q., Weiner, H., & Crabb, D. W. (1996). The mutation in the mitochondrial aldehyde dehydrogenase (ALDH2) gene responsible for alcohol-induced flushing increases turnover of the enzyme tetramers in a dominant fashion. *Journal of Clinical Investigation, 98*(9), 2027–2032.

Yahn, S. L., Watterson, L. R., & Olive, M. F. (2013). Safety and efficacy of acamprosate for the treatment of alcohol dependence. *Substance Abuse, 7*, 1–12. doi:10.4137/SART.S9345

Yonker, J. E., Nilsson, L. G., & Herlitz, A. (2005). Sex Differences in Spatial Visualization and Episodic Memory as a Function of Alcohol Consumption. *Alcohol and Alcoholism, 40*(3): 201–207. Retrieved June 30, 2014.

Young, A., Grey, M., & Abbey, A. (2008). Alcohol-related sexual assault victimization among adolescents: Prevalence, characteristics, and correlates. *Journal of Studies on Alcohol and Drugs, 69*(1), 39–48.

Zamboanga, B. L., Tomaso, C. C., & Cloutier, R. M. (2016). Drinking games participation among high school and incoming college students: A narrative review. *Journal of Addictions Nursing, 27*(1), 24–E1. doi:10.1097/JAN.0000000000000108

Zinberg, N. E. (1986). *Drug, Set, and Setting: The Basis for Controlled Intoxicant Use*. New Haven, CT: Yale Univeristy Press.

Zung, B. J. (1982, April). Evaluation of the Michigan Alcoholism Screening Test (MAST) in assessing lifetime and recent problems. *Journal of Clinical Psycholology, 38*(2), 425–439.

2
Amphetamines and Cocaine

The "amphetamines" and "cocaine" are two major subclasses of the psychostimulants[1] that are commonly used by adolescents and young adults in the U.S., particularly homeless adolescents and undergraduate university/college students. Although children are not as likely to "recreationally" use these two subclasses of the psychostimulants, they are likely to be exposed to them by their: (1) pediatricians, in the context of the medical management of attention-deficit/hyperactivity disorder (ADHD); and (2) parent(s), siblings, and others, who illicitly produce, deal, or use these psychostimulants. Unfortunately, regarding the latter, many fetuses and neonates, whose mothers use amphetamines or cocaine, are placed at significant risk for harmful effects and toxicities, primarily through in utero exposure and/or breastfeeding. In addition, young children may suffer serious harmful effects and toxicities due to unintentional poisonings and overdosages, which may be fatal.

In order to provide health and social care professionals with a comprehensive understanding of child, adolescent, and young adult exposure to and use of the amphetamines and cocaine, the following topics are presented and discussed separately for each of these major psychostimulants in their own section:

1. Discovery, or synthesis;
2. Chemistry;
3. Pharmacology: pharmacodynamics; pharmacokinetics; drug–drug interactions; and undesired, or harmful, effects and toxicities—including physical and psychological dependence or use disorder; overdosage; pediatric poisoning; and effects on pregnancy, lactation, and mothering;
4. Medical Use;
5. New millennial trends and factors associated with: (1) neonatal, infant, and child exposure; and (2) adolescent and young adult use;
6. Age-appropriate assessment and diagnosis;
7. Common contemporaneous diagnoses;
8. Pharmacotherapy and psychotherapy/counseling.

We begin with the amphetamines.

Amphetamines

The amphetamines (see Table 2.1) include the: (1) licit, prescription amphetamines (e.g., amphetamine; dextroamphetamine, Dexedrine®; mixed amphetamines, Adderall®),[2] which are

1 See Chapter 3, "Caffeine and Nicotine," for a discussion of two other major subclasses of the psychostimulants.

2 The psychostimulant, methylphenidate (Ritalin®)—"The Smart Drug"—although not an amphetamine, is a closely related "chemical cousin" of the amphetamines (i.e., they are both "substituted phenethylamines"). Like the amphetamines, methylphenidate, is also widely used medically for the management of ADHD among children, adolescents, and young adults in the U.S. It is also widely "illicitly" used by adolescents and young adults. Consequently, a discussion of methylphenidate is included in this section.

Table 2.1 Amphetamines and Closely Related Psychostimulants

Psychostimulant Subclassification	*Generic Name*	*Brand/ Trade Names*[3]	*Common Street Names*[4]
Amphetamines			
	Amphetamine[5]	Adzenys XR-ODT®;[6] Evekeo®	"Ace;" "Amp;" "Co-Pilot"
	Dextroamphetamine	Dexedrine®	"Co-Pilots;" "Dex;" "Dexies;" "Hearts"
	Methamphetamine[7]	Desoxyn®	"Crank;" "Crystal Meth;" "Glass;" "Hillbilly Crack;" "Ice;" "Jib;" "Meth;" "Speed;" "Stove Top;" "Tina"
	Mixed Amphetamines[8]	Adderall®	"Addies;" "Blueberries;" "Oranges;" "Tic-Tac"
Closely Related Psychostimulants			
	Methylphenidate	Concerta®; Ritalin®	"JIF;" "MPH;" "Rs;" "The Smart Drug"

often medically prescribed to manage ADHD; and (2) illicitly produced and illicitly obtained amphetamines (e.g., "Speed;" "Uppers"), particularly methamphetamine (i.e., "Crank;" "Crystal Meth;" "Glass;" "Meth;" "Tweak"), which are generally readily available "on-the-street."

Chemistry, Synthesis, and History of Medical Use

> There has been only one addition to the original seven deadly sins, and that one is speed.
> (Grinspoon & Hedblom, 1975, attributed to *Aldous Huxley, 1894–1963*)

The amphetamines are chemically related to ephedrine, the active ingredient of the ancient herb, Ephedra,[9] which was first medically used more than 5,000 years ago in China (Pagliaro &

3 Examples of common Brand/Trade names of related prescription drugs.

4 Partial list. Examples of the most common street names are provided. See Pagliaro and Pagliaro (2009) for a comprehensive listing of the drugs and substances of abuse and their common street names.

5 Amphetamine, in its salt forms (i.e., amphetamine aspartate; amphetamine sulfate) is only legally available in the U.S. in the combination, mixed amphetamine product, Adderall®.

6 Adzenys XR-ODT® is an extended-release (XR), orally disintegrating tablet (ODT) approved for the medical treatment of ADHD.

7 Methamphetamine is a commonly used contraction for N-methylamphetamine.

8 This product contains the amphetamine salt forms, amphetamine aspartate and amphetamine sulfate. It also contains dextroamphetamine.

9 Ephedrine is found in many of the over 50 species of Ephedra, including: *Ephedra equisetina; Ephedra Sinica;* and *Ephedra vulgaris*.

Pagliaro, 2004; Schaneberg, Crockett, & Bedir, 2003).[10] Ephedrine was chemically isolated from the plant form, *Ephedra vulgaris*, in 1885 by the Japanese organic chemist, Nagai Nagayoshi. However, its sympathomimetic actions were not generally recognized until the early 1920s when its use, as an alternative to epinephrine (i.e., adrenaline) for the treatment of nasal congestion and bronchoconstriction, were explored (Lee, 2011).

Ephedrine was soon touted as being superior to epinephrine because it: (1) could be ingested or inhaled; (2) had a longer duration of action; and (3) displayed predictable actions with fewer related harmful effects and toxicities. However, as medical use increased, concerns about depleting the natural supplies of ephedrine began to be raised. These concerns encouraged researchers in Europe, Japan, and the U.S. to search for a synthetic substitute. The divergent research directions taken by these scientists led to the subsequent synthesis of the amphetamines—amphetamine sulfate, dextroamphetamine, and methamphetamine.

The psychostimulant action of amphetamine was discovered in Los Angeles by Gordon Alles, who, at that time, was a young research chemist. Having reviewed ephedrine research, he concluded that phenylisopropylamine, a volatile base synthesized during the late 1800s, provided the best direction for further research.[11] In 1932, performing animal experiments, as well as experimenting on himself, he discovered that Benzedrine® (i.e., racemic or dextro-levo-amphetamine) and Dexedrine® (i.e., the "right-handed" isomer of Benzedrine®) had powerful psychostimulant actions, in addition to, the peripheral alpha-adrenergic and beta-adrenergic actions characteristic of the indirectly acting sympathomimetics.[12] The Benzedrine® inhaler was introduced for use, in the U.S., by Smith, Kline, and French as an over-the-counter product in the early 1930s. It quickly became a "huge" success.[13]

More commonly injected intravenously, the amphetamines also could be ingested or inhaled with the latter surpassing the former in alleviating fatigue, enhancing alertness, and creating "euphoric confidence" (Grinspoon & Hedblom, 1975). Methamphetamine, the N-methyl analogue of dextro rotatory amphetamine, was synthesized by Japanese scientists in 1919. This form of amphetamine has remained the most potent member of this class of psychostimulants.

Since their synthesis, amphetamines, commonly known on-the-street as "Bennies," "Bombers," "Cartwheels," "Crystal," "Dexies," "Ice," and "Pep Pills," have been, and continue to be, widely used in the U.S., and other countries, for their psychostimulant actions that include: enhanced alertness; increased psychomotor abilities; and suppression of feelings of drowsiness, fatigue, or hunger. These actions have also made the amphetamines attractive as "performance enhancers" for aircraft pilots, athletes, entertainers, parents, soldiers, surgeons, teachers, truck drivers, university/college students, and others.

Pharmacology

The amphetamines are synthetic drugs that produce dose-dependent actions on both the central and peripheral (i.e., sympathetic) nervous systems (Pagliaro & Pagliaro, 2009). As psychostimulants, their actions are similar to those produced by the endogenous

10 Ephedrine, the primary constituent of the medicinal herb *Ma huang*, was brewed and ingested as a tea in ancient China and continues to be widely used in Traditional Chinese Medicine.

11 Phenylisopropylamine (i.e., amphetamine) was initially synthesized in Germany in 1887 by the Romanian chemist, Lazar Edeleanu.

12 Amphetamine is also chemically known as, alpha-methylphenethylamine (AMPH).

13 By the late 1930s, adolescents and young adults were commonly removing the amphetamine impregnated paper or cotton strips from the Benzedrine® inhalers and placing them into a cup of coffee, or simply chewing and swallowing the strips, to get "high" (Pagliaro & Pagliaro, 2004).

catecholamine excitatory neurotransmitters: dopamine; epinephrine; norepinephrine; and serotonin. Peripherally, they promote the actions of the sympathetic nervous system that, consequently, increase heart rate and constrict blood vessels, thus elevating blood pressure. However, the amphetamines, being more potent than natural ephedrine (see also the related discussion in the earlier amphetamine subsection, "Chemistry, Synthesis, and History of Medical Use") achieve higher levels of central and peripheral nervous system stimulation resulting in significantly heightened alertness, psychomotor abilities, and diminished feelings of drowsiness and fatigue. It is these actions that make the amphetamines attractive as "performance enhancers."

Pharmacodynamics: Mechanism of Action

The amphetamines are "non-catecholamine" sympathomimetics. The sympathomimetics are drugs that mimic the actions of the sympathetic nervous system, which is involved with the homeostatic regulation of: blood pressure; bronchial airway tone; carbohydrate and fatty acid metabolism, particularly during periods of physical activity or psychological stress; force of cardiac contraction; heart rate; and vasomotor tone. These responses are usually endogenously mediated by circulating levels of the hormones—epinephrine (adrenaline) and norepinephrine (noradrenaline)—which act at five adrenergic receptors: alpha one (α_1); alpha two (α_2); beta one (β_1); beta two (β_2); and beta three (β_3).

Agonist actions at "alpha" adrenergic receptors include: decreased gut motility; glycogenolysis; mydriasis; piloerection; sweating; urinary retention; and vasoconstriction. Agonist actions at "β_1-receptors," which are predominant in the heart, are associated with: decreased gut motility and secretions; increased heart rate; increased lipolysis; and increased renin release.[14] Agonist actions at "β_2-receptors," which are predominant in the lungs, include: bronchodilation; fine skeletal muscle tremor; glycogenolysis; mast cell stabilization; and vasodilation.[15] Agonist actions at "β_3-receptors," which are are predominant in adipose tissues and which appear to upregulate during cardiovascular diseases, include lipolysis and potential cardiodepressant effects on human ventricles (Dessy & Baligand, 2010; Skeberdis, 2004).

The amphetamines, as well as methylphenidate, are indirect-acting psychostimulants. As such, they stimulate the release of the biogenic amines (i.e., dopamine, norepinephrine, and serotonin) from the presynaptic nerve terminal storage vesicles that are primarily located in the midbrain and mesolimbic dopamine pathway (Pagliaro & Pagliaro, 2004; Rothman, Baumann, & Dersch, 2001). They also inhibit the reuptake of the biogenic amines, primarily by blocking the neuronal dopamine transporter (DAT) and the vesicular monoamine transporter-2[16] (Faraone, 2018; Fleckenstein, Volz, & Riddle, 2007). These actions result in an increase in synaptic extracellular neurotransmitters, particularly dopamine and norepinephrine. Figure 2.1 provides a simplified, stylized representation of the principal sites and mechanisms of these psychostimulant actions.

Pharmacokinetics: Absorption, Distribution, Metabolism, and Excretion

The amphetamines and methylphenidate are licitly available in several ingestible formulations including: capsules; chewable tablets; and liquid products. However, they are commonly

14 The agonist actions at the β_1-receptors are primarily mediated by the stimulation of adenyl cyclase enzyme activity which, in turn, facilitates the conversion of ATP to cAMP with resultant "opening" of calcium channels.

15 The agonists actions at the β_2-receptors also are primarily mediated by stimulation of adenyl cyclase enzyme activity in association with the resultant "closing" of calcium channels.

16 Also referred to as the norepinephrine transporter (NET).

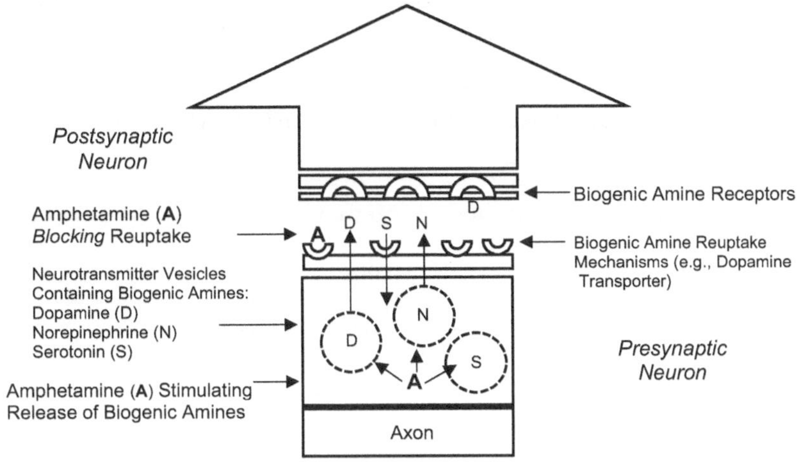

Figure 2.1 Amphetamines: Mechanism of Psychostimulant Action

illicitly self-administered by means of: intravenous (IV) injection; nasal insufflation, or "snorting;" and pulmonary inhalation (i.e., "smoking;" "vaporizing" [or "vaping"]). Like all drugs, the amphetamines are immediately and completely absorbed following IV injection. They are also well-absorbed following ingestion. In addition, because of their high lipid solubility, they are well-absorbed following: nasal insufflation and pulmonary inhalation.[17] Transmucousal absorption, after rectal or vaginal insertion, is also high. Following absorption, the amphetamines are widely distributed throughout body tissues, and, due to their lipid solubility, readily cross the blood-brain barrier.[18]

Related Professional Reminder: ***When considering plasma protein binding, it is important to keep in mind that only "free," or unbound, drugs can readily cross biological membranes including, the "blood-brain barrier." Consequently, and of clinical significance, plasma protein binding is—in the vast majority of clinical contexts—only of concern for drugs that are highly protein bound (i.e., in excess of 98%) because seemingly small changes in the concentration of unbound drugs can have profound therapeutic or toxic consequences. For example, a 1% change in plasma protein binding (i.e., from 99% to 98%) would result in a 50% increase in free drug plasma concentrations.***

Urinary excretion of the amphetamines is pH-dependent with acidic urine (pH lower than 7) increasing excretion and alkaline urine (pH higher than 7) decreasing excretion. These differences in urinary pH and associated changes in excretion rates explain why regular, long-term amphetamine users, commonly ingest antacids (e.g., calcium carbonate, Tums®) to alkalinize their urine. This action both enhances and prolongs the desired pharmacologic actions of the amphetamines. The half-life of elimination of the various amphetamines is approximately 10 hours, with slight variations among amphetamine sulfate, dextroamphetamine, and methamphetamine (Pagliaro & Pagliaro, 2009).[19] (See Table 2.2)

17 Interestingly, when methamphetamine is smoked, it is significantly degraded to amphetamine due to pyrolysis by means of N-demethylation (Sato, Hida, & Nagase, 2004).

18 Because of the addition of a methyl (-CH_3) chemical group to the amphetamine molecule, methamphetamine has greater lipophilicity and, consequently, crosses the blood-brain barrier more rapidly than the other amphetamines do.

19 An exception is "lisdexamfetamine." Lisdexamfetamine is a prodrug that is rapidly converted to dextroamphetamine by an aminopeptidase present within erythrocytes. Consequently, the mean half-life of elimination of lisdexamfetamine is approximately 30 minutes (Ermer, Pennick, & Frick, 2016).

Table 2.2 Comparative Pharmacokinetic Values Following Ingestion of Dextroamphetamine, Methamphetamine, and the Closely Related Psychostimulant, Methylphenidate[20]

Pharmacokinetic Processes Following Ingestion	*Pharmacokinetic Values for Dextroamphetamine, Methamphetamine, and Methylphenidate*		
Absorption	**Dextroamphetamine**	**Methamphetamine**	**Methylphenidate**
Bioavailability	Good	Good (~ 60% pulmonary) (~ 80% intranasal)	Low (F = 0.3)
Time to Peak Blood Concentration	~ 3.5 hours	~ 5 hours	~ 2 hours
Distribution			
Volume of Distribution	5.4 L/kg	4.2 L/kg	2.25 L/kg
Plasma Protein Binding	Low (~ 25%)	Low (~ 15%)	Low (~ 15%)
Metabolism	Hepatic (primarily involving CYP2D6)	Hepatic (primarily involving CYP2D6)[21]	Hepatic (primarily by carboxylesterase)
Total Body Clearance	0.7 L/kg/hour	~ 270 L/kg/hour	~ 10 L/kg/hour
Mean Half-Life of Elimination	~ 12 hours	~ 10 hours	~ 22 hours
Excretion			
Urinary Excretion	pH dependent	pH dependent (parent drug and metabolites)	< 1% in unchanged form

Sources: Pagliaro & Benet (1975); Pagliaro & Pagliaro (2009); Roberts, Cook, & Stockmann (2015); Schepers, Oyler, & Joseph (2003).

Common Misbelief. The half-life of elimination of a specific amphetamine (e.g., methamphetamine) depends on its method of use (i.e., route of administration).

20 Pharmacokinetic values presented in this table are from human studies only. Blank cells indicate that related valid and reliable values for these cells are *not* currently available.

21 Amphetamine is a major active metabolite of methamphetamine.

The stated common misbelief is simply not true. While the method of use may affect the rate of absorption and, consequently, the onset of action, it does not affect the half-life of elimination.

Table 2.3 Amphetamines: Major Potential Drug–Drug Interactions[22]

Drugs that Interact with Amphetamines	*Comments*
Adrenergic Blockers (e.g., atenolol; prazosin; propranolol)	Amphetamines inhibit the actions of the adrenergic blockers, both alpha and beta (see the earlier amphetamines pharmacology subsection, "Pharmacodynamics: Mechanism of Action")
Antidepressants Monoamine Oxidase Inhibitors (MAOIs) (e.g., phenelzine; tranylcypromine)	MAOIs, when used with amphetamines, increase the possibility of a hypertensive crisis (i.e., noradrenergic/serotonergic syndrome)
Selective Serotonin Reuptake Inhibitors (SSRIs) (e.g., fluoxetine; paroxetine; sertraline)	SSRIs, when used with amphetamines, increase the possibility of the occurrence of the noradrenergic/serotonergic syndrome
Tricyclic Antidepressants (e.g., amitriptyline; nortriptyline)	Tricyclic antidepressants, when used with amphetamines, can potentially enhance the actions of both drugs (see the earlier amphetamine pharmacology subsection, "Pharmacodynamics: Mechanism of Action")
Antipsychotics (e.g., chlorpromazine; haloperidol)	Antipsychotics inhibit the psychostimulant actions of the amphetamines (see the earlier amphetamine pharmacology subsection, "Pharmacodynamics: Mechanism of Action")
Proton Pump Inhibitors (e.g., omeprazole; rabeprazole)	Proton pump inhibitors decrease gastric acid production and, consequently, may facilitate a shortened time to maximal amphetamine serum concentration resulting in a more rapid onset of amphetamine action
Psychodepressants (e.g., opiate analgesics; sedative-hypnotics)	Psychodepressants, when used with amphetamines, antagonize the psychostimulant actions of the amphetamines
Psychostimulants (e.g., caffeine; cocaine; nicotine)	Psychostimulants, when used with amphetamines, cause additive psychostimulant actions

(*Continued*)

22 The clinical significance of these potential drug–drug interactions depends upon several factors, including the: (1) dosage of each drug; (2) characteristics of the adolescent or young adult (e.g., age; gender; genetics); (3) concomitant physical health status (e.g., hepatic and renal function); and (4) concomitant mental health status.

Table 2.3 (Cont.)

Drugs that Interact with Amphetamines	*Comments*
Urinary Acidifiers (e.g., ammonium chloride)	Urinary acidifiers, when used with amphetamines, increase the urinary excretion of amphetamines (see the earlier related discussion in the amphetamines pharmacology subsection, "Pharmacokinetics—Excretion")
Urinary Alkalinizers (e.g., sodium bicarbonate)	Urinary alkalinizers, when used with amphetamines, decrease the urinary excretion of amphetamines (see the related discussion in the earlier amphetamines pharmacology subsection, "Pharmacokinetics—Excretion")

Table 2.4 Methylphenidate: Major Potential Drug–Drug Interactions[23]

Drugs that Interact with Methylphenidate	*Comments*
Monoamine Oxidase Inhibitors (MAOIs) (e.g., phenelzine; tranylcypromine)	MAOIs, when used with methylphenidate, increase the possibility of a hypertensive crisis (i.e., noradrenergic/serotonergic syndrome)
Psychodepressants (e.g., opiate analgesics; sedative-hypnotics)	Psychodepressants, when used with methylphenidate, antagonize the psychostimulant actions of methylphenidate
Psychostimulants (e.g., amphetamines; caffeine; nicotine)	Psychostimulants, when used with methylphenidate, cause additive psychostimulant actions

Amphetamine and Methylphenidate Drug–Drug Interactions

The amphetamines and methylphenidate have been involved in several drug–drug interactions. The major clinically significant drug–drug interactions involving these psychostimulants are presented and briefly discussed in Tables 2.3 and 2.4, respectively.

Undesired, or Harmful, Effects and Toxicities

Amphetamine use is associated with several undesired, or harmful, effects and toxicities that can be acute[24] or chronic, direct or indirect, minor or major, and physical or mental. These

23 The clinical significance of these possible drug–drug interactions depends upon several factors, including the: (1) dosage of each drug; (2) characteristics of the adolescent or young adult (e.g., age; gender; genetics); (3) concomitant physical health status (e.g., hepatic and renal function); and (4) concomitant mental health status.

24 Following ingestion, the acute toxicities associated with the use of amphetamines generally begin within 20 to 60 minutes. However, following intravenous (IV) injection or pulmonary inhalation, toxicities can begin within 30 to 60 seconds.

"adverse effects" involve virtually every major body system (Pagliaro & Pagliaro, 2009). The frequency and severity of these effects are generally related to:

1. Dosage used (e.g., 40 mg versus 1,000 mg);
2. Method of use (e.g., ingestion versus IV injection—see later discussion);
3. Frequency of use (e.g., every hour over one or two days versus twice a week);
4. Pattern of use (e.g., occasional use versus regular, long-term use);
5. Mental health status at the time of use (e.g., an adolescent who has a contemporaneous mental disorder versus one who does not);
6. Physical health status at the time of use (e.g., a child or adolescent who has a significant cerebral aneurysm versus one who does not);
7. Specific personality characteristics (e.g., a young adult who has a risk-taking personality trait versus one who does not);
8. Interactions associated with concurrent use of licit or illicit, prescription and nonprescription drugs and substances of abuse (see also the related discussion in the previous subsection, "Amphetamine and Methylphenidate Drug–Drug Interactions" and Tables 2.3 and 2.4).

The "acute" toxicities that are related to amphetamine use are more likely to occur among adolescents and young adults, who are novice or occasional amphetamine users, rather than regular, long-term users—even though the latter, being more tolerant to the amphetamines, typically use higher dosages. (See also the later Amphetamine subsection, "Overdosage.") The "chronic" toxicities are usually related to the regular, long-term use of amphetamines. These undesired, or harmful, effects and toxicitites are presented and discussed, in alphabetical order, in the following sections:

- Amphetamine Psychosis;
- Cardiotoxicities;
- Diminished Executive Function;
- Excessive dosage;
- Fatalities;
- Human Immunodeficiency Virus Infection and Acquired Immune Deficiency Syndrome (HIV/AIDS);
- Intravenous Toxicities;
- "Meth Mouth;"
- Miscellaneous Toxicities;
- Physical and Psychological Dependence.

We begin with "Amphetamine Psychosis."

AMPHETAMINE PSYCHOSIS

Amphetamine-induced psychosis is usually associated with the continuous use of amphetamines over several weeks or months (Curran, Byrappa, & McBride, 2004; Pagliaro & Pagliaro, 2009). It also may occur within 24 hours of amphetamine use or within two days following the ingestion of a single, large dose of amphetamine by a sensitive user.[25] As noted by Berman, Kuczenski, and McCracken (2009):

25 N.B. Adolescents and young adults, who experience an episode of amphetamine psychosis, are at increased risk for its recurrence. This increased sensitivity to amphetamine psychosis is thought to be associated with a lowering of the threshold for this effect. In fact, amphetamine psychosis may recur in some adolescents and young adults following the single ingestion of as little as 75 mg of amphetamine (Pagliaro & Pagliaro, *Clinical Patient Data Files*).

> High doses of amphetamines can produce psychotic behavior indistinguishable from schizophrenia in asymptomatic schizophrenics and in some healthy human subjects.
> (p. 131)

Adolescents and young adults with amphetamine psychosis display behaviors that resemble the signs and symptoms of paranoid schizophrenia. Relatively more common during an "amphetamine run," aggressive and violent behavior, may also occur when users—experiencing acute paranoia—often can be found holding a loaded handgun or rifle, peeking from behind closed curtains for the "enemy"—perhaps a "narc" (i.e., drug enforcement officer). This behavior is well-documented and has been recognized for some time in medical, psychological, and legal contexts of practice (Pagliaro & Pagliaro, *Clinical Patient Data Files*).

Efforts have been made to differentiate the clinical similarities and differences between amphetamine psychosis and schizophrenia (e.g., Bramness & Rognli, 2016). Although both conditions may be associated with delusional thinking, a flattened affect, hallucinations, mental depression, and paranoia, they generally differ in etiology and duration.

Generally, adolescents and young adults, who develop mild forms of psychotic-like behavior associated with their amphetamine use, can be treated by "talking them down." However, acute or severe forms of psychosis usually require medical management with a sedative-hypnotic (i.e., diazepam, Valium®) in combination with an antipsychotic (e.g., chlorpromazine, Thorazine®; haloperidol, Haldol®), which can promptly reverse many of the signs and symptoms of the psychosis (Buxton & Dove, 2008). Untreated, the psychosis generally resolves within two to 14 days. (See also the later amphetamine subsection, "Other Toxicities Associated with Amphetamine Use.")

CARDIOTOXICITIES

Amphetamine use, in general, and methamphetamine use, in particular, have long been associated with cardiotoxicity, including sudden death, which may occur as a direct result of the mechanism of action of the amphetamines (see related discussion in the earlier amphetamines pharmacology subsection, "Pharmacodynamics: Mechanism of Action").[26]

As found by Kaye, McKetin, and Duflou (2007, p. 1204), in their review of methamphetamine and cardiovascular pathology:

1. Methamphetamine users are at higher risk of cardiac pathology.
2. Risk is unlikely to be limited to the duration of their methamphetamine use because of its associated chronic pathology.
3. Risk of cardiac pathology is highest among regular, long-term methamphetamine users.
4. Pre-existing cardiac pathology, due to methamphetamine use or other factors, increases the risk of an acute cardiac event.
5. Methamphetamine use is likely to exacerbate the risk of cardiac pathology associated with other factors and may, therefore, lead to premature mortality.

A significant number of methamphetamine-related cardiac events occur among adolescents and young adults, who appear to be at particular risk for dysrhythmias and hemorrhagic stroke (Huang, Yang, & Lin, 2016). Associated findings (e.g., Huang, Yang, & Lin, 2016; Jafari, 2017; Lappin, Darke, & Farrell, 2017) include:

26 Consequently, the psychostimulants are not recommended for use among children and adolescents with known serious, structural cardiac abnormalities.

1. For younger patients, poorer prognosis for methamphetamine-related hemorrhagic stroke;
2. For adolescent boys and young men, greater likelihood for methamphetamine-related cardiotoxicity;
3. For males, increased probability to present with late, severe dilated cardiomyopathy;
4. For females, increased probability to present with stress-induced Takotsubo cardiomyopathy.

For example, regarding the latter, Alsidawi, Muth, and Wilkin (2011, p. 910) reported that a:

> 19-year-old female was brought to the Emergency Department after ingesting 30 Adderall® tablets ... diagnosed with inverted-Takotsubo cardiomyopathy.

And, as presented by Toce, Farias, and Bruccoleri (2017, p. 385):

> A 15-year-old adolescent girl who was found to have a Takotsubo cardiomyopathy after acute amphetamine/dextroamphetamine ingestion...

Other cardiac and related physical toxicities associated with the use of amphetamines, include:

- Cardiac dysrhythmias;
- Chest pain;
- Heart failure;
- Heart palpitations;
- Hypertension;
- Myocardial infarction;
- Tachycardia.

DIMINISHED EXECUTIVE FUNCTION AND OTHER NEUROTOXICITIES

Higher order, cognitive performance is controlled by executive function—mental processes associated with integration, synthesis, and problem solving—which are typically required for goal- or task-oriented behaviors, including consciously planning, implementing, monitoring, and ceasing goal-directed behaviors. Minor and temporary deficits and fluctuations in executive function are largely situational. For example, while occurring among most people at some time in their lives, theses deficits and fluctuations are more likely to occur when a person is: (1) extremely tired; (2) under extreme psychological stress; (3) experiencing reactive depression following a significant loss; or (4) acutely intoxicated with alcohol or another psychodepressant drug or substance of abuse (Pagliaro & Pagliaro, *Clinical Patient Data Files*).

Additionally, significant deficits in executive function among children, adolescents, and young adults are associated with several mental and neurological disorders, including:

- ADHD;
- Autism;
- Fetal Alcohol Syndrome/Fetal Alcohol Spectrum Disorder (FAS/FASD);
- Major depressive disorder (MDD);
- Obsessive-compulsive disorder (OCD);
- Psychotic disorder;
- Tourette's syndrome.

Moreover, diminished executive function has been identified as both a "cause" and "result" of drug and substance use (e.g., Goldstein & Volkow, 2011; Pagliaro & Pagliaro,

2012). As found by Ersche, Clark, and London (2006), in their study of both regular, long-term amphetamine and opiate analgesic users:

> Chronic drug users display pronounced neurophysiological impairment in the domains of executive and memory function. Impairment persists after several years of drug abstinence and may reflect neuropathology in frontal and temporal cortices ... Compared to opiate users, amphetamine users showed more pronounced deficits on tasks of executive function ...
>
> (p. 1036)

(Also see the related discussion of executive function in Chapter 1, "Alcohol," Chapter 4, "Cannabis and Other Psychodelics," and Chapter 5, "Prescription Opiate Analgesics and Heroin.")

Methamphetamine-related diminished cognitive and executive function also includes deficits in abstract thinking, learning, memory, and psychomotor speed (Dean, Kohno, & Morales, 2015). These deficits appear to be related to neurotoxicity associated with the dopamine terminals. Specifically, this neurotoxicity has long been associated with methamphetamine-induced damage to: (1) dopaminergic neurons[27] in the basal ganglia; and (2) reduced dopamine transporter density in the caudate/putamen, nucleus accumbens, and prefrontal cortex (see Figure 2.2).

Although not as well characterized, methamphetamine-induced damage to serotonergic neurons, which may be mediated by the formation of reactive oxygen species, also has been identified (Hanson, Rau, & Fleckenstein, 2004). In addition, methamphetamine neurotoxicity may be mediated by downregulation (i.e., temporary neuroadaptive changes). Consequently, in this context, the associated neurotoxicity may be reversible with long-term abstinence from methamphetamine use.

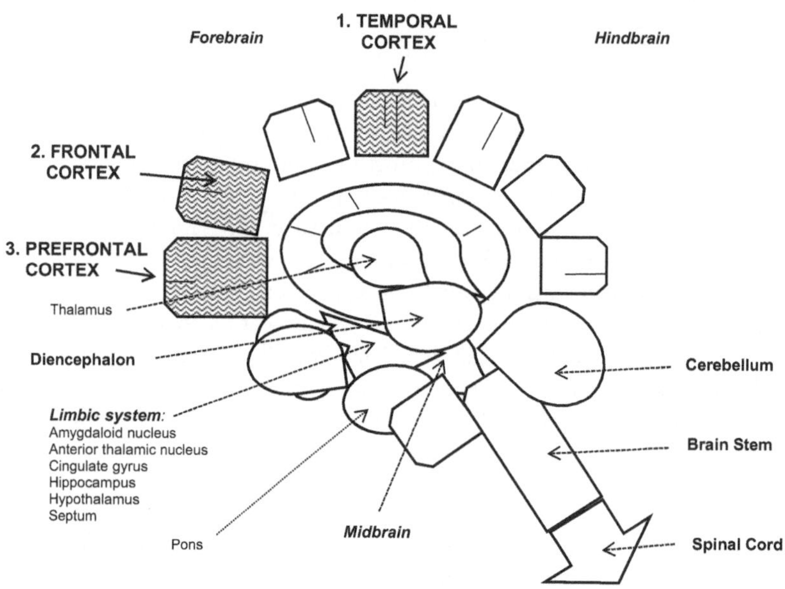

Figure 2.2 Three Major Sites of Amphetamine Toxicity in the CNS

27 Several researchers (e.g., Shin, Tran, & Nguyen, 2017) have suggested that the damage to dopaminergic neurons may be mediated by impairment of mitochondrial function.

Of concern, however, is the observation that some of the neurotoxic effects appear to be permanent. For example, research findings indicate that regular, long-term high dosage methamphetamine use can selectively damage the striatal dopaminergic axons in the substantia nigra. This methamphetamine neurotoxicity has been associated with permanent parkinsonian-like signs (e.g., pill-rolling tremor; shuffling gait) (Ares-Santos, Granado, & Espadas, 2014; Ares-Santos, Granado, & Moratalla, 2013; Matthew & Gedzior, 2015; Todd, Noyes, & Flavel, 2013).[28, 29]

EXCESSIVE DOSAGES

As the dosage of amphetamine is increased, abdominal pain (severe); anorexia, with loss of body weight; blurred vision; chest pain; dizziness; emotional lability; headache; nausea; palpitations; punding; tremor; and urinary retention may be experienced. A further increase in amphetamine dosage may culminate in amphetamine psychosis (see the earlier discussion in the amphetamine subsection, "Undesired, or Harmful, Effects and Toxicities—Amphetamine Psychosis").

FATALITIES ASSOCIATED WITH AMPHETAMINE USE

Although relatively uncommon, the use of amphetamines can "directly" or "indirectly" result in death. For example, amphetamine use has been "directly" related to death due to: myocardial infarctions (Kaye, McKetin, & Duflou, 2007); cerebrovascular accidents; and overdosages (see the later amphetamine subsection, "Amphetamine Overdosage"). Yet, these fatal toxicities rarely occur among otherwise healthy adolescents and young adults, who are regular, long-term amphetamine users. However, for these adolescents and young adults, the most severe, and potentially fatal, acute physical toxicities associated with amphetamine use are:

1. "Hypertensive crisis," which is characterized by a drastic increase in blood pressure;
2. "Hyperpyretic crisis," which is characterized by a sustained elevated body temperature exceeding 106° F [41° C]).

These two acute physical toxicities require emergency medical support, including appropriate medical intervention and monitoring of body systems.

"Indirectly," amphetamine use has been related to deaths due to: (1) fatal hepatitis C infection or HIV/AIDS—usually contracted through the use of contaminated needles and syringes; (2) fatal IV injection of an adulterated or contaminated form of amphetamine, or an unknown toxic substance thought to be amphetamine; (3) fatal injuries due to amphetamine induced psychotic episodes and homicidal rages; and (4) fatal accidents related to amphetamine use (Pagliaro & Pagliaro, *Clinical Patient Data Files*).

> In Nebraska, two 20-year-olds, who were high on meth, froze to death after getting lost in a snowstorm in January.
>
> (Irvine, 2005, p. 1)

28 This affected area of the substantia nigra, when visualized by transcranial sonography, assumes an abnormally enlarged and bright appearance. This change in appearance is referred to as "hyperechogenicity" (Todd, Noyes, & Flavel, 2013).

29 Although these chronic, amphetamine use-related neurotoxic effects typically appear during "old age," several researchers (e.g., Park & Haning, 2016), including ourselves, have expressed concern that, because brain development does not typically conclude until early adulthood, the use of amphetamines, particularly methamphetamine, during adolescence and early adulthood is potentially significantly more neurotoxic than use during later adulthood.

HUMAN IMMUNODEFICIENCY VIRUS (HIV) INFECTION AND ACQUIRED IMMUNE DEFICIENCY SYNDROME (AIDS)

In addition to significantly increasing risk for HIV infection among adolescent and young adults by means of sharing contaminated needles and syringes (see the following section, "Intravenous Toxicities"), amphetamine use also increases risky sexual behavior among adolescents and young adults. Several studies and reviews (e.g., Pagliaro & Pagliaro, 2000, 2012, 2018; Pagliaro, Pagliaro, & Thauberger, 1990, 1993) have described and documented this risk for 30 years. The use of amphetamines—particularly the use of methamphetamine in moderate to high dosages—significantly increases sexual pleasure for adolescents and young adults by means of its associated action on neurotransmitters (see the earlier amphetamines pharmacology subsection, "Pharmacodynamics: Mechanism of Action"). As reported by Zapata, Hillis, and Marchbanks (2008):

> Lifetime methamphetamine use (among a nationally representative sample of U.S. 9th- to 12th-grade students) was associated with recent sexual intercourse, having two or more recent sexual partners, and ever being pregnant or getting someone pregnant.
>
> (p. 641)

As found by Lorvick, Bourgois, and Wenger (2012, p. 385), in the responses of the participants in their qualitative/quantative, mixed method study of women (18 years-of-age to 50+ years-of-age), who used methamphetamine:

- "I love the way it makes me feel sexually;"
- "It prolongs, um, my orgasms;"
- "It makes me uninhibited;"
- "It makes me feel sexy."

Consequently, methamphetamine use, commonly places adolescent girls and young women at significantly increased risk for HIV infection and AIDS—directly because of engaging in high-risk sexual behavior, particularly unprotected sexual intercourse with multiple partners. Also of concern are the related tragic outcomes for young mothers (e.g., neonatal in utero HIV infection; negative effects on mothering). (See also the related discussion in the later Amphetamine subsection, "Pregnancy, Lactation, and Mothering.")

In addition, among adolescent boys and young adult men, who identify as bisexual, homosexual, or transsexual, the use of methamphetamine, in particular, as well as other psychostimulants, has long been associated with increased risky sexual behaviors—multiple sexual partners; sex with adolescent boys, young adult men, and older men who are HIV positive or who have AIDS; and unprotected anal intercourse—particularly in the context of attendance at "bath houses" and/or "circuit parties." Accordingly, we have cautioned adolescent boys and young men, since the late 1980s, regarding this drug-related risky sexual behavior and the significant spread of HIV infection and other STDs (e.g., Pagliaro & Pagliaro, *Clinical Patient Data Files;* Pagliaro, Pagliaro, & Thauberger, 1993).

More recently, the use of psychostimulants (i.e., amphetamine; methamphetamine) and other illicit drugs and substances of abuse (e.g., alcohol; methylenedioxymethamphetamine [Ecstasy; MDMA]) before and during bisexual, homosexual, and transgender sex among men—including adolescent boys and young men—has become inculcated among these subcultures. This sexualized drug use has become colloquially known as "party and play," or, more commonly, as "chemsex" (Melendez-Torres & Bourne, 2016; Pakianathan, Lee, & Kelly, 2016). Of increasing concern, chemsex, in addition to related-substance use disorders and other undesired effects associated with amphetamine and methamphetamine abuse, has been associated with a documented higher incidence of: (1) acute bacterial sexually transmitted diseases (STDs); (2) hepatitis C; (3) HIV infection; and (4) rectal STDs (e.g., Bourne, Reid, & Hickson, 2015; Hegazi, Lee, & Whittaker, 2017; Sewell, Miltz, & Lampe, 2017).

INTRAVENOUS TOXICITIES

Direct acute toxicities have been related to both the early and late phases of intravenous amphetamine use. Commonly, during the "early phase," which generally occurs following the IV injection of 20 to 40 mg of amphetamine, a desired "flash," or "rush," is experienced that is reportedly characterized by:

1. Extreme euphoria—a sense of increased physical energy, mental capacity, and self-confidence;
2. Heightened sexual orgasm.

During the "later phase," or "run," users frequently inject increasingly higher dosages of amphetamine in an effort to achieve the desired actions that they experienced during the early phase. Unable to achieve these actions, primarily due to the development of tolerance (see the related discussion in the later amphetamine subsection, "Physical and Psychological Dependence—Tolerance," they typically remain awake and, while generally eating little, if at all, continue to inject their amphetamine every one to three hours, for several days—around the clock—until their run ends, typically when they:

1. Deplete their amphetamine supplies (e.g., the total available supply is used);
2. Are unable to obtain additional amphetamines because their funds are exhausted;
3. Become so mentally disorganized, or paranoid, that they cannot continue their amphetamine use.

Finally, incapable of continuing their amphetamine use, they usually fall into a deep, but restless, sleep that lasts for 12 to 18 hours, or more. Upon awakening, they typically feel tired, weak, depressed, and hungry (Pagliaro & Pagliaro, *Clinical Patient Data Files*).

Also of concern, the IV injection (i.e., "mainlining") of amphetamines, or any other drug or substance of abuse, is associated with several well-identified toxicities, including:

- Abscesses at the injection site;
- Aneurysms;
- Bacteremia;
- Cellulitis;
- Cutaneous venous ulcers;
- Endocarditis;
- Gangrene;
- Hepatitis B;
- Hepatitis C;
- HIV infection;[30]

30 See the earlier related discussion in the amphetamines pharmacology subsection, "Undesired, or Harmful, Effects and Toxicities—Human Immunodeficiency Virus (HIV) Infection and Acquired Immune Deficiency Syndrome (AIDS)."

- Myonecrosis;
- Myositis;
- Necrotizing fasciitis;
- Scarring of skin (i.e., "railroad tracks");
- Septicemia;
- Tetanus;
- Thrombophlebitis;
- Thrombosis;
- Venous sclerosis;
- Wound botulism.

It is important to note that these serious toxicities do not occur "directly" because of the pharmacology of the amphetamines, but rather occur "indirectly" as a result of: (1) adulterants added to the amphetamine product; (2) improper/poor IV injection techniques; and (3) using/sharing contaminated needles and syringes. Thus, they do not occur when the amphetamines are administered by other routes, such as: ingestion; nasal insufflation; or pulmonary inhalation.

Related Professional Reminder: ***The use of "safe injection sites" are associated with harm reduction,* not *harm prevention. Consequently, many of the toxicities that are associated with IV injection will* not *be prevented or reduced by the use of "safe injection sites"—even with the provision of sterile needles and syringes.***[31]

METH MOUTH

The condition of meth mouth is associated with the regular, long-term use of methamphetamine and prolonged neglect of oral hygiene, both of which contribute to the loss of teeth and the associated distinctive appearance commonly referred to as "meth mouth" (e.g, Brown, Morisky, & Silverstein, 2013; Pagliaro & Pagliaro, *Clinical Patient Data Files*; Rommel, Rohleder, & Koerdt, 2016). This condition also is characterized by "rampant caries, periodontal diseases, and excessive tooth wear" (Rommel, Rohleder, & Wagenpfeil, 2016, p. 469). In addition, several researchers, such as Boyer, Thompson, and Hill (2015) have noted that:

> For missing teeth, there was a significant methamphetamine race/ethnicity interaction (p = 0.028) among Whites, who used methamphetamine, compared to Whites, who did *not* use methamphetamine.
>
> (p. 119)[32]

In their study of 100 chronic methamphetamine users and 100 matched-pair controls, Rommel, Rohleder, and Wagenpfeil (2016) found that total saliva production among the methamphetamine users was significantly lower and had a lower pH than that found for controls. These findings led Rommel and colleagues to posit that the noted differences in saliva production and pH contribute to the increased risk for dental caries and erosions that are seen among regular, long-term methamphetamine users.

OTHER TOXICITIES ASSOCIATED WITH AMPHETAMINE USE

Other toxicities associated with amphetamine use include both mental and physical toxicities.
Other "mental" toxicities, include:

31 In addition, an unanticipated consequence of safe injection sites is that they often promote, or, at least, "enable," drug and substance abuse that, consequently, can result in the continuation of regular, long-term use with associated harmful effects and toxicities—both to the user and others (Pagliaro & Pagliaro, *Clinical Patient Data Files*).

32 It should be kept in mind that this observation may be influenced by the fact that, in the U.S., the highest percentage of methamphetamine users are of European continental descent.

- Aggression;
- Agitation;
- Anxiety;
- Compulsive behavior;
- Confusion;
- Delirium;
- Emotional lability;
- Euphoric grandiosity;
- Formication;[33]
- Hallucinations;
- Hyperactivity;
- Hypervigilance;
- Impaired judgment;
- Insomnia;
- Irritability;
- Loquacity extending to pressured speech;
- Mania;
- Nervousness;
- Obsessive behavior;
- Panic attacks;
- Paranoia;
- Preoccupation with thinking processes and philosophical concerns about meaning;
- Punding;
- Restlessness;
- Suicidal ideation.

Other "physical" toxicities, include:

- Acute renal failure;
- Anorexia;
- Bruxism, which usually occurs during sleep, is associated with involuntary contraction, or spasm, of the jaw muscles;
- Cerebrovascular accident;
- Coma;
- Cramps;
- Diaphoresis;
- Dizziness;
- Dysuria;
- Headache;
- Hyperglycemia;
- Hyperthermia;
- Local skin burns, which are often associated with methamphetamine production;
- Metabolic acidosis;
- Rhabdomyolysis;
- Seizures;

33 Touching and picking at the arms and face, which is usually related to the delusional sensation of something (e.g., "bugs") crawling under the skin. Over time, the associated scratching and picking at the skin often results in extensive disfiguration due to associated infections and scarring. The characteristic facial appearance resembles severe acne, with open sores, or lesions (Mullin, 2016; Pagliaro & Pagliaro, *Clinical Patient Data Files*).

- Tachypnea;
- Tremor;
- Urinary retention;
- Vomiting;
- Weight loss.

Physical and Psychological Dependence

In the U.S., the inability to discontinue the use of amphetamines, particularly methamphetamine, has led to over a million people across the lifespan, to seek professional assistance from mental health care professionals, physicians, psychiatrists, psychologists, and other health and social care professionals for the management of amphetamine dependence, or amphetamine use disorder, and related tolerance and withdrawal. A stark reflection of this situation is found in the outcomes of a national study analyzing trends in methamphetamine treatment among almost 250,000 pregnant women, including adolescents, from 1994 to 2006:

> Methamphetamine has become the *primary* substance compelling treatment during pregnancy.
>
> (Terplan, Smith, & Kozloski, 2009)[34]

AMPHETAMINE TOLERANCE

Regular, long-term use of the amphetamines results in a tolerance to their desired psychostimulant actions. Thus, in an effort to achieve desired effects, including associated euphoria, users often increase their dosages to several grams per day (Pagliaro & Pagliaro, *Clinical Patient Data Files*). Tolerance also affects other related actions, particularly those that are centrally mediated, including cardiovascular effects and hyperthermia. However, tolerance to the occurrence of chronic toxicities, such as amphetamine psychosis, does not generally occur. Thus, regular, long-term users of the amphetamines, particularly those who are tolerant and increase their dosages in an effort to achieve desired effects, inevitably increase their risk for amphetamine psychosis (see the related discussion in the earlier subsection, "Amphetamine Psychosis").

AMPHETAMINE WITHDRAWAL SYNDROME

A true or classic withdrawal syndrome—such as that which occurs following the abrupt discontinuation of the regular, long-term use of alcohol, opiate analgesics, or nicotine, and which can be immediately relieved with the resumed use of the drug or substance of abuse—has not been documented for any of the amphetamines, including methamphetamine. However, the abrupt discontinuation of regular, long-term patterns of high dosage amphetamine or methamphetamine use may result in the signs and symptoms of "early-phase" amphetamine or methamphetamine withdrawal, which includes:

- Anxiety;
- Apathy;
- Cognitive impairment;
- Depressed mood (which may be severe);
- Drug craving (often quite intense);
- Fatigue;
- Increased appetite;
- Sleep disturbance (i.e., excessive sleep).

34 See also the related discussion in the later pharmacology subsection, "Pregnancy, Lactation, and Mothering."

The early phase of amphetamine or methamphetamine withdrawal largely resolves within one week of the discontinuation of amphetamine or methamphetamine use, respectively. Of note, it is during early-phase amphetamine or methamphetamine withdrawal, that most users perpetrate acts of violence against others, including their children or other family members (Hamilton & Goeders, 2010; Pagliaro & Pagliaro, *Clinical Patient Data Files*). A "later-phase" amphetamine withdrawal follows, characterized by similar, but significantly less severe signs and symptoms, that may last for two additional weeks (McGregor, Srisurapanont, & Jittiwutikarn, 2005). There is no specific pharmacotherapy for the management of the signs and symptoms associated with amphetamine or methamphetamine withdrawal (Shoptaw, Kao, & Heinzerling, 2009). Medical management remains symptomatic (Pagliaro & Pagliaro, 2009, 2018).

Pregnancy, Lactation, and Mothering

In an analysis of self-reported data obtained from the *Infant Development, Environment, and Lifestyle (IDEAL) Study*, Arria, Derauf, and LaGasse (2006) estimated that approximately 5% of pregnant adolescent girls and young women, in the U.S., used methamphetamine. Based on a further analysis of data from the *IDEAL Study*, Della Grotta, LaGasse, and Arria (2010) found that over 40% of these adolescent girls and young women continued methamphetamine use during their third trimester of pregnancy. As later reported by the Committee on Health Care for Underserved Women (2011, p. 751):

> Among pregnant women, admissions for the treatment of methamphetamine abuse *increased* from 8% of federally funded treatment admissions in 1994 to 24% by 2006, with 73% of these admissions occurring in the western states.

Maternal methamphetamine placental transfer to the embryo or fetus has been demonstrated by measurable neonatal levels (Garcia-Bournissen, Rokach, & Karaskov, 2007). Fortunately, the use of methamphetamine by adolescent girls or young women during pregnancy, as well as the use of dextroamphetamine or methylphenidate, has not been conclusively associated with teratogensis, or major physical birth defects (Pagliaro & Levin, 1979; Pagliaro & Pagliaro, 2009, 2012). However, the use of methamphetamine by pregnant adolescent girls and young women has been associated with an increased risk for expected toxicities including:

1. Placental abruption;
2. Premature birth;
3. Low neonatal birth weight;
4. Reduced neonatal size, "small-for-gestational-age;"
5. Neonatal death.

(e.g., Gorman, Orme, & Nguyen, 2014; Pagliaro & Pagliaro, 2018; Ross, Graham, & Money, 2015; Wright, Schuetter, & Tellei, 2015).

Additionally, a significant number of researchers suggest that intrauterine exposure of embryos and fetuses to methamphetamine, may result in neurodevelopmental abnormalities during childhood, including:

1. Decreased "neurobehavioral disinhibition;"
2. Increased externalizing behavior, including aggressive behavior;
3. Increased "rule-breaking" behavior.

(e.g., Eze, Smith, & LaGasse, 2016; Himes, LaGasse, & Derauf, 2014; Pagliaro & Pagliaro, 2012; Roos, Kwiatkowski, & Fouche, 2015).[35]

***Related Professional Reminder:* As a precautionary measure, adolescent girls and young women, who are pregnant, should be advised not to use amphetamines, including methamphetamines.**

The amphetamines are excreted in breast milk (e.g., Bartu, Dusci, & Ilett, 2009; Chomchai, Chomchai, & Kitsommart, 2016)—often in concentrations that are two to three times higher than those found in maternal plasma. Consequently, breastfed neonates and infants may experience expected psychostimulant effects, including: agitation; crying; decreased body weight (generally associated with poor feeding behaviors and/or poor maternal-infant attachment); and irritability (Pagliaro & Pagliaro, 2009, 2012, 2018).

***Related Professional Reminder:* Young mothers, who are breastfeeding, should be advised not to use the amphetamines. Conversely, young mothers, who are unable to discontinue their amphetamine use (i.e., for therapeutic or other reasons), should not breastfeed.**[36]

Nair, Schuler, and Black (2003) also noted that, "when drug use occurs in the context of multiple other risks, it may interfere with the mothers' ability to care for their children" (p. 3). In addition, methamphetamine use by young mothers, particularly those who have neonates, infants, and young children in their custodial care, has been found, in several studies, to adversely affect both: (1) maternal-infant bonding; and (2) positive mothering behaviors (Pagliaro & Pagliaro, 2012, 2018). As identified by Derauf, LaGasse, and Smith (2007), "methamphetamine using women are more likely to have multiple, intertwined psychosocial risks that may result in maladaptive parenting and caregiving" (p. 281). Contributing factors, identified by the researchers, which could potentially increase "parenting problems and negative child outcomes" among "drug abusing mothers" include:

- Absence of a boyfriend, girlfriend, fiancé, fiancée, husband, wife, or other intimate partner (e.g., being a "single mother");
- Domestic violence, including intimate partner violence (IPV), psychological abuse, and sexual abuse;
- Family size (i.e., a large number of children);
- Homelessness, or "living on the street;"
- Incarceration, particularly with longer sentences;
- MDD or other mental disorders;
- Severity of disorders associated with drug and/or substance use.

As identified in the analysis of data involving methamphetamine use on the Navajo Nation, from the Tuba City Health Facility, one-half of the cases involved women and, of these women, a significant number were pregnant young mothers. This situation resulted in significant negative consequences for the American Indian community. As shared by the director of the facility, it "creates a serious problem at home and in the community because children are neglected" (First Nations Centre, 2006, p. 20).

35 See also the related discussion of methamphetamine-related neurotoxicity in the earlier amphetamines pharmacology subsection, "Undesired, or Harmful, Effects and Toxicities—Diminished Executive Function."

36 However, for young mothers, who require medically prescribed methylphenidate (e.g., for the medical management of ADHD) and are breastfeeding, the dose reportedly received by nursing infants is generally less than 1% of the maternal dose (Bolea-Alamanac, Green, & Verma, 2013). Thus, for these young mothers, the use of methylphenidate appears to be a relatively safer choice in terms of reducing the associated risk for breastfed infants.

It must be noted that this tragic situation, which involves child neglect and other serious problems related to methamphetamine use by young mothers, is not restricted to the American Indian community. As reported by the Associated Press (2018):

> A Florida woman was arrested after police say she left her child in a car while she shoplifted items from a market . . . According to an arrest report, sheriff's deputies broke into the car to help the crying child and called emergency medical personnel in to administer first aid . . . While searching her [i.e., the mother] police say they found methamphetamine laced with cocaine . . .
> (p. 1)

As also illustrated in another case related to maternal methamphetamine use:

> Atom Bomb was born inside of a compact car on New Year's Day, while his mother Jessica Dawn Killian sat in the passenger seat, WSOC reported.
>
> Police said Killian ran a drug trafficking operation from the same 2011 Cheverolet Cruze where she gave birth to Atom Bomb, Gaston County's first baby of 2019, according to the Gaston Gazette . . .
>
> Jail records show Killian was arrested on similar charges on Dec. 13, less than three weeks before giving birth to Atom Bomb.
>
> In addition to Atom Bomb, Killian has three other children, WSOC reported. That includes a five-year-old daughter who was in the back seat of the car when she gave birth early New Year's Day . . .
>
> From her Dec. 13 arrest [a little over two weeks earlier], records show Killian was charged with possession with the intent to manufacture, sell and deliver methamphetamine; maintaining a vehicle for a controlled substance; manufacturing drugs; in addition to misdemeanor charges of possession of drug paraphernalia and failure to appear.
> (Feit, 2019, p. 1)

For adolescent girls and young women, who are mothers, and who use methamphetamine—as well as for their children—the abuse typically culminates in outcomes that are both unanticipated and undesired. For example, as reported by Schabner (2004):

> "I didn't have to deal with everyday life," the mother of two said. "I felt energetic. I felt like I could do everything." She said she realized how false that impression was when the local child protective services took her children away.
> (p. 2)

Or, as further illustrated by Calhoun (2012):

> Kimbrough talked about her arrest following the death of her child, Timmy Jr. Born premature at 25 weeks on April 29, 2008, Timmy Jr. weighed 2 pounds 1 ounce, and lived only 19 minutes. When Kimbrough tested positive for methamphetamine, her two daughters were swiftly removed from her custody, and for 90 days, she was allowed only supervised visits. Social services mandated parenting classes and drug treatment.
> (p. 1)[37]

37 Three months after being released on bond, Kimbrough was back in jail on charges of selling oxycodone (see Chapter 5, "Prescription Opiate Analgesics and Heroin") to a confidential informant (Calhoun, 2012).

Mothering by adolescents and young women, who abuse amphetamines and other drugs and substances of abuse, can ultimately have the most extreme and horrific of consequences—as sadly reported in the following case:

> Three people [with histories of drug and substance abuse, including the abuse of methamphetamine] have been charged in the brutal sexual assault, murder and dismemberment of a 10-year-old girl, including the girl's mother. The mother's boyfriend and his cousin were also charged ... Police say Victoria [the child victim] was injected with methamphetamine, sexually assaulted, strangled, and stabbed before being dismembered [and her body burned].
>
> (Contrearas & Montoya Bryan, 2016, p. 1)

Or, as distressingly reported in a news story by NBC News/Reuters:

> A baby in Oklahoma died after her mother, high on methamphetamine and opioids, put the 10-day-old girl in a washing machine with a load of dirty laundry.
>
> (Wilson & Shiffman, 2015, p. 3)

Amphetamine Overdosage[38]

Overdosages involving the amphetamines are common, particularly when obtained illicitly "on-the-street" for IV injection (i.e., methamphetamine) or pulmonary inhalation (i.e., "smoking" or "vaping" "Crystal Meth").[39] Zosel, Bartelson, and Bailey (2013), in their analysis of data collected from the *Researched Abuse Diversion and Addiction-Related Surveillance (RADAR®) System*, found that, between 2007 and 2009:

1. A total of 16,209 intentional adolescent exposers to prescription drugs were reported;
2. The mean age for the intentionally exposed adolescents was 16.6 years-of-age;
3. Over half of these adolescent exposures (i.e., 52.4%) involved adolescent girls;[40]
4. 18% of these exposures involved amphetamines;
5. 14% of these exposures involved methylphenidate.

In the U.S., psychostimulant-related deaths increased three-fold during the first decade of the new millennium from 0.2 per 100,000 person-years in 2000, to 0.6 per 100,000 person-years in 2009 (Calcaterra & Binswanger, 2013, p. 11). The rates of psychostimulant deaths were highest among individuals of European continental descent, American Indian descent, and those who resided in the western states (Calcaterra & Binswanger, 2013; Kerley, Leban, & Copes, 2014). As identified by

38 See also the related discussion in the later amphetamines pharmacology subsection, "Pediatric Amphetamine Poisoning."

39 Illicit street purchase of the amphetamines is particularly problematic in terms of overdosage because, what is purchased, generally cannot be verified as: (1) actually being an amphetamine (e.g., methamphetamine); (2) not containing adulterants or other illicit drugs; and (3) being the actual dosage, or strength, claimed by the dealer.

40 Later, Mercado, Holland, and Leemis (2017, p. 1931), in their 2001 to 2015 study of self-inflicted injuries among youth that resulted in emergency department visits, identified three interesting, but disturbing related findings:

1. Youth suicide rates trended upward throughout the new millennium;
2. "Poisoning was the most commonly reported method of self-inflicted injury for females;"
3. After 2006, "females aged 10 to 14 years experienced the greatest increase."

Calcaterra and Binswanger (2013), who utilized the *CDC Wonder Database* for their comprehensive review of all deaths in the U.S. from 1999 to 2009:

> Accidental poisoning, was the most frequently listed cause of death among those who died with psychostimulants.
>
> (p. 1)

From 2015 to 2016, the largest change in the rate of psychostimulant overdosage deaths in the U.S.—by age cohort—was noted in the 15 to 24 years-of-age group (i.e., 44.4%) (Seth, Scholl, & Rudd, 2018). In 2016, the overall death rate associated with psychostimulant use in the U.S. increased, overall, by 33% (Orciari Herman, 2018).

Amphetamine poisoning can be unintentional (i.e., accidental)[41] or intentional (i.e., attempted or completed suicide).[42] Most cases of amphetamine poisoning are associated with the ingestion of oral amphetamine formulations (i.e., capsules; tablets) that are easily ingested. These posisonings are generally treated with slurries of activated charcoal that, when appropriately administered, can prevent the further absorption of the ingested amphetamines from the stomach. In these cases, the use of emetics to induce vomiting are contraindicated because of the risk for: (1) precipitating seizures; and (2) aspirating the vomitus that may subsequently result in the development of aspiration pneumonia, or death.

Children, who have unintentionally ingested methamphetamine, typically present with the following signs and symptoms: agitation; irritability; tachycardia; and vomiting (Kolecki, 1998;[43] Pagliaro & Pagliaro 2009, 2012). As identified by Matteucci, Auten, and Crowley (2007, p. 638), in their retrospective review of cases of acute methamphetamine poisoning that involved children younger than six years-of-age:

1. Agitation was the most frequent presenting sign or symptom;
2. Tachycardia, with a mean heart rate of 171 beats/minute, was common;
3. Benzodiazepine pharmacotherapy was successfully used to treat the majority of cases.

Signs and symptoms of acute amphetamine overdosage, include:

41 See also the related discussion in the following Amphetamines pharmacology subsection, "Embryo, Fetus, Infant, and Child Amphetamine Exposure."

42 Several studies of methamphetamine users in outpatient treatment (e.g., Glasner-Edwards, Mooney, & Marinelli-Casey, 2008; Zweben, Cohen, & Christian, 2004) provide strong evidence to support a significant association with suicide attempts. For example, in their related review and study of a "large sample of treatment-seeking methamphetamine users," Durrell, Kroutil, and Crits-Christoph (2008), identified that 27% reported a previous suicide attempt, and 43% reported violent behavior problems" (p. 2). In addition, as found by Kaland and Klein-Schwartz (2015), regarding amphetamine exposures reported to U.S. poison centers, for "both adolescents and adults, the most common reasons were suicide attempts" (p. 477).

We, too, have noted this relationship in our own clinical practice (Pagliaro & Pagliaro, *Clinical Patient Data Files*). However, based on other available data, we would suggest that the relationship between methamphetamine use and suicide is more tangential—being related, for example, to an underling intervening variable such as, MDD. The mental depression also may be a mediating factor contributing to both IPV and suicide ideation or attempts. That said, it is important to consider this relationship in the context of the significantly increasing incidence of suicide thoughts/attempts among adolescents and young adults. As found by Ahrnsbrak, Bose, and Hedden (2017), in their analysis of the 2016 *National Survey on Drug Use and Health* for the Substance Abuse and Mental Health Services Administration (SAMHSA):

> The percentage of young adults aged 18 to 25 with serious thoughts of suicide was higher in 2016 than in 2008 to 2014.
>
> (p. 3)

43 Kolecki (1998), based upon a retrospective chart review of methamphetamine poisoning in pediatric patients, found that "the most common complication of methamphetamine poisoning was rhabdomyolysis" (p. 385).

1. Agitation;
2. Constipation;
3. Hallucinations;
4. Panic;
5. Paranoia;
6. Restlessness;
7. Seizures;
8. Tachycardia;
9. Tachypnea;
10. Tremor.

Depression and fatigue usually follow the initial psychostimulation phase (see earlier related discussion). Other signs and symptoms, include:

- Abdominal cramps;
- Circulatory collapse;
- Diarrhea;
- Dysrhythmias;
- Hypertension or hypotension;
- Nausea;
- Vomiting.

Hyperthermia and rhabdomyolysis also can occur (see previous footnote). In addition, as noted by Vallersnes, Dines, and Wood (2016), amphetamine psychosis is commonly observed among cases of amphetamine poisoning (see also the earlier related discussion in the amphetamines subsection, "Undesired, or Harmful, Effects and Toxicities—Amphetamine Psychosis").

Amphetamine overdosages, including overdosages involving dextroamphetamine, lisdexamphetamine, and methamphetamine—as well as methylphenidate—require appropriate: (1) supportive medical treatment to maintain vital body organ functions; and (2) pharmacotherapy to manage troublesome signs and symptoms. Various antipsychotics have been effectively used to antagonize many of the toxic effects associated with overdosages involving the amphetamines, including:

- Haloperidol (Haldol®), a butyrophenone antipsychotic;
- Chlorpromazine (Thorazine®), a phenothiazine antipsychotic;
- Olanzapine (Zyprexa®), an atypical antipsychotic.

Diazepam (Valium®), a benzodiazepine sedative-hypnotic/anticonvulsant, is generally effective for managing associated agitation and seizures. Ammonium chloride also may be used to acidify the urine to increase amphetamine renal excretion (see the related discussion in the earlier amphetamines pharmacology subsection, "Pharmacokinetics—Excretion"). There is no known antidote for amphetamine overdosage (Pagliaro & Pagliaro, 2009; Ruha & Yarema, 2006).

Embryo/Fetus, Neonate, Infant, and Child Amphetamine Exposure[44]

Currently, embryos/fetuses, neonates, and infants are exposed to the amphetamines primarily by: (1) in utero exposure; and (2) breastfeeding. As with children, infants also can be exposed by unintentional poisoning, often associated with the illicit production of methamphetamine

44 See also the previous amphetamines pharmacology subsection, "Pregnancy, Lactation, and Mothering" and the later amphetamines pharmacology subsection, "Methamphetamine."

in "home labs." These unintentional pediatric amphetamine poisonings are presented and discussed in the following subsections with particular attention to injuries associated with illicit methamphetamine production in the home.

Pediatric Amphetamine Poisoning[45]

Pediatric amphetamine poisonings reported to the Toxicology Investigators Consortium (TOXIC),[46] from 2010 through 2012, indicate that amphetamine poisonings occur, but are relatively uncommon, particularly among children (Wiegand, Wax, & Smith, 2013). Subsequent related analyses provide similar findings (e.g., Rhyee, Farrugia, & Campleman, 2015; Rhyee, Farrugia, & Wiegand, 2014). However, we caution that most pediatric amphetamine poisonings occur in the context of the illicit home production of methamphetamine and go largely unreported because of related parental "fears," including:

1. Being arrested;
2. Having their children taken into custody by social services

(Pagliaro & Pagliaro, *Clinical Patient Data Files*).

In the context of methamphetamine production in the home, infants and children are frequently exposed to the chemicals used in the production process. As identified by Messina, Marinelli-Casey, and West (2014):

> Approximately 55% of children removed from home-based methamphetamine labs test positive for toxic levels of chemicals in their bodies.
>
> (p. 1872)

Farst, Duncan, and Moss (2007) first reported the unintentional poisoning of children associated with the illicit production of methamphetamine in home laboratories, identifying "cases of children harmed by ingesting caustic substances used in the production of methamphetamine in the home" (p. 341). (See also the related discussion in the later amphetamines embryo/fetus, infant and child exposures subsection, "Illicit Methamphetamine Production"). Since then, others have reported similar findings. For example, Burge, Hunsaker, and Davis (2009) reported "the death of an unattended toddler, who ingested sulfuric acid drain cleaner [used in the production of methamphetamine] in his home" (p. 298). (See also the related discussion in the earlier amphetamines pharmacology subsection, "Amphetamine Overdosage.")

In a study of the impact of parental methamphetamine abuse on the development and well-being of school-aged children, Haight, Jacobsen, and Black (2005) found that:

> Children are brought by their methamphetamine abusing parents into a rural drug culture characterized by distinct antisocial beliefs and practices. Children's experience of this culture includes environmental danger, chaos, neglect, abuse, loss, and isolation ... children develop antisocial beliefs and practices such as lying, stealing, drug use, and violence through direct teaching by their parents and indirectly, through observing [their] parents' own antisocial behavior.
>
> (p. 949)

45 See also the related discussion in the earlier amphetamines pharmacology subsection, "Amphetamine Overdosage."

46 TOXIC, is a case registry for reported toxic exposures, which was established in 2010, by the American College of Medical Toxicology.

As identified by Grant (2007):

> The illicit manufacturing and use of methamphetamine continues to be a significant and growing problem in the United States. Children are often found in homes where this activity is occurring and are affected by it on many levels.
>
> (p. 31)

Also of concern is the associated involvement of the criminal justice system that typically results in severe negative effects on young mothers and their children. For example, the prolonged mother-child separation due to the mother's arrest and incarceration (Gold, 2016) can have serious adverse effects on later mothering and often also directly contribute to child neglect and physical, psychological, and sexual abuse.

Illicit Methamphetamine Production

Illicit methamphetamine (i.e., "Crystal Meth") is generally chemically synthesized in sophisticated, large scale clandestine "super labs" for sale "on-the-street." The so-called "super labs," which are primarily controlled and directed by Mexican criminal organizations in Mexico and in Los Angeles, California, can generally produce 10 or more pounds of methamphetamine per day. Other super labs are operated by major Asian and other criminal organizations, including outlaw motor-cycle gangs (e.g., the Hells Angels Motorcycle Club) (Pagliaro & Pagliaro, 2009; Shukla, Crump, & Chrisco, 2012).[47]

> Common Misbelief. Only minimal chemistry knowledge and experience are needed to illicitly produce methamphetamine.

Actually, no chemistry knowledge or experience is needed. Methamphetamine is relatively easy to illicitly synthesize from inexpensive, over-the-counter ingredients and commonly

47 In addition, in parts of the U.S., illicit methamphetamine—produced in Mexico (i.e., "Mexican Meth")—significantly replaced that produced in illicit home laboratories (i.e., "home-cooked meth"). This change became established by 2007 and, since that time, the average purity of Mexican Meth has increased from approximately 37% to approximately 100% (Berkes, 2007; Buie & Tamburin, 2014) while the street price has significantly decreased (Pagliaro & Pagliaro, *Clinical Patient Data Files*). As identified by Shukla, Crump, and Chrisco (2012, p. 426):

> Transnational [criminal] organizations now control much of the methamphetamine supply in the U.S. and methamphetamine remains widely available.

> Super-strength methamphetamine from Mexico super labs is flooding streets in the United States.
>
> (Mammoser, 2017, p. 1)

During the second decade of the new millennium, Mexican drug smugglers increasingly turned to shipping "liquid meth" into the U.S. Liquid meth is simply methamphetamine crystals that have been dissolved in water (note that methamphetamine base is a colorless, volatile oil that is insoluble in water) resulting in a dark yellow, syrupy fluid that can be stored in sealed liquor bottles (or other larger containers) in order ot avoid detection at U.S. ports of entry along the U.S.-Mexico border (e.g., Cheromcha, 2018; D'Angelo, 2018; Eldridge, 2016; The United States Attorney's Ofice, 2018). Once successfully transported across the border to its intended destination, which is often several states away from the border crossing point, the liquid meth is converted back to methamphetamine crystals prior to sale to users (Pagliaro & Pagliaro, *Clinical Patient Data Files*).

available supplies.[48] It is often synthesized in small, unsophisticated, clandestine labs across the U.S., which range from small basement laboratories (e.g., "mom and pop labs") to larger, more sophisticated laboratories on college/university campuses. Methamphetamine also is synthesized in kitchens, bathrooms, and other places in the family home, including those where infants and children are often exposed to production fumes and methamphetamine while they entertain themselves by watching TV or playing their favorite android and computer games.

The "easiest" methods of methamphetamine production (i.e., the "anhydrous ammonia method" or the "red phosphorus method") frequently utilize precursor drugs, such as amphetamine, phenylalanine, phenylpropanolamine, or pseudoephedrine.[49, 50, 51, 52] To prevent, or at least significantly diminish, the wide-spread diversion of these precursor drugs for the illicit production of methamphetamine, the *Comprehensive Methamphetamine Control Act* of 1996 was passed. In 2005, Congress passed a related law, the *Combat Methamphetamine Epidemic Act* (CMEA), that was followed by the *Methamphetamine Production Prevention Act of 2008*, which was implemented in 2011 (DEA, 2011).[53]

SHAKE AND BAKE METHOD

The increasing adoption of the "shake and bake" method of methamphetamine production has largely nullified the past regulatory efforts aimed at controlling methamphetamine production (Hamilton, 2010; Pagliaro & Pagliaro, *Clinical Patient Data Files*). The "shake and bake" method only requires: a few packages of "common cold pills;" several corrosive, or flammable chemicals, which can be readily purchased at most hardware, farm supply, Walmart®, and similar stores; water; and an empty, 32- or 64-ounce plastic soda bottle to quickly and easily produce enough methamphetamine for an adolescent's use or sale on a very small scale (Carnevale Associates, 2011; Hall & Dunham, 2013; ONDCP, 2010; Pagliaro & Pagliaro, 2009).

48 These ingredients and supplies include: acetone; anhydrous ammonia; common cold and allergy tablets that contain pseudoephedrine; coffee filters; drain cleaner; isopropyl (rubbing) alcohol; lithium batteries; lye; Mason® jars; pillow cases; and toluene. (Also see later list of supplies in text associated with the "shake and bake" method of production.)

49 Alterations to the licit pharmaceutical formulations of pseudoephedrine have been used in an attempt to impede the illicit production of methamphetamine from pseudoephedrine. For example, the Nexafed® pseudoephedrine tablet maintains bioequivalence with Sudafed® pseudoephedrine tablets, while utilizing the Impede® technology to limit the extraction of pseudoephedrine and its subsequent conversion to methamphetamine (Brzeczko, Leech, & Stark, 2013).

50 Also, commonly referred to as either the "Birch Method" or the "Nazi Method" because this method of production was used during World War II to supply German soldiers with methamphetamine to increase their alertness (Pagliaro & Pagliaro, 2004).

51 N.B. Generally, amphetamine (i.e., dextroamphetamine) is only legally available by prescription while phenylalanine and pseudoephedrine, which are commonly found in common cold products, are generally legally available without a prescription (i.e., over-the-counter ["OTC"]).

52 The anhydrous ammonia method is more often used in the production of large quantities of methamphetamine because of the ready and unregulated availability of nitrogen farm fertilizer (i.e., the source of anhydrous ammonia).

53 In this context, various state and federal regulations have been enacted, including: (1) prior to sale, keeping these and other related products (e.g., ephedrine; pseudoephedrine) "behind the counter" in pharmacies; (2) limiting the amount of related product sold; and (3) for several states, such as Oregon and Mississippi, requiring a prescription for the purchase of related products. As identified by Messina, Marinelli-Casey, and West (2014):

> A review of state bills and regulations on over-the-counter purchases of these products reveals that as of 2005, 34 of the 50 states have passed bills to restrict access to and/or purchase of "cold medications" that include pseudoephedrine.
>
> (p. 1874)

As noted by the National Drug Intelligence Center (2006, p.1), these changes had an unanticipated consequence:

> Law enforcement pressure and strong precursor chemical sales restrictions have achieved marked success in decreasing domestic methamphetamine production. Mexican DTOs, however, have exploited the vacuum created by rapidly expanding their control over methamphetamine distribution—even to eastern states—as users and distributors, who previously produced the drug, have sought new, consistent sources.

Various detailed lists of the typical supplies needed for the "Shake and Bake Method" of illicit methamphetamine production can be found on the internet. For example, the following list is from "Some Chick's Blog" (Shake and bake, no date, p. 2):

- Two 32 oz. Gatorade® bottles;
- Two Mason® jars;
- three–four ft. of aquarium tubing;
- aquarium air pump (optional);
- fine coffee filters;
- a funnel;
- 75g 100% lye;
- 130g 15-0-15 fertilizer (no week killers);
- Two 96 ct. Pseudophedrine capsules or tablets (emptied and crushed into fine powder);
- Coleman® lantern fuel;
- 1.5g Ice;
- Two AA lithium batteries;
- Iodized Salt;
- Liquid Lightning® (drain cleaner);
- Pipe cutter;
- Needle nose pliers;
- Xacto® knife/Scissors.

Illicit methamphetamine producers generally identify three benefits of the "Shake and Bake Method," when compared to other methods of illicit methamphetamine production (Pagliaro & Pagliaro, *Clinical Patient Data Files*):

1. Ease of preparation (i.e., no need for basic knowledge, skills, or techniques in chemistry);
2. Less expenditure (i.e., no need for costly, specialized chemical laboratory equipment);
3. Quick "cooking time" (i.e., using this method, a "batch" of methamphetamine can be easily produced in as little as 30 minutes).

The identification of illicit "meth labs" is crucial for law enforcement, as well as for mental health care professionals, public health nurses, and social workers. Thus, various lists of related signs[54] of the presence of a possible meth lab have been compiled (e.g., Bartos, 2005). From these lists, we have provided three main areas for inspection: (1) inside; (2) outside; and (3) around meth labs and drug houses.

Positive "Inside Meth Lab" inspections include the presence of:

- Basic laboratory equipment (e.g., clear glass jugs; glassware; rubber tubing);
- Camp stoves, heat plates, or other heat sources;
- Coolers or thermos bottles;
- Cookware that contains powdery substances;
- Empty cold/allergy medication packaging;
- Strong odor of urine or unusual chemical odors such as acetone, ammonia, or ether;
- Used coffee filters that have a white or red pasty or powdery coating;
- Various drugs or chemicals in plain sight (e.g., cold/allergy medications, or ether).

54 It should be kept in mind that the signs included in these listings are indicative of, but not definitive for, methamphetamine production activity.

Positive "Outside Meth Lab" inspections include the presence of:

- Empty containers of: acetone; antifreeze; drain cleaners (e.g., Draino®); Freon®; Heet®; lye; starting fluids; or paint thinner;
- Empty propane tanks.

Positive "Around Meth Lab" and "Drug House" inspections include the presence of:

- Heavily covered windows;
- Little or no traffic during the day, but a large amount of traffic at night;
- Never putting out the trash;
- Reinforced doors;
- Renters who pay landlords in cash;
- Renters who are unfriendly, paranoid, or secretive;
- Unemployed people who seem to have plenty of cash.

CHILD EXPOSURE, PARENTAL NEGLECT, AND PHYSICAL, PSYCHOLOGICAL, AND SEXUAL ABUSE

Children are frequently "found at the scene" of methamphetamine production "laboratories," which are often located in the kitchen, or bathroom, of their apartment, home, or house trailer. As a result, they are exposed to a countless number of toxic chemicals, including: (1) chemicals used in the production of methamphetamine; (2) methamphetamine, itself; and (3) toxic wastes that are the "by-products" of the methamphetamine production process (Hohman, Oliver, & Wright, 2002, p. 373).[55] These children also are susceptible to various physical injuries (e.g., burns) related to laboratory explosions and fires—injuries that may be severe and, sometimes, fatal (e.g., Winslow, Voorhees, & Pehl, 2007; Pagliaro & Pagliaro, 2012, 2018).

Adults, who produce, sell, and abuse methamphetamine in their homes, often have young children who reside with them, and who, consequently, may be inadvertently exposed to the toxic fumes associated with the production of methamphetamne. Signs and symptoms of exposure to these toxic fumes often include:

- Abdominal pain;
- Amber or dark-colored urine;
- Blurred vision;
- Chemical burns;
- Chest pain;
- Cognitive impairment;
- Coughing;
- Diarrhea;
- Eye pain;
- Fever;
- Hallucinations;
- Headaches;
- Irritability;
- Loss of body weight;
- Skin irritation;

55 Citing U.S. DEA data, Winslow, Voorhees, and Pehl (2007) noted that, for each pound of methamphetamine produced in "home laboratories," over six-pounds of toxic waste are produced.

- Sneezing;
- Tachycardia;
- Watery eyes, tearing, or eye discharge;
- Vomiting.

(e.g., Horton, Berkowitz, & Kaye, 2003; Pagliaro & Pagliaro, 2012).[56]

Children, who live in households in which their parents, and others, produce methamphetamine, also may suffer from serious parental neglect identified by: various infections (e.g., particularly those involving the respiratory and urinary tracts); infestations (e.g., body and head lice); malnutrition; and poor hygiene. They also may suffer various forms of direct physical, psychological, or sexual abuse. Physical abuse is often identified by patterns of bruising, broken bones, burns, and other physical injuries perpetrated by their mothers or others (e.g., father; mother's boyfriend or fiancé) living in the home—often, as previously noted, an abandoned residence, apartment, camper truck, hotel or motel room, house trailer, or remote, rural residence (Pagliaro & Pagliaro, *Clinical Patient Data Files*). In this regard, the CDC (2007) cautioned that:

> Illegal methamphetamine production results in fires, explosions, spills, or air releases of hazardous chemicals (meth-chemical incidents), placing the meth producer and others nearby, including children, workers, and responders, at risk of injury or death and causing environmental contamination.
>
> (p. 910)

In 2015, the CDC noted that:

> During 2001–2012, a total of 1,325 meth-related incidents were reported in five states (Louisiana, Oregon, Utah, New York, and Wisconsin).
>
> (Melnikova, Orr, & Wu, 2019, p. 1)

Children, whose mothers abuse and illicitly produce amphetamines, may also suffer various types of psychological abuse commonly identified by behavioral problems, learning difficulties, and mental depression:

> The on-call social worker had been summoned to evaluate the 6-year-old son [of a 23-year-old, single mother who has a history of methamphetamine abuse]. She learns that the boy not only has had irregular school attendance but also has been experiencing academic difficulties and behavioral outbursts.
>
> (Lineberry & Bostwick, 2006, p. 81)

As identified by Connell-Carrick (2007), "Methamphetamine use and production is changing child welfare practice" (p. 125). To better deal with the significant risks posed to these children, several states (e.g., California) have created special "drug-endangered children's units" (Messina, Marinelli-Casey, & West, 2014). These units generally involve some degree of cooperation among various concerned agencies including, for example, child protective services (CPS), district attorney's offices, health and social care professionals, and police departments (also see the related discussion in the earlier amphetamine subsection, "Amphetamine Production").

56 N.B. It must be emphasized that these signs and symptoms are not unique to, or pathognomonic for, harmful exposure to toxic fumes produced by methamphetamine production. However, when not readily accounted for by other factors, they should be a reminder for clinicians to rule-out this potential etiology. They also may serve to alert teachers and others (e.g., social workers) to potential child exposure to methamphetamine production in the home.

In addition, several states have formally developed and adopted specific, related guidelines. For example, the state of Georgia, in a collaborative project with the Georgia Poison Center, developed a 15-page report entitled, *Guidelines for Managing Children Found at Clandestine Methamphetamine Laboratory Sites*. The explicit stated goals of these "Guidelines" are:

> 1. To assure the safety of the children found at meth laboratories;
> 2. To assure the safety of law enforcement, health care providers, state agency personnel and the public interacting with and caring for children found at meth laboratories;
> 3. To minimize the psychosocial trauma to the children while protecting their health and safety.
>
> (Geller, 2005, p. 5)

Adolescent and Young Adult Amphetamine Use

Purchased from classmates and street dealers, stolen from family members, or obtained from the illicit diversion of medical prescriptions, the amphetamines are commonly used by adolescents and young adults—particularly college/university students. We begin with the medical prescription of amphetamines and their illicit diversion by adolescents and young adults.

Medical Prescription and Illicit Diversion of Amphetamines and Related Drugs

> Psychostimulants, including amphetamines and methylphenidate, are first line pharmacotherapies for individuals with attention-deficit/hyperactivity disorder (ADHD).
>
> (Faraone, 2018, p. 255)

Indeed, psychostimulants have been widely recognized as the principal form of pharmacotherapy (i.e., the "gold standard") for the treatment and management of ADHD—at least in the U.S. (e.g., Pagliaro & Pagliaro, 1999, 2009, 2012). However, we would hasten to emphasize that: (1) psychostimulant pharmacotherapy is not indicated for the treatment of all children, adolescents, or young adults with ADHD; and (2) if clinical improvement of the presenting signs and symptoms of ADHD are not observed within one month—at an adequate therapeutic dosage—then the pharmacotherapy should be discontinued.

The prescription psychostimulants used for the treatment and management of ADHD include:[57]

1. Amphetamine (Adzenys XR-ODT®), an extended-release, orally disintegrating tablet approved by the FDA in 2016 for the treatment of ADHD among children six years-of-age and older (Fellner, 2016);
2. Mixed-Amphetamines (Adderall®; "Addies;" "Tic Tacs"), a combination drug that contains amphetamine and dextroamphetamine, as well as their salt forms;
3. Lisdexamfetamine (Vyvanse®; LDX), a more recently developed amphetamine that is a dextroamphetamine prodrug of the phenethylamine and amphetamine classes and that is beginning to be more widely used to treat ADHD (Blick & Keating, 2007; Boellner, Stark, & Krishnan, 2010; Popovic, Bhattacharya, & Sivaswamy, 2009);

57 Interestingly, and as probably expected–given the nature of ADHD, prescription rates for the psychostimulants are highest in all 50 states for children and adolescents—in comparison to adults (e.g., Pagliaro & Pagliaro, 2012; Paulozzi, Strickler, & Kreiner, 2015).

4. Methylphenidate (Ritalin®; "Rs;" "The Smart Drug"), a psychostimulant of the phenethylamine and piperidine classes that is closely related to the amphetamines and, for decades (i.e., since the 1960s), has been extensively used, and continues to be used, to treat ADHD among children six years-of-age and older, adolescents, and adults;
5. Racemic Amphetamine Sulfate (Evekeo®), an extended-release, disintegrating tablet approved by the FDA for the treatment of: ADHD among children three years-of-age and older, as well as adults; narcolepsy for children six years-of-age and older, as well as adults; and obesity (short-term treatment) for children 12 years-of-age and older, as well as adults (Abramowicz, 2015; Pagliaro & Pagliaro, 2009).

Since the 1990s, adolescents and young adults have been increasingly attracted to the illicit use of the amphetamines and closely related drugs that are primarily prescribed for the medical management of ADHD.[58]

> She told Women's Health US, "Eventually, I was snorting it in the bathroom of my high school. And I knew it wasn't good, but I couldn't stop."
>
> (Keegan, 2018, p. 1)

Prescriptions for the medical management of ADHD among children and adolescents has increased constantly and significantly during the new millennium, particularly among boys in the U.S. of European continental descent. This pattern of prescribing appears to be unrelated to the true incidence of ADHD, particularly when compared and contrasted with the rates reported by other developed countries (Pagliaro & Pagliaro, 2012). In addition, most medical prescriptions (virtually all) are written based almost entirely upon observations (complaints) provided by the mother or teacher of the child or adolescent and only rarely include direct observation by the prescriber in the home or classroom environment (Pagliaro & Pagliaro, *Clinical Patient Data Files*).[59] Unfortunately, these trends in increased prescription and use of the psychostimulants to treat ADHD has extended into the new millennium and continues to be of significant concern (Burcu, Zito, & Metcalfe, 2016).

> Over the 8-year period [1990 to 1997], the prescribing rates of amphetamines increased significantly, ranging from 380% for children 2–4 years to 817% for teenagers older than 14 years.
>
> (Lin, Crawford, & Lurvey, 2005, p. 617)

In this regard, Berman, Kuczenski, and McCracken (2009) further noted that:

> Insufficient physician follow-up care for stimulant-treated children contributes to the problem.
>
> (p. 30)

58 During the last half of the 20th century, the amphetamines (e.g., dextroamphetamine, Dexedrine®) were extensively prescribed in the U.S.—almost exclusively for women—to manage exogenous obesity (Pagliaro & Pagliaro, 2004). Due to their wide-spread abuse and limited, long-term efficacy, the medical use of the amphetamines for this indication, although still legal, has virtually disappeared from mainstream medical practice.

59 We are concerned here, not only with the potential for subsequent amphetamine abuse by the child or adolescent for whom the psychostimulants were prescribed, but also (and as importantly) for the long-term (i.e., often many years or decades, particularly since ADHD has become to be viewed as a "life-long" disorder and not one that is simply "outgrown" during adolescence) unanticipated consequences of the "medical use" of these drugs by children and adolescents (e.g., neurotoxicity). (Also see related discussion in the earlier amphetamines pharmacology subsection, "Undesired, or Harmful, Effects and Toxicities—Neurotoxicity.")

Later, McDonald and Kuck Jalbert (2013, p. 1079) recognized:

> Wide variations in treatment prevalence signal disparities between established clinical practice guidelines and actual practice, especially for primary care, where most patients prescribed stimulants are managed. Better education and training for physicians may improve identification and treatment, thereby reducing disparities in care for attention-deficit/hyperactivity disorder.

As noted by Brahmbhatt, Hilty, and Hah (2016):

> Diagnostic challenges [in relation to ADHD] include ... limited training and time for primary care providers to conduct thorough evaluations.
>
> (p. 135)

Additionally, as further identified in a clinical report by two psychiatric residents:

> The patient went so far as to feign illness, by mimicking symptoms and presenting himself as a textbook case of attention deficit hyperactivity disorder to a psychiatrist to secure a prescription ... What does this all mean? What should be extremely crucial is for clinicians to conduct a thorough evaluation to ensure that they make an appropriate, non-pressured, correct diagnosis and before considering prescribing a medication as a first resort.
>
> (Ahmed & Virani, 2017, p. 11–12)

It should be noted that feigning illness (i.e., "faking bad") by adolescents and young adults in order to receive a prescription for psychostimulants is a rather common practice (Pagliaro & Pagliaro, *Clinical Patient Data Files*). For example, as shared by two high school students—both of whom abused prescription psychostimulants and also sold them to their classmates:

> "I lie to my psychiatrist—I express feelings I didn't really have, knowing the consequence of it," he said, standing in a park a few miles from the high school. "I tell the doctor, 'I find myself very distracted, and I feel this really deep pain inside, like I'm anxious all the time,' or something like that." He coughed out a chuckle and added proudly, "Generally, if you keep playing the angsty-teen role, you'll get something good."
>
> Christine, a junior sitting nearby, said she followed the well-known lines to get her drugs directly and legally, a script for scripts. "I'm not able to focus on schoolwork," she said in a mockingly anxious voice. "I'm constantly looking out the window." Although she often uses the drugs herself, snorting them for a faster and more intense effect, she said she preferred to save them for when her customers crave them most.
>
> (Schwarz, 2012, p. 7)

***Related Professional Reminder:* Changes in the diversion and nonmedical use of the prescription psychostimulants (i.e., amphetamines; methylphenidate) generally directly parallel changes in medical prescription trends.**

Some children and adolescents, who have ADHD, misuse their prescription drugs in order to get "high." Others, who do not have ADHD and want to get "high," often buy or steal medically prescribed drugs from their classmates or siblings, who have ADHD (Wilens, Adler, & Adams, 2008). In comparison, adolescents and young adults, generally, obtain their illicit prescription amphetamines by:

1. Diverting drugs prescribed for legitimate medical conditions (e.g., ADHD);
2. Stealing them from family members (e.g., siblings; parents) and friends;
3. Engaging in sex-for-drug exchanges (usually adolescent girls and gay/bisexual adolescent boys);
4. Purchasing from "street dealers," including classmates at school;
5. Purchasing them over the "dark net."

As illustrated in a related ABC news report:

> Stone began misusing Ritalin after being diagnosed with ADHD as a sixth-grader, and later sold the prescription drug to fellow high school students, charging $5 for three blue 10-milligram pills or one orange 30-milligram pill.
>
> (ABC, 2003, p.1)

Over the first two decades of the new millennium, the problem of ADHD prescription drug abuse by adolescents and young adults has been significant (Pagliaro & Pagliaro, 2004, 2009, 2012, 2018). As reported by Clemow and Walker (2014), in their related literature review:

> Overall, the data suggest that ADHD medication misuse and diversion are common health care problems for stimulant medications, with the prevalence believed to be approximately 5% to 10% of high school students and 5% to 35% of college students.
>
> (p. 64)

As significant and troubling as these numbers are, we believe that the actual incidence of ADHD psychostimulant abuse may be closer to 20% of high school students and 50% of undergraduate college/university students (Pagliaro & Pagliaro, *Clinical Patient Data Files*).

This observation is made particularly in the light of the significant increase in the use of the amphetamines and methylphenidate by high school students—often from prestigious high schools—as "study aids" to increase their GPA and performance on college/university entrance examinations in order to improve their competitive academic performance and, consequently improve their chances of being admitted to the college/university of their choice (e.g., Cadwalladr, 2015; Huffpost Staff, 2012; Schwarz, 2012). As noted by Schwarz (2012) in his comprehensive related exposé that was published in the New York Times:

> "Now I have to worry about this, too? Really? This shouldn't be what they need to do to get where they want to," said Dodi Sklar, after listening to her ninth-grade son, Jonathan, describe how some classmates abuse stimulants ...
>
> [In the high school parking lot] he twisted open a capsule of orange powder and arranged it in a neat line on the armrest. He leaned over, closed one nostril and snorted it.
>
> Throughout the parking lot, he said, eight of his friends did the same thing.
>
> The drug was not cocaine or heroin, but Adderall, an amphetamine prescribed for attention deficit hyperactivity disorder that the boy said he and his friends routinely shared to study late into the night, focus during tests and ultimately get the grades worthy of their prestigious high school in an affluent suburb of New York City. The drug did more than just jolt them awake for the 8 a.m. SAT; it gave them a tunnel focus tailor-made for the marathon of tests long known to make or break college applications.
>
> "Everyone in school either has a prescription or has a friend who does," the boy said.
>
> At high schools across the United States, pressure over grades and competition for college admissions are encouraging students to abuse prescription stimulants, according to interviews with students, parents and doctors ... "It's throughout all the private schools here,"

> said DeAnsin Parker, a New York psychologist who treats many adolescents from affluent neighborhoods like the Upper East Side. Its not as if there is one school where this is the culture. "This is the culture."
>
> (pp. A1–A2)

For further discussion, see the following subsection, "Undergraduate College/University Students."

As identified by Rabinber (2013):

> As prescriptions for stimulant medication to treat ADHD have increased, so have concerns about the nonmedical use and diversion of stimulant medication.
>
> (p. 375)

Further to this situation, and consistent with our own recommendations, Tapscott and Schepis (2013) suggested that prescribing clinicians "may want to consider prescribing fewer pills and refills and scheduling less time between follow-up appointments" (p. 7). In this clinical context, others, such as Brahmbhatt, Hilty, and Hah (2016, p. 135), also recommend that "providers should be cognizant of prevention, early identification, and treatment of conditions associated with ADHD that emerge during adolescence, such as substance use disorders."

***Related Professional Reminder:* Given the tremendous over-prescription of drugs for the treatment of ADHD in the U.S., we recommend that these drugs only be prescribed for severe cases in which the behavior has been directly observed and diagnosed by the prescriber.**

Undergraduate College/University Students

Regarding the amphetamines and other psychostimulant drugs, undergraduate college/university students comprise a "special case" in terms of both type and frequency of amphetamine and other psychostimulant use, as well as, reasons for their use. In fact, undergraduate college/university students are the largest group, who report the illicit use of prescription amphetamines (i.e., drugs that are primarily prescribed for the management of ADHD, both for children and adults in the U.S.). This subsection presents and discusses this special case of amphetamine use by college/university students. We begin with illicit prescription use and diversion.

As identified by Kondrotas (2006):

> Without the generosity of students diagnosed with ADHD there would be no speed around for others to use illicitly [at Harvard and MIT].
>
> (p. 1)

ILLICIT PRESCRIPTION USE AND DIVERSION

College/university students reportedly comprise the *largest* group that acknowledges illicit use of prescription amphetamines, particularly the mixed amphetaines (Adderall®) and methylphenidate (Ritalin®), in the U.S. (e.g., Clemow & Walker, 2014; Pagliaro & Pagliaro, *Clinical Patient Data Files*; Varga, 2012; Weyandt, Marraccini, & Gudmundsdottir, 2013). As identified by Frances (2015):

> College students are using and abusing *Adderall*—the drug commonly used to treat attention-deficit/hyperactivity disorder (ADHD)—in record numbers. Adderall may not yet be in the water supply, but it's part of the fabric of life on modern American college campuses.
>
> (p. 1)

For example:

- 43% of 1,550 undergraduate students reported using prescription stimulants illicitly (Advokat, Guidry, & Martino, 2008);
- 31% of 115 undergraduate students from two universities, who were receiving prescriptions for ADHD, reported misuse during attendance at college (Rabiner, Anastopoulos, & Costello, 2009, p. 144);
- 20% of 1,023 undergraduate students reported past-year nonmedical use of prescription stimulants (Dussault & Weyandt, 2013, p. 87);[60]
- Half of the [college] students reported they took stimulant drugs to study or improve their academic performance (Haelle, 2014, p. 1).

> The first time I took Adderall, I was a sophomore at Brown University, lamenting to a friend the impossibility of my plight: a five-page paper due the next afternoon on a book I had only just begun reading. "Do you want an Adderall?" she asked. "I can't stand it—it makes me want to stay up all night doing cartwheels in the hallway." Could there be a more enticing description? . . .
>
> Adderall wiped away the question of willpower. Now I could study all night, then run 10 miles, then breeze through that week's New Yorker, all without pausing to consider whether I might prefer to chat with classmates or go to the movies. It was fantastic. I lost weight. That was nice, too.
>
> (Schwartz, 2016, p. 1)

In this context of use, DeSantis and Curtis Hane (2010) conducted in-depth interviews with 175 undergraduate students to determine their reasons for "non-medically" using psychostimulants that are generally medically used to treat ADHD:

> Lisa, for example, a third-year business major, who told us that "Adderall is definitely not a drug. No way, It is a study tool. You don't get high or anything like that, I take it to do good in school. How can that be bad? So its all good." (p. 35)
>
> Lauren, a junior Spanish major, also claimed to only take stimulants during finals: "No I don't feel bad because I only take it when I really need to take it. Finals is just too crazy not to. But as long as I don't abuse it like everday, I think it's fine." (p. 39)
>
> I don't feel like there is any difference in me taking it [Adderall] and me taking a caffeine pill," explained Jason. "Whats the difference. Basically, it is just a way to stay awake. There're both pills . . . Katie told us that "During finals, it was either NoDoz, you know, or Adderall and it is just easier for me to take Adderall. I would've had to drive to the store . . . It was easy, a girl in my [sorority] house had some, so. But I really think it is all the same."
>
> (p. 41)

60 In regard to this "lower" reported overall percentage, it should be recognized that:

> The sample, overall, was consistent with the demographics of the individual university population with respect to age, ethnicity, and social sorority membership. [However,] gender and social membership was not representative of the individual university population; a disproportionate number of participants identified as female (n = 723) rather than male (n = 300).

These sample biases may have contributed to the "lower" reported percentage of use in this study. Additionally, as demonstrated by Palamar and Le (2017) adolescents and young adults may under-report use of amphetamines because they are "unaware" that Adderall® is an amphetamine.

Finally, as concluded by DeSantis and Curtis Hane (2010):

> With the multifaceted demands placed on college students (e.g., grades, social life, finance, etc.) and the increasingly competitive work force that awaits them after graduation, these students believe they have found the "magic bullet." "It works!" explained Lisa, a senior pre-med major. "Why wouldn't you use it if it works? The stuff is great. Great!"
>
> (p. 43)

Several researchers have observed a significant increase in subsequent psychostimulant abuse among those, who as children and adolescents, received psychostimulant pharmacotherapy to treat a chronic mental disorder—most often ADHD. As noted by Berman, Kuczenski and McCracken (2009):

> A survey of over 9,000 Midwestern college students found that those who initiated prescribed use of stimulant medication for ADHD in secondary school were three times as likely as students never prescribed stimulant medication to report illicit use of prescription stimulants, and that those who initiated such medication in college were seven times as likely to report illicit use.
>
> (p. 131)

In addition, diversion of amphetamines and methylphenidate, which have been prescribed for the management of ADHD, is common among this group (e.g., Bogle & Smith, 2009; Cepeda, Fife, & Berwaerts, 2015; Clemow & Walker, 2014; Pagliaro & Pagliaro, *Clinical Patient Data Files*; Wilens, Adler, & Adams, 2008). For example, from a random sample of 1,738 university students, Sepulveda, Thomas, and McCabe (2011), found that, among a cohort of 55 past-year "prescription stimulant users:"

> Diversion of prescription stimulants was common (36%) and occurred more frequently among stimulant users (57%).
>
> (p. 551)

Rabiner, Anastopoulos, and Costello (2009) found that 26% of their sample of undergraduate students diverted their psychostimulant prescriptions to peers. While among those, who had never been prescribed a psychostimulant for the treatment of ADHD, diversion from family (e.g., younger siblings) and friends (e.g., college classmates) are the most common sources for the prescription psychostimulants (e.g., Cassidy, McNaughton, & Varughese, 2015; Novak, Kroutil, & Williams, 2007). In a later study, Gallucci, Martin, and Usdan (2015) found that 59% of 151 current undergraduate students with current prescriptions for psychostimulants had "given away or sold their stimulant medication during their lifetime ... The most common motivations reported for both lifetime and current diversion were 'to make extra money' and to 'help [others] during a time of high academic stress'" (p. 154).

The prescription formulation, mixed amphetamines (Adderall®), is generally more frequently used by college/university students than is the more closely related "chemical cousin," methylphenidate (Concerta®, Metadate®, Ritalin®) (e.g., Brandt, Taverna, & Hallock, 2014). For example, in a web-based survey of a random sample of 4,580 college/university students, Teter, McCabe, and LaGrange (2006) found that, among the past-year illicit prescription psychostimulant users, approximately 75% reported use of mixed amphetamines while only approximately 25% reported use of methylphenidate. In addition, among those who illicitly ingested prescription amphetamines, "immediate release" formulations were significantly more likely to be used than the "extended-release" formulations (Cassidy, Varughese, & Russo, 2015; Upadhyaya, Kroutil, & Deas, 2010).[61]

Undergraduate college/university students, who also abuse prescription amphetamines and other prescription psychostimulant drugs, can be generally distinguished by one or more of the following characteristics:

- Attend a "noncommuter college;"
- Belong to a fraternity or sorority;
- Have been diagnosed with ADHD;
- Engage in weekly partying that is significantly related to prescription amphetamine or other prescription psychostimulant use;
- Frequently attend clubs;
- Have a medical history of prescription psychotropic use;
- Have a Jewish religious affiliation;
- Are more likely to be of European continental descent than of African or Asian continental descent or Hispanic descent;
- Are more likely to be males;
- Are more likely to have lower/average GPAs;
- Are more likely to report increased rates of undesired, or harmful, effects and toxicities (e.g., insomnia and restlessness) associated with the use of prescription amphetamine or other prescription psychostimulant use;
- Have a higher incidence of concomitant poly-drug and substance abuse (e.g., Benson, Flory, & Humphreys, 2015; Dussault & Weyandt, 2013; Esteban-McCabe, West, & Teter, 2014; Kelly, Wells, & Leclair, 2013).

Several reasons, as previously noted, have been identified by undergraduate college/university students for their use and abuse of the prescription amphetamines and other prescription psychostimulants, as well as the abuse of illicit amphetamines (e.g., methamphetamine). These reasons also include to:

- Achieve euphoria;
- Be more energetic;
- Get "high;"
- Increase athletic/sport performance;[62]
- Increase confidence, or self-esteem;
- Increase sexual arousal and pleasure;
- Increase wakefulness;
- Initially experience the effects of using a specific psychostimulant;

61 Although illicit amphetamines are usually ingested, a significant and increasing number of college/university students report intranasal use (Pagliaro & Pagliaro, *Clinical Patient Data Files*). For example, Teter, McCabe, and LaGrange (2006), in their web-based survey of 4,580 college students, found that:

> Nearly every illicit user (95.3%) reported oral administration, and 38.1% reported snorting prescription stimulants. (p. 1501)

62 This reason for adolescent and young adult use, particularly in the context of participation in high school and college/university sports, is significant, but has not been adequately addressed (Pagliaro & Pagliaro, *Clinical Patient Data Files*; Veliz, Boyd, & McCabe, 2013; Wolf, 2015).

- Intensify alertness;
- Lose body weight;
- Self-medicate in an attempt to relieve or manage a mental disorder (e.g., mental depression);
- Stay awake to "party" through the night or to go "clubbing" (e.g., Pagliaro & Pagliaro, *Clinical Patient Data Files*; Teter, McCabe, & Cranford, 2005; Varga, 2012; Wilens, Adler, & Adams, 2008).

However, the primary reason provided by undergraduate college/university students for their illicit use of the prescription amphetamines and other psychostimulants (i.e., methylphenidate) is reportedly to improve academic performance by being able to:

- Focus better in class;
- Complete academic assignments;
- Perform better on schoolwork;
- Achieve higher marks on tests (e.g., DuPont, Coleman, & Bucher, 2008; Dussault & Weyandt, 2013; Pagliaro & Pagliaro, *Clinical Patient Data Files*; Rabiner, Anastopoulos, & Costello, 2009).

> Adderall became my study buddy and I owe many successful all-nighters to those tiny capsules.
>
> (Workman & Eells, 2010, p. 2)

As noted by a MIT student:

> The current attitude is one of opportunism, not opposition, so while amphetamines themselves haven't changed, 60s-era connotations of crime and speed freak are absent today. Rather, students feel justified in their desire for drugs that make their work salient and absorbing, allowing them to push limits of academic aptitude, efficiency, and exhaustion. In fact, speed is hardly a drug anymore—it's a tool.
>
> (Kondrotas, 2006, p. 2)

Illicit Methamphetamine Use among Adolescents and Young Adults[63]

During the 1980s, the use of the amphetamines among adolescents and young adults was largely replaced by the use of cocaine (see the next major section of this chapter, "Cocaine"). However, by the mid-1990s, there was a renewed interest in the use of the amphetamines as an economic alternative to cocaine, particularly illicit methamphetamine, which was significantly less expensive.

This renewed interest in the use of amphetamines was further fostered by the increased availability of both its "powdered" form (e.g., "chalk") and "crystalline" form (i.e., "Crystal Meth," "Glass," or "Ice"). The use of "Crystal Meth"—the "smokable" form—had its origin in Hawaii from where it quickly spread to California (hence, one of its common street names, "West Coast"). Subsequently, it quickly spread across the U.S. (Pagliaro & Pagliaro, 2009, 2012, 2018), where its use became particularly widespread across urban and rural areas in the midwestern and southern states—hence, another common street name, "Hillbilly Crack" (Gonzales, Mooney, & Rawson, 2010; Hauer, 2010; Sexton, Carlson, & Siegal, 2006; Winslow, Voorhees, & Pehl, 2007).

63 N.B. When considering the amphetamines, particularly methamphetamine, it is important to keep in mind that an overwhelming majority of users (i.e., approximately 90%) concurrently use other drugs and substances of abuse (e.g., Glover-Kerkvliet, 2009; Pagliaro & Pagliaro, *Clinical Patient Data Files*).

The spread of methamphetamine across the U.S. was profoundly affected by changing sociocultural norms with the use of methamphetamine being consistently highest among adolescents and young adults of European continental descent. Another troubling trend that developed during the first decade of the new millennium was the increased use of methamphetamine by adolescent girls, 16 to 17 years-of-age (Wu, Schlenger, & Galvin, 2006).

The use of methamphetamine, primarily the use of the crystalline form—"Crystal Meth,"—soared, from 2000 to 2010, because of its ready availability, relatively low cost, and rapid achievement of high methamphetamine blood concentrations (along with desired psychostimulant effects)—without IV injection. "Crystal Meth," smoked in much the same way as Crack cocaine,[64] also could produce a longer duration of desired psychostimulant effects than Crack cocaine (i.e., four to eight hours versus 15 to 60 minutes). During the same period of time, a new method of methamphetamine use, "parachuting," increased in popularity.

"Parachuting" and other related techniques became established around 2006 to enable adolescents and young adults to ingest their methamphetamine. There are generally, two major methods of parachuting:

1. Placing the methamphetamine dose in a small plastic baggie that has been punctured with "pin-holes," and swallowing it;
2. Placing the methamphetamine in the middle of a 1- to 2-inch square of toilet paper, pulling up the corners and twisting them to make a "parachute," and then swallowing the "parachute."

(Hendrickson, Horowitz, & Norton, 2006; Pagliaro & Pagliaro, *Clinical Patient Data Files*)

By 2010, the use of illicit methamphetamine began to be slowly replaced with cocaine (e.g., Johnston, O'Malley, & Bachman, 2013).[65] (See the next major section of this chapter, "Cocaine.") It may seem ironic, or even surprising, to some readers that the same attributes that made methamphetamine so popular—its widespread availability, cheaper price, and longer duration of action in comparison to cocaine—subsequently contributed to its decline in popularity as it increasingly became known as, the "Poor Kid's Drug" or the "White Trash Drug" (Pagliaro & Pagliaro, *Clinical Patient Data Files*) (See Table 2.5).

Throughout the first two decades of the new millennium, methamphetamine use became entrenched among U.S. adolescents—particularly in areas of the country where it was readily available:

> In Oregon, officials recently reported that meth is second only to marijuana—surpassing alcohol—as the drug that sends the most teens to treatment there.
>
> (Irvine, 2005, p. 1)

64 "Crystal Meth" is most often smoked by adolescents (and others) with a small glass pipe that is commonly referred to as a "bubble," "pizzo," or "tweak pipe" (Pagliaro & Pagliaro, *Clinical Patient Data Files*).

65 N.B. When discussing methamphetamine—or any other drug or substance of abuse—related usage statistics often appear contradictory, or in opposition. However, often they all may be "factually correct." Apparently different, even contradictory, statistics are most often the result of differences in: (1) sampling (e.g., all adolescents versus only those currently enrolled in high school); and (2) definitions (e.g., is "current use" defined by use within the previous day, week, month, or year?). A prime example is the often-cited annual series of national survey results on drug use (i.e., *Monitoring the Future*) by Johnston and colleagues at the University of Michigan. This annual survey of adolescent drug use, is based on sampled self-reports obtained from questionnaires administered to a national representative group of "8th, 10th, and 12th graders" (see Table 2.6). Thus, by definition, these survey results are limited to, and, consequently, only reflect adolescents who are currently enrolled in, and attending, high school.

Table 2.5 General Comparison between Methamphetamine and Cocaine

Methamphetamine	*Cocaine*
Classification: Psychostimulant (amphetamine), Synthetic	**Classification:** Psychostimulant, Natural
Available Form: Powdered crystal	**Available Forms:** Cocaine base ("Crack;"[66] "Rocks") and Cocaine hydrochloride (powdered crystal)
Desired Effects: Produces long-lasting euphoria, sexual stimulation, and other desired effects due to its relatively long half-life of elimination	**Desired Effects:** Produces a brief euphoria, sexual stimulation, and other desired effects due to its relatively short half-life of elimination
Medical Use: Not legally available in the U.S.	**Medical Use:** Limited dental and medical use as a local anesthetic for short surgical and other procedures
Child, Adolescent, and Young Adult Use: "Poor Kid's Drug" primarily used by adolescents and young adults in the U.S. of European continental descent	**Child, Adolescent, and Young Adult Use:** "Rich Kid's Drug" primarily used by adolescents and young adults in the U.S. of African continental descent
Methods of Use: Methamphetamine is ingested; dissolved and IV injected; or nasally insufflated ("snorted"). It is also heated, and the fumes inhaled from a glass pipe, the top of a discarded soda pop can, or on a piece of tin foil	**Methods of Use:** Cocaine HCl powder can be dissolved and IV injected; or nasally insufflated ("snorted"). Cocaine Base is heated, and the fumes inhaled with a crack pipe, on the top of a discarded soda pop can, or on a piece of tin foil
Mechanism of Action: Acts by increasing dopamine release and blocking its reuptake	**Mechanism of Action:** Acts by blocking dopamine re-uptake
Metabolism/Elimination: 50% of methamphetamine is excreted in unchanged form in the urine over approximately 12 hours (pH dependent)	**Metabolism/Elimination:** 50% of cocaine is excreted in unchanged form in the urine over approximately one hour (pH dependent)
Abuse Potential: High abuse potential with a characteristic methamphetamine withdrawal syndrome that is not relieved with resumed use. Methamphetamine does not display a true,	**Abuse Potential:** High abuse potential with extreme psychological craving and a characteristic cocaine withdrawal syndrome that cannot be relieved with the resumed use of cocaine.

(*Continued*)

66 "Crack" is cocaine base that has been prepared from the salt form of cocaine (i.e., cocaine hydrochloride) utilizing the addition of sodium bicarbonate. The associated chemical reaction is:

$$\textbf{Cocaine HCl} + \textbf{NaHCO}_3 \rightarrow \textbf{Cocaine} + \textbf{H}_2\textbf{O} + \textbf{CO}_2 + \textbf{NaCl}$$

(i.e., cocaine hydrochloride and sodium bicarbonate produce cocaine base + water + carbon dioxide + sodium chloride).

Table 2.5 (Cont.)

Methamphetamine	*Cocaine*
or classical, withdrawal syndrome such as that which occurs with the opiate analgesics and that is immediately relieved with resumed use. Dependence is primarily psychological	Cocaine does not display a true, or classical, withdrawal syndrome such as alcohol and opiate analgesics, which can be immediately relieved with resumed use. Dependence is primarily psychological.
Street Names: "Crank;" "Crystal;" "Glass;" "Ice;" "Meth;" "Speed;" "Tina;" "Tweak"	**Street Names:** Cocaine Hydrochloride—"Blow;" "C;" "Coke;" "Nose Candy;" "Powder;" "Snow;" "Toot" Cocaine Base—"Crack;" "Freebase"

Lifetime prevalence of methamphetamine use among men and women in the U.S. is approximately 8% (Durrell, Kroutil, & Crits-Christoph, 2008). However, as noted previously in this chapter section, the use of methamphetamine, waxes and wanes over time. As identified by Calcaterra and Binswanger (2013), "methamphetamine use declined significantly [in the U.S.] from 2002 to 2008, but rose again in 2009" (p. 2).[67] Consequently, treatment statistics vary over the years—obviously, falling behind use statistics (see Table 2.6). Data available from the SAMHSA (2014), indicate that adolescent girls and women, from 15 years-of-age to 55 years-of-age, significantly outnumber (by %) adolescent boys and men in terms of methamphetamine being the primary drug responsible for treatment admissions. This trend is expected to continue.[68]

Regarding this trend, it also is important to recognize that adolescent girls and young women use amphetamines for some of the same, as well as for significantly different, reasons than do adolescent boys and young men. Often introduced to the use of amphetamines by their boyfriends, adolescent girls and young women primarily use amphetamines:

1. For their euphorigenic effects;
2. To decrease social inhibitions;
3. To enhance sexual pleasure;
4. To gain acceptance, or to "fit in," with their peers;
5. To get "high;"
6. To feel more attractive and sexy;
7. To self-medicate their mental depression—usually subconsciously;
8. To maintain or lose body weight as an appetite suppressant.

(e.g., Lyons, 2014; Pagliaro & Pagliaro, 2018; Schabner, 2004; Schulzke, 2013)

67 This general trend also was identified by Johnston, O'Malley, and Bachman (2013) in their survey, *Monitoring the Future*, in which they identified a significant decline in self-reported methamphetamine use by 8th and 12th graders beginning in 2005 until a significant increase "among 12th graders in 2011." (p. 19)

68 In addition, as with the use of other drugs and substances of abuse, the use of methamphetamine—while naturally varying slightly across the U.S. from year to year—can spike in particular areas (i.e., neighborhoods, cities, counties, or states) because of unique facilitating factors (e.g., availability, price, social trends). For example, as noted by Irvine (2005):

> In Minnesota, one-fifth of addicts who entered treatment for meth use last year were younger than 18 . . . Another recent state survey found that one-fourth of girls and one-fifth of boys in Minnesota's alternative learning schools had used meth at least once in the past year. Ten percent had used it 10 times or more.
>
> (p. 1)

Table 2.6 Percentage of Methamphetamine Use among 8th, 10th, and 12th Graders

Drug	*Use Period*	*Percentage of Use by Grade*		
		8th Graders	**10th Graders**	**12th Graders**
Methamphetamine	Past Month	0.3%	0.2%	0.3%
	Past Year	0.4 %	0.4%	0.8%
	Lifetime	0.6%	0.7%	1.2%

Modified from: Johnston, O'Malley, & Miech (2017, pp. 25–26)

> There were 225,000 past year initiates of methamphetamine aged 12 or older in 2015, which, averages to about 600 people per day who initiated methamphetamine use. In 2015, an estimated 24,000 adolescents aged 12 to 17, 91,000 young adults aged 18 to 25, and 110,000, adults aged 26 or older used methamphetamine for the first time in the past year.
>
> (Lipari, Williams, & Copello, 2016, p. 14)

Interestingly, when the data were analyzed in terms of meeting the *Diagnostic and Statistical Manual of Mental Disorders* (i.e., DSM-5) criteria for "methamphetamine use disorder"—in comparison to undifferentiated "methamphetamine use"—Ahrnsbrak, Bose, and Hedden (2017) found that:

> In 2016, an estimated 684,000 people aged 12 or older had a methamphetamine use disorder . . . which represents about 10,000 adolescents and approximately 135,000 young adults aged 18 to 25.
>
> (p. 29)

Several risk factors have been identified for methamphetamine use among adolescents and young adults (e.g., Herman-Stahl, Krebs, & Kroutil, 2007; Russell, Dryden, & Liang, 2008). (See Table 2.7)

Other significant, methamphetamine-related trends include adolescent and young adult involvement in the drug trade and exchanging sex for methamphetamine.

DRUG TRADE INVOLVEMENT

Up to 25% of adolescents, who abuse methamphetamine, are actively involved in the drug trade, filling many diverse roles (Semple, Strathdee, & Zians, 2012). These roles include:

- "Look-out;"
- Manufacturer;
- "Mule;"
- "Runner;"
- Street-level dealer;
- Wholesale/high-level dealer.

Table 2.7 Risk Factors for Adolescent and Young Adult Methamphetamine Use

Adolescents (10 to 20 Years-of-Age)	*Young Adults (18 to 25 Years-of-Age)*
• Female gender	• Female gender
• Family history of drug and substance abuse	• Family history of drug and substance abuse
• Alcohol use	• Not enrolled in college/university
• Opiate analgesic use	• History of arrest
• Tobacco use	

> A woman attempted to smuggle methamphetamine into Texas from Mexico by hiding the drugs under her clothing and those of her infant child.
>
> (Price, 2016, p. 1)

A more common, and more successful method of smuggling drugs and substances of abuse across borders or into closed/locked facilities (e.g., juvenile detention centers), which is used by both adolescents and young adults, is "body packing" or "body stuffing" (Hendrickson, Horowitz, & Norton, 2006; Kashani & Ruha, 2004; Pagliaro & Pagliaro, *Clinical Patient Data Files*; West, McKeown, & Hendrickson, 2010). This method involves secreting a drug or substance of abuse (such as methamphetamine or cocaine) within the body by:

1. Swallowing plastic "baggies" or "condoms" filled with the drug or substance of abuse;[69]
2. Inserting the drug or substance of abuse into the rectum after "packaging" (i.e., wrapping it in plastic or a condom);
3. Inserting the drug or substance of abuse into the vagina after "packaging" (i.e., wrapping it in plastic or a condom).

(Pagliaro & Pagliaro, *Clinical Patient Data Files*)

These methods, although often successful—in terms of smuggling—also have been associated with unintentional overdosages that may be fatal. These overdosages are related to burst or torn packages that release the drug or substance of abuse into the stomach, rectum, or vagina, where it is absorbed into the systemic circulation and distributed throughout the body.

Several reasons for becoming involved in the drug trade have been shared by adolescents and young adults, who use illicit methamphetamine, including: (1) monetary incentives; (2) to please a boyfriend, girlfriend, or other significant person; (3) to achieve a feeling or sense of accomplishment and control; and (4) to satisfy criminal youth gang membership requirements/duties (Boeri, 2013; Pagliaro & Pagliaro, *Clinical Patient Data Files*; Semple, Strathdee, & Zians, 2012).

69 Before swallowing, the "baggies" are simply sealed shut while the "condoms" are tied shut with a knot.

SEX-FOR-DRUG EXCHANGES

Several researchers examining the phenomenon of exchanging sex-for-methamphetamine (e.g., Corsi & Booth, 2008; Mimiaga, Fair, & Mayer, 2008; Watanabe-Galloway, Ryan, & Hansen, 2009) have identified that up to one-third of women, including adolescent girls and young women, who use methamphetamine, exchange sex for the drug (e.g., Pagliaro & Pagliaro, *Clinical Patient Data Files*; Semple, Strathdee, & Zians, 2011).[70] For related discussion involving adolescent boys and young men, see the earlier subsection, "Undesired, or Harmful, Effects and Toxicities—Human Immunodeficiency Virus Infection and AIDS."

Assessment and Diagnosis of Adolescent Amphetamine Dependence or Use Disorder

The assessment and diagnosis of amphetamine dependence, or use disorder, among adolescents begins with a clinical interview appropriately based on the age and mental capacity of the adolescent—generally with the presence, and/or consent, of a parent.[71] In addition, past medical records, relevant school reports, and court/police referral documents, when available, require careful inspection and interpretation regarding the adolescent's situation—prior to the clinical interview in order to: (1) help to identify any relevant "data gaps;" and (2) plan the clinical interview, including identification of specific interview data that need to be confirmed or refuted. Rarely, adolescents, self-diagnose and present to a mental health care or other professional with a complaint of a SUD. More often, they are accompanied by a parent, or legal guardian, or referred to the health professional by a court judge; school counselor; or other adult for an assessment of suspected drug and substance abuse in the context of significant related signs and symptoms, including, for example:

1. Academic problems (e.g., significant decline in school attendance and/or performance);
2. Aggressive behavior;
3. Arrest for amphetamine-related charges/offenses (e.g., possession; trafficking);
4. Delinquent or criminal behavior (e.g., "break and entry");
5. ED admission for overdosage or suspected suicide attempt involving amphetamines;
6. Engagement in uncharacteristic and risky sexual or other behavior;
7. Parental discovery of a "hidden stash" of amphetamines;
8. Found by an undercover police, or school resource officer (SRO), to be in the possession of amphetamines or related drug paraphernalia (e.g., glass pipe), or caught selling amphetamines.

70 The actual percentage of adolescent girls, who exchange sex-for-methamphetamine, may actually be significantly higher because, most oftenly, the "exchange" is never made explicit. For example, these adolescent girls may be attracted to, go out with, and, subsequently, have sex with someone (female or male)—not because they "are in love" or find that their date has "a nice car," or is "particularly good looking," "popular," or "rich"—but, because the date has, or can readily obtain, methamphetamine (Pagliaro & Pagliaro, *Clinical Patient Data Files*).

71 The term "parent" is used in this context to denote the primary care provider or guardian—be he or she a mother, father, foster parent, grandparent, older sibling, or other person, who is legally responsible for an adolescent's care.

Reflecting the professional's personal style and experience, a typical clinical "workup" is used to form an accurate diagnosis. This clinical work-up[72] includes, a clinical interview with the adolescent, as well as her or his parent(s), depending on the adolescent's age and developmental level, mental functioning, reading ability, and other relevant factors. The adolescent is usually the primary source of related data/information.

These data are collected using standard clinical interview approaches and, when deemed appropriate, facilitated by the use of DSM criteria or the administration of one or more psychometric screening tests that are available for detecting amphetamine use among adolescents and young adults. In addition, further related assessment of sexual health (e.g., laboratory testing for STDs and, for adolescent girls and young women, pregnancy). Physical examination for undesired, or harmful, effects and toxicities associated with amphetamine or methamphetamine use, such as significant loss of body weight and "meth mouth" are also required (see the earlier related discussion in the amphetamines pharmacology subsection, "Undesired, or Harmful, Effects and Toxicities, Chronic Toxicities—Meth Mouth").

***Related Professional Reminder:* As appropriate, a direct clinical interview and physical examination of adolescents is required, including laboratory testing. Additionally, the use of DSM criteria or quick-screen psychometric tests to identify patterns of amphetamine use, including those indicative of amphetamine or methamphetamine dependence or use disorder should be completed. Also, always required is the confirmation/reconfirmation of all related data collected from: interviews with parent(s); reports from police, social services, school counselors and teachers; and, when available, electronic medical records from other health care professionals, including colleagues.**

Psychometric Testing[73]

Although there are several valid psychometric screening tests available for detecting harmful patterns of alcohol (see Chapter 1, "Alcohol"), nicotine (see Chapter 3, "Caffeine and Nicotine"), and psychodelic use, particularly cannabis (see Chapter 4, "Cannabis and Other Psychodelics"), there are no specifically designed and validated quick-screen psychometric tests for the detection of harmful patterns of amphetamine use, particularly for children, adolescents, and young adults. However, seven general quick-screen psychometric tests, which were designed for detecting harmful patterns of adolescent drug and substance abuse—including amphetamines—are currently available:

1. "Drug Abuse Screening Test" (DAST)—four versions for which testing process, number of items, and average time for administration are listed in Table 2.8;
2. "Drug Use Disorders Identification Test" (DUDIT);
3. "Problem Oriented Screening Instrument for Teenagers" (POSIT);
4. "Severity of Dependence Scale" (SDS).

72 We generally prefer and recommend casting a "wide net" regarding assessment and diagnosis—particularly because adolescents, in this clinical context, often present with multiple drug and substance use disorders as well as related contemporaneous diagnoses. Utilizing the extensively adopted process of "multiple working hypotheses" we consider all possible clinical diagnoses that are compatible with the observed presenting signs and symptoms. Then, utilizing a hypothetical-deductive process, we identify relevant "data gaps" and seek to appropriately fill these "data gaps." Subsequently, based upon the best fit with the data collected, we rule out diagnoses until we are left with the one (or more) that appears to be the most probable.

73 For a general definition of terms, discussion of testing statistics, and approaches for test administration for both the tester and test-taker, see also the related overview and discussion of quick-screen psychometric tests in Chapter 1, "Alcohol."

Table 2.8 Seven "Non-Specific" Quick-Screen Psychometric Tests That Can Be Used to Detect Adolescent and Young Adult Amphetamine Abuse

Test Name Abbreviation/Acronym	*Testing Process*	*Number of Items*	*Average Completion Time (Minutes)*
Drug Abuse Screening Test DAST	Self-administered or structured interview	20	5
Drug Abuse Screening Test—Adolescent DAST-A	Self-administered	20	5
Drug Abuse Screening Test (Short Form) DAST-10	Self-administered	10	3
Drug Abuse Screening Test (Revised) DAST-20	Self-administered or structured interview	20	5
Drug Use Disorders Identification Test DUDIT	Self-administered	11	3
Problem Oriented Screening Instrument for Teenagers POSIT	Self-administered	17	5
Severity of Dependence Scale SDS	Self-administered	5	1

Each of these screening tests (see Table 2.8) are presented and discussed in the following subsections.

DRUG ABUSE SCREENING TEST—REVISED (DAST-20)

The DAST (Revised) is a 20-item quick-screen psychometric test (Table 2.9 DAST [Revised]) that was developed by Skinner (1982) to detect problem use of the drugs and substances of abuse, excluding alcohol. The DAST (Revised) was adapted from the original 28-item version of the DAST, which was adapted from the "Michigan Alcoholism Screening Test" (MAST) (see Chapter 1, "Alcohol"). A significant noted difference between the DAST and the MAST is that the DAST items refer to patterns of drug and substance use during the past 12 months while the MAST items refer to patterns of drug and substance use over a lifetime. As a self-administered, quick-screen psychometric test, the DAST minimally requires a 6th-grade reading level. The revised and shortened 20-item version of the DAST (i.e., 20-item DAST [Revised]) has: (1) excellent correlation (i.e., $r = 0.99$) with the original 28-item version; and (2) a more complete set of available test statistics. Thus, it is included in this subsection.

Other versions of the DAST also have been developed and used, including the Drug Abuse Screening Test, Short Form (DAST-10) and the DAST-A for adolescents. The DAST-10 was developed as a 10-item brief version of the original 28-item DAST using

Table 2.9 Drug Abuse Screening Test—Revised (DAST-20)

Item/Question	*Scoring Criteria [Point Allocation]*
Over the last 12 months:	
1. Have you used drugs other than those required for medical reasons?	No, [0]; Yes, [1]
2. Have you abused prescription drugs?	No, [0]; Yes, [1]
3. Do you abuse more than one drug at a time?	No, [0]; Yes, [1]
4. Can you get through the week without using drugs (other than those required for medical reasons)?	No, [1]; Yes, [0]
5. Are you always able to stop using drugs when you want to?	No, [1]; Yes, [0]
6. Have you had blackouts or flashbacks as a result of drug use?	No, [0]; Yes, [1]
7. Do you ever feel bad or guilty about your drug use?	No, [0]; Yes, [1]
8. Does your spouse or parents ever complain about your involvement with drugs? [The DAST-A replaces "spouse" with "boyfriend/girlfriend."]	No, [0]; Yes, [1]
9. Has drug use ever created problems between you and your spouse or your parents? [The DAST-A replaces "spouse" with "boyfriend/girlfriend."]	No, [0]; Yes, [1]
10. Have you ever lost friends because of your use of drugs?	No, [0]; Yes, [1]
11. Have you ever neglected your family because of your use of drugs?	No, [0]; Yes, [1]
12. Have you ever been in trouble at work (or school, or missed school assignments) because of drug abuse?	No, [0]; Yes, [1]
13. Have you ever lost a job because of drug abuse? [The DAST-A replaces "ever" with "ever been kicked out of school or"]	No, [0]; Yes, [1]
14. Have you gotten into fights when under the influence of drugs?	No, [0]; Yes, [1]
15. Have you engaged in illegal activities in order to obtain drugs?	No, [0]; Yes, [1]
16. Have you ever been arrested for possession of illegal drugs?	No, [0]; Yes, [1]
17. Have you ever experienced withdrawal symptoms (felt sick) when you stopped taking drugs?	No, [0]; Yes, [1]
18. Have you had medical problems as a result of your drug use (e.g., memory loss, hepatitis, convulsions, bleeding, etc.)?	No, [0]; Yes, [1]
19. Have you ever gone to anyone for help for a drug problem?	No, [0]; Yes, [1]
20. Have you ever been involved in a treatment program specifically related to drug use?	No, [0]; Yes, [1]

Modified from: Skinner (1982).

items: 1, 3, 5, 6, 7, 9, 11, 15, 17, and 18. Grekin, Svikis, and Lam (2010) examined the ability of the DAST-10 to identify prenatal drug use among a sample of 300 low-income, postpartum women of African continental descent. The sample was comprised of women who were recruited from their hospital rooms shortly after giving birth. Hair and urine samples were utilized as criterion variables to assess the measured sensitivity of the DAST-10, which was found to be only 47%

In an earlier study, Cranford, Esteban McCabe, and Boyd (2006) found that, although the prevalence of illicit drug use did not differ as a function of gender, undergraduate men were significantly more likely to endorse DAST-10 items than were undergraduate women. For this reason, and until additional data are available, we do not generally recommend the use of the DAST-10 for adolescent girls or young women, particularly those who are college/university students. (Also see later subsection, "Available Test Statistics and Recommendations.")

The DAST-A was developed to detect the use of drugs and substances of abuse among adolescents who were psychiatric inpatients (Martino, Grilo, & Fehon, 2000). Other than some relatively minor wording changes (e.g., replacing "work" with "school"), the DAST-A is exactly the same as the 20-item DAST (Revised). (See Table 2.9.)

SCORING THE DAST. Each "yes" or "no" response on the DAST is assigned a zero or one point (see Table 2.9, DAST, for scoring criteria). The scores are summed for a possible maximal score of 20. A total score of 6, or higher, indicates the likelihood of harmful patterns of drug or substance abuse (i.e., that DSM criteria have been met.) The DAST-A is scored exactly like the DAST.

AVAILABLE TEST STATISTICS AND RECOMMENDATIONS. Data on specificity and sensitivity, as well as validity and reliability, are available and are presented, followed by our recommendations.

SPECIFICITY AND SENSITIVITY The DAST has a high specificity of approximately 81% to 91% (Staley & el-Guebaly, 1990). Reportedly, its sensitivity ranges from 82% to 96% (McCann, Simpson, & Ries, 2000; Staley & el-Guebaly, 1990). For a clinical sample of participants with first-episode psychosis, Cassidy, Schmitz, and Mailla (2008) obtained a specificity of 73% and a sensitivity of 85% using a criterion value, or cutoff score, of 3.

VALIDITY AND RELIABILITY The DAST has very good concurrent and discriminant validity and can achieve 85% overall accuracy, or efficacy, in classifying subjects who are tested per DSM criteria (Gavin, Ross, & Skinner, 1989; Yudko, Lozhkina, & Fouts, 2007). Reportedly, the DAST has high internal consistency, or reliability (i.e., 0.92) (El-Bassel, Schilling, & Schinke, 1997; McCann, Simpson, & Ries, 2000; Staley & el-Guebaly, 1990) and test-retest reliability (i.e., 0.85) (Yudko, Lozhkina, & Fouts, 2007). Skinner (1982) reported a Cronbach's alpha coefficient of 0.92 for the DAST and 0.95 for the 20-item DAST (Revised). In fact, all available versions of the DAST have been found to have satisfactory measures of validity and reliability (Yudko, Lozhkina, & Fouts, 2007).

RECOMMENDATIONS Based upon acceptable psychometric evaluations, we generally recommend the use of the DAST-A as a quick-screen psychometric test for detecting adolescent amphetamine (or cocaine) use, as well as other drugs and substances of abuse, excluding alcohol.

DRUG USE DISORDERS IDENTIFICATION TEST (DUDIT)

The DUDIT is an 11-item, self-administered quick-screen psychometric test (Table 2.10) developed by Swedish researchers (Berman, Bergman, & Palmstierna, 2005). It is used to

Table 2.10 Drug Use Disorders Identification Test (DUDIT)

Here are a few questions about drugs. Please answer as correctly and honestly as possible by indicating which answer is right for you.

☐ **Man** ☐ **Woman** ☐ **Age**

Item or Question	**Scoring Criteria** [Point Allocation]
1. How often do you use drugs other than alcohol?	Never, [0]; once a month, or less often, [1]; two to four times a month, [2]; two to three times a week, [3]; four times a week, or more often, [4]
2. Do you use more than one type of drug on the same occasion?	Never, [0]; once a month, or less often, [1]; two to four times a month, [2]; two to three times a week, [3]; four times a week, or more often, [4]
3. How many times do you take drugs on a typical day when you use drugs?	0 times, [0]; one or two times, [0]; three or four times, [1]; five or six times, [2]; seven or more times, [4]
4. How often are you influenced heavily by drugs?	Never, [0]; less often than once a month, [1]; every month, [2]; every week, [3]; daily or almost every day, [4]
5. Over the past year, have you felt that your longing for drugs was so strong that you could not resist it?	Never, [0]; less often than once a month, [1]; every month, [2]; every week, [3]; daily, or almost every day, [4]
6. Has it happened, over the past year, that you have not been able to stop taking drugs once you started?	Never, [0]; less often than once a month, [1]; every month, [2]; every week, [3]; daily, or almost every day, [4]
7. How often over the past year have you taken drugs and then neglected to do something you should have done?	Never, [0]; less often than once a month, [1]; every month, [2]; every week, [3]; daily, or almost every day, [4]
8. How often over the past year have you needed to take a drug the morning after heavy drug use the day before?	Never, [0]; less often than once a month, [1]; every month, [2]; every week, [3]; daily, or almost every day, [4]
9. How often over the past year have you had guilt feelings or a bad conscience because you used drugs?	Never, [0]; less often than once a month, [1]; every month, [2]; every week, [3]; daily, or almost every day, [4]
10. Have you or anyone else been hurt (mentally or physically) because you used drugs?	No, [0]; Yes, but not over the past year, [2]; Yes, over the past year, [4]
11. Has a relative or a friend, doctor or a nurse, or anyone else, been worried about your drug use or said to you that you should stop using drugs?	No, [0]; Yes, but not over the past year, [2]; Yes, over the past year, [4]

Source: Berman, Bergman, & Palmstierna (2005).

detect dependence on virtually all of the commonly available drugs and substances of abuse, excluding alcohol. The DUDIT is somewhat unique in that a printed list of over 100 generic and brand/trade names, divided into pharmacological categories, is included on the reverse side of the single-page questionnaire to facilitate self-administration.

SCORING THE DUDIT. The scoring of the DUDIT is generally more involved than that for other quick-screen psychometric tests. In this regard, it is similar to the "Alcohol Use Identification Test" (AUDIT) (see Chapter 1, "Alcohol") in terms of both the response set and scoring. For items 1 through 9, responses are coded "1," "2," "3," or "4." For items 10 and 11, responses are coded "0," "2," or "4" (see Table 2.10). The maximal score possible for the 11-item quick-screen psychometric test is 44. A cutoff score of 2, for women, and 6, for men, likely indicates a SUD. A score of 25, or higher, indicates "heavy dependence" on drugs or substances of abuse.

AVAILABLE TEST STATISTICS AND RECOMMENDATIONS. Data are available for specificity and sensitivity, as well as, validity and reliability. These data, and our recommendations, are discussed in the following subsections.

SPECIFICITY AND SENSITIVITY Among a sample of heavy drug users selected from Swedish inpatient detoxification settings, prisons, and probation offices, the DUDIT's specificity for predicting drug dependence was 78% when compared to established DSM-IV criteria and 88% when compared to established ICD-10 criteria. Sensitivity for the DUDIT was 90% for both sets of criteria (Berman, Bergman, & Palmstierna, 2005).

VALIDITY AND RELIABILITY The DUDIT has good face validity and its criterion-related validity, as noted in the previous subsection, is good when predicting drug dependence based on the DSM-IV or ICD-10 criteria. The DUDIT's reliability also is good as indicated by its inter-item consistency that yielded a Cronbach's alpha coefficient of 0.80 (Berman, Bergman, & Palmstierna, 2005). In a review of 18-related research publications, Hildebrand (2015) reported high, consistent reliability estimates with Cronbach's alpha coefficient generally reported as greater than 0.90.

RECOMMENDATIONS The DUDIT has good statistical results in relation to its psychometric analysis. We generally recommend its use. However, until additional data are available concerning its validity and use with various population samples of adolescents and young adults in the U.S., caution is warranted.

PROBLEM ORIENTED SCREENING INSTRUMENT FOR TEENAGERS (POSIT)

The POSIT, a 139-item psychometric screening test, was developed by Elizabeth Rahdert of the NIDA in 1991. It was designed to identify 10 different problem areas of adolescent behavior and health, including mental health, physical health, social skills, and substance abuse. The substance use and abuse area, addressed by 17 specific items, has been used as an independent questionnaire (see Table 2.11). The POSIT, which minimally requires a 5th-grade reading level, was developed to be self-administered by adolescents. A computerized version also is available.

SCORING THE POSIT. The entire POSIT is scored using a scoring system available from the NIDA. Empirically derived cutoff scores detect low, medium, or high risk for each of the

Table 2.11 Problem Oriented Screening Instrument for Teenagers (POSIT)

Item/Question	*Scoring Criteria [Point Allocation]*
1. Do you get into trouble because you use drugs or alcohol at school?	No, [0]; Yes, [1]
2. Have you accidently hurt yourself or someone else while high on alcohol or drugs?	No, [0]; Yes, [1]
3. Do you miss out on activities because you spend too much money on drugs or alcohol?	No, [0]; Yes, [1]
4. Do you ever feel you are addicted to alcohol or drugs?	No, [0]; Yes, [1]
5. Have you started using more and more drugs or alcohol to get the effect you want?	No, [0]; Yes, [1]
6. Do you ever leave a party because there is no alcohol or drugs?	No, [0]; Yes, [1]
7. Do you have a constant desire for alcohol or drugs?	No, [0]; Yes, [1]
8. Have you had a car accident while high on alcohol or drugs?	No, [0]; Yes, [1]
9. Do you forget things you did while drinking or using drugs?	No, [0]; Yes, [1]
10. During the past month have you driven a car while you were drunk or high?	No, [0]; Yes, [1]
11. Does alcohol or drug use cause your moods to change quickly like from happy to sad or vice versa?	No, [0]; Yes, [1]
12. Do you miss school or arrive late because of your alcohol or drug use?	No, [0]; Yes, [1]
13. Do your family or friends ever tell you to cut down on your drinking or drug use?	No, [0]; Yes, [1]
14. Do you have serious arguments with friends or family members because of your drinking or drug use?	No, [0]; Yes, [1]
15. Does your alcohol or drug use ever make you do something you would not normally do like breaking rules, missing curfew, or breaking the law?	No, [0]; Yes, [1]
16. Do you have trouble getting along with any of your friends because of your alcohol or drug use?	No, [0]; Yes, [1]
17. Do you ever feel you can't control your alcohol or drug use?	No, [0]; Yes, [1]

Modified from: Rahdert (1991).

10 identified problem areas addressed by the POSIT. For the 17-item substance use and abuse scale, each affirmative response is assigned 1 point for a possible maximal score of 17. (See Table 2.11 for scoring criteria for the POSIT.) A cutoff score of 2 or higher is recommended for the detection of alcohol or drug abuse problems (Latimer, Winters, & Stinchfield, 1997).

AVAILABLE TEST STATISTICS. The test statistics (i.e., specificity and sensitivity; validity and reliability) that have been reported for the POSIT, as well as our recommendations, are discussed in the following subsections.

SPECIFICITY AND SENSITIVITY Using the recommended cutoff score of 2 or higher, the POSIT substance use and abuse scale was reported to have an efficacy of 84% with a specificity of 79% and a sensitivity of 95% (Latimer, Winters, & Stinchfield, 1997). Knight, Sherritt, and Harris (2003), using a cutoff score of 1, obtained a mean sensitivity of 84% with a 95% confidence interval of 79% to 90%. Using a sample of adolescent mothers, Scafidi, Field, and Prodromidis (1997) found that the POSIT scales correctly detected 75% of mothers who were drug abusing (i.e., sensitivity) and 84% of mothers who were not drug abusing (i.e., specificity).

VALIDITY AND RELIABILITY Criterion-related validity has been found to be moderate to high (Dembo, Schmeidler, & Borden 1996; McLaney, Del Boca, & Babor, 2009). Regarding reliability, Dembo, Schmeidler, and Borden (1996) reported high test-retest reliability among adolescents, who were incarcerated on more than one occasion, and were tested at the time of initial incarceration and at subsequent times of incarceration, varying from one to 33 weeks. In a later study, Knight, Goodman, and Pulerwitz (2001) found test-retest reliability to be greater than 0.70 after one week.

RECOMMENDATIONS The POSIT has good statistical results in relation to its psychometric analysis and was developed and normed for adolescents in the U.S. Consequently, we generally recommend its use as a quick-screen psychometric test for adolescents to detect drug and substance abuse, including that involving amphetamine (or cocaine).[74]

SEVERITY OF DEPENDENCE SCALE (SDS)

The SDS is a five-item quick-screen psychometic test (Table 2.12 SDS) that requires less than one minute to complete. It was developed by Gossop, Darke, and Griffiths (1995) to detect the degree of dependence experienced by users of different drugs and substances of abuse. The SDS was originally tested in the contexts of amphetamine, cocaine, and heroin use in Australia and England. It has since been used for many different drugs and substances of abuse, particularly cannabis, to evaluate dependence among:

- Australian adolescent cannabis users (Martin, Copeland, & Gates, 2006);
- Spanish heroin users (Iraurgi Castillo, Gonzalez Saiz, & Lozano Rojas, 2010);
- Dutch cannabis users (van der Pol, Liebregts, & de Graaf, 2013);
- Italian adolescent cannabis users (Bastiani, Siciliano, & Curzio, 2013);
- Spanish adolescent cannabis users (Thanki, Domingo-Salvany, & Barrio Anta, 2013).

74 When used to detect amphetamine or cocaine use, we substitute "amphetamine" or "cocaine" for "alcohol or drug" in the wording of each question.

Table 2.12 Severity of Dependence Scale (SDS)

Item/Question	*Scoring Criteria [Point Allocation]*
Over the last three months:	
1. Did you ever think your use of [insert drug name] was out of control?	Never or almost never [0]; Sometimes [1]; Often [2]; Always or nearly always [3]
2. Did the prospect of missing the use of [insert drug name] make you very anxious or worried?	Never or almost never [0]; Sometimes [1]; Often [2]; Always or nearly always [3]
3. Did you worry about your use of [insert drug name]?	Never or almost never [0]; Sometimes [1]; Often [2]; Always or nearly always [3]
4. Did you wish you could stop using [insert drug name]?	Never or almost never [0]; Sometimes [1]; Often [2]; Always or nearly always [3]
5. How difficult would you find it to stop or go without [insert drug name]?	Not difficult [0]; Quite difficult [1]; Very difficult [2]; Impossible [3]
	Total SDS Score:/15

Modified from: Gossop, Darke, & Griffiths (1995).

The SDS also has been recommended for use by the World Health Organization (WHO). It has been produced in several different language versions, including Chinese (Chen, Chen, & Lin, 2008) and Portuguese (Ferri, Marsden, & de Araujo, 2000). The items comprising the SDS are explicitly concerned with psychological components of dependence and, using principal components analysis, load significantly on a single factor.

SCORING THE SDS. Each item/question of the SDS is given a score of "0," "1," "2," or "3" (see Table 2.12 for scoring criteria). The scores are summed for a possible maximal total score of 15. For adolescents and young adults, a total score of 4, or higher, indicates the likelihood of a significant degree of "psychological" dependence.

AVAILABLE TEST STATISTICS AND RECOMMENDATIONS. Published data on specificity, sensitivity, positive predictive value, negative predictive value, as well as, validity and reliability, are available and are presented and discussed in the following subsections. We conclude with our recommendations in relation to the use of the SDS for the detection of psychological dependence for the various drugs and substances of abuse.

SPECIFICITY, SENSITIVITY, AND POSITIVE AND NEGATIVE PREDICTIVE VALUE The specificity and sensitivity of the SDS is variable, but generally high. For example, van der Pol, Liebregts, and de Graaf (2013) reported a specificity of 63.5% and a sensitivity of 61.3% for the SDS while Iraurgi Castillo, Gonzalez Saiz, and Lozano Rojas (2010) reported a specificity of 84.5% and a sensitivity of 83.2%.

Reported variance in specificity and sensitivity has been associated with both the population sampled and the drug or substance of abuse being evaluated. However, the major determining factor, as per other quick-screen psychometric tests, is the chosen cutoff score (i.e., as the cutoff score increases, specificity increases while sensitivity correspondingly decreases). Generally, the optional cutoff score is 4 (e.g., Bastiani, Siciliano, & Curzio, 2013; Gossop, Darke, & Griffiths, 1995; Martin, Copeland, & Gates, 2006).[75]

In their study of cannabis dependence among German adults, Steiner, Baumeister, and Kraus (2008) reported a positive predictive value of 44% and a negative predictive value of 89% when using a cutoff score of 4 for the SDS. In addition, as the cutoff score increased from 1 to 6, the positive predictive value increased from 22% to 72% while the negative predictive value decreased, although not as significantly, from 100% to 95%.

VALIDITY AND RELIABILITY Whereas the face validity of the SDS is good, the content validity is limited by its sole focus on psychological measures of dependence and lack of evaluation of physical measures of dependence. However, overall, the SDS has good validity.

Criterion-related validity of the total SDS score compared with other independent indicators including DSM-III-R, DSM-IV, DSM-5, and ICD-10 ranges from moderate to good (e.g., Cuenca-Royo, Sanchez-Niubo, & Forero, 2012; Hides, Dawe, & Young, 2007; Martin, Copeland, & Gates, 2006; Swift, Copeland, & Hall, 1998).

The item reliability for the SDS, as a measure of internal consistency has ranged from good—Cronbach's alpha = 0.70 (e.g., Cuenca-Royo, Sanchez-Niubo, & Forero, 2012; van der Pol, Liebregts, & de Graaf, 2013)—to moderate—Cronbach's alpha = 0.80 to 0.85 (e.g., Martin, Copeland, & Gates, 2006; Steiner, Baumeister, & Kraus, 2008).

The test-retest reliability of the SDS is satisfactory ranging fron 0.80 to 0.89 (e.g., Cuenca-Royo, Sanchez-Niubo, & Forero, 2012; Gossop, Best, & Marsden, 1997; Martin, Copeland, & Gates, 2006).

RECOMMENDATIONS Based upon acceptable psychometric evaluations in regard to several drugs and substances of abuse, particularly cannabis, we generally recommend the use of the SDS as an initial quick-screen psychometric test to detect psychological dependence. However, because of the paucity of published U.S. adolescent psychometric data, caution is required.

Related Professional Reminder:* *Obtaining a positive outcome from a quick-screen psychometric test does not confirm a diagnosis of amphetamine or other alcohol or substance use disorder per se. The results simply indicate that an amphetamine or other alcohol or substance use disorder is "likely." Consequently, positive outcomes must be supported or confirmed by the relevant data obtained from a clinical interview and other relevant sources (e.g., laboratory toxicology results).

Treating Adolescent and Young Adult Amphetamine Dependence or Use Disorder

Once a professional assessment and diagnosis of amphetamine, methamphetamine, or methylphenidate dependence, or use disorder—are made for an adolescent or young adult, the development of an individualized age-appropriate intervention plan is required. This plan requires the involvement of the adolescent or young adult and, for the former, parent(s), with attention to the selection and implementation of generally two major categories of appropriate treatment that can be used individually or together: (1) pharmacotherapy; and (2) psychotherapy/counseling. Apropriately combined therapy has been generally associated with more efficatious outcomes for children, adolescents, and young adults (see the related discussion in Chapter 1, "Alcohol").

75 Hides, Dawe, and Young (2007) evaluated the utility of the SDS in the assessment of cannabis dependence among a sample of Australian adult in-patients with schizophrenia. Using a SDS cutoff score of 2 and DSM-IV criteria for cannabis dependence, they found a specificity of 83%, sensitivity of 86%, positive predictive value of 83%, and negative predictive value of 86%.

Unfortunately, to date, no published research studies have identified effective treatment interventions—"best practices"—for adolescents and young adults (or other adults) with amphetamine, methamphetamine, or methylphenidate dependence or use disorder (Harada, Tsutomi, & Mori, 2014). However, we begin with an overview of what is known regarding related pharmacotherapy for amphetamine dependence or use disorder focusing primarily on published studies involving adults.

Pharmacotherapy

Currently, no prescription drugs have been approved by the FDA for the treatment or management of amphetamine dependence, or use disorder, including relapse prevention (e.g., Ballester, Valentine, & Sofuoglu, 2017; Cao, Shi, & Hao, 2016; Lee, Jenner, & Nielsen, 2014; Morley, Cornish, & Faingold, 2017). Consequently, as noted by Ballester, Valentine, and Sofuoglu (2017):

> Clinical trials examining the potential for pharmacotherapies of methamphetamine use disorder have largely been negative.
>
> (p. 305)

And, as further identified by Morley, Cornish, and Faingold (2017):

> Effective management for methamphetamine dependence remains elusive and the large majority of methamphetamine users relapse following treatment.
>
> (p. 563)

However, several prescription drugs have been used in an "off label" context to treat amphetamine use disorder. While several research studies have been published regarding the efficacy of many of these drugs, most report a lack of efficacy for treating amphetamine dependence or use disorders, particularly those for managing methamphetamine use or withdrawal. Some, however, show potential promise for some patients (see Table 2.13).

Reasons for this lack of success are varied and range from poor research design and execution to inattention to the occurrence of confounding variables, or co-morbidities (e.g., other concurrent mental disorders, including SUDs). Unfortunately, these research design flaws, examples of which are presented in the following bullet list, negatively affect the reliability of research findings and severely limit their generalizability:

- High rate of subject/participant attrition;
- Inadequate or inconsistent identification of amphetamine use among study participants;
- Inadequate sample size;
- Lack of control group;
- Lack of long-term follow-up;
- Lack of objective outcome criteria;
- Lack of placebo control;
- Non-blinded study;
- Nonrandom sample selection (e.g., use of convenience sampling);
- Nonrandom assignment of subject/participant to "treatment" groups;
- Reliance on self-report;
- Short duration of research study.

In addition, little or no attention has been given to the study of the prevention and treatment of "relapsed use," which often occurs subsequent to "successful" treatment of

Table 2.13 Examples of the Efficacy of Pharmacotherapy in Relation to Amphetamine Dependence, Program Retention, and/or Withdrawal Syndrome

Pharmacotherapy	*Efficacy*	*Sources*
Amlodipine (Norvasc®) *Calcium channel blocker*	Ineffective	Karilla, Wienstein, & Aubin, 2010
Aripiprazole (Abilify®) *Antipsychotic, atypical*	Increased amphetamine use	Elkashef, Vocci, & Hanson, 2008
	Ineffective May increase methamphetamine use	Karilla, Wienstein, & Aubin, 2010
Baclofen (Lioresal®) *Antispastic, GABA receptor agonist*	Ineffective	Elkashef, Vocci, & Hanson, 2008
	Ineffective in reducing methamphetamine use	Karilla, Wienstein, & Aubin, 2010
Benzodiazepines (e.g., Ativan®, Valium®) *Sedative-Hypnotics*	Ineffective in the treatment of amphetamine withdrawal	Lee, Jenner, & Nielsen, 2014
Bupropion (Wellbutrin®) *Antidepressant*	Limited efficacy in limited populations	Brensilver, Heinzerling, & Shoptaw, 2013
	Limited efficacy among "light" methamphetamine users May reduce signs and symptoms of methamphetamine withdrawal	Karilla, Wienstein, & Aubin, 2010
	Limited efficacy for treating amphetamine dependence among "low frequency" users (less than 18 days/month)	Lee, Jenner, & Nielsen, 2014
	Ineffective	Perez-Mana, Castells, & Torrens, 2013
Dextroamphetamine (Dexedrine®) *Psychostimulant, amphetamine*	Limited efficacy Potential for addiction to dextroamphetamine	Elkashef, Vocci, & Hanson, 2008
	Increased retention in treatment group/program	Karilla, Wienstein, & Aubin, 2010

(*Continued*)

Table 2.13 (Cont.)

Pharmacotherapy	*Efficacy*	*Sources*
	Limited efficacy in reducing methamphetamine use Potential for addiction to dextroamphetamine	
	May be effective for reducing signs and symptoms of the methamphetamine withdrawal syndrome Limited efficacy for increasing retention in treatment for amphetamine dependence	Lee, Jenner, & Nielsen, 2014
	Effective for: Increasing treatment program retention Decreasing methamphetamine use	Longo, Wickes, & Smout, 2010
	Ineffective	Perez-Mana, Castells, & Torrens, 2013
Fluoxetine (Prozac®) *Antidepressant, selective serotonin reuptake inhibitor [SSRI]*	Ineffective	Karilla, Wienstein, & Aubin, 2010
Gabapentin (Neurontin®) *Non-Selective GABA agonist*	Ineffective for reducing methamphetamine use	Karilla, Wienstein, & Aubin, 2010
Imipramine (Tofranil®) *Antidepressant, tricyclic*	Ineffective	Elkashef, Vocci, & Hanson, 2008
Lobeline *Naturally occurring alkaloid, partial nicotinic receptor antagonist*	Possibly effective	Karilla, Wienstein, & Aubin, 2010
Methylphenidate (Ritalin®) *Psychostimulant, amphetamine-like*	Limited efficacy in limited populations	Brensilver, Heinzerling, & Shoptaw, 2013
	Limited efficacy in reducing methamphetamine use Potential for addiction to methylphenidate	Elkashef, Vocci, & Hanson, 2008

Pharmacotherapy	*Efficacy*	*Sources*
	Limited efficacy among IV amphetamine users Potential for addiction to methylphenidate	Karilla, Wienstein, & Aubin, 2010
	Limited efficacy for treatment of amphetamine dependence	Lee, Jenner, & Nielsen, 2014
	Ineffective	Perez-Mana, Castells, & Torrens, 2013
Mirtazapine (Remeron®) *Antidepressant, atypical*	Limited efficacy in limited populations	Brensilver, Heinzerling, & Shoptaw, 2013
	Ineffective	Karilla, Wienstein, & Aubin, 2010
	Possibly effective in reducing signs and symptoms of the methamphetamine withdrawal syndrome	Lee, Jenner, & Nielsen, 2014
Modafinil (Provigil®) *Psychostimulant, non-amphetamine*	Limited efficacy in *decreasing*: Methamphetamine use Severity of the methamphetamine withdrawal syndrome	Karilla, Wienstein, & Aubin, 2010
	May be effective in reducing the signs and symptoms of the methamphetamine withdrawal syndrome	Lee, Jenner, & Nielsen, 2014
	Ineffective	Perez-Mana, Castells, & Torrens, 2013
Naltrexone (ReVia®) *Opiate analgesic receptor antagonist*	Limited efficacy in limited populations	Brensilver, Heinzerling, & Shoptaw, 2013
	Possibly effective in both decreasing: Craving for amphetamines Using amphetamines	Karilla, Wienstein, & Aubin, 2010
	Limited efficacy for: Amphetamine treatment program retention Reducing craving	Lee, Jenner, & Nielsen, 2014

(*Continued*)

Table 2.13 (Cont.)

Pharmacotherapy	*Efficacy*	*Sources*
Ondansetron (Zofran®) *Antiemetic, serotonin receptor antagonist*	Ineffective	Elkashef, Vocci, & Hanson, 2008
	Ineffective	Johnson, Ait-Daoud, & Elkashef, 2008
	Ineffective	Karilla, Wienstein, & Aubin, 2010
Paroxetine (Paxil®) *Antidepressant, selective serotonin reuptake inhibiter [SSRI]*	Ineffective	Karilla, Wienstein, & Aubin, 2010
Risperidone (Risperdal®) *Antipsychotic, atypical*	Possibly effective in reducing methamphetamine use	Karilla, Wienstein, & Aubin, 2010
Rivastigmine (Exelon®) *Parasympathomimetic, cholinesterase inhibitor*	Possibly effective	Karilla, Wienstein, & Aubin, 2010
Sertraline (Zoloft®) *Antidepressant, selective serotonin reuptake inhibitor [SSRI]*	Ineffective	Elkashef, Vocci, & Hanson, 2008
	Ineffective	Karilla, Wienstein, & Aubin, 2010
Topiramate (Topamax®) *Anticonvulsant, sulfamate substituted monosaccharide*	Ineffective May increase methamphetamine plasma concentrations	Karilla, Wienstein, & Aubin, 2010
Tyrosine *Amino acid*	Ineffective	Elkashef, Vocci, & Hanson, 2008
Vigabatrin (Sabril®) *GABA agonist, Inhibitor of GABA-aminotransferase*	Possibly effective for reducing methamphetamine use	Karilla, Wienstein, & Aubin, 2010

amphetamine dependence or use disorder (e.g., Brackins, Brahm, & Kissack, 2011; Lee, Jenner, & Nielsen, 2014; Morley, Cornish & Faingold, 2017; Petit, Karila, & Chalmin, 2012).

We now turn to the psychotherapy/counseling approaches used for amphetamine use disorder and related disorders.

Psychotherapy/Counseling

> At this time, the most effective treatments for methamphetamine addiction are behavioral interventions. These approaches are designed to help to modify the patient's expectancies and behaviors related to drug use, and to increase skills in coping with various life stressors.
>
> (NIDA/NIH, 2005, p. 8)

This situation has not changed over the ensuing 15 years of the new millennium. Psychotherapy/Counseling continues to be the mainstay for the treatment of amphetamine dependence or use disorder, including the management of the amphetamine withdrawal syndrome. However, overall success has been limited and, consequently, a significant number of patients with amphetamine dependence or disorder fail to successfully respond to these interventions. The most common psychotherapy/counseling approaches,[76] which have been used for adolescents and young adults with these disorders, include:

- 12-Step/Facilitation Programs (12-Step);
- Cognitive-Behavioral Therapy (CBT);
- Contingency Management Programs (CM);
- Family Therapy (FT);
- Interpersonal Therapy (IT);
- Matrix Model (MM);
- Motivational Interviewing (MI);
- Residential Treatment Programs (RTP).

Virtually, all of the research studies aimed at the treatment of amphetamine dependence or use disorder have involved the application of either CBT and/or CM (e.g., Harada, Tsutomi, & Mori, 2014; Lee & Rawson, 2008). Related randomized controlled studies have consistently, at least for adults, resulted in several positive outcomes that include:

- Increased treatment retention;
- Reduced amphetamine use;
- Increased abstinence at follow-up;
- More amphetamine-free urine samples;
- Longer periods of abstinence.

It also has been found that positive outcomes are more likely to persist post-CBT treatment rather than post-CM treatment.

BRIEF COGNITIVE-BEHAVIORAL THERAPY (BCBT)

Brief cognitive behavioral therapy has no published empirical evidence of success for the treatment of SUDs among adolescents.[77] Thus, we do not recommend its use for the treatment of amphetamine-related disorders among adolescents.

76 For a detailed discussion of each of these approaches, see the subsection, in Chapter 1, "Alcohol," "Psychotherapy/Counseling."

77 However, among adults, including young adults, the results of several empirical studies (e.g., Baker, Lee, & Claire, 2005) have indicated that BCBT (i.e., two to four sessions) was associated with a significant *increase* in abstinence at six months among regular amphetamine users in comparison to either "placebo" or a control consisting of structured assessment and use of a self-help booklet.

COGNITIVE BEHAVIORAL THERAPY (CBT)

Cognitive behavioral therapy does not have a "good track record" of documented use and associated success in the treatment of amphetamine related disorders. In one of the few empirical studies of CBT for methamphetamine dependence, Keoleian, Stalcup, and Poicin (2013)—noting that "psychosocial treatments for methamphetamine dependence are of limited effectiveness" (p. 434)—developed and tested a "CBT-based text messaging intervention" that was used in conjunction with standard CBT group therapy. Although concluding that the texted messages were rated as useful by the participants, a re-analysis of their data indicated a lack of clinical significance and a reported *increase* in "craving" following the receipt of the text messages.

***Related Professional Reminder:* Although therapeutic success for amphetamine dependence or use disorder is limited, when successful, it almost always involves the combination of pharmacotherapy and psychotherapy/counseling.**

Additionally, we, and others (e.g., Krueger & Glass, 2013; Minozzi & Saulle, 2016), have generally recommended the combination of *two*, or *more*, of the psychotherapy/counseling techniques (e.g., "cognitive-behavioral therapy" and "12-step program"). In addition, as deemed appropriate for the specific adolescent or young adult patient and her or his specific amphetamine use or other related disorder, we often add pharmacotherapy to this combination (see related discussion of "pharmacotherapy" in the proceeding section of this chapter).

Contemporaneous Diagnoses[78]

Adolescents and young adults are susceptible to, and experience, virtually every form of contemporaneous diagnoses (Pagliaro & Pagliaro, 2012; Riggs, 2003; Wise, Cuffe, & Fischer, 2001). However, the most often reported contemporaneous diagnosis, particularly in the context of adolescent amphetamine depenendence or use disorder, is major depressive disorder (Pagliaro & Pagliaro, *Clinical Patient Data Files*).

As identified by Ahrnsbrak, Bose, and Hedden (2017):

> The 333,000 adolescents in 2016 who had a co-occurring MDE [major depressive episode] and an SUD in the past year represent about one third (33.0 percent) of the 1.1 million adolescents who had a past year SUD.
>
> (p. 43)

Amphetamine dependence or use disorder among adolescents and young adults also has been associated with several other mental disorders:

- ADHD;
- AUD;
- Conduct disorder;
- Eating disorders;
- PTSD;
- SUD(s).

For example, it has been reported that over 50% of adolescents, who illicitly use prescription amphetamines, including methylphenidate, report an associated alcohol or other dependence

78 See also the related overview and discussion in Chapter 1, "Alcohol," "Common Contemporaneous Diagnoses Among Children and Adolescents."

use disorder, particularly, cannabis use disorder (Chen, Crum, & Strain, 2015). In addition, for adolescents diagnosed with methamphetamine dependence or use disorder, the most commonly involved mental disorder, as previously noted, is MDD (Pagliaro & Pagliaro, *Clinical Patient Data Files*). Although various prescription antidepressants have been used in an attempt to simultaneously treat both the MDD and the methamphetamine use disorder, these attempts have been largely unsuccessful. For example, as found by Hellem, Lundberg, and Renshaw (2015) in their detailed integrative review of related studies:

> Psychological approaches and [the] combination of psychological with pharmacological approaches have *not* been shown to be effective in treating these co-occurring conditions [i.e., MDD and methamphetamine use disorder].
>
> (p. 1)

We now turn to "cocaine."

Cocaine

Widely available across the U.S., cocaine is commonly used by adolescents and young adults for such desired psychostimulant effects as euphoria and heightened sexual experiences. For a significant number of adolescents and young adults, who use cocaine, the cocaine "high" often becomes the only—or, at least, primary—reason for living (i.e., cocaine use being preferred to personal likes, desires, or needs—including family, food, friends, recreation, sex, or future career aspirations/goals, such as plans to go to college/university). This pattern of cocaine use results in significant adverse social consequences for these adolescents and young adults—and/or for their families and friends. In this major section of Chapter 2, we begin with the botany and pharmacology of cocaine. We then present and discuss embryo/fetal, infant, and child exposure to cocaine and its patterns of use among adolescents and young adults, in the U.S., during the first two decades of the new millennium. We also present and discuss the contemporaneous diagnoses that are commonly detected among adolescents and young adults, who use cocaine. The section concludes with an overview of the assessment, diagnosis, and treatment of adolescent and young adult cocaine dependence or use disorder.

Cocaine Botany

Cocaine (benzoylmethylecgonine) is a natural liquid alkaloid that is extracted from the leaves of two cultivated species of the coca plant,[79] which are indigenous to South America—(1) *Erythroxylum coca* and (2) *Erythroxylum novogranatense.*

Erythroxylum coca has two varieties:

1. *Coca variety* (i.e., Bolivian or Huanuco coca), which is found primarily in the moist, tropical mountaneous forest regions of the eastern Andes with cultivation extending from Ecuador south to Bolivia. It is a large shrub, typically three to nine feet in height, and grows primarily at elevations between 1,500 and 4,500 feet;
2. *Ipadu variety* (i.e., Amazonian coca), which is found primarily in the lowland Amazon Basin regions of Brazil, Colombia, and Peru, where it has been cultivated for many centuries.

79 The name for this alkaloid (i.e., cocaine) was derived from the plant's name, "coca," and the alkaloid suffix, "ine."

Erythroxylum novogranatense also has two varieties:

1. *Novogranatense variety* (i.e., Colombian coca), which is primarily found in the drier regions throughout Colombia. An adaptable plant, it also is grown in both high- and low-land areas. In comparison to *E. coca, E. novogranatense* has several distinct differences, including, for example: *E. novogranatense*: (1) grows well in arid regions in which *E. coca* generally would not survive; and (2) leaves also contain methyl salicylate, whereas, *E. coca* leaves do not;
2. *Truxillense* variety (i.e., Trujillo coca) is a drought-resistant shrub, that is tall and bushy and grown primarily in Columbia and Peru (Pagliaro & Pagliaro, 2004; Plowman, 1985).

Cocaine, which is indigenous to South America, has been cultivated there since the pre-Columbian era. During the 20th and 21st centuries, coca leaves were, and continue to be, the major cash crop for the South American countries of Argentina, Bolivia, Colombia, Ecuador, and Peru. The green leaves ("matu") are harvested by hand, and are initially spread in thin layers to dry in the sun. The dried leaves are then packed into sacks, which are kept dry until ready for sale. The Native Indigenous Peoples of South America, traditionally chew the cocaine leaves, much like tobacco is chewed, or grind the leaves into a powder to make tea. Coca tea or "mate de coca," is also made by brewing raw or dried leaves much like other herbal teas. Mate de coca also is made with commercially available mate de coca teabags. Drug traffickers typically purchase the sacks of dried cocaine leaves leaves and then chemically extract the cocaine alkaloid utilizing a variety of organic solvents—a process that typically occurs in unsophisticated "jungle laboratories."

Leaves from coca plants typically contain, by weight, about 1% cocaine. However, reported concentrations have ranged from 0.25% to 1.5%. Other natural alkaloids found in these leaves include benzoylecgonine and ecgonine. Concentrations are primarily dependent on the: (1) species and variety of the coca plant; (2) region of cultivation; and (3) growing conditions. The presence of cocaine in coca leaves purportedly serves as a natural insecticide for the plant (Lewis, 1994).

Pharmacology

Cocaine is generally produced for illicit distribution and sale in two forms: (1) cocaine hydrochloride (HCl), a white powder; and (2) "crack cocaine," small white or light tan- to-brownish "rocks." Each of these forms has its own distinct pharmacologic characteristics and patterns of use. The pharmacology of both of these forms of cocaine—pharmacodynamics; pharmacokinetics; undesired, or harmful, effects and toxicities; drug–drug interactions; and overdosage—is presented and discussed. Attention also is given to the teratogenic risks and toxicities associated with neonatal and infant exposure by adolescent girls and young women, who are pregnant or breastfeeding.

Cocaine Hydrochloride

Cocaine hydrochloride, the salt form of cocaine, is a white crystaline powder that is highly water solubility (i.e., one gram in 0.5 ml). This high solubility allows cocaine powder to readily dissolve for IV injection. It also allows it to be rapidly absorbed from the moist mucous membranes that line the oral,[80] nasal, rectal, and vaginal cavities. For these reasons, cocaine hydrochloride is commonly intranasally insufflated ("snorted") or inserted rectally or vaginally.

Crack Cocaine

Crack Cocaine (i.e., cocaine base, or freebase cocaine), is produced from the natural form of cocaine that is directly extracted from the coca leaves (see Figure 2.3). Only slightly soluble in water (i.e., one gram in 1,300 ml), crack cocaine readily dissolves in ethanol (i.e., one gram in seven ml), ether (i.e., one gram in four ml), and chloroform (i.e., one gram in 0.5 ml).[81] The melting point of crack cocaine is significantly lower than that for cocaine hydrochloride (i.e., 98° Celsius versus 195° Celsius). Thus, when heated, crack cocaine, as compared to cocaine hydrochloride, vaporizes much more readily and is involved in less pyrolysis, or heat-related chemical destruction.[82] Accordingly, pulmonary inhalation of the vaporized crack cocaine can achieve blood cocaine concentrations that are equal to those achieved by the IV injection of cocaine hydrochloride.

In addition, because of the mechanisms inherent in pulmonary absorption (i.e., extremely large surface area provided by approximately 500 million alveoli), the onset of action for pulmonary inhalation is more rapid than for IV injection and it produces a more intense desired action—at least as subjectively reported by crack cocaine users. For these and other reasons (e.g., convenience; lower cost; avoidance of infections, such as HIV infection associated with IV injection), adolescents and young adults generally prefer the pulmonary inhalation of vaporized crack cocaine to any other method of cocaine use.

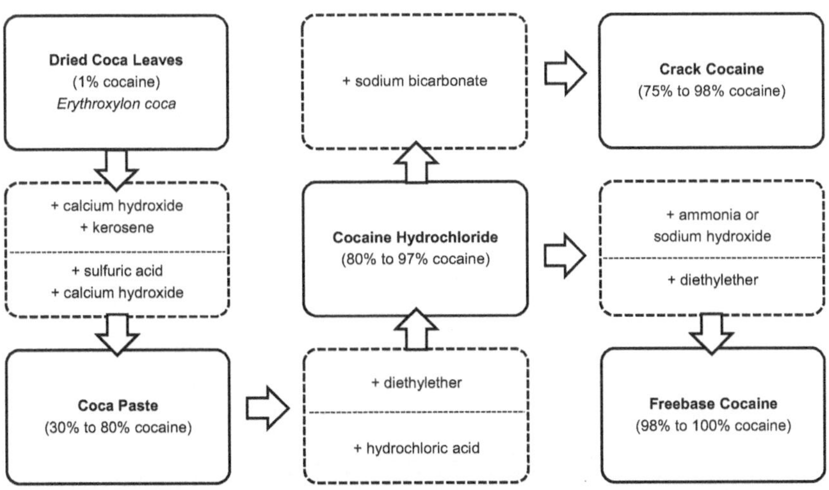

Figure 2.3 Production of Cocaine

80 Cocaine hydrochloride, because of its high-water solubility, also is used for selected medical and dental purposes, such as local anesthesia of the membranes of the oral, laryngeal, and nasal cavities. In illicit drug deals, it also is commonly rubbed on the gums, numbing them—thus, serving as "proof" that the product actually is cocaine hydrochloride (although any "caine"-based local anesthetic would produce the same numbing effect).

81 Thus, the requisite use of organic solvents (e.g., acetone; gasoline; kerosene) in South American "jungle" laboratories to extract the cocaine from harvested cocaine leaves.

82 The common street name, "Crack," originates from the "crackling" sound produced when "crack rocks" are heated and vaporized by holding a cigarette lighter under a crack pipe, a piece of aluminum foil, or the lid of a soft drink can.

Pharmacodynamics: Mechanism of Action

After absorption into the systemic circulation, cocaine can be found in virtually all areas of the brain. However, it appears to preferentially accumulate in the "caudate nucleus," the "nucleus accumbens," and the "ventral tegmental area." Cocaine decreases the dopamine transporter (DAT) clearance of dopamine from the synaptic cleft by blocking its reuptake into the presynaptic cells. It also appears to block the reuptake of other monoamines, including serotonin and norepinephrine. Consequently, cocaine increases the accumulation and activity of neurotransmitters in the synaptic cleft. A simplified representation of the proposed principal site and mechanism of the action of cocaine is shown in Figure 2.4.

Common Misbelief: Acting at different brain centers, the actions of crack cocaine are much stronger than those of cocaine hydrochloride.

Actually, once absorbed into the systemic circulation, both crack cocaine and cocaine hydrochloride share exactly the same mechanism of action and, at equivalent dosages, produce exactly the same effects. As reported by Grabus (2017), NIH-funded research has demonstrated that in addition to increasing dopamine concentration in the synaptic cleft by blocking the dopamine transporter, cocaine stimulates the production of the endocannabinoid molecule, 2-arachidonoylglycerol (2-AG). In turn, 2-AG is reportedly associated with a significant increase in dopamine concentration within the nucleus accumbens (see related discussion in Chapter 4, "Cannabis and Other Psychodelics").

The ability of cocaine to increase neurotransmitter activity in the brain causes several desired effects that contribute to its continued use. These effects, include:

1. Intense euphoria;
2. Feelings of increased energy and competence;
3. Heightened sociability and sexual desire;
4. Decreased feelings of fatigue and hunger;
5. Indifference to pain and discomfort.

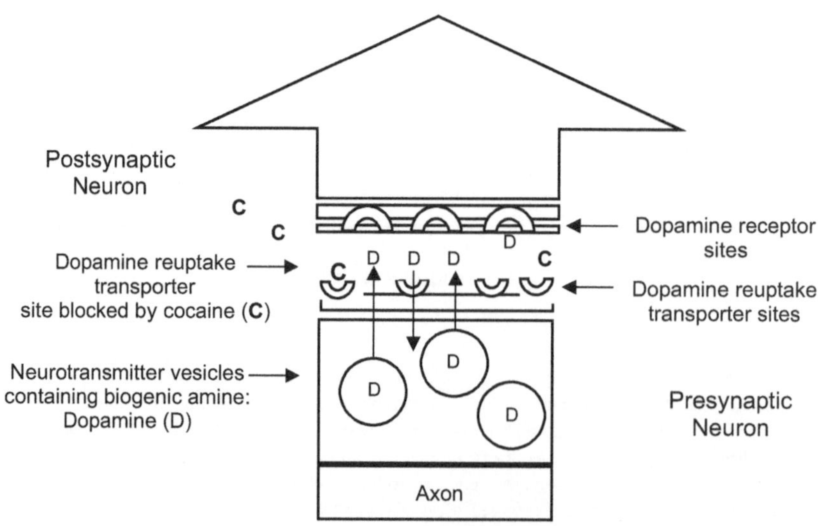

Figure 2.4 Cocaine: Mechanism of Action

Table 2.14 Cocaine Pharmacokinetics

Cocaine Pharmacokinetics	
Absorption	
• Bioavailability	33% oral 70% intranasal ≥ 90% pulmonary
• Time to Peak Blood Concentration	~ 45 minutes, oral ~ 10 minutes, intranasal 1 minute, intravenous or pulmonary
Distribution	
• Volume of Distribution	~ 3 L/kg
• Plasma Protein Binding	Moderate (~90%)
Metabolism (Hydrolysis and metabolism primarily occur in the liver)[83]	
• Total Body Clearance	~ 1 L/minute
• Mean Half-Life of Elimination	1.25 hours
Excretion	
• Urinary Excretion	1% to 5% (influenced by urinary pH with lower excretion in alkaline urine and higher excretion in acidic urine)

Sources: Laizure, Mandrell, & Gades (2003); Pagliaro & Benet (1975); Pagliaro & Pagliaro (2009).

Approximately 30 years ago, Dackis and Gold (1990) identified that, during cocaine use episodes, the CNS actions of cocaine and associated effects could be divided into three phases: Phase 1: "Mild Stimulation;" Phase 2: "Excitation;" and Phase 3: "Depression." During "Phase 1," cocaine stimulates the CNS, beginning with the cerebral cortex, by decreasing the re-uptake of neurotransmitters (e.g., dopamine and serotonin). These actions generally result in euphoria and mild stimulation. As the amount of cocaine is increased, for example, by continued inhalation of vaporized crack cocaine, IV injection of dissolved cocaine hydrochloride, or nasal insufflation of more lines of cocaine powder, "Phase 2"—the excitation phase—begins. During Phase 2, CNS stimulation becomes more pronounced with various associated effects (e.g., anxiety; hypertension; mydriasis; pressured speech; tachycardia; tremors; vomiting). However, as cocaine use continues, the endogenous neurotransmitters in the CNS (i.e., dopamine and serotonin) become depleted and "Phase 3," the depression phase, begins.

Phase 3 is characterized by a depression of the cortical areas of the CNS, which may progress to medullary depression and associated respiratory failure. This phase spontaneously resolves, but not until after the depleted endogenous neurotransmitters have sufficient time to be naturally replenished. The associated mental depression experienced during this phase is colloquially referred to as the "cocaine blues" (Pagliaro & Pagliaro, 2009). (Also see the later

83 Carboxylesterases, present in several tissues, including the liver, catalyze the hydrolysis of cocaine to its two major metabolites: (1) benzyl ecgonine; and (2) ecgonine methyl ester.

cocaine subsection, "Undesired, or Harmful, Effects and Toxicities—Physical and Psychological Dependence.")

Pharmacokinetics: Absorption, Distribution, Metabolism, and Excretion

The absorption, distribution, metabolism, and excretion of cocaine is affected by its: (1) formulation—cocaine hydrochloride versus crack cocaine; (2) purity; and (3) method of use, or route of administration (see Table 2.14).

ABSORPTION

After oral ingestion the mean bioavailability of cocaine hydrochloride is low, approximately only 33%. Thus, adolescents and young adults rarely use this method of administration. Following intranasal insufflation, or "snorting," the bioavailability of cocaine is increased to approximately 70%, but is still reduced because the rate of intranasal absorption is constrained by the: (1) limited surface area provided by the nasal mucosa; and (2) local nasal vasoconstriction due to the actions of cocaine. However, with IV injection, the bioavailability of cocaine hydrochloride—as with other drugs and substances of abuse—is 100%.

In comparison, when crack cocaine is vaporized and inhaled into the lungs, pulmonary bioavailability is very high (i.e., over 90%). However, the use of a glass crack pipe may affect overall bioavailability because: (1) a small portion of the dose can be destroyed by pyrolysis;[84] and (2) a relatively larger portion of the dose, often remains adhered to the inner surfaces of the crack pipe.

Peak serum cocaine concentrations occur approximately: 45 minutes after ingestion; 10 minutes after intranasal insufflation (i.e., "snorting"); and one minute after IV injection (i.e., "mainlining") and pulmonary inhalation (e.g., inhaling vapors from a crack pipe, piece of aluminum foil, or soft drink can).[85]

METABOLISM

Cocaine is hydrolyzed and metabolized primarily in the liver to several metabolites, including: benzoylecgonine; ecgonine; ecgonine methyl ester; hydroxycocaine; hydroxybenzoylecgonine; and norcocaine. Esterases found in the plasma are predominately responsible for the formation of the major metabolite, benzoylecgonine. Esterases also are found in many other body tissues, including the brain, liver, lungs, and pancreas.

EXCRETION

The mean half-life of elimination for cocaine is 1.25 hours. However, the urinary elimination of cocaine appears to be influenced by urinary pH (as observed with the amphetamines—see earlier related discussion in the amphetamine section of this chapter). Consequently, cocaine elimination is increased in acidic urine (i.e., pH below 7) and decreased in alkaline urine (i.e., pH above 7). In addition, the total body clearance of cocaine may be significantly reduced with the concurrent use of alcohol (see also the related discussion of cocaethylene in the later subsection, "Cocaine Drug–Drug Interactions").

84 The major product of the pyrolysis of crack cocaine is "methylecgonidine." The amount of methylecgonidine that is produced, generally ranges from 1% to 5%, depending upon the temperature and rate of air flow in the crack pipe. The presence of methylecgonidine (i.e., anhydroecgonine methyl ester) has been used as a biological marker to differentiate (e.g., in forensic biological samples) crack cocaine smoking from other methods of cocaine use.

85 Interestingly, passive "side-stream" exposure to freebase cocaine vapors does *not* generally result in the absorption of clinically significant amounts of cocaine (Cone, Yousefnejad, & Hillsgrove, 1995)—contrary to the passive "side-stream" exposure to nicotine that has been associated with e-cigarette vapor (e.g., Czogala, Goniewicz, & Fidelus, 2014). (See Chapter 3, "Caffeine and Nicotine").

Common Misbelief: The half-life of elimination of crack cocaine is significantly shorter than that of cocaine hydrochloride.

In fact, the half-life of elimination of cocaine is exactly the same regardless of the form of cocaine that is used or its route of administration.

Cocaine Drug–Drug Interactions

A metabolic interaction exclusively involving the concomitant use of cocaine and alcohol may result in approximately 23% of the systemically available cocaine being converted to "cocaethylene," a psychoactive ethyl homologue of cocaine (Harris, Everhart, & Mendelson, 2003; Herbst, Harris, & Everhart, 2011). Adolescents and young adults, who concomitantly use alcohol and cocaine, often share that their use of alcohol and cocaine appears to: (1) enhance, or prolong, the euphoria they experience with cocaine alone; and (2) mitigate the undesired effects associated with the use of alcohol (e.g., sedation) (Pagliaro & Pagliaro, *Clinical Patient Data Files*). These effects may be explained, at least in part, by the formation of cocaethylene.

Several other drugs and substances have been involved in clinically significant cocaine drug–drug interactions. These major related drug–drug interactions are presented and briefly discussed in Table 2.15.

Undesired, or Harmful, Effects and Toxicities

According to the National Drug Abuse Warning Network (DAWN), cocaine is involved in most of the admissions related to illegal drug and substance abuse reported by EDs across the U.S. Approximately 0.5% of *all* ED admissions, on an annual basis, involve the use of cocaine (ONDCP, 2010).

The use of cocaine has been commonly associated with several "acute" toxicities that are directly related to its specific pharmacologic actions on various body systems. The regular, long-term use of cocaine also has been implicated with the development of "chronic" toxicities,

Table 2.15 Cocaine: Major Potential Drug–Drug Interactions[86, 87]

Drugs that Interact with Cocaine	*Comments*
Monoamine Oxidase Inhibitors (MAOIs) (e.g., phenelzine [Nardil®]; tranylcypromine [Parnate®])	MAOIs, when used with cocaine, increase the possibility of a hypertensive crisis (noradrenergic syndrome)
Psychodepressants (e.g., opiate analgesics; sedative-hypnotics)	Psychodepressants, when used with cocaine, ameliorate the psychostimulant effects of cocaine
Psychostimulants (e.g., caffeine; cocaine; nicotine)	Psychostimulants, when used with cocaine, cause additive psychostimulant effects

86 The clinical significance of these drug–drug interactions depends upon several factors, including the: (1) dosage of each drug; (2) characteristics of the adolescent or young adult (e.g., age; gender; genetics); (3) concomitant physical health (e.g. hepatic and renal function); and (4) concomitant mental health status.

87 Topical drug interactions for cocaine are *not* included.

including physical and psychological dependence or use disorder, and, when used by adolescent girls and women during pregnancy, teratogenesis. Other toxicities have been specifically related to its adulteration and methods of use—intranasal insufflation, or "snorting;" pulmonary inhalation of the vaporized form; and IV injection, or "mainlining" or "shooting-up." These common toxicities are presented and discussed in the following sections.

ACUTE TOXICITIES

The use of cocaine has been associated with several acute toxicities that are primarily related to its psychostimulant actions, including:

- Agitation;
- Anxiety;
- Apathy;
- Cerebrovascular accidents;
- Difficulty concentrating;
- Hallucinations;
- Headache;
- Hyperpnea;
- Hyperthermia;
- Hypertension;
- Insomnia;
- Irritability;
- Loss of sexual desire;
- Memory impairment;
- Muscle twitching/tics;
- Mydriasis;
- Myocardial infarction;
- Panic attacks;
- Premature ventricular contractions;
- Pressured Speech;
- Restlessness;
- Seizures;
- Suicide attempts;
- Tachycardia;
- Tachypnea;
- Tremors.

The acute toxicities of cocaine, which are directly related to its pharmacologic actions, primarily depend upon the dosage used (i.e., the larger the dosage, the larger the associated effect—in this context, toxicity).[88] However, because cocaine is predominantly used in an illicit context and, consequently, predominantly illicitly produced without stringent quality control standards (as used with pharmaceutical-grade cocaine), the dose used depends upon the purity of the cocaine. Studying the correlation between cocaine purity and trends in emergency department (ED) visits (i.e., as a measure of toxicity), Zhu, Wilson, and Stimpson (2014) found that:

88 The health status of the user, age, and concomitant use of other drugs or substances of abuse, both illicit and licit, also can significantly affect the nature, extent, and consequent impact of acute cocaine toxicity.

> Cocaine purity is positively correlated with cocaine-related ED visits, and our findings suggest decreases in powder cocaine purity were associated with significant declines in ED visits.[89]
> (p. 1015)

CHRONIC TOXICITIES

Regular, long-term use of cocaine has been associated with the development of additional toxicities, including: mental depression, paranoia, and psychological dependence (e.g., Pagliaro & Pagliaro, *Clinical Patient Data Files*; Pagliaro, Jaglalsingh, & Pagliaro, 1992). Increasing attention also is being given to data that suggest an association between regular, long-term use of cocaine with cognitive impairment—particularly, deficits in executive, or high-level, cognitive function that involves decision making and problem solving abilities (Bickel, Franck, & Moody, 2013; Moody, Franck, & Jarmolowicz, 2014).

Cocaine psychosis and IPV are two other troubling undesired, or harmful, effects that are commonly associated with cocaine abuse (see the following subsections for further discussion).

COCAINE PSYCHOSIS. Cocaine psychosis is virtually indistinguishable from amphetamine psychosis, although it is usually of shorter duration (see the related discussion in the major amphetamines subsection of this chapter). Cocaine psychosis also shares, together with amphetamine psychosis, a similarity to paranoid schizophrenia. Both cocaine psychosis and amphetamine psychosis are often characterized by hypervigilance and paranoia and have been associated with an increased incidence of aggressive and violent behavior, including homicide (Pagliaro & Pagliaro, *Clinical Patient Data Files*).

INTIMATE PARTNER VIOLENCE (IPV). In a retrospective analysis of data from 96 related studies, Moore, Stuart, and Meehan (2008) found that, of all the drugs and substances of abuse, cocaine had the strongest relationship with IPV. Although associated factors (e.g., personality traits; concurrent mental disorders; concomitant use of alcohol or other drugs and substances of abuse) are likely major contributing factors (Pagliaro & Pagliaro, *Clinical Patient Data Files*), IPV has been consistently found to be strongly associated with cocaine use (e.g., Ernst, Weiss, & Enright-Smith, 2008; Smith, Homish, & Leonard, 2012; Winhusen & Lewis, 2013)—and this IPV has commonly been associated with significant injurious effects, including fatalities that frequently involve children and adolescents, who live in this environment (see the later cocaine subsection, "Cocaine and Mothering").

POTENTIALLY FATAL TOXICITIES

Cocaine use has been directly related to four potentially fatal toxicities that can occur regardless of age or method of use:

1. Cardiotoxicity;
2. Cerebrovascular Accidents;
3. Hyperthermia;
4. Seizures.

It also has been indirectly associated with potentially fatal toxicities related to the: (1) inadvertent contamination, or deliberate adulteration, of street supplies of cocaine prior to their distribution, sale, and use; and (2) concomitant use of other drugs and substances of abuse, particularly drug–drug interactions involving alcohol and heroin (Bernstein, Bucciarelli, & Piper, 2007; Pagliaro & Pagliaro, 2009). (See later section, "Adulterants.") We begin with cardiotoxicity.

89 The finding was in the context of the related finding, which indicated that the average purity for cocaine powder in the greater Chicago area/market, fell from 65.2% in 2004 to 37% in 2010 (Zhu, Wilson, & Stimpson, 2014, p. 1013).

CARDIOTOXICITY. The actions of cocaine on the cardiovascular system have been associated with both an increase in heart rate and blood pressure. These actions, in turn, may lead to increased risk for dysrhythmias, end-stage renal disease, myocardial infarction, and cerebral vascular asccident, or stroke (e.g., Norris, Thornhill-Joynes, & Robinson, 2001; Phillips, Luk, & Soor, 2009; Pilgrim, Woodford, & Drummer, 2013). For example, Diercks, Kirk, and Turnipseed (2007) reported a significantly high rate of CAD among cocaine-using patients.

These severe, and potentially fatal,[90] cardiotoxicities (Phillips, Luk, & Soor, 2009) appear to occur, in part, because of the decrease in blood pH that is associated with cocaine use. The acidemia has been reported to cause scarring and disruption of the cardiac electrical conduction system with prolongation of the QRS complex and QTc (i.e., corrected QT interval) duration on the electrocardiogram (Wang, 1999). However, others have suggested molecular mechanisms of action for the cardiovascular effects associated with cocaine use, including: (1) interaction with cardiac calcium, potassium, and sodium (i.e., cation) channels (Turillazzi, Bello, & Neri, 2012); and (2) oxidative stress and resultant antioxidant cellular system injuries (Cerretani, Fineschi, & Bello, 2012).

***Related Professional Reminder:* These different purported mechanisms of cocaine-induced cardiotoxicity are not mutually exclusive.**

***Related Professional Reminder:* When evaluating, or caring for, adolescents or young adults, who are sudden cardiac arrest survivors, always inquire about illicit use of drugs or substances of abuse, particularly the psychostimulants—amphetamines and cocaine—and, if necessary, recommend appropriate follow-up care regarding their SUD prior to discharge.**

CEREBROVASCULAR ACCIDENTS. CNS hemorrhage, or stroke, results from the combined effects of the vasoconstriction and increased cardiac output associated with cocaine use. Ischemic stroke has long been documented in the context of cocaine use among adolescents and young adults (as well as older adults). For example, in their study of the relationship of cocaine use and young-onset ischemic stroke, Cheng, Ryan, and Qadwai (2016) found that "acute cocaine use in the previous 24 hours was strongly associated with increased risk for stroke" (p. 918). In addition, Shoamanesh, Catanese, and Romero (2016) identified an increased incidence of cerebral microbleeds—as assessed by magnetic resonance imaging (MRI)—among "young stroke patients," who had a "positive serum toxicology for cocaine" (p. 733).

Cerebrovascular accidents occur more often among adolescents who have cerebral aneurysms. Although it is estimated that approximately one in 20 people have a cerebral aneurysm (e.g., Rinkel, Djibuti, & Algra, 1998), most adolescents, who use cocaine, are unaware of this risk. This risk reportedly increases with age, irrespective of the previous length of time that cocaine was used.[91]

90 For example, "sudden death" in the young has been associated with cocaine use and is likely due to "myocardial ischemia and infarction" (Fischbach, 2017, p. S75).

91 Among hospitalized patients with aneurysmal subarachnoid hemorrhage, cocaine users are three times more likely to die than are non-users (Chang, Kowalski, & Caserta, 2013). In a large retrospective analysis of patients admitted to a stroke service from 2004 to 2007, Martin-Schild, Albright, and Hallevi (2010) similarly found that:

> Patients with cocaine-associated intracerebral hemorrhage were nearly three times more likely to die during their acute hospitalization when compared to cocaine-negative patients.
>
> (p. 680)

HYPERTHERMIA. Cocaine-induced hyperthermia, a body temperature exceeding 104° Fahrenheit (41° Celsius), is usually caused by the combined effects of: (1) excessively stimulated body metabolism; and (2) vasoconstriction, which significantly impairs the ability of the body to cool itself (i.e., thermoregulation).[92] A body temperature of this magnitude can cause seizures and coma, and may be fatal in up to 20% of cases—more, if left untreated. In non-fatal cases, irreversible brain damage may occur. Hyperpyrexia also is an associated symptom that is observed in both cocaine-induced fatal excited delirium and cocaine-induced rhabdomyolysis (Bauwens, Boggs, & Hartwell, 1989; Crandell, Vongpatanasin, & Victor, 2002).

SEIZURES. Seizures,[93] which may terminate in cardiovascular collapse, can be caused by several actions associated with cocaine use, including: (1) anoxia; (2) heightened psychostimulation; and (3) hyperthermia. On a molecular level, it has been proposed that the seizures associated with cocaine use are mediated by the enhancement of monoamine, particularly dopamine and serotonin, activity (Lason, 2001). This cocaine-induced seizure activity appears to be modulated by the stimulantion of dopamine D_1 receptors and the inhibition of gamma-aminobutyric acid ($GABA_A$) receptors. Subsequently, Rolland, Karila, and Geoffroy (2011) extended this hypothesis by suggesting that the activation of the D_1 receptor produces a neurological kindling process involving the NMDA receptor phosphorylation state. Utilizing the case history of a 21-year-old woman, who chronically abused cocaine, they further postulated that the mechanism underlying cocaine-induced seizures could overlap with the mechanism underlying cocaine-induced psychosis.

ADULTERANTS

Due to the lack of stringent quality control that would otherwise occur with the Good Manufacturing Practices, which guide licit pharmaceutical production in the U.S., the potential risk for unique and unexpected toxicities can occur whenever an illicitly manufactured drug or substance of abuse is prepared, sold, bought, or used. Adulterants (e.g., arsenic; benzocaine; corn starch; lactose; quinine; sodium bicarbonate) are also often purposely used by illicit drug dealers to "cut" various drugs and substances of abuse prior to their sale—most often to increase their bulk/volume and, consequently, to increase dealer profits. Several unique toxicities, which can be even more serious than those directly associated with the particular drug or substance of abuse that is adulterated, have been associated with the use of many of these adulterants—including those used to adulterate cocaine. (See also, for example, the related discussions in Chapter 5, "Prescription Opiate Analgesics and Heroin.")

For example, during 2008–2009, a specific adulterant, "levamisole" (Ergamisol®),[94] was found in approximately two-thirds of all of the cocaine samples that were seized and analyzed by the U.S. government (Pagliaro & Pagliaro, 2009). Probably added to illicit cocaine to boost its effects or to increase its weight and, consequently, the related profits for the distributor/seller, it resulted in significant toxicity among users. For example, as reported by Lee, Ladizinski, and Federman (2012):

92 Currently, it is believed that impaired heat dissipation (i.e., cocaine-induced impairment of both sweating and cutaneous vasodilation) is the primary mechanism underlying the development of cocaine-induced hyperthermia (Crandell, Vongpatanasin, & Victor, 2002).

93 Cocaine seizures, colloquially referred to as "doing the chicken," are commonly experienced (Pagliaro & Pagliaro, *Clinical Patient Data Files*). "The DEA also has noted a bump in cocaine seizures" (Leonard, 2017, p. 1).

94 Levamisole, a veterinary anthelminthic, that also has psychostimulant action, was experimentally used for the treatment of some types of human cancers (Larocque & Hoffman, 2012). It was withdrawn from U.S. markets, in 2005, because of reports of agranulocytosis (Buxton, Omura, & Kuo, 2015).

> Complications associated with the use of levamisole-laced cocaine include neutropenia, agranulocytosis, arthralgias, retiform purpura, and skin necrosis.
>
> (p. 1033)

TOXICITIES ASSOCIATED WITH METHOD OF USE

Several toxicities have been commonly associated with four specific methods of cocaine use:

1. Intranasal insufflation, or "snorting;"
2. IV injection, or "mainlining;"
3. Pulmonary inhalation, or "vaping" (i.e., inhaling crack cocaine vapor);
4. Subcutaneous injection and "Coke Burns;"

The toxicities associated with each of these methods of use are presented and discussed in the following subsections.

INTRANASAL INSUFFLATION, OR "SNORTING". Intranasal insufflation of cocaine hydrochloride is associated with both minor irritation and severe injury to nasal mucous membranes and to other related underlying structures (e.g., nasal septum). Although less serious effects may occur, such as rhinitis and eczema in and around the nostrils, more serious effects, such as nasal erosion and perforation of the nasal septum, also may occur, particularly with regular, long-term use (Vilela, Langford, & McCullagh, 2002).

The minor irritation, as well as the more serious injuries to the nose, are caused by: (1) the direct action of cocaine (i.e., vasoconstriction) on the surrounding skin and mucous membranes; and (2) the direct irritation caused by the hydrochloride salt-form of cocaine, which, when it encounters nasal secretions, forms a dilute, but irritating, solution of hydrochloric acid. The occurrence of these local effects, together with the relatively small surface area of the nasal mucosa, which effectively restricts absorption rates to begin with, have helped to increase the popularity of the pulmonary inhalation, or smoking, of cocaine in its freebase, or crack, form—currently, the most popular method of cocaine use in the U.S.[95] Unfortunately, this method of use (i.e., "smoking," or "vaping") is associated with its own toxicities, particularly those associated with the pulmonary system (see the later subsection, "Pulmonary Inhalation, or Vaping").

INTRAVENOUS INJECTION, OR "MAINLINING". The IV injection of cocaine has been related to the development of abscesses at injection sites, local infections, and, phlebitis when injected veins become irritated and inflamed as a response to being pierced with a needle and injected with an irritating solution of cocaine. IV injection of cocaine also is associated with the development of thrombosis, which may be fatal.

It is important to note that these effects commonly occur with the intravenous use of *any* drug or substances of abuse (See also the related discussion in the amphetamines pharmacology subsection, "Undesired, or Harmful, Effects and Toxicities—Intravenous Toxicities"). It also is important to note that the IV injection of cocaine was a major contributing factor to the spread of the HIV infection during the late 1980s and 1990s (Pagliaro, Pagliaro, & Thauberger, 1990, 1993; Pagliaro & Pagliaro, 2000).

95 Freebase and crack cocaine are essentially the same forms of cocaine—at least in terms of their purity and method of use. However, freebase is more difficult and dangerous to produce because of the need to "heat-off" a flammable solvent prior to use (See Figure 2.3) with the resultant risk of fire (Feaver, 1986; People Staff, 1980).

PULMONARY INHALATION, OR "VAPING". The toxicities associated with inhaling cocaine vapor result in both irritation and damage to the lungs, including pneumomediastinum, pneumonia, and pulmonary infiltrates. Acute exacerbation of asthma and bronchitis also may occur among adolescents and young adults who already have these chronic obstructive pulmonary diseases (Ali, Krugar, & Houghton, 2002; Gatof & Albert, 2002). In addition, the regular, long-term smoking of crack cocaine has been associated with alveolar and microvascular lung damage at the microscopic level—a condition that has been commonly referred to as "crack lung" (e.g., Bulbena-Cabre, Ramos Dunn, & Gorman Swift, 2015; Shah, Patel, & Mousa, 2015).

Finally, adolescents and young adults are known to often use crack cocaine in groups in which the crack pipe (commonly referred to as a "bubble") is shared among users (Pagliaro & Pagliaro, *Clinical Patient Data Files*). As noted by Cheng, Wood, and Nguyen (2015):

> Crack pipe sharing is a risky practice that has been associated with the transmission of hepatitis C and other harms [e.g., hepatitis A; HIV].
>
> (p. 259)

SUBCUTANEOUS INJECTION AND "COKE BURNS". "Coke burns," which are associated with the repeated inadvertent subcutaneous injection of cocaine by intravenous cocaine users, who "miss the vein." Caused in much the same way as intranasal irritation and damage occurs with snorting cocaine (see the discussion in the previous subsection), coke burns are associated with the formation of dilute hydrochloric acid when the dissolved cocaine hydrochloride interacts with the subcutaneous body fluids.

Physical and Psychological Dependence

It has been estimated that, of a group of 100 people who try cocaine, 30 of them will become "abusive users" and 10 will become "compulsive users" (Pagliaro & Pagliaro, *Clinical Patient Data Files*). However, over the last two decades, the consensus has been that there is no true physical dependence associated with the regular, long-term use of cocaine as classically defined by the existence of both: (1) the development of tolerance with regular, long-term use; and (2) when use is abruptly discontinued, the occurrence of a withdrawal syndrome that is immediately relieved when the use of the drug or substance of abuse is resumed.

Similar to the amphetamines, cocaine does not fit this classic definition of physical dependence because the endogenous neurotransmitters—which become depleted with continued cocaine use—must be naturally replenished before desired effects can, once again, be achieved or undesired effects be relieved. (See also the discussion in the earlier pharmacology subsection, "Pharmacodynamics: Mechanism of Action").

Although, cocaine does not fit the classic definition of "physical" dependence, the abrupt discontinuation of cocaine, following regular, long-term use, may result in "psychological" dependence, or a "cocaine withdrawal syndrome." This syndrome is characterized by several undesired effects, including:

- Anhedonia;
- Anxiety;
- Apathy;
- Dysphoria;
- Fatigue, both mental and physical;
- Headaches;
- Increased appetite;

- Irritability;
- Mental depression;
- Muscle cramps;
- Somnolence;
- Vivid and unpleasant dreams.

These signs and symptoms may begin within a few hours of discontinuing cocaine use and generally resolve within 24 hours (Walsh, Stoops, & Moody, 2009). However, as previously noted, they *cannot* be immediately relieved by resuming cocaine use.

The underlying cellular mechanism involved regarding the cocaine withdrawal syndrome appears to be related to a decrease in mesolimbic dopamine activity (Hu, 2007; Kuhar & Pilotte, 1996). Dopamine modulates neuronal activity in the prefrontal cortex, which is necessary for optimal cognitive functioning (Nogueira, Kalivas, & Lavin, 2006). The decrease in dopamine activity, associated with the cocaine withdrawal syndrome, has been related to severe psychological dependence with intense craving for cocaine, and, consequently, the occurrence of resumed cocaine use (Kuhar & Pilotte, 1996; Pagliaro & Pagliaro, *Clinical Patient Data Files*; Walsh, Stoops, & Moody, 2009). Interestingly, women are more likely than men to report craving for cocaine within one hour of discontinuing its use (Kennedy, Epstein, & Phillips, 2013).

Although based largely on data obtained from animal studies, as reported by the NIH (2017), females appear to be more likely to develop cocaine dependence than males, as demonstrated by: (1) reportedly more intense "highs;" and (2) a proclivity for developing cocaine dependence more rapidly (i.e., "telescoping effect"). Based on these findings, the NIH posited that these effects are due to the female hormone estradiol and are mediated by activation of the mGluR5 receptor on neurons that, in turn, stimulate the release of endocannabinoid neurotransmitters. (See also the earlier cocaine pharmacology subsection, "Pharmacodynamics: Mechanism of Action.")

Cocaine Overdosage

During the second decade of the new millennium, cocaine, after the opiate analgesics (see Chapter 5, "Prescription Opiate Analgesics and Heroin"), was involved in most of the overdosage deaths in the U.S.[96] For example, from 2015 to 2016 the annual number of cocaine overdosage deaths among young adults, 15 to 24 years-of-age, in the U.S. significantly increased by 1% (Seth, Scholl, & Rudd, 2018). A significant contributor was the increasing use of "speedballs"—the use of cocaine in combination with an opiate analgesic (e.g., fentanyl; heroin; or morphine).[97] As noted, for example, by Leonard (2017):

> An examination of CDC data show that 6,784 people died of a cocaine-involved overdose in 2015. Of these 2,565 also had heroin as a contributing cause of death and 1,077 had a prescription pain reliever. In 1,542 cases, fentanyl contributed to the cause of

96 As reported by Herman (2017), among ethnic groups, "cocaine was the greatest contributor to deaths among blacks" (p. 1).

97 This appears to continue a trend that became significant two decades earlier (Pagliaro & Pagliaro, *Clinical Patient Data Files*). For example, as noted by Li, Zhang, and Levine (2011):

> The Office of the Chief Medical Examiner of Maryland recorded a total of 149 drug abuse deaths of teenagers aged 13–19 between 1991 and 2006. Of these . . . 19.5% by both narcotics and cocaine and 4.0% by cocaine only.
>
> (p. 1029)

> death, and some of these drugs overlapped, meaning that about 63 percent of cases involved an opioid.
>
> (p. 1)

In 2017, the CDC reported 14,556 overdosage deaths in the U.S. related to cocaine use (NIH, 2018, p. 1). This was the highest reported number of cocaine overdosage deaths at any time during the preceding years of the new millennium.

Cocaine overdosage may be fatal with death being generally a result of: cardiac dysrhythmias; hyperthermia; intracranial hemorrhage; respiratory arrest; or status epilepticus (see related discussion in the earlier amphetamine subsection, "Undesired, or Harmful, Effects and Toxicities—Potentially Fatal Toxicities"). Acute cocaine overdosage requires emergency medical support of body systems, with attention to increasing cocaine elimination (see related discussion of urinary pH in the earlier pharmacology subsection, "Pharmacokinetics—Excretion.") Medical management is primarily directed at preventing related body organ damage and ameliorating associated signs and symptoms. Many of the associated signs and symptoms (e.g., aggressive behavior; anxiety; insomnia; irritability; panic attacks; seizures; temors) respond well to benzodiazepine (e.g., diazepam [Valium®]) pharmacotherapy. There is no known antidote for cocaine overdosage (Pagliaro & Pagliaro, 2009, 2012).

Pregnancy, Breastfeeding, and Mothering

The use of cocaine by adolescent girls and young women during pregnancy, when breastfeeding, or when mothering neonates, infants, and young children can result in many harmful effects, which are presented and discussed in the following sections.

COCAINE USE DURING PREGNANCY

Cocaine use by women, who are pregnant, is a significant problem in most major cities across the U.S. The three major factors associated with high rates of cocaine use during pregnancy are: (1) African continental descent; (2) poor education; and (3) lower socioeconomic status (e.g., Barthelemy, Richardson, & Rose-Jacobs, 2016; Pagliaro & Pagliaro, 2018; Pagliaro & Pagliaro, *Clinical Patient Data Files*). Numerous studies have documented sex-for-drug exchanges that involve crack cocaine, particularly among pregnant women of African continental descent.[98] (For additional related discussion, see also the later cocaine subsection, "Adolescent and Young Adult Sex-For-Drug Exchanges.")

In their review of the published literature related to fetal exposure to drugs and substances of abuse, Ross, Graham, and Money (2015) identified that the effects associated with in utero exposure to cocaine are complex and varied:

> Overall, fetal cocaine exposure can affect fetal and long-term growth patterns, as well as cause language deficits, behavior defects, and executive functioning abnormalities.
>
> (p. 67)

However, these noted effects appear to be significantly affected, in terms of both incidence and severity, by: (1) dosage; (2) gestational timing; (3) duration of exposure; (4) exposure to

98 For example, Sharpe (2001), in an ethnographic study of "34 poor Black women, who exchanged sex for crack," found that "18 reported sex-for-crack pregnancies, and more than half of that number became pregnant this way more than once" (p. 612).

"co-teratogens;" (5) genetics;[99] and (6) postnatal care—which is largely related to socio-economic status (Pagliaro & Pagliaro, 2002). We expand on these in regard to fetal cocaine exposure in the following discussion.

The use of cocaine by adolescent girls and young women during pregnancy is associated with: intrauterine death, including spontaneous abortion; preterm delivery; and a variety of fetal physical anomalies, including cerebral hemorrhages or infarctions, and intrauterine growth retardation (e.g., smaller head circumference). However, a causal relationship between cocaine use and the various observed fetal abnormalities has not been definitively established (i.e., there is no consensus in terms of common characteristics or features of the so-called "crack baby"—in stark contrast to the FAS/FASD, see Chapter 1, "Alcohol") (e.g., Pagliaro & Pagliaro, *Clinical Patient Data Files*; Schiller & Allen, 2005; Vidaeff & Mastrobattista, 2003). This lack of a definitive relationship is due, in part, to the observation that adolescent girls and young women, who use cocaine while pregnant, are over 50 times more likely to also use other drugs and substances of abuse, including alcohol and nicotine—both of which have been recognized as human teratogens (See Chapter 1, "Alcohol," and Chapter 3, "Caffeine and Nicotine"). In fact, the NIDA (2018) noted that, among those with cocaine dependence or use disorder, 60% have concurrent alcohol dependence or use disorder and 50% have concurrent nicotine dependence or use disorder.

In addition, cocaine use by pregnant adolescent girls and young women has been associated with low birth weight, seizures, and tachycardia among neonates and a significantly higher rate of developmental delays and learning disorders among preschoolers and school-age children (Pagliaro & Pagliaro, 2012). It also has been suggested by several researchers (e.g., Meyer & Zhang, 2009) that intrauterine cocaine exposure also may result in a later increased risk for heart disease during adulthood, as well as deficits in executive function (e.g., Ross, Graham, & Money, 2015).

<u>Common Misbelief</u>: Intrauterine exposure to cocaine clearly results in later developmental neurotoxicity.

The available research data, which appear to be both valid and reliable, indicate that neurobehavioral toxicity is significantly more likely to occur in infants, children, adolescents, and young adults after prenatal exposure to "alcohol" or "amphetamines" rather than cocaine. (See also the earlier amphetamine subsection in this chapter and Chapter 1, "Alcohol.") As identified by Viteri, Soto, and Bahado-Singh (2015):

> In summary, the literature available evaluating long-term effects on growth and neurodevelopment in children exposed to cocaine in utero is contradictory and likely subject to confounding bias as a result of the adverse social environment in which these children live. (p. 408)[100]

Interestingly, Minnes, Min, and Short (2016), in their study of executive function among "children who were primarily African American and of low socioeconomic status," concluded that:

> Girls with PCE [prenatal cocaine exposure] were perceived by caregivers to have more behavioral regulation problems at age 12 ($p < 0.005$) and more metacognitive problems at

99 In this context, we have long noted–as in the case of FAS/FASD (see Chapter 1, "Alcohol")—that a major genetic variable, which is central to the significance of related executive functional deficits, is expressed as the intelligence quotient (IQ) of the exposed offspring (Pagliaro & Pagliaro, *Clinical Patient Data Files*).

100 We would add "use of multiple drugs and substances of abuse" by pregnant adolescents and young women—as previously documented—as another major "confounding" factor (Pagliaro & Pagliaro, *Clinical Patient Data Files*).

> age 12 (p < 003) than NCE [non-prenatal cocaine exposure] females, but there was no association for males.
>
> (p. 79)

However, a further and closer examination of the researchers' data and results, revealed that:

> Compared to PCE girls living with biologic mothers/relatives, those living in foster/adoptive care were rated as having more behavioral regulations and metacognitive executive function problems at 12 and 15 years.
>
> (p. 83)

This finding is congruent with, and supports, the earlier findings of Viteri, Soto, and Bahado-Singh (2015).

Because these issues are currently unresolved, we compiled Table 2.16, which presents research findings, published over the last decade, regarding prenatal exposure to cocaine, reported effects, and mediating variables for children and adolescents. Diametrically opposed results regarding the effects associated with prenatal cocaine exposure and, subsequently, effects identified among infants, children, adolescents, and young adults are common. A number of variables appear to contribute to this observation. As noted by Molnar, Levitt, and Eiden (2014):

> One possible explanation for these mixed findings may be due to differences in amount, duration, and timing of [prenatal cocaine] exposure that are difficult to determine. A second explanation is variations in quality of care including custody changes and type of foster care across different studies. A third explanation may be differences in sample size that may lead to non-significant findings for small effects, and control for different covariates. Finally, a fourth explanation may be the role of cumulative caregiving environmental risk and the possibility of indirect pathways in the absence of direct associations.
>
> (p. 522)

Additionally, the greater the lapsed time since intrauterine cocaine exposure (e.g., noted effects among infants versus noted effects among adolescents or young adults) allows for the increasing effect of intervening/modifying variables.

Neonates, whose mothers used large amounts of cocaine near term, also may experience CNS excitation (e.g., increased crying; irritability; and tremulousness). Thus, despite the lack of definitive confirmatory data, but with an abundance of caution, we strongly recommend that adolescents and young women, who are pregnant, should not use cocaine.[101]

101 N.B. During the new millennium, an overwhelming body of knowledge has accumulated in support of the claim that maternal cocaine use during pregnancy has the potential to cause serious harm to developing embryos and fetuses. To protect the unborn, many states have enacted legislation to mandate treatment aimed at adolescent girls and women, who use/abuse cocaine and are pregnant (Pagliaro & Pagliaro, 2012). For example, as reported by Chung (2017):

> Wisconsin's *Unborn Child Protection Act*, enacted in 1998, gives courts power over any expectant mother who "habitually lacks self-control" over drugs or alcohol, placing an unborn child at risk. The law allows officials to hold the pregnant woman in custody if she refuses treatment. [This law was upheld by the U.S. Supreme Court in July 2017].
>
> (p.1)

Table 2.16 Prenatal Cocaine Exposure: Effects on Infants, Children, Adolescents, and Young Adults

Subjects/ Participants	*Research Design*	*Effects*	*Mediating Variables*	*References*
Children, six years-of-age and older	Literature review	Increased "negative associations with sustained attention and behavioral self-regulation"	Noted, but modified by "environmental variables"	Ackerman, Riggins, & Black (2010)
Children, eight to 11 years-of-age, primarily of African continental descent	Experimental research study	Increased caregiver reports of "aggressive behavior"	Appears to be primarily mediated by "postnatal social environment"	Barthelemy, Richardson, & Rose-Jacobs (2016)
Children, birth through mid-adolescence	Longitudinal study	Decreased attention, behavior regulation, executive function, and language function—including delays	Noted, but mediated by prenatal "alcohol and tobacco exposure, lead exposure, maternal/care-giver education, IQ, depression, quality of the caregiving environment, and violence exposure"	Singer, Minnes, & Min (2015)
Children, birth through late adolescence	Prospective longitudinal study	Increased number of SUDs	Appears to be primarily mediated by "earlier substance initiation, exposure to violence, and to household substance use"	Frank, Kuranz, & Appugliese (2014)
Children and Adolescents, birth through 14.5 years-of-age	Longitudinal study	Increased "adolescent delinquent behaviors"	Appears to be primarily mediated by intrauterine tobacco/nicotine exposure and exposure to violence during childhood	Gerteis, Chartrand, & Martin (2011)
Adolescents, 12.4 to 15.9 years-of-age			Appears to be primarily mediated by:	Liebschultz, Crooks, &

(*Continued*)

Table 2.16 (Cont.)

Subjects/ Participants	*Research Design*	*Effects*	*Mediating Variables*	*References*
	Prospective longitudinal study	Decreased "behavioral resilience"	caregiver supervision in early adolescence; higher violence exposure in childhood; and intrauterine tobacco exposure	Rose-Jacobs (2015)
Adolescents, 14 to 16 years-of-age	Diffusion Tensor Imaging study	Decreased attention, behavior regulation, and executive function	Noted, but modified by prenatal concurrent "cocaine and alcohol exposure"	Lebel, Warner, & Colby (2013)
Mother-Child dyads assessed at birth through four years-of-age, primarily of African continental descent	Longitudinal study	Increased "deficits in arousal/attention regulatory system" (i.e., "self-regulation")	Noted, but modified by "caregiving experience" (e.g., "maternal harshness")	Eiden, Godleski, & Schuetze (2015)
Mother-Child dyads with children assessed at birth through six years-of-age, primarily boys of African continental descent	Longitudinal study	Increased "externalizing problems"	Noted, but modified by "maternal negative affect"	Molnar, Levitt, & Eiden (2014)

COCAINE AND BREASTFEEDING

Cocaine is excreted in breast milk. Thus, breast-fed neonates and infants may display characteristic CNS stimulation (e.g., irritability; seizures; tremulousness) and other expected effects (e.g., mydriasis). Consequently, we recommend that adolescent girls and young women, who use cocaine, should not breastfeed their neonates and infants (Pagliaro & Pagliaro, 2002, 2009, 2012, 2018).

> The [4-month-old] baby was taken to the hospital on May 15 after being breastfed and appearing to be in distress ... According to the police report, the couple admitted to using cocaine at a party the night before. Krystin Lisaius also admitted that she had breastfed the child the next morning because she didn't think he would be affected by the drug.
>
> (Fox News, 2016, p. 1)

COCAINE AND MOTHERING

The disruption of maternal-infant bonding and child attachment because of a young mother's cocaine use may result in many harmful effects (Eiden, Schuetze, & Coles, 2011; Parolin & Simonelli, 2016), including placing infants and children at extreme risk for neglect and abuse (Pagliaro & Pagliaro, *Clinical Patient Data Files*; Strathearn & Mayes, 2010).

In addition, as found by Mansoor, Morrow, and Accornero (2012), in their study of the relationship between prenatal maternal cocaine use and mother-child interactions:

> Prenatal and past-year maternal cocaine use seems to be associated with poorer quality in mother-child interaction during early childhood.
>
> (p. 32)

Further, as described by Strathearn and Mayes (2010, p. 9) and Ryder and Brisgone (2013, p. 40), of increasing concern, particularly regarding alcohol and marijuana abuse—as well as cocaine abuse—is the apparent significant potential for "intergenerational transmission" of drug abuse and drug-related problems, particularly among daughters.

Medical/Licit Prescription Cocaine Use

In the U.S., the only currently approved medical use for cocaine is its use as a local anesthetic. A topical solution of cocaine (4% or 10%) is applied to accessible mucous membranes of the oral, laryngeal, or nasal cavities, where it blocks the initiation and conduction of nerve impulses and, thus, elicits local anesthetic action. As noted in the position statement of the American Academy of Otolaryngology—Head and Neck Surgery, "No other single drug combines the anesthetic and vasoconstriction properties of cocaine" (2013, p. 1). The cocaine solution is not generally prescribed, nor is it particularly attractive to users who prefer the use and effects of cocaine hydrochloride crystalline powder and crack cocaine.[102]

Embryo/Fetus, Neonate, Infant, and Child Cocaine Exposure

For discussion of prenatal, postnatal, and child cocaine exposure, including unintentional child poisonings associated with cocaine, see the earlier pharmacology subsection, "Pregnancy, Breastfeeding, and Mothering." We now turn to adolescent and young adult, including undergraduate college/university student, cocaine use.

Adolescent and Young Adult Cocaine Use[103]

> With a crack hit, five minutes later you're running and chasing that feeling, that high.
>
> (Ryder & Brisgone, 2013, p. 48)

Various U.S. studies and reports estimate that the annual use of cocaine by adults is approximately 2%. In comparison, the estimate for "past year use" of cocaine by university/college students is

102 An exception that we have noted in our clinical practices has included several dentists, who were abusing pharmaceutical grade cocaine topical solution administered through refilled, disposable nasal spray containers (e.g., empty Dristan® nasal spray containers)—kept readily available in their dental jacket pocket or hung from a chain or cord around their neck—reportedly, "to treat nasal congestion." Additionally, we have encountered cases of pharmacists, including pharmacy students, who have diverted the cocaine solution from pharmacies where they were employed and, subsequently, sold, "shared with friends," or self-injected the drug intravenously (Pagliaro & Pagliaro, *Clinical Patient Data Files*).

103 N.B. Variance in the rates of cocaine use reported in this subsection reflect several prominent variables including: (1) subject age or grade level; (2) subject gender and gender orientation; (3) subject continental descent and ethnicity; (4) sampling procedures; (5) month/year sampled; (6) city/state/region sampled; and (7) period of use sampled (e.g., past month; past year; lifetime). Thus, while of interest in a global sense and informative in relation to popular trends in cocaine use, none of the reported statistics can be validly and reliably generalized across the U.S.—or to specific individual practice sites.

approximately 5% (University of Michigan, 2008).[104] More recently, Johnston and colleagues, who have surveyed and also published associated findings in annual summary reports regarding the use of drugs and substances of abuse for over 40 years in the U.S., have noted variances in patterns of cocaine use among adolescents in relation to both age and grade[105] Their published 2016 survey of cocaine and crack cocaine use are presented in Tables 2.17 and 2.18.

In addition, it is estimated that approximately 40 million people in the U.S., 12 years-of-age and older (i.e., approximately 15% of the population), have used cocaine at least once in their lifetimes—a number that is generally maintained with approximately one million new users initiating cocaine use annually (ONDCP, 2010). It also has been estimated that 5.3 million people in the U.S. (i.e., 1.6%), 12 years-of-age and older, including an estimated two million parents, have used cocaine during the previous year (NIDA, 2013b). As reported by the NIDA (2016):

> In 2014, there were an estimated 1.5 million current (past month) cocaine users aged 12 or older (0.6 percent of the [U.S.] population) . . . 1.1 percent of 12th graders reported using cocaine in the past month.
>
> (p. 5)

Finally, in terms of "cocaine use disorder," which meets DSM diagnostic criteria, Ahrnsbrak, Bose, and Hedden (2017) found that:

> About 867,000 people aged 12 or older had a cocaine use disorder in the past year . . . An estimated 0.1 percent of adolescents aged 12 to 17 in 2016 had a cocaine use disorder in the past year, or about 29,000 adolescents.
>
> (p. 27)

***Related Professional Reminder:* Reported general trends in the use of various drugs and substances of abuse may not accurately reflect those found for individual clinics or private practices because of local "biases," particularly in regard to: (1) demographic factors; and (2) availability and cost of drugs and substances of abuse.**

Demographic Factors

Throughout the U.S. during the new millennium, a high incidence of adolescent and young adult cocaine use was found to be related to several demographic factors, including:

- Age;
- Continental or other decent;
- Criminal youth gang affiliation/membership;
- Family history of alcoholism;

104 Using data obtained from a convenience sample of 4,580 undergraduate students from a major Midwestern research university, McCabe, Morales, and Cranford (2007)—utilizing the data from the female students only—found that the highest reported use of cocaine was among female students of European continental descent and Hispanic descent (i.e., 3.5%). The lowest reported use of cocaine was among female students of African and Asian continental descents (i.e., approximately 1%).

105 As previously noted for the amphetamines (see the "Amphetamine" subsection of this chapter) and other drugs and substances of abuse, significant variances in reported usage rates are commonly encountered in the published literature. These variances most likely reflect "differences in the population sampled" rather than "errors in research design and methods." For example, Bracken, Rodolico, and Hill (2013) reported that "lifetime" use of cocaine by adolescents, in the U.S., was estimated to be: (1) approximately 35% among adolescents admitted for substance abuse treatment between 1995 and 2010; and (2) approximately 5% among adolescents, enrolled in high school, who had completed the Johnson and colleagues surveys between 1995 and 2010.

Table 2.17 Percentage of Cocaine Hydrochloride Use and Crack Cocaine Use by Grade

Drug	*Period of Use*	*Percentage of Use by Grade*		
		8th Graders	**10th Graders**	**12th Graders**
Cocaine Hydrochloride	Past Month	0.30 %	0.40 %	0.90 %
	Past Year	0.80 %	1.30 %	2.30 %
	Lifetime	1.40 %	2.10 %	3.70%
Crack Cocaine	Past Month	0.20 %	0.20 %	0.50 %
	Past Year	0.50 %	0.40 %	0.80 %
	Lifetime	0.90 %	0.80 %	1.40 %

Modified from: Johnston, O'Malley, & Miech (2017, pp. 19–22)

Table 2.18 Percentage of Cocaine Hydrochloride Use and Crack Cocaine Use by Age

Drug	*Period of Use*	*Percentage of Use by Age*			
		12 Years-of-Age or Older	**12 to 17 Years-of-Age**	**18 to 25 Years-of-Age**	**26 Years-of-Age**
Cocaine Hydrochloride	Past Month	0.70 %	0.10 %	1.60 %	0.60 %
	Past Year	1.90 %	0.50 %	5.60 %	1.40 %
	Lifetime	14.40 %	0.90 %	11.30 %	16.60 %
Crack Cocaine	Past Month	0.20 %	0.00 %	0.00 %	0.20 %
	Past Year	0.30 %	0.00 %	0.30 %	0.40 %
	Lifetime	3.30 %	0.10 %	1.10 %	4.00 %

Modified from: Schulenberg, Johnston, & O'Malley (2017, p. 48)

- Homelessness and socioeconomic status;
- Involvement in drug dealing and trafficking;
- Sex-for-drug exchanges.

(e.g., John & Wu, 2017; Pagliaro & Pagliaro, *Clinical Patient Data Files*; Pope, Falck, & Carlson, 2011)

Related research findings for each of these factors are highlighted in the following subsections.

AGE

For adolescents, both boys and girls, the median age of first use for cocaine is approximately 15 years-of-age (e.g., Bracken, Rodolico, & Hill, 2013; Pagliaro & Pagliaro, 2012). For adolescents, who are homeless, the median age for initial use is reduced to 12 years-of-age (e.g., Rew & Taylor-Seehafer, 2001).

Consistently, club-going adolescent girls and young women (16 to 30 years-of-age)—who are usually poly-drug and substance of abuse users—reportedly have one of the highest rates of cocaine use (e.g., Grov, Kelly, & Parsons, 2009; Parsons, Grov, & Kelly, 2009; Ramo, Grov, & Delucchi, 2010). Lifetime cocaine use among U.S. high school students decreased from 9.54% in 1999 to 5.19% in 2015 (Schneider, Krawczyk, & Xuan, 2018).

Participants in a cohort study of 200 "African American crack-using women," generally reported that their use of crack cocaine began in their mid-twenties (Wechsberg, Lam, & Zule, 2003, p. 669).

CONTINENTAL OR OTHER DESCENT

A preference for cocaine or amphetamine (i.e., methamphetamine) appears to be generally divided in the U.S. largely by continental descent. As found by several researchers, adolescents and young adults, who abuse "crack cocaine," are predominantly of African continental descent, while adolescents and young adults, who abuse "methamphetamine," are predominantly of European continental descent (e.g., Esteban McCabe, Morales, & Cranford, 2007; Pagliaro & Pagliaro, 2009, 2012, 2018).

In this regard, Palamar, Davies, and Ompad (2015), in their secondary analysis of data from the *National Survey on Drug Use and Health, 2009–2012*, also identified that, in the U.S.:

1. Cocaine hydrochloride was primarily used by Americans of European continental descent;
2. Crack cocaine (i.e., cocaine base) was primarily used by Americans of African continental descent.

In addition, Schneider, Krawczyk, and Xuan (2018), in their analysis of data from the *National Youth Risk Behavior Surveys* (NYRBS) from 1999 to 2015, found that U.S. high school students of American Indian, Alaskan Native, Native Hawaiian, Pacific Islander, or Hispanic decsent had the highest rates of lifetime cocaine use.

Although available data appear to support arguments that preferences for cocaine (or amphetamines) among adolescents of different continental descents may be primarily related to genetic differences, the noted preferences may also be related to socioeconomic and sociocultural differences. In addition, they may use cocaine to self-medicate their depression, as reported by Pagliaro, Jaglalsingh, and Pagliaro (1992) and, more recently, Hammond, Lai, and Wright (2016), who concluded that the use of cocaine, in their study, was associated with "nearly twofold increased odds of depression" (p. 345). See also the related discussion in the earlier cocaine pharmacology subsection, "Pharmacodynamics: Mechanism of Action"—Phase 3.

FAMILY HISTORY OF ALCOHOLISM

During the last decades of the 20th Century, a positive history of alcoholism in an immediate family member was noted to be associated with a risk for initiating cocaine use and subsequent psychological dependence (Pagliaro & Pagliaro, *Clinical Patient Data Files*). However, the full nature of the genetic and/or sociocultural relationship has not yet been determined (Compton, Cottler, & Ridenour, 2002).[106]

HOMELESSNESS AND SOCIOECONOMIC STATUS

Homeless adolescents and young adults have been widely noted to:

1. Concurrently use multiple drugs and substances of abuse;
2. Use significantly more, and higher dosages of, individual drugs and substances of abuse than comparable cohort groups of adolescents and young adults (Pagliaro & Pagliaro, 2012; Pagliaro & Pagliaro, *Clinical Patient Data Files*).

As found by Petering (2016), in a study of "gang-involved homeless youth," cocaine use was approximately 10% in the "non-involved" group and approximately 20% in the "affiliated" and "member" groups.

INVOLVEMENT IN DRUG DEALING AND TRAFFICKING

During the new millennium, adolescents and young adults became increasingly involved in drug dealing and trafficking. Typical characteristics of these adolescents and young adults include that they:

- Are members or affiliates of a criminal youth gang;[107]
- Are socioeconomically disadvantaged;
- Deal from their homes or apartments;
- "Front" for an adult (i.e., if arrested, courts tend to be *more* lenient with adolescents than adults, who also may have extensive criminal records);
- Have a poor education;
- Live in an ethnic "ghetto" or enclave;
- Receive social assistance;
- Sell relatively small amounts of cocaine to support their own use, rather than using sex-for-drug exchanges;
- Use cocaine.

106 In a more recent study, Marks, Pike, and Stoops (2015) identified an interesting relationship between alcohol and cocaine use—although the mechanism has *not* yet been discerned. Recognizing that "alcohol consumption is a known antecedent to cocaine relapse," they conducted a double-blind, placebo-controlled, within-subjects study with 20 current cocaine users. The purpose of their study was to evaluate the effect of three different doses of alcohol on cocaine cue attentional bias. The result was that "alcohol administration increased craving for cocaine in a dose-dependent manner" (p. 1823). (See also the related discussion of cocaethylene in the earlier cocaine pharmacology subsection, Pharmacokinetics—Metabolism").

107 Increasingly, these "criminal youth gangs" include cross-over membership in primarily adult criminal gangs, such as MS-13, where adolescent gang members can often commit crimes and, because they are "underage," will receive much more lenient sentencing if caught and convicted (Pagliaro & Pagliaro, *Clinical Patient Data Files*). For example:

> Eight MS-13 gang members in the notorious crew's "Sailors Clique" faction participated in a violent racketeering conspiracy in and around Maryland, engaging in a terrifying campaign of murder, drug trafficking (cocaine and marijuana), and extortion ...
>
> The state attorney's office identified the eight men [ranging in age from 18 to 22] in custody as: "Krusty," 20; "Stop," 20; "Daffy," 22; "Hyper," 21; "Trankilo," 20; "Insoportable," 22; "Pinguino," 18; and "Choucky," 18.
>
> (Associated Press, 2017, pp. 1 & 2)

SEX-FOR-DRUG EXCHANGES[108]

Drug and substance abuse has always had some association with sexual activity (e.g., use of date rape drugs—see, for example, Chapter 1, "Alcohol"). However, sex-for-drug exchange came to its zenith in the U.S. during the 1990s when it became inextricably ingrained in the crack cocaine subculture—particularly that affecting inner city neighborhoods primarily comprised of families of African continental descent (Pagliaro & Pagliaro, 2000). Since that time, numerous studies and reports have documented the degradation and dehumanization of adolescent girls and young women (i.e., "crack whores") by men within, and beyond, "crack houses." Unfortunately, this damaging degradation and dehumanization of adolescent girls and young women continued into the new millennium (Pagliaro & Pagliaro, *Clinical Patient Data Files*). Sadly, as noted by Ryder and Brisgone (2013):

> Neither the mothers nor the daughters of the Crack Era have fared well, and to ignore their stories is to watch the repetition of destructive patterns in future generations, regardless of the next "drug of choice."
>
> (p. 58)

Adolescent and young adults, who exchange sex-for-drugs, particularly cocaine, are at a significant risk for contracting HIV infection and, as documented by several researchers (e.g., Pagliaro, Pagliaro, & Thauberger, 1993), are at significant risk for spreading HIV to others. For example, Nilsson Schonnesson, Atkinson, and Williams (2008), in their study of "African-American crack cocaine smokers with HIV infection," found that, in direct relation to their cocaine use:

1. Numbers of sexual partners increased;
2. Use of condoms became more inconsistent.

In addition, Harzke, Williams, and Bowen (2009), in their study of African-American HIV-positive crack cocaine users, found that cocaine "bingers" were more likely to report:

1. Lifetime trading of sex-for-drugs;
2. Binges, on average, lasting for 3.7 days;
3. For 72% of bingers, smoking, on average, 40 crack cocaine "rocks" during a binge;
4. During their last binge, having sex, on average, with 3.1 different sexual partners (female and male).

Also, during the new millennium, a new group of youth became widely recognized as being at risk for involvement in sex-for-drug exchanges—"trans*female youth." Often socially marginalized, trans*female youths are generally homeless and commonly engage in the sex trade and/or sex-for-drug exchanges in order to obtain: (1) cocaine; and (2) money necessary for "living" (Pagliaro & Pagliaro, *Clinical Patient Data Files*). Unfortunately, this lifestyle also places them at extremely high risk for HIV infection. As noted by Turner, Santos, and Araytasirikul (2017):

> Trans-female youth carry a disproportionate burden of HIV ... Those who reported recent crack/cocaine use ... had significantly higher odds of condom-less receptive anal intercourse.
>
> (p. 258)

108 See also the earlier related discussion in the cocaine pharmacology subsection, "Undesired, or Harmful, Effects and Toxicities—Cocaine Use During Pregnancy."

In addition, in order to obtain the money needed to maintain their crack cocaine use, many trans (and other adolescents) have resorted to involvement in the drug trade, including drug dealing. (See the related discussion in the earlier cocaine subsection, "Involvement in Drug Dealing and Trafficking").

Treating Cocaine Dependence or Use Disorder

Similar to the amphetamines (see the earlier amphetamine subsection, "Treating Amphetamine Dependence or Use Disorder"), the treatment of cocaine dependence or use disorder among adolescents and young adults has involved various approaches, particularly: (1) pharmacotherapy; and/or (2) psychotherapy/counseling.

Pharmacotherapy

Although a number of different classes of drugs—anticonvulsants, antidepressants, antihypertensives, and antipsychotics—have been used in an attempt to effectively treat cocaine use disorder, antipsychotic pharmacotherapy has been the major focus of research and treatment during the last decade. Unfortunately, results generally have been disappointing. For example, as identified by Howell and Cunningham (2015):

> Although cocaine abuse is a significant public health problem, *no* effective pharmacotherapeutics are available to treat this disorder.
>
> (p. 192)

As summarized by Indave, Minozzi, and Pani (2016), based on their review of 14 studies representing a combined total of 719 participants and seven different drugs—five antipsychotics (i.e., aripiprazole; haloperidol; olanzapine; quetiapine; and risperidone), one antihypertensive (i.e., reserpine), and one anticonvulsant (i.e., lamotrigine):

> At present, there is *no* evidence supporting the clinical use of antipsychotic medications in the treatment of cocaine dependence.
>
> (p. 1)

And, as concluded by Davidson (2016):

> Despite many years of research, there are *no* approved medications for stimulant dependence, and treatment is focused on psychotherapy and abstinence.
>
> (p. 52)

In addition, as we, and others (e.g., Tobin, 2017) have noted, preventing "relapsed use" of cocaine is another major area of concern related to successful treatment that, unfortunately, has proved to be equally resistant to efficacious pharmacotherapeutic intervention (see Table 2.19).[109]

109 Interestingly, and of clinical relevance, is the observation by Parvaz, Moeller, and Goldstein (2016) that both subjective measures of craving (e.g., self-reports of "liking cocaine" and "wanting cocaine") and findings from measures of EEG cue reactivity demonstrated a linear decline from two days of abstinence (rated lowest at a rating of 1 on a scale of 0 to 5)—this rating persisted among those abstinent, formerly "cocaine dependent" adults sampled at one year of abstinence.

Table 2.19 Cocaine Dependence or Use Disorder: Representative Studies of Pharmacotherapeutic Efficacy[110]

Pharmacotherapy Drug Names / Classification	*Participants / Sample*[111]	*Study / Design*	*Findings / Conclusions*	*Source*
Acamprosate (Campral®) *Alcohol withdrawal and Abstinence maintenance drug*	60 subjects with cocaine dependence	Double-blind, placebo-controlled study	Lack of efficacy, [112] "no more efficacious than placebo"	Kampman, Dackis, & Pettinati (2011)
Amantadine (Symmetrel®) *Anti-viral drug*	69 subjects with cocaine dependence	Double-blind, placebo-controlled study	Lack of efficacy	Shoptaw, Kintaudi, & Charuvastra (2002)
Amantadine	10 "cocaine smokers"	In-patient, double-blind, cross-over study	Lack of efficacy, "amantadine maintenance did *not* modify the choice to self-administer smoked cocaine"	Collins, Vosburg, & Hart (2003)
Amantadine	199 cocaine dependent subjects	Random, placebo-controlled study	Lack of efficacy	Kampman, Dackis, & Lynch (2006)
Anticonvulsants				
Carbamazepine Gabapentin Lamotrigine Phenytoin Tiagabine Topiramate	2,068 total participants	Systematic review of 20 studies	Lack of efficacy	Minozzi, Cinquini, & Amato (2015)

(*Continued*)

110 See also Table 2.20, "Cocaine Dependence or Use Disorder: Representative Studies of Psychotherapeutic Efficacy," for a discussion of the efficacy of related combinations of pharmacotherapy and psychotherapy/counseling.

111 Only human studies are included in this table. Because of the lack of published research aimed at child and adolescent drug and substance abuse due to the inherent difficulties in obtaining ethical approval and convenience samples from established treatment programs, the research subjects for the studies included in this table are adults.

112 "Lack of efficacy" indicates that, according to our assessment and interpretation of the presented data, results in terms of cocaine use fail to demonstrate statistical significance in comparison to no pharmacotherapy or placebo intervention. Note that our assessment is generally more critical/stringent than that of the study authors, who in many cases have equivocated on the results with descriptors such as "moderate support," "may reduce," "possibly helpful," and "further study is needed."

Table 2.19 (Cont.)

Pharmacotherapy Drug Names/ Classification	*Participants/ Sample*	*Study/Design*	*Findings/Conclusions*	*Source*
Vigabatrin				
Gabapentin (Neurontin®)	—	Double-blind, crossover design study	Lack of efficacy	Hart, Ward, & Collins, 2004
Gabapentin	12, "nontreatment-seeking" cocaine abusers	Inpatient/outpatient study	Lack of efficacy	Hart, Haney, & Vosburg (2007)
Gabapentin	Six "nontreatment seeking" cocaine dependent subjects	Double-blind, crossover design study	Lack of efficacy	Hart, Haney, & Collins (2007)
Tiagabine (Gabitril®)	141 cocaine-dependent subjects	Double-blind, placebo-controlled, outpatient trial	Lack of efficacy, "in changing cocaine use"	Winhusen, Somoza, & Ciraulo (2007)
Topiramate (Topamax®)	170 cocaine and alcohol dependent subjects	Double-blind, placebo-controlled study	Lack of efficacy, "topiramate was no better than placebo in reducing cocaine use"	Kampman, Pettinati, & Lynch (2013)
Topiramate	171 cocaine-dependent methadone maintenance patients	Double-blind, placebo-controlled clinical study	Lack of efficacy, "no significant difference in cocaine abstinence between topiramate and placebo conditions"	Umbricht, DeFulio, & Winstanley (2014)
Antidepressants				
Bupropion (Wellbutrin®) *Antidepressant/smoking cessation drug*	70 chronic cocaine users	Randomized, double-blind, placebo-controlled, out-patient study	Lack of efficacy	Shoptaw, Heinzerling, & Rotheram-Fuller (2008)
Bupropion		Systematic review of five studies	Lack of Efficacy, "efficacy of bupropion appears to be	Stoops & Rush (2013)

Table 2.19 (Cont.)

Pharmacotherapy Drug Names/ Classification	*Participants/ Sample*	*Study/Design*	*Findings/Conclusions*	*Source*
			limited to when it is combined with robust behavioral treatments or administered to *lighter users*"	
Citalopram (Celexa®) *Antidepressant*	76 cocaine-dependent patients	Double-blind, placebo-controlled study	Possibly effective, "Citalopram treated subjects showed a significant reduction in cocaine-positive urines during treatment compared to placebo"	Moeller, Schmitz, & Steinberg (2007)
Antihypertensives				
Reserpine (Serpasil®) *Antihypertensive/ Antipsychotic*	119 cocaine dependent subjects	Double-blind, placebo-controlled, outpatient trial	Lack of efficacy	Winhusen, Somoza, Sarid-Segal (2007)
Antipsychotics				
Aripiprazole (Abilify®) Haloperidol (Haldol®) Olanzapine (Zyprexa®) Quetiapine (Seroquel®) Risperidone (Risperdal®) and the antihypertensive, Reserpine (Serpasil®)	719 total participants	Systematic review of 14 studies comparing antipsychotic drugs to placebo	Lack of efficacy, "comparing any antipsychotic drug versus placebo, we found that antipsychotics reduced dropout... We found no other significant differences"	Indave, Minozzi, & Pani (2016)
Olanzapine (Zyprexa®) Risperidone (Risperdal®) and the anti-hypertensive,	562 subjects with "primary cocaine dependence"	Meta-analysis of 10 studies comparing selected antipsychotics to placebo	"Antipsychotics did not differ from placebo in regard to cocaine use days, abstinence, or craving"	Kishi, Matsuda, & Iwata (2013)

Table 2.19 (Cont.)

Pharmacotherapy Drug Names/ Classification	*Participants/ Sample*	*Study/Design*	*Findings/Conclusions*	*Source*
Reserpine (Serpasil®)				
Baclofen (Lioresal®) *Muscle relaxant drug*	Seven non-treatment seeking, recent cocaine users	Double-blind, placebo-controlled study	Lack of efficacy, "pretreatment with baclofen had no effect on any cocaine-related measure"	Lile, Stoops, & Allen (2004)
Baclofen	160 subjects with "severe cocaine dependence"	Multi-site, double-blind study	Lack of efficacy, (no significant differences between baclofen-treated and placebo groups)	Kahn, Biswas, & Childress (2009)
Buspirone (Buspar®) *Anti-anxiety drug*	Nine current cocaine users	Repeated measures, inpatient study	Lack of efficacy	Bolin, Lile, & Marks (2016)
Citicoline (Ceraxon®) *Anti-Alzheimer drug*	130 with bipolar disorder *and* cocaine dependence	Randomized double-blind, placebo-controlled, outpatient study	Lack of efficacy	Brown, Todd, & Schmitz (2015)
Disulfiram (Antabuse®) *Acetaldehyde dehydrogenase Inhibitor/ Alcohol abstinence maintenance drug*	121 cocaine-dependent subjects	Randomized, double-blind, placebo-controlled, factorial study	Possibly effective, "participants assigned to disulfiram reduced their cocaine use significantly more than those assigned to placebo"	Carroll, Fenton, & Ball (2004)
Disulfiram	492 total participants	Systematic review of seven studies	Lack of efficacy	Pani, Trogu, & Vacca (2010)
Disulfiram	112 cocaine dependent subjects	Randomized, double-blind, placebo-controlled study	Lack of efficacy, "no significant main effects for disulfiram versus placebo"	Carroll, Nich, & Shi (2012)
Modafinil (Provigil®)	62 cocaine dependent	Randomized, double-blind,	"Modafinil improves clinical outcome	Dackis, Kampman,

Table 2.19 (Cont.)

Pharmacotherapy Drug Names/ Classification	*Participants/ Sample*	*Study/Design*	*Findings/Conclusions*	*Source*
Dopamine re-uptake inhibitor (wakefulness promoting drug)	patients, predominately of African continental descent	placebo-controlled study	when combined with psychosocial treatment for cocaine dependence"	& Lynch (2005)
Modafinil	Eight "non-treatment-seeking," cocaine-dependent subjects	Double-blind, crossover design study	Modafinil attenuated the "subject-effect ratings" associated with cocaine self-administration	Hart, Haney, & Vosburg (2008)
Modafinil	210 cocaine dependent "treatment-seekers"	Double-blind, placebo-controlled study	"Modafinil, in combination with individual behavioral therapy" demonstrated an *increase* in the maximum number of consecutive non-use days for cocaine and a reduction in craving. However, there was *no* significant difference between modafinil and placebo "in average weekly percent of cocaine non-use days"	Anderson, Reid, & Li (2009)
Modafinil	210 subjects, "who were actively using cocaine"	Randomized, double-blind, placebo-controlled study	Lack of efficacy, "No significant difference between modafinil and placebo"	Dackis, Kampman, & Lynch (2012)
Modafinil		Systematic review of three studies	Lack of efficacy, "Analysis showed little difference between placebo and modafinil"	Stoops & Rush (2013)
Modafinil	94 cocaine-dependent subjects	Double-blind, placebo-	In comparison to placebo, modafinil significantly increased	Kampman, Lynch, &

(*Continued*)

Table 2.19 (Cont.)

Pharmacotherapy Drug Names/ Classification	*Participants/ Sample*	*Study/Design*	*Findings/Conclusions*	*Source*
		controlled, clinical trial	abstinence and reduced self-reported "levels of cocaine craving"	Pettinati (2015)
Naltrexone (ReVia®) *(Opiate analgesic receptor blocker)*	164 patients "with co-occurring cocaine and alcohol dependence"	Randomized, double-blind, placebo- controlled study	Lack of efficacy, (when added to psycho-social treatment—possibly effective for men, but *not* for women)	Pettinati, Kampman, & Lynch (2008b)
Naltrexone	208 patients "with co-occurring cocaine and alcohol dependence"	Randomized, double-blind, placebo-controlled study	Lack of efficacy	Pettinati, Kampman, & Lynch (2008a)
Naltrexone	87 subjects "with both cocaine and alcohol dependence"	Randomized, double-blind, placebo-controlled study	Lack of efficacy	Schmitz, Lindsay, & Green (2009)
Progesterone *Hormone*	45 male methadone-stabilized cocaine users	Randomized, double-blind, placebo-controlled study	Lack of efficacy	Sofuoglu, Poling, & Gonzalez (2007)
Progesterone	25 cocaine-dependent women "recruited from obstetrical clinics"	Randomized, double-blind, placebo-controlled study	Lack of efficacy	Yonkers, Forray, & Nich (2014)
Psychostimulants				
Methylphenidate (Ritalin®)	—	Systematic review of four studies	Lack of efficacy, "generally, does *not* reduce cocaine use"	Stoops & Rush (2013)

Pharmacotherapy Drug Names/ Classification	*Participants/ Sample*	*Study/Design*	*Findings/Conclusions*	*Source*
Six Selected Psychostimulants: Dexamphetamine (Dexedrine®) Lisdexamfetamine (Vyvanse®) Mazindol (Sanorex®) Methamphetamine Methylphenidate (Ritalin®) Mixed-Amphetamines (Adderall®); and One Dopamine Reuptake Inhibitor: Modafinil (Provigil®)	2,366 total participants	Systematic review of 26 studies	Lack of efficacy	Castells, Cunill, & Perez-Mana (2016)

Psychotherapy/Counseling

Various psychotherapy/counseling approaches have been utilized in an attempt to treat cocaine use disorder (i.e., cocaine dependence). However, although some approaches have shown potential, or partial success (e.g., increasing the number of days in treatment versus "non-intervention" control), the overall results have been disappointing. Currently, there are no established "best practices" (i.e., empirically validated and reliable psychotherapeutic approaches) for treating cocaine use disorder among adolescents and young adults—or older adults. However, as identified by Vocci and Montoya (2009), "Psychosocial and behavioral treatments, notably CBT and contingency management, of cocaine and methamphetamine users are moderately effective" (also see the earlier Amphetamine section). An overview of the findings from related published research studies is presented in Table 2.20 in order to highlight the nature and extent of past attempted interventions and identify for the reader potentially efficacious psychotherapeutic approaches.

Related Professional Reminder:* *The lack of an identifiable "best practice" does* not *mean that: (1) patients should* not *be treated; or (2) some patients will* not *respond well to some psychotherapeutic interventions.

Also, as noted in the earlier related discussion of the psychotherapeutic approaches utilized for the treatment of amphetamine-related disorders (Vocci & Montoya, 2009):

> There is currently no evidence for a differential treatment effect of any psychosocial treatment in the management of cocaine and methamphetamine users in treatment.
>
> (p. 6)

Table 2.20 Cocaine Dependence or Use Disorder: Selected Representative Studies of Psychotherapeutic Efficacy[113]

Psychotherapy	*Sample*	*Study/ Design*	*Findings/ Conclusions*	*Source*
Cognitive-Behavioral Therapy (CBT)				
CBT; CM; CBT & CM	193 cocaine dependent methadone-maintained outpatients	Randomized treatment study	CBT "showed no main effects on any of the cocaine-related outcome measures." CM "had robust main effects on all cocaine-related outcome measures" Combined CBT & CM was more effective than CBT alone, although initial therapeutic effects were "briefly [initially] dampened if CM was augmented with CBT"	Epstein, Hawkins, & Covi (2003)
CBT & disulfiram; CBT & placebo; Interpersonal therapy (IPT) & disulfiram; IPT & placebo	121 cocaine dependent subjects (non-alcoholics)	Randomized placebo-controlled, double-masked, factorial trial	Possibly effective, CBT reduced cocaine use more than IPT; and disulfiram reduced cocaine use more than placebo	Carroll, Fenton, & Ball (2004)
CBT		Literature review	Lack of efficacy, "in longitudinal studies where, long-term abstinence is the primary outcome of interest"	Penberthy, Ait-Daoud, & Vaughan (2010)
CBT; CM	Five studies	Literature review examining CBT and CM effects on cocaine dependence	Possibly effective, with CBT being less effective than CM in the acute treatment phase, but having a	Farronato, Dursteler-Macfarland, & Wiesbeck (2013)

113 Behavioral treatment approaches that include pharmacotherapeutic approaches also are presented in this table.

Psychotherapy	*Sample*	*Study/ Design*	*Findings/ Conclusions*	*Source*
			more lasting effect in the post-treatment phase	
CBT; disulfiram	434 total cocaine-dependent subjects	Literature review of clinical trials for treating cocaine dependence	Possibly effective, CBT is possibly effective for both men and women; disulfiram is possibly effective, but less so among women	DeVito, Babuscio, & Nich (2014)
Contingency Management (CM)				
CM; CBT; CM & CBT; Methadone maintenance, alone	120 cocaine-dependent patients, who were receiving methadone maintenance therapy	Randomized treatment study	Possibly effective, those in the CM and CM & CBT groups "had significantly superior in-treatment urinalysis results." CBT "in-treatment urinalysis results" were *not* significantly different than those obtained with methadone alone	Rawson, Huber, & McCann (2002)
CM; "Day Treatment;" CM & "Day Treatment"	127 "homeless persons with crack/ cocaine disorders"	Randomized treatment study	Possibly effective, "CM & day treatment was 2.1 times more likely to have a positive treatment outcome than day treatment [alone]"	Schumacher, Milby, & Wallace (2003)
CM; Group Therapy (GT); CM & GT	77 cocaine-dependent methadone patients	Randomized treatment study	Possibly effective, "Patients in the CM condition submitted more cocaine-negative [urine] samples and attended more groups than patients in standard treatment [i.e. group therapy]"	Petry, Martin, & Simcic (2005)

(*Continued*)

Table 2.20 (Cont.)

Psychotherapy	*Sample*	*Study/ Design*	*Findings/ Conclusions*	*Source*
CM; CM & bupropion; CM & placebo; Voucher control & bupropion; Voucher control & placebo	106 cocaine abusing, methadone-maintained outpatients	Randomized, double-blind, placebo-controlled trial	Possibly effective, CM & bupropion, "proportion of cocaine-positive samples significantly decreased during weeks three to 13." CM & placebo, "significantly *increased* cocaine use during weeks three to 13." Voucher control & bupropion or placebo "showed *no* significant improvement in cocaine use"	Poling, Oliveto, & Petry (2006)
CM; CRA & 12-Step facilitation (TSF); Voucher control	145 cocaine dependent women (with children or pregnant)	Randomized, 2X2 study	Possibly effective, "CM was associated with significantly greater duration of cocaine abstinence;" and CRA and TSF "were *not* significant for any measures"	Schottenfeld, Moore, & Pantalon (2011)
CM; GT; CM & GT (abstinence, negative urine); CM & GT (attendance)	333 cocaine-negative patients	Randomized treatment study	Possibly effective, "both attendance and abstinence-based CM resulted in improvements in some measures"	Petry, Barry, & Alessi (2012)
CM	1,664 total subjects	Literature review of 19 studies	Possibly effective, CM appears to: (1) *increase* cocaine abstinence; (2) improve treatment retention; and (3) "may act synergistically with pharmacotherapy"	Schierenberg, van Amsterdam, & van Den Brink (2012)

Psychotherapy	*Sample*	*Study/ Design*	*Findings/ Conclusions*	*Source*
Community Reinforcement Approach (CRA)				
CRA; CRA & Vouchers	70 cocaine-dependent outpatients	Randomized treatment study	Possibly effective, "Abstinence-contingent incentives [i.e., vouchers] significantly increased cocaine abstinence during treatment and at one year of follow-up compared with non-contingent incentives"	Higgins, Wong, & Badger (2000)
CRA; CRA & Vouchers; Vouchers only	100 cocaine-dependent outpatients	Randomized treatment study	Possibly effective, "patients treated with CRA & vouchers were retained better in treatment, used cocaine at a lower frequency during treatment, but *not* follow-up"	Higgins, Sigmon, & Wong (2003)
CRA	11 studies with 812 total subjects	Systematic review of four studies focusing on "cocaine treatment"	Possibly effective, "CRA with incentives is more effective than usual care or CRA without incentives in the treatment of cocaine abuse or dependence"	Roozen, Boulogne, & van Tulder (2004)

Finally, as difficult and problematic as treatment for cocaine use disorder is, in general, several other factors have been identified that further contribute to the poor prognosis for treatment outcomes. For example, as found by Savage, Durant, and Clark (2015), in their study of the effects of motherhood on substance use treatment program outcomes for adolescent girls and young women:

> Adolescent mothers were *less* likely to successfully complete the treatment program than nonmothers. Adolescent women with reliance on family or friends for financial support, lower education status, and cannabis and cocaine use disorders had *worse* treatment program outcomes.
>
> (p. 478)

References

ABC News. (2003, February 25). Ritalin abuse. *ABC News Features*, 1–2. New York: ABC News.

Abramowicz, M. (2015, September 28). Racemic amphetamine sulfate (Evekeo) for ADHD. *The Medical Letter on Drugs and Therapeutics*, *57*(1478), 137–139.

Ackerman, J. P., Riggins, T., & Black, M. M. (2010, March). A review of the effects of prenatal cocaine exposure among school-aged children. *Pediatrics*, *125*(3), 554–565. doi:10.1542/peds.2009-0637.

Advokat, C. D., Guidry, D., & Martino, L. (2008). Licit and illicit use of medications for attention-deficit hyperactivity disorder in undergraduate college students. *Journal of College Health*, *56*(6), 601–606. doi:10.3200/JACH.56.6.601-606

Ahmed, S., & Virani, S. (2017, September 1). Case report: Stimulant overprescribing, abuse, and diversion. *The American Journal of Psychiatry Residents' Journal*, 11–12. doi: 10.1176/appi.ajp-rj.2017.120905

Ahrnsbrak, R., Bose, J., & Hedden, S. L. (2017). *Key Substance Use and Mental Health Indicators in the United States: Results from the 2016 National Survey on Drug Use and Health*. Rockville, MD: Center for Behavioral Health Statistics and Quality, Substance Abuse and Mental Health Services Administration. Retrieved from www.samhsa.gov/data/

Ali, S. R., Krugar, M., & Houghton, J. (2002). Upper airway obstruction and acute lung injury associated with cocaine abuse. *International Journal of Clinical Practice*, *56*(6), 484–485.

Alsidawi, S., Muth, J., & Wilkin, J. (2011). Adderall induced inverted-Takotsubo cardiomyopathy. *Catheterization and Cardiovascular Interventions*, *78*(6), 910–913. doi:10.1002/ccd.23036

American Academy of Otolaryngology-Head and Neck Surgery. (2013, May 6). *Position statement: Medical use of cocaine*. Retrieved March 11, 2016, from entnet.org, pp. 1–3: www.entnet.org/content/medical-use-cocaine

Anderson, A. L., Reid, M. S., & Li, S. H. (2009, September 1). Modafinil for the treatment of cocaine dependence. *Drug and Alcohol Dependence*, *104*(1–2), 133–139. doi:10.1016/j.drugalcdep.2009.04.015

Ares-Santos, S., Granado, N., & Espadas, I. (2014). Methamphetamine causes degeneration of dopamine cell bodies and terminals of the nigrostriatal pathway evidenced by silver staining. *Neuropsychopharmacology*, *39*(5), 1066–1080. doi:10.1038/np.2013.307

Ares-Santos, S., Granado, N., & Moratalla, R. (2013). The role of dopamine receptors in the neurotoxicity of methamphetamine. *Journal of Internal Medicine*, *273*(5), 437–453. doi:10.1111/joim.12049

Arria, A. M., Derauf, C., & LaGasse, L. L. (2006). Methamphetamine and other substance use during pregnancy: Preliminary estimates from the Infant Development, Environment, and Lifestyle (IDEAL) Study. *Materal and Child Health Journal*, *10*, 293–302.

Associated Press. (2017). *MS-13 Gang Members Charged in Series of Murders, Drug Crimes, Authorities Say*. Fox News.

Associated Press. (2018, January 22). Florida mom arrested for leaving child in car, shoplifting. *FoxNews.com*, 1. Vero Beach, FL. Retrieved from www.foxnews.com/us/2018/01/22/florida-mom-arrested-for-leaving-child-in-car

Baker, A., Lee, N. K., & Claire, M. (2005). Brief cognitive behavioural interventions for regular amphetamine users: A step in the right direction. *Addiction*, *100*, 367–378. doi:10.1111/j.1360-0443.2005.001002.x

Ballester, J., Valentine, G., & Sofuoglu, M. (2017). Pharmacological treatments for methamphetamine addiction: Current status and future directions. *Expert Review of Clinical Pharmacology*, *10*(3), 305–314. doi:10.1080/17512433.2017.1268916

Barthelemy, O. J., Richardson, M. A., & Rose-Jacobs, R. (2016, May-June). Effects of intrauterine substance and postnatal violence exposure on aggression in children. *Aggressive Behavior*, *42*(3), 209–221. doi:10.1002/ab.21607

Bartos, L. (2005, July). Meth production is toxic to communities (methtoxic). *NEBLINE Newsletter*, 1–4. Lincoln, NE: University of Nebraska-Lincoln. Retrieved November 2, 2016, from http://lancaster.uni.edu/family/meth toxic.shtml

Bartu, A., Dusci, L. J., & Ilett, K. F. (2009). Transfer of methylamphetamine and amphetamine into breast milk following recreational use of methylamphetamine. *British Journal of Clinical Pharmacology*, *67*(4), 455–459. doi:10.1111/j.1365-2125.2009.03366.x

Bastiani, L., Siciliano, V., & Curzio, O. (2013). Optimal scaling of the CAST and the SDS scale in a national sample of adolescents. *Addictive Behaviors*, *38*(4), 2060–2067. doi:10.1016/j.addbeh.2012.12.016

Bauwens, J. E., Boggs, J. M., & Hartwell, P. S. (1989). Fatal hyperthermia associated with cocaine use. *WJM, Western Journal of Medicine*, *150*(2), 210–212.

Benson, K., Flory, K., & Humphreys, K. L. (2015, March). Misuse of stimulant medication among college students: A comprehensive review and meta-analysis. *Clinical Child and Family Psychology Review*, *18*(1), 50–76. doi:10.1007/s10567-014-0177-z

Berkes, H. (2007, April 4). *Mexican "ice" replaces home-cooked meth in U. S.* Retrieved from National Public Radio (NPR), pp. 1–15: www.npr.org/templates/story/story.php?storyId=9193186

Berman, A. H., Bergman, H., & Palmstierna, T. (2005). Evaluation of the Drug Use Disorders Identification Test (DUDIT) in criminal justice and detoxification settings and in Swedish population sample. *European Addiction Research*, *11*, 22–31. doi:10.1159/000081413

Berman, S. M. Kuczenski, R., & McCracken, J. T. (2009). Potential adverse effects of amphetamine treatment on brain and behavior: A review. *Molecular Psychiatry, 14*(2),123–142. doi: 10.1038/mp.2008.90

Bernstein, K. T., Bucciarelli, A., & Piper, T. M. (2007, March 9). Cocaine- and opiate-related fatal overdose in New York City, 1990-2000. *BMC Public Health, 7*, 31. doi:10.1186/1471-2458-7-31

Bickel, W. K., Franck, C. T., & Moody, L. (2013). Executive dysfunction among alcohol- and cocaine-dependent women: 2013. *APA 121st Annual Convention Proceedings* (p. NP). Honolulu, Hawai'i: American Psychological Association. doi:10.1037/e612522013-001

Blick, S. K., & Keating, G. M. (2007). Lisdexamfetamine. *Paediatric Drugs, 9*(2), 129–135.

Boellner, S. W., Stark, J. G., & Krishnan, S. (2010, February). Phamacokinetics of lisdexamfetamine dimesylate and its active metabolite, d-amphetamine, with increasing oral doses of lisdexamfetamine dimesylate in children with attention-deficit/hyperactivity disorder. *Clinical Therapeutics, 32*(2), 252–264. doi:10.1016/j.clinthera.2010.02.011

Boeri, M. (2013). *Women on Ice: Methamphetamine Use among Suburban Women*. New Brunswick, NJ: Rutgers University.

Bogle, K. E., & Smith, B. H. (2009). Illicit methylphenidate use: A review of prevalence, availability, pharmacology, and consequences. *Current Drug Abuse Reviews, 2*(2), 157–176.

Bolea-Alamanac, B. M., Green, A., & Verma, G. (2013). Methylphenidate use in pregnancy and lactation: A systemic review of evidence. *British Journal of Clinical Pharmacology*, 77(1), 96–101. doi:10.1111/bcp.12138

Bolin, B. L., Lile, J. A., & Marks, K. R. (2016, June). Buspirone reduces sexual risk-taking intent but not cocaine self-administration. *Experimental and Clinical Psychopharmacology, 24*(3), 162–173. doi:10.1037/pha0000076

Bourne, A., Reid, D., & Hickson, F. (2015). Illicit drug use in sexual settings ("chemsex") and HIV/STI transmission risk behaviour among gay men in South London: Findings from a qualitative study. *Sexually Transmitted Infections, 91*(8), 564–568. doi:10.1136/sextrans-2015-052052

Boyer, E. M., Thompson, N., & Hill, T. (2015). The relationship between methamphetamine use and dental caries and missing teeth. *Journal of Dental Hygiene, 89*(2), 119–131.

Bracken, B. K., Rodolico, J., & Hill, K. P. (2013). Sex, age, and progression of drug use in adolescents admitted for substance use disorder treatment in the northeastern United States: Comparison with a national survey. *Substance Abuse, 34*(3), 263–272. doi:10.1080/08897077.2013.770424

Brackins, T., Brahm, N. C., & Kissack, J. C. (2011, December). Treatments for methamphetamine abuse: A literature review for the clinician. *Journal of Pharmacy Practice, 24*(6), 541–550. doi:10.1177/0897190011426557

Brahmbhatt, K., Hilty, D. M., & Hah, M. (2016, August). Diagnosis and treatment of ADHD during adolescence in the primary care setting: Review and future directions. *Journal of Adolescent Health, 59*(2), 135–143. doi:10.1016/j.jadohealth.2016.03.025

Bramness, J. G., & Rognli, E. B. (2016). Psychosis induced by amphetamines. *Current Opinion in Psychiatry, 29*(4), 236–241. doi:10.1097/YCO.0000000000000254

Brandt, S. A., Taverna, E. C., & Hallock, R. M. (2014, October 1). A survey of nonmedical use of tranquilizers, stmulants, and pain relievers among college students: Patterns of use among users and factors related to abstinence in non-users. *Drug and Alcohol Dependence, 143*, 272–276. doi:10.1016/j.drugalcdep.2014.07.034

Brensilver, M., Heinzerling, K. G., & Shoptaw, S. (2013, September). Pharmacotherapy of amphetamine-type stimulant dependence: An update. *Drug and Alcohol Review, 32*(5), 449–460. doi:10.1111/dar.12048.

Brown, E. S., Todd, J. P., & Schmitz, J. M. (2015). A randomized, double-blind, placebo-controlled trial of citicoline for cocaine dependence in bipolar I disorder. *The American Journal of Psychiatry, 172*(10), 1014–1021. doi:10.1176/appi.ajp.2015.14070857

Brown, R. E., Morisky, D. E., & Silverstein, S. J. (2013). Meth mouth severity in response to drug-use patterns and dental access in methamphetamine users. *Journal of the California Dental Association, 41*(6), 421–428.

Brzeczko, A. W., Leech, R., & Stark, J. G. (2013, September). The advent of a new pseudoephedrine product to combat methamphetamine abuse. *American Journal of Drug and Alcohol Abuse, 39*(5), 284–290. doi:10.3109/00952990.2013.821476

Buie, J., & Tamburin, A. (2014, November 17). *Meth-lab busts down; dealers getting drug from Mexico*. Retrieved from The Tennessean: www.story/news/crime/2014/11/16/meth-labs-tn-dealers-turning-mexico/19141893/

Bulbena-Cabre, A., Ramos Dunn, N., & Gorman Swift, R. (2015). "Crack Lung": A pulmonary complication of crack cocaine case. *Journal of Addiction Medicine*, 164–165. doi:10.1097/ADM.0000000000000172

Burcu, M., Zito, J. M., & Metcalfe, L. (2016, September). Trends in stimulant medication use in commercially insured youths and adults, 2010–2014. *JAMA Psychiatry, 73*(9), 992–993.

Burge, M., Hunsaker, J. C., & Davis, G. J. (2009, December). Death of a toddler due to ingestion of sulfuric acid at a clandestine home methamphetamine laboratory. *Forensic Science, Medicine, and Pathology, 5*(4), 298–301. doi:10.1007/s12024-009-9127-3

Buxton, H. A., & Dove, N. A. (2008). The burden and management of crystal meth use. *CMAJ, Canadian Medical Association Journal, 178*(12), 1537–1539. doi:10.1503/cmaj.071234

Buxton, J. A., Omura, J., & Kuo, M. (2015, June 13). Genetic determinants of cocaine-associated agranulocytosis. *BMC Research Notes, 8*, 240. doi:10.1186/s13104-015-1219-4

Cadwalladr, C. (2015, February 15). Students used to take drugs to get high: Now they take them to get higher grades. *The Guardian*, 1–10.

Calcaterra, S., & Binswanger, I. A. (2013). Psychostimulant-Related deaths as reported by a large national database. *Substance Abuse*, *34*(2), 1–17. doi:10.1080/08897077.2012.726959

Calhoun, A. (2012, April 5). *The criminalization of bad mothers*. Retrieved July 12, 2016, from The New York Times: www.nytimes.com/2012/04/29/magazine/the-criminalization-of-bad-mothers.html?_r=0

Cao, D. N., Shi, J. J., & Hao, W. (2016, June 5). Advances and challenges in pharmacotherapeutics for amphetamine-type stimulants addiction. *European Journal of Pharmacology*, *780*, 129–135. doi:10.1016/j.ejphar.2016.03.040

Carnevale Associates. (2011, March). Update: The changing landscape of the methamphetamine epidemic. *Policy Brief*. Gaithersburg, MD: Carnevale Associates.

Carroll, K. M., Fenton, L. R., & Ball, S. A. (2004). Efficacy of disulfiram and cognitive behavioral therapy in cocaine-dependent outpatients: A randomized placebo-controlled trial. *Archives of General Psychiatry*, *61*(3), 264–272. doi:10.1001/archpsyc.61.3.264

Carroll, K. M., Nich, C., & Shi, J. M. (2012, November 1). Efficacy of disulfiram and Twelve Step Facilitation in cocaine-dependent individuals maintained on methadone: A randomized placebo-controlled trial. *Drug and Alcohol Dependence*, *126*(1–2), 224–231. doi:10.1016/j.drugalcdep.2012.05.019

Cassidy, C. M., Schmitz, N., & Mailla, A. (2008, January 1). Validation of the alcohol use disorders identification test and the drug abuse screening test in first episode psychosis. *The Canadian Journal of Psychiatry*. doi:10.1177/070674370805300105

Cassidy, T. A., McNaughton, E. C., & Varughese, S. (2015). Nonmedical use of prescription ADHD stimulant medications among adults in a substance abuse treatment population: Early findings from the NAVIPPRO surveillance system. *Journal of Attention Disorders*, *19*(4), 275–283. doi:10.1177/1087054713493321

Cassidy, T. A., Varughese, S., & Russo, L. (2015). Nonmedical use and diversion of ADHD stimulants among U. S. adults ages 18–49: A national internet survey. *Journal of Attention Disorders*, *19*(7), 630–640. doi:10.1177/1087054712468486

Castells, X., Cunill, R., & Perez-Mana, C. (2016, September 27). Psychostimulant drugs for cocaine dependence. *The Cochrane Database of Systematic Reviews*, *9*, CD007380. doi:10.1002/14651858.CD007380.pub4

CDC, Centers for Disease Control and Prevention. (2007, January). Methamphetamine use and risk for HIV/AIDS. Retrieved from www.cdc.gov/hiv

Cepeda, M. S., Fife, D., & Berwaerts, J. (2015). Doctor shopping for medications used in the treatment of attention deficit hyperactivity disorder: Shoppers often pay in cash and cross state lines. *The American Journal of Drug and Alcohol Abuse*, *41*(3), 226–229.

Cerretani, D., Fineschi, V., & Bello, S. (2012). Role of oxidative stress in cocaine-induced cardiotoxicity and cocaine-related death. *Current Medicinal Chemistry*, *19*(33), 5619–5623.

Chang, T. R., Kowalski, R. G., & Caserta, F. (2013). Impact of acute cocaine use on aneurysmal subarachnoid hemorrhage. *Stroke*, *44*(7), 1825–1829. doi:10.1161/STROKEAHA.111.000749

Chen, L. Y., Crum, R. M., & Strain, E. C. (2015, October). Patterns of concurrent substance use among adolescent nonmedical ADHD stimulant users. *Addictive Behaviors*, *49*, 1–6. doi:10.1016/j.addbeh.2015.05.007

Chen, V. C., Chen, H., & Lin, T. Y. (2008). Severity of heroin dependence in Taiwan: Reliability and validity of the Chinese version of the Severity of Dependence Scale (SDS[Ch]}. *Addictive Behaviors*, *33*(12), 1590–1593. doi:10.1016/j.addbeh.2008.06.001

Cheng, T., Wood, E., & Nguyen, P. (2015, May). Crack pipe sharing among street-involved youth in a Canadian setting. *Drug and Alcohol Review*, *34*(3), 259–266. doi:10.111/dar.12180.

Cheng, Y. C., Ryan, K. A., & Qadwai, S. A. (2016). Cocaine use and risk of ischemic stroke in young adults. *Stroke*, *47*(4), 918–922. doi:10.11651/STROKEAHA.115.011417

Cheromcha, K. (2018, October 29). Cops find 1,200 pounds of liquid meth worth $4.4M hidden in semi-truck fuel tank. *Time Magazine*.

Chomchai, C., Chomchai, S., & Kitsommart, R. (2016, May). Transfer of methamphetamine (MA) into breast milk and urine of postpartum women who smoked MA tablets during pregnancy: Implications for initiation of breastfeeding. *Journal of Human Lactation*, *32*(2), 333–339. doi:10.1177/0890334415610080

Chung, A. (2017, July 7). Supreme Court lifts block on Wisconsin "cocaine mom" law during appeal. *US News & World Report*, 1–2. Retrieved from www.usnews.com/news/us/articles/2017-07-07/supreme-court-lifts-block-on-wisconsin-cocaine-mom-law-during-appeal#

Clemow, D. B., & Walker, D. J. (2014, September). The potential for misuse and abuse of medications in ADHD: A review. *Postgraduate Medicine*, *126*(5), 64–81. doi:10.3810/pgm.2014.09.2801

Collins, E. D., Vosburg, S. K., & Hart, C. L. (2003, December). Amantadine does not modulate reinforcing, subjective, or cardiovascular effects of cocaine in humans. *Pharmacology, Biochemistry, and Behavior*, *76*(3–4), 401–407.

Committee on Health Care for Underserved Women. (2011). Methamphetamine abuse in women of reproductive age (Committee Opinion No. 479). *Obstetrics & Gynecology*, *117*, 751–755.

Compton, W. M., Cottler, L. B., & Ridenour, T. (2002). The specificity of family history of alcohol and drug abuse in cocaine abusers. *The American Journal on Addictions*, *11*(2), 85–94.

Cone, E. J., Yousefnejad, D., & Hillsgrove, M. J. (1995, October). Passive inhalation of cocaine. *Journal of Analytical Toxicology, 19*(6), 399–411.

Connell-Carrick, K. (2007, May-June). Methamphetamine and the changing face of child welfare: Practice principles for child welfare workers. *Child Welfare, 86*(3), 125–144.

Contreäras, R., & Montoya Bryan, S. (2016, August 26). *Mother, 2 others arrested after horrific rape and murder of 10-year-old girl.* Retrieved August 26, 2016, from National | Globalnews.ca: http://globalnews.ca/news/2904176/mother-2-others-arrested-after-horrific-rape-and-murder-of-10-year-old-girl/

Corsi, K. F., & Booth, R. E. (2008). HIV sex risk behaviors among heterosexual methamphetamine users: Literature review from 2000 to present. *Current Drug Abuse Reviews, 1*(3), 292–296.

Crandell, C. G., Vongpatanasin, W., & Victor, R. G. (2002). Mechanism of cocaine-induced hyperthermia in humans. *Annals of Internal Medicine, 136*(11), 785–791.

Cranford, J. A., Esteban McCabe, S., & Boyd, C. J. (2006, October). A new measure of binge drinking: Prevalence and correlates in a probability sample of undergraduates. *Alcoholism: Clinical & Experimental Research.* doi:10.1111/j.1530-0277.2006.00234.x

Cuenca-Royo, A. M., Sanchez-Niubo, A., & Forero, C. G. (2012). Psychometric properties of the CAST and SDS scales in young adult cannabis users. *Addictive Behaviors, 37*(6), 709–715. doi:10.1016/j.addbeh.2012.02.012

Curran, C., Byrappa, N., & McBride, A. (2004, September). Stimulant psychosis: Systematic review. *British Journal of Psychiatry, 185*, 196–204. doi:10.1192/bjp.185.3.196

Czogala, J., Goniewicz, M. L., & Fidelus, B. (2014, June). Secondhand exposure to vapors from electronic cigarettes. *Nicotine & Tobacco Research, 16*(6), 655–662. doi:10.1093/ntr/ntt203

D'Angelo, B. (2018, May 20). North Carolina deputies find nearly $91 million of liquid meth on truck. *Dayton Daily News.* Cox Media Group.

Dackis, C. A., & Gold, M. S. (1990). Addictiveness of central stimulants. *Advances in Alcohol & Substance Abuse, 9*(1–2), 9–26. doi:10.1300/J251v09n01_02

Dackis, C. A., Kampman, K. M., & Lynch, K. G. (2005). A double-blind, placebo-controlled trial of modafinil for cocaine dependence. *Neuropsychopharmacology, 30*(1), 205–211. doi:10.1038/sj.np.1300600

Dackis, C. A., Kampman, K. M., & Lynch, K. G. (2012, October). A double-blind, placebo-controlled trial of modafinil for cocaine dependence. *Journal of Substance Abuse Treatment, 43*(3), 303–312. doi:10.1016/j.jsat.2011.12.014

Davidson, C. (2016, June). Developing treatments for stimulant abuse: A brief overview. *East Asian Archives of Psychiatry, 26*(2), 52–59.

DEA, Drug Enforcement Administration. (2011, December 1). Implementation of the Methamphetamine Production Prevention Act of 2008. Final rule. *Federal Register, 76*(231), 74696–74699.

Dean, A., Kohno, M., & Morales, A. M. (2015, June 1). Denial in methamphetamine users: Associations with cognition and functional connectivity in brain. *Drug and Alcohol Dependence, 151*, 84–91. doi:10.1016/j.drugalcdep.2015.03.004

Della Grotta, S., LaGasse, L. L., & Arria, A. M. (2010). Patterns of methamphetamine use during pregnancy: Results for the Infant Development, Environment, and Lifestyle (IDEAL) Study. *Maternal and Child Health Journal, 14*, 519–527.

Dembo, R., Schmeidler, J., & Borden, P. (1996). Use of the POSIT among arrested youths entering a juvenile assessment center: A replication and update. *Journal of Child & Adolescent Substance Abuse, 6*(3), 19–42.

Derauf, C., LaGasse, L. L., & Smith, L. M. (2007). Demographic and psychosocial characteristics of mothers using methamphetamine during pregnancy: Preliminary results of the Infant Development, Environment, and Lifestyle Study (IDEAL). *The Journal of Drug and Alcohol Abuse, 33*(2), 281–289. doi:10.1080/00952990601175029

DeSantis, A. D., & Curtis Hane, A. (2010). "Adderall is definitely not a drug": Justifications for the illegal use of ADHD stimulants. *Substance Use & Misuse, 45*, 31–46. doi:10.3109/10826080902858334

Dessy, C., & Baligand, J.-L. (2010). Beta3-adrenergic receptors in cardiac and vascular tissues: Emerging concepts and therapeutic perspectives. *Advances in Pharmacology, 59*, 135–163. doi:10.1016/s1054-3589(10)5900-7

DeVito, E. E., Babuscio, T. A., & Nich, C. (2014, December 1). Gender differences in clinical outcomes for cocaine dependence: Randomized clinical trials of behavioral therapy and disulfiram. *Drug and Alcohol Dependence, 145*, 156–167. doi:10.1016/j.drugalcdep.2014.10.007

Diercks, D. B., Kirk, J. D., & Turnipseed, S. D. (2007, December). Evaluation of patients with methamphetamine- and cocaine-related chest pain in a chest pain observation unit. *Critical Pathways in Cardiology, 6*(4), 161–164.

DuPont, R. L., Coleman, J. J., & Bucher, R. H. (2008, May-June). Characterisitics and motives of college students who engage in nonmedical use of methylphenidate. *The American Journal on Addictions, 17*(3), 167–171. doi:10.1080/10550490802019642

Durrell, T. M., Kroutil, L. A., & Crits-Christoph, P. (2008). Prevalence of nonmedical methamphetamine use in the United States. *Substance Abuse Treatment, Prevention, and Policy, 3*, 1–10. doi:10.1186/1747-597X-3-19

Dussault, C. L., & Weyandt, L. L. (2013). An examination of prescription stimulant misuse and psychological variables among sorority and fraternity college populations. *Journal of Attention Disorders, 17*(2), 87–97. doi:10.1177/1087054711428740

Eiden, R. D., Godleski, S., & Schuetze, P. (2015, September). Prenatal substance exposure and child self-regulation: Pathways to risk and protection. *Journal of Experimental Child Psychology, 137*, 12–29. doi:10.1016/j.jecp.2015.02.007

Eiden, R. D., Schuetze, P., & Coles, C. D. (2011). Maternal cocaine use and mother-infant interactions: Direct and moderated associations. *Neurotoxicology & Teratology, 1*, 120–128. doi:10.1016/j.ntt.2010.08.005

El-Bassel, N., Schilling, R. F., & Schinke, S. (1997). Assessing the utility of the Drug Abuse Screening Test in the workplace. *Research on Social Work Practice*, 7(1), 99–114.

Eldridge, E. (2016, March 3). Cops: Drug smugglers disguise liquid meth as beer, use tour buses. *The Atlantic Journal-Constitution*. Cox Media Group.

Elkashef, A., Vocci, F., & Hanson, G. (2008). Pharmacotherapy of methamphetamine addiction: An update. *Substance Abuse, 29*(3), 31–49. doi:10.1080/08897070802218554

Epstein, D. H., Hawkins, W. E., & Covi, L. (2003, March). Cognitive-behavioral therapy plus contingency management for cocaine use: Findings during treatment and across 12-month follow-up. *Psychology of Addictive Behaviors, 17*(1), 73–82.

Ermer, J. C., Pennick, M., & Frick, G. (2016). Lisdexamfetamine dimesylate: Prodrug delivery, amphetamine exposure and duration of efficacy. *Clinical Drug Investigation, 36*, 341–356. doi:10.1007/s40261-015-0354-y

Ernst, A. A., Weiss, S. J., & Enright-Smith, S. (2008). Perpetrators of intimate partner violence use significantly more methamphetamine, cocaine, and alcohol than victims: A report by victims. *The American Journal of Emergency Medicine, 26*(5), 592–596. doi:10.1016/j.ajem.2007.09.015

Ersche, K. D., Clark, L., & London, M. (2006). Profile of executive and memory function associated with amphetamine and opiate dependence. *Neuropsychopharmacology, 31*(5), 1036–1047. doi:10.1038/sj.np.1300889

Esteban McCabe, S., Morales, M., & Cranford, J. A. (2007). Race/Ethnicity and gender differences in drug use and abuse among college students. *Journal of Ethnicity in Substance Abuse, 6*(2), 75–95.

Esteban-McCabe, S., West, B. T., & Teter, C. J. (2014, July). Trends in medical use, diversion, and nonmedical use of prescription medications among college students from 2003 to 2013: Connecting the dots. *Addictive Behaviors, 39* (7), 1176–1182. doi:10.1016/j.addbeh.2014.03.008

Eze, N., Smith, L. M., & LaGasse, L. L. (2016). School-aged outcomes following prenatal methamphetamine exposure: 7.5-year follow-up from the Infant Development, Environment, and Lifestyle Study. *Journal of Pediatrics, 170*, 34–38. doi:10.1016/j.peds.2015.11.070

Faraone, S. V. (2018). The pharmacology of amphetamine and methylphenidate: Relevance to the neurobiology of attention-deficit/hyperactivity disorder and other psychiatric comorbidities. *Neuroscience and Biobehavioral Reviews, 87*, 255–270. doi:10.1016/j.neubiorev.2018.02.001

Farronato, N. S., Dursteler-Macfarland, K. M., & Wiesbeck, G. A. (2013). A systematic review comparing cognitive-behavioral therapy and contingency management for cocaine dependence. *Journal of Addictive Diseases, 32*(3), 274–287. doi:10.1080/10550887.2013.824328

Farst, K., Duncan, J. M., & Moss, M. (2007). Methamphetamine exposure presenting as caustic ingestions in children. *Annals of Emergency Medicine, 49*(3), 341–343. doi:10.1016/j.annemergmed.2006.05.020

Feaver, D. B. (1986, January 15). Drug-related fire suspected in Rick Nelson plane crash. *The Washington Post*.

Feit, N. (2019, January 22). Woman in speeding car gives birth to Atom Bomb, then gets arrested, NC police say. *The State*. Gaston, NC.

Fellner, C. (2016). Pharmaceutical approval update. *P&T, Pharmacy and Therapeutics, 41*(3), 162–163.

Ferri, C. P., Marsden, J., & de Araujo, M. (2000). Validity and reliability of the Severity of Dependence Scale (SDS) in a Brazilian sample of drug users. *Drug and Alcohol Review, 19*(4), 451–455.

First Nations Centre. (2006, May). *The Emerging Issue of Crystal Methamphetamine Use in First Nations Communities*. National Aboriginal Health Organization. Retrieved November 2, 2016.

Fischbach, P. (2017, January). The role of illicit drug use in sudden death in the young. *Cardiology in the Young, 27*(S1), S75–S79. doi:10.1017/S1047951116002274

Fleckenstein, A. E., Volz, T. J., & Riddle, E. L. (2007). New insights into the mechanism of action of amphetamines. *Annual Review of Pharmacology & Toxicology, 47*, 681–698. doi:10.1146/annurev.pharmtox.47.120505.105140

Fox News. (2016, June 29). Ex-Arizona TV reporters face drug, child abuse charges after cocaine found in infant's system. *TucsonNewsNow.com*. Tucson, AZ: Fox News.

Frances, A. J. (2015, November 8). Why are so many American youth abusing Adderall? *Psychology Today*, 1–4.

Frank, D. A., Kuranz, S., & Appugliese, D. (2014, September 1). Prolematic substance use in urban adolescents: Role of intrauterine exposures to cocaine and marijuana and post-natal environment. *Drug and Alcohol Dependence, 142*, 181–190. doi:10.1016/j.drugalcdep.2014.06.014.

Gallucci, A. R., Martin, R. J., & Usdan, S. L. (2015, March). The diversion of stimulant medications among a convenience sample of college students with current prescriptions. *The Psychology of Addictive Behaviors, 29*(1), 154–161. doi:10.1037/adb0000012

Garcia-Bournissen, F., Rokach, B., & Karaskov, T. (2007, September). Methamphetamine detection in maternal and neonatal hair: Implications for fetal safety. *Archives of Disease in Childhood. Fetal and Neonatal Edition, 92*(5), F351–F355. doi:10.1136/adc.2006.100156

Gatof, D., & Albert, R. K. (2002). Bilateral thumb burns leading to the diagnosis of crack lung. *Chest, 121*(1), 289–291.

Gavin, D. R., Ross, H. E., & Skinner, H. A. (1989). Diagnostic validity of the drug abuse screening test in the assessment of DSM-III drug disorders. *British Journal of Addiction, 84*(3), 301–307.

Geller, R. (2005, July 19). *Guidelines for Managing Children Found at Clandestine Methamphetamine Laboratory Sites* (pp. 1–15). Atlanta, GA: Georgia Bureau of Investigation.

Gerteis, J., Chartrand, M., & Martin, B. (2011, June). Are there effects of intrauterine cocaine exposure on delinquency during ealy adolescence? A preliminary report. *Journal of Developmental & Behavioral Pediatrics, 32*(5), 393–401. doi:10.1097/DBP.0b013e318218d9f2

Glasner-Edwards, S., Mooney, L. J., & Marinelli-Casey, P. (2008). Risk factors for suicide attempts in methamphetamine-dependent patients. *The American Journal on Addictions, 17*(1), 24–27. doi:10.1080/10550490701756070

Glover-Kerkvliet, J. (2009). The methamphetamine crisis in American Indian and Native Alaskan Communities: Toward a new research agenda. *Student Pulse, 1*(12), 1–11. Retrieved from Student Pulse: www.studentpulse.com/a?id=77

Gold, J. (2016, August 16). *California Court Helps Kids By Healing Parents' Addictions.* Retrieved from Shots—Health News: NPR: www.npr.org/sections/health-shots/2016/08/16/480960622/california-court-helps-kids-by-healing-parents-addiction

Goldstein, R. Z., & Volkow, N. D. (2011, November). Dysfunction of the prefrontal cortex in addiction: Neuroimaging findings and clinical implications. *Nature Reviews | Neuroscience, 12*, 652–669. Retrieved from). www.nature.com/reviews/neuro

Gonzales, R., Mooney, L., & Rawson, R. A. (2010). The methamphetamine problem in the United States. *Annual Review of Public Health, 31*, 385–398. doi:10.1146/annurev.publhealth.012809.103600

Gorman, M. C., Orme, K. S., & Nguyen, N. T. (2014, October). Outcomes in pregnancies complicated by methamphetamine use. *AJOG, American Journal of Obstetrics & Gynecology, 211*(4), 429. doi:10.1016/j.ajog.2014.06.005

Gossop, M., Best, D., & Marsden, J. (1997). Test-retest reliability of the Severity of Dependence Scale. *Addiction, 92*(3), 353–354. doi:10.1080/09652149738439

Gossop, M., Darke, S., & Griffiths, P. (1995). The Severity of Dependence Scale (SDS): Psychometric properties of the SDS in English and Australian samples of heroin, cocaine and amphetamine users. *Addiction, 90*(5), 607–614.

Grabus, S. (2017, March 22). *Endocanabinoid regulates cocaine reward.* Retrieved December 13, 2017, from National Institute on Drug Abuse (NIDA): www.drugabuse.gov/news-events/nida-notes/2017/03/endocannabinoid-regulates-cocaine-reward

Grant, P. (2007, February). Evaluation of children removed from a clandestine methamphetamine laboratory. *Journal of Emergency Nursing, 33*(1), 31–41. doi:10.1016/j.jen.2006.12.003

Grekin, E. R., Svikis, D. S., & Lam, P. (2010, December). Drug use during pregnancy: Validating the Drug Abuse Screening Test against physiological measures. *Psychology of Addictive Behaviors, 24*(4), 719–723. doi:10.1037/a0021741

Grinspoon, L., & Hedblom, P. (1975). *The Speed Culture: Amphetamine Use and Abuse in America.* Cambridge: Harvard University Press.

Grov, C., Kelly, B. C., & Parsons, J. T. (2009). Polydrug use among club-going young adults recruited through time-space sampling. *Substance Use & Misuse, 44*(6), 848–864. doi:10.1080/10826080802484702

Haelle, T. (2014, November 13). ADHD stimulant drug abuse common among young adults: Survey. *HealthDay*, 1–2.

Haight, W., Jacobsen, T., & Black, J. (2005). "In these bleak days": Parent methamphetamine abuse and child welfare in the rural Midwest. *Children and Youth Services Review, 27*(8), 949–971.

Hall, K., & Dunham, T. (2013, November 11). *The methiest states in the U. S. (Infographic).* Retrieved from HOFFPOST CRIME: www.huffingtonpost.com/2013/10/07/meth-states_n_4057372.html

Hamilton, A. B., & Goeders, N. E. (2010). Violence perpetrated by women who use methamphetamine. *Journal of Substance Use, 15*(5), 313–329. doi:10.3109/14659890903431611

Hamilton, K. (2010, May 19). *Methology 101: Old-school meth labs give way to "shake and bake".* Retrieved November 2, 2016, from St Lewis News and Events | Riverfront Times: www.riverfronttimes.com/stlouis/methology-101-old-school-mth-labs-give-way-to-shake-and-bake/Cont?mode=print&old=2483461

Hammond, E. R., Lai, S., & Wright, C. M. (2016). Cocaine use may be associated with increased depression in persons infected with HIV. *AIDS and Behavior, 20*(2), 345–352. doi:10.1007/s10461-015-1187-7

Hanson, G. R., Rau, K. S., & Fleckenstein, A. E. (2004). The methamphetamine experience: A NIDA partnership. *Neuropharmacology, 47*(Supplement 1), 92–100. doi:10.1016/j.neuropharm.2004.06.004

Harada, T., Tsutomi, H., & Mori, R. (2014). Cognitive-behavioural treatments for amphetamine-type stimulants (ATS) use disorders (Protocol). *Cochrane Database of Systematic Reviews, 10*(CD011315), 1–9. doi:10.1002/14651858.CD011315

Harris, D. S., Everhart, E. T., & Mendelson, J. (2003, November). The pharmacology of cocaethylene in humans following cocaine and ethanol administration. *Drug and Alcohol Dependence, 72*(2), 169–182.

Hart, C. L., Haney, M., & Collins, E. D. (2007, January). Smoked cocaine self-administration by humans is not reduced by large gabapentin maintenance doses. *Drug and Alcohol Dependence, 86*(2–3), 274–277. doi:10.1016/j.drugalcdep.2006.05.028

Hart, C. L., Haney, M., & Vosburg, S. K. (2007, February). Gabapentin does not reduce smoked cocaine self-administration: Employment of a novel self-administration procedure. *Behavioral Pharmacology, 18*(1), 71–75. doi:10.1097/FBP.0b013e328014139d

Hart, C. L., Haney, M., & Vosburg, S. K. (2008, March). Smoked cocaine self-administration is decreased by modafinil. *Neuropsychopharmacology, 33*(4), 761–768. doi:10.1038/sj.np.1301472

Hart, C. L., Ward, A. S., & Collins, E. D. (2004, March 8). Gabapentin maintenance decreases smoked cocaine-related subjective effects, but not self-administration by humans. *Drug and Alcohol Dependence, 73*(3), 279–287. doi:10.1016/j.drugalcdep.2003.10.015

Harzke, A. J., Williams, M. L., & Bowen, A. M. (2009, December). Binge use of crack cocaine and sexual risk behaviors among African-American, HIV-positive users. *AIDS and Behavior, 13*(6), 1106–1118. doi:10.1007/s10461-008-9450-9

Hauer, P. (2010). Systemic affects of methamphetamine use. *South Dakota Medicine, 63*(8), 285–287.

Hegazi, A., Lee, M. J., & Whittaker, W. (2017, March). Chemsex and the city: Sexualised substance use in gay bisexual and other men who have sex with men attending sexual health clinics. *International Journal of STD & AIDS, 28* (4), 362–366. doi:10.1177/0956462416651229

Hellem, T. L., Lundberg, K. J., & Renshaw, P. F. (2015). A review of treatment options for co-occurring methamphetamine use disorders and depression. *Journal of Addictions Nursing, 26*(1), 14–E1. doi:10.1097/JAN.0000000000000058

Hendrickson, R. G., Horowitz, B. Z., & Norton, R. L. (2006). Parachuting" meth: A novel delivery method for methamphetamine and delayed-onset toxicity from "body stuffing". *Clinical Toxicology (Phila), 44*(4), 379–382. doi:10.1080/15563650600671746

Herbst, E. D., Harris, D. S., & Everhart, E. T. (2011, April). Cocaethylene formation following ethanol and cocaine administration by different routes. *Experimental and Clinical Psychopharmacology, 19*(2), 95–104. doi:10.1037/a0022950

Herman, A. O. (2017, December 5). *Physician's first watch.* (D. G. Fairchild & J. E. Hefner, Editors) Retrieved from NEJM Journal Watch: www.jwatch.org/fw113601/2017/12/05/cocaine-accounts-substantial-overdose-burden-among-black?query=pfw&jwd=0000200002443&jspvc=

Herman-Stahl, M., Krebs, C. P., & Kroutil, L. A. (2007, May). Risk and protective factors for methamphetamine use and nonmedical use of prescription stimulants among young adults aged 18 to 25. *Addictive Behaviors, 32*(5), 1003–1015. doi:10.1016/j.addbeh.2006.07.010

Hides, L., Dawe, S., & Young, R. M. (2007). The reliability and validity of the Severity of Dependence Scale for detecting cannabis dependence in psychosis. *Addiction, 102*(1), 35–40.

Higgins, S. T., Sigmon, S. C., & Wong, C. J. (2003). Community reinforcement therapy for cocaine-dependent outpatients. *Archives of General Psychiatry, 60*(10), 1043–1052. doi:10.1001/archpsych.60.9.1043

Higgins, S. T., Wong, C. J., & Badger, G. J. (2000, February). Contingent reinforcement increases cocaine abstinence during outpatient treatment and 1 year of follow-up. *Journal of Consulting and Clinical Psychology, 68*(1), 64–72.

Hildebrand, M. (2015, June). Psychometric propertis of the Drug Use Disorders Identification Test: A review of recent research. *Journal of Substance Abuse Treatment, 53*, 52–59. doi:10.1016/j.jsat.2015.01.008

Himes, S. K., LaGasse, L. L., & Derauf, C. (2014, August). Risk of neurobehavioral disinhibition in prenatal methamphetamine-exposure young children with positive hair toxicology results. *Therapeutic Drug Monitoring, 36*(4), 535–543. doi:10.1097/FTD.0000000000000049

Hohman, M., Oliver, B. A., & Wright, W. (2002). Methamphetamine abuse and manufacture: The child welfare response. *Oxford Journals-Social Sciences-Social Work, 49*(3), 373–381.

Horton, D. K., Berkowitz, Z., & Kaye, W. E. (2003). The acute health consequences to children exposed to hazardous substances used in illicit methamphetamine production, 1996 to 2001. *Journal of Children's Health, 1*(1), 99–108.

Howell, L. L., & Cunningham, K. A. (2015, January). Serotinin 5-HT2 receptor interactions with dopamine function: Implications for therapeutics in cocaine use disorder. *Pharmacological Reviews, 67*, 176–197. doi:10.1124/PR.114.009514

Hu, X. T. (2007). Cocaine withdrawal and neuro-adaptations in ion channel function. *Molecular Neurobiology, 35*(1), 95–112.

Huang, M. C., Yang, S. Y., & Lin, S. K. (2016). Risk of cardiovascular diseases and stroke events in methamphetamine users: A 10-year follow-up study. *Journal of Clinical Psychiatry*, 77(10), 1396–1403. doi:10.4088/JCP.15m09872

Huffpost Staff. (2012, June 12). High school students turn to study drugs to enhance academic performance. *Huffpost.* Huffpost.com.

Indave, B. I., Minozzi, S., & Pani, P. P. (2016, March 19). Antipsychotic medications for cocaine dependence. *Cochrane Database of Systematic Reviews, 3*, CD006306. doi:10.1002/14651858.CD006306.pub3

Iraurgi Castillo, I., Gonzalez Saiz, F., & Lozano Rojas, O. (2010). Estimation of cutoff for the Severity Dependence Scale (SDS) for opiate dependence by ROC analysis. *Actas Espanalas De Psiquiatric, 38*(5), 270–277.

Irvine, M. (2005, April 25). Teenage meth addicts struggle to stay clean. *Los Angeles Times*, pp. 1–3.

Jafari, G. M. (2017). Exposure to amphetamine leads to development of amphetamine type stimulants associated cardiomyopathy (ATSAC). *Cardiovascular Toxicology, 17*(1), 13–24. doi:10.1007/s12012-016-9385-8

John, W. S., & Wu, L. (2017). Trends and correlates of cocaine use and cocaine use disorder in the United States from 2011 to 2015. *Drug and Alcohol Dependence, 180*, 376–384. doi:10.1016/j.drugalcdep.2017.08.031

Johnson, B. A., Ait-Daoud, N., & Elkashef, A. M. (2008, February). A preliminary randomized, double-blind, placebo-controlled study of the safety and efficacy of ondansetron in the treatment of methamphetamine dependence. *International Journal of Neuropsychopharmacology, 11*(1), 1–14. doi:10.1017/S1461145707007778

Johnston, L. D., O'Malley, P. M., & Bachman, J. G. (2013). *Monitoring the Future: National Survey Results on Drug Use 1975–2012*. Institute for Social Research. Ann Arbor, MI: The University of Michigan.

Johnston, L. D., O'Malley, P. M., & Miech, R. A. (2017). *Monitoring the Future National Survey Results on Drug Use, 1975–2016: Overview, Key Findings on Adolescent Drug Use*. Ann Arbor, MI: Institute for Social Research, The University of Michigan.

Kahn, R., Biswas, K., & Childress, A. R. (2009, July 1). Multi-center trial of baclofen for abstinence initiation in severe cocaine-dependent individuals. *Drug and Alcohol Dependence, 103*(1–2), 59–64. doi:10.1016/j.drugalcdep.2009.03.011

Kaland, M. E., & Klein-Schwartz, W. (2015, June). Comparison of lisdexamfetamine and dextroamphetamine exposures reported to U.S. poison centers. *Clinical Toxicology (Phila), 53*(5), 477–485. doi:10.3109/15563650.2015.1027903

Kampman, K. M., Dackis, C., & Lynch, K. G. (2006, November 8). A double-brind, placebo-controlled trial of amantadine, propranolol, and their combination for the treatment of cocaine dependence in patients with severe cocaine withdrawal symptoms. *Drug and Alcohol Dependence, 85*(2), 129–137. doi:10.1016/j.drugalcdep.2006.04.002

Kampman, K. M., Dackis, C., & Pettinati, H. M. (2011). A double-blind, placebo-controlled pilot trial of acamprosate for the treatment of cocaine dependence. *Addictive Behaviors, 36*(3), 217–221. doi:10.1016/j.addbeh.20210.11.003

Kampman, K. M., Lynch, K. G., & Pettinati, H. M. (2015, October 1). A double-blind, placebo controlled trial of modafinil for the treatment of cocaine dependence without co-morbid alcohol dependence. *Drug and Alcohol Dependence, 155*, 105–110. doi:10.1016/j.drugalcdep.20215.08.005

Kampman, K. M., Pettinati, H. M., & Lynch, K. G. (2013, November 1). A double-blind, placebo-controlled trial of topiramate for the treatment of comorbid cocaine and alcohol dependence. *Drug and Alcohol Dependence, 133*(1), 94–99. doi:10.1016/j.drugalcdep.2013.05.026

Karilla, L., Wienstein, A., & Aubin, H.-J. (2010). Pharmacological approaches to methamphetamine dependence: A focused review. *British Journal of Clinical Pharmacology, 69*(6), 578–592. doi:10.1111/j.1365-2125.2010.03639.x

Kashani, J., & Ruha, A. M. (2004). Methamphetamine toxicity secondary to intravaginal body stuffing. *Journal of Toxicology: Clinical Toxicology, 42*(7), 987–989.

Kaye, S., McKetin, R., & Duflou, J. (2007). Methamphetamine and cardiovascular pathology: A review of the evidence. *Addiction, 102*(8), 1204–1211. doi:10.1111/j.1360-0443.2007.01874.x

Keegan, N. (2018, February 18). Girl whose drug overdose landed her in the hospital explains the story behind the viral photo. *The Sun*, 1–3. Nashville, TN: The Sun.

Kelly, B. C., Wells, B. E., & Leclair, A. (2013). Prevalence and correlates of prescription drug misuse among socially active young adults. *International Journal of Drug Policy, 24*(4), 297–303. doi:1016/j.drugpo.2012.09.002

Kennedy, A. P., Epstein, D. H., & Phillips, K. A. (2013). Sex differences in cocaine/heroin users: Drug-use triggers and craving in daily life. *Drug and Alcohol Dependence, 132*(1–2), 29–37. doi:10.1016/j.drugalcdep.2012.12.025

Keoleian, V., Stalcup, A., & Poicin, D. (2013). A cognitive behavioral therapy-based text messaging intervention for methamphetamine dependence. *Journal of Psychoactive Drugs, 45*(5), 434–442.

Kerley, K. R., Leban, L., & Copes, H. (2014). Methamphetamine using careers of White and Black women. *Deviant Behavior, 35*(6), 477–495. doi:10.1080/01639625.2013.859046

Kishi, T., Matsuda, Y., & Iwata, N. (2013, December). Antipsychotics for cocaine or psychostimulant dependence: Systematic review and meta-analysis of randomized placebo-controlled trials. *Journal of Clinical Psychiatry, 74*(12), e1169–e1180. doi:10.4088/JCP.13r08525

Knight, J. R., Goodman, E., & Pulerwitz, T. (2001, August). Reliability of the Problem Oriented Screening Instrument for Teenagers (POSIT) in adolescent medical practice. *The Journal of Adolescent Health, 29*(2), 125–130.

Knight, J. R., Sherritt, L, & Harris, S. K. (2003). Validity of brief alcohol screening tests among adolescents: A comparison of the AUDIT, POSIT, CAGE, and CRAFFT. *Alcoholism: Cinical & Experimental Research, 27* (1), 67–73.

Kolecki, P. (1998). Inadvertent methamphetamine poisoning in pediatric patients. *Pediatric Emergency Care, 14*(6), 385–387.

Kondrotas, O. (2006, May 15). Speed culture in the digital generation: A commentary on amphetamine use at MIT and colleges nationwide. *"hero" Course Paper*, 1–9. Retrieved October 25, 2017, from https://studylib.net/doc136471

Krueger, S. J., & Glass, C. R. (2013). Integrative psychotherapy for children and adolescents: A practice-oriented literature review. *Journal of Psychotherapy Integration, 23*(4), 331–344. doi:10.1037/a0034949

Kuhar, M. J., & Pilotte, N. S. (1996). Neurochemical changes in cocaine withdrawal. *Trends in Pharmacological Sciences, 17*(7), 260–264.

Laizure, S. C., Mandrell, T., & Gades, N. M. (2003). Cocaethylene metabolism and interation with cocaine and ethanol: Role of carboxylesterases. *Drug Metabolism and Disposition, 31*(1), 16–20.

Lappin, J. M., Darke, S., & Farrell, M. (2017). Stroke and methamphetamine use in young adults: A review. *Journal of Neurology, Neurosurgery, and Psychiatry, 88*(12), 1079–1091. doi:10.1136/jnnp-2017-316071

Larocque, A., & Hoffman, R. S. (2012). Levamisole in cocaine: Unexpected news from an old acquaintance. *Clinical Toxicology, 50*(4), 231–241. doi:10.3109/15563650.2012.665455

Lason, W. (2001). Neurochemical and pharmacological aspects of cocaine-induced seizures. *Polish Journal of Pharmacology, 53*(1), 57–60.

Latimer, W. W., Winters, K. C., & Stinchfield, R. D. (1997). Screening for drug abuse among adolescents in clinical and correctional settings using the Problem-Oriented Screening Instrument for Teenagers. *The American Journal of Drug and Alcohol Abuse, 23*(1), 79–98. doi:10.3109/00952999709001689

Lebel, C., Warner, T., & Colby, J. (2013, August 30). White matter microstructure abnormalities and executive function in adolescents with prenatal cocaine exposure. *Psychiatry Research, 213*(2), 161–168. doi:10.1016/j.psychresna.2013.04.002

Lee, K. C., Ladizinski, B., & Federman, D. G. (2012). Complications associated with use of levamisole-contaminated cocaine: An emerging public health challenge. *Mayo Clinic Proceedings, 87*(6), 581–586.

Lee, M. R. (2011). The history of Ephredra (ma-huang). *The Journal of the Royal College of Physicians of Edinburgh, 41*, 78–84. doi:10.4997/JRCPE.2011.116

Lee, N., Jenner, L., & Nielsen, S. (2014). *Medication Treatment: Options for Amphetamine-type Stimulant Users.* Canberra: Australian National Council on Drugs. Retrieved October 24, 2017.

Lee, N. K., & Rawson, R. A. (2008, May). A systematic review of cognitive and behavioural therapies for methamphetamine dependence. *Drug and Alcohol Reviews, 27*, 309–317. doi:10.1080/09595230801919494

Leonard, K. (2017, January 3). What's behind the rise in cocaine-linked deaths? *US News & World Report*, 1–5. Retrieved from www.usnews.com/topics/subjects/cocaine

Lewis, D. (1994, January 12). Cocaine and other botanical insecticides. *Horticulture and Home Pest News*, 1–2. Iowa State University.

Li, L., Zhang, X., & Levine, B. (2011, July). Trends and pattern of drug abuse deaths in Maryland teenagers. *Journal of Forensic Sciences, 56*(4), 1029–1033. doi:10.111/j.1556-4029.2011.01743.x

Liebschultz, J. M., Crooks, D., & Rose-Jacobs, R. (2015, June). Prenatal substance exposure: What predicts behavioral resilience by early adolescence? *Psychology of Addictive Behaviors, 29*(2), 329–337. doi:10.1037/adb0000082

Lile, J. A., Stoops, W. W., & Allen, T. S. (2004, February). Baclofen does not alter the reinforcing, subject-rated or cardiovascular effects of intranasal cocaine in humans. *Psychopharmacology (Berlin), 171*(4), 441–449. doi:10.1007/s00213-003-1598-4

Lin, S. J., Crawford, S. Y., & Lurvey, P. L. (2005, February). Trend and area variation in amphetamine prescription usage among children and adolescents in Michigan. *Social Science & Medicine, 60*(3), 617–626. doi:10.1016/j.socscimed.2004.06.002

Lineberry, T. W., & Bostwick, J. M. (2006). Methamphetamine abuse: A perfect storm of complications. *Mayo Clinic Proceedings, 81*(1), 77–84.

Lipari, R. N., Williams, M., & Copello, E. A. (2016). *Risk and Protective Factors and Estimates of Substance Use Initiation: Results from the 2015 National Survey on Drug Use and Health.* Substance Abuse and Mental Health Services Administration, SAMHSA. Retrieved from www.samhsa.gov/data/sites/default/files/NSDUH-PreventionandInit-20215.htm

Longo, M., Wickes, W., & Smout, M. (2010). Randomized controlled trial of dexamphetamine maintenance for the treatment of methamphetamine dependence. *Addiction, 105*(1), 146–154. doi:10.111/j.1360-0443.2009.02727.x

Lorvick, J., Bourgois, P., & Wenger, L. D. (2012). Sexual pleasure and sexual risk among women who use methamphetamine: A mixed methods study. *International Journal of Drug Policy, 23*(5), 385–392. doi:10.1016/j.drugpo.2012.07.005

Lyons, K. (2014, February 27). *How young women desperate to be slim are using crystal meth to control their weight.* Retrieved July 4, 2014, from MailOnline: www.dailymail.co.uk/news/article-2568929/The-dangerous-weight-loss-drug-Young-..

Mammoser, G. (2017, December 17). Latest "street meth" coming from labs in Mexico. *Healthline*, 1–3. Healthline.

Mansoor, E., Morrow, C. E., & Accornero, V. H. (2012). Longitudinal effects of prenatal cocaine use on mother-child interactions at ages 3 and 5 years. *Journal of Developmental and Behavioral Pediatrics, 33*(1), 32–41. doi:10.1097/DBP.0b013e31823968ab

Marks, K. R., Pike, E., & Stoops, W. W. (2015). Alcohol administration increases cocaine craving but not cocaine cue attentional bias. *Alcoholism: Clinical & Experimental Research, 39*(9), 1823–1831. doi:10.111/acer.12824

Martin, G., Copeland, J., & Gates, P. (2006, June 9). The Severity of Dependence Scale (SDS) in an adolescent populaltion of cannabis users: Reliability, validity and diagnostic cut-off. *Drug and Alcohol Dependence, 83*(1), 90–93.

Martino, S., Grilo, C., & Fehon, D. C. (2000). Development of the drug abuse screening test for adolescents. *Addictive Behaviors, 25*(1), 57–70. doi:10.1016/S0306-4603(99)00030.1

Martin-Schild, S., Albright, K. C., & Hallevi, H. (2010). Intracerebral hemorrhage in cocaine users. *Stroke, 41*(4), 680–684. doi:10.1161/STROKEAHA.109.573147

Matteucci, M. J., Auten, J. D., & Crowley, B. (2007). Methamphetamine exposures in young children. *Pediatric Emergency Care, 207*(9), 638–640. doi:10.1097/PEC.0b013e31814a6a79

Matthew, B. J., & Gedzior, J. S. (2015). Drug-induced parkinsonism following chronic methamphetamine use by a patient on haloperidol decanoate. *The International Journal of Psychiatry in Medicine, 50*(4), 405–411. doi:10.1177/0091217415612736

McCabe, S. E., Morales, M., & Cranford, J. A. (2007). Race/ethnicity and gender differences in drug use and abuse among college students. *Journal of Ethnicity in Substance Abuse, 6*(2), 75–95.

McCann, B., Simpson, T., & Ries, R. (2000). Reliability and validity of screening instruments for drug and alcohol abuse in adults seeking evaluation for attention-deficit/hyperactivity disorder. *The American Journal on Addictions, 9*, 1–9.

McDonald, D. C., & Kuck Jalbert, S. (2013). Geographic variation and disparity in stimulant treatment of adults and children in the United States in 2008. *Psychiatric Services, 54*(11), 1079–1086. doi:10.1176/appi.ps.004442012

McGregor, C., Srisurapanont, M., & Jittiwutikarn, J. (2005). The nature, time course, and severity of methamphetamine withdrawal. *Addiction, 100*(9), 1320–1329. doi:10.1111/j.1360-0443.2005.01160.x

McLaney, M. A., Del Boca, F., & Babor, T. (2009, July). A validation study of the Problem Oriented Screening Instrument for Teenagers (POSIT). *Journal of Mental Health, 3*(3), 363–376. doi:10.3109/09638239408997947

Melendez-Torres, G. J., & Bourne, A. (2016, February). Illicit drug use and its assciation with sexual risk behavior among MSM: More questions than answers? *Current Opinion In Infectious Diseases, 29*(1), 58–63. doi:10.1097/QCO.0000000000000234

Melnikova, N., Orr, M. F., & Wu, J. (2019, February 12). Injuries from methamphetamine-related chemical incidents: Five states, 2001–2012. *Medscape.*

Mercado, M. C., Holland, K., & Leemis, R. W. (2017). Trends in emergency department visits for nonfatal self-inflicted injuries among youth aged 10 to 24 years in the United States, 2001–2015. *JAMA, Journal of the American Medical Association, 318*(19), 1931–1933. doi:10.1001/jama.2017.13317

Messina, N., Marinelli-Casey, P., & West, K. (2014). Children exposed to methamphetamine use and manufacture. *Child Abuse & Neglect, 38*(11), 1872–1883. doi:10.1016/j.chiabu.2006.06.009

Meyer, K. D., & Zhang, L. (2009). Short- and long-term adverse effects of cocaine abuse during pregnancy on the heart development. *Theapeutic Advances in Cardiovascular Disease, 3*(1), 7–16. doi:10.1177/1753944708099877

Mimiaga, M. J., Fair, A. D., & Mayer, K. H. (2008). Experiences and sexual behaviors of HIV-infected MSM who acquired HIV in the context of crystal methamphetamine use. *AIDS Education & Prevention, 20*(1), 30–41.

Minnes, S., Min, M. O., & Short, E. J. (2016). Executive function in children with prenatal cocaine exposure (12–15 years). *Neurotoxicology and Teratology, 57*, 79–86. doi:10.1016/j.ntt.2016.07.002

Minozzi, S., Cinquini, M., & Amato, L. (2015, April 17). Anticonvulsants for cocaine dependence. *Cochrane Database of Systematic Reviews, 4*, CD006754. doi:10.1002/146451858.CD006754.pub4

Minozzi, S., & Saulle, R. D. (2016, September 29). Psychosocial interventions for psychostimulant misuse. *Cochrane Database of Systematic Reviews, 9*, CD011866. doi:10.1002/14651858.CD011866.pub2.

Moeller, F. G., Schmitz, J. M., & Steinberg, J. L. (2007). Citalopram combined with behavioral therapy reduces cocaine use: A double-blind, placebo-controlled trial. *The American Journal of Drug and Alcohol Abuse, 33*(3), 367–378. doi:10.1080/00952990701313686

Molnar, D. S., Levitt, A., & Eiden, R. D. (2014, May). Prenatal cocaine exposure and trajectories of externalizing behavior problems in early childhood: Examining the role of maternal negative affect. *Development and Psychopathology, 26*(2), 515–528. doi:10.1017/S0954579414000091.

Moody, L., Franck, C., & Jarmolowicz, D. P. (2014). Executive functioning deficits in cocaine-dependent individuals. *Drug and Alcohol Dependence, 140*, e155.

Moore, T. M., Stuart, G. L., & Meehan, J. C. (2008). Drug abuse and aggression between intimate partners: A meta-analytic review. *Clinical Psychology Review, 28*(2), 247–274.

Morley, K. C., Cornish, J. L., & Faingold, A. (2017). Pharmacotherapeutic agents in the treatment of methamphetamine dependence. *Expert Opinion on Investigational Drugs, 26*(5), 563–578. doi:10.1080/13543784.2017.1313229

Mullin, G. (2016, January 28). *Faces of Crystal Meth: Shocking before and after Pictures Reveal Damage of Prolonged Drug Use.* Retrieved from World news.

Nair, P., Schuler, M. E., & Black, M. M. (2003). Cumulative environmental risk in substance abusing women: Early intervention, parenting stress, child abuse potential and child development. *Child Abuse & Neglect, 27*(9), 993–995.

National Drug Intelligence Center. (2006). *National methamphetamine threat assessment 2007*. Johnstown, PA: U.S. Department of Justice. Retrieved June, 30, 2018.

NIDA, National Institute on Drug Abuse. (2013, December). *Cocaine*. Retrieved from Cocaine | National Institute on Drug Abuse (NDA), pp. 1–6: www.drugabuse.gov/drugs-abuse/cocaine

NIDA, National Institute on Drug Abuse. (2016). *Cocaine*. National Institute on Drug Abuse. Retrieved from www.drugabuse.gov/drugs-abuse/cocaine

NIDA, National Institute on Drug Abuse. (2018). *Common Comorbidities with Substance Use Disorders*. Bethesda, MD: NIDA.

NIDA/NIH, National Institute on Drug Abuse/National Institutes of Health. (2005). *Medications Development Research for Treatment of Amphetamine and Methamphetamine Addiction*. Bethesda, MD: Department of Health and Human Services. Retrieved October 24, 2017.

NIH, National Institutes on Health. (2017, August 3). *Why females are more sensitive to cocaine*. Retrieved from National Institute on Drug Abuse News & Events: www.drugabuse.gov/news-events/nida-notes/2017/08/why-females-are-more-sensitive-to-cocaine

NIH, National Institutes on Health. (2018, August). Overdose death rates. *National Overdose Deaths*, 1–7. NIH.

Nilsson Schonnesson, L., Atkinson, J., & Williams, M. L. (2008, September). A cluster analysis of drug use and sexual HIV risks and their correlates in a sample of African-American crack cocaine smokers with HIV infection. *Drug and Alcohol Dependence*, *97*(1–2), 44–53. doi:10.1016/j.drugalcdep.2008.03.023

Nogueira, L., Kalivas, P. W., & Lavin, A. (2006). Long-term neuroadaptations produced by withdrawal from repeated cocaine treatment: Role of dopaminergic receptors in modulating cortical excitability. *The Journal of Neuroscience*, *26*(47), 12308–12313. doi:10.1523/JNEUROSCI.3206-06.2006

Norris, K. C., Thornhill-Joynes, M., & Robinson, C. (2001). Cocaine use, hypertension, and end-stage renal disease. *American Journal of Kidney Diseases*, *38*(3), 523–528. doi:10.1053/ajkd.2001.26845

Novak, S. P., Kroutil, L. A., & Williams, R. L. (2007, October 31). The nonmedical use of prescription ADHD medications: Results from a national internet panel. *Substance Abuse Treatment, Prevention, and Policy*, *2*, 32. doi:10.1186/1747-597X-2-32

ONDCP, Office of National Drug Control Policy. (2010, July). *Fact Sheet: Methamphetamine Trends in the United States*. Retrieved April 5, 2016, from www.WhiteHouseDrugPolicy.gov

Orciari Herman, A. (2018, March 30). Drug overdose deaths still increasing, opioids largely to blame. *NEJM Journal Watch*, 1.

Pagliaro, A. M., & Pagliaro, L. A. (2000). *Substance Use among Women: A Reference and Resource Guide*. Philadelphia, PA: Brunner/Mazel.

Pagliaro, A. M., & Pagliaro, L. A. (2018). *Women's Drug and Substance Abuse: A Comprehensive Analysis and Reflective Synthesis*. New York: Routledge.

Pagliaro, A. M., Pagliaro, L. A., & Thauberger, P. C. (1990). AIDS and injection drug use: Changing dimensions of the epidemic. *Alberta Psychology*, *19*(5), 5–7.

Pagliaro, A. M., Pagliaro, L. A., & Thauberger, P. C. (1993). Knowledge, behaviours, and risk perception of intravenous drug users in relation to HIV infection and AIDS: The PIARG projects. *Advances in Medical Psychotherapy*, *6*, 1–28.

Pagliaro, L. A., & Benet, L. Z. (1975). Critical compilation of terminal half-lives, percent excreted unchanged, and changes in renal and hepatic dysfunction for studies in adults with references. *Journal of Pharmacokinetics and Biopharmaceutics*, *3*, 333–383.

Pagliaro, L. A., Jaglalsingh, L. H., & Pagliaro, A. M. (1992). Cocaine use and depression. *Canadian Medical Association Journal*, *147*, 1636–1637.

Pagliaro, L. A., & Levin, R. H. (Eds.). (1979). *Problems in Pediatric Drug Therapy* (1st ed.). Hamilton, IL: Drug Intelligence.

Pagliaro, L. A., & Pagliaro, A. M. (1999). *PPDR: Psychologists' Psychotropic Drug Reference*. Philadelphia, PA: Brunner/Mazel.

Pagliaro, L. A., & Pagliaro, A. M. (Eds.). (2002). *Problems in Pediatric Drug Therapy* (4th ed.). Washington, DC: American Pharmaceutical Association.

Pagliaro, L. A., & Pagliaro, A. M. (2004). *Pagliaros' Comprehensive Guide to Drugs and Substances of Abuse* (1st ed.). Washington, DC: American Pharmacists Association.

Pagliaro, L. A., & Pagliaro, A. M. (2009). *Pagliaros' Comprehensive Guide to Drugs and Substances of Abuse* (2nd ed.). Washington, DC: American Pharmacists Association.

Pagliaro, L. A., & Pagliaro, A. M. (2012). *Handbook of Child and Adolescent Drug and Substance Abuse*. Hoboken, NJ: Wiley & Sons.

Pakianathan, M. R., Lee, M. J., & Kelly, B. (2016, December). How to assess gay, bisexual and other men who have sex with men for chemsex. *Sexually Transmitted Infections*, *92*(8), 568–570. doi:10.10365/sextrans-2015-052405.

Palamar, J. J., Davies, S. H., & Ompad, D. C. (2015). Powder cocaine and crack use in the United States: An examination of risk for arrest and socioeconomic disparities in use. *Drug and Alcohol Dependence*, *149*, 108–116. doi:10.1016/j.drugalcdep.2015.01.029

Palamar, J. J., & Le, A. (2017, December 1). Discordant reporting of nonmedical amphetamine use among Adderall-using high school seniors in the US. *Drug and Alcohol Dependence*, *181*, 208–212. doi:10.1016/j.drugalcdep.2017.09.033.

Pani, P. P., Trogu, E., & Vacca, R. (2010, January 20). Disulfiram for the treatment of cocaine dependence. *Cochrane Database of Systematic Reviews, 1*, CD007024. doi:10.1002/146541858.CD007024.pub2.

Park, T. M., & Haning, 3rd, W. F. (2016). Stimulant use disorders. *Child & Adolescent Psychiatric Clinics of North America, 25*(3), 461–471. doi:10.1016/j.chc.2016.02.004

Parolin, M., & Simonelli, A. (2016, August). Attachment theory and maternal drug addiction: The contribution to parenting interventions. *Frontiers in Psychiatry*, 7(Article 152), 1–14. doi:10.3389/fpsyt.2016.00152

Parsons, J. T., Grov, C., & Kelly, B. C. (2009). Club drug use and dependence among young adults recruited through time-space sampling. *Public Health Reports, 124*(2), 246–254.

Parvaz, M. A., Moeller, S. J., & Goldstein, R. Z. (2016). Incubation of cue-induced craving in adults addicted to cocaine measured by electroencephalography. *JAMA Psychiatry, 673*(11), 1127–1134.

Paulozzi, L. J., Strickler, G. K., & Kreiner, P. W. (2015, October 16). Controlled substance prescribing patterns—Prescription behavior surveillance system, eight states, 2013. *MMWR, Morbidity and Mortality Weekly Report, 64* (SS09), 1–14.

Penberthy, J. K., Ait-Daoud, N., & Vaughan, M. (2010, March). Review of treatment for cocaine dependence. *Current Drug Abuse Reviews, 3*(1), 49–62.

People Staff. (1980, June 30). Richard Pryor's tragic accident spotlights a dangerous drug craze: Freebasing. *People*, 1–4.

Perez-Mana, C., Castells, X., & Torrens, M. (2013, September 2). Efficacy of psychostimulant drugs for amphetamine abuse or dependence. *Cochrane Database of Systematic Reviews, 9*, CD009695. doi:10.1002/14651858.CD009695.pub2

Petering, R. (2016, April). Sexual risk, substance use, mental health, and trauma experiences of gang-involved homeless youth. *Journal of Adolescence, 48*, 73–81. doi:10.1016/j.adolescence.2016.01.009

Petit, A., Karila, L., & Chalmin, F. (2012). Methamphetamine addiction: A review of the literature. *Journal of Addiction Research & Therapy*, S1(006), 1–6. doi: 10.4172/2156-6105.S1-006

Petry, N. M., Barry, D., & Alessi, S. M. (2012, April). A randomized trial adapting contingency management targets based on initial abstinence status of cocaine-dependent patients. *Journal of Consulting and Clinical Psychology, 80*(2), 276–285. doi:10.1037/a0026883

Petry, N. M., Martin, B., & Simcic, F. (2005). Prize reinforcement contingency management for cocaine dependence: Integration with group therapy in a methadone clinic. *Journal of Consulting and Clinical Psychology, 73*(2), 354–359. doi:10.1037/0022-006X.73.2.354

Pettinati, H. M., Kampman, K. M., & Lynch, K. G. (2008a). A double-blind, placebo-controlled trial that combines disulfiram and naltrexone for treating co-occurring cocaine and alcohol dependence. *Addictive Behaviors, 33*(3), 651–667. doi:10.1016/j.addbeh.2007.11.011

Pettinati, H. M., Kampman, K. M., & Lynch, K. G. (2008b, June). Gender differences with high-dose naltrexone in patients with co-occurring cocaine and alcohol dependence. *Journal of Substance Abuse Treatment, 34*(4), 378–390. doi:10.1016/j.jsat6.2007.05.011

Phillips, K., Luk, A., & Soor, G. S. (2009). Cocaine cardiotoxicity: A review of the pathophysiology, pathology, and treatment options. *American Journal of Cardiovascular Drugs, 9*(3), 177–196. doi:10.2165/00129784-200909030-00005

Pilgrim, J. L., Woodford, N., & Drummer, O. H. (2013). Cocaine in sudden and unexpected death: A review of 49 post-mortem cases. *Forensic Science International, 227*(1–3), 52–59. doi:10.1016/j.forsciint.2012.08.037

Plowman, T. (1985). Coca chewing and the botanical origins of coca (Erythroxylum spp.) in South America. In D. Pacini & C. Franquemont (Eds.), *Coca and Cocaine: Effects on People and Policy in Latin America* (pp. 1–31). Peterborough: Transcript Printing.

Poling, J., Oliveto, A., & Petry, N. (2006). Six-month trial of bupropion with contingency management for cocaine dependence in a methadone-maintained population. *Archives of General Psychiatry, 63*(2), 219–228. doi:10.1001/archpsyc.63.2.219

Pope, S. K., Falck, R. S., & Carlson, R. G. (2011). Characteristics of rural crack and powder cocaine users: Gender and other correlates. *The American Journal of Drug and Alcohol Abuse, 37*(6), 491–496. doi:10.3109/00952990.2011.600380

Popovic, B., Bhattacharya, P., & Sivaswamy, L. (2009). Lisdexamfetamine: A prodrug for the treatment of attention-deficity/hyperactivity disorder. *American Journal of Health-System Pharmacy, 66*(22), 2005–2012. doi:10.2146/ajhp080353

Price, B. (2016, August 10). *Texas woman uses infant child to smuggle meth from Mexico*. Retrieved August 16, 2016, from Breitbart.com: www.breitbart.com/texas/2016/08/10/texas-woman-uses-infant-child-smuggle-meth-mexico/

Rabinber, D. L. (2013). Stimulant prescription cautions: Addressing misuse, diversion and malingering. *Current Psychiatry Reports, 15*(7), 375. doi:10.1007/s11920-013-0375-2

Rabiner, D. L., Anastopoulos, A. D., & Costello, E. J. (2009). The misuse and diversion of prescribed ADHD medications by college students. *Journal of Attention Disorders, 13*(2), 144–153. doi:10.1177/1087054708320414

Rahdert, E. R. (1991). *The Adolescent Assessment/Referral System Manual*. USDHHS. Rockville, MD: NIDA.

Ramo, D. E., Grov, C., & Delucchi, K. (2010). Typology of club drug use among young adults recruited using time-space sampling. *Drug and Alcohol Dependence, 107*(2–3), 119–127. doi:10.1016/j.drugalcdep.2009.09.014

Rawson, R. A., Huber, A., & McCann, M. (2002). A comparison of contingency management and cognitive-behavioral approaches during methadone maintenance treatment for cocaine dependence. *Archives of General Psychiatry, 59*(9), 817–824.

Rew, L., & Taylor-Seehafer, M. (2001). Sexual abuse, alcohol and other drug use, and suicidal behaviors in homeless adolescents. *Comprehensive Pediatric Nursing, 24*(4), 225–240. doi:10.1080/014608601753260326

Rhyee, S. H., Farrugia, L., & Campleman, S. L. (2015, December). The Toxicology Investigators Consortium Case Registry—The 2014 experience. *Journal of Medical Toxicology, 11*(4), 388–409. doi:10.1007/s13181-015-0507-7

Rhyee, S. H., Farrugia, L., & Wiegand, T. (2014, December). The Tocicology Investigators Consortium Case Registry —The 2013 experience. *Journal of Medical Toxicology, 10*(4), 342–359. doi:10.1007/s13181-014-0417-0

Riggs, P. D. (2003). Treating adolescents for substance abuse and comorbid psychiatric disorders. *Science Practice & Perspectives, 2*(1), 18–29.

Rinkel, G. J., Djibuti, M., & Algra, A. (1998). Prevalence and risk of rupture of intracranial aneurysms: A systematic review. *Stroke, 29*, 251–256.

Roberts, J. K., Cook, S. F., & Stockmann, C. (2015, October). A population pharmacokinetic analysis of dextroamphetamine in the plasma and hair of healthy adults. *Clinical Drug Investigation, 35*(10), 633–643. doi:10.1007/s40261-015-0323-5

Rolland, B., Karila, L., & Geoffroy, P. A. (2011). Shared vulnerability between seizures and psychosis in cocaine addiction? *Epilepsy & Behavior, 22*(3), 596–598. doi:10.1016/j.yebeh.2011.08.004

Rommel, N., Rohleder, N. H., & Koerdt, S. (2016, May 26). Sympathomimetic effects of chronic methamphetamine abuse on oral health: A cross-sectional study. *BMC Oral Health, 16*(1), 59. doi:10.1186/s12903-016-0218-8

Rommel, N., Rohleder, N. H., & Wagenpfeil, S. (2016, April). The impact of the new scene drug "crystal meth" on oral health: A case-control study. *Clinical Oral Investigations, 20*(3), 469–475. doi:10.1007/s00784-015-1527-z

Roos, A., Kwiatkowski, M. A., & Fouche, J. P. (2015). White matter integrity and cognitive performance in children with prenatal methamphetamine exposure. *Behavioural Brain Research, 279*, 62–67. doi:10.1016/j.bbr.2014,11.005

Roozen, H. G., Boulogne, J. J., & van Tulder, M. W. (2004). A systematic review of the effectiveness of the community reinforcement approach in alcohol, cocaine and opioid addiction. *Drug and Alcohol Dependence, 74*(1), 1–13.

Ross, E. J., Graham, D. L., & Money, K. M. (2015). Developmental consequences of fetal exposure to drugs: What we know and what we still must learn. *Neuropsychopharmacology Reviews, 40*, 61–87. doi:10.1038/np.2014.147

Rothman, R. B., Baumann, M. H., & Dersch, C. M. (2001). Amphetamine-type central nervous system stimulants release norepinephrine more potently than they release dopamine and serotonin. *Synapse, 39*(1), 32–41. doi:10.1002/1098-2396(20010101)39:1<32::AID-SYN5>3.0.CO:2-3

Ruha, A. M., & Yarema, M. C. (2006). Pharmacologic treatment of acute pediatric methamphetamine toxicity. *Pediatric Emergency Care, 22*(12), 782–785. doi:10.1097/01.pec.0000245179.51535.ab

Russell, K., Dryden, D. M., & Liang, Y. (2008, October). Risk factors for methamphetamine use in youth: A systematic review. *BMC Pediatrics, 8*, 1–10. doi:10.1186/1471-2431-8-48.

Ryder, J. A., & Brisgone, R. E. (2013). Cracked perspectives: Reflections of women and girls in the aftermath of the crack cocaine era. *Feminist Criminology, 8*(1), 40–62. doi:10.1177/1557085112444899

SAMHSA, Substance Abuse and Mental Health Services Administration. (2014, April 3). *The TEDS Report: Gender Differences in Primary Substance of Abuse across Age Groups*. Rockville, MD: U. S. Department of Health and Human Services, Center for Behavioral Health Statistics and Quality.

Sato, M., Hida, M., & Nagase, H. (2004, November-December). Analysis of pyrolysis products of methamphetamine. *Journal of Analytical Toxicology, 28*(8), 638–643.

Savage, R. J., Durant, N., & Clark, C. B. (2015). The adverse effects of motherhood on substance use treatment program outcomes among adolescent women. *Journal of Addiction Medicine, 9*(6), 478–484. doi:10.1097/ADM.0000000000000165

Scafidi, F. A., Field, T., & Prodromidis, M. (1997, Spring). Psychosocial stressors of drug-abusing disadvantaged adolescent mothers. *Adolescence, 32*(125), 93–100.

Schabner, D. (2004, October 25). *Meth use by women on the rise*. Retrieved July 4, 2014, from ABC News: http://abcnews.go.com/US/print?id=185310

Schaneberg, B. T., Crockett, S., & Bedir, E. (2003, March). The role of chemical fingerprinting: Application to Ephedra. *Phytochemistry, 62*(6), 911–918.

Schepers, J. F., Oyler, J. M., & Joseph, R. E. (2003). Methamphetamine and amphetamine pharmacokinetics in oral fluid and plasma after controlled oral methamphetamine administration to human volunteers. *Clinical Chemistry, 49*(1), 121–132. doi:10.1373/49.1.121

Schierenberg, A., van Amsterdam, J., & van Den Brink, W. (2012, December). Efficacy of contingency management for cocaine dependence treatment: A review of the evidence. *Current Drug Abuse Reviews, 5*(4), 320–331.

Schiller, C., & Allen, P. J. (2005). Follow-up of infants prenatally exposed to cocaine. *Pediatric Nursing, 31*(5), 427–436.

Schmitz, J. M., Lindsay, J. A., & Green, C. E. (2009, September–October). High-dose naltrexone therapy for cocaine-alcohol dependence. *The American Journal on Addictions, 18*(5), 356–362. doi:10.3109/10550490903077929

Schneider, K. E., Krawczyk, N., & Xuan, Z. (2018, February 1). Past 15-year tends in lifetime cocaine use among US high school students. *Drug and Alcohol Dependence, 183*, 69–72. doi:10.1016/j.drugalcdep.2017.10.028

Schottenfeld, R. S., Moore, B., & Pantalon, M. V. (2011, October 1). Contingency management with community reinforcement approach or twelve-step facilitation drug counseling for cocaine dependent pregnant women or women with young children. *Drug and Alcohol Dependence, 118*(1), 48–55. doi:10.1016/j.drugalcdep.2011.02.019

Schulenberg, J. E., Johnston, L. D., & O'Malley, P. M. (2017). *Monitoring the Future National Survey Results on Drug Use, 1975–2016: Volume II, College Students and Adults Ages* (pp. 19–55). Ann Arbor, MI: Institute for Social Research, The University of Michigan.

Schulzke, E. (2013, May 24). *Mothers on meth: New book highlights family struggles in the suburbs.* Retrieved July 4, 2014, from Deseret News: https://www.deseretnews.com/article/865580620/Mothers-on-meth-New-book-highlights-family-struggles-in-the-suburbs.html

Schumacher, J. E., Milby, J. B., & Wallace, D. (2003, May). Diagnostic compared with abstinence outcomes of day treatment and contingency management among cocaine-dependent homeless persons. *Experimental and Clinical Psychopharmacology, 11*(2), 146–157.

Schwartz, C. (2016, October 12). Generation Adderall. *The New York Times*, 1–12. Retrieved from https://nyti.ms/2dVnYcF

Schwarz, A. (2012, June 12). Risky rise of the good-grade pill. *The New York Times*, A1–A11. The New York Times.

Semple, S. J., Strathdee, S. A., & Zians, J. (2011). Correlates of trading sex for methamphetamine in a sample of HIV-negative heterosexual methamphetamine users. *Journal of Psychoactive Drugs, 43*(2), 79–88.

Semple, S. J., Strathdee, S. A., & Zians, J. (2012). Correlates of drug dealing in female methamphetamine users. *Journal of Urban Health: Bulletin of the New York Academy of Medicine, 90*(3), 529–541. doi:10.1007/s11524-012-9748-9

Sepulveda, D. R., Thomas, L. M., & McCabe, S. E. (2011). Misuse of prescribed stimulant medication for ADHD and associated patterns of substance use: Preliminary analysis among college students. *Journal of Pharmacy Practice, 24*(6), 551–560. doi:10.1177/0897190011426558

Seth, P., Scholl, L., & Rudd, R. A. (2018, March 30). Overdose deaths involving opioids, cocaine, and psychostimulants —United States, 2015–2016. *MMWR, Morbidity and Mortality Weekly Report, 67*(12), 349–358.

Sewell, J., Miltz, A., & Lampe, F. C. (2017, May). Poly drug use, chemsex drug use, and associations with sexual risk behaviour in HIV-negative men who have sex with men attending sexual health clinics. *The International Journal of Drug Policy, 43*, 33–43. doi:10.1016/j.drugpo.2017.01.001

Sexton, R. L., Carlson, R. G., & Siegal, H. (2006). The role of African-American clergy in providing informal services to drug users in the rural South: Preliminary ethnographic findings. *Journal of Ethnicity in Substance Abuse, 5*(1), 1–21. doi:10.1300/J233v05n01_01

Shah, R., Patel, A., & Mousa, O. (2015). Crack lung: Cocaine-induced lung injury. *QJM: an International Journal of Medicine, 108*(9), 749. doi:10.1093/qjmed/hcv064

Shake and Bake or One Pot Meth Making. (n.d.). Retrieved November 2, 2016, from Some Chick's Blog All About Meth, pp. 1–11: http://somechicksblog.com/make-meth/shake-and-bake-or-one-pot-meth-making

Sharpe, T. T. (2001). Sex-for-crack-cocaine exchange, poor black women, and pregnancy. *Qualitative Health Research, 11*(5), 612–630.

Shin, E. J., Tran, H. Q., & Nguyen, P. T. (2017, June 7). Role of mitochondria in methamphetamine-induced dopaminergic neurotoxicity: Involvement in oxidative stress, neuroinflammation, and pro-apoptosis—A review. *Neurochemical Research.* doi:10.1007/s11064-017-2318-5

Shoamanesh, A., Catanese, L., & Romero, J. R. (2016). High prevalence of cerebral microbleeds in inner city young stroke patients. *Journal of Stroke & Cerebrovascular Diseases, 25*(4), 733–738. doi:10.1016/j.jstrokecerebrovascdis.2015.11.022

Shoptaw, S., Heinzerling, K. G., & Rotheram-Fuller, E. (2008). Bupropion hydrochloride versus placebo, in combination with cognitive behavioral therapy, for the treatment of cocaine abuse/dependence. *Journal of Addictive Diseases, 27*(1), 13–23. doi:10.1300/J069v27n01_02

Shoptaw, S., Kintaudi, P. C., & Charuvastra, C. (2002, May 1). A screening trial of amanatadine as a medication for cocaine dependence. *Drug and Alcohol Dependence, 66*(3), 217–224.

Shoptaw, S. J., Kao, U., & Heinzerling, K. (2009, April 15). Treatment for amphetamine withdrawal. *Cochrane Database of Sytematic Reviews, 2009*(2), CD003021. doi:10.1002/14651858.CD003021.pub2

Shukla, R. K., Crump, J. L., & Chrisco, E. S. (2012, November). An evolving problem: Methamphetamine production and trafficking in the United States. *The International Journal on Drug Policy, 23*(6), 426–435. doi:10.1016/_drugpo.2012.07.004

Singer, L. T., Minnes, S., & Min, M. O. (2015, July). Prenatal cocaine exposure and child outcomes: A conference report based on a prospective study from Cleveland. *Human Psychopharmacology: Clinical & Experimental, 30*(4), 285–289. doi:10.1002/hup.2454.

Skeberdis, V. A. (2004). Structure and function of beta3-adrenergic receptors. *Medicina (Kaunas), 40*(5), 407–413.

Skinner, H. A. (1982). The drug abuse screening test. *Addictive Behaviors*, 7(4), 363–371.

Smith, P. H., Homish, G. G., & Leonard, K. E. (2012). Intimate partner violence and specific substance use disorders: Findings from the National Epidemiologic Survey on Alcohol and Related Conditions. *Psychology of Addictive Behaviors, 26*(2), 236–245. doi:10.1037/a0024855

Sofuoglu, M., Poling, J., & Gonzalez, G. (2007, October). Progesterone effects on cocaine use in male cocaine users maintained on methadone: A randomized, double-blind, pilot study. *Experimental and Clinical Psychopharmacology, 15*(5), 454–460. doi:10.1037/1064-1297.15.5.453

Staley, D., & el-Guebaly, N. (1990). Psychometric properties of the Drug Abuse Screening Test in a psychiatric patient population. *Addiction Behaviors, 15*, 257–264.

Steiner, S., Baumeister, S. E., & Kraus, L. (2008). Severity of Dependence Scale: Establishing a cut-off point for cannabis dependence in the German adult population. *Sucht, 54*(Supplement 1), S57–S63. doi:10.1463/2008.07.07

Stoops, W. W., & Rush, C. R. (2013). Agonist replacement for stimulant dependence: A review of clinical research. *Current Pharmaceutical Design, 19*(40), 7026–7035.

Strathearn, L., & Mayes, L. C. (2010). Cocaine addiction in mothers: Potential effects on maternal care and infant development. *Annals of the New York Academy of Sciences, 1187*(1), 172–183. doi:10.1111/j.1749-6632.2009.05142.x

Swift, W., Copeland, J., & Hall, W. (1998). Choosing a diagnostic cut-off for cannabis dependence. *Addiction, 93*(11), 1681–1692. doi:10.1080/09652149834504

Tapscott, M. A., & Schepis, T. S. (2013, December). Nonmedical use of prescription medications in young adults. *Adolescent Medicine: State of the Art Reviews, 24*(3), 597–610.

Terplan, M., Smith, E. J., & Kozloski, M. J. (2009). Methamphetamine use among pregnant women. *Obstetrics & Gynecology, 113*(6), 1285–1291. doi:10.1097/AOG.0b013e3181a5ec6f

Teter, C. J., McCabe, S. E., & Cranford, J. A. (2005). Prevalence and motives for illicit use of prescription stimulants in an undergraduate student sample. *Journal of American College Health, 53*(6), 253–262. doi:10.3200/JACH.53.6.253-262

Teter, C. J., McCabe, S. E., & LaGrange, K. (2006). Illicit use of specific prescription stimulants among college students: Prevalence, motives, and routes of administration. *Pharmacotherapy: the Journal of Human Pharmacology and Drug Therapy, 26*(10), 1501–1510. doi:10.1592/phco.26.10.1501

Thanki, D., Domingo-Salvany, A., & Barrio Anta, G. (2013). The choice of screening instruments matters: The case of problematic cannabis use screening in Spanish population of adolescents. *Addiction, (2013*(723131), 1–13. doi:10.1155/2013/723131

Tobin, S. C. (2017). EEG indicates that cocaine relapse vulnerability peaks 1 to 6 months into abstinence. *National Intitute on Drug Abuse. Retrieved November, 5*, 2017.

Toce, M. S., Farias, M., & Bruccoleri, R. (2017, March). A case report of reversible Takotsubo cardiomyopathy after amphetamine/dextroamphetamine ingestion in a 15-year-old adolescent girl. *The Journal of Pediatrics, 182*, 385–388. doi:10.1016/j.peds.2016.11.038

Todd, G., Noyes, C., & Flavel, S. C. (2013). Illicit stimulant use is associated with abnormal substantia nigra morphology in humans. *PLoS One, 8*(2), e56438. doi:10.1371/journal.pone.0056438

Turillazzi, E., Bello, S., & Neri, M. (2012). Cardiovascular effects of cocaine: Cellular, ionic and molecular mechanisms. *Current Medicinal Chemistry, 19*(33), 5664–5676.

Turner, C. M., Santos, G. M., & Araytasirikul, S. (2017, March 1). Brief report: Psychosocial predictors of engagement in sexual risk behavior among trans*female youth aged 16–24 years in San Francisco. *Journal of Acquired Immune Deficiency Syndrome, 74*(3), 258–264. doi:10.1097/QAI.0000000000001246

Umbricht, A., DeFulio, A., & Winstanley, E. L. (2014, July 1). Topiramate for cocaine dependence during methadone maintenance treatment: A randomized controlled trial. *Drug and Alcohol Dependence, 140*, 92–100. doi:10.1016/j.drugalcdep.20124.03.033

The United States Attorney's Office. (2018, August 7). Man sentenced for smuggling liquid methamphetamine to Kansas. *Press Release*. Kansas City, MO: Department of Justice.

University of Michigan. (2008, October). *Monitoring the future: National survey results on drug use, 1975–2007: Volume II: College students and adults ages 19–45, 2007*. Ann Arbor, MI: Author.

Upadhyaya, H. P., Kroutil, L. A., & Deas, D. (2010). Stimulant formulation and motivation for nonmedical use of prescription attention-deficit/hyperactivity disorder medications in a college-aged population. *The American Journal of Addictions, 19*(6), 569–577. doi:10.1111/j.1521-0391.2010.00078.x

Vallersnes, O. M., Dines, A. M., & Wood, D. M. (2016, August 18). Psychosis associated with acute recreational drug toxicity: A European case series. *BMC Psychiatry, 16*, 293. doi:10.1186/s12888-016-1002-7

van der Pol, P., Liebregts, N., & de Graaf, R. (2013, June). Reliability and validity of the Severity of Dependence Scale for detecting cannabis dependence in frequent cannabis users. *International Journal of Methods in Psychiatric Research, 22*(2), 138–143. doi:10.1002/mpr.1385

Varga, M. D. (2012). Adderall abuse on college campuses: A comprehensive literature review. *Journal of Evidence-Based Social Work, 9*(3), 293–313. doi:10.1080/15433714.2010.525402

Veliz, P., Boyd, C., & McCabe, S. E. (2013, September). Adolescent athletic participation and nonmedical Adderall use: An exploratory analysis of a performance-enhancing drug. *Journal of Studies on Alcohol and Drugs, 74*(5), 714–719.

Vidaeff, A. C., & Mastrobattista, J. M. (2003). In utero cocaine exposure: A thorny mix of science and mythology. *American Journal of Perinatology, 20*(4), 165–172.

Vilela, R. J., Langford, C., & McCullagh, L. (2002). Cocaine-induced oronasal fistulas with external nasal erosion but without palate involvement. *Ear, Nose, & Throat Journal, 81*(8), 562–563.

Viteri, O. A., Soto, E. E., & Bahado-Singh, R. A. (2015). Fetal anomalies and long-term effects associated with substance abuse in pregnancy: A literature review. *Amercian Journal of Perinatology, 32*(5), 405–416. doi:10.1055/s-0034-1393932

Vocci, F. J., & Montoya, I. D. (2009, May). Psychological treatments for stimulant misuse, comparing and contrasting those for amphetamine dependence and those for cocaine dependence. *Current Opinion in Psychiatry, 22*(3), 263–268. doi:10.1097/YCO.0b013e32832a3b44

Walsh, S. L., Stoops, W. W., & Moody, D. E. (2009). Repeated dosing with oral cocaine in humans: Assessment of direct effects, withdrawal, and pharmacokinetics. *Experimental and Clinical Psychopharmacology, 17*(4), 205–216. doi:10.1037/a0016469

Wang, R. Y. (1999). pH-dependent cocaine-induced cardiotoxicity. *The American Journal of Emergency Medicine, 17*(4), 364–369.

Watanabe-Galloway, S., Ryan, S., & Hansen, K. (2009). Effects of methamphetamine abuse beyond individual users. *Journal of Psychoactive Drugs, 41*(3), 241–248.

Wechsberg, W. M., Lam, W. K., & Zule, W. (2003). Violence, homelessness, and HIV risk among crack-using African-American women. *Substance Use & Misuse, 38*(3–6), 669–700.

West, P., McKeown, N. J., & Hendrickson, R. G. (2010). Methamphetamine body stuffers: An observational case series. *Annals of Emergency Medicine, 55*(2), 190–197. doi:10.1016/j.annemergmed.2009.08.005

Weyandt, L. L., Marraccini, M. E., & Gudmundsdottir, B. G. (2013, October). Misuse of prescription stimulants among college students: A review of the literature and implications for morphological and cognitive effects on brain functioning. *Experimental & Clinical Psychopharmacology, 21*(5), 385–407. doi:10.1037/a0034013

Wiegand, T., Wax, P., & Smith, E. (2013). The Toxicology Investigators Consortium Case Registry—The 2012 experience. *Journal of Medical Toxicology, 9*, 380–404. doi:10.1007/s13181-013-0352-5

Wilens, T. E., Adler, L. A., & Adams, J. (2008). Misuse and diversion of stimulants prescribed for ADHD: A systematic review of the literature. *Journal of the American Academy of Child & Adolescent Psychiatry, 47*(1), 21–31. doi:10.1097/chi.0b013e31815a56f1

Wilson, D., & Shiffman, J. (2015). Newborns die after being sent home with mothers struggling to kick drug addictions. *Lehighton: Reuters. Retrieved February, 10*, 2019.

Winhusen, T., & Lewis, D. (2013). Sex differences in disinhibition and its relationship to physical abuse in a sample of stimulant-dependent patients. *Drug and Alcohol Dependence, 129*(1–2), 158–162. doi:10.1016/j.drugalcdep.2012.09.014

Winhusen, T., Somoza, E., & Ciraulo, D. A. (2007, December 1). A double-blind, placebo-controlled trial of tiagabine for the treatment of cocaine dependence. *Drug and Alcohol Dependence, 91*(2–3), 141–148. doi:10.210216/j.drugalcdep.2007.05.028

Winhusen, T., Somoza, E., & Sarid-Segal, O. (2007, December 1). A double-blind, placebo-controlled trial of reserpine for the treatment of cocaine dependence. *Drug and Alcohol Dependence, 91*(2–3), 205–212. doi:10.1016/j.drugalcdep.2007.05.021

Winslow, B. T., Voorhees, K. I., & Pehl, K. A. (2007). Methamphetamine abuse. *American Family Physician, 76*(8), 1169–1174.

Wise, B. K., Cuffe, S. P., & Fischer, T. (2001, October). Dual diagnosis and successful participation of adolescents in substance abuse treatment. *Journal of Substance Abuse Treatment, 21*(3), 161–165.

Wolf, A. (2015, August 31). The risks of Adderall abuse in sports. *Fox 40*. Sacramento, CA: Fox News.

Workman, T. A., & Eells, G. (2010). Assessing the risks and issues: Prescription drug abuse on campus. *2010 National Conference for Law and Higher Education* (pp. 1–17). Orlando, FL: Stetson University College of Law.

Wright, T. E., Schuetter, R., & Tellei, J. (2015, March-April). Methamphetamines and pregnancy outcomes. *Journal of Addiction Medicine, 9*(2), 111–117. doi:10.1097/ADM.0000000000000101

Wu, L. T., Schlenger, W. E., & Galvin, D. M. (2006). Concurrent use of methamphetamine, MDMA, LSD, ketamine, GHB, and flunitrazepam among American youths. *Drug and Alcohol Dependence, 84*(1), 102–113.

Yonkers, K. A., Forray, A., & Nich, C. (2014, October 1). Progesterone reduces cocaine use in postpartum women with a cocaine use disorder: A randomized, double-blind study. *Lancet Psychiatry, 1*(5), 360–367. doi:10.1016/S2215-0366(14)70333-5

Yudko, E., Lozhkina, O., & Fouts, A. (2007, March). A comprehensive review of the psychometric properties of the Drug Abuse Screening Test. *Journal of Substance Abuse Treatment, 32*(2), 189–198. doi:10.1016/j.jsat.2006.08.002

Zapata, L. B., Hillis, S. D., & Marchbanks, P. (2008). Methamphetamine use is independently associated with recent risky sexual behaviors and adolescent pregnancy. *The Journal of School Health, 78*(12), 641–648. doi:10.1111/j.1746-1561.2008.00360.x

Zhu, H., Wilson, F. A., & Stimpson, J. P. (2014). Correlation between cocaine prices and purity with trends in emergency department visits in a major metropolitan area. *Journal of Urban Health: Bulletin of the New York Academy of Medicine, 91*(5), 1009–1018. doi:10.1007/s11524-014-9899-y

Zosel, A., Bartelson, B., & Bailey, E. (2013). Characterization of adolescent prescription drug abuse and misuse using the Researched Abuse Diversion and Addiction-Related Surveillance (RADARS) System. *Journal of the American Academy of Child and Adolescent Psychiatry, 52*(2), 196–204. doi:10.1016/j.jaac.2012.11.014

Zweben, J. E., Cohen, J. B., & Christian, D. (2004). Psychiatric symptoms in methamphetamine users. *The American Journal on Addictions, 13*(2), 181–190.

3
Caffeine and Nicotine

Caffeine and nicotine—the most widely used psychostimulants in the world[1]—are "natural" psychostimulants that are commonly used by adolescents and young adults to:

- Achieve a sense of well-being;
- "Fit in," or conform, with peers;
- Facilitate "cramming" for tests or studying;
- Improve sport performance;
- Increase attentiveness/concentration;
- "Just relax;"
- "Keep going" during a long day at school or work;
- Lose, or maintain, body weight;
- Prevent, or self-manage, the caffeine or nicotine withdrawal syndromes;
- Wake-up, or "get going," in the morning.
  (e.g., Cormier, Reid, & Hammond, 2018; Fulgoni, Keast, & Lieberman, 2015; Lieberman, Stavinoha, & McGraw, 2012; Pagliaro & Pagliaro, 2012)

In fact, adolescents and young adults often use these two psychostimulants together—drink a cup of coffee and smoke a cigarette: (1) before going to school or work; (2) during breaks between classes; (3) during coffee breaks at work; or (4) during or after a meal. Both caffeine and nicotine have interesting histories, botany, pharmacology, and patterns of use by children, adolescents, and young adults. We begin with "caffeine."

Caffeine

Caffeine, in the form of coffee (e.g., "Brew;" "Java;" "Joe"), is ingested world-wide by millions of people every morning upon awakening to "get them going," and during school or work breaks, throughout the day, to "keep them going." For many, coffee also is ingested throughout the evening—to complete an enjoyable dinner, relax from a hectic day, to keep awake while cramming for a test, to watch movies "till dawn," or to "party" with friends until late into the night. In fact, over 97% of the daily caffeine intake among adolescents and young

1 For an overview and discussion of two other psychostimulants, which are also commonly used by adolescents and young adults in the U.S., see Chapter 2, "Amphetamines and Cocaine".

adults is attributed to the ingestion of caffeine-containing beverages (Chen, Bell, & Browne, 2014; Mitchell, Knight, & Hockenberry, 2014; Somogyi, 2010).[2] These beverages include: coffee; tea; cocoa; and carbonated drinks, including colas (see the later related discussion in the Caffeine subsection, "Caffeinated Beverages"). Also popular among adolescents and young adults, are energy drinks and energy shots, which, much like colas, are sometimes mixed into alcoholic beverages (see the later related discussion it the Caffeine subsection, "Energy Drinks"). See also Table 3.1.

During the second decade of the new millennium, several researchers reported the following facts and statistics regarding caffeine use among children and adolescents in the U.S.:

- ~50% of children (two to five years-of-age) consume caffeine (Ahluwalia & Herrick, 2015);
- ~75% of children and adolescents (two to 19 years-of-age) ingest caffeine on a given day (Ahluwalia, Herrick, & Moshfegh, 2014; Branum, Rossen, & Schoendorf, 2014);
- Children and adolescents ingest caffeine primarily in the form of caffeinated beverages (Branum, Rossen, & Schoendorf, 2014; Tran, Barraj, & Bi, 2016);
- Primary sources of caffeine for children and adolescents, in order of contribution, are: coffee; tea; carbonated soft drinks; and energy drinks (Ahluwalia & Herrick, 2015; Drewnowski & Rehm, 2016; Martyn, Lau, & Richardson, 2018; Tran, Barraj, & Bi, 2016);
- Adolescents ingest most of their daily caffeine in the morning rather than the afternoon and evening (Martyn, Lau, & Richardson, 2018);

Table 3.1 Average Caffeine Content for Selected Caffeinated and Decaffeinated Beverages

Caffeinated Beverage	*Average Caffeine Content*
Brewed Coffee	65 to 200 mg per eight oz
Carbonated Sodas	25 to 40 mg per 12 oz
Chocolate Milk	2 to 8 mg per eight oz
Cocoa	11 to 15 mg per eight oz[3]
Energy Drinks	200 mg per 12 oz
Energy Shots	200 mg two oz
Tea	20 to 80 mg per eight oz
Decaffeinated Beverage	*Average Caffeine Content*
Decaffeinated Coffee	2.5 to 10 mg per eight oz

2 Less than 5% of daily caffeine intake in the U.S. is associated with the ingestion of foods, including chocolate candies and desserts and other food products to which caffeine has been "selectively" added—such as: beef jerky (e.g., Perky Jerky®); chewing gum (e.g., Jolt® gum); gummy bears (Energy® gummy bears); jelly beans (e.g., Jelly Belly Extreme Sport Beans®); lollipops (Javapop®); maple syrup (Wired Wyatt's Caffeinated Maple Syrup®); marshmallows (Caffex®); sunflower seeds (Energized® sunflower seeds); and waffles (Wired Waffles®).

3 Made with two tablespoonsful of cocoa powder.

- Rates of caffeine ingestion increase with increasing age from childhood through early adulthood (Ahluwalia & Herrick, 2015; Ahluwalia, Herrick, & Moshfegh, 2014; Pagliaro & Pagliaro, 2012).

An analysis of data from the *NHANES*, a nationally representative survey of the civilian noninstitutionalized population in the U.S., from 1999 to 2010, indicated that 70% of children (two to 11 years-of-age) and 75% of adolescents (12 to 22 years-of-age) "consumed caffeine" (Branum, Rossen, & Schoendorf, 2014). Overall, approximately 90% of adolescents and young adults in the U.S. use caffeine with 25% using it on a regular, daily basis. Generally, these adolescents and young adults consider caffeine to be totally harmless (Pagliaro & Pagliaro, *Clinical Patient Data Files*).

The FDA considers caffeine to be "generally regarded as safe," or "GRAS" (Wikoff, Welsh, & Henderson, 2017). However, caffeine, like other drugs and substances of abuse, is associated with several undesired, or harmful, effects and toxicities, including physical and psychological dependence. Although most mental health care professionals seldom encounter adolescents or young adults whose major presenting problem is caffeine dependence,[4] they often encounter adolescents and young adults who—in addition to using other drugs and substances of abuse—socially, habitually, abusively, or compulsively use caffeine.

Caffeine Plant Botany—Coffee, Tea, and Cocoa

Although caffeine is found in over 60 different plants, the major natural sources of the caffeine that is used in the U.S. are:

- Beans of two species of coffee, *Coffea arabica* and *Coffea robusta*;
- Leaves of one species of tea, *Camellia sinensis* (*Thea sinensis*);
- Beans of *Theobroma cocoa*, from which cocoa is obtained and chocolate is made.

Coffea arabica, which is native to Ethiopia, is now widely grown in Brazil and Colombia. *Coffea robusta*, which is native to Saudi Arabia, also is currently widely grown in Brazil, as well as, Africa and Indonesia. The caffeine content in a cup of coffee (generally, 65 to 150 mg) primarily depends on: (1) the type of coffee bean selected; and (2) its method of roasting. For example, *Arabica* coffee generally contains less caffeine than the *Robusta* variety and "dark roast" coffee generally contains less caffeine than "light-roast" coffee.[5, 6]

Camellia sinensis, a tea bush native to China and India, continues to be grown primarily in these two countries. Black tea, green tea, oolong tea, white tea, and yellow tea all come from the leaves of the *Camellia sinensis* plant. Fresh tea leaves contain approximately 4% caffeine and the average cup of tea contains approximately 20 to 80 mg per cup. The differences in color and flavor of these teas are due to their methods of processing and the associated chemical reaction

4 For various reasons, "caffeine use disorder" is not included in the DSM-5. However, both "caffeine intoxication disorder" and "caffeine withdrawal disorder" are included (APA, 2013). (For further related discussion, see the later caffeine pharmacology subsection, "Undesired, or Harmful, Effects and Toxicities—Physical and Psychological Dependence.")

5 The roasting process reduce*s* caffeine content (Somogyi, 2010). Thus, light roast coffee beans typically have 10% to 20% more caffeine per bean than do dark roast coffee beans. On average, roasted coffee beans contain between 1% and 3% caffeine (Pagliaro & Pagliaro, 2004).

6 N.B. It should be noted that additional caffeine often is added to augment the caffeine content found in coffee. Starbucks® significantly increases the natural caffeine content of several of their coffees. For example, a Solo Shot® of espresso contains 75 mg of caffeine, while a Caffe Americano® has 225 mg of caffeine, and a Pikes Place® drip coffee has 310 mg of caffeine (Appelbaum, 2017). Other coffee producers also commonly add caffeine to their products. For example, Maxwell House adds 1.5 times more caffeine to produce their MAX Boost® coffee.

(i.e., oxidation). Indian tea ("Assam" and "Darjeeling"—named after the regions in which they are produced) also are made from *Camellia sinensis*, but from a different variety of the plant (e.g., *Camellia sinensis assamica*). Although tea is the most widely consumed prepared beverage in the world, significantly more adolescents and adults in the U.S. drink coffee (Martyn, Lau, & Richardson, 2018).

Coffee and tea grow best in the "coffee bean belt," the area within 1000 miles of the equator, or the band that encircles the earth between the Tropic of Capricorn and the Tropic of Cancer. The well-known "Kona" coffee, grown on coffee plantations in the Hawaiian Islands, particularly the big island of Oahu, is the only coffee grown in the U.S. Most teas, sold in cans of loose tea leaves or packages of tea bags, are composed of various tea blends. Scents and flavorings also may be added to improve taste and to distinguish a brand or type of tea from another. For example, "Earl Grey" tea contains oil of bergamot, while "Jasmine" tea contains jasmine flowers or jasmine oil.

Theobroma cocoa, which is native to South America, now grows in several parts of the world, although South America, continues to be the primary source of cocoa beans. Cocoa is commonly ingested by children and adolescents in chocolate candy, cakes, ice cream, and hot chocolate.[7] In addition to cocoa, children and adolescents in the U.S., also ingest caffeine in the form of caffeinated beverages.

Artificially-Caffeinated Beverages

There are three major artificially-caffeinated beverages that are consumed in the U.S.: (1) caffeinated carbonated colas; (2) caffeinated energy drinks and shots; and (3) caffeinated alcoholic beverages. These artificially-caffeinated sources contain considerable amounts of caffeine because they are made with:

- Caffeine-containing extracts of the nuts of the *Cola acuminata* (i.e., guru nuts that are traditionally chewed by indigenous peoples of the Sudan for their psychostimulant effects);
- Guarana, which naturally contains higher concentrations of caffeine than found in cocoa, coffee, kola, or tea;
- Additional caffeine that is added during their production.

Caffeinated Carbonated Colas

Caffeinated carbonated colas are non-alcoholic, naturally or artificially sweetened beverages to which caffeine has been added or included as a natural derivative of the ingredients used in the preparation of the cola beverage. Carbonated colas typically contain approximately 40 mg of caffeine per 12 ounces of beverage.[8]

7 The generally mild psychostimulant effects associated with the ingestion of cocoa is primarily due to its generally low-level amount of caffeine (i.e., 11 to 15 mg in a typical 1-ounce chocolate bar). Other methylxanthines (i.e., theobromine and theophylline) found in cocoa also may contribute to the observed psychostimulation associated with the ingestion of chocolate.

8 It is interesting that carbonated cola drinks were initially referred to as "soft drinks" to differentiate them from those that contained high percentages of alcohol (i.e., "hard liquor"). During the late 19th and early 20th centuries, one of the earliest carbonated cola "soft drinks" produced in the U.S., Coca-Cola®, contained cocaine as its active psychostimulant until it was replaced by caffeine in 1903 (Pagliaro & Pagliaro, 2004). (See for related discussion, Chapter 2, "Amphetamines and Cocaine"). Although not yet available in the U.S., the Coca-Cola® company, in 2018, introduced in Japan a new carbonated drink product, Lemon-Do®, which contains between 3% and 7% alcohol (Adelstein, 2018).

Caffeinated Energy Drinks and Shots

Carbonated or non-carbonated, sweetened or unsweetened, "caffeinated energy drinks" (e.g., Monster®; NOS®; Red Bull®; Rock Star®) are, non-alcoholic beverages to which caffeine, vitamins, and various herbs (e.g., guarana, taurine) are added to improve alertness and physical performance—to provide additional "energy."[9] Caffeinated energy drinks typically contain approximately 200 mg of caffeine per 12 ounces of beverage.

> When to Drink: On the road, during lectures & study sessions, at work, while doing sports, playing video games, or going out day and night.
>
> (RedBull.COM, 2018)

"Caffeinated energy shots" (e.g., 5-Hour Energy®) are concentrated versions of energy drinks and typically contain approximately 200 mg of caffeine per two ounces of beverage.

Caffeinated Alcoholic Beverages

Caffeinated alcoholic beverages are alcoholic beverages to which significant amounts of caffeine have been added. The caffeine can be added: (1) during commercial production (e.g., Four Loko®; Joose®; Moonshot®);[10] (2) by a bartender while mixing a cocktail (e.g., vodka Red Bull®);[11] or (3) by the drinker (e.g., mixing a shot of Jägermeister® in a pint glass filled with an energy drink to create a "Jager Bomb"). When compared to the use of caffeine or alcoholic beverages alone, the use of caffeinated alcoholic beverages potentially increases the risk for alcohol dependence; binge drinking;[12] impaired driving; risky sexual behavior; and sexual assault (Marczinski, 2015; Marczinski & Fillmore, 2014).

Despite these concerns, adolescents and young adults, who choose to drink caffeinated alcoholic beverages (i.e., alcohol mixed with energy drinks), do so because they generally endorse the explanation that, "the experience of drinking alcohol appears to be more rewarding when combined with energy drinks" (Marczinski, 2015, p. 96). Specifically, these individuals reported that the ingestion of caffeinated alcoholic beverages "increased stimulation and alertness, offset fatigue from drinking, and facilitated drinking" (McKetin, Coen, & Kaye, 2015, p. 15). The reported "stimulation and alertness" associated with the ingestion of caffeinated alcoholic beverages was primarily limited to altered perceptions or interpretations (Marczinski, Fillmore, & Bardgett, 2011; Marczinski, Fillmore, & Henges, 2012). (For additional related discussion, See Chapter 1, "Alcohol.")

9 Of interest, a significant number of medical students reported favorable attitudes toward the use of cognitive performance enhancing drugs, including, "high caffeine products" (Kudlow, Naylor, & Xie, 2013, p. 360).

10 In November 2010, the FDA expressed concerns about the safety of these products and the commercial preparations were subsequently removed from the U.S. market. Four Loko® was subsequently reformulated without caffeine, guarana, and taurine, but maintained the alcohol content (i.e., Four Loko Bartender Series® with 10% alcohol and Four Loko Shots® with 35% alcohol). It is no longer marketed in the U.S. as an "energy drink."

11 The standard caffeinated alcohol cocktail contains a favorite energy drink/shot mixed with a favorite variety of vodka (Pagliaro & Pagliaro, *Clinical Patient Data Files*).

12 Interestingly, Watson, Sweeney, and Louis (2014) identified that binge-drinkers and caffeinated alcoholic beverage consumers both reported higher and similar measures of "sensation-seeking" and "drinking-induced disinhibition" behaviors—suggesting the potential interaction of certain personality traits with the psychodepressants and the psychostimulants (e.g., psychodepressants that "suppress" conscious fear of known consequences of behavior—STD infection, pregnancy, getting into fights—and psychostimulants that "encourage" such behaviors).

Common Misbelief: When you ingest energy drinks, you can drink all the alcohol you want, and you won't get drunk.

Although caffeine, as a psychostimulant, can reduce some of the psychodepressant actions associated with low blood alcohol concentrations (BACs) (see Chapter 1, "Alcohol"), as the BAC increases, the only thing that caffeine can do is to create a "wide-a-wake drunk" (O'Brien, McCoy, & Rhodes, 2008; Pagliaro & Pagliaro, *Clinical Patient Data Files*). In fact, the mental impairment associated with the ingestion of alcohol (e.g., diminished judgment and problem solving) are unaffected by any caffeine that may be ingested. Thus, adolescents and young adults, who believe this "Common Misbelief," and practice it, are cautioned that, as a "wide-awake drunk," they are more likely to engage in hazardous behavior (e.g., drunk driving; physical assault; unsafe sex), which may cause harm to themselves and to others (Bigard, 2010; Cleary, Levine, & Hoffman, 2012; Pagliaro & Pagliaro, 2012). Additionally, energy drink consumption by adolescents has been associated with subsequent drug use during young adulthood (Arria, Caldeira, & Bugbee, 2017).

Other "Specialized" Caffeine Sources

Three more recent products have been marketed for the convenient oral, inhalable, and intranasal delivery of caffeine:

1. "AeroShot® Energy," an orally ingested product that was initially advertised as an inhalable product;
2. "SurgeStix®," an inhalable product;
3. "TurboSnort®," an intranasal spray.

AeroShot® Energy, Surge Stix®, and Turbo Snort® were not developed as drug delivery systems. Thus, their production, in the U.S., did not require the submission of new drug application (NDA) data to the Food and Drug Administration (FDA) prior to marketing. Because of this "loop hole," related pharmacokinetic data, such as the effect of the associated methods of administration (i.e., oral ingestion, pulmonary inhalation, or intranasal insufflation) on the absorption of caffeine, are not available. However, to help to assure that health and social care professionals are aware of these products and their use, they are briefly discussed in the following sections.

AeroShot® Energy

To facilitate and quickly obtain a "caffeine fix," Dave Edwards, a professor at Harvard University, invented, "AeroShot® Energy." AeroShot® Energy, released for commercial sale early in 2012, is a small canister about the size and shape of a tube of lipstick. It contains 100 mg of caffeine combined with a mixture of B vitamins.

Common Misbelief: AeroShot® Energy is an "inhalable" form of caffeine.

This common misbelief began with the name of the U.S. company that produces AeroShot® Energy—*Breathable Foods, Inc.* The associated confusion that developed regarding the product's method of use necessitated a warning letter from the FDA (2012) expressing concerns over both: (1) labeling; and (2) safety issues. Specific concerns were related to the AeroShot® Energy advertising claims that:

- "Should be inhaled;"
- "Is not intended for people under 12" (which implies that it is okay, or safe, to use for tweens, adolescents, and adults);
- Might possibly be used "in combination with alcohol" (FDA, 2012; Jalonick, 2012; Jaslow, 2012; Roosevelt, 2012).

AeroShot® Energy is primarily marketed in and around college campuses in both convenience and campus stores as a novel, convenient, and readily available source of "breathable energy, any time, any place" (Aubrey, 2012). Each single-use canister delivers up to six "shots," or puffs, of a fine, green apple-, lime-, or raspberry-flavored—and calorie-free—powder-form of caffeine. As presented on the website for AeroShot® Energy (2017):

- Pull the colored cap to open, put the other end between your lips, and draw the powder gently into your mouth;
- No calories; No liquids; No limits; Each AeroShot® Energy delivers a unique blend of 100 mg of caffeine and B vitamins;
- AeroShot® Energy gives you the energy to go forth and conquer.

Thus, although promoted in the literature, and perceived by most users as a product used by pulmonary inhalation, AeroShot® Energy is *not* delivered to the lungs for absorption. The fine powder is released and delivered into the mouth along with the caffeine and vitamins. There it dissolves in the saliva and is swallowed and absorbed from the GI tract into the circulatory system (Aubrey, 2012). Once dissolved in the saliva, the caffeine also may undergo buccal, sublingual, and transmucosal absorption.

SurgeStix®

Whereas AeroShot® Energy does *not* deliver caffeine to the lungs by pulmonary inhalation for absorption, another non-prescription product does—"SurgeStix®." Designed, produced, and marketed to resemble tobacco cigarettes, a SurgeStix® delivers caffeine to the lungs in much the same way as tobacco cigarettes deliver nicotine. Created and marketed primarily with adolescents and young adults in mind, we also believe that the use of this product will also be attractive to children for whom use may prove particularly problematic. As noted by the SurgeStix® website advertisement retrieved from www.thinkgeek.com (SurgeStix, 2012, p. 1):

> You don't actually light *SurgeStix®*, that's too 1990, instead you bend them (like a glow stick) until you hear a snap. This will send the caffeine solution flowing into the filter-looking end. Wait five seconds for the "filter" to absorb the solution. You will notice a slight temperature increase as the solution reacts with the harmless chemicals in the "filter" which causes the caffeine to vaporize. Then, take a drag. Each "puff" will suck roughly 18 mg of caffeine into your lungs (and right into your bloodstream!) With about 10 "tokes" per *SurgeStix®*, you'll get 180 mg of caffeine in just a few breaths. That more caffeine than a really strong cup of coffee just by breathing. Ouch.

TurboSnort®

A "caffeine energy nasal spray," "TurboSnort®" contains caffeine in the form of "caffeinated herbs" (i.e., green tea; guarana; and kola nut) and an amino acid complex containing "creatine, glutamine, and taurine" (Castle, 2011). Like "AeroShot®" and similar energy products, this product—to avoid related FDA regulations and testing (e.g., the need to provide pharmacokinetic data)—claims to be a "nutritional" product, as opposed to a "drug" product.

The delivery device for TurboSnort® resembles many similar nasal pump devices that are used to deliver both prescription and non-prescription drugs to the nasal cavity. Data provided on the product labeling and website, state:

- Worlds' 1st Caffeinated Nasal Spray.
- Works Instantly with No Crash.
- No Calories, Sugars, or Carbs.TurboSnort® delivers one mg of caffeine per metered [dose] spray ... There are approximately 223 metered sprays per bottle. (About TurboSnort, 2014, November, p. 1)[13]

Caffeine Pharmacology

Caffeine, 1,3,7-trimethylxanthine, is a mild, natural psychostimulant. It was identified by the German analytical chemist, Friedrich Ferdinand Runge (1795–1867), who first isolated it from the coffee bean in 1819. The dose-dependent actions of caffeine first affect the cerebral cortex, the most sensitive part of the CNS, followed by the medulla oblongata. The spinal cord is affected last, and only after extremely high doses of caffeine are ingested (see the later caffeine subsection, "Undesired, or Harmful, Effects and Toxicities"). In addition to the CNS, caffeine also affects other body systems, particularly the cardiovascular and pulmonary systems.

Desired Psychostimulant and Other Body System Effects

The ingestion of caffeine produces such desired psychostimulant effects as: increased mental attentiveness; a faster, clearer flow of thoughts; and wakefulness without disrupting coordinated intellectual or psychomotor performance (Hindmarch, Rigney, & Stanley, 2000; McLellan, Caldwell, & Lieberman, 2016; van Duinen, Lorist, & Zijdewind, 2005). Subsequently, unlike most psychodepressants and psychodelics, the use of caffeine (as well as nicotine and other psychostimulants) can improve, under specific conditions, dose-dependent performance on vigilance tasks (Smith, 2002).

For example, in one of the few studies of its kind, Sharwood, Elkington, and Meuleners (2013, p. 1) evaluated the use of caffeine by over 1,000 long distance commercial truck drivers (both men and women) and its relationship to crashes that were attended by police. 43% of the commercial drivers consumed caffeine products "for the express purpose of staying awake." When compared to drivers who did not use caffeine to stay awake, the caffeine consuming drivers "had a 63% *reduced* likelihood of crashing."

The use of caffeine can also affect attention, learning, and memory in various ways. For example, the ingestion of as little as 100 to 200 mg of caffeine, or one to two cups of coffee, can sustain intellectual effort, including that associated with studying for a test or final

13 TurboSnort® is self-described as a "homeopathic formulation" (Castle, 2011) and, given its insignificant amount of caffeine per each metered spray (i.e., one mg), it is likely to be totally devoid of any actual pharmacologic activity—any observed response associated with its use is most likely due to a "placebo response." The manufacturer recommends, "2 to 4 sprays in each nostril to increase energy, alertness, and performance."

examination.[14] Primarily, by improving attention, it also can facilitate learning, particularly, among users who are tired, sleepy, or otherwise in a less than optimal state of attentiveness (Lorist & Tops, 2003; Nehlig, 2010; Pagliaro & Pagliaro 2012). In addition, caffeine may also enhance memory (Pagliaro & Pagliaro, 2012) and, as found by Borota, Murray, and Keceli (2014), and memory consolidation, that consequently, enhances performance for up to 24 hours after use.

In addition to its psychostimulant actions, caffeine also: (1) "directly" affects the cardiovascular and pulmonary systems; and (2) "indirectly" affects other body systems. Cardiovascular effects include: (1) a marginal increase in heart rate; (2) increased cardiac contractility; and (3) increased blood pressure, particularly diastolic pressure. Together, these three effects increase cardiac output. Caffeine also produces the dilation of the coronary arteries and, thus, increases the amount of oxygen that is delivered to the myocardium. These effects result in an increase in cardiac work capacity, or performance. By increasing cardiac performance, caffeine increases renal blood flow causing a mild diuretic effect (Maughan & Griffin, 2003). In addition, caffeine decreases blood flow to the brain by constricting cerebral blood vessels providing relief for both hypertensive and certain migraine headaches—conditions for which caffeine has been medically used for over a century.

Caffeine also stimulates the respiratory center in the lower brain stem, or medulla oblongata, particularly in response to functional changes in the body associated with disease or injury (e.g., respiratory depression associated with opiate analgesic overdosage). Caffeine appears to increase the sensitivity of the respiratory center to the stimulant action of carbon dioxide. This action, in turn, increases the volume of air that is inhaled or exhaled in one minute. In addition, caffeine also affects the smooth muscles of the bronchi resulting in mild bronchodilation and, consequently, making breathing easier and facilitating air exchange.

In a review of over 200 published meta-analyses, Herman (2017, p. 1) found several positive benefits associated with coffee consumption:

- Daily consumption of three cups of coffee—regular or decaffeinated—was associated with a 17% lower risk for all-cause mortality, relative to no coffee consumption.
- Caffeinated coffee was linked to lower risks for cardiovascular disease, coronary heart disease, and stroke with benefits highest at three to five cups daily.
- Caffeinated coffee was associated with lower risks for cancer and hepatic disorders.
- Both regular and decaffeinated coffee appeared to lower risk for type 2 diabetes.

<u>Related Professional Reminder:</u> Generally, meta-analyses, because of their very nature, "collapse" data across subgroups. Consequently, although the overall reported finding(s) may be factually correct—the possible occurrence of an "interaction effect" or of a "selective effect" within a particular subgroup—is left unaddressed and unanswered (e.g., "Would a different result have occurred if analyses included only: children; adolescent boys of Hispanic descent; or young adult women attending college/university?").

14 Hence, the rationale for the development and use of traditional nonprescription, solid oral dosage forms of caffeine (e.g., 200 mg NoDoz® caplets; Stay Awake® tablets) that have been available and used for over 50 years as aids to increase alertness and forestall sleep.

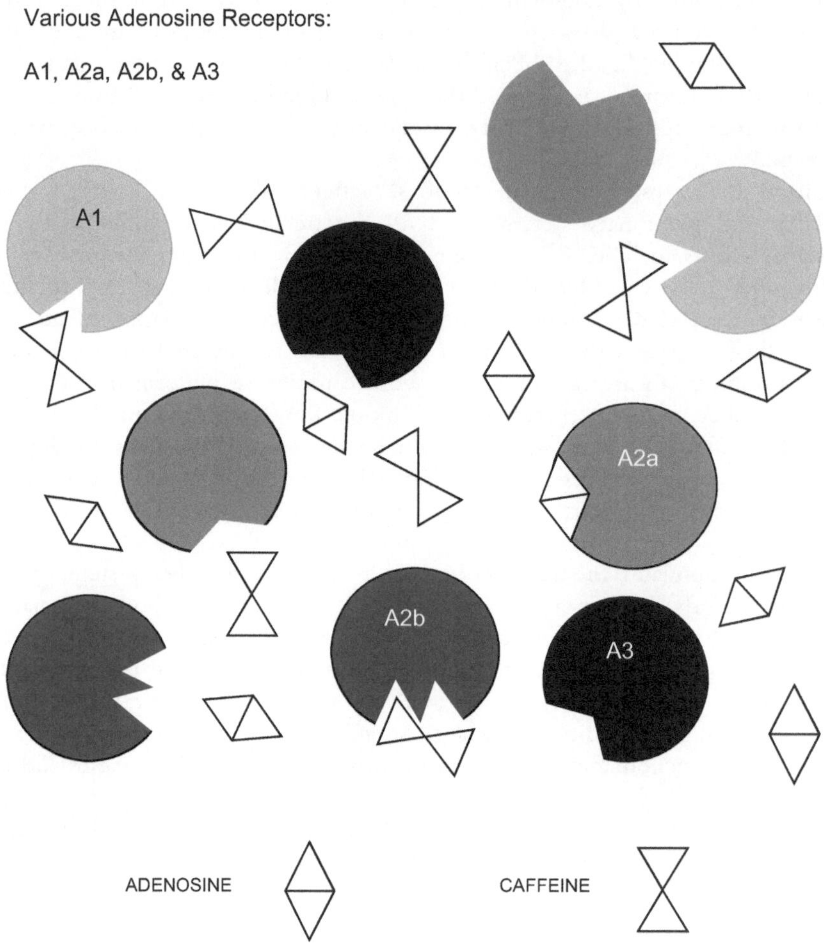

Figure 3.1 Caffeine: Mechanism of Action

Pharmacodynamics: Mechanism of Action

Caffeine, having no receptor sites of its own and being similar to adenosine in chemical structure, produces its psychostimulant actions by competitively binding to adenosine receptor site subtypes (i.e., A_1; A_{2A}; A_{2B}; A_3), which are present in the CNS (Nehlig, Daval, & Debry, 1992; Ribeiro & Sebastiao, 2010). These receptor site subtypes are found in many body organs, particularly the brain, where adenosine functions as an inhibitory neurotransmitter that promotes sedation. Acting as an antagonist, caffeine blocks endogenous adenosine and, consequently, the inhibitory effects of adenosine (see Figure 3.1).

The A_1 adenosine receptor site subtype is present throughout the brain with the highest density found in the cerebellum, cortex, hippocampus, and hypothalamus. The highest density of A_{2A} receptor site subtype is found within the amygdala, nucleus accumbens, olfactory tubercles, and the striatum (McLellan, Caldwell, & Lieberman, 2016). The A_1 adenosine receptor site subtype is coupled to "inhibitory" G proteins while the A_{2A} adenosine receptor site subtype is coupled to "stimulatory" G proteins (Temple, 2009).

The adenosine A_{2A} receptors are colocalized with the dopamine D1 and D2 receptors. "Presynaptic" adenosine inhibits dopamine and glutamate release by actions on adenosine A_1

receptors that are localized in nerve terminals. "Postsynaptic" adenosine causes an antagonistic interaction between adenosine and dopamine receptors that results in decreased dopaminergic activity (Solinas, Ferre, & You, 2002). Consequently, as an adenosine antagonist, caffeine is able to directly potentiate dopamine neurotransmission by stimulating dopamine release and potentiating the effects of dopamine receptor stimulation. (Temple, 2009).

Acting as an adenosine antagonist, caffeine blocks inhibitory actions of adenosine (Fisone, Borgkvist, & Usiello, 2004; Pagliaro & Pagliaro, 2009). Consequently, within 30 minutes of ingesting a low to moderate dose of caffeine, the following desired excitatory effects are produced, which can last for approximately three hours:

1. Heightened alertness, because of increased CNS neuron activity;
2. A sense of well-being, or mild euphoria, because of the increased release of dopamine.

ERGOGENIC ACTIONS

The use of caffeine has long been known to produce energy and endurance, which have often been associated with increased work output—particularly at moderate levels of ~3mg/kg (McLellan, Caldwell, & Lieberman, 2016). These actions have contributed to the establishment of the now traditional "coffee break" that, in the U.S., is inculcated at specific times during the day in almost every work setting.[15] Several possible mechanisms have been proposed to explain these effects, including the ergogenic actions of caffeine that:

1. Antagonize adenosine-mediated fatigue, pain perception, and sleep induction;
2. Enhance calcium release from the sarcoplasmic reticulum;
3. Enhance muscle metabolism by increasing lipolysis and the availability of free fatty acids (FFAs);
4. Increase epinephrine concentrations in the blood plasma
(Beedie, 2010; Davis & Green, 2009; Tarnopolsky, 2010).

Lower dosages of caffeine also enhance athletic performance by releasing more calcium in muscles allowing them to contract and relax more efficiently (Tarnopolsky, 2008). In addition, lower dosages of caffeine inhibit an enzyme that ordinarily breaks down cyclic adenosine monophosphate (cyclic AMP) to its inactive end product. The increased intracellular glucose production makes more energy available to allow higher rates of cellular activity. Thus, the use of caffeine can enable athletes to train at greater power output and can increase the speed required for running races (Graham, 2001).

As identified by Tarnopolsky (2010):

> Scientifically, the balance of the evidence indicates that the consumption of caffeine at 2–6 mg/kg before exercise or 0.75–2.0 mg/kg during exercise will enhance endurance exercise performance.
>
> (p. 7)

15 During the new millennium, a "new" related phenomenon was identified, particularly among adolescents and young adults—the increasing use of energy drinks to facilitate athletic performance. As identified by Ballard, Wellborn-Kim, and Clauson (2010), the "observed ergogenic benefits of energy drinks are likely attributable to caffeine and glucose content" (p. 107).

Caffeine was classified by the international Olympic Committee (IOC) as a "doping agent" (Keisler & Armsey, 2006) because of its ergogenic actions.[16] However, it continued to be widely used by athletes, particularly body builders and weight lifters, and several studies have demonstrated significant performance gains associated with caffeine use. For example, Lara, Gonzalez-Millan, and Salinero (2014) found that—for 18 young women, who were soccer players—the ingestion of an energy drink, equivalent to three mg of caffeine/kg body weight, resulted in a significant increase in their: (1) total running distance; (2) number of sprints/ bouts; and (3) running distance covered over 18 km/hr.

Conversely, other researchers have not reported significant performance gains. For example, Astorino, Matera, and Basinger (2012) found *no* significant ergogenic benefit in repeated sprint performance among young women athletes, when one serving of Red Bull® was administered at a dosage of 1.3 mg of caffeine/kg body weight. However, examining these two studies, it is obvious that the differences in caffeine dosages reported for each of the studies may explain the differences in reported findings. As well, other researchers also have postulated other reasons for the observed differences found in caffeine-related ergogenic studies. For example, the ergogenic effects of caffeine have been explained, at least in part, as a "placebo effect" (Duncan, Lyons, & Hankey, 2009).

Several major amateur and professional sports regulatory organizations (e.g., World Anti-Doping Agency [WADA]) established "urinary thresholds" for caffeine in order to distinguish between caffeine use associated with "doping attempts" and caffeine use associated with "social use." The criterion threshold value for caffeine urinary measurements was set at 12 mcg/ml. However, as emphasized by Del Coso, Munoz, and Munoz-Guerra (2011):

> The inefficiency of the urinary threshold to distinguish between the social use and the abuse of caffeine in sports forced the World Anti-Doping Agency (WADA) to remove caffeine from the prohibited list in January 2004. Currently, athletes can freely consume caffeine before or during competition without fear of violating the WADA Code or being penalized by anti-doping organizations.
>
> (p. 556)

Pharmacokinetics: Absorption, Distribution, Metabolism, and Excretion

Caffeine, in its various beverage, edible, and pharmaceutical forms, is usually ingested. However, within the last decade, several novel caffeine delivery systems and products have been developed. These alternative methods of caffeine use (e.g., AeroShot® Energy; Surge Stix®; Turbo Snort®) may affect the rate and extent of caffeine absorption, distribution, metabolism, and excretion (see the earlier caffeine subsection, "Other 'Specialized' Caffeine Sources"). However, most studies (e.g., Laizure, Meibohm, & Nelson, 2017; White, Padowski, & Zhong, 2016) suggest that, generally, the pharmacokinetics of caffeine are not significantly affected by the source of caffeine or its methods of use.

ABSORPTION

Following ingestion, caffeine is well-absorbed (i.e., 75% to 90%), primarily from the small intestine. Peak plasma concentrations generally occur within 45 to 90 minutes.

16 The IOC subsequently reversed this ban predicated upon a decision of the WADA in 2004 (see later related discussion in this subsection). However, it remains as a banned substance by the National College Athletic Association (NCAA) (Turner, 2018).

DISTRIBUTION

Following absorption, caffeine is distributed to all body tissues with an apparent volume of distribution of 0.6 L/kg. It readily crosses the blood-brain-barrier and the fetal-placental barrier. (See also the later caffeine pharmacology subsection, "Undesired, or Harmful, Effects and Toxicities—Pregnancy and Lactation.")

METABOLISM

Caffeine is extensively metabolized in the liver by the cytochrome P450 oxidase enzyme system, particularly the CYP1A2 isoenzyme, to three major active metabolites (i.e., "paraxanthine," "theobromine," and "theophylline").[17]

The mean half-life of elimination for caffeine is approximately seven hours (White, Padowski, & Zhong, 2016). Thus, for example, if an adolescent drinks a Starbucks® Grande brewed coffee containing 320 mg of caffeine in the morning on the way to school or work, half of the caffeine ingested from that beverage (in this case, 160 mg of caffeine) will still be working in the body at the end of the normal school/workday. This half-life of elimination is the reason why consuming caffeine in the evening (i.e., up to seven hours before retiring to bed) can result in one of the most common undesired pharmacological effects of caffeine—"insomnia."

The half-life of elimination may be increased by several factors including age-related changes in liver function.[18] In regard to adolescents and young adults, severe liver diseases (e.g., hepatitis C) can increase the half-life of elimination for caffeine to up to 100 hours. The half-life of elimination for caffeine also may be increased from seven hours to 16 hours among adolescent girls and young women, who are pregnant or who are using oral contraceptives (Temple, Bernard, & Lipshultz, 2017). However, the half-life of elimination of caffeine, can be significantly decreased for adolescents and young adults who smoke nicotine tobacco cigarettes, which can increase the production of the hepatic isoenzyme, CYP1A2 (Zevin & Benowitz, 1999).

EXCRETION

Less than 2% of ingested caffeine is excreted in unchanged form in the urine. The active metabolites of caffeine (see the previous "Metabolism" section) are further metabolized and are also excreted in the urine.

Caffeine Drug–Drug Interactions

Although, literally hundreds of drug–drug interactions related to caffeine consumption can be found in the published literature, these interactions can be reduced to: (1) pharmacodynamic drug–drug interactions; and (2) pharmacokinetic drug–drug interactions.

17 Children, adolescents, and young adults, who possess a variant genotype for the CYP1A2 isoenzyme, have a slower rate of caffeine metabolism. Consequently, they may be at increased risk for caffeine-induced toxicities such as hypertension and myocardial infarction (Meredith, Juliano, & Hughes, 2013). (See also the following caffeine subsection, "Undesired, or Harmful, Effects and Toxicities.")

18 For example, the half-life of elimination among neonates can be increased to over 100 hours because of immature hepatic function (Temple, Bernard, & Lipshultz, 2017).

PHARMACODYNAMIC DRUG–DRUG INTERACTIONS

Caffeine, as a psychostimulant, can interact with: (1) other psychostimulants (e.g., amphetamines; cocaine; nicotine) resulting in "additive" psychostimulation; and (2) psychodepressants (e.g., alcohol; opiate analgesics; and prescription sedative-hypnotics) resulting in the moderation of related effects.[19]

PHARMACOKINETIC DRUG–DRUG INTERACTIONS

Drugs that induce or inhibit the production of CYP1A2 can significantly affect caffeine metabolism and, consequently, its effects, because caffeine is primarily metabolized by the hepatic microsomal enzyme system, particularly CYP1A2. Primary "inducers" of CYP1A2 include: carbamazepine (Tegretol®); rifampin (Rifadin®); and tobacco smoking. Primary "inhibitors" of CYP1A2 include: cimetidine (Tagamet®); ciprofloxacin (Cipro®); ethinylestradiol; and fluvoxamine (Luvox®) (Horn & Hansten, 2007).

Undesired, or Harmful, Effects and Toxicities

Undesired, or harmful, effects and toxicities have been reported by approximately one-third of caffeinated beverage drinkers, including those who drink energy drinks and energy shots. These dose-related effects and toxicities are "directly" associated with blood caffeine concentrations, and include:

- Agitation;
- Anxiety;
- Chest pain;
- Dizziness;
- Dyspepsia;
- Fever;
- Headache;
- Heart palpitations;
- Hyperventilation;
- Insomnia;
- Jitters, or nervousness;
- Nausea;
- Tachycardia;
- Tremors;
- Vomiting.

"Indirect" effects associated with caffeine use, include: accidents and related injuries; motor vehicle crashes; and seizures, which are more likely to be related to the concurrent use of other psychostimulants—particularly, cocaine and methamphetamine (e.g., Mora-Rodriguez & Pallares, 2014; Peacock, Pennay, & Droste, 2014; Roemer & Stockwell, 2017; Wikoff, Welsh, & Henderson, 2017).

Whereas low to moderate daily caffeine use (i.e., the ingestion of less than 400 mg per day) is usually not associated with significant harmful effects or toxicities among healthy adolescents

19 In addition, adolescents and young adults, who regularly drink alcohol in combination with caffeinated energy drinks, are at significantly greater risk for becoming physically dependent on alcohol than are adolescents and young adults, who do not drink alcohol in combination with caffeinated energy drinks (Arria, Caldeira, & Kasperski, 2011).

and young adults (Nawrot, Jordan, & Eastwood, 2003), more serious toxicities are associated with high to extremely high daily caffeine use. Caffeine use also has been associated with cancer and cardiovascular disease.

LOW TO MODERATE CAFFEINE USE[20]

Undesired effects associated with low to moderate caffeine use are relatively minor and include:

- Anxiety;
- Diuresis;
- Excitement;
- Facial flushing;
- GI disturbances (e.g., abdominal pain; dyspepsia);
- Insomnia, particularly when caffeine beverages are ingested later in the day or prior to retiring for bed in the evening;
- Nervousness or restlessness (i.e., "the jitters"), particularly at the end of a busy work day during which caffeine beverages or other products were ingested throughout the day.

HIGH TO EXTREMELY HIGH CAFFEINE USE

High to extremely high daily doses of caffeine is usually associated with more serious toxicities. For example, the ingestion of:

- 12 or more cups of coffee a day (1.5 gm of caffeine) can cause intense psychostimulation characterized by: anxiety; cardiac dysrhythmias; headache; heart palpitations; hyperventilation; insomnia; irritability; tachycardia; and tremors;
- 20 to 50 cups of coffee a day (i.e., two to five gm of caffeine) can excite the spinal cord causing increased stimulation of the spinal reflexes;
- 100 cups of coffee a day, or more (i.e., over 10 gm of caffeine), can cause seizures and death. However, fatalities are relatively rare because of the large amounts of coffee, or other common caffeine-containing beverages (e.g., colas, teas), that need to be ingested. As the availability of energy drinks—and other more recently produced high caffeine-content products (e.g., caffeinated edible bars)—become more popular among adolescents and young adults, additional caution is required.

20 As recognized by Wikoff, Welsh, and Henderson (2017):

> Consumption of up to 400 mg of caffeine per day in healthy adults in *not* associated with overt, adverse cardiovascular effects, behavioral effects, reproductive and developmental effects, acute effects, or bone status. Evidence also supports consumption of up to 300 mg per day in healthy pregnant women as an intake that is generally *not* associated with adverse reproductive and developmental effects. Limited data were identified for child and adolescent populations; the available evidence suggests that 2.5 mg of caffeine per kg of body weight per day remains an appropriate recommendation.
>
> (p. 585)

CAFFEINE AND CANCER

Theories regarding the relationships among caffeine use and various cancers (e.g., breast; colon; endometrial; or rectal) have been widely studied for several decades. However, the preponderance of available published research data and reported findings (e.g., Dik, Bueno-de-Mesquita, & Van Oijen, 2014; Gierach, Freedman, & Andaya, 2012; Oh, Sandin, & Strom, 2015; Yang, Crowe, & Cairns, 2015) indicate that the proposed relationships, if they do exist, are tenuous at best and that any relationships found, are probably best accounted for by individual genetic and/or environmental variables.

CAFFEINE AND CARDIOVASCULAR DISEASE

The ingestion of low to moderate amounts of caffeine has not been associated with the increased risk for cardiac toxicities—even among adolescents and young adults who have pre-existing heart disease (Klatsky, Hasan, & Armstrong, 2011; Pelchovitz & Goldberger, 2011; Turnbull, Rodricks, & Mariano, 2017). However, high daily amounts of caffeine—usually in the form of the ingestion of coffee—may cause various cardiac toxicities, including: cardiac dysrhythmias; heart palpitations; and tachycardia.

Atrial or supraventricular tachycardia has been associated with the concurrent ingestion of various amounts of caffeine-containing products, including: candies, coffee, cola drinks, and teas. For adolescents and young adults, who are at risk (i.e., those who have a pre-existing heart disease, including dysrhythmias), low dosages of caffeine may be sufficient to cause these effects. However, in most reported cases, the caffeine doses are high (e.g., more than one pot of coffee daily) (Kinugawa, Kurita, & Nohara, 2011; Pagliaro & Pagliaro, *Clinical Patient Data Files*; Sanchis-Gomar, Pareja-Galeano, & Cervellin, 2015).[21]

During the past decade, the use of caffeinated energy drinks and energy shots by adolescents and young adults has resulted in an increased number of cases of atrial fibrillation. If not medically treated, this cardiac condition can progress to the lower chambers of the heart causing ventricular fibrillation and death.

Reported cases of caffeine-induced cardiac toxicity also have been increasing among adolescents and young adults, who do not have previous significant histories of heart disease (Di Rocco, During, & Morelli, 2011; Gunja & Brown, 2012; Seifert, Schaechter, & Hershorin, 2011). The overwhelming majority of these cases, generally, spontaneously return to normal rhythm when the acute ingestion of caffeine is discontinued. However, in some cases, it may be fatal (e.g., Artin, Singh, & Richeh, 2010; Mostofsky, Schlaug, & Mukamal, 2010).

> Fourteen-year-old Anais Founier downed two 24-ounce Monster energy drinks ... the Maryland teenager went into cardiac arrest [and died] ... Anais and her family knew she had a common heart condition called mitral valve prolapse, which caused one of the heart's valves to malfunction.
>
> (TODAY, 2012, p. 1)

In addition, the oily lipid components of coffee contain both "cafestol" and "kahweol." These components appear to raise serum cholesterol levels, which increase the risk for myocardial

21 See also the related discussion of the increased risk for cardiotoxicity associated with variation of the CYP1A2 gene, which is primarily responsible for the metabolism of caffeine (see earlier caffeine pharmacology subsection, "Pharmacokinetics: Metabolism").

infarction and cerebral vascular accidents (Butt & Sultan, 2011). This risk would be particularly significant among adolescents and young adults who both:

1. Have familial hypercholesterolemia;
2. Regularly consume large amounts of coffee daily.

***Related Professional Reminder:* Generally, no significant undesired, or harmful, effects and toxicities have been associated with the ingestion of 2.5 mg/kg/day (or less) of caffeine by children, or the ingestion of 100 mg/day (or less) of caffeine by adolescents. Consequently, according to the FDA, caffeine use is "generally recognized as safe"—GRAS.**[22]

Physical and Psychological Dependence

Common Misbelief: Caffeine has little, or no, abuse liability.

Not true. The regular, long-term use of caffeine is associated with both physical and psychological dependence.[23] Regarding physical dependence, both the development of: (1) tolerance to the desired effects of caffeine; and (2) a caffeine withdrawal syndrome—which occurs when: (a) regular, long-term caffeine use is abruptly discontinued; and (b) is immediately relieved with the resumed use of caffeine—have been identified. With physical dependence, preventing the occurrence of withdrawal symptoms may influence continued caffeine use. With the development of psychological dependence, craving becomes the primary reason for continued use and, generally, for those who wish to quit caffeine use, is the major reason given for resuming caffeine use (Pagliaro & Pagliaro, 2009).

Several specific terms have been used as diagnostic labels to denote the occurrence of caffeine physical and psychological dependence. These terms include, for example:

- Caffeine addiction;
- Caffeine dependence (WHO);
- Caffeine dependence syndrome (ICD-10);
- Caffeine use disorder (DSM-5 [included as a "condition for further study"]);
- Substance use disorder (DSM-IV).

Although, "caffeine use disorder," is not officially listed in the DSM-5, "Caffeine Intoxication" and "Caffeine Withdrawal" are listed.[24]

Common Misbelief: Caffeine is primarily a nutrient.

22 We would caution that, due to the possible stimulation of gastric acid secretion, any amount of caffeine use (e.g., ingesting as little as 12 ounces of a caffeinated cola drink) can be risky for adolescents or young adults, who have severe, untreated stomach ulcers.

23 A study of 94 regular caffeine users, who identified as being physically or psychologically dependent upon caffeine and sought treatment, reported a daily caffeine consumption range of 120 mg to 2667 mg (mean, 548 mg; median, 388 mg) (Juliano, Evatt, & Richards, 2012.)

24 Additionally, DSM-5 includes "Caffeine-Induced Anxiety Disorder" and "Caffeine-Induced Sleep Disorder."

Not true. First, caffeine is exactly like the other drugs and substances of abuse because it meets the general criteria required for this classification:

- Caffeine is primarily used for its major psychotropic actions (i.e., psychostimulation);
- Regular, long-term use of caffeine is associated with both physical and psychological dependence.

Second, caffeine—although commonly found in several popular beverages, foods, candies, gums, and other edible products—is not a nutrient and does not provide the body with any elements that are necessary for growth and the maintenance of life.

Tolerance

The regular, long-term use of small amounts of caffeine is associated with the development of a low degree of tolerance, particularly in regard to the psychostimulant actions of caffeine (Temple, 2009; Watson, Deary, & Kerr, 2002). Correspondingly, the regular, long-term use of large amounts of caffeine is associated with a high degree of tolerance.

Caffeine Withdrawal Syndrome

The regular, long-term use of moderate amounts of caffeine (e.g., approximately five or more cups of caffeinated coffee daily) may result in the caffeine withdrawal syndrome when caffeine use is abruptly discontinued (Addicott, 2014; Juliano & Griffiths, 2004). Up-regulation of the adenosine receptor system is suggested as the primary mechanism underlying the caffeine withdrawal syndrome (Meredith, Juliano, & Hughes, 2013) (see also the related discussion in the earlier caffeine pharmacology subsection, "Pharmacodynamics: Mechanism of Action").

The caffeine withdrawal syndrome is characterized by:

- Anxiety;
- Drowsiness;
- Dysphoria;
- Fatigue (marked);
- Headache;
- Impaired concentration;
- Increased appetite;
- Irritability;
- Muscle pain and stiffness;
- Nausea;
- Weakness (Addicott, 2014; Dews, O'Brien, & Bergman, 2002; Meredith, Juliano, & Hughes, 2013).

These signs and symptoms: (1) are generally mild and begin within 12 to 24 hours after the last use of caffeine; (2) peak between 24 and 48 hours after onset; and (3) are generally short-lived, but may last for up to one week.

The caffeine withdrawal syndrome is immediately relieved by the ingestion of caffeine (Pagliaro & Pagliaro, 2009). In the past, those who had relatively mild dose-related signs and symptoms of caffeine withdrawal, tended to manage them with a cup of coffee, "first thing in the morning," and periodically throughout the day while at home, school, or work. However, the caffeine concentrations now available in many beverages, foods, and other products contain several times the amount of caffeine that was available at the beginning of the new millennium. These sources of caffeine, particularly the more recently developed dosage forms (e.g., "Blast® caffeine powder" and various energy shots), contain such high amounts of caffeine per serving that they can produce blood caffeine concentrations high enough to result in a pronounced caffeine withdrawal syndrome if regular, long-term use is abruptly discontinued.

In fact, in the past, these blood caffeine levels would require drinking approximately 50 cups of coffee a day. Thus, mental health care professionals may be confronted with a new population that requires assistance with the prevention and management of harmful patterns of caffeine use. They also need to be aware that, like other drugs and substances of abuse, genetic and other factors may affect both the incidence and severity of the caffeine withdrawal syndrome experienced by adolescents and young adults. Mental health care professionals also are reminded that when helping adolescents and young adults who are trying to "cut down" or "quit" their use of caffeine, individual and novel treatment approaches may be required because of the following factors:

- Different signs and symptoms of caffeine withdrawal (e.g., dose-related moderate to severe effects; prolonged withdrawal period) that are primarily mediated by genetic factors;
- Multiple-drug and substance abuse withdrawal syndromes that may or may not be concomitant with caffeine withdrawal (e.g., alcohol; nicotine), and with each other, or otherwise related in ways that would affect positive treatment outcomes. For example, adolescents and young adults who have specific mental disorders (i.e., anorexia nervosa; anxiety disorders; MDD; panic disorder) have a significantly high correlation with caffeine tolerance and withdrawal (i.e., they possess shared genetic liability—see earlier related discussion) (Bergin & Kendler, 2012);
- Several unsuccessful attempts to decrease or totally discontinue caffeine use (i.e., several attempts to maintain resumed nonuse with several returns to relapsed use) (Juliano, Evatt, & Richards, 2012);
- Expense associated with the daily/weekly purchase of caffeinated beverages, foods, or other caffeine products;
- Persistent dyspepsia or gastric ulcer disease that are aggravated by the continued use of caffeine (Juliano, Evatt, & Richards, 2012; Pagliaro & Pagliaro, *Clinical Patient Data Files*).

Caffeine Overdosage/Unintentional Poisoning

Fatalities associated with caffeine overdosage are relatively rare (Temple, Bernard, & Lipshultz, 2017). When reported—generally in the context of "case reports"—the following features are noted:

- Most victims are middle-aged;
- The overwhelming majority of cases of fatal caffeine overdosage are associated with deliberate suicide attempts, usually involving the powder and tablet forms of caffeine rather than caffeinated beverages;
- The median fatal blood caffeine concentration is approximately 200 mg/L (Banerjee, Ali, & Levine, 2014; Bonsignore, Sblano, & Pozzi, 2014; Jabber & Hanly, 2013; Jones, 2017).

There are, of course, noted exceptions reflecting unintentional poisoning:

> James Stone, a 19-year-old from Wallingford, Conn., died in 2006 after he took nearly two dozen NoDoz® tablets. Each tablet has about 200 mg of caffeine.
>
> (Stokes, Fox, & Carroll, 2012, p. 1)

> A 16-year-old boy died from a caffeine overdose after drinking caffeine-laden soft drinks, coffee and an energy drink, a South Carolina coroner said Monday . . . "On this particular day within the two hours prior to his death, we know [he] had consumed a large diet Mountain Dew, a cafe latte from McDonalds and also some type of energy drink" . . . . The autopsy was performed and there was nothing there to indicate any type of . . . undiagnosed heart condition . . . [only] arrhythmia caused by caffeine.
>
> (Fox, 2017, pp. 1–2)

As noted by the SAMHSA (2011), regarding emergency department (ED) visits that involved caffeinated energy drinks between 2005 and 2009:

- Visits increased ten-fold to over 13,000 visits annually in the U.S.;[25]
- 52% of the visits (i.e., over half) by young adults, 18 to 25 years-of-age (36% women, 64% men), also involved other drugs and substances of abuse that, for women, were more likely to be pharmaceuticals, and for men, alcohol;
- 67% of visits were for undesired, or harmful, effects and toxicities that did not involve other drugs or substances of abuse.

Seifert, Seifert, and Schaechter (2013), in their analysis of energy-drink toxicities—in the context of related exposures reported to the U.S. National Poison Data System (NPDS) between October 1, 2010 and September 30, 2011—found that:

> About half the cases of energy drink-related toxicity involved unintentional exposures by children < 6 years old.
>
> (p. 566)

Additionally, it has been commonly identified that the introduction of energy drinks to the U.S. market has profoundly influenced the nature and extent of caffeine overdosage, particularly among children and adolescents:

> More than 5,000 cases of people who got sick from energy drinks were reported to the U.S. poison control centers between 2010 and 2013 and almost half of those cases were in children . . .
>
> Lipshyltz [Chair of Pediatrics at the Children's Hospital of Michigan] and his colleagues analyzed case reports from all U.S. poison control centers between October 2010 and September 2013. They found that 5,156 cases had been reported to the centers, with about 40 percent involving kids younger than age 6.
>
> (Ghose, 2014, p.1)

25 This trend has continued into the second decade of the new millennium. As identified by Mattson (2013), using data from the Drug Abuse Warning Network (DAWN):

> The estimated number of ED visits involving energy drinks doubled from 10,068 visits in 2007 to 20,783 visits in 2011.
>
> (p. 1)

As reported by Cleary, Levine, and Hoffman (2012), in a case series study of 11 ED visits for alcohol intoxication associated with the use of the caffeinated alcoholic beverage, "Four Loko®:"

> All arrived by emergency medical services (EMS) . . . patients were found in high-risk settings, with altered mental status on subway tracks, in public buildings, or parks after dark . . .
>
> (p. 67)

Additionally, the SAMHSA (2014) reported that:

- One in 10 energy drink-related ED visits resulted in hospitalization

The management of caffeine overdosage depends on its severity. Mild signs and symptoms of caffeine overdosage, such as anxiety, diaphoresis, dizziness, headache, increased heart rate, insomnia, irritability, mild heart palpitations, restlessness, and tremor, are generally self-managed, until the signs and symptoms resolve, by:

1. Discontinuing caffeine use;
2. Drinking adequate amounts of water;
3. Executing mild exercise.

More severe signs and symptoms (e.g., cardiac dysrhythmias; chest pain; seizures) require medical assessment and appropriate treatment in a hospital ED setting. Adjunctive pharmacotherapy may include, for example, the use of a: (1) cardioselective beta-blocker (e.g., esmolol [Brevibloc®]); and (2) benzodiazepine sedative-hypnotic (e.g., diazepam [Valium®]). There is no specific antidote for the treatment of caffeine overdosage.

New Millennial Trends in Caffeine Use

Medical use of caffeine, embryo/fetus and neonate caffeine exposure, and child, adolescent, and young adult social/recreational caffeine use are presented and discussed in the following sections. We begin with the medical use of caffeine.

Medical Use of Caffeine

Caffeine is used as a medical respiratory stimulant. For example, caffeine (generally in the form of caffeine citrate) is therapeutically indicated for the treatment of neonates, who are born significantly earlier than their estimated due date, and who are diagnosed with "apnea of prematurity," a respiratory condition characterized by a temporary cessation of breathing (Aranda, Beharry, & Valencia, 2010; Koch, Datta, & Jost, 2017; Lemke, 2002).

Classic pharmacologic studies of caffeine published during the first half of the 20th century confirmed the stimulant actions that were associated with caffeine use, including an elevated mood, decreased fatigue, and increased capacity for work. These studies also revealed that methylxanthines, such as caffeine, theobromine, and theophylline possess other important pharmacologic properties. These properties were exploited for many years in in a variety of therapeutic applications (e.g., treatment of COPD) that are now being generally treated with more specific and effective pharmacotherapy.

Embryo/Fetus, Neonate, and Infant Caffeine Exposure

This section presents and discusses fetal exposure to caffeine related to maternal use of caffeine during pregnancy. It also presents and discusses neonatal and infant exposure associated with maternal use of caffeine during lactation.

CAFFEINE USE DURING PREGNANCY

Caffeine has been associated with teratogenic effects among certain animal species, such as mice and rats (Nehlig & Debry, 1994). However, teratogenic effects (i.e., major congenital anomalies) have not been reported among neonates whose mothers used caffeine during pregnancy (Brent, Christian, & Diener, 2011; Browne, Hoyt, & Feldkamp, 2011; Pagliaro & Pagliaro, 2012, 2018; Wikoff, Welsh, & Henderson, 2017). The most commonly reported fetotoxic effect associated with maternal caffeine use during pregnancy is small for gestational age (SGA) live births (i.e., intrauterine growth restriction) among neonates born to mothers who daily ingested three, or more, cups of coffee (i.e., 300+ mg of caffeine) (Bracken, Triche, & Belanger, 2003; Hoyt, Browne, & Richardson, 2014; Pagliaro & Pagliaro, 2002; Rhee, Kim, & Kim, 2015).

In their comprehensive meta-analysis of data obtained from 53 published studies, 1966–2010, Greenwood, Thatcher, and Ye (2014) found significant associations between the ingestion of caffeine during pregnancy and the risk of: spontaneous abortion; stillbirth, and SGA. Hahn, Wise, and Rothman (2015), in their large Danish study, found that the ingestion of caffeine—during the first trimester of pregnancy—was associated with an increased risk for spontaneous abortion. However, the size of the relationship effect was small and not linear. In another meta-analysis of 26 related studies, published during the same year, Li, Zhao, and Song (2015) also found that the "consumption of caffeine and coffee during pregnancy seems to increase the risk for pregnancy loss" (p. 116). More recently, Herman (2017), following a comprehensive review of over 200 published meta-analyses of observational or interventional research into coffee consumption, concluded that:

> In terms of harms, high coffee consumption in pregnancy was tied to pregnancy loss, low birth weight, and preterm birth.
>
> (p. 1)

Consequently, to reduce any associated risk for preterm birth or low birth weight among neonates—however small—study guidelines, over the new millennium, suggest that the use of caffeine during pregnancy be limited to approximately two cups of coffee per day (i.e., less than 200 mg per day) (Food Standards Agency, 2008; Rubin, 2008).[26]

A positive trend in the U.S. during the new millennium appears to be that, in comparison to other adult groups, lower coffee consumption and, consequently, lower daily ingestion of caffeine, have been reported among women of childbearing age (e.g., Somogyi, 2010). As found by Chen, Bell, and Browne (2014), in their large retrospective review of pregnant women in the U.S., from 1997 to 2007:

> Most mothers stopped or decreased their caffeinated beverage consumption during pregnancy.
>
> (p. 2446)

26 If the mother has a history of miscarriage, we would recommend total abstinence from coffee and other foods and beverages that are high in caffeine content until after delivery.

However, as reported by Svikis, Berger, and Haug (2005) in their earlier study of "44 women seeking obstetrical care in an office-based practice:"

> Fifty percent of the women with both a lifetime diagnosis of caffeine dependence and a family history of alcoholism continued to use caffeine in amounts greater than those considered safe during pregnancy (>300 mg/day).
>
> (p. 2344)

CAFFEINE USE AND BREASTFEEDING

Following maternal ingestion, caffeine is transferred into breast milk and, subsequently is excreted during breastfeeding. The peak breast milk caffeine concentration (i.e., ~ 1% of the maternal serum caffeine concentration) is, generally, achieved within 60 to 90 minutes following maternal caffeine ingestion. Once the breast milk is ingested by neonates and infants, the caffeine is absorbed, distributed, metabolized, and eliminated. It is important to note that neonates and infants have a prolonged half-life of caffeine elimination when compared to their mothers (see also the earlier caffeine pharmacology subsection, "Pharmacokinetics: Metabolism") and depending on caffeine serum concentrations, may display: agitation; irritability; restlessness; and sleeplessness (Berlin, Denson, & Daniel, 1984; Oo, Burgio, & Kuhn, 1995; Pagliaro & Pagliaro, 2002; Ryu, 1985).

Child, Adolescent, and Young Adult Social/Recreational Caffeine Use

Coffee, and other caffeinated beverages and food products, are deliberately selected and ingested by children, adolescents, and young adults across the U.S. and are used for various reasons. As previously reported, it is estimated that, in the U.S., approximately 90% of the population, 18 years-of-age and older, ingest caffeine products daily with males, on average, ingesting one-third more than females.[27] Mitchell, Knight, and Hockenberry (2014) also found that males, on average, ingest more milligrams of caffeine daily in comparison to females. However, after adjusting for body weight (i.e., mg/kg), the daily ingestion of caffeine was actually higher for women. Regardless, for all groups, including adolescents and young adults, coffee is the major contributor to daily caffeine use.

CHILD CAFFEINE EXPOSURE AND USE

Definitive national surveys and research studies that examine caffeine consumption among children in the U.S. are currently lacking. The research design and ethical difficulties in conducting research studies involving children are readily self-apparent and include:

- Access to a sufficiently large representative sample of children one to 10 years-of-age, particularly including those under five years-of-age, who have not yet begun attendance at public grammar school;
- Obtaining appropriate consent from all involved including, for example, child participants, parent(s) or legal guardians, school administrators, and universities;

27 Even when including those two years-of-age or older, the % of the U.S. population that consumes at least one caffeinated beverage on a daily basis, remains quite high (i.e., ~ 85%). For example, among those two to five years of age, the mean is 43% while, for those over 65 years-of-age, the mean is 99% (Mitchell, Knight, & Hockenberry, 2014).

- Reliance on self-reports;
- Accuracy of estimates of total caffeine intake from a variety of generally unstandardized caffeine sources (e.g., caffeine content differs from coffee to carbonated coca drinks as well as from coffee type or brand to coffee type or brand and from soft drink brand to soft drink brand).

However, even with these challenges, some limited data are available. For example: Mitchell, Knight, and Hockenberry (2014), in their study utilizing a naturally representative sample from the *Kantar World Panel (KWP) Beverage Consumption Panel Survey* of caffeinated beverage consumers in the U.S. two years-of-age or older, found that:

- Among caffeinated beverage consumers two to five years-of-age:
  - Approximately 25 mg of caffeine was consumed daily;
  - The primary source of caffeine was tea.

- Among caffeinated beverage consumers six to 12 years-of-age:
  - Approximately 35 mg of caffeine was consumed daily;
  - The primary source of caffeine was from carbonated soft drinks.

Branum, Rossen, and Schoendorf (2014), in their study[28] of caffeine consumption from all sources (i.e., various beverages and foods), found that:

1. Approximately 73% of children consumed caffeine on a given day;
2. Percentage of consumers increased from 1999 to 2010: by 63% among children two to five years-of-age; and by 75% among older children and adolescents;
3. Coffee, as a percent of caffeine consumption among children and adolescents, from 1999 to 2010, increased from 10% to 24%;
4. Energy drinks, as a percentage of caffeine consumption among children and adolescents, from 1999 to 2010, increased from 0% to 6%;
5. Among children two to five years-of-age: approximately 65% consume caffeine with a mean caffeine intake of 16 mg/day;
6. Among children six to 11 years-of-age: approximately 75% consume caffeine with a mean caffeine intake of 32 mg/day;
7. The main source of caffeine intake for children, five to 11 years-of-age, is carbonated soda drinks.

Burnham, Matiak, and Makrigiorgos (2015), in a study of 315 mother-infant dyads to determine coffee consumption among infants and children in Boston less than two years-of-age, found that:

- 2.5% of one-year-olds had consumed coffee;
- 15% of two-year-olds consumed coffee with approximately one out of seven drinking ½ cup (i.e., four ounces) of coffee daily.

28 This study analyzed data, which were obtained annually from the *National Health and Nutrition Examination Study* (NHANES) for the years 1999–2010, to examine associated caffeine consumption and usage patterns. The NHANES is a nationally representative survey, which is composed of an interview at home followed by a telephone interview, of subjects from the civilian, noninstitutionalized population in the U.S.

Variables associated with coffee consumption at two years-of-age included:

- Breastfeeding at one year-of-age;
- Infant female gender;
- Lower maternal education;
- Maternal Hispanic ethnicity;
- Non-U.S. maternal place of birth.

> Alicia Diaz started drinking coffee at age 2, sitting on her dad's lap and stealing sips of his café Cubano.
>
> (McGinnis, 2018, p. 1)

> Kamyra L. Harding never gives her son coffee or soda, and rarely opts for treats such as chocolate cupcakes. But about twice a month, the mom does give in to her 4-year-old son Garrett David Brand's request for a Chai tea latte from Starbucks [95 mg caffeine].
>
> (Linn, 2007, p. 1)

Common Misbelief: Adolescents drink coffee primarily to "calm down" and "relax."

Not true. Generally, adolescents, who say that they drink coffee "to calm down and relax," are actually most likely drinking coffee to relieve the common signs and symptoms of the caffeine withdrawal syndrome (see the earlier caffeine pharmacology subsection, "Physical and Psychological Dependence—Caffeine Withdrawal Syndrome"). In fact, among adolescents who are regular, coffee drinkers, this statement signifies that they are probably physically dependent on caffeine and that their attempts "to calm down and relax" are, actually, an attempt to manage the signs and symptoms of caffeine withdrawal (i.e., because caffeine is a psychostimulant, it is counter-intuitive to think that it would "calm users down"—unless they are experiencing withdrawal).

ADOLESCENT SOCIAL/RECREATIONAL CAFFEINE USE

Temple, Dewey, and Briatico (2010), in their survey of 52 adolescents (12 to 17 years-of-age) enrolled in local middle and high schools in Buffalo, New York, found that caffeine was used to:

- Increase athletic performance;
- Increase energy (get a "rush");
- Stay awake.

> The National Coffee Association is celebrating "the most robust increase in coffee consumption among Americans ages 13 to 18."
>
> (McGinnis, 2018, p. 1)

Two new millennial trends helped to maintain and augment coffee consumption among U.S. high school students:

1. Availability of attractive local coffee shops and expresso bars to stop in before school, during open campus lunch periods, and after school (e.g., Dunkin'®; Mc Cafe®; Starbucks®; Tim Hortons®);
2. Installation of deluxe coffee vending machines and specialized coffee shops within many large high schools (Pagliaro & Pagliaro, *Clinical Patient Data Files*).

For example:

> Melody Esteves, 13, visits Starbucks a few times a week, often with friends. The New York City resident said she has been a regular since she was 11, often opting for white chocolate mochas [75–150 mg caffeine] or flavored iced tea [30–50 mg caffeine].
> Even some local schools are getting into the act, selling coffee to students with in-school coffee shops or vending machines.
>
> (McGinnis, 2018, p. 2)

The exact percentage of adolescents, in the U.S., who use caffeine or are physically dependent on caffeine, is unknown. However, it is estimated to be between 20% and 50% of adolescents (Pagliaro & Pagliaro, *Clinical Patient Data Files*).

COLLEGE AND UNIVERSITY STUDENTS

Analyzing data from a convenience sample of 1,248 college students, across the U.S., Mahoney, Giles, and Marriott (2018) identified several reasons for college student caffeine use, which are listed by percentage of endorsed responses:

- "Feel awake" (79%);
- "Enjoy the taste" (68%);
- Socialize (39%);
- Improve mental concentration (31%);
- Increase physical energy (27%);
- Improve mood (18%);
- Alleviate stress—"to relax" (9%).

Other Sources of Caffeine

The other major source of caffeine, for both adolescents and young adults, is energy drinks.

ENERGY DRINKS

Over the last two decades, caffeinated energy drinks (e.g., Monster®; NOS®; Red Bull®; Rockstar®), primarily, and other caffeinated beverages, foods, and products, have become increasingly popular sources of caffeine for adolescents and young adults. These products are "attractive" because of their:

1. Relatively high caffeine content when compared to common traditional sources (e.g., coffee; colas; teas);
2. Marketing and advertising campaigns that specifically target adolescents and young adults with promises of relief of fatigue and improved athletic and sexual performance.

(Oddy & O'Sullivan, 2009; Pagliaro & Pagliaro, 2009)

See also the related discussion in the earlier caffeine pharmacology subsection, "Caffeine Overdosage/Unintentional Poisoning."

In a meta-analysis of published studies involving the use of energy drinks among adolescents, Visram, Cheetham, and Riby (2016) identified that:

> Taste and energy-seeking were identified as key drivers [of energy drink use] and branding and marketing were highlighted as major influences on young people's consumption choices.
>
> (p. 1)

It is currently estimated that approximately 30% to 50% of adolescents and young adults (16 to 23 years-of-age) ingest caffeine-containing energy drinks on a regular basis (i.e., at least weekly) (Mahoney, Giles, & Marriott, 2018; Maynard, 2015; Poulos & Pasch, 2015; Seifert, Schaechter, & Hershorin, 2011). Use of these caffeine-containing drinks largely has been a phenomenon associated with the new millennium. In fact, the sale and use of energy drinks, alone, increased over 500% from 2002 to 2006 (Reissig, Strain, & Griffiths, 2009).[29] Over one-third of the annual U.S. energy drink market share is controlled by Red Bull® (Somogyi, 2010).[30]

Another contributing factor associated with the increased popularity of energy drinks is related to the assertion that caffeinated alcoholic beverages—or combining caffeine with beverage alcohol—enable users to drink for longer periods of time (Attwood, Rogers, & Ataya, 2012). Even if this assertion was completely accurate, this pattern of alcohol use would be associated with an exacerbation of AUD and other related disorders. (See related discussion in Chapter 1, "Alcohol.") Additionally, the use of alcohol mixed with energy drinks (AmED) has consistently been associated with an increased risk for such adverse consequences as:

1. Being involved in a physical or sexual assault—as a perpetrator or as a victim;
2. Driving a motor vehicle while intoxicated—or riding as a passenger with an intoxicated driver

   (e.g., O'Brien, McCoy, & Rhodes, 2008; Pagliaro & Pagliaro, *Clinical Patient Data Files*).

Approximately 33% of young adults report concurrent use of energy drinks and alcohol (Caviness, Anderson, & Stein, 2017). In comparison, using a large nationally representative sample of ~ 6,500 12th-grade students, Martz, Patrick, and Schulenberg (2015) found that approximately 25% reported concurrent use of energy drinks and alcohol. A similar percentage (i.e., 24%) was reported by O'Brien, McCoy, and Rhodes (2008) in their earlier study using a stratified random sample of college/university students, who were from 10 different colleges/universities and who reported alcohol use within the past 30 days. In a more recent study, Patrick, Macuada, and Maggs (2015) found that 27% of their sample of 614 second-year college/university students reported AmED use in the past 30 days.

29 The use of caffeinated energy drinks has become so ubiquitous that it is added to U.S. army rations to help maintain cognitive performance among soldiers (Lieberman, Stavinoha, & McGraw, 2012)—in a somewhat similar manner and purpose as providing amphetamines to soldiers and aircraft pilots during WWII (see Chapter 2, "Amphetamines and Cocaine," for related discussion).

30 In April 2019, in direct response to the popularity of Red Bull®—particularly among adolescent boys, the Sonic® fast food chain added a "Red Bull slushie" to its menu (Brown, 2019).

Regardless, the use of caffeine-containing energy drinks has been associated with an associated increase in several negative health outcomes, including:[31]

- Adverse cardiovascular effects (e.g., hypertension; tachycardia);[32]
- Aggressive behavior (e.g., bullying; fighting; truancy);
- Conduct disorder;
- GI irritation (e.g., aggravation of gastric ulcers; dyspepsia);
- Insomnia;
- Risk taking behavior (e.g., increased incidence or association with: cigarette smoking [see the related discussion in the following nicotine subsection of this chapter]; illicit psychostimulant use [see the related discussion in Chapter 2, "Amphetamines and Cocaine"]; unprotected sex).

(e.g., Leal & Jackson, 2017; Marmorstein, 2016; Owens, Mindell, & Baylor, 2014; Polak, Dillon, & Koch, 2016)

Assessment and Diagnosis of Caffeine Dependence, or Use Disorder[33, 34]

The assessment and diagnosis of caffeine dependence is limited in clinical practice by the social normalization of caffeine use in the U.S. (and other countries) and a lack of consistent clinical criteria for its detection. For example, caffeine use disorder is not listed in the DSM-5 (2012)—although "Caffeine Intoxication" and "Caffeine Withdrawal" are included.[35] For these and other reasons, there are, currently, no available valid and reliable quick-screen psychometric tests to detect caffeine dependence, or use disorder, among children, adolescents, and young adults.

Given the current lack of consensus regarding diagnostic criteria upon which to establish a formal diagnosis of "caffeine dependence," "or use disorder," among children, adolescents, and young adults, we recommend the use of the following basic three criteria:

1. Unsuccessful attempts to restrict or discontinue caffeine use—often due to signs and symptoms of caffeine withdrawal;
2. Continued caffeine usage despite risk for, or experiencing, undesired, or harmful, effects and toxicities associated with caffeine use (e.g., cardiovascular effects; nervousness);
3. Presence of the signs and symptoms of caffeine tolerance or the caffeine withdrawal syndrome (see the earlier caffeine pharmacology subsection, "Physical and Psychological Dependence").

Consequently, assessment and diagnosis mainly rely on clinical assessment, including a child's, adolescent's, or young adult's interview/history that addresses caffeine use. The

31 See also the related discussion of the undesired, or harmful, effects and toxicities of caffeine use in the earlier caffeine subsection, "Pharmacotherapy—Undesired, or Harmful, Effects and Toxicities."

32 This risk may be exacerbated among adolescents with eating disorders (e.g., anorexia nervosa) because of the high propensity for electrolyte disturbances associated with purging behaviors (Seifert, Schaechter, & Hershorin, 2011).

33 For a general overview of the clinical processes of assessment and diagnosis of the SUDs see the related discussion in Chapter 1, "Alcohol."

34 See also the related discussion in the earlier caffeine pharmacology subsection: "Physical and Psychological Dependence—Caffeine Withdrawal Syndrome."

35 The DSM-5 does, however, formally recognize a "Caffeine Use Disorder" as a "research diagnosis" that may be considered for inclusion in a future revision of the DSM. Similarly, the ICD does not include a category for "Caffeine Dependence."

diagnosis is often confirmed with the assistance of related clinical laboratory tests (i.e., toxicology analysis for caffeine blood concentrations).[36] Additionally, the use of "generic" quick-screen psychometric tests may be of assistance (see Chapter 2, "Amphetamines and Cocaine," for a presentation and discussion of these tests). As with all drugs and substances of abuse, individual "expectancies" play a major role in the initiation and continuation of caffeine use. For example, Huntley and Juliano (2012), who developed the "Caffeine Expectancy Questionnaire," found that:

> The frequency and quantity of caffeine use were associated with greater expectancies for withdrawal/dependence, energy/work enhancement, appetite suppression, social/mood enhancement, and physical performance enhancement and lower expectancies for anxiety/negative physical effects and sleep disturbance. Caffeine expectancies predicted various caffeine-associated features of substance dependence (e.g., use despite harm, withdrawal incidence and severity, perceived difficulty stopping use, tolerance). Expectancies for caffeine consumed via coffee were stronger than for caffeine consumed via soft drinks or tea.
>
> (p. 592)

Adolescent and Young Adult Treatment for Caffeine Dependence or Use Disorder

Empirically-based treatment approaches for caffeine dependence, or use disorder, are extremely limited because of a general "lack" of:

1. Formal, official recognition of caffeine dependence or use disorder;
2. Concern for the clinical significance of caffeine dependence or use disorder.

No pharmacotherapeutic approaches have been developed, demonstrated to be of use, or approved by the FDA for the treatment of caffeine dependence, or use disorder. Consequently, therapeutic intervention—with little empirical validation—has focused on psychotherapy/counseling approaches (e.g., Evatt, Juliano, & Griffiths, 2016). In our own practice, we have found cognitive therapy to be effective for adolescents and young adults, who are well motivated to actively address their caffeine dependence or use disorder. We

36 The DSM-5 criteria for the diagnosis of "caffeine intoxication" requires the identification of five, or more, of the following signs and symptoms in an adolescent or young adult, who has recently ingested a large amount of caffeine:

- Diuresis;
- Excitement;
- Flushed face;
- GI disturbance;
- Insomnia;
- Muscle twitching;
- Nervousness;
- Periods of inexhaustibility;
- Psychomotor agitation;
- Rambling flow of thought and speech;
- Restlessness;
- Tachycardia.

Additionally, the signs and symptoms must be associated with significant physical, psychological, and social distress (Meredith, Juliano, & Hughes, 2013).

also embed the following therapeutic auxiliary behavioral techniques as individually required:

- Use a diary to track date, time, and price of each caffeine purchase/use;
- Avoid coffee bars and expresso shops (e.g., Starbucks®);
- Limit caffeine (i.e., coffee, tea) use to specific locations and times (e.g., first thing in the morning at home);
- Substitute decaffeinated coffee (~ 5 mg of caffeine per eight ounces) for caffeinated coffee (~ 100 mg caffeine per eight ounces);
- Substitute caffeine-free carbonated soda (0 mg per 12 ounces) for caffeinated soda (e.g., ~ 30 mg per 12 ounces);
- Substitute milk chocolate (20 mg caffeine per 100 gm) for dark chocolate (40 mg caffeine per 100 gm).

Rather than obtaining complete abstinence from caffeine, our therapeutic goal is generally to reduce caffeine consumption to controlled levels and, consequently, significantly decrease problems related to caffeine use.

Contemporaneous Diagnoses[37]

In addition to caffeine dependence or use disorder, adolescents and young adults are also susceptible to concurrent alcohol and other drug and substance abuse dependence or use disorders, as well as, one or more other mental disorders and physical medical disorders. Together, these disorders comprise more serious and complicated contemporaneous diagnoses that often require more complex interdisciplinary mental health care planning and management (Pagliaro & Pagliaro, 2012; Riggs, 2003; Wise, Cuffe, & Fischer, 2001). For adolescents diagnosed with caffeine dependence, or use disorder, other mental disorders that are commonly involved in—or significantly correlated with—the formulation of contemporaneous diagnoses are:

- Anxiety Disorders;
- Alcohol Dependence or Use Disorder;
- Conduct Disorder;
- MDD;
- Nicotine Dependence or Use Disorder (Nicotine [Tobacco] Use Disorder, NUD);
- Psychotic Disorders (Schizophrenia).

We now turn to nicotine.

Nicotine

Nicotine is a widely available, and relatively safe, psychostimulant that is often "tried" by inquisitive children and enjoyed by adolescents and young adults across the U.S. In fact, as noted by the U.S. surgeon general—nearly nine out of 10 cigarette smokers in the U.S. first tried smoking before 18 years-of-age (USDHHS, 2014). However, the general method of nicotine use, "tobacco cigarette smoking," is identified as the largest single cause of

37 See also the related overview and discussion in Chapter 1, "Alcohol," "Contemporaneous Diagnoses Among Children, Adolescents, and Young Adults."

premature death worldwide and is estimated to kill more than five million people each year. As reported by the U.S. Preventive Services Task Force:

> Tobacco use is the leading preventable cause of disease, disability, and death in the United States.
>
> (Patnode, Henderson, & Thompson, 2015a, p.1)

As emphasized by Siqueira (2017) on behalf of the Committee on Substance Use and Prevention of the American Academy of Pediatrics:

> Tobacco exposure, whether through personal use, second- or thirdhand smoke exposure, or unintentional exposure, is the most important preventable cause of illness, disability, and death among adults in the United States.
>
> (p. e1)

Nicotine is only one of approximately 5000 chemicals found in tobacco smoke (Streller & Roth, 2014). Although it is less toxic than many of these other chemicals, it is the only chemical in tobacco smoke that is associated with physical and psychological dependence. We begin with the natural source of nicotine, the tobacco plant.

Tobacco Plant Botany

The tobacco plant (*Nicotiana tobaccum*), the primary source of nicotine,[38] is a member of the family *Solanaceae,* or Nightshade, which is indigenous in both North and South America—but is currently cultivated worldwide.[39] The principal alkaloid found in tobacco plants is nicotine—approximately 95%.[40] Nicotine is produced in the roots of the tobacco plant where it is transported throughout the plant by the xylem, particularly to the leaves (i.e., approximately 5% in the flowers, 13% in the root, 18% in the stem, and 64% in the leaves). Depending on the type and brand of tobacco, the concentration of nicotine varies from 15 to 20 mg of nicotine per gram of tobacco leaf (Malson, Sims, & Murty, 2001).

Nicotine, a natural occurring liquid alkaloid,[41] was first isolated from the leaves of the tobacco plant (*Nicotiana tabacum*) by two German students at the university of Heidelberg—Wilhelm Heinrich Posselt (1806–1877) and Karl Ludwig Reimann (1804–1872).[42] Finding the pure chemical salt form of nicotine bitter to the taste, they considered it to be a poison (Pagliaro & Pagliaro, 2004).[43] Later, nicotine was correctly identified as a psychostimulant.

38 Nicotine is also found in significantly lower concentrations in related plants from the family, Solanaceae. These plants include: cauliflower; eggplant; green pepper; potato; and tomato (Domino, Hornbach, & Demana, 1993; Sheen, 1988).

39 There are over 70 species of tobacco plants. *Nicotiana rustica* (i.e., Aztec tobacco; wild tobacco) has a higher nicotine content than *Nicotiana tobacum* and was used, primarily by ancient (e.g., Mayan) and rural, isolated peoples (e.g., Russian farmers/peasants). Current use is generally limited to some ethnobotanical shamanism (Pagliaro & Pagliaro, 2004).

40 In addition to nicotine, the tobacco plant contains another psychotropic, "harmine," a harmala alkaloid (Streller & Roth, 2014).

41 The nicotine naturally found in the tobacco plant is, primarily (i.e., > 99%), in the form of the levorotary (s)-isomer.

42 The plant and its alkaloid were named in honor of the French diplomat, Jean Nicot de Villemain, who brought the seeds and leaves of the plant to France from Brazil in 1556.

43 Nicotine can be harmful to humans (e.g., Rogers, Denk, & Wax, 2004) (See also the later nicotine subsection, "Pharmacology—Undesired, or Harmful, Effects and Toxicities"). Although, nicotine has been used as an insecticide, it has now been largely replaced by a related, and more potent class of insecticides—the "neonicotinoids" (Tomizawa & Casida, 2005, 2009).

Nicotiana tabacum, which does not grow wild in nature, is an annual herbaceous plant that requires cultivation. After the tobacco leaves are harvested, usually by hand, they are cured/ dried by air, fire, flue, or sun methods for a period of several days to several weeks. The leaves are then aged for up to three years to enhance their flavor and aroma.[44]

During the first decade of the new millennium, tobacco smoking, particularly cigarette smoking, continued to be the most common method of nicotine use. However, during the second decade of the new millennium, another method of use became popular—"e-cigarette vaping." The pharmacology of nicotine is discussed in the following subsections, with attention to these and other methods of use.

Nicotine Pharmacology

A tobacco cigarette usually contains 1% to 2% nicotine by weight. After smoking one to two cigarettes, the plasma concentration of neurotransmitters—particularly, noradrenaline, dopamine, and the amino acid, glutamate—increase significantly in specific areas of the central nervous, cardiovascular, and pulmonary systems. In the CNS, nicotine stimulates the cerebral cortex, where it causes increased cognitive activity with observed attention-enhancing effects (Hahn, 2015), followed by CNS depression.[45] It also stimulates the ventral tegmental area, where it causes the release of dopamine and further stimulates the release of glutamate. These actions, in turn, trigger additional dopamine release in the limbic system causing feelings of euphoria (Zickler, 2003).

Cardiovascular effects associated with nicotine use include tachycardia, vasoconstriction, and, consequently, hypertension, associated with the action of nicotine on the sympathetic ganglia, adrenal medulla, and aortic and carotid chemoreceptors. The actions of nicotine on motor neurons in the muscular-skeletal system lead to a marked reduction in muscle tone, associated feelings of relaxation, and a decrease in the muscle tone of some skeletal muscles (e.g., rectus femoris muscles of the thighs)—actions that are often reported by tobacco smokers. In addition to decreasing deep-tendon reflexes, nicotine also typically causes an increase in hand tremor and an alerting pattern on the electroencephalogram. These effects are thought to involve Renshaw cell stimulation in the spinal cord.

Pharmacodynamics: Mechanism of Action

The psychostimulant action of nicotine is dose-dependent. At lower dosages, nicotine acts as an agonist and stimulates the autonomic ganglia. At higher dosages, it acts as an antagonist and blocks the autonomic ganglia (Heeschen, Weis, & Aicher, 2002; Kimura, Ushiyama, & Fujii, 2003). Interestingly, for regular, long-term nicotine users, agonistic actions may vary according to the degree of their nicotine tolerance. (For related discussion, including signs and symptoms, see the later nicotine subsection, "Pharmacology—Nicotine Overdosage and Unintentional Poisoning.")

Nicotine exerts its psychostimulant actions by stimulating nicotinic acetylcholine (cholinergic) receptors (nAChRs). The nAChRs are ligand-gated ion channels, or "pores" in cell plasma membranes, which open and close when stimulated.[46] Nicotine rapidly increases the cellular

44 During the aging period, the process of fermentation occurs resulting in the degradation of some proteins and the reduction in nicotine concentration. Additionally, numerous new chemicals are produced (Streller & Roth, 2014).

45 The associated CNS depression appears to be related to nicotine-induced changes in nAChR function. However, the exact cause and relationship between nicotine use and CNS depression is variable and not yet fully understood (e.g., Fluharty, Taylor, & Grabski, 2017; Mineur & Picciotto, 2010).

46 To elicit an action, a ligand binds, or attaches, to a chemical—in this case, acetylcholine or nicotine.

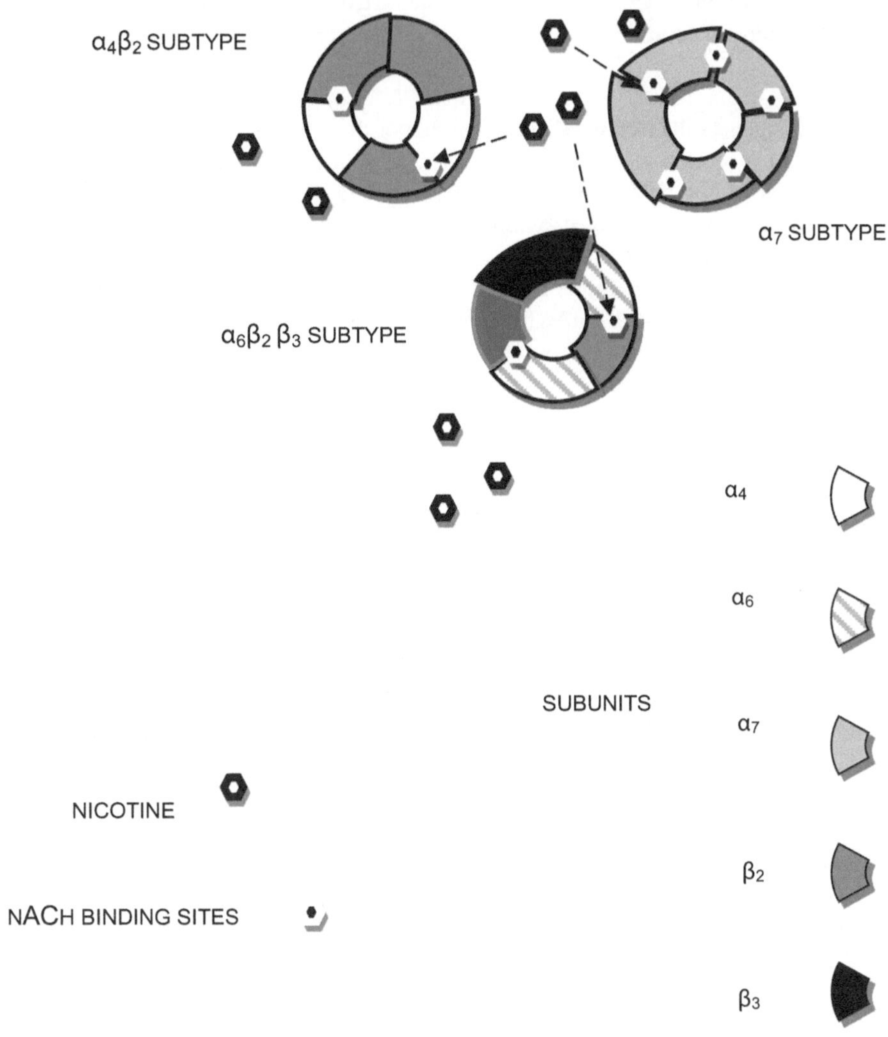

Figure 3.2 Nicotine: Mechanism of Action

permeability of nAChRs to sodium (Na^+) and calcium (Ca^{++}) ions, which results in their depolarization and resultant excitation. For nAChR subunit combinations located at skeletal neuromuscular junctions (e.g., α1-ε-α1-β1-δ), depolarization primarily affects muscle tone by producing muscular contraction. For nAChR combinations located at synapses between neurons in the CNS (e.g., α4-β2-α4-β2-β2), associated depolarization and associated excitation primarily produce: (1) arousal; (2) enhanced cognitive functioning—including learning and memory; and (3) reward.

There are five types of structurally diverse subunits of nAChRs: (1) alpha (α); (2) beta (β); (3) delta (δ); (4) epsilon (ε); and (5) gamma (γ). These subunits are found in six different combinations. In the CNS, combinations of α subunits and β subunits appear to be particularly relevant to the achievement of both the desired and undesired actions of nicotine (Figure 3.2). For example, the α4 and β2 subunits appear to contribute to the euphoria associated with nicotine use, whereas the α3, α5, and β3 subunits appear to be responsible for determining both the risk for, and severity of, nicotine use disorder, or nicotine physical dependence (Whitten, 2009).

Subunits in autonomic ganglia also affect depolarization and firing of postganglionic neurons. In the adrenal medulla, they also affect the secretion of catecholamines, because of the opening of cation channels and the influx of calcium ions through the depolarized membrane pores of the nAChRs (Araki, Suemaru, & Gomita, 2002).

Thought to be genetically influenced, the response of the nAChRs to nicotine helps to explain various patterns of nicotine use among adolescents and young adults, including the development of nicotine physical and psychological dependence, or NUD. It also helps to explain the signs and symptoms of the nicotine withdrawal syndrome, which occur as nicotine blood concentrations decline when regular, long-term nicotine use is abruptly discontinued.[47] For example, collectively, "the protective effects of progesterone on craving in nicotine-dependent women may be mediated through its inhibitory effect on β2-nAChR function" (Moran-Santa Maria, Flanagan, & Brady, 2014, p. 5). Whereas, individually, women "inherit different forms of half a dozen genes that dictate the features of the brain receptor to which nicotine binds" (Whitten, 2009, p. 1).

Pharmacokinetics: Absorption, Distribution, Metabolism, and Excretion

The pharmacokinetics of nicotine are presented and discussed in the following subsections.

ABSORPTION AND DISTRIBUTION

Chemically, nicotine is a weak base (pka = 8.0). Consequently, its transfer across biological membranes is pH dependent.[48] Thus, the buccal and sublingual absorption of nicotine can significantly vary because of pH differences in tobacco products. For example, American cigarettes, which are usually produced using "flue cured" tobacco, have an "acidic" pH. The acidic pH results in the nicotine existing predominantly in an ionized form that has "minimal" buccal or sublingual absorption. Conversely, some European cigarettes, as well as cigar and pipe tobacco, which are usually produced using "air cured" tobacco, have an "alkaline" pH. The alkaline pH, in turn, results in "maximal" buccal and sublingual absorption of nicotine (Hukkanen, Jacob, & Benowitz, 2005).

An average American tobacco cigarette, when smoked, delivers only about one mg of nicotine because approximately 90% of the nicotine is destroyed by pyrolysis. Regardless, adolescents and young adults, who smoke tobacco cigarettes, can achieve relatively high blood nicotine concentrations due to the relatively large surface area of their lungs and its excellent blood supply that results in the high pulmonary absorption of nicotine (F = 0.9). Bioavailability also can be increased several-fold by smoking techniques, for example:

1. Increasing the number of puffs per tobacco cigarette;
2. Inhaling the smoke more deeply into the lungs;
3. Holding the inhaled smoke in the lungs for a longer period of time before exhaling.

When nicotine is inadvertently ingested, its absorption into the circulatory system is low (i.e., F = 0.3, or approximately 30%). It also undergoes significant "first-pass" hepatic metabolism (see following section) that results in its rapid and extensive inactivation. In comparison, the nicotine in buccal absorption spray products (e.g., Nicorette, Quick Mist®) and lozenges

47 More recent research (e.g., Gamaleddin, Trigo, & Gueye, 2015) suggests a significant role of endocannabinoids and the associated CB_1 receptors in modulating the effects of nicotine—both the reinforcing effects, as well as, those involved with nicotine withdrawal. (For additional related discussion of the endocannabinoids and their receptors, See Chapter 4, "Cannabis and Other Psychodelics").

48 For additional related discussion of the effects of pH on absorption and excretion, see Chapter 2, "Amphetamines and Cocaine," amphetamine subsection, "Pharmacology—Pharmacokinetics."

(e.g., Thrive® lozenges), is rapidly absorbed from the inner cheeks of the mouth and, consequently, avoids first-pass hepatic metabolism. Buccally absorbed chewing tobacco and nicotine chewing gum formulations (e.g., Nicorette®), when chewed and the juices held in the mouth before being spat out, achieve blood nicotine concentrations that approximate those obtained by smoking a regular tobacco cigarette (i.e., F = 0.9). Interestingly, the nicotine in chewing gum products, which is bound to an ion-exchange resin, is only released by chewing. Thus, the amount of nicotine released from the chewing gum, and the resultant blood nicotine concentrations that are achieved, are related to the rate and vigor of chewing.

Transdermal nicotine delivery systems (i.e., "nicotine patches") are well-absorbed (i.e., ~ 80%) through intact skin sites following topical application. However, the rate of absorption is significantly slower than that associated with pulmonary inhalation or other methods of use. Regardless of the method of use, once nicotine is absorbed, it is only slightly bound to plasma proteins (i.e., less than 5%). Having a low affinity for adipose tissue, it is distributed to, and preferentially binds to, brain, renal, hepatic, and pulmonary tissues (Benowitz, Hukkanen, & Jacob, 2009). The volume of distribution of nicotine is approximately two to three L/kg.

METABOLISM

Nicotine is primarily metabolized (i.e., ~ 90%) by the hepatic microsomal enzymes CYP2A6[49] and CYP2B6 to several metabolites—the most important of which is the "inactive" metabolite, cotinine.[50] Cotinine is subsequently metabolized to 3-hydroxycotinine—the major nicotine metabolite that is detected in the urine of tobacco smokers (i.e., accounting for ~ 50% of the administered nicotine dose).[51]

The hepatic clearance rate of nicotine is approximately 1.2 L/minute, which means that the liver is very efficient at clearing and, hence, removing nicotine from the circulatory system.[52] However, nicotine clearance displays large interindividual variation being highly correlated with age, continental or other descent, diet, and gender (e.g., Hukkanen, Jacob, & Benowitz, 2005; Johnstone, Benowitz, & Cargill, 2006). For example:

1. African or Asian continental descent is generally associated with slower metabolism of nicotine (e.g., Hukkanen, Jacob, & Benowitz, 2005; Schoedel, Hoffmann, & Rao, 2004);
2. Females generally metabolize nicotine faster than males (e.g., Benowitz, Lessov-Schlaggar, & Swan, 2006; Piper, Cook, & Schlam, 2010);
3. Adolescent girls and young adult women, who use oral contraceptives, generally metabolize nicotine faster than those who do not (e.g., Berlin, Gasior, & Moolchan, 2007).

In addition, genetic variation in the multiple alleles of the CYP2A6 has been associated with the slow, intermediate, and normal metabolism of nicotine (e.g., Nakajima, Kuroiwa, & Yokoi, 2002; Nakajima & Yokoi, 2005). Interestingly, slow metabolizers, have generally demonstrated: (1) lower rates of smoking; (2) decreased risk of developing nicotine

49 Differences in the observed rates of nicotine metabolism have been directly related to identified variations in the CYP2A6 gene (St Helen, Dempsey, & Wilson, 2013).

50 It also is metabolized, albeit, to a significantly lesser extent, in the brain, kidneys, and lungs (Sobkowiak & Lesicki, 2013).

51 Over 20 different metabolites of nicotine have been identified. These metabolites are not as pharmacologically active as their parent drug, nicotine.

52 In addition to hepatic clearance, nicotine also undergoes renal clearance, but at a significantly lower rate (i.e., ~ 75 ml/min).

dependence, or NUD; and (3) greater success in smoking cessation (e.g., Ho & Tyndale, 2007; Malaiyandi, Sellers, & Tyndale, 2005; Mwenifumbo & Tyndale, 2007; Tanner, Chenoweth, & Tyndale, 2015).

However, Rubinstein, Shiffman, and Moscicki (2013), in a study of 164 adolescent smokers, 13 to 17 years-of-age, found—seemingly paradoxically—that slow metabolizers smoked more cigarettes per day than intermediate or normal metabolizers. They posited that this observation may be mediated by high levels of nicotine exposure per cigarette smoked, particularly in the context of the "early phase of their smoking careers." Additionally, they noted a more generally observed relationship between the nicotine metabolism rate and the number of cigarettes smoked per day as the adolescents enter into the "later phase of their smoking careers."

The mean half-life of elimination for nicotine is two hours.[53] Consequently, regular, long-term smokers of tobacco cigarettes will need to "light-up," on average, at least every two hours to maintain blood nicotine concentrations that are needed to avoid the occurrence of the signs and symptoms of the nicotine withdrawal syndrome (see the related discussion in the later nicotine Pharmacology subsection, "Undesired, or Harmful, Effects and Toxicities, Physical and Psychological Dependence—Nicotine Withdrawal Syndrome").

EXCRETION

Nicotine and its metabolites are rapidly excreted in the urine (approximately 10% to 15% in unchanged form). Affected by urinary pH, nicotine excretion is decreased in alkaline urine (i.e., urine pH above 7.4), and increased in acidic urine (i.e., urine pH below 7.4). In fact, the acidification of the urine to below a pH of 5 can result in up to 30% of a dosage of nicotine being excreted in the urine in unchanged form. A small percentage of nicotine (i.e., ~ 1%) and its metabolites are excreted in the feces and sweat (Hukkanen, Jacob, & Benowitz, 2005).

Nicotine and Tobacco Smoke Drug–Drug Interactions

Nicotine, primarily in the form of e-cigarettes, tobacco cigarettes, and nicotine replacement products (e.g., buccal sprays; chewing gums; transdermal delivery systems) is often concurrently used with over-the-counter drugs, or "OTCs" (e.g., acetaminophen, Tylenol®), and prescription drugs (e.g., estrogens; insulins; theophylline, Theolair®). Nicotine also is concurrently used with other drugs and substances of abuse—alcohol, benzodiazepines, caffeine, and opiate analgesics (Cross, Lotfipour, & Leslie, 2017; Pagliaro & Pagliaro, 2009, 2012, 2018; Verplaetse & McKee, 2017).

The clinical significance of potential drug–drug interactions involving nicotine and tobacco smoke—along with OTC drugs and other drugs and substances of abuse—is generally subtler and more complex than generally expected because these drug interactions are predicated upon several factors including the method, context, and pattern of nicotine use. Nicotine and tobacco smoke drug–drug interactions may be associated with, for example:

- Initiating and gradually increasing use;
- Maintaining regular, long-term use;
- Decreasing or ceasing use, including use of nicotine replacement therapy.

53 By comparison, the mean half-life of elimination for cotinine, nicotine's first and principal metabolite, is approximately 18 hours. Cotinine concentrations can be readily measured in biological samples (e.g., hair; saliva; serum; and urine) to determine tobacco exposure/use (Pagliaro & Pagliaro, 2004).

Table 3.2 Drug–Drug Interactions Involving Nicotine and Tobacco Smoke[54]

Drugs and substances that interact with nicotine or tobacco smoke	*Comments*
Acetaminophen (e.g., Tylenol®)	Concurrent acetaminophen use with tobacco smoking may require an increase in the acetaminophen dosage due to the: (1) induction of hepatic microsomal enzymes (e.g., CYP1A2) associated with tobacco smoking; and (2) resultant increased metabolic clearance of acetaminophen
Alcohol[55]	Concurrent alcohol use with tobacco smoking appears to have a reciprocal effect resulting in increased craving for and increased use of alcohol and tobacco smoking
Benzodiazepines (e.g., oxazepam, Serax®)	Concurrent benzodiazepine use with tobacco smoking may require an increase in benzodiazepine dosage due to the: (1) induction of hepatic microsomal enzymes (e.g., CYP1A2) associated with tobacco smoking; and (2) resultant increase in the metabolic clearance[56] of the benzodiazepine
Caffeine	Concurrent caffeine use with tobacco smoking may increase the usual amount of caffeine ingested due to the: (1) induction of hepatic microsomal enzymes (e.g., CYP1A2) associated with tobacco smoking; and (2) resultant increased metabolic clearance of caffeine
Estrogens	Estrogens (e.g., oral contraceptives) can induce the production of CYP2A6—of which nicotine is a substrate—resulting in lower nicotine concentrations
Insulin	Nicotine related cutaneous vasoconstriction may slow the rate of insulin absorption when injected subcutaneously. Conversely, with smoking cessation, a decrease in insulin dosage may be required due to the associated increase in insulin subcutaneous absorption

(*Continued*)

54 The clinical significance of these potential nicotine drug–drug interactions depends upon several factors, including the: (1) dosage of each drug; (2) characteristics of the adolescent or young adult (e.g., age; gender; genetics); (3) concomitant physical health status (e.g., hepatic and renal function); and (4) concomitant mental health status.

55 As identified by Yardley, Mirbaba, and Ray (2015):

> The link between heavy drinking and smoking is thought to be driven by many factors including genetics, neurobiological mechanisms, conditioning processes, and psychosocial influences.
>
> (p. 834)

56 N.B. Nicotine-related tobacco exposure/use is a special case that requires consideration. Polycyclic aromatic hydrocarbons that are present in tobacco smoke reduce the production of the hepatic microsomal enzymes that are responsible for the metabolism of many drugs (Anderson & Chan, 2016; Schaffer, Yoon; & Zadezensky, 2009; Zevin & Benowitz, 1999).

Table 3.2 (Cont.)

Drugs and substances that interact with nicotine or tobacco smoke	*Comments*
Opiate Analgesics[57] (e.g., pentazocine, Talwin®; propoxyphene, Darvon®)	Concurrent pentazocine use and tobacco smoking may require an increase in the opiate analgesic dosage due to the: (1) *induction* of hepatic microsomal enzymes (e.g., CYP1A2) associated with tobacco smoking; and (2) resultant increase in metabolic clearance of the opiate analgesic
	Concurrent propoxyphene use during tobacco smoking cessation, may require a decrease in the propoxyphene dosage due to the reduction of first pass hepatic metabolism associated with smoking cessation
Theophylline (e.g., Theolair®)	Concurrent theophylline use with tobacco smoking may require an increase in the theophylline dosage due to the: (1) induction of the hepatic microsomal enzymes (e.g., CYP1A2) associated with tobacco smoking; and (2) resultant increased metabolic clearance of theophylline

In this regard, "tobacco smoking" presents a special case. Not directly associated with nicotine, itself, polycyclic aromatic hydrocarbons present in tobacco smoke induce the production of the hepatic microsomal enzyme CYP1A2, which affects the metabolism of many drugs (Anderson & Chan, 2016; Schaffer, Yoon, & Zadezensky, 2009; Zevin & Benowitz, 1999). An overview of other major potentially clinically significant nicotine drug–drug interactions, including those associated with tobacco smoking, and for which more published data also are available, is presented in Table 3.2.

Undesired, or Harmful, Effects and Toxicities

The major undesired, or harmful, effects and toxicities associated with nicotine are related to its "direct" effects on the CNS and other body systems, which can be acute or chronic, mild or severe, and, rarely, fatal.

DIRECT EFFECTS OF NICOTINE

Although many of the acute psychostimulant effects related to nicotine use are desired effects—including euphoria, increased cognitive abilities, and vigilance—undesired effects

57 Most opiate analgesic users, including those participating in methadone maintenance programs, smoke tobacco cigarettes (Pagliaro & Pagliaro, *Clinical Patient Data Files*). Smoking cessation is particularly difficult to achieve for these nicotine users regardless of pharmacological, psychological/counseling, or other treatment approaches (e.g., Stein, Weinstock, & Herman, 2006; Zirak Zadeh, Shuman, & Stauter, 2013).

related to nicotine use occur, and include: anorexia;[58] diarrhea; dizziness; edema; flushing; GI cramps; headache; heart palpitations; hypertension; hypoglycemia (in insulin-dependent diabetics); hyperventilation; increased salivation; insomnia;[59] irritability; lightheadedness; nausea; tachycardia; tinnitus; tremors; and vomiting (e.g., Mishra, Chaturvedi, & Datta, 2015; Pagliaro & Pagliaro, 2004).

TOBACCO SMOKING

> Tobacco use is the leading preventable cause of disease, disability, and death in the United States. According to the Centers for Disease Control and Prevention (CDC), cigarette smoking results in more than 480,000 premature deaths in the United States each year—about one in every five U.S. deaths—and.... for every one person who dies from smoking, about 30 more suffer from at least one serious tobacco-related illness.
>
> (NIDA, 2016, p. 1)

As emphasized by Carter, Abnet, and Feskanich (2015), "mortality among current smokers is 2 to 3 times as high as that among persons who never smoked" (p. 631).

The chemicals present in tobacco smoke include: (1) chemicals naturally found in tobacco leaves (e.g., heavy metals, such as arsenic, chromium, and lead); (2) chemicals added during the farming (e.g., insecticides) and curing processes (e.g., menthol flavoring); and (3) chemicals produced by pyrolysis (e.g., carbon dioxide; tar). For example, carbon dioxide can be found in concentrations 200 to 300 times that found in normal room air. The high concentrations of carbon dioxide (i.e., approximately 13%) have been associated with an inflammatory response in pulmonary tissues (Guais, Brand, & Jacquot, 2011; Schwartz, Guais, & Chaumet-Riffaud, 2010). The two major classes of carcinogens present in tobacco smoke are: (1) "polycyclic aromatic hydrocarbons" (PAHs), including benzo(a)pyrene, chrysene, and naphthalene;[60] and (2) nicotine-derived nitrosamines (NDNs).[61]

These chemicals are present in various physical forms (i.e., gases, liquids, and solids) in tobacco smoke. In addition, their concentrations can vary significantly as a result of several factors, including the:

- Type of tobacco used in the preparation of cigarettes, cigars, pipe tobacco, and other tobacco products;
- Conditions under which tobacco plants are grown (e.g., soil content);
- Process of fermentation;
- Additives used in the preparation of the tobacco leaves (e.g., menthol);
- Processing of the tobacco leaf after harvesting;
- Type of paper/wrap used for preparing cigarettes and cigars;

58 Anorexia can be a "desired" effect of nicotine use for those adolescents and young adults who want to lose, or maintain, body weight.

59 Insomnia can be a "desired" effect of nicotine use for those adolescents and young adults who want to stay awake in order to, for example, study, work, or "party."

60 Several studies have found that "flue-cured" tobacco typically can deliver more PAHs than other tobacco types (e.g., Ding, Yan, & Jain, 2006, p. 1133).

61 In the published literature, NDNs also are referred to as "tobacco-specific nitrosamines" (TSNAs) (Wu, Zhang, & Jain, 2005). Two major TSNAs that are present in tobacco and tobacco smoke are 4-(methylnitrosamino)-1-(3-pyridyl)-1-butanone (NNB) and N-nitrosonornicotine (NNN) (Hecht, 2014; Pfeifer, Denissenko, & Olivier, 2002; Vu, Taylor, & Holman, 2015; Wang, Li, & Guo, 2016).

- Type of filter, if any;
- Smoking technique used by the smoker.

All smoke, regardless of the source, is comprised of colorless gases (e.g., carbon dioxide; carbon monoxide; nitrogen; oxygen), which contain particulate, or solid, matter. The generally warm gases and particulate matter dispersed in tobacco smoke, irritate and dry the pulmonary system leading to a characteristic dry, non-productive cough (i.e., "smokers cough"). Regular, long-term exposure to tobacco smoke also leads to the loss of muscle mass and the development of related respiratory dysfunction even before the development of overt, symptomatic pulmonary toxicity (Degens, Gayan-Ramirez, & van Hees, 2015). In addition, particulate matter that makes its way into the alveolar sacs can get "trapped" and compromise alveolar function.

In addition to premature aging of the skin and other undesired effects, tobacco smoke has been associated with increased occurrence of coronary heart and pulmonary diseases, as well as cancers involving several body systems (see the following subsections). In fact, as previously noted, during the first decade of the new millennium, tobacco smoking was identified as the major single preventable cause of illness and disease in the U.S., where it contributes to an estimated 1,500 deaths every day[62] (NIDA, 2016; USDHHS, 2010).

CARDIOVASCULAR DISEASES. As identified in an expert consensus statement from the American College of Cardiology:

> Tobacco use, especially cigarette smoking, is a major risk factor for cardiovascular disease and mortality.
>
> (Barua, Rigotti, & Benowitz, 2018, p. 3332)

The association between tobacco smoke and coronary heart disease was identified over 80 years ago by English, Willius, and Berkson in 1940—cited by Paul (1989). It is now recognized that tobacco smoke is associated with a two- to four-fold increased risk for coronary heart disease among regular, long-term tobacco smokers. Several interrelated factors contribute to the complex cardiovascular toxicity associated with tobacco smoke. As explained by D'Allessandro, Boeckelmann, and Hammwhoner (2012), regarding cardiac dysrhythmias, the:

> Profibrotic effect of nicotine on myocardial tissue with consequent increased susceptibility to catecholamine might play a role. In addition, other constituents of tobacco smoke, such as carbon monoxide and oxidative stress, are likely to contribute to the generation of cardiac dysrhythmias. Finally, tobacco smoke may induce coronary artery disease and chronic obstructive pulmonary disease, which may cause dysrhythmias independently.
>
> (p. 297)

62 N.B. The specific contributions of cigarette smoking to illness and death are often difficult to properly identify. Consequently, the actual rate of illness and death may be higher than what is presented. For example, O'Cleirigh, Valentine, and Pinkston (2015), in their study of people living in the U.S. with HIV, found that the tobacco smoking rate among participants in the study was triple that reported for the general population (i.e., 57% versus 19%). They also identified several confounding findings when they compared smokers to non-smokers in their study. Smokers were identified as having: lower adherence to anti-AIDS medication regimens; higher detectable viral load; fewer routine medical visits; more recent hospitalization; and more concurrent drug and substance abuse, particularly alcohol, cocaine, heroin, and/or marijuana abuse (p. 178). Thus, for example, the total impact of smoking on the health of those with HIV is significant and complex. Consequently, it is extremely difficult to directly quantify.

Interestingly, Hackshaw, Morris, & Boniface (2018), in their large-scale meta-analysis of 141 cohort studies, identified that among adults, both men and women, the pooled relative risk for coronary heart disease was estimated to be 50% higher among those who smoked "one cigarette per day."[63]

PULMONARY DISEASES. Pulmonary toxicity associated with tobacco smoke (i.e., cancer of the lungs, bronchi, and trachea; chronic obstructive pulmonary disease [COPD]) is associated with three major factors: (1) the direct irritant and damaging effects of tobacco smoke; (2) carcinogens present in tobacco and/or produced by the pyrolysis of tobacco leaves and wrapping paper; and (3) other chemicals that are present in tobacco smoke.[64] In addition, nicotine, itself, "induces" the formation of oxygen radicals and "reduces" the antioxidant capacity of the lungs (Henley, Thomas, & Sharapova, 2016; Maritz, 2008).

> Becky started smoking cigarettes in 1976 as an exchange student when she was living with a host family in Germany... At age 45, Becky was diagnosed with chronic obstructive pulmonary disease... Today, Becky needs continuous oxygen to help her breathe...
>
> (CDC, 2016c, p. 1)

Given the demonstrated and long-known respiratory toxicity that is directly related to tobacco smoke (and nicotine itself) it is perplexing that adolescents with asthma have long been identified as being at a higher risk for the initiation and continuation of tobacco cigarette smoking than adolescents without asthma (Pagliaro & Pagliaro, 2012). As noted by the CDC, this observation appears to be continuing:[65]

> Current use of all tobacco product types and multiple tobacco products was significantly higher among students with asthma than among those without asthma.
>
> (Reid, Forrest, & Porter, 2018, p. 599)

LUNG CANCER. Tobacco smoke is clearly associated with an increased risk for lung cancer. In most of these cases, the risk for developing lung cancer is directly related to the number of cigarettes smoked per day—with due consideration of genetic contributions. However, in the U.S., for cigarette smokers of African continental descent, when compared to those of European continental descent:

1. The incidence of lung cancer is higher;
2. Lung cancer occurs in association with a significantly lower rate of daily tobacco cigarette smoking.

Several researchers (e.g., Benowitz, Dains, & Dempsey, 2011; St Helen, Dempsey, & Wilson, 2013) suggest that the associated increased risk for lung cancer may be due to the

63 N.B. The study evaluated cohorts of adults (45, 55, and 65 years-of-age) and did not include adolescents or young adults.

64 See the related discussion in the earlier nicotine subsection, "Tobacco Plant Botany."

65 Although not substantiated, we have long thought that the increased risk for cigarette use among children and adolescents with asthma is due entirely to psychological factors (i.e., the need to appear normal and to also demonstrate "strength" to their peers—much like Hispanic adolescents demonstrate their "machismo" by the use of phencyclidine (PCP) (Pagliaro & Pagliaro, *Clinical Patient Data Files*). (See also the related discussion in Chapter 4, "Cannabis and Other Psychodelics").

noticeable, significant differences in cigarette smoking techniques between smokers of African and European continental descents (i.e., related to the former's inhalation of larger amounts of carcinogens per tobacco cigarette smoked).

> Rose started smoking at age 13 and continued for many years, smoking two packs a day. Rose developed lung cancer from smoking cigarettes and... had chemotherapy, surgery, radiation, and a painful drainage tube in her left chest... She died in January 2015, at age 60 from cancer caused by smoking.
>
> (CDC, 2016d, p. 1)

OTHER CANCERS. Tobacco smoke also has been associated with cancers of the: breast; cervix; colon; esophagus; head; kidneys and renal pelvises; larynx; liver; neck; mouth and oropharynx; ovaries; pancreas; rectum; stomach; and urinary bladder (e.g., Beral, Gaitskell, & Hermon, 2012; Gallaway, Henley, & Steele, 2018; Kuper, Boffetta, & Adami, 2002; Thun, Henley, & Calle, 2002), and acute myeloid leukemia. However, for many of these cancers, a direct cause-and-effect relationship with tobacco smoke remains tentative.

Research findings increasingly suggest a significant genetic contribution to the relationship between tobacco smoke and cancer. However, this putative relationship is complex, and findings are not always consistent (e.g., Fagan, Moolchan, & Pokhrel, 2015). For example, tobacco smokers with higher CYP2A6 activity have higher rates of nicotine metabolism. Thus, they smoke more extensively and, consequently, are exposed to more carcinogens in tobacco smoke that, in turn, places them at higher related risk for developing cancer (Derby, Cuthrell, & Caberto, 2008).

PASSIVE SMOKE

We have consistently emphasized, for over four decades, that the nicotine, which is a constituent of tobacco, has a relatively low level of toxicity in comparison to tobacco "smoke"—that is unsafe at any level of exposure due to the constitution of "smoke" (i.e., the therapeutic index for tobacco smoke is "zero").

As noted by the World Health Organization (WHO, 2009):

> There is *no* safe level of exposure to tobacco smoke. All people should be protected from such exposure.
>
> (p. 14)

As further noted by the CDC:

> There is no risk-free level of exposure to tobacco smoke, and there are no safe tobacco products.
>
> (USDHHS, 2010, p. 1)

As such, tobacco smoke is identified as the leading cause of preventable and unnecessary deaths adding up to over 500,000 deaths annually with approximately 50,000 of these indirect deaths due to passive exposure, secondhand, or side-stream smoke (Carter, Abnet, & Feskanich, 2015; CDC, 2010; Danaei, Ding, & Mozaffarian, 2009; Wang, Tynan, & Hallett, 2017). As identified by the CDC (2010):

> Secondhand exposure to tobacco smoke causes heart disease and lung cancer in nonsmoking adults and sudden infant death syndrome, acute respiratory infections, middle ear

disease, exacerbated asthma, respiratory symptoms, and decreased lung function in children.

(p. 1)

Unfortunately, cigarette, cigar, and pipe smoking continues to be widespread in the U.S. and appears to be increasing in certain population groups (e.g., adolescent girls; members of the military; individuals who have mental disorders) despite cautions and wide publicity of the harmful effects and toxicities associated with its use.[66] (See also the later discussion in the nicotine subsection, "New Millennial Trends in Nicotine Use").

E-CIGARETTES

The increased public awareness of the serious toxicities associated with nicotine tobacco smoking—in addition to the successful outcomes of major lawsuits for previous tobacco cigarette smokers and their families (e.g., CBC News, 2015; Reuters, 2015)—has been associated with decreased rates of tobacco smoking in the U.S. It also has been the basis for a significant refocusing by cigarette manufacturers, during the new millennium, regarding the research and development of "smoke-free" nicotine products. This attention has involved research with various concentrations and flavors of liquid nicotine products along with convenient delivery systems, which, in general, are both attractive and similar in shape and style to traditional cigarettes (i.e., electronic cigarettes, or e-cigarettes) (Pagliaro & Pagliaro, 2009).

E-Cigarettes were introduced to the U.S. market in 2006/2007. Their delivery systems produce an inhalable liquid nicotine vapor[67] rather than the smoke produced by "lighting-up" and burning the leaf tobacco of a typical tobacco cigarette, cigar, or pipe that, in addition to nicotine, delivers significantly more harmful and toxic chemicals to the pulmonary system (Czogala, Goniewicz, & Fidelus, 2014; Oh & Kacker, 2014; Rom, Pecorelli, & Valacchi, 2015). In the U.S., during the new millennium, a major new and developing trend among adolescents and young adults began—e-cigarette[68] (e.g., "Smoke Stik®") vaping. E-Cigarette vaping, particularly among adolescents and young adults, increased significantly throughout the second decade of the new millennium. For example, as identified by Barrington-Trimis and Leventhal (2018):

In 2011, less than 2% of U.S. high school students reported having used e-cigarettes in the previous month. But by 2015, the percentage had jumped to 16%.

(p. 1099)

66 In a government sponsored attempt to reduce the toxicity associated with tobacco cigarette smoking, the composition of cigarettes was significantly changed in the U.S. during the last half of the 20th century. As identified by Hoffmann and Hoffmann (1997):

In the United States the sales-weighted average "tar" and nicotine yields have declined from a *high* of 38 mg *tar* and 2.7 mg *nicotine* in 1954 to 12 mg and 0.95 mg in 1992, respectively.

(p. 307)

67 Consequently, the use of e-cigarettes is commonly referred to as "vaping." See also the related discussion of "vaping" in the cannabis subsection of Chapter 4, "Cannabis and Other Psychodelics."

68 The prototype for the current e-cigarette was developed by the Chinese pharmacist, Hon Lik, in 2003 and was first introduced into the U.S. in 2006/2007. Currently, over 500 different brands of e-cigarettes are available.

As later reported by the National Academies (2018):

> In 2016 youth e-cigarette use was substantially higher than cigarette smoking or use of any other tobacco product.
>
> (p. 51)

The CDC also noted that:

> Electronic cigarettes/e-cigarettes were the most commonly used tobacco product among U.S. middle school and high school students in 2016.
>
> (Tsai, Walton, & Coleman, 2018, p. 196)

E-Cigarettes, also known as, "electronic nicotine delivery systems" (ENDS),[69] generally resemble common tobacco cigarettes,[70] which makes them attractive to traditional cigarette smokers and to adolescents and young adults who have not yet begun to smoke. However, because there is no tobacco or cigarette wrap to burn, with "vaping" there is no odor and, more importantly, there is little, or no, cancer-producing chemicals—carbon monoxide, tars, and other carcinogens—to inhale.[71]

> E-cigarette aerosol contains fewer and lower levels of most toxicants than smoke from combustible tobacco cigarettes do.
>
> (National Academies, 2018, p. S1)

However, as identified by the U.S. Surgeon General:

> Although e-cigarettes generally emit fewer toxicants than combustible tobacco products, we know that aerosol from e-cigarettes is not harmless.
>
> (USDHHS, 2016b, p. vii)[72]

Typically, e-cigarettes have several basic components (Brown & Cheng, 2014; Pagliaro & Pagliaro, 2009):[73]

69 ENDS broadly encompass several related products variously known as: "cigalikes;" "e-cigs;" "e-cigarettes;" "e-hookahs;" "electronic cigarettes;" "e-Pods;" "mods;" "pod mods;" "tank systems;" "vape pens;" and "vapes."

70 A noted exception to the typical look of e-cigarettes is the JUUL®, which is shaped like a USB flash drive. A single JUUL® pod can contain as much nicotine (i.e., 42 mg) as a package of 20 regular tobacco cigarettes. JUUL® became available for sale in the U.S. in 2015 and by 2017 it became the top-selling e-cigarette brand among adolescents and young adults—capturing ~ 50% of the e-cigarette market by 2018. The use of the JUUL® is commonly referred to as "JULLing" (Goniewicz, Gupta, & Lee, 2015; Kavuluru, Han, & Hahn, 2018; USDHHS, 2016b; Willett, Bennett, & Hair, 2018).

71 Even when concerns are raised, and some issues remain unresolved (e.g., the risk posed by products that are high in nitrosamines), the consensus is that "smokeless" tobacco products cause less than 10% of the toxicity associated with equivalent tobacco cigarette smoking—in terms of nicotine exposure (e.g., National Academies, 2018; Pagliaro & Pagliaro, 2012; Varlet, 2016; Warner & Pollack, 2014).

72 The aerosol "vaper" from e-cigarettes contains nicotine, carbonyl compounds, glycerol (i.e., glycerin), heavy metals (e.g., lead; nickel; tin), propylene glycol, and volatile organic compounds. When heated, glycerol and propylene glycol can be converted to acrolein, acetaldehyde, and formaldehyde—compounds that are both irritating to the respiratory system and possible carcinogens (Shields, Berman, & Brasky, 2017; USDHHS, 2016a).

73 Most of these systems can be considered to be "open-systems" (i.e., various components can be replaced, and the nicotine solution can be refilled). An exception is the "Vype ePod®," which is a "closed-system" resembling a small insulin pen. It consists of two components—a central sealed unit and a sealed e-Pen cartridge. The closed-system minimizes leakage and mess that are associated with open-systems.

- LED light cover to resemble a burning cigarette and to also indicate that the product is activated;
- Rechargeable battery (and external battery charger) in portable models, to provide an energy source so that it can be conveniently used almost anywhere;
- Storage unit/space to contain a solution of nicotine (i.e., a refill cartridge);
- Atomizer, or heating element, to vaporize the liquid nicotine;[74]
- Flow sensor that controls the amount of nicotine delivered to the atomizer;
- Cartridge mouthpiece that is placed between the lips (like a traditional cigarette) to provide a familiar and convenient means for inhaling the vaporized nicotine into the lungs.

The liquid nicotine refill cartridges (i.e., "e-liquid;" "e-juice") are available in several strengths ranging from 0 mg to 24 mg of nicotine per refill cartridge.[75] The cartridges typically last as long as a standard package of 20-tobacco cigarettes. Further increasing the attractiveness of e-cigarettes to adolescents and young adults, e-cigarette refill cartridges come in a vast variety of flavors, including, for example: apple; Boston cream pie; caramel; cherry; chocolate; clove; cookies and milk; coffee; cola; crème brûlée; menthol; pear; peppermint; spearmint; strawberry daiquiri; tobacco; and vanilla. In fact, approximately, 10,000 different e-cigarette flavors are currently available. In response to the increasing use of flavored tobacco products during the first decade of the new millennium, the FDA banned their use in 2009.[76] Additionally, several states (e.g., Arizona; Maryland; New Hampshire; New Jersey) also banned the sale of electronic cigarettes to minors. However, these bans may *not* be as effective as anticipated because the e-cigarettes, as well as their liquid nicotine cartridges, are widely available for purchase over the internet.

Interestingly, as identified by Zhu, Sun, and Bonnevie (2014):

> Older brands [of e-cigarettes] tend to highlight their advantages over conventional cigarettes while newer brands emphasize consumer choice in multiple flavors and product versatility.
>
> (p. iii3)

In this context, it is also interesting to note that the most common reasons cited by U.S. adolescents and young adults for using e-cigarettes include:

- Curiosity;
- Flavor/taste;
- Safety (i.e., safer than use of conventional tobacco cigarettes);

74 Propylene glycol, glycerol (glycerin), and water are generally the major pharmaceutical vehicles for most e-liquid nicotine solutions (Grana, Benowitz, & Glantz, 2014). Consequently, e-cigarettes typically aerosolize and deliver to the smoker a chemical mixture consisting primarily of: (1) nicotine; (2) propylene glycol; and (3) various flavoring agents (Chun, Moazed, & Calfee, 2017; Durmowicz, 2014).

75 More than 500 different brands of e-cigarettes are available in smoke/vapor shops or over the internet, and every major commercial tobacco manufacturer actively markets these products (Shields, Berman, & Brasky, 2017). Whereas several e-cigarette components, including nicotine solution containing cartridges, are interchangeable among similar products, others are not. Unapproved and inappropriate use of components made for one e-cigarette product for another product may subject users to potential harm, including improper delivery of nicotine (i.e., too much or too little) and fires/explosions.

76 In 2009, Congress passed the *Family Smoking Prevention and Tobacco Control Act of 2009* that extended the regulatory authority of the FDA to include the manufacturing, distribution, and marketing of e-cigarettes. The final related rule was published in the Federal Register by the FDA in May 2016 (FDA, 2016a).

- Convenience (e.g., avoidance of indoor smoking restrictions associated with the production of secondhand tobacco smoke) (USDHHS, 2016b, p. 7).

Among U.S. middle and high school respondents to the *National Youth Tobacco Survey*, the CDC found that the most commonly selected reasons for use of e-cigarettes were:

- Used by a "friend or family member" (39%);
- Availability of "flavors such as mint, candy, fruit, or chocolate" (31%);
- Belief that e-cigarettes "are less harmful than other forms of tobacco such as cigarettes" (17%).

(Tsai, Walton, & Coleman, 2018, p. 196)

Although not approved for smoking cessation by the FDA, many adults report using e-cigarettes to help them decrease or quit their tobacco smoking (Foulds, Veldheer, & Berg, 2011; Pagliaro & Pagliaro, *Clinical Patient Data Files*). In addition, as identified by several researchers (e.g., Pacifici, Pichini, & Graziano, 2015; Perkins, Karelitz, & Michael, 2017), when compared to "placebo-e-cigarettes," nicotine-containing e-cigarettes (i.e., "regular" e-cigarettes) can relieve smoking abstinence symptoms (i.e., the nicotine withdrawal syndrome) in a manner similar to the Food and Drug Administration-approved nicotine replacement therapy products. (See the related discussion in the later nicotine subsection, "Pharmacotherapy, Nicotine Replacement Therapy.")

***Related Professional Reminder:* Health and social care professionals need to be fully aware that—because the e-cigarettes can deliver as much nicotine as a traditional tobacco cigarette—users are at risk for initial, or continued, nicotine physical and psychological dependence, or NUD. This concern becomes increasingly significant when considering that the sale and use of "e-cigarettes" is projected to increase by over 10-fold (i.e., 1,000 %) by 2030 (Electronic nicotine delivery systems, 2014).**

Physical and Psychological Dependence[77]

Prior to the 1970s, the medical and scientific communities generally, and erroneously, agreed that the regular, long-term use of nicotine, as a component of tobacco smoke, was *not* associated with "physical" dependence. However, they generally, and correctly, agreed that tobacco smoking was associated with "psychological" dependence (i.e., "craving;" "habitual use"). These views were strongly supported by the large tobacco companies and the research—including much university-based research—that they financially supported.[78] Over the 1970s and 1980s, scientific data accumulated that increasingly supported a change in view that the regular, long-term use of nicotine caused both physical and psychological dependence. A decade later, Collins (1990, p. 84) summarized the 20th Report of the Surgeon General on the health

77 The previous DSM categories of "nicotine abuse" and "nicotine dependence" were replaced in the DSM-5 with the category, "Tobacco Use Disorder." This terminology reflects other related DSM-5 categories, including "alcohol use disorder" (AUD) and the more general "substance use disorder" (SUD). In response to the identification that nicotine is the addictive component of tobacco smoke and the increased use by adolescents and young adults of "tobacco-free," smokeless products—such as e-cigarettes—which quickly developed during the second decade of the new millennium, we suggest the use of the term, "nicotine use disorder (NUD)." Reflecting the fact that nicotine is associated with both physical and psychological dependence, we use the preferred terminology, "nicotine dependence or use disorder."

78 Prior to, and during this period of time, it was common to observe patients and health care professionals—particularly, nurses, pharmacists, and physicians—smoking cigarettes in health care facilities, including offices and hospital settings (e.g., cafeteria; nursing desk) during working breaks and when providing medical and other health services to patients (Pagliaro & Pagliaro, *Clinical Patient Data Files*).

consequences of tobacco smoking, which was entitled, "Nicotine Addiction." The summary, a 500-page comprehensive review of over 1,000 published studies, led to the conclusions that:

1. Tobacco products are associated with the development of physical dependence;
2. The nicotine in tobacco products is the substance identified as causing the physical dependence;
3. Nicotine physical dependence is similar to that observed for "classic" alcohol, opiate analgesic, and sedative-hypnotic physical dependence;
4. Nicotine physical dependence also occurs with the use of all smokeless tobacco products because they can achieve the same blood nicotine concentrations as tobacco smoking.

Since the publication of this report in 1990, it has been generally agreed upon that nicotine is, in fact, the component of tobacco smoke that is responsible for the development of physical dependence related to the use of tobacco smoking products (Benowitz, 1999; Dani & De Biasi, 2001; Pagliaro & Pagliaro, 2004, 2009). Based on a sample of over 30,000 adults drawn from the 2001–2002 *National Epidemiological Survey of Alcoholism and Related Conditions* (NESARC), Goodwin, Keyes, and Hasin (2009) found that, although the overall rate of tobacco cigarette use declined significantly between 1964 and 2002, the rate of nicotine dependence did not decline. In addition, they reported that:

> The group most at risk of nicotine dependence among cigarette users is women in poverty in the most recent birth cohort [i.e., new millennial adolescent girls and young women], whose risk is substantially higher than that calculated for the overall population.
>
> (p. 1476)

In addition, most researchers, in this area of study (e.g., Vetulani, 2001), agree that the development of nicotine physical dependence is caused by the release of brain dopamine.[79] The dopamine, subsequently, interacts at neural reward centers in the brain that are primarily located in the limbic system—predominately the amygdala and the insula (Sutherland, Carroll, & Salmeron, 2013). However, other researchers have suggested that any, or all, of the following four proposed mechanisms of action could play a major role in the development of nicotine physical dependence:

1. Nicotine-induced alteration in nAChR synaptic plasticity (e.g., Dani & De Biasi, 2001; Dani, Ji, & Zhou, 2001);
2. Nicotine-induced release of other neurotransmitters and neuromodulators (e.g., Kenny & Markou, 2001);
3. Up-regulation of nAChRs following prolonged exposure to nicotine (e.g., Buisson & Bertrand, 2002);
4. Interaction with, or modification by, the activation of the endogenous cannabinoid receptor, CB_1 (e.g., Gamaleddin, Trigo, & Gueye, 2015).

Regardless of the actual mechanism(s) involved, physical dependence is characterized by: (1) the development of "tolerance" with the regular, long-term nicotine use by any method of

79 For additional details, see also the earlier nicotine pharmacology subsection, "Pharmacodynamics: Mechanism of Action."

use; and (2) a classic "nicotine withdrawal syndrome" that: (a) occurs when the regular, long-term use of nicotine is abruptly discontinued; and (b) immediately resolves when the use of nicotine is resumed.

NICOTINE TOLERANCE. The regular, long-term use of nicotine—in the form of tobacco smoking (e.g., smoking tobacco cigarettes, cigars, or pipes), e-cigarette vaping, or using other smokeless tobacco products (e.g., chewing tobacco; pharmaceutical nicotine replacement products; snuff or snus[80] tobacco)—can result in the development of tolerance to nicotine as respectively occurs with other drugs and substances of abuse (e.g., alcohol; opiate analgesics; prescription sedative-hypnotics). Thus, with the regular, long-term use of nicotine, adolescents and young adults, characteristically, increase the number of cigarettes they smoke, change the brand of the nicotine product that they use to another that contains higher levels of nicotine, or change their tobacco smoking, or e-cigarette vaping, techniques (e.g., increase the number of puffs per tobacco cigarette; inhale the tobacco smoke, or e-cigarette vapor, more deeply, and hold it in the lungs for a longer period of time). These changes in techniques associated with nicotine use are made, generally unconsciously, in an effort to increase the amount of nicotine absorbed into the systemic circulation for distribution to nicotinic receptors in the brain, and, consequently, achieve, once again (or almost) the original desired nicotine experience, or effects (Pagliaro & Pagliaro, *Clinical Patient Data Files*).

Tolerance also develops to most of the undesired effects associated with nicotine use (e.g., dizziness, nausea, vomiting), but not all. For example, after one or two cigarettes, even a regular, long-term cigarette smoker exhibits an increase in blood pressure, pulse rate, and hand tremor. Tobacco cigarette smokers and e-cigarette vapers metabolize nicotine more rapidly than nonsmokers or non-vapers, respectively. Thus, it is likely that tolerance to nicotine is due primarily to "pharmacodynamic" changes (e.g., neuroadaptation of nicotine receptors) rather than to "pharmacokinetic" changes. There also are conflicting reports on the duration of tolerance. In human smokers, some aspects of tolerance wax and wane repeatedly with the first tobacco cigarette or e-cigarette of the day producing a much greater cardiovascular and subjective response than subsequent tobacco cigarettes or e-cigarettes subsequently smoked or vaped later in the day. This response may also be due, at least in part, to the need to manage the nicotine withdrawal associated with the low nicotine blood concentrations that occur overnight when smokers are generally sleeping.

NICOTINE WITHDRAWAL SYNDROME. Both central and peripheral groups of nAChRs are involved in mediating the affective and somatic signs and symptoms of nicotine withdrawal. Many adolescents and young adults, who use nicotine for its psychostimulant effects, find that after a period of continued use, they are unable to completely cease, or control, their nicotine use without the occurrence of undesired effects. Consequently, they often seek professional help (e.g., from a counselor, mental health care professional, nurse, pediatrician, pharmacist, or psychologist). However, even with professional help, 33% of these adolescents and young adults are unable to cease nicotine use for more than a few days and only 20% to 30% are able to be "nicotine free" 12 months later.

A classic nicotine withdrawal syndrome has been clearly identified and appears to be influenced by both genetic and environmental factors (McLaughlin, Dani, & De Biasi, 2015).

80 "Snus," unlike snuff, which is dry tobacco powder, is moist tobacco powder that is usually placed under the lip (Pagliaro & Pagliaro, 2004).

For example, adolescents and young adults, who are fast metabolizers of nicotine, report more frequent and serious signs and symptoms of nicotine withdrawal (Hartz, Short, & Saccone, 2012). Consequently, they are more likely to, subconsciously, "self-medicate"—smoke a tobacco cigarette or vape an e-cigarette to immediately relieve the undesired signs and symptoms of withdrawal (Mathew, Wahlquist, & Garrett-Mayer, 2014; Piper, McCarthy, & Bolt, 2008).

Common signs and symptoms of the nicotine withdrawal syndrome, include:

- Anxiety;
- Bradycardia;
- Dizziness;
- Fatigue;
- Headache;
- Hunger;
- Inability to concentrate;
- Insomnia;
- Irritability;
- Lack of energy;
- Mental depression;
- Memory impairment;
- Nightmares;
- Restlessness;
- Weight gain.

These signs and symptoms generally begin within four to 24 hours of discontinuing regular, long-term tobacco cigarette smoking or other nicotine use because of nicotine's relatively short half-life of elimination (i.e., approximately two hours). To forestall or ameliorate nicotine withdrawal, adolescent and young adult smokers, who are physically dependent on nicotine, will generally display various behaviors associated with boosting their blood nicotine concentrations, including the following (see also the earlier nicotine pharmacology subsection, "Pharmacokinetics"):

- Smoking first thing in the morning when they awaken;
- Going out in a stormy night to buy a pack of cigarettes when they find they have none in the house;
- Taking a "break" as soon as they can during the school/work day to "have a smoke."

The nicotine withdrawal syndrome may intensify over two to four days and, then, gradually dissipate over one to three weeks. The aversive aspects of nicotine withdrawal often contribute to resumed nicotine use. Many adolescents and young adults attempt to manage nicotine withdrawal by gradually decreasing nicotine use by cutting down the number of cigarettes smoked daily and while some may be successful, many others are not. To aid nicotine withdrawal, several pharmacotherapeutic approaches have been developed and approved, including nicotine-containing products, such as NicoDerm® transdermal delivery systems ("patches") and Nicorette® chewing gum and buccal/mouth spray products (e.g., Nicorette Quick Mist®). Non-nicotine containing products, such as bupropion (Zyban®) and varenicline (Chantix®) also are available. (See the related discussion in the later nicotine subsection, "Pharmacotherapy—Nicotine Replacement Therapy.")

The argument that nicotine is the active substance in tobacco smoke that is responsible for continued regular use, also is supported by several studies of both the use of low-yield nicotine cigarettes and high-yield nicotine cigarettes (Benowitz & Jacob, 1984; Nakazawa, Shigeta, & Ozasa, 2004). For example, low-yield cigarette smokers have been found to smoke more cigarettes per day than high-yield cigarette smokers (i.e., smoke in a manner that satisfies their internal individual nicotine cravings) (CDC, 2018a; Pagliaro & Pagliaro, 2004). In addition, "brand-switching" studies have reported that when smokers are changed from high- to low-yield cigarettes, they may unconsciously change their smoking behavior to maintain their blood nicotine concentration by increasing the:

1. Number of cigarettes smoked;
2. Depth of puffs or rate of puffing;
3. Duration of inhalation.

For example, although light smokers are traditionally considered to be less dependent on nicotine, the findings of Krebs, Chen, and Zhu (2016) suggest that light smokers "are exposed to more nicotine per cigarette than are heavy smokers due to more frequent, intensive puffing" (p. 48). Additionally, Benowitz and colleagues (e.g., Benowitz, Dains, & Dempsey, 2011; Perez-Stable, Herrera, & Jacob, 1998) identified that U.S. tobacco cigarette smokers of African continental descent "smoke cigarettes differently" than those of European continental descent, inhaling "on average" 30% more nicotine per individual cigarette smoked (St Helen, Dempsey, & Wilson, 2013, p. 2)

Consequently, in response to the observations that low-yield tobacco cigarettes: (1) are not generally safer to use than high-yield cigarettes; and (2) were deliberately being labelled as "light," "low," or "mild," by their manufacturer to make their product more marketable—related regulatory changes were enacted in the U.S.:

> The Family Smoking Prevention and Tobacco Control Act of 2009 now prohibits manufacturers from selling or distributing any tobacco products that have "light," "low," or "mild" on their labels.
>
> (FDA, 2010, p. 1)

An area that requires more study are the individual differences reported regarding the nicotine withdrawal experience. These experiences have been largely ignored. The assumption is generally made that, for example, a regular, long-term tobacco smoker is physically dependent on tobacco. This assumption may be as incorrect as is the assumption that all those who drink alcohol daily are physically dependent on alcohol. It may be that some adolescents and young adults who smoke tobacco can regularly use nicotine for longer periods of time without becoming physically dependent on nicotine (Pagliaro & Pagliaro, *Clinical Patient Data Files*). In addition to the contribution of factors, such as personality and the co-occurrence of other mental disorders, genetic variability appears to explain the majority of the variance noted in this context (e.g., De Biasi & Dani, 2011; Paolini & De Biasi, 2011). Because smokers often use other drugs and substances of abuse (e.g., alcohol; caffeine; marijuana), the synergistic effects of concurrent drug and substance use, also may play a significant role in the experience of the nicotine withdrawal syndrome.

Nicotine Overdosage/Unintentional Poisoning

The regular, long-term use of tobacco cigarettes or that of other tobacco products, has not been associated with the occurrence of overdosage. However, it has been associated with unintentional nicotine poisoning. In fact, for adolescents and young adults, 50 mg to 60 mg of nicotine may be fatal,[81] and, for young children, as little as 10 mg of nicotine may be fatal. Fortunately, nicotine overdose and related deaths rarely occur because:

1. When tobacco leaf is smoked, ~ 90% of the nicotine in the tobacco product is destroyed by pyrolysis (see the earlier discussion in the nicotine subsection, "Pharmacology, Pharmacokinetics—Absorption");
2. Oral bioavailability of nicotine from tobacco products is low (i.e., F = 0.3) when tobacco is ingested;
3. Nicotine stimulates vomiting as blood nicotine concentrations increase. Thus, tobacco products that are ingested often are vomited—offering some protection against fatal nicotine poisoning.

Unfortunately, unintentional poisonings have occurred when nicotine tobacco products are chewed or ingested by infants and children, or pets. It also has been reported with inadvertent access of infants and young children to cigarette butts or other nicotine products (e.g., Bassett, Osterhoudt, & Brabazon, 2014; Novotny, Hardin, & Hovda, 2011; Seo, Kim, & Yu, 2016). For example, poisonings have been associated with:

- Simultaneously chewing, or chewing in rapid succession, more than the recommended number of nicotine chewing gum squares (e.g., Cantrell, 2005);
- Simultaneously applying several transdermal delivery systems or chewing and swallowing these systems (Pagliaro & Pagliaro, *Clinical Patient Data Files*; Woolf, Burkhart, & Caraccio, 1997).

Of growing concern, in relation to the increased use of e-cigarettes in the U.S., are calls made to poison control centers regarding unintentional poisonings involving nicotine liquid refills, which:

1. Have been significantly increasing over the new millennium;
2. Are associated with more severe sequelae (e.g., respiratory failure; death) in comparison to traditional tobacco cigarettes;
3. Primarily involve children younger than five years-of-age
(e.g., Chatham-Stephens, Law, & Taylor, 2016; Weiss, Tomasallo, & Meiman, 2016).

As noted by Kamboj, Spiller, and Casavant (2016), in their analysis of the calls made to the National Poison Data System from January 2012 through April 2015 in regard to nicotine and tobacco product exposure among children younger than six years-of-age:

> Children exposed to e-cigarettes had 5.2 times higher odds of a health care facility admission and a 2.6 times higher odds of having a severe outcome than children exposed to cigarettes.
>
> (e20160041)

81 Several researchers, most notably Mayer (2014), questioned the LD_{50} for nicotine arguing that it is erroneously based on unreliable data that are:

- Outdated, being 50 to100 years-old;
- Inconsistent with the findings of documented cases of nicotine overdosages and unintentional poisonings.

While, agreeing that nicotine is a toxic substance that is potentially lethal, they argue that the LD_{50} for humans is five-fold to ten-fold higher than the current estimate—an argument that is interesting and plausible, but not yet substantiated.

The signs and symptoms of nicotine overdosages and unintentional poisonings associated with nicotine gums, transdermal delivery systems, and other tobacco smoking cessation products are characterized by a biphasic pattern with an initial phase of psychostimulation ("Phase 1") followed by a second phase of psychodepression ("Phase 2"). (See also the related discussion in the earlier nicotine pharmacology subsection, "Pharmacodynamics: Mechanism of Action").

- Phase 1 signs and symptoms of "psychostimulation" include: abdominal pain; agitation; cold sweat; confusion; diarrhea; diaphoresis; dizziness; headache; hearing and vision disturbances; hypertension; nausea; pallor; salivation (excessive); seizures; tachycardia; tremor; and vomiting.
- Phase 2 signs and symptoms of "psychodepression" include: bradycardia; confusion; circulatory collapse; drowsiness; dyspnea; faintness and prostration; hypotension; lethargy; muscle weakness; rapid, weak, irregular pulse; and respiratory failure due to paralysis of the muscles of respiration, which, within minutes, can result in death.

Suspected, or actual, nicotine overdosage/unintentional poisoning requires immediate discontinuation of the use of the involved nicotine product and emergency medical support of body systems, with particular attention to maintaining adequate respiratory function and increasing nicotine elimination. For example, a slurry of activated charcoal may be administered to decrease GI absorption of nicotine or, for transdermal delivery system, removing the transdermal delivery system[82] and flushing the skin with water (soap should *not* be used, because it may increase nicotine absorption from the skin site). Additionally, for example, a benzodiazepine (e.g., diazepam, Valium®) can be used to prevent or manage associated phase 1 seizures, while atropine can be used to manage phase 2 bradycardia. Severe respiratory failure may necessitate the use of mechanical ventilation. There is no known specific antidote for nicotine overdosage/unintentional poisoning.

Pregnancy and Lactation

This subsection presents and discusses the use of nicotine and tobacco smoking during pregnancy and lactation with particular attention to adolescent girls and young women.

Pregnancy

In a report on cigarette smoking among pregnant women, which was prepared on behalf of the CDC, Driscoll and Mathews (2018, p. 1) identified that:[83]

1. 7.2% of women who gave birth, smoked cigarettes during pregnancy;
2. Prevalence of smoking during pregnancy was highest among women aged 20–24 (10.7%), followed by women aged 15–19 (8.5%) and 25–29 (8.2%);

82 N.B. Nicotine will continue to be delivered into the bloodstream for several hours after removal of the transdermal system—because of the depot of nicotine that is formed in the skin as part of the mechanism of action designed for nicotine transdermal delivery systems.

83 Interestingly, as also has been reported to us, a small number of pregnant women "keep smoking through pregnancy just because they want to give birth to a smaller baby" (Adams, 2011, p. 1).

3. Non-Hispanic American Indian or Alaska Native women had the highest prevalence of smoking during pregnancy (16.7%); non-Hispanic Asian women had the lowest (0.6%);
4. The prevalence of smoking during pregnancy was highest among women with a completed high school education (12.2%), and second-highest among women with less than a high school education (11.7%).

Approximately 13% of women in the U.S., report smoking tobacco cigarettes during the last three months of pregnancy (CDC, 2012, p. 1).[84] In this regard, disparity of tobacco smoking rates has been reported among pregnant women in the U.S. of various continental descents. For example, Wright and Tam (2010) found in their study that significantly more women, who were Native Hawaiians (21% versus 8%), continued to smoke through pregnancy to within one week of admission for labor. For another example, in a study of 690 pregnant women, participants of African (62%) and European (38%) continental descents at an urban prenatal clinic, De Genna, Goldschmidt, and Day (2016) found that:

1. Rates of chronic smoking and nonsmoking were roughly equivalent (i.e., approximately 33%);
2. Younger pregnant women were more likely to smoke than older pregnant women;
3. Pregnant women of European continental descent were more likely to be chronic smokers;
4. Significant co-variants included: educational level; socioeconomic status; and the drugs and substances of abuse that were prenatally used.

In addition, the CDC evaluated rates of tobacco smoking and cessation among women during the first and second trimesters of pregnancy in 46 states and in the District of Columbia (Mathews, 2016). The data pool accounted for 3,819,113 births and represented 95% of all U.S. births in 2014. On average, 20.6% of pregnant women smoked during the first and second trimesters of pregnancy. Regarding smoking cessation during pregnancy, among the 46 states, Dakota had the highest cessation rate (i.e., 31.3%) while Kentucky had the lowest (i.e., 11.4%). In another study, which examined the course of smoking among pregnant women who also had a concurrent history of other drug and substance abuse, Forray, Gotman, and Kershaw (2014) found that:

> Women were able to discontinue or decrease smoking during pregnancy but were likely to resume or increase smoking postpartum.
>
> (p. 749)

The relationship between maternal use of nicotine during pregnancy and physical birth defects, or teratogenesis, have not been well-substantiated. However, smoking tobacco cigarettes has been related to increased rates of spontaneous abortion, stillbirth, pre-term delivery, and neonatal death. It has been hypothesized that the in-utero exposure of the embryo/fetus to nicotine, together with other components of tobacco smoke (e.g., carbon monoxide), can cause vasoconstriction and an associated decrease in blood flow to the uterus/placenta that may result in, or contribute to, these toxic effects (Ernst, Moolchan, & Robinson, 2001; Phelan, 2014; Shea & Steiner, 2008). In-utero

84 Other factors may significantly increase this percentage. For example, Goodwin, Cheslack-Postava, and Nelson (2017) found that depression increased the percentage of women, who smoked while pregnant, from 13% to 32.5% (see the related discussion in the later nicotine subsection, "Contemporaneous Diagnoses—Major Depressive Disorder").

exposure to nicotine (e.g., in the context of maternal tobacco smoking) may also result in genetic changes that subsequently produce accelerated lung aging and increased susceptibility to the development of chronic obstructive lung diseases in the exposed offspring later in life (Maritz & Harding, 2011).

In addition, neonates born to mothers who smoke tobacco cigarettes[85] during pregnancy, have lower birth weights (Pagliaro & Pagliaro, 2002, 2012). They also are twice as likely to die during early infancy due to the "Sudden Infant Death Syndrome" (SIDS) (Abbot & Winzer-Serhan, 2012). The SIDS is thought to be related to the infant's exposure to sidestream and environmental tobacco smoke in the home where the mother, father, or other household members and caregivers, smoke tobacco cigarettes or other tobacco products.

> Avoid [tobacco] exposure during pregnancy and after birth. Both maternal smoking during pregnancy and smoke in the infant's environment after birth are major risk factors for SIDS.
>
> (Moon, Darnall, & Goodstein, 2011, p. 1034)

Finally, several studies (e.g., Holbrook 2016; Keyes, Davey Smith, & Susser, 2014; Kovess, Keyes, & Hamilton, 2015) have suggested an association between in utero exposure to nicotine and risk for the subsequent development of ADHD among offspring—as has been noted in relation to prenatal exposure to other psychostimulants (see the related discussion in Chapter 2, "Amphetamines and Cocaine"). In their comprehensive review of this topic, Tiesler and Heinrich (2014) concluded that:

> In summary, the majority of studies, and especially several recent epidemiological studies, observed a higher likelihood for ADHD or ADHD symptoms in subjects prenatally exposed to nicotine. However, both human and animal studies have failed to provide clear evidence on causality.
>
> (p. 923)

Some of the noted concern regarding causality is related to the observation that paternal smoking during pregnancy also appears to be related to an increased risk for the subsequent development of ADHD among children (e.g., Kovess, Keyes, & Hamilton, 2015; Langley, Heron, & Smith, 2012). We would suggest that a likely explanation of this observation lies with the secondhand exposure of pregnant, "non-smoking" mothers (and, consequently, their developing fetuses) to tobacco smoke from smoking fathers or others living in the household. See also the related discussion in the later subsection, "Contemporaneous Diagnoses."

85 Although the maternal use of nicotine replacement products may be safer for the embryo/fetus than tobacco smoking (i.e., the fetus is not exposed to additional chemicals that are present in tobacco smoke), the use of nicotine products has been associated, as has tobacco smoking, with spontaneous abortion. Long-term expected pharmacologic actions associated with nicotine may be observed among neonates, including physical dependence and the signs and symptoms of the nicotine withdrawal syndrome. Adolescent girls and women who are pregnant should not smoke tobacco and should avoid the use of nicotine replacement products. These products should be used during pregnancy only if the risks to the mother and embryo/fetus or neonate is justified in comparison to the risks related to the continued maternal use of nicotine. If nicotine replacement pharmacotherapy is required, pregnant adolescent girls and young women should be advised of the potential benefits and possible risks to themselves and their embryo, fetus, or neonate.

Lactation

Nicotine, whether obtained from tobacco cigarette smoking or other methods of use—including e-cigarette vaping or use of nicotine replacement products—is excreted in breast milk. Concentrations of nicotine, and its metabolite, cotinine, in breast milk may be as much as three times the maternal plasma concentration (Dahlstrom, Lundell, & Curvall, 1990). Signs of nicotine/cotinine ingestion among these breastfed neonates and infants may include: colic; diarrhea; decreased sleep time; excessive crying; irritability; restlessness; tachycardia; and vomiting (Banderali, Martelli, & Landi, 2015; Mennella, Yourshaw, & Morgan, 2007). Additionally, odor and taste of cigarettes transfer to the breast milk of mothers who smoke tobacco cigarettes or other tobacco products (Mennella & Beauchamp, 1998). However, it does not appear to significantly affect infant breast milk intake (Mennella, Yourshaw, & Morgan, 2007).

Regardless, adolescent girls and young women, who are breastfeeding, should be advised of the potential risks to their neonates and infants. If tobacco cigarette smoking, vaping, or other methods of nicotine use is continued, or if nicotine replacement products are required, breastfeeding should be discontinued.

New Millennial Trends in Nicotine Use

Millennial trends in relation to: (1) the medical use of nicotine; (2) embryo/fetal, neonate, infant, and child nicotine exposure; and (3) adolescent and young adult nicotine use—including passive smoke exposure—are presented and discussed in this nicotine subsection. We begin with patterns of the medical use of nicotine.

Medical Use of Nicotine

For most of its history, the pharmacotherapeutic use of nicotine received little medical attention because of its early—and correct—identification as a poison. However, during the late 1970s, amidst the accumulation of research data supporting a relationship between tobacco smoking and lung cancer, nicotine replacement therapy (NRT) was medically initiated as an aid to facilitate the cessation of tobacco smoking among those who wanted to "kick-the-habit" (Hyde, Paxton, & Carr, 1982). (See the later nicotine subsection, "Adolescent and Young Adult Treatment for Nicotine Dependence or Use Disorder—Pharmacotherapy").

Embryo/Fetal, Neonate, Infant, and Young Child Nicotine and Tobacco Smoke Exposure

Nicotine and tobacco smoke exposure among infants and young children primarily occurs in the context of: (1) prenatal, or in utero, exposure; (2) exposure associated with breastfeeding; and (3) unintentional poisonings. For related discussion, see the earlier nicotine subsections, "Pregnancy and Lactation" and "Nicotine Overdosage/Unintentional Poisoning."

Child, Adolescent, and Young Adult Tobacco Smoke Exposure and Nicotine Use

New millennial trends regarding: (1) passive tobacco smoke exposure; (2) tobacco cigarette smoking and other leaf-tobacco use; (3) e-cigarette vaping and vapor exposure; and (4) hookah smoking and exposure are presented and discussed in this nicotine subsection.

PASSIVE TOBACCO SMOKE EXPOSURE

Nabi-Burza, Regan, and Drehmer (2012), in their study of "981 smoking parents" from eight states, found that "the majority of smoking parents exposed their children to tobacco smoke in cars" (p. e1471). More recently, in their secondary analysis of data from over 7,000 adolescents, who completed the *Population Assessment of Tobacco and Health Study*, Merianos, Jandarov, and Mahabee-Gittens (2018, p. 1) found that adolescents, who were exposed to secondhand tobacco smoke, "were at increased risk of reporting shortness of breath, finding it hard to exercise, wheezing during or after exercise, and dry cough at night."

Passive exposure to tobacco smoke varies among adolescents and young adults of different continental and other descents. For example, the CDC (2015a, p. 103), based on an analysis of data for the years 2011 and 2012, found that approximately 50% of "Black nonsmokers," 25% of "Mexican-American nonsmokers," and 20% of "Non-Hispanic White nonsmokers" were exposed to secondhand smoke. Most exposure to secondhand smoke occurs in the home and in workplaces. However, significant exposure still occurs across the U.S. in various public places, including bars, casinos, and restaurants (CDC, 2016a). The CDC goes on to emphasize that:

> Separating smokers from nonsmokers, opening windows, or using air filters does *not* prevent people from breathing secondhand smoke.
>
> (2016a, p. 1)

As shared in "Ellie's Story:"

> Ellie is an active member of the LGBT communities. In her mid-thirties, Ellie was diagnosed with asthma. Ellie never smoked but worked [as a young adult] in a bar [in her LGBT community] that allowed smoking. Her doctor said her asthma attacks were triggered by secondhand smoke [exposure that occurred while working in the bar] . . .
>
> (CDC, 2016b, p. 1)

TOBACCO CIGARETTE SMOKING

Common Misbelief: When compared to other adolescents and young adults in the U.S., adolescents and young adults of American Indian descent generally have lower rates of tobacco use because they primarily respect and smoke tobacco as a part of their traditional American Indian ceremonies.

Not true—on both counts. As found by Odani, Armour, and Agaku (2018)—on behalf of the CDC:

> During 2014–2017, ever-use and current use of any tobacco product among U.S. middle and high school students were highest among Native Hawaiians/Other Pacific Islanders and American Indians/Alaska Natives and lowest among Asians.
>
> (p. 952)

It should be noted that tobacco smokers, overall, cannot be generally defined as belonging preferentially to any continental or other descent, ethnic, or socioeconomic group. They include approximately one-fourth of the adult population in the U.S.,[86] most of whom began to smoke before they were 14 years-of-age.

As reported by the FDA Commissioner:

> Almost all adult smokers started smoking when they were kids. Nearly 90 percent started smoking before the age of 18, and 95 percent by age 21. Only about 1 percent of cigarette smokers begin at age 26 or older.
>
> (Gottlieb, 2018, p. 2)

It is estimated that, every day of the year in the U.S., over 3000 children and adolescents—mostly girls—begin to smoke tobacco (Pagliaro & Pagliaro, 2009), and over an additional 2000 adolescents and young adults, become daily cigarette smokers (USDHHS, 2014).[87]

Birge, Duffy, and Astrid Miler (2018), in their meta-analysis of the initiation of tobacco cigarette use, found that:

> Over two-thirds of people who try one cigarette become, at least temporarily, daily smokers.
>
> (p. 1427)

86 N.B. Tobacco smoking rates in the U.S. are difficult to fully compare and evaluate because different surveys define the sample measures in a variety of ways that generally preclude collapsing, or often even directly comparing, data from various studies. For example, in the often cited 2015 *National Health Interview Survey* (NHIS), which is a nationally representative, in-person survey of the noninstitutionalized adult (i.e., 18 years-of-age or older) U.S. civilian population conducted on behalf of the CDC, "current cigarette smokers" are defined as "adults who smoked 100 or more cigarettes during their lifetime and, at the time of the interview, smoked every day or on some days" (CDC, 2016f, p. 1205).

In that study, "current cigarette smoking among U.S. adults [was reported to have] declined from 20.9% in 2005 to 15.1% in 2015" (p. 1205). The trend (i.e., decline in cigarette smoking) appears to be accurate and substantiated by (i.e., consistent with) data from other related studies. For example, the CDC identified that tobacco cigarette smoking among U.S. adults decreased from 42% in 1965 to its record low of 14% in 2017 (LaVito, 2018). However, the magnitude (i.e., as based on reported percentages) is less reliable because of the related definition of "cigarette smoking" and the defined characteristics of the samples. In addition, other tobacco use—such as the use of cigars and pipe tobacco—as well as "e-cigarette" use (see later discussion in the section, "E-Cigarette Vaping"), were not included.

However, in this context, a more recent study, which used data from Wave 1 (i.e., September 2013 through December 2014) of the *Population Assessment of Tobacco and Health (PATH) Study*, and determined prevalence estimates for the use of 12 different forms of tobacco products in the U.S., found that:

> More than a quarter (27.6%) of adults were current users of at least one type of tobacco product in 2013 and 2014 ... [In addition,] approximately 40% of tobacco users, adults and youths alike, used multiple tobacco products; cigarettes plus e-cigarettes was the most common combination.
>
> (Kasza, Ambrose, & Conway, 2017, p. 342)

In addition, Odani, Agaku, and Graffunder (2018), in their study of tobacco product use among U.S. military veterans from 2010 to 2015, found that the highest use of tobacco products (i.e., 56.8%)—in their sample—was among young adults, 18 to 25 years-of-age.

87 This behavior has significant health implications well beyond those solely associated with nicotine/tobacco use (see earlier related discussion in this chapter, particularly in the section, "Undesired, or Harmful, Effects and Toxicities"). For example, Keyes, Hamilton, and Kandel (2016), in their analysis of data collected from high school students from 1991 to 2008, noted that:

> Lifetime rates of 8th and 10th grade cigarette use was significantly associated with subsequent lifetime rates of marijuana and cocaine use.
>
> (p. 1143)

Several pertinent, summary findings were reported in the SAMHSA-sponsored *2016 National Survey on Drug Use and Health*. As identified by Ahrnsbrak, Bose, and Hedden (2017, pp. 6–11):

- 885,000 adolescents, 12 to 17 years-of-age, smoked tobacco cigarettes in the past month;
- 8.1 million young adults, 18 to 25 years-of-age, smoked tobacco cigarettes in the past month;
- 67% of current tobacco users, 12 years-of-age and older, only smoked tobacco cigarettes;
- 40% of young adults, 18 to 25 years-of-age, smoked tobacco cigarettes daily in the past month;
- 35.4% of adolescents, who were current tobacco users, used tobacco products other than tobacco cigarettes (i.e., did not smoke tobacco cigarettes);[88]
- 25% of adolescents and young adults, who were current tobacco users, both smoked cigarettes and used other tobacco products;
- 20% of adolescents, 12 years-of-age or older, were current cigarette smokers (i.e., smoked within the past month);
- 15% of adolescents, 12 to 17 years-of-age, smoked tobacco cigarettes daily in the past month;
- 9% of young adults, 18 to 25 years-of-age, smoked tobacco during the past month;
- 5.2 % of young adults, 18 to 25 years-of-age, used smokeless tobacco (e.g., chewing tobacco; snuff or snus tobacco) during the past month;
- 2% of adolescents, 12 to 17 years-of-age, smoked tobacco cigars during the past month;
- 2% of young adults, 18 to 25 years-of-age, smoked pipe tobacco during the past month;
- 1.4% of adolescents, 12 to 17 years-of-age, used smokeless tobacco (e.g., chewing tobacco; snuff or snus) during the past month;
- 0.5% of adolescents, 12 to 17 years-of-age, smoked pipe tobacco during the past month.

E-CIGARETTE VAPING[89]

Regarding e-cigarettes, formal studies and related estimates of use among adolescents in the U.S. (e.g., USDHHS, 2016b) have confirmed a definite and significant positive trend. Sutfin, McCoy, and Morrell (2013), in an earlier large, web-based survey of 4500 college students from eight colleges conducted in 2009, found that 5% of respondents endorsed e-cigarette use. We estimate that, currently, approximately 30% of adolescents have used e-cigarettes (Pagliaro & Pagliaro, *Clinical Patient Data Files*) because: (1) e-cigarette use steadily increased during the intervening years (e.g., Adams, 2018; Clapp & Jaspers, 2017; McConnell, Barrington-Trimis, & Wang, 2017; Miech, Johnston, & O'Malley, 2018); and (2) adolescents have higher e-cigarette use rates. In addition:

> As reported by the Centers for Disease Control and Prevention, e-cigarette experimentation and recent use among US middle and high school students doubled from 2011 to 2012 and has increased significantly since then. It is now estimated that 1.78 million students have ever used e-cigarettes.
>
> (Siqueira, 2017, p. e1)

88 We, and others (e.g., Sherburne Hawkins, Bach, & Baum, 2018), have suggested that this number will significantly increase over the next decade—particularly, in response to states increasing cigarette taxes without a commensurate increase in taxes on other tobacco products (e.g., chewing tobacco; cigars) and e-cigarettes.

89 See also the related discussion in the earlier nicotine subsection, "E-Cigarettes."

> Among middle and high school students, both ever and past-30-day e-cigarette use have more than tripled since 2011. Among young adults 18–24 years-of-age, ever e-cigarette use more than doubled from 2013 to 2014.
>
> (USDHHS, 2016b, p. 7)

Based upon an analysis of data obtained from the *2015 National Youth Survey* and the *2016 Monitoring the Future Survey* (as reported by the National Academies [2018]), we also estimate rates of e-cigarette use as approximately:

- 20% among 8th grade students;[90]
- 32% among 10th grade students;
- 40% among 12th grade students.

Variability in rates of e-cigarette use within each of these grade levels appears to be largely related to:

1. Gender, with higher use among boys;
2. Continental or other descent, with higher use among students of European continental descent;[91, 92]
3. Geographic location, with higher use on each coast versus the central part of the U.S.

Additionally, as found by Goldbach, Mereish, and Burgess (2017), sexual orientation is significantly associated with e-cigarette use among adolescent middle and high school students. Those adolescents, who identified as LGB, were twice as likely to report lifetime e-cigarette use in comparison to the heterosexual adolescents in their sample.

As emphasized by Zhu, Sun, and Bonnevie (2014), "E-cigarettes are largely unregulated and internet sales are substantial" (p. iii3). Thus, some additional and largely unresolved concerns accompany the current use of e-cigarettes. These concerns include:

1. Fires and explosions caused by the e-cigarette devises (National Academies, 2018; Roger, Abayon, & Elad, 2016);[93]
2. Irritation of the mouth and throat with a related dry cough associated with the glycerol and propylene glycol present in the e-cigarette aerosol, or vapor (Callahan-Lyon, 2014; Shields, Berman, & Brasky, 2017);
3. Toxicity associated with the metal nanoparticles from the vaporizing mechanism (National Institute on Drug Abuse, 2016; USDHHS, 2016b);
4. Possible secondhand exposure, particularly to infants and children, of aerosols containing relatively high concentrations of nicotine (i.e., higher than that found in typical

90 In comparison, for example, Westling, Rusby, and Crowley (2017), in their analysis of data from seven school districts in Oregon, found that: (1) 27.7% of eight graders had used e-cigarettes; and (2) 16.8% of eight graders were current e-cigarette users (i.e., within the past 30 days). Similarly, Gentzke, Creamer, and Cullen (2019), in their analysis of data from the *National Youth Tobacco Survey*, found that 4.9% of middle school students and 27.1% of high school students reported current e-cigarette use.

91 According to the U.S. Surgeon General's report on e-cigarettes, use was: (1) highest among adolescents of European continental descent and Hispanic descent; and (2) lowest among adolescents of African continental descent (USDHHS, 2016b, p. 5).

92 Regarding the initiation of e-cigarette use among "minority youth in the U.S.," Hammig, Daniel-Dobbs, and Blunt-Vinti (2017) reported similar findings with the highest "minority" initiation and usage rates occurring among Hispanic youth.

93 Because of this concern, the U.S. Department of Transportation in 2015 banned e-cigarette devices from being packed in checked airline baggage (Roger, Abayon, & Elad, 2016).

tobacco cigarette smoke) (Callahan-Lyon, 2014; Czogala, Goniewicz, & Fidelus, 2014; Wang, Marynak, & Agaku, 2017);[94]

5. Nicotine physical and psychological dependence associated with e-cigarette use (National Academies, 2018; Schroeder & Hoffman, 2014; USDHHS, 2016b);
6. Thirdhand exposure to nicotine because of e-cigarette use (Goniewicz, Gupta, & Lee, 2015);[95]
7. Increased incidence of COPD (e.g., McConnell, Barrington-Trimis, & Wang, 2017).[96]

<u>Related Professional Reminder:</u> Nicotine concentrations vary among the different brands of tobacco cigarettes. However, this variance is significantly more pronounced among the different brands of e-liquid solutions available for use with e-cigarettes (i.e., from 0% to 24%).

Since the development and release of e-cigarettes in the U.S. during the new millennium, we have consistently predicted the increased use of e-cigarettes among adolescents and, consequently, the eventual later "supremacy" of e-cigarettes as the predominant form of recreational nicotine delivery (i.e., the steady and ultimate replacement of tobacco cigarettes with e-cigarettes) (Pagliaro & Pagliaro, *Clinical Patient Data Files*). Over the years, our prediction has been supported by several authors and researchers (e.g., Huang, Kowitt, & Sutfin, 2016; Kamat & Van Dyke, 2017; Rom, Pecorelli, & Valacchi, 2015).

As reported by the director of the CDC:

> In recent years, e-cigarette use by youth and young adults has increase at an alarming rate. E-cigarettes are now the most commonly used tobacco product among youth in the United States.
>
> (USDHHS, 2016b, p. v)

As further reported by the U.S. Surgeon General:

> E-cigarette use increased considerably in recent years, growing an astounding 900% among high school students from 2011 to 2015. These products are now the most commonly used form of tobacco products, including cigarettes, cigars, chewing tobacco, and hookahs.
>
> (USDHHS, 2016b, p. vii)

In addition, during the new millennium, it has consistently been demonstrated that adolescents, who use e-cigarettes, are significantly:

94 Because the e-cigarette delivery systems vary from manufacturer to manufacturer, or brand to brand, some systems produce and deliver higher or lower secondhand nicotine aerosol, or vapor, concentrations than others (e.g., Trehy, Ye, & Hadwiger, 2011). However, in their analysis of secondhand exposure utilizing three different brands of e-cigarettes, Czogala, Goniewicz, and Fidelus (2014) found that, in comparison to traditional tobacco cigarettes, e-cigarettes produced no combustion toxicants and one-tenth the level of nicotine secondhand exposure.

95 Thirdhand nicotine exposure refers to the nicotine vapor that remains on various surfaces (e.g., carpets; couches; curtains; floors; tables) in areas where e-cigarette use is significant (National Academies, 2018).

96 Interestingly, as previously noted in this chapter, Clapp and Jaspers (2017) found that:

> Adolescents with asthma had a higher prevalence of current e-cig use (12.4%) compared to their non-asthmatic peers (10.2%).
>
> (p. 79)

1. Less likely to abstain from tobacco use for a prolonged period of time (i.e., for six months or longer);
2. More likely to subsequently initiate tobacco cigarette use

(e.g., Huang, Kowitt, & Sutfin, 2016; Soneji, Barrington-Trimis, & Wills, 2017)

DRIPPING. Dripping involves "dripping" e-liquids directly onto heated e-cigarette atomizers to produce a vapor that is quickly inhaled. In a study of over 7,000 students from eight Connecticut high schools, Krishnan-Sarin, Morean, and Kong (2017) found that "a substantial portion (one in four) of high school adolescents, who had ever used e-cigarettes, also reported using the device for dripping."

Reasons given for "dripping" primarily include:

- Curiosity;
- Enhancement of the taste of flavored vapors;
- Production of a stronger "throat hit;"
- Production of thicker clouds of vapor.

(Krishnan-Sarin, Morean, & Kong, 2017, p. e20163224)

HOOKAH USE

The hookah, or water-pipe,[97] is an ancient smoking device that filters and cools inhaled smoke by drawing it through cold water. It was originally developed in the Middle East to smoke opium and cannabis, particularly hashish, or hash. Following the introduction of tobacco to the Middle East from the U.S. during the 17th and 18th centuries, the hookah was readily adapted for smoking tobacco, including mixtures of cannabis and tobacco (Pagliaro & Pagliaro, 2004).

The use of hookahs in the U.S. was relatively uncommon until its popularity increased among "hippies"—the predominant youth culture—during the 1960s and 1970s. Even then, their use was never particularly significant until the beginning of the new millennium when "hookah cafes" began to flourish near college/university campuses across the U.S. together with the growth of middle-eastern communities. The tobacco traditionally smoked in a hookah is called *mu'assel* (maassel) and generally consists of a syrupy mixture of shredded tobacco leaf, flavored molasses or dried fruit, and vegetable glycol, or honey. Typical flavors include: apple, banana, coconut, grape, guava, lemon, licorice, mint, peach, rose, strawberry, and watermelon. In the U.S., the wet, flavored and sweetened smoking mixture of tobacco is often called, *shisha* (Morris, Fiala, & Pawlak, 2012).

Common Misbelief: The use of a hookah eliminates virtually all the toxicities associated with smoking tobacco cigarettes because the smoke is filtered through water before being inhaled.

97 The hookah, or water-pipe, has been used for centuries throughout the world, particularly in Moslem countries. Hence, it is known by a large variety of names (and alternative spellings) including: argile; argileh; argyleh; bong; chillim; galyan; hookah; hubble-bubble; huqqa; huqqo; nargila; nargilah; narghile; narguile; qaelyan; qalyan; and water-pipe. "Shisha" ("Sheesha"), another common term for the hookah, also refers to the flavored tobacco that is smoked through a hookah. (See also the related discussion in the "cannabis" subsection—"Hookah Use," in Chapter 4, "Cannabis and Other Psychodelics").

Not true. Several undesired, or harmful, effects and toxicities are associated with smoking tobacco through a hookah, including:

1. Risk of exposure to several harmful chemicals (e.g., acrolein; carbon monoxide; heavy metals; and tobacco-specific nitrosamines) that are not filtered-out by the water in the hookah (Kassem, Kassem, & Liles, 2018; Shihadeh, 2003);
2. Risk of exposure to infectious diseases (e.g., helicobacter pylori; hepatitis; influenza; oral herpes; and tuberculosis), particularly when shared with others (e.g., Masadeh, Hussein, & Alzoubi, 2015);
3. Risk of exposure to several harmful chemicals (e.g., nicotine; polycyclic aromatic hydrocarbons; tobacco specific nitrosamines) in secondhand hookah smoke (e.g., Moon, Rule, & Magid, 2018).

In addition, smoking tobacco with a hookah does not filter out the nicotine from the inhaled smoke. Therefore, hookah smokers are at risk for any nicotine-related toxicity, including physical and psychological dependence, or NUD. Despite these documented toxicities, most adolescents and young adults, who smoke tobacco using a hookah, believe it is significantly safer than smoking tobacco cigarettes (Asfar, Ward, & Eissenberg, 2005; Pagliaro & Pagliaro, *Clinical Patient Data Files*). The method of hookah smoking also contributes to other potential toxicities associated with nicotine. For example, hookah smokers typically "puff" more often, inhale more deeply, and smoke for longer periods of time during each smoking session.[98] In fact, a typical 1-hour hookah smoking session has been estimated to involve approximately 200 puffs, or ten times the puffs inhaled when smoking a typical tobacco cigarette (i.e., a typical hookah smoking session is, in this regard, equivalent to smoking approximately 10 filter-tipped tobacco cigarettes) (Hays, 2015; Sathya, 2014).

In comparison to adolescent and young adult use of e-cigarettes (see previous subsection, "E-Cigarette Vaping"), data related to hookah usage statistics in the U.S. are relatively sparse. However, over the new millennium, it has been generally observed that, hookah use has steadily and significantly increased (e.g., Siqueira, 2017). For example, Sutfin, McCoy, and Reboussin (2011), in their study of 3,770 college students from eight universities, found that "forty percent of the sample reported ever having smoked tobacco from a waterpipe" (p. 131). In another example based on a comprehensive literature review, Grekin and Ayna (2012) reported that "1 in 5 American college students reported past-year waterpipe use" (p. 244).

In the U.S., several factors have been identified that significantly correlate with hookah smoking by adolescents and young adults, including:

- Alcohol use;
- Arab ethnicity;
- Belief that hookah use is significantly less harmful than cigarette smoking;[99]

98 The methods used for smoking tobacco through a hookah are similar, in many ways, to those used for smoking cannabis through a hookah (see also the related discussion in the "cannabis" subsection of Chapter 4, "Cannabis and Other Psychodelics.")

99 This erroneous belief is commonly held among adolescents and young adults in the U.S. For example, as noted by Cornacchione, Wagoner, and Wiseman (2016):

> Use of hookah and little cigars/cigarillos (LCCs) is high among adolescents and young adults. Although these products have health effects similar to cigarettes, adolescent and young adults believe them to be safe.
>
> (p. 818)

- Cigarette smoking;
- Freshman college/university class membership;
- Having a commercial "waterpipe" venue (e.g., hookah bar) close to campus;
- Male gender;
- Marijuana use.

(Grekin & Ayna, 2012; Sutfin, McCoy, & Reboussin, 2011)

Hookah smoking of tobacco and cannabis, alone, or in combination, is relatively common in the U.S., with approximately 20% of high school seniors and up to 40% of U.S. college/ university students reporting hookah use within the past year (Palamar, Zhou, & Sherman, 2014; Sathya, 2014). However, the CDC estimated hookah use among U.S. high school students to be less than 5% (CDC, 2015b, 2018b). Hookah smoking is highest among young adults, 18 to 24 years-of-age and, within this group, particularly those of European continental descent and those of Middle-Eastern descent (American Lung Association, 2007).[100]

In response to the steady and rapid increase in the use of both e-cigarettes and hookahs for the delivery of nicotine during the new millennium, the FDA extended its full control over the devices in 2016 (FDA, 2016a). Consequently, nationwide tobacco regulations currently extend to *all* tobacco products, including:

- Cigarettes;
- Cigars;
- E-Cigarettes and their liquid nicotine solutions;
- Hookah tobacco;
- Pipe tobacco.

(NIDA, 2016)

Assessment and Diagnosis of Nicotine Dependence or Use Disorder

Assessment and diagnosis of nicotine physical and psychological dependence, or NUD, among adolescents and young adults requires a detailed clinical interview and examination of presenting signs and symptoms that addresses both the:

1. Use of tobacco smoking products and e-cigarettes, including the extent and duration of use;
2. Clinical sequelae that are commonly associated with their use (e.g., COPDs; oral cancers; smoker's cough, particularly with the regular, long-term use of nicotine tobacco cigarettes, cigars, and little cigars and cigarillos (LCCs)—as well as that associated with the regular, long-term use of e-cigarettes (e.g., irritation of the mouth and throat; dry cough associated with the glycerol and propylene glycol present in the e-cigarette aerosol, or vapor).

The use of DSM criteria for detecting NUD, or specific quick-screen psychometric tests, can assist with the determination of the nature and extent of nicotine use—among adolescents and young adults. However, to date, there are no specific available tests to assist with the determination of the nature and extent of nicotine use in the form of e-cigarettes.[101]

100 Recent trends in preferred smoking methods, for both tobacco and cannabis, suggest a consistent and dominant move, particularly among adolescents and young adults, to the use of vaping devices—e-cigarettes and e-hookahs (see the related discussion in the earlier nicotine subsection, "E-Cigarette Vaping").

101 N.B. A major related concern is that, based on an analysis of data from the *National Survey on Drug Use and Health*, less than 50% of adolescents, who visited a physician within the past year, reported being screened for tobacco use (Collins, Smiley, & Moore, 2017).

Table 3.3 The AUTOS

Item #	*Question*	*This statement describes me…*			
1.	When I go too long without a cigarette or a dip, I get impatient.	Not at all	A little	Pretty well	Very well
2.	When I see other people smoking or using dip, I want a cigarette or a dip.	Not at all	A little	Pretty well	Very well
3.	I rely on smoking or dip to focus my attention.	Not at all	A little	Pretty well	Very well
4.	When I smell cigarette smoke or dip, I want a cigarette or dip.	Not at all	A little	Pretty well	Very well
5.	I rely on smoking or dipping to take my mind off being bored.	Not at all	A little	Pretty well	Very well
6.	When I go too long without a cigarette or a dip, I get strong urges to smoke or dip that are hard to get rid of.	Not at all	A little	Pretty well	Very well
7.	After eating I want a cigarette or dip.	Not at all	A little	Pretty well	Very well
8.	I would go crazy if I couldn't smoke or use dip.	Not at all	A little	Pretty well	Very well
9.	When I go too long without a cigarette or a dip, I lose my temper more easily.	Not at all	A little	Pretty well	Very well
10.	When I feel stressed, I want a cigarette or a dip.	Not at all	A little	Pretty well	Very well
11.	I rely on smoking or dipping to deal with stress.	Not at all	A little	Pretty well	Very well
12.	When I go too long without a cigarette or a dip, I feel nervous or anxious.	Not at all	A little	Pretty well	Very well

Source: DiFranza, Wellman, & Ursprung (2009).

Quick-Screen Psychometric Tests

Three specific quick screen psychometric tests are predominantly used to assess the nature and extent of nicotine dependence associated with tobacco smoking, the: (1) "Autonomy Over Tobacco Scale" (AUTOS); (2) the "Fagerström Test for Nicotine Dependence" (FTND); and (3) the "Brief Wisconsin Inventory of Smoking Dependence" (Brief WISDM). The use of these tests for adolescents and young adults, as well as their psychometric properties, when available, are discussed in the following nicotine subsections.

AUTONOMY OVER TOBACCO SCALE (AUTOS)

The AUTOS, a 12-item, quick-screen psychometric test (Table 3.3, The AUTOS), is comprised of 12 possible signs and symptoms of nicotine dependence. It was developed by DiFranza, Wellman, and Ursprung (2009) to provide a more reliable screening test for detecting nicotine dependence than the Fagerström Test for Nicotine Dependence (see the later nicotine subsection, "Fagerström Test for Nicotine Dependence," and Table 3.4). The AUTOS is an updated version of the "Hooked on Nicotine Checklist," which was developed by the lead author's research group (DiFranza, Savageau, & Rigotti, 2002). Based on confirmatory factor analysis, the AUTOS appears to be unidimensional in adult smokers (Wellman, DiFranza, & O'Loughlin, 2015) "with a single factor solution explicating 59% of the variance in adults and 61% to 74% of the variance in adolescents" (Kim, 2017, p. 67).

DiFranza, Wellman, and Ursprung (2009, p. 656) claim 16 specific advantages, or "attractive features," associated with the AUTOS. As follows, it:

1. Is theory-based;
2. Has excellent internal reliability, retest reliability, and concurrent validity;
3. Is tested and recommended for all ages;
4. Is tested and recommended for tobacco smokers and buccal tobacco users;
5. Can be used with daily and non-daily tobacco users;
6. Is invulnerable to cultural measurement bias caused by differences in the affordability of tobacco, or racial measurement bias caused by differences in nicotine metabolism;
7. Can be used before and after cessation (i.e., during active tobacco use as well as during abstinence);
8. Can be used in longitudinal studies to track the development of nicotine dependence;
9. Can be used in cessation studies to track the persistence or resolution of signs and symptoms;
10. Measures nicotine withdrawal (i.e., nicotine physical dependence);
11. Measures psychological dependence;
12. Measures cue-induced urges, or craving, to use tobacco;
13. Can be used in cessation settings to guide anticipatory counseling and relapse prevention;
14. Can be easily scored;
15. Can be self-administered in less than three minutes;
16. Is currently available for use in Dutch, English, French, German, and Spanish.

SCORING THE AUTOS. Each of the 12 questions is scored, per response, from 0 to 3,[102] and summed to provide a total AUTOS score. The potential total score can range from 0 to 36. In addition, outcomes regarding three correlated, lower-order symptom domains are determined as follows:

1. "Withdrawal score"—sum of the total score for questions one through four;
2. "Psychological dependence"—sum of the total score for questions five through eight;
3. "Cue-induced urges to use tobacco"—sum of the total score for questions nine through 12.

The potential "total score" from each of the three domains can range from 0 to 12.

102 "Scoring criteria" and "point allocations" are as follows: "not at all," 0; "a little," 1; "pretty well," 2; and "very well," 3.

AVAILABLE TEST STATISTICS AND RECOMMENDATIONS. There were no published data found for the AUTOS regarding specificity and sensitivity. However, published data were found regarding validity and reliability. These data are followed by our recommendations.

VALIDITY AND RELIABILITY The questions comprising the AUTOS are derived from symptoms of nicotine dependence and, consequently, have good face validity. In addition, as identified by DiFranza, Savageau, and Wellman (2012), based on their study of 422 adult smokers (62% women; 57% daily smokers):

> The AUTOS and its subscales correlated with all measures of concurrent validity (r = .70, between AUTOS and FTND). The AUTOS correlated better than the FTND with the "Hooked on Nicotine Checklist," the longest period of abstinence, latency to wanting, percentage of time a person smokes because of momentary need, pleasure from smoking, days smoked per month, and concern about deprivation. The measures showed similar correlations with the latencies to craving and needing.
>
> (p. 856)

In addition, Wellman, Edelen, and DiFranza (2015) evaluated the reliability of the full AUTOS across "the range of diminished autonomy" among a sample of 777 adults, 18 to 78 year-of-age, and found an acceptable reliability of greater than 0.70 (p. 195).

The "internal reliability," or item reliability, of the AUTOS is high with "inter-item correlations range from 0.65 to 0.89 (mean = 0.79)" (Wellman, DiFranza, & Morgenstern, 2012, p. 76). Again, as found by DiFranza, Savageau, and Wellman (2012a, p. 856): "Cronbach's alpha was 0.94 for the AUTOS and greater than 0.75 for each of the three subscales; 0.73 for the FTND."[103]

RECOMMENDATIONS The validity and reliability of the AUTOS, as reported, appear to be satisfactory. They also appear to be superior to the FTND (see discussion in later section, "Fagerström Test for Nicotine Dependence"). In addition, several studies have included adolescent participants. However, other than validity and reliability data, *no* other published statistical data (e.g., specificity and sensitivity) were included. Thus, we generally do not recommend the use of the AUTOS for screening adolescents.

FAGERSTRÖM TEST FOR NICOTINE DEPENDENCE (FTND)

The FTND is a six-item quick-screen psychometric test (Table 3.4) that was developed by Heatherton, Kozlowski, and Frecker (1991) as an improved version of the original "Fagerström Tolerance Questionnaire" (FTQ). The FTQ was originally developed by Kari Fagerström, in 1978, to determine if nicotine replacement therapy (NRT) was required for the management of nicotine withdrawal. It was later found to be a useful test for measuring nicotine dependence. However, as determined by DiFranza, Wellman, and Savageau (2013), and others, the FTND correlated significantly greater with nicotine withdrawal than with nicotine dependence.

The FTND, which should only be completed by current, active tobacco smokers, has been translated into several languages. It also has been tested and used to measure nicotine dependence in several countries, including: Brazil, Canada, China, France, Germany, Holland, Japan, Mexico, Spain, Switzerland, Turkey, United States, and Yemen (de Meneses-Gaya,

103 Similar values for internal reliability (i.e., Cronbach's alpha of 0.94 was obtained when the AUTOS was used with a sample of 1541 U.S. adolescents (mean, 16 years-of-age) (DiFranza, Sweet, & Savageau, 2012).

Zuardi, & Loureiro, 2009; Etter, Duc, & Perneger, 1999; Huang, Lin, & Wang, 2006; Mikami, Akechi, & Kugaya, 1999; Moreno-Coutino & Villalbos-Gallegos, 2017; Nakajima, al'Absi, & Dokam, 2012; Perez-Rios, Santiago-Perez, & Alonso, 2009; Pomerleau, Carton, & Lutzke, 1994; Richardson & Ratner, 2005; Uysal, Kadakai, & Karsidag, 2004; Uysal, Oztuna, & Bahadir, 2015). The FTND also has been tested and used for detecting nicotine dependence among smokers who have post-traumatic stress disorder (PTSD), schizophrenia, or other mental disorders (e.g., Buckley, Mozley, & Holohan, 2005; Weinberger, Reutenauer, & Allen, 2007).

Piper, McCarthy, and Baker (2008), using data from three randomized placebo-controlled smoking cessation studies, found that the FTND was a better predictor of smoking cessation outcomes at one week and six months "post quit" than the WISDM (see the later discussion in the nicotine subsection, "Brief Wisconsin Inventory of Smoking Dependence").

Several modified versions of the FTND have been developed, including: (1) The "Modified-FTND," a version to which additional possible responses, such as, "I have never smoked cigarettes," were added to each question, as well as, an additional question concerning "inhaling smoke" (Prokhorov, Koehly, & Pallonen, 1998); and (2) the "FTND-ST" (Ebbert, Patten, & Schroeder, 2006), which is used to assess nicotine dependence among users of smokeless tobacco products (e.g., chewing tobacco; snuff or snus tobacco).[104]

Table 3.4 The FTND[105]

Item/question	*Scoring Criteria [Point Allocation]*
1. How soon after you wake up do you have your first cigarette?	Within five minutes, [3]; six to 30 minutes, [2]; 31 to 60 minutes, [1]; after 60 minutes, [0]
2. Do you find it difficult to refrain from smoking in places where it is forbidden such as church, the library or movie theaters?	Yes, [1]; No [0]
3. Which cigarette would you hate most to give up?	The first one in the morning, [1]; all others, [0]
4. How many cigarettes do you smoke? (20 cigarettes per pack)	10 or less, [0]; 11 to 20, [1]; 21 to 30, [2]; 31 or more, [3]
5. Do you smoke more frequently during the first hours after waking than the rest of the day?	Yes, [1]; No [0]
6. Do you smoke if you are so ill that you are in bed most of the day?	Yes, [1]; No [0]

104 Poor psychometric statistical performance was reported for both modified versions of the FTND by Ebbert, Patten, and Schroeder (2006), and others—consequently, precluding us from recommending either of the "modified" versions for clinical use. Thus, copies of these quick-screen tests and further discussion are not included in this chapter.

105 Source: Heatherton, Kozlowski, & Frecker, (1991).

SCORING THE FTND. Each of the six questions in the FTND is assigned 0 to 3 points depending on the selected response (see Table 3.4). All the scores are summed for a possible maximal score of 10. Total scores are generally evaluated as follows: 0 to 2, "very low" dependence; 3 or 4, "low dependence;" 5, "medium" dependence; 6 or 7, "high" dependence; and 8 to 10, "very high" dependence.

AVAILABLE TEST STATISTICS AND RECOMMENDATIONS. Data regarding specificity, sensitivity, positive and negative predictive values, and validity and reliability are available. These data are followed by our recommendations.

SPECIFICITY, SENSITIVITY, AND POSITIVE AND NEGATIVE PREDICTIVE VALUES Data are unavailable for tobacco smokers in the U.S. However, a Japanese study (i.e., Mikami, Akechi, & Kugaya, 1999) reported a specificity of 0.80 and a sensitivity of 0.75 when a cutoff score of 5 was used. A Brazilian study (i.e., de Meneses-Gaya, Zuardi, & Loureiro, 2009) reported a specificity of 0.74 and a sensitivity of 0.80 when a cutoff score of 4 was used. This study also reported a positive predictive value of 0.95 and a negative predictive value of 0.30. A Spanish study (i.e., Chabrol, Niezborala, & Chastan, 2005), which involved 398 cigarette-smoking women, reported a specificity of 0.97 and a sensitivity of 0.81. The study also reported a positive predictive value of 78% and a negative predictive value of 97%.

VALIDITY AND RELIABILITY Studies of the criterion-related validity of the FTND, in comparison to selected biological markers (e.g., carbon monoxide blood concentrations; saliva cotinine concentrations), among regular tobacco smokers have been performed (e.g., Buckley, Mozley, & Holohan, 2005; Burling & Burling, 2003; Huang, Lin, & Wang, 2006). The mean criterion-related validity coefficient was 0.5 (i.e., a moderate, but generally unacceptable result). A similar low concurrent validity (i.e., r ~ 0.45) was obtained when FTND and AUTOS scores were correlated (Kim, 2017). Similarly, measures of concurrent and convergent validity (e.g., when comparing results from the FTND to those obtained using DSM criteria) have been disappointing. In this regard, it has been suggested that the FTND and DSM criteria measure different aspects of nicotine dependence with the FTND providing a stronger measure of physical dependence (Moolchan, Radzius, & Epstein, 2002).[106]

The mean of the reported Cronbach's alpha coefficients of item reliability for the FTND is 0.68, range 0.58 to 0.72 (e.g., Etter, 2005; Fagan, Pohkrel, & Herzog, 2015; Haddock, Lando, & Klesges, 1999; Okuyemi, Pulvers, & Cox, 2007),[107] indicating moderate, but generally unacceptable, internal consistency for the psychometric test.[108] In this regard, it has been suggested that the deletion of items two and three (see Table 3.4) may increase the internal consistency of the FTND (de Leon, Diaz, & Becona, 2003; Etter, Duc, & Perneger, 1999; Uysal, Kadakai, & Karsidag, 2004).

106 Regarding the use of the FTND among U.S. subjects of African continental descent, St Helen, Dempsey, and Wilson (2013) noted that:

> Biomarkers per CPD [cigarettes per day] decreased with FTND in Blacks but remained flat among Whites. Blacks appear to smoke cigarettes more intensely than Whites, particularly at lower FTND scores and CPD, suggesting a greater degree of nicotine compensation when smoking fewer CPD. This suggests that Blacks at the lower level of FTND have a greater level of nicotine dependence than the FTND scale reveals.
>
> (p. 7)

107 A Brazilian study (i.e., de Meneses-Gaya, Zuardi, & Loureiro, 2009) reported a Cronbach's alpha coefficient of 0.83.

108 Similarly, Kim (2017), in an analysis of data from Korean-American women, also found unacceptably low item-to-total score correlation coefficients ranging from 0.21 to 0.63 (mean $\alpha = 0.32$).

Test-retest reliability was reported as ranging from 0.82 (Weinberger, Reutenauer, & Allen, 2007) to 0.92 (de Meneses-Gaya, Zuardi, & Loureiro, 2009) for tobacco smokers who did not have co-occurring disorders, or a contemporaneous diagnosis. For a sample of USAF recruits (average age, 19 years), the reported test-retest reliability at six weeks was 0.87 (Haddock, Lando, & Klesges, 1999). Inter-rater reliability has been reported as being extremely high (i.e., 0.99) (de Meneses-Gaya, Zuardi, & Loureiro, 2009). In another study, Cohen's kappa was reported at 0.76 (Chabrol, Niezborala, & Chastan, 2005).

RECOMMENDATIONS Overall, given the: (1) higher correlation of the FTND with nicotine withdrawal—in comparison to nicotine dependence; (2) relatively low validity and reliability reported for the FTND;[109] and (3) dearth of test statistics for adolescents in the U.S.; we do not recommend its use.

BRIEF WISCONSIN INVENTORY OF SMOKING DEPENDENCE (BRIEF WISDM)

The Brief WISDM is a 37-item quick-screen psychometric test (see Table 3.5) that was developed by Smith, Piper, and Bolt (2010) as an improved shortened version (i.e., subset) of the original 68-item, "Wisconsin Inventory of Smoking Dependence Motives" (WISDM). The WISDM was originally developed by Piper, Piasecki, and Federman (2004) to determine the factors that may contribute to:

1. Smoking (nicotine) dependence;
2. Motivation to continue use;
3. Relapse following an attempt to quit smoking.

As summarized by Smith, Piper, and Bolt (2010, p. 489), in the Brief WISDM:

- The "Behavioral Choice/Melioration" subscale in the original 68-item WISDM has been dropped from the Brief WISDM due to lack of support for its predictive validity;
- The "Negative Reinforcement" and the "Positive Reinforcement" subscales have been merged into a new subscale called, "Affective Enhancement."

Consequently, the Brief WISDM has 11 subscales rather than the 13 original scales found in the WISDM.

The WISDM and the Brief WISDM have been tested and used with several identified diverse groups of subjects including:

- Adults with ADHD;
- Americans of African continental descent;
- Hungarian smokers;
- Italian smokers;
- Pregnant smokers.

109 In order to address the poor reliability of the FTND, Korte, Capron, and Zvolensky (2013) suggested changing the scoring procedure for items #2, #5, and #6 to a 4-point Likert response set (i.e., 0 = never; 1 = sometimes; 2 = most of the time; 3 = always). Significant improvement in scale reliability and enhanced convergent validity were reported. However, these findings have not been subsequently replicated.

Table 3.5 Brief WISDM

Below are a series of statements about cigarette smoking. Please rate your level of agreement for each using the following scale:

STATEMENTS	**LEVEL OF AGREEMENT**						
	Not True of Me at All						*Extremely True of Me*
	1	2	3	4	5	6	7
1. I often smoke without thinking about it	1	2	3	4	5	6	7
2. Cigarettes control me	1	2	3	4	5	6	7
3. I usually want to smoke right after I wake up	1	2	3	4	5	6	7
4. It's hard to ignore an urge to smoke	1	2	3	4	5	6	7
5. The flavor of a cigarette is pleasing	1	2	3	4	5	6	7
6. I frequently smoke to keep my mind focused	1	2	3	4	5	6	7
7. I rely upon smoking to control my hunger and eating	1	2	3	4	5	6	7
8. My life is full of reminders to smoke	1	2	3	4	5	6	7
9. Smoking helps me to feel better in seconds	1	2	3	4	5	6	7
10. I smoke without deciding to	1	2	3	4	5	6	7
11. Cigarettes keep me company, like a close friend	1	2	3	4	5	6	7
12. There are particular sights and smells that trigger strong urges to smoke	1	2	3	4	5	6	7
13. Smoking helps me to stay focused	1	2	3	4	5	6	7
14. I frequently light cigarettes without thinking about it	1	2	3	4	5	6	7
15. Most of my daily cigarettes taste good	1	2	3	4	5	6	7
16. Sometimes I feel like cigarettes rule my life	1	2	3	4	5	6	7
17. Frequently I crave cigarettes	1	2	3	4	5	6	7
18. Most of the people I spend time with are smokers	1	2	3	4	5	6	7

(*Continued*)

Table 3.5 (Cont.)

Below are a series of statements about cigarette smoking. Please rate your level of agreement for each using the following scale:							
19. Weight control is a major reason that I smoke	1	2	3	4	5	6	7
20. Some of the cigarettes I smoke taste great	1	2	3	4	5	6	7
21. I am really hooked on cigarettes	1	2	3	4	5	6	7
22. Sometimes I feel like cigarettes are my best friends	1	2	3	4	5	6	7
23. My urges to smoke keep getting stronger if I don't smoke	1	2	3	4	5	6	7
24. Seeing someone smoke makes me really want a cigarette	1	2	3	4	5	6	7
25. I find myself reaching for cigarettes without thinking about it	1	2	3	4	5	6	7
26. I would feel alone without my cigarettes	1	2	3	4	5	6	7
27. A lot of my friends or family smoke	1	2	3	4	5	6	7
28. Other smokers would consider me a heavy smoker	1	2	3	4	5	6	7
29. When I haven't been able to smoke for a few hours, the craving gets intolerable	1	2	3	4	5	6	7
30. Most of my friends and acquaintances smoke	1	2	3	4	5	6	7
31. I smoke within the first 30 minutes of awakening in the morning	1	2	3	4	5	6	7
32. Smoking helps me think better	1	2	3	4	5	6	7
33. Smoking really helps me feel better if I've been feeling down	1	2	3	4	5	6	7
34. Smoking keeps me from overeating	1	2	3	4	5	6	7
35. My smoking is out of control	1	2	3	4	5	6	7
36. I consider myself a heavy smoker	1	2	3	4	5	6	7
37. Even when I feel good, smoking helps me feel better	1	2	3	4	5	6	7

Modified from Smith, Piper, & Bolt, (2010).

However, the majority of studies involved U.S. adults, 18 to 65 years-of-age, of European continental descent (e.g., Mitchell, McIntyre, & McClernon, 2013; Pancani, D'Addario, & Cappelletti, 2015; Parrott, Rathnataka, & Blalock, 2014; Piper, McCarthy, & Baker, 2008; Sato, Sato, & Nozawa, 2012).

SCORING THE BRIEF WISDM. Scoring for each of the 37 items is completed with a seven-point Likert scale, which ranges from 1, "Not true of me at all," to 7, "Extremely true of me." In order to calculate the scores on the 11 subscales, the mean of the items that load onto each subscale is used. The total scale score is the sum of all of the 11 subscale scores, or the sum of the means for each subscale (see Table 3.6).

AVAILABLE TEST STATISTICS AND RECOMMENDATIONS. Published data regarding validity and reliability are available and are discussed in the following sections. These data are followed by our recommendations.

Table 3.6 Brief WISDM Scoring Procedure

Brief WISDM Subscale	*Scoring Procedure*
Affiliated Attachment	Mean of 11, 22, 26
Automaticity	Mean of 1, 10, 14, 25
Loss of Control	Mean of 2, 16, 21, 35
Cognitive Enhancement	Mean of 6, 13, 32
Craving	Mean of 4, 17, 23, 29
Cue Exposure/Associative Processes	Mean of 8, 12, 24
Social/Environmental Goals	Mean of 18, 27, 30
Taste	Mean of 5, 15, 20
Tolerance	Mean of 3, 28, 31, 36
Weight Control	Mean of 7, 19, 34
Affective Enhancement	Mean of 9, 33, 37
Primary Dependence Motives Scale	Mean of means for "Automaticity," "Loss of Control," "Craving," and "Tolerance"
Total Score	**Sum of means** for the 11 subscales (Do not include the "Primary Dependence Motives" scale)

Modified from Smith (2018).

VALIDITY Concurrent validity of the Brief WISDM has been assessed by correlating each of the subscales with the FTND and Heaviness of Smoking Index (HSI). Correlations with the FTND/HSI, ranged from a low of 0.2/0.1 for the "weight control" subscale to a high of 0.7/0.7 for the "tolerance" scale. Overall, for all of the Brief WISDM scales combined, the correlation with the FTND was 0.6 and with the HSI was 0.45 (Adkison, Rees, & Bansal-Travers, 2016). Additionally, Adkison, Rees, and Bansal-Travers (2016) noted concerns and limitations in regard to both the discriminant and convergent validity of several of the subscales.

Ma, Li, and Payne (2012) found unacceptable low correlations between the 11 subscales of the Brief WISDM (i.e., ranging from 0.05 to 0.36 among "European Americans") and the FTND and CPD (cigarettes smoked per day).[110] Consequently, concurrent validity of the Brief WISDM was *not* supported.

Similarly, Smith, Piper, and Bolt (2010) found low correlations between the 11 subscales of the Brief WISDM (i.e., ranging from 0.02 to 0.68) and the CPD, HSI, and FTND. In addition, two particular subscales (i.e., "Social/Environmental Goals" and "Weight Control") had consistently low correlations ranging from 0.00 to 0.18.

RELIABILITY The reported Cronbach's alpha coefficient of item reliability for each of the 11 scales of the Brief WISDM was higher than 0.7 (Ma, Li, & Payne, 2012) indicating moderate, generally acceptable, internal consistency.[111] Smith, Piper, and Bolt (2010) reported Cronbach's alpha at baseline (i.e., internal consistency) to be moderate to high (i.e., ranging from 0.63 to 0.93) for the 11 subscales. Fagan, Pohkrel, and Herzog (2015) reported a Cronbach's alpha of 0.90 for quitting behaviors among both menthol and non-menthol tobacco smokers.

The Brief WISDM demonstrates good to excellent text-retest reliability. Adkison, Rees, and Bansal-Travers (2016) reported Cronbach's alpha for total score test-retest reliability at three months as 0.89 (range, 0.80 to 0.91, over the 11 different dependence motive subscales). Smith, Piper, and Bolt (2010) reported a one-year stability of the 11 subscales that ranged from 0.61 to 0.81.

RECOMMENDATIONS Overall, given the: (1) lack of published test statistics regarding specificity and sensitivity; and (2) low to moderate results regarding validity and reliability, we do not recommend the use of the Brief WISDM for detecting nicotine dependence or use disorder for adolescents.

Common Adolescent and Young Adult Contemporaneous Diagnoses[112]

Adolescents and young adults are susceptible to, and often experience, nicotine and other dependence, or use disorders, at the same time as one or more other mental disorders. Together, these disorders comprise more serious and complicated contemporaneous diagnoses that often require more complex interdisciplinary professional health and social care treatment planning and management (Pagliaro & Pagliaro, 2012; Riggs, 2003; Wise, Cuffe, & Fischer, 2001). For adolescents diagnosed with nicotine dependence or use disorder, the most common mental disorders involved in—or significantly correlated with—the formulation of a contemporaneous diagnosis are:

110 Interestingly, the correlations were consistently higher for Americans of African continental descent (i.e., 0.17 to 0.43), but still unacceptable.

111 In comparison, Piper, Piasecki, and Federman (2004) reported significantly better internal consistency for the subscales of the original WISDM (i.e., Cronbach's alpha higher than 0.87 for each of the 13 subscales).

112 For a related overview and discussion, see also Chapter 1, "Alcohol," subsection, "Contemporaneous Diagnoses Among Children, Adolescents, and Young Adults."

- ADHD;
- Anxiety Disorders;
- Bipolar Disorder;
- Eating Disorders;
- MDD;
- Other Dependence or Use Disorders;
- Psychotic Disorder (Schizophrenia).

Attention Deficit Hyperactivity Disorder (ADHD)

Several researchers (e.g., Fuemmeler, Kollins, & McClernon, 2007) have identified a significant positive relationship between ADHD and tobacco smoking progressing from adolescence through early adulthood. As explained by Modesto-Lowe, Danforth, and Neering (2010):

> Childhood ADHD increases risk for early smoking during adolescence… [and] ADHD in adolescence increases the risk for daily smoking in adulthood.
>
> (p. 229)

In their study of the relationships between ADHD and adolescent smoking behaviors, Rhodes, Pelham, and Gnagy (2016) found that—in comparison to adolescents without ADHD:

- 11 to 14 year-olds with ADHD were significantly more likely to have "tried a cigarette" and be "daily smokers;"
- 15 to 17 year-olds with ADHD were significantly more likely to have "smoked a cigarette" and be "daily smokers;"
- 18 to 20 year-olds with ADHD were significantly more likely to be "daily smokers;"
- The noted associations were greater in girls than boys.

Elkins, Saunders, and Malone (2018), in their study of ADHD among same-sex twin samples, found that children diagnosed with severe ADHD were: (1) more likely to initiate smoking; and (2) start smoking younger as adolescents. In addition, the noted associations were greater for girls than boys.

Bipolar Disorder

Bipolar disorder and nicotine dependence or use disorder, frequently occur together. As with virtually all of the other contemporaneous diagnoses, the relationship has been demonstrated to differ among individuals with nicotine dependence or use disorder preceding bipolar disorder in some cases and following it in others (e.g., Martinez-Ortega, Goldstein, & Gutierrez-Rojas, 2013).

Eating Disorders

Among adolescents, particularly girls and young adult women, cigarette smoking has been widely recognized as a commonly used method to control weight (i.e., maintain or lose weight) (e.g., Cavallo, Duhig, & McKee, 2006; Harakeh, Engels, & Monshouwer, 2010; Johnson, Eaton, & Pederson, 2009; Lanza, Grella, & Chung, 2014). Smoking cessation is frequently accompanied by weight gain and is a significant therapeutic impediment to maintaining abstinence (Farley, Hajek, & Lycett, 2012; Pagliaro & Pagliaro, 2012; Thorner-Bantug, Jaszyna-Gasior, & Schroeder, 2009).

Major Depressive Disorder (MDD)

Major depressive disorder has been associated with nicotine use (e.g., tobacco smoking) and the use of all of the other major psychostimulants. When MDD precedes nicotine dependence, it is often characterized as an attempt to "self-medicate" the condition. Goodwin, Cheslack-Postava, and Nelson (2017), for example, noted that, among pregnant women, depression was associated with an almost three-fold increase in tobacco smoking (i.e., from 13% to 32.5%).

Martinez-Ortega, Franco, and Rodriguez-Fernandez (2017), in their analysis of data from the *National Epidemiologic Survey on Alcohol and Related Conditions*, found that these individuals were more likely to have a history of suicide attempts and an earlier age of onset of their first depressive episode.

As illustrated in "Rebecca's Story:"

> Rebecca, age 57, started smoking cigarettes at age 16... At age 33, Rebecca was diagnosed with depression. She smoked frequently when she felt depressed because she felt smoking might help her cope with her feelings. Rebecca felt ashamed when she smoked, so when she tried to quit and couldn't, she felt even more depressed. "That was just a vicious, vicious cycle", she said ...
>
> (CDC, 2016e, p. 1)

Psychotic Disorder: Schizophrenia

The high prevalence of nicotine use (e.g., tobacco cigarette smoking; e-cigarette vaping) among individuals with schizophrenia has long been noted. The most plausible explanation for this contemporaneous diagnosis is the use of nicotine as an attempt to self-medicate the signs and symptoms of schizophrenia, particularly the "negative" symptoms, such as apathy, avolition, difficulty concentrating, impaired attention, and social withdrawal (e.g., Dalack, Healy, & Meador-Woodruff, 1998; Pagliaro & Pagliaro, *Clinical Patient Data Files*; Williams & Gandhi, 2008).

Nicotine and Other Dependence or Use Disorders[113]

The concurrent use of several drugs and substances of abuse is extremely common among adolescents and young adults who use various sources of nicotine. The abusable psychotropics that are most frequently and concurrently used include: alcohol; amphetamines; caffeine; cocaine; marijuana; and opiate analgesics, particularly, heroin (e.g., Cross, Lotfipour, & Leslie, 2017; Harrell, Trenz, & Scherer, 2012; Kohut, 2017; Pagliaro & Pagliaro, *Clinical Patient Data Files*).

A significant and common contemporaneous diagnosis involves the association of nicotine dependence or use disorder and alcohol dependence and use disorder (Littleton, Barron, & Prendergast, 2007; Ostroumov, Thomas, & Dani, 2015). Alcohol and nicotine appear to have reciprocal effects upon each other resulting in increased craving and use. These reciprocal

113 See also the related discussion in the earlier nicotine pharmacology subsection—"Nicotine Drug–Drug Interactions."

Table 3.7 Relationship between Menstrual Cycle Phase and Nicotine Withdrawal Syndrome

Menstrual phase	*Outcome*	*Source*
Follicular Phase	Less favorable outcome in relation to tobacco smoking cessation	Allen, Bade, & Center, 2008
	Greater success in tobacco smoking cessation when initiated during this phase	Franklin, Ehrman, & Lynch, 2008
	Greater nicotine craving upon awakening that may contribute to "smoking first thing in the morning"	Allen, Allen, & Widenmier, 2009
	Increased stress and arousal	Saladin, Wray, & Carpenter, 2015
Luteal Phase	Greater success in tobacco smoking cessation and continued abstinence with bupropion sustained release formulation (Wellbutrin SR®) when initiated during this phase	Mazure, Toll, & McKee, 2011
	Decreased subjective effects of nicotine and increased cognition	DeVito, Herman, & Waters, 2014
	Greater increase in stimulation and greater decrease in urge to smoke following use of nicotine nasal spray (Nicotrol NS®)	Allen, Lunos, & Heishman, 2015
	Improved nicotine tobacco smoking cessation outcomes following nicotine or varenicline (Chantix®) pharmacotherapy	Saladin, McClure, & Baker, 2015
	Greater craving for nicotine among women during this phase when compared to men	Saladin, Wray, & Carpenter, 2015
	Greater nicotine withdrawal symptomatology	Weinberger, Smith, & Allen, 2015

effects also have significant implications for treatment. However, unfortunately, as identified by Yardley, Mirbaba, & Ray (2015, p. 833):

> There are currently *no* available treatment protocols tailored to this comorbid condition [i.e., alcohol use disorder and nicotine use disorder].

Several researchers have hypothesized a number of possible explanations for this associated phenomenon. Many of these explanations have involved overlapping, or commonly shared, receptor systems. For example, in explaining contemporaneous diagnoses involving dependence on alcohol and nicotine, or other psychostimulants, Cross, Lotfipour, and Leslie (2017) suggest that:

> Cholinergic and serotonergic systems underlie reward-related behaviors, including drug intake, preference, and dependence to all three drugs of abuse.
>
> (p. 185)

Adolescent and Young Adult Treatment for Nicotine Dependence or Use Disorder

The treatment of nicotine dependence or use disorder, primarily involves two approaches —pharmacotherapy and psychotherapy/counseling. Each of these treatment approaches, alone or in combination, has demonstrated particular efficacy in the: (1) cessation of nicotine tobacco smoking; and, once achieved; (2) prevention of "resumed" tobacco smoking. We begin with an overview of factors that may affect treatment approaches for nicotine dependence or use disorder. We then present and discuss current approved pharmacotherapy approaches for adolescents and young adults followed by approved psychotherapy/counseling approaches.

Factors Affecting Treatment

Women are often identified as responding less favorably to the various pharmacotherapeutic interventions aimed at facilitating cigarette smoking cessation (e.g., Pagliaro & Pagliaro, 2018; Pagliaro & Pagliaro, *Clinical Patient Data Files*; Smith, Kasza, & Hyland, 2015). In this context, several researchers have examined the relationship between menstrual cycle phase and signs and symptoms of the nicotine withdrawal syndrome among women—from menarche to menopause—including adolescent girls and young women (see Table 3.7). In addition, several other researchers have studied recognized relationships among various treatment outcomes and the follicular and luteal menstrual phases. These findings are briefly presented and discussed in the following section.

OVARIAN CYCLE EFFECTS ON TREATMENT OUTCOMES

In terms of ovarian effects, the normal menstrual cycle consists of three phases:

1. "Follicular phase" (days 0 to 14);
2. "Ovulatory phase" (days 13 to 15); and
3. "Luteal phase" (days 15 to 28).

Uterine effects also occur in three distinct phases:

1. "Menstrual phase" (days 0 to 6);
2. "Proliferative phase" (days 6 to 14); and
3. "Secretory phase" (days 14 to 28).

Both estrogens, primarily estradiol, and progestins, primarily progesterone, are present throughout the 28 days of the menstrual cycle. Estrogens predominate, in terms of hormone levels, during the first half of the menstrual cycle and progestins, during the second half (i.e., estradiol is predominant during the late follicular, or pre-ovulation, phase, while progesterone is dominant during the luteal, or premenstrual phase). The normal menstrual cycle is significantly changed when women are either pregnant or are using oral contraceptives (Pagliaro & Pagliaro, 1986). The menstrual cycle has been demonstrated, in numerous studies (for examples, see Table 3.7), to significantly impact the efficacy of the results associated with pharmacologic prevention and treatment efforts.

As identified by Wetherill, Franklin, and Allen (2016):

> Although progesterone and estradiol are primarily involved in sexual maturation and reproductive functions, they also produce direct effects on the reward-related mesolimbic dopaminergic system and influence addiction-related processes.
>
> (p. 1)

Regarding nicotine tobacco smoking prevention and treatment, estradiol may enhance drug reward and increase tobacco smoking behavior while progesterone may decrease drug reward, nicotine craving, and tobacco smoking behavior (Saladin, McClure, & Baker, 2015; Wetherill, Franklin, & Allen, 2016). Consequently, among adolescent girls and young women, it has been reported that the luteal phase is generally associated with:

1. Better smoking cessation outcomes;
2. A longer period of smoking cessation with a decreased craving for nicotine and an associated decreased urge to smoke
   (e.g., Allen, Allen, & Widenmier, 2009; Allen, Bade, & Center, 2008; Allen, Lunos, & Heishman, 2015; Franklin, Ehrman, & Lynch, 2008).

While the reported relationships are significant, they are not universal. Other co-variables may play a major contributory role, such as mental depression (e.g., Allen, al'Absi, & Lando, 2013; Pang, Bello, & Stone, 2016)—particularly the premenstrual dysphoric disorder (PMDD), which is most specific to the luteal phase (Pinkerton, Guico-Pabia, & Taylor, 2010; Steiner, 2000). (See also the related discussion in the later nicotine subsection, "Contemporaneous Diagnoses.")

Others (e.g., Huttlin, Allen, & Tosun, 2015) posited a significant role for related endogenous adrenocortical activity. When, for example, nicotine nasal spray was administered to women smokers during the follicular phase, higher morning cortisol levels were associated with decreases in negative affect and withdrawal symptomatology coincident with increases in reported feelings of relaxation. Conversely, when nicotine nasal spray was administered during the luteal phase, higher morning cortisol levels were associated with decreases in reported "head rush" and "urge to smoke."

Finally, several researchers, including Bowker, Lewis, and Coleman (2014), suggest possible explanations related to increased metabolism during pregnancy:[114]

> Our findings are significant and consistent with the hypothesis that NRT (Nicotine Replacement Therapy) patches deliver an inadequate dose of nicotine to aid smoking cessation during pregnancy.
>
> (p. 895)

In general support of this hypothesis, Gray, McClure, and Baker (2015), in their study of oral varenicline versus transdermal nicotine delivery system (i.e., "patch") use among women, 18 to 45 years-of-age, found that varenicline was significantly more effective than the nicotine patch.

114 This relationship is purportedly mediated by the effect of estrogens on nicotine metabolism (see the related discussion in the earlier nicotine pharmacology subsection, "Nicotine Drug–Drug Interactions").

Pharmacotherapy

Two major areas of focus for the treatment of adolescent and young adult nicotine dependence or use disorder are: (1) tobacco smoking cessation; and (2) nicotine maintenance, or nicotine replacement therapy (NRT). Often used together as combination pharmacotherapy, each of these approaches are presented and discussed in the following sections.

TOBACCO SMOKING CESSATION

Various pharmacological approaches have been used to achieve tobacco smoking cessation (i.e., achieving abstinence)—bupropion (Wellbutrin SR®; Zyban®), varenicline (CHANTIX®), nicotine replacement therapy (NRT), and combination pharmacotherapy. Bupropion and varenicline are the principal components of pharmacotherapy approved by the FDA for facilitating smoking cessation and achieving tobacco smoking abstinence (Patnode, Henderson, & Thompson, 2015a, 2015b). The pharmacotherapeutic approaches to ND/NUD focus on the: (1) cessation of nicotine use; and (2) management of the signs and symptoms associated with the disorder.

BUPROPION. Two decades ago, bupropion, an antidepressant of the aminoketone class, was approved for the management of the nicotine withdrawal syndrome associated with cessation of tobacco smoking (Corelli & Hudmon, 2006; Pagliaro & Pagliaro, 1999).[115] Since its approval, bupropion pharmacotherapy has been associated with several benefits, including:

- Decreasing the reward associated with smoking;
- Relieving the signs and symptoms of nicotine withdrawal;
- Decreasing post-cessation weight gain.

(Barua, Rigotti, & Benowitz, 2018)

The mechanism by which bupropion facilitates tobacco smoking cessation has not yet been clearly identified. Bupropion pharmacotherapy generally is initiated approximately one week before the patient's identified "quit date" in order to allow sufficient time to achieve steady-state blood concentrations. Bupropion pharmacotherapy is continued for two to three months while monitoring patient response and progress in terms of smoking cessation.[116] The sustained-release tablets should be swallowed whole and not crushed, divided, or chewed.

Buproprion has also been used in combination with NRT, including the use of nicotine transdermal systems. Published research findings and reviews of tobacco smoking cessation approaches and the management of the signs and symptoms of nicotine withdrawal (e.g., Anthenelli, Benowitz, & West, 2016; Cahill, Stevens, & Perera, 2013) generally indicate that bupropion pharmacotherapy and NRT are equally efficacious—with each being significantly superior to placebo in regard to facilitating and maintaining tobacco smoking cessation. In addition, it is recommended that patients receive related counseling support throughout treatment.

Limited adolescent clinical trials regarding tobacco smoking cessation have generally produced results consistent with those reported for adults. For example, Upadhyaya, Brady, and Wang (2004), in their pilot study of 16 adolescents, found that the administration of bupropion sustained release (SR) tablets, at a dosage of 150 mg twice daily (together with brief counseling), was efficacious in promoting a significant decrease in the average number of cigarettes smoked.

115 Although commonly used for both adults and adolescents, formal clinical trials for bupropion generally do not include subjects under 18 years-of-age. Consequently, the use of bupropion to achieve tobacco smoking cessation is not FDA approved for adolescents and, therefore, must be undertaken with due caution.

116 N.B. Adolescents, who have been unable to quit smoking after 12 weeks of bupropion pharmacotherapy, are unlikely to respond positively to further continued bupropion pharmacotherapy.

In a later example, Muramoto, Leischow, and Sherrill (2007), in their study of 312 adolescent tobacco cigarette smokers, found similar results:

> Sustained-release buproprion hydrochloride, 300 mg/d, plus brief counseling, demonstrated short-term efficacy for adolescent smoking cessation.
>
> (p. 1068)

In this context, Leischow, Muramoto, and Matthews (2016) noted that:

> Effectiveness of bupropion for adolescent smoking cessation is contingent on achieving high rates of medication adherence.
>
> (p. 1202)

Several studies (e.g., Cox, Nollen, & Mayo, 2012; Robles, Singh-Franco, & Ghin, 2008) have failed to demonstrate long-term smoking cessation with bupropion use among smokers of African continental descent, particularly those who smoke: (1) menthol cigarettes; (2) fewer than 10 cigarettes per day; and/or (3) within 30 minutes of waking. These observations may have more to do with the menthol in the cigarettes than to continental or other descent (Ahijevych & Garrett, 2010). For example, Wickham (2015, p. 279) suggests four distinct biological mechanisms by which menthol can possibly affect smoking behavior and, consequently, the response to smoking cessation interventions:

1. Menthol acts to reduce the initially aversive experiences associated with tobacco smoking.
2. Menthol can serve as a highly reinforcing sensory cue when associated with nicotine and promoting smoking behavior.
3. Menthol's actions on nicotinic acetylcholine receptors may change the reinforcing value of nicotine.
4. Menthol can alter nicotine metabolism, thus increasing nicotine bioavailability.

Bupropion is contraindicated among patients undergoing abrupt discontinuation of the sedative-hypnotics, including: alcohol; barbiturates; and benzodiazepines. Associated undesired, or harmful, effects and toxicities, which have been identified in over 10% of patients, include: anxiety disorders; insomnia; and nausea. The most undesired, or harmful, effects and toxicities associated with buproprion pharmacotherapy for smoking cessation, include:

- Activation of mania/hypomania;
- Angle closure glaucoma;
- Hypersensitivity;
- Hypertension;
- Psychosis;
- Seizures;[117]
- Suicidal thoughts and behaviors.[118]

117 The risk for seizure appears to be dose-related. Consequently, seizure disorders are a contraindication to the use of bupropion.

118 As noted in the FDA "black box" warning:

> Antidepressants increase the risk of suicidal thoughts and behaviors in children, adolescents, and young adults in short term trials.
>
> (FDA, 2009, p. 1)

Long-term efficacy of bupropion for the facilitation of cigarette smoking cessation among adolescents and adults, has generally not been formally evaluated because:

1. Pharmacotherapy is not recommended beyond 12 weeks;
2. It is generally agreed that, if smoking cessation is not achieved by 12 weeks, it is highly unlikely to be achieved with further continued use.

VARENICLINE. Varenicline (Chantix®) was approved by the FDA in 2006 as first-line pharmacotherapy aimed at facilitating smoking cessation.[119] An alternative to NRT (Fant, Buchhalter, & Buchman, 2009; Frishman, 2009), varenicline use is associated with, on average, a 1.5 times greater efficacy in smoking cessation success (Cahill, Stevens, & Perera, 2013).

A partial nicotine antagonist, varenicline competitively binds to the nicotinic acetylcholine receptors (nAChRs), particularly the $\alpha_4\beta_2$ subtype where it helps to stop smoking by its actions as a:

1. Partial "agonist," reducing the signs and symptoms of nicotine withdrawal by maintaining moderate levels of dopamine;
2. Partial "antagonist," blocking nicotine from binding to the receptor sites and reducing its desired actions, including smoking satisfaction.

Consequently, the ability of nicotine to stimulate the mesolimbic dopamine system is significantly reduced.

Varenicline is available as an oral tablet that is ingested once or twice daily,[120] after meals, for generally three to six months (FDA, 2016b). Varenicline pharmacotherapy is generally initiated one to four weeks prior to the identified "quit date." The most common undesired effect associated with varenicline pharmacotherapy is nausea, which is usually mild to moderate and subsides over time (Cahill, Stead, & Lancaster, 2012; Faessel, Obach, & Rollema, 2010; Garrison & Dugan, 2009; Hays, Croghan, & Schroeder, 2010). The use of varenicline also can lower the seizure threshold.

The FDA required a "black box" warning for the official labeling of Chantix® that includes the statement, "Some people have had changes in behavior, hostility, agitation, depressed mood, and suicidal thoughts" (FDA, 2009). The risk for these less common undesired, or harmful, effects and toxicities is reportedly greater for those who have a positive history of mental disorders (Ahmed, Ali, & Kramers, 2013). However, in late 2016, the FDA officially removed this "black box" warning from varenicline's official labeling (FDA, 2016b).

Adolescents and young adults generally are cautioned to limit their ingestion of alcohol until they have monitored and evaluated the effects associated with their varenicline use (and the associated decreased tobacco smoking) on their drinking patterns. However, the results from a large scale, double-blind, triple-dummy, placebo-controlled study indicate that varenicline's associated risk for undesired neuropsychiatric effects and toxicities was not significantly greater than that associated with the use of a placebo (Anthenelli, Benowitz, & West, 2016).

119 N.B. Although commonly used as an aid for smoking cessation among adolescents and although several published "clinical" studies have included adolescent subjects, varenicline is not currently FDA approved for use among tobacco smokers under 18 years-of age.

120 Optimal therapeutic response generally appears to be associated with a dosage of one mg twice daily. However, among adolescents weighing less than 55 kg, it has been recommended—based on pharmacokinetic data—that the dosage be reduced to 0.5 mg twice daily (Faessel, Obach, & Rollema, 2010; Faessel, Ravva, & Williams, 2009).

Serious cardiovascular events also have been reported to be related to varenicline pharmacotherapy, including congestive heart failure, dysrhythmias, and myocardial infarction (Singh, Loke, & Spangler, 2011). However, a comprehensive meta-analysis failed to substantiate either the clinical or statistical significance of these concerns (Prochaska & Hilton, 2012), particularly in the context of use by adolescents and young adults.

Although generally associated with nausea and a need for cautious use, varenicline pharmacotherapy for tobacco smoking cessation is well established as a suitable alternative to NRT, particularly for adolescents and young adults who smoke tobacco and who have been unsuccessful in achieving smoking cessation with NRT. Several studies (e.g., Baker, Piper, & Stein, 2016; Gonzales, Rennard, & Nides, 2006; Nides, Oncken, & Gonzales, 2006; Tonstad, Tonnesen, & Hajek, 2006) have demonstrated significant increases in the achievement of smoking cessation with the use of varenicline when compared to placebo and/or bupropion pharmacotherapy.

For example, Jorenby, Hays, and Rigotti (2006) found that, after one year, the rate of continuous abstinence for varenicline was 23% in comparison to 15% for bupropion and 10% for placebo. Cahill, Lindson-Hawley, and Thomas (2016), in their meta-analysis of 39 trials that tested varenicline, found that:

> Varenicline at standard dose increased the chances of successful long-term smoking cessation between two- and three-fold compared with pharmacologically unassisted quit attempts.
>
> (p. 1)

In addition, Aubin, Bobak, and Britton (2008) reported that:

> The outcomes of this trial established that abstinence from smoking was greater and craving, withdrawal symptoms and smoking satisfaction were less at the end of treatment with varenicline than with transdermal NRT.
>
> (p. 717)

In a systematic review of approximately 20 random, controlled studies that compared varenicline pharmacotherapy with placebo, bupropion, nicotine replacement therapy, or counseling, varenicline was found to increase the overall chances of long-term smoking cessation by two to three-fold (Cahill, Stead, & Lancaster, 2012). Zhu, Cummins, and Gamst (2016) reported similar findings, but cautioned that after three months of varenicline pharmacotherapy, the relapse rate did not significantly differ from that associated with other related pharmacotherapies.

COMBINATION VARENICLINE PHARMACOTHERAPY. Chang, Chiang, and Ho (2015) found that combined varenicline and NRT has been recommended and touted as being more efficacious than varenicline alone.[121] In addition, it has been found that the efficacy of varenicline can be increased significantly with combination varenicline pharmacotherapy and appropriate cognitive-behavioral psychotherapy (Ebbert, Wyatt, & Zirakzadeh, 2009; Ebbert, Wyatt, & Hays, 2010; Hays, Croghan, & Schroeder, 2010).

NICOTINE REPLACEMENT THERAPY (NRT)

Nicotine replacement therapy, in its various formulations (e.g., buccal sprays, chewing gums, intranasal sprays, oral inhalers, oral lozenges, and transdermal delivery systems—see Table 3.8),

121 Because of the increased undesired, or harmful, effects associated with the combined use of varenicline and NRT, we do not generally recommend this combination of pharmacotherapy.

Table 3.8 Nicotine Replacement Therapy (NRT) Formulations

Formulation	*Usual adult dosage*	*Administration*	*Advantages/ Disadvantages*
Buccal Spray Nicorette Quick-Mist® Each buccal spray delivers one mg; each spray pump bottle delivers 150 sprays. OTC	Weeks one to six: One to two sprays every half hour. Weeks seven to nine: Reduce number of sprays per day by half. Weeks 10 to 12: Two to four sprays per day. After 12 weeks: Stop using Quick-Mist®. Maximum: Two sprays at a time; Four sprays per hour; 64 sprays per day.	No food or drink 15 minutes prior to use and during use. Directions: 1. Push the black button down until you can push it lightly inwards. 2. While pushing the button in, slide upwards and continue until the top of the dispenser locks into place. 3. Before using for the first time, prime the pump by pressing the top firmly into a tissue until a fine mist appears. If you don't use the spray for a couple of days, you may need to repeat this step. 4. Place the dispenser as close as possible to your open mouth, avoiding the lips. 5. Press the top of the dispenser firmly to release one spray into your mouth. For best results, wait a few seconds before swallowing. Do not inhale the spray. Avoid spraying directly onto your lips or throat. 6. Repeat dose (i.e., step #5) once if craving is still present after one minute. 7. To close the dispenser, slide the button down until it can be pushed lightly inwards. Then, while pushing in, slide down to lock. Use for three to six months, as needed.	• If inadvertently sprayed into the eye, immediately flush with copious amounts of plain water.

(Continued)

Table 3.8 (Cont.)

Formulation	*Usual adult dosage*	*Administration*	*Advantages/ Disadvantages*
Chewing Gum (nicotine polacrilex) Nicorette Gum® Thrive Gum® two & four mg per piece OTC	If first cigarette is $\leq$ 30 minutes of waking: Four mg. Use one piece per hour. If first cigarette is $\geq$ 30 minutes of waking: Two mg. Use one piece per hour. Average: Nine pieces per day. Maximum: 24 pieces per day.	No food or drink 15 minutes prior to use and during use. Do not chew more than one piece of gum at a time (i.e., do not use two pieces to make-up for a missed dose). Directions: 1. Chew briefly until mouth tingles, then "park" gum inside cheek until tingle fades. 2. Repeat chew-and-park each time tingle fades. 3. Discard gum after 30 minutes of use. 4. Repeat use when craving to smoke returns. Use for three to six months, as needed.	• Oral substitute for cigarettes. • User controls nicotine dose. • Not chewed in same way as regular gum; requires careful instruction. • Can damage dental work and be difficult to use with dentures. • Vigorous chewing may strain jaw and neck muscles resulting in jaw/neck pain and migraine headaches.
Intranasal Spray Nicorette Nasal Spray® Nicotrol NS® 10 mg/ml Each intranasal spray delivers 0.5 mg; each intranasal spray bottle delivers 200 sprays. Rx	Use one spray in each nostril, every one to two hours. Maximum: Two sprays in each nostril per hour; 64 sprays per day.	Directions: 1. Wash your hands. 2. Gently blow your nose to clear your nasal passages. 3. Remove the cap of the nasal spray by pressing in the circles on the side of the bottle. 4. To prime the pump before the first use, hold the bottle in front of a tissue or paper towel. Pump the spray bottle six to eight times until a fine spray appears. Throw away the tissue or towel.	• Of all NRT products, has most rapid delivery of nicotine. • User controls nicotine dose. • Some users cannot tolerate local irritation to nasal mucosa.

		5. Tilt your head back slightly. 6. Insert the tip of the bottle as far as you comfortably can into one nostril, pointing the tip toward the back of your nose. 7. Breathe through your mouth. 8. Pump the spray firmly and quickly one time. Do not sniff, swallow, or inhale while spraying. 9. If your nose runs, gently sniff to keep the nasal spray in your nose. Wait two to three minutes before blowing your nose. 10. Repeat steps six to eight for the second nostril. 11. Replace the cover on the spray bottle. 12. Anytime you have not used the nasal spray for 24 hours, prime the pump in a tissue one or two times. However, do not prime too much as it will decrease the amount of medication in the container. Use for three to six months, as needed.	
Oral Inhaler Nicorette Inhaler® Nicotrol Inhaler® four & 10 mg per cartridge; each cartridge delivers ~ 80 puffs. Rx	Up to 12 weeks: A minimum of six cartridges to a maximum of 12 cartridges per day. 12 to 24 weeks: Gradually reduce the number of cartridges. Maximum: 16 puffs per day.	Do not inhale into the lungs. Puff into mouth or back of throat until cravings subside. Use one cartridge every one to two hours. Change cartridge when nicotine taste disappears. Directions: 1. Line up the markers and pull each end in the opposite direction. 2. Insert the cartridge into the mouthpiece and twist to close securely. 3. Bring the mouthpiece to your mouth.	• Frequent puffing required for over 20 minutes. • Each cartridge lasts for approximately 20 minutes of frequent puffing. • User controls nicotine dose. • Nicotine cartridge and mouthpiece look

(*Continued*)

Table 3.8 (Cont.)

Formulation	*Usual adult dosage*	*Administration*	*Advantages/ Disadvantages*
		4. Inhale deeply into the back of your throat, or puff in short breaths. Use for three to six months, as needed.	similar to a tobacco cigarette. • Mimics hand-to-mouth ritual of smoking cigarettes.
Oral Lozenge (nicotine bitartrate) Commit Lozenge® Nicorette Lozenge® Nicorette Mini Lozenge® Thrive Lozenge® two & four mg per lozenge OTC	If first cigarette is ≤ 30 minutes of waking: Four mg. If first cigarette is ≥ 30 minutes of waking: Two mg. Weeks one to six: One lozenge every one to two hours. Weeks seven to nine: One lozenge every two to four hours. Weeks 10 to 12: One lozenge every four to eight hours. Maximum: Five lozenges per six hours; 20 lozenges per 24 hours.	No food or drink 15 minutes prior to use and during use. Do not chew, crush, or swallow lozenge. Do not use more than one lozenge at a time. Directions: 1. Place lozenge between gum and cheek, let it dissolve slowly. Use for three to six months, as needed.	• User controls nicotine dose. • Easier to use than gum for those with dental work or dentures.
Transdermal Delivery System Nicoderm CQ Patch® Nicotrol Patch® 5, 7, 10, 14, 15, 21, & 25 mg per patch	Usual Initial Dose: For ≥ 10 cigarettes per day: 21 or 25 mg. For ≤ 10 cigarettes per day: 14 or 15 mg.	Directions: 1. Apply a new patch at the same time each morning to a clean, dry, hairless skin site on the chest, shoulder, upper arm, or hip as instructed by the package insert.	• Easiest nicotine product to use. • Provides a steady nicotine level for 16–24 hours, depending on brand.

OTC or Rx	After six weeks: Option to taper to lower doses (i.e., five, seven, or 10 mg patch) for two to six weeks; or to continue original dose (either option is acceptable).	2. Avoid placing patch over areas of broken, irritated, oily, or scarred skin. 3. Do not shave the application site. If necessary, clip hair from the site before applying patch. 4. Do not cut patch 5. Never wear two patches at the same time. 6. To avoid skin irritation, rotate application sites daily—may reuse previous site in three to seven days. 7. Can wear patch while bathing or showering but avoid exposure of applied patch to a direct heat source (e.g., heated water bed; hot tub; sauna) that may increase drug release from the patch. 8. If using a 16-hour patch, remove patch before going to sleep (see comments in "Advantages/Disadvantages" column). 9. Wash your hands with plain water after applying patch—do not use soap because it can increase nicotine absorption from the skin. 10. Do not wear the same patch for longer than 24 hours.	• User cannot alter dose if cravings occur during the day. • If use of a 24-hour patch causes vivid dreams or interferes with sleep, then a 16-hour patch may be indicated. • If user of a 16-hour patch wakes up craving cigarettes, then a 24-hour patch may be indicated. • User may display an allergy to the adhesive tape used in the patch.
		Use for three to six months, as needed.	

Modified from[123, 124] FDA-approved prescription drug monographs; official manufacturer package inserts; and web sites for the products listed.

has become the medical mainstay of tobacco smoking cessation because of its: (1) safety and efficacy in regard to reducing the undesired signs and symptoms associated with nicotine withdrawal; and (2) enhancement of associated successful outcomes regarding "quitting" nicotine use (see related discussion in the earlier nicotine subsection, "Pharmacotherapy"). The noted success and related relative safety of these products have encouraged their conversion from prescription to nonprescription status (Crain & Bhat, 2010; Fant, Buchhalter, & Buchman, 2009; Pagliaro & Pagliaro, 2012).[122]

Whereas methadone maintenance, in the context of opiate analgesic dependence, is just that, maintenance, it is generally expected that nicotine replacement products, or substitutes, be used for short periods of time (e.g., up to 12 weeks).[125] The nicotine substitutes help older adolescents and young adults to slowly discontinue their regular, long-term nicotine use while experiencing diminished signs and symptoms of the nicotine withdrawal syndrome (Cahill, Stevens, & Perera, 2013; Frishman, 2007). The transdermal nicotine delivery systems (e.g., Habitrol®, Nicoderm®), nicotine nasal sprays (Nicotrol NS®), and other products have become important adjuncts to smoking cessation programs and have demonstrated positive results in relation to decreasing or ceasing tobacco smoking. In this context, the use of e-cigarettes (see earlier Nicotine subsection, "E-cigarettes") has been suggested as another possible intervention to facilitate tobacco smoking cessation and the management of nicotine withdrawal. However, sufficient published research regarding e-cigarette nicotine replacement therapy is not currently available to formally support this potential intervention (Shields, Berman, & Brasky, 2017; USDHHS, 2016b).

Although NRT was neither intended nor approved by the FDA for long-term use (i.e., maintenance pharmacotherapy) several clinicians and researchers have suggested that this approach may secure a significant degree of "harm reduction" for those who cannot obtain complete abstinence. In their comprehensive systematic review of this topic, including consideration of the use of e-cigarettes, Lindson-Hawley, Hartmann-Boyce, and Fanshawe (2016) found that people, who do not wish to [or cannot] quit tobacco cigarette smoking, in the long-term, can be helped to cut down on the: (1) number of tobacco cigarettes smoked daily; and (2) exposure to toxic tobacco smoke—with the aid of long-term NRT and/or e-cigarettes.

122 N.B. None of the various dosage forms available for NRT have consistently provided superior results (Yardley, Mirbaba, & Ray, 2015). Consequently, we recommend the use of the nicotine replacement product that is most preferred by the patient (i.e., that the patient finds most affordable, comfortable, convenient, or "user friendly").

123 N.B. The data in this table are current and accurate. However, different manufacturers of similar products, particularly those that are OTC, have some slight variance in their exact package directions. When disagreement is encountered, always follow the directions on the current package insert for the specific brand product that is being used.

124 Whether the use of e-cigarettes are efficacious as a means for NRT has not yet been demonstrated. However, we generally recommend the use of e-cigarettes (i.e., vaping) as an efficacious harm reduction strategy for those who would not—or cannot with repeated attempts—otherwise quit tobacco smoking (for related discussion, see earlier nicotine subsection, "E-Cigarettes"). E-Cigarette use as a mode of NRT has not been FDA approved.

125 N.B. While this is the current, and probably ideal, recommendation regarding the length of nicotine pharmacotherapy, it should be noted that a significant number of (former) tobacco smokers continue the use of nicotine pharmacotherapy well beyond this recommended time period. While we welcome the associated health benefits, which are related to the cessation of tobacco smoking (see earlier discussion in this chapter, particularly in the section, "Undesired, or Harmful, Effects and Toxicities"), we recognize that physical dependence to nicotine is maintained in this context of use. Additionally, the efficacy and safety of long-term use, particularly among adolescents and young adults, has not been evaluated.

In a study of the use of NRT for U.S. adolescents of African continental descent, Botello-Harbaum, Schroeder, and Collins (2010) found that adolescents of African continental descent were significantly *less* likely to use NRT than were adolescents of European continental descent. The reason(s) for this significant difference is unknown. Although most adolescents of African continental descent smoke mentholated cigarettes, this preference did not appear to be directly related to their *lower* use of NRT (Hyland, Garten, & Giovino, 2002).

While NRT is of potential benefit, studies over the last 30 years (e.g., Grimshaw & Stanton, 2006) have repeatedly demonstrated that the use of nicotine substitutes is, in most cases, only significantly effective when combined with appropriate counseling or other psychotherapeutic approaches. For example, as noted by Covey and Glassman (1991):

> Evidence of the addictive nature of chronic tobacco use suggests that pharmacologic interventions, in conjunction with behaviorally oriented therapy, may present the best hope for achieving smoking cessation in refractory smokers.
>
> (p. 69)

Or, as noted by Generali (1992):

> Smoking cessation rates associated with nicotine transdermal patch therapy have varied in clinical trials. However, appropriate patient instruction and an extensive behavioral modification program ensure optimal response to transdermal nicotine therapy.
>
> (p. 34)

In addition, as noted by Laniado-Laborin (2010):

> The rate of successful smoking cessation at 1 year is 3% to 5% when the patient simply tries to stop, 7% to 16% if the smoker undergoes behavioral intervention, and up to 25% when receiving pharmacologic treatment and behavioral support.
>
> (p. 74)

And, finally, as noted by Stead, Koilpillai, and Fanshawe (2016), in their retrospective meta-analysis of 53 studies including a total of over 25,000 participants:

> Interventions that combine pharmacotherapy and behavioral support increase smoking cessation success.
>
> (p. 1)

Psychotherapy/Counseling

Several forms of psychotherapy/counseling have been successfully used to treat adolescents and young adults, who have been diagnosed with nicotine dependence or use disorder. For example, CBT has demonstrated particular success (for further related discussion of CBT, see the adolescent and young adult treatment section in Chapter 1, "Alcohol"—"Psychotherapy/Counseling"). In addition, other forms of behavioral interventions, including motivational interviewing and the use of "financial incentives" (i.e., "cash" or "vouchers") have been successfully utilized in this treatment context (Barua, Rigotti, & Benowitz, 2018; Lasser, Quintiliani, & Truong, 2017). Community-based support-service programs also can be used to augment the psychotherapeutic approaches selected for the management of nicotine dependence or use disorder. For example, the use of:

1. Telephone quit lines (e.g., 1-800-QUIT-NOW [1-800-784-8669];
2. Text messaging programs for use with cell phones or personal computers (e.g., Smokefree TXT that is available from the National Cancer Institute website);
3. Web-based programs (e.g., BecomeAnEx.org that was developed by the Truth Initiative in collaboration with the Mayo Clinic).

***Related Professional Reminder:* Regardless of which therapeutic intervention(s) are chosen for a specific adolescent, or young adult, who wants to quit smoking, it should be generally noted that: (1) combination therapeutic interventions, as previously discussed, usually provide the most favorable results; and (2) although the optimal duration of therapy must be individually determined for each smoker, based on experience with most smokers, therapy should be maintained for a minimal period of three to six months.**

References

Abbot, L. C., & Winzer-Serhan, U. H. (2012). Smoking during pregnancy: Lessons learned from epidemiological studies using animal models. *Critical Reviews in Toxicology, 42*(4), 279–303. doi:10.3109/10408444.2012.658506

About Turbo Snort Caffenated Nasal Spray. (2014, December 27). Retrieved December 27, 2016, from Turbo Snort, p. 1: www.turbosnort.com/About_Turbo_Snort.html

Adams, J. (2018). *Surgeon General's Advisory on E-Cigarette Use among Youth*. Centers for Disease Control and Prevention, U.S. Department of Health and Human Services. Atlanta: National Center for Chronic Disease Prevention and Health Promotion.

Adams, S. (2011, July 7). *Mothers-to-be Smoking for Smaller Babies*. Retrieved March 5, 2016, from Telegraph Media Group, pp. 1–2: www.telegraph.co.uk/news/health/news/8623267/Mothers-to-be-smoking-for-smaller-babies.html

Addicott, M. A. (2014). Caffeine use disorder: A review of the evidence and future implications. *Current Addiction Reports, 1*(3), 186–192. doi:10.1007/s40429-014-0024-9

Adelstein, J. (2018, April 26). Coca-cola experiments with new boozy drinks as Japan's beverage market becomes "saturated". *Forbes*, 1–4.

Adkison, S. E., Rees, V. W., & Bansal-Travers, M. (2016). Psychometric characteristics of the Brief Wisconsin Inventory of Smoking Dependence Motives among a nonclinical sample of smokers. *Nicotine & Tobacco Research, 18*(4), 470–476. doi:10.1093/ntr/ntv113

AeroShot Energy, green apple, lime and raspberry (pack of 12). (2017, December 23). *Amazon.com*. Retrieved December 23, 2017, from www.amazon.com/AeroShot-Energy-Green-Apple-Raspberry/dp/B007Y4BIBK?th=1

Ahijevych, K., & Garrett, B. E. (2010, December). The role of menthol in cigarettes as a reinforcer of smoking behavior. *Nicotine & Tobacco Research, 12*(Supplement 2), S110–S116. doi:10.1093/ntr/ntq203

Ahluwalia, N., & Herrick, K. (2015). Caffeine intake from food and beverage sources and trends among children and adolescents in the United States: Review of national quantitative studies from 1999 to 2011. *Advances in Nutrition, 6*, 102–111. doi:10.3945/an.114.007401

Ahluwalia, N., Herrick, K., & Moshfegh, A. (2014, October). Caffeine intake in children in the United States and 10-y trends: 2001–2010. *American Journal of Clinical Nutrition, 100*(4), 1124–1132. doi:10.3945/ajcn.113.082172

Ahmed, A., Ali, A. N., & Kramers, C. (2013). Neuropsychiatric adverse events of varenicline: A systematic review of published reports. *Journal of Clinical Psychopharmacology, 33*(1), 55–62. doi:10.1097/JCP.0b013e31827c0117

Ahrnsbrak, R., Bose, J., & Hedden, S. L. (2017). *Key Substance Use and Mental Health Indicators in the United States: Results from the 2016 National Survey on Drug Use and Health*. Substance Abuse and Mental Health Services Administration, Center for Behavioral Health Statistics and Quality. Rockville, MD: U.S. Department of Health and Human Services.

Allen, A. M., al'Absi, M., & Lando, H. (2013). Menstrual phase, depressive symptoms, and allopregnanolone during short-term smoking cessation. *Experimental and Clinical Psychopharmacology, 21*(6), 427–433. doi:10.1037/a0034075

Allen, A. M., Allen, S. S., & Widenmier, J. (2009). Patterns of cortisol and craving by menstrual phase in women attempting to quit smoking. *Addictive Behaviors, 34*(8), 632–635. doi:10.1016/j.addbeh.2009.03.024

Allen, A. M., Lunos, S., & Heishman, S. J. (2015, April). Subjective response to nicotine by menstrual phase. *Addictive Behaviors, 43*, 50–53. doi:10.1016/j.addbeh.2014.12.008

Allen, S. S., Bade, T., & Center, B. (2008). Menstrual phase effects on smoking relapse. *Addiction, 103*(5), 809–821. doi:10.1111/j.1360-0443.2008.02146.x

American Lung Association. (2007, February). *Tobacco Policy Trend Alert. An Emerging Deadly Trend: Waterpipe Tobacco Use*. Retrieved June 12, 2016, from lungusa.org, pp. 1–8: www.lungusa.org

Anderson, G. D., & Chan, L. N. (2016). Pharmacokinetic drug interactions with tobacco, cannabinoids and smoking cessation products. *Clinical Pharmacokinetics, 55*(11), 1353–1368. doi:10.1007/s40262-016-0400-9

Anthenelli, R. M., Benowitz, N. L., & West, R. (2016). Neuropsychiatric safety and efficacy of varenicline, bupropion, and nicotine patch in smokers with and without psychiatric disorders (EAGLES): A double-blind, randomised, placebo-controlled clinical trial. *The Lancet*. doi:PIISO140-6736(16)30272-0

APA, American Psychiatric Association. (2013). *Diagnostic and Statistical Manual of Mental Disorders, DSM-5*. Washington, D.C.: American Psychiatric Association.

Appelbaum, C. (2017, November 15). 10 popular Starbucks coffees, ranked by how much caffeine they have. *Business Insider*, 1–6.

Araki, H., Suemaru, K., & Gomita, Y. (2002). Neuronal nicotinic receptor and psychiatric disorders: Functional and behavioral effects of nicotine. *The Japanese Journal of Pharmacology, 88*(2), 133–138.

Aranda, J. V., Beharry, K., & Valencia, G. B. (2010). Caffeine impact on neonatal morbidities. *The Journal of Maternal-Fetal & Neonatal Medicine, 23*(Supplement 3), 20–23. doi:10.3109/14767058.2010.517704

Arria, A. M., Caldeira, K. M., & Bugbee, B. A. (2017, October 1). Trajectories of energy drink consumption and subsequent drug use during young adulthood. *Drug and Alcohol Dependence, 179*, 424–432. doi:10.1016/j.drugalcdep.2017.06.008

Arria, A. M., Caldeira, K. M., & Kasperski, S. J. (2011). Energy drink consumption and increased risk for alcohol dependence. *Alcoholism: Clinical and Experimental Research, 35*(2), 365–375. doi:10.1111/j.1530-0277.2010.01352.x

Artin, B., Singh, M., & Richeh, C. (2010). Caffeine-related atrial fibrillation. *American Journal of Therapeutics, 17*(5), e169–e171. doi:10.1097/MJT.0b013e3181df8cf8

Asfar, T., Ward, K. D., & Eissenberg, T. (2005, February 25). Comparison of patterns of use, beliefs, and attitudes related to waterpipe between beginning and established smokers. *BMC Public Health, 5*, 19.

Astorino, T. A., Matera, A. J., & Basinger, J. (2012). Effects of red bull energy drink on repeated sprint performance in women athletes. *Amino Acids, 42*(5), 1803–1808.

Attwood, A. S., Rogers, P. J., & Ataya, A. F. (2012). Effects of caffeine on alcohol-related changes in behavioural control and perceived intoxcication in light caffeine consumers. *Psychopharmacology (Berlin), 221*(4), 551–560. doi:10.1007/s00213-02112-2601-0

Aubin, H. J., Bobak, A., & Britton, J. R. (2008). Varenicline versus transdermal nicotine patch for smoking cessation: Results from a randomized open-label study. *Thorax, 63*(8), 717–724. doi:10.1136/thx2007.090647

Aubrey, A. (2012, March 7). *Inhalable Caffeine Maker Gets Warning Letter from FDA*. Retrieved October 6, 2016, from The Salt: NPR: www.npr.org/sections/thesalt/2012/03/07/1481611621/inhalable-caffeine-maker-gets-warning-letter-from-fda

Baker, T. B., Piper, M. E., & Stein, J. H. (2016). Effects of nicotine patch vs varenicline vs combination nicotine replacement therapy on smoking cessation at 26 weeks: A randomized clinical trial. *JAMA, Journal of the American Medical Association, 315*(4), 371–379. doi:10.1001/jama.2015.19284

Ballard, S. L., Wellborn-Kim, J. J., & Clauson, K. A. (2010). Effects of commercial energy drink consumption on athletic performance and body composition. *The Physician and Sportsmedicine, 38*(1), 107–117. doi:10.3810/psm.2010.04.1768

Banderali, G., Martelli, A., & Landi, M. (2015). Short and long term health effects of parental tobacco smoking during pregnancy and lactation: A descriptive review. *Journal of Trasactional Medicine, 13*, 327–337. doi:10.1186/s12967-015-0690-y

Banerjee, P., Ali, Z., & Levine, B. (2014, May). Fatal caffeine intoxication: A series of eight cases from 1999 to 2009. *Journal of Forensic Sciences, 59*(3), 865–868. doi:10.1111/1556-4029.12387

Barrington-Trimis, J. L., & Leventhal, A. M. (2018, September 20). Adolescents' use of "pod mod" e-cigarettes—Urgent concerns. *The New England Journal of Medicine, 379*, 1099–1102. doi:10.1056/NEJMp1805758

Barua, R. S., Rigotti, N. A., & Benowitz, N. L. (2018). 2018 ACC expert consensus decision pathway on tobacco cessation treatment. *Journal of the American College of Cardiology, 72*(25), 3332–3365. doi:10.1016/j.jacc.2018.10.027

Bassett, R. A., Osterhoudt, K., & Brabazon, T. (2014). Nicotine poisoning in an infant. *The New England Journal of Medicine, 370*, 2249–2250. doi:10.1056/NEJMc1403843

Beedie, C. J. (2010). All in the mind? Pain, placebo effect, and ergogenic effect of caffeine in sports performance. *Open Access Journal of Sports Medicine, 1*, 87–94.

Benowitz, N. L. (1999). Biomarkers of environmental tobacco smoke exposure. *Environmental Health Perspectives, 107* (Supplement 2), 349–355.

Benowitz, N. L., Dains, K. M., & Dempsey, D. (2011, September). Racial differences in the relationship between number of cigarettes smoked and nicotine and carcinogen exposure. *Nicotine & Tobacco Research, 13*(9), 772–783. doi:10.1093/ntr/ntr072

Benowitz, N. L., Hukkanen, J., & Jacob, P. (2009). Nicotine biochemistry, metabolism, kinetics, and biomarkers. *Handbook of Experimental Pharmacology, 192*, 29–60. doi:10.1007/978-3-540-69248-5_2

Benowitz, N. L., & Jacob, P. (1984). Daily intake of nicotine during cigarette smoking. *Clinical Pharmacology and Therapeutics, 35*(4), 499–504.

Benowitz, N. L., Lessov-Schlaggar, C. N., & Swan, G. E. (2006). Female sex and oral contraceptive use accelerate nicotine metabolism. *Clinical Pharmacology and Therapeutics, 79*(5), 480–488.

Beral, V., Gaitskell, K., & Hermon, C. (2012). Ovarian cancer and smoking: Individual participant meta-analysis including 28,114 women with ovarian cancer from 51 epidemiological studies. *The Lancet Oncology, 13*(9), 946–956. doi:10.1016/S1470-2045(12)70322-4

Bergin, J. E., & Kendler, K. S. (2012). Common psychiatric disorders and caffeine use, tolerance, and withdrawal: An examination of shared genetic and environmental effects. *Twin Research and Human Genetics, 15*(4), 473–482. doi:10.1017/thg.2012.25

Berlin, C. M., Denson, H. M., & Daniel, C. H. (1984). Disposition of dietary caffeine in milk, saliva, and plasma of lactating women. *Pediatrics, 73*, 59–63.

Berlin, I., Gasior, M. J., & Moolchan, E. T. (2007). Sex-based and hormonal contraception effects on the metabolism of nicotine among adolescent tobacco-dependent smokers. *Nicotine & Tobacco Research, 9*(4), 493–498.

Bigard, A. X. (2010). Risks of energy drinks in youths. *Archives De Pediatrie, 17*(11), 1625–1631. doi:10.1016/j.arcped.2010.08.001

Birge, M., Duffy, S., & Astrid Miler, J. (2018, November 215). What proportion of people who try one cigarette become daily smokers? A meta-analysis of representative surveys. *Nicotine & Tobacco Research, 20*(12), 1427–1433. doi:10.1093/ntr/ntx243

Bonsignore, A., Sblano, S., & Pozzi, F. (2014, September). A case of suicide by ingestion of caffeine. *Forensic Science, Medicine, and Pathology, 10*(3), 448–451. doi:10.1007/s120254-014-9571-6

Borota, D., Murray, E., & Keceli, G. (2014). Post-study caffeine administration enhances memory consolidation in humans. *Nature Neuroscience, 17*(2), 201–203. doi:10.1038/nn.3623

Botello-Harbaum, M., Schroeder, J. R., & Collins, C. C. (2010). Nicotine replacement therapy among adolescent smokers seeking cessation treatment. *Ethnicity & Disease, 20*(2), 180–184.

Bowker, K. A., Lewis, S., & Coleman, T. (2014). Comparison of cotinine levels in pregnant women while smoking and when using nicotine replacement therapy. *Nicotine & Tobacco Research, 16*(6), 895–898. doi:10.1093/ntr/ntu029

Bracken, M. B., Triche, E. W., & Belanger, K. (2003). Association of maternal caffeine consumption with decrements in fetal growth. *American Journal of Epidemiology, 157*(5), 456–466.

Branum, A. M., Rossen, L. M., & Schoendorf, K. C. (2014, March). Trends in caffeine intake among US children and adolescents. *Pediatrics, 133*(3), 386–393. doi:10.1542/peds.2013-2877

Brent, R. L., Christian, M. S., & Diener, R. M. (2011). Evaluation of the reproductive and developmental risks of caffeine. *Birth Defects Research. Part B, Developmental and Reproductive Toxicology, 92*(2), 152–187.

Brown, A. (2019, March 27). Sonic brings Red Bull to fast food menus. *Bloomberg*.

Brown, C. J., & Cheng, J. M. (2014). Electronic cigarettes: Product characterisation and considerations. *Tobacco Control, 23*(Supplement 2), 4–10. doi:10.1136/tobaccocontrol-2013-051476

Browne, M. L., Hoyt, A. T., & Feldkamp, M. L. (2011). Maternal caffeine intake and risk of selected birth defects in the National Birth Defects Prevention Study. *Birth Defects Research Part A: Clinical and Molecular Teratology, 91*(2), 93–101. doi:10.1002/bdra.20752

Buckley, T. C., Mozley, S. L., & Holohan, D. R. (2005). A psychometric evaluation of the Fagerstrom Test for Nicotine Dependence in PTSD smokers. *Addictive Behaviors, 30*(5), 1029–1033.

Buisson, B., & Bertrand, D. (2002). Nicotine addiction: The possible role of functional upregulation. *Trends in Pharmacological Sciences, 23*(3), 130–136. doi:10.1016/S0165-6147(00)01979-9

Burling, A. S., & Burling, T. A. (2003). Comparison of self-report measures of nicotine dependence among male drug/alcohol-dependent cigarette smokers. *Nicotine & Tobacco Research, 5*(5), 625–633.

Burnham, L., Matiak, S., & Makrigiorgos, G. (2015, May). Breastfeeding and coffee consumption in children younger than 2 years in Boston, Massachusetts, USA. *Journal of Human Lactation, 31*(2), 267–272. doi:10.1177/0890334415570971

Butt, M. S., & Sultan, M. T. (2011). Coffee and its consumption: Benefits and risks. *Critical Review Food Science and Nutrition, 51*(4), 363–373. doi: 10.1080/10408390903586412

Cahill, K., Lindson-Hawley, N., & Thomas, K. H. (2016, May 9). Nicotine receptor partial agonists for smoking cessation. *Cochrane Database of Systematic Reviews, 0*(5), CD006103. doi:10.1002/14651858.CD006103.pub7

Cahill, K., Stead, L. F., & Lancaster, T. (2012, April 18). Nicotine receptor partial agonists for smoking cessation. *Cochrane Database of Systematic Reviews, 0*(4), CD006103. doi:10.1002/14651858.CD006103.

Cahill, K., Stevens, S., & Perera, R. (2013, May 31). Pharmacological interventions for smoking cessation: An overview and network meta-analysis. *Cochrane Database of Systematic Reviews, 0*(5), CD009329. doi:10.1002/14651858.CD009329.

Callahan-Lyon, P. (2014). Electronic cigarettes: Human health effects. *Tobacco Control, 23*(Supplement 2), 36–40. doi:10.1136/tobaccocontrol-2013-051470

Cantrell, L. (2005, June 20). Nicotine poisoning. *California Poison Control System Newsletter*, 1–2.

Carter, B. D., Abnet, C. C., & Feskanich, D. (2015). Smoking and mortality–Beyond established causes. *The New England Journal of Medicine, 372*(7), 631–640. doi:10.1056/NEJMsa1407211

Castle, D. (2011, November 29). Turbo Snort nasal spray gives caffeine heads a new way to wake up. *PRWeb*. Clifton Park, New York. Retrieved December 23, 2017, from www.Greensations.com

Cavallo, D. A., Duhig, A. M., & McKee, S. (2006). Gender and weight concerns in adolescent smokers. *Addictive Behaviors, 31*(11), 2140–2146.

Caviness, C. M., Anderson, B. J., & Stein, M. D. (2017). Energy drinks and alcohol-related risk among young adults. *Substance Abuse, 38*(4), 376–381. doi:10.1080/08897077.2017.1343217

CBC News. (2015, June 1). Tobacco companies ordered to pay $15B in damages. CBC News.

CDC, Centers for Disease Control and Prevention. (2010). Vital signs: Nonsmokers' exposure to secondhand smoke—United States, 1999–2008. *MMWR, Morbidity and Mortality Weekly Report, 59*(35), 1141–1146. Retrieved October 7, 2016, from www.cdc.gov/mmwr/preview/mmwrhtml/mm5935a4.htm

CDC, Centers for Disease Control and Prevention. (2012, January 25). *PRAMS and Smoking*. Atlanta, GA: Division of Reproductive Health, National Center for Chronic Disease Prevention and Health Promotion.

CDC, Centers for Disease Control and Prevention. (2015a). Vital signs: Disparities in nonsmokers' exposure to secondhand smoke—United States, 1999–2012. *MMWR, Morbidity and Mortality Weekly Report, 64*(4), 103–108. Retrieved from www.cdc.gov/mmwr/preview/mmwrhtml/mm6404a7.htm?s_cid=mm6404a7_w

CDC, Centers for Disease Control and Prevention. (2015b). Flavored tobacco product use among middle and high school students—United States, 2014. *MMWR, Morbidity and Mortality Weekly Report, 64*(38), 1066–1070.

CDC, Centers for Disease Control and Prevention. (2016a, February 17). Secondhand Smoke (SHS) Facts. *Fact Sheets*. Retrieved from www.cdc.gov/chronicdisease/)

CDC, Centers for Disease Control and Prevention. (2016b, October 5). *Ellie's Story. 1*. Centers for Disease Control and Prevention. Retrieved November 11, 2016, from www.cdc.gov/tobacco/campaign/tips/quit-smoking/index.html?s_cid=OSH_tips_D9317

CDC, Centers for Disease Control and Prevention. (2016c, September 28). Becky's Story. 1. Centers for Disease Control and Prevention. Retrieved November 11, 2016, from www.cdc.gov/tobacco/campaign/tips/quit-smoking/index.html?s_cid=OSH_tips_D9317

CDC, Centers for Disease Control and Prevention. (2016d, October 22). Rose's Story. 1. Retrieved November 11, 2016, from www.cdc.gov/tobacco/campaign/tips/quit-smoking/index.html?s_cid=OSH_tips_D9317

CDC, Centers for Disease Control and Prevention. (2016e, October 12). Rebecca's Story. 1. Centers for Disease Control and Prevention. Retrieved November 11, 2016, from http://www.cdc.gov/tobacco/campaign/tips/quit-smoking/index.html?s_cid=OSH_tips_D9317

CDC, Centers for Disease Control and Prevention. (2016f, December 30). National Health Interview Survey. CDC/National Center for Health Statistics. Retrieved from www.cdc.gov/nchs/nhis/nhis_listserv.htm

CDC, Centers for Disease Control and Prevention. (2018a, January 17). Low-yield cigarettes. Office on Smoking and Health, National Center for Chronic Disease Prevention and Health Promotion.

CDC, Centers for Disease Control and Prevention. (2018b). Tobacco use among middle and high school students—United States, 2011–2017. *MMWR, Morbidity and Mortality Weekly Report, 67*(22), 629–633.

Chabrol, H., Niezborala, M., & Chastan, E. (2005). Comparison of the heavy smoking index and of the Fagerstrom test for nicotine dependence in a sample of 749 cigarette smokers. *Addictive Behaviors, 30*(7), 1474–1477. doi:10.1016/j.addbeh.2005.02.001

Chang, P. H., Chiang, C. H., & Ho, W. C. (2015). Combination therapy of varenicline with nicotine replacement therapy is better than varenicline alone: A systematic review and meta-analysis of randomized controlled trials. *BMC Public Health, 15*, 689. doi:10.1186/s12889-015-2055-2055-0

Chatham-Stephens, K., Law, R., & Taylor, E. (2016, December). Exposure calls to U. S. Poison centers involving electronic cigarettes and conventional cigarettes—September 2010–December 2014. *Journal of Medical Toxicology, 12*(4), 350–357. doi:10.1007/s13181-016-0563-7

Chen, L., Bell, E. M., & Browne, M. L. (2014). Exploring maternal patterns of dietary caffeine consumption before conception and during pregnancy. *Maternal and Child Health Journal, 18*(10), 2446–2455. doi:10.1007/s10995-014-1483-2

Chun, L. F., Moazed, F., & Calfee, C. S. (2017, August 1). Pulmonary toxicity of e-cigarettes. *American Journal of Physiology, Lung Cellular and Molecular Physiology, 13*(2), L193–L206. doi:10.1152/ajplung.00071.2017

Clapp, P. W., & Jaspers, I. (2017, October 5). Electronic cigarettes: Their constituents and potential links to asthma. *Current Allergy and Asthma Reports, 17*(11), 79. doi:10.1007/s11882-017-0747-5

Cleary, K., Levine, D. A., & Hoffman, R. S. (2012). Adolescents and young adults presenting to the emergency department intoxicated from a caffeinated alcoholic beverage: A case series. *Annals of Emergency Medicine, 59*(1), 67–69. doi:10.1016/j.annemergmed.2011.06.015

Collins, A. C. (1990). An analysis of the addiction liability of nicotine. *Advances in Alcohol & Substance Abuse, 9*(1–2), 83–101. doi:10.1300/J251v09n01_06

Collins, L., Smiley, S. L., & Moore, R. A. (2017). Physician tobacco screening and advice to quit among U.S. adolescents—National Survey on Drug Use and Health, 2013. *Tobacco Induced Diseases*, 1–7. doi:10.1186/s12971-016-0107-6

Corelli, R. L., & Hudmon, K. S. (2006). Pharmacologic interventions for smoking cessation. *Critical Care Nursing Clinics of North America, 18*(1), 39–51.

Cormier, B., Reid, J. L., & Hammond, D. (2018). *Perceptions of Caffeinated Drinks among Youth and Young Adults in Canada.* Health Promotion and Chronic Disease Prevention. Ottawa: Government of Canada. Retrieved May 16, 2018, from https://doi.org/10.24095/hpcdp.28.5.04

Cornacchione, J., Wagoner, K. G., & Wiseman, K. D. (2016). Adolescent and young adult perceptions of hookah and little cigars/cigarellos: Implications for risk messages. *Journal of Health Communication, 21*(7), 818–825. doi:10.1080/10810730.2016.1177141

Covey, L. S., & Glassman, A. H. (1991). New approaches to smoking cessation. *Physician Assistant, 15*, 69, 70, 73, 74, 77.

Cox, L. S., Nollen, N. L., & Mayo, M. S. (2012). Bupropion for smoking cessation in African American light smokers: A randomized controlled study. *Journal of the National Cancer Institute, 104*(4), 290–298. doi:10.1093/jnci/djr513

Crain, D., & Bhat, A. (2010). Current treatment options in smoking cessation. *Hospital Practice (Minneapolis), 38*(1), 53–61.

Cross, S. J., Lotfipour, S., & Leslie, F. M. (2017, March). Mechanisms and genetic factors underlying co-use of nicotine and alcohol or other drugs of abuse. *The American Journal of Drug and Alcohol Abuse, 43*(2), 171–185. doi:10.1080/00952990.2016.1209512

Czogala, J., Goniewicz, M. L., & Fidelus, B. (2014, June). Secondhand exposure to vapors from electronic cigarettes. *Nicotine & Tobacco Research, 16*(6), 655–662. doi:10.1093/ntr/ntt203

D'Allessandro, A., Boeckelmann, I., & Hammwhoner, M. (2012). Nicotine, cigarette smoking and cardiac arrhythmia: An overview. *European Journal of Preventive Cardiology, 19*(3), 297–305.

Dahlstrom, A., Lundell, B., & Curvall, M. (1990). Nicotine and cotinine concentrations in the nursing mother and her infant. *Acta Paediatrica Scandinavica, 79*(2), 142–147.

Dalack, G. W., Healy, D. H., & Meador-Woodruff, J. H. (1998). Nicotine dependence in schizophrenia: Clinical phenomena and laboraory findings. *American Journal of Psychiatry, 155*(11), 1490–1501. doi:10.1176/ajp.155.11.1490

Danaei, G., Ding, E. L., & Mozaffarian, D. (2009). The preventable causes of death in the United States: Comparative risk assessment of dietary, lifestyle, and metabolic risk factors. *PLoS Medicine, 6*(4), e1000058. doi:10.1371/journal.pmed.1000058

Dani, J. A., & De Biasi, M. (2001). Cellular mechanisms of nicotine addiction. *Pharmacology Biochemistry and Behavior, 70*(4), 439–446.

Dani, J. A., Ji, D., & Zhou, F. M. (2001). Synaptic plasticity and nicotine addiction. *Neuron, 31*(3), 349–352.

Davis, J. K., & Green, J. M. (2009). Caffeine and anaerobic performance: Ergogenic value and mechanisms of action. *Sports Medicine, 39*(10), 813–832. doi:10.2165/11317770-000000000-00000

De Biasi, M., & Dani, J. A. (2011). Reward, addiction, withdrawal to nicotine. *Annual Review of Neuroscience, 34*, 105–130. doi:10.1146//annurev-neuro-061010-113734

De Genna, N. M., Goldschmidt, L., & Day, N. L. (2016). Maternal trajectories of cigarette use as a function of maternal age and race. *Addictive Behaviors, 65*, 33–39. doi:10.1016/j.addbeh.2016.09.011

de Leon, J., Diaz, F. J., & Becona, E. (2003). Exploring brief measures of nicotine dependence for epidemiological surveys. *Addictive Behaviors, 28*(8), 1481–1486.

de Meneses-Gaya, C., Zuardi, A. W., & Loureiro, S. R. (2009). Is the Fagerstrom Test for Nicotine Dependence a good instrument to assess tobacco use in patients with schizophrenia? *Revista Brasileira De Psiquiatria, 31*(3), 281–292.

Degens, H., Gayan-Ramirez, G., & van Hees, H. W. (2015). Smoking-induced skeletal muscle dysfunction: From evidence to mechanisms. *American Journal of Respiratory and Critical Care Medicine, 191*(6), 620–625. doi:10.1164/rccm.201410-1830PP

DeVito, E. E., Herman, A. L.. & Waters, A. J. (2014). Subjective, physiological, and cognitive responses to intravenous nicotine: Effects of sex and menstrual cycle phase. *Neuropsychopharmacology, 39*(6), 1431–1440. doi: 10.1038/npp.2013.339

Del Coso, J., Munoz, G., & Munoz-Guerra, J. (2011). Prevalence of caffeine use in elite athletes following its removal from the World Anit-Doping Agency list of banned substances. *Applied Physiology, Nutrition, and Metabolism, 36*, 555–561. doi:10.1139/H11-052

Derby, K. S., Cuthrell, K., & Caberto, C. (2008). Nicotine metabolism in three ethnic/racial groups with different risks of lung cancer. *Cancer Epidemiology, Biomarkers & Prevention, 17*(12), 3526–3535. doi:10.1158/1055-9965.EPI-08-0424

Dews, P. B., O'Brien, C. P., & Bergman, J. (2002). Caffeine: Behavioral effects of withdrawal and related issues. *Food and Chemical Toxicology, 40*(9), 1257–1261.

Di Rocco, J. R., During, A., & Morelli, P. J. (2011). Atrial fibrillation in healthy adolescents after highly caffeinated beverage consumption: Two case reports. *Journal of Medical Case Reports, 5*, 18. doi:10.1186/1752-1947-5-18

DiFranza, J. R., Savageau, J. A., & Rigotti, N. A. (2002). Development of symptoms of tobacco dependence in youths: 30 month follow up data from the DANDY study. *Tobacco Control, 11*, 228–235. doi:10.1136/tc.11.3.228

DiFranza, J. R., Savageau, J. A., & Wellman, R. J. (2012a). A comparison of the autonomy over tobacco scale and the Fagerstrom test for nicotine dependence. *Addictive Behaviors, 37*(7), 856–861. doi:10.1016/j.addbeh.2012.03.013

DiFranza, J. R., Sweet, M., & Savageau, J. A. (2012b). The assessment of tobacco dependence in young users of smokeless tobacco. *Tobacco Control, 21*(5), 471–476. doi:10.1136/tc.2011.043810

DiFranza, J. R., Wellman, R. J., & Savageau, J. A. (2013). What aspect of dependence does the Fagerstrom Test for Nicotine Dependence measure?. *Addiction, Article ID, 906276*, 1–8.

DiFranza, J. R., Wellman, R. J., & Ursprung, S. (2009). The Autonomy over Smoking Scale. *Psychology of Addictive Behaviors, 23*, 656–665.

Dik, V. K., Bueno-de-Mesquita, H. B., & Van Oijen, M. G. (2014). Coffee and tea consumption, genotype-based CYP1A2 and NAT2 activity and colorectal cancer risk-results from the EPIC cohort study. *International Journal of Cancer, 135*(2), 401–412. doi:10.1002/ijc.28655

Ding, Y. S., Yan, X. J., & Jain, R. B. (2006). Determination of 14 polycyclic aromatic hydrocarbons in mainstream smoke from U. S. brand and non-U. S. brand cigarettes. *Environmental Science & Technology, 40*(4), 1133–1138.

Domino, E. F., Hornbach, E., & Demana, T. (1993). The nicotine content of common vegetables. *The New England Journal of Medicine, 329*, 437. doi:10.1056/NEJM199308053290619

Drewnowski, A., & Rehm, C. D. (2016, March 10). Sources of caffeine in diets of US children and adults: Trends by beverage type and purchase location. *Nutrients, 8*(3), 154. doi:10.3390/nu8030154

Driscoll, D. P., & Mathews, T. J. (2018, February). Cigarette smoking during pregnancy: United States, 2016. *NCHS Data Brief*, (305), 1–5.

Duncan, M. J., Lyons, M., & Hankey, J. (2009). Placebo effects of caffeine on short-term resistance exercise to failure. *International Journal of Sports Physiology and Performance, 4*(2), 244–253.

Durmowicz, E. L. (2014). The impact of electronic cigarettes on the paediatric population. *Tob Control, 23*, ii41–ii46. doi:10.1136/tobaccocontrol-2013-051468

Ebbert, J. O., Patten, C. A., & Schroeder, D. R. (2006). The Fagerstrom Test for Nicotine Dependence-Smokeless Tobacco (FTND-ST). *Addictive Behaviors, 31*(9), 1716–1721. doi:10.1016/j.addbeh.2005.12.015

Ebbert, J. O., Wyatt, K. D., & Hays, J. T. (2010). Varenicline for smoking cessation: Efficacy, safety, and treatment recommendations. *Patient Preference and Adherence, 4*, 355–362.

Ebbert, J. O., Wyatt, K. D., & Zirakzadeh, A. (2009). Clinical utility of varenicline for smokers with medical and psychiatric comorbidity. *International Journal of Chronic Obstructive Pulmonary Disease, 4*, 421–430.

Electronic nicotine delivery systems. (2014, July 21). *World Health Organization to 6th Session of the Conference of the Parties to the WHO Framework Convention on Tobacco Control*, (pp. 2–3). doi:fctc/PDF/cop6/fctc_COP6_10-en. pdf?ua=1

Elkins, I. J., Saunders, G. R., & Malone, S. M. (2018). Increased risk of smoking in female adolescents who had childhood ADHD. *The American Journal of Psychiatry, 175*(1), 63–70. doi:10.1176/appi.ajp.2017.17010009

Ernst, M., Moolchan, E. T., & Robinson, M. L. (2001). Behavioral and neural consequences of prenatal exposure to nicotine. *Journal of the American Academy of Child & Adolescent Psychiatry, 40*(6), 630–641.

Etter, J. F. (2005). A comparison of the content-, construct- and predictive validity of the cigarette dependence scale and the Fagerstrom test for nicotine dependence. *Drug and Alcohol Dependence*, 77(3), 259–268. doi:10.1016/j.drugalcdep.2004.08.015

Etter, J. F., Duc, T. V., & Perneger, T. V. (1999). Validity of the Fagerstrom test for nicotine dependence and of the heaviness of smoking index among relatively light smokers. *Addiction, 94*(2), 269–281.

Evatt, D. P., Juliano, L. M., & Griffiths, R. R. (2016). A brief manualized treatment for problematic caffeine use: A randomized control trial. *Journal of Consulting and Clinical Psychology, 84*(2), 113–121. doi:10.1037/ccp0000064

Faessel, H., Ravva, P., & Williams, K. (2009). Pharmacokinetics, safety, and tolerability of varenicline in healthy adolescent smokers: A multicenter, randomized, double-blind, placebo-controlled, parallel-group study. *Clinical Therapeutics, 31*(1), 177–189. doi:10.1016/j.clinthera.2009.01.003

Faessel, H. M., Obach, R. S., & Rollema, H. (2010). A review of the clinical pharmacokinetics and pharmacodynamics of varenicline for smoking cessation. *Clinical Pharmacokinetics, 49*(12), 799–816. doi:10.2165/11537850-00000000-00000

Fagan, P., Moolchan, E. T., & Pokhrel, P. (2015). Biomarkers of tobacco smoke exposure in racial/ethnic groups at high risk for lung cancer. *American Journal of Public Health, 105*(6), 1237–1245. doi:10.2105/AJPH.2014.302492

Fagan, P., Pohkrel, P., & Herzog, T. (2015, April 1). Comparisons of three nicotine dependence scales in a multiethnic sample of young adult menthol and non-menthol smokers. *Drug and Alcohol Dependence, 149*, 203–211. doi:10.1016/j.drugalcdep.2015.02.005

Fant, R. V., Buchhalter, A. R., & Buchman, A. C. (2009). Pharmacotherapy for tobacco dependence. *Handbook of Experimental Pharmacology, 192*, 487–510.

Farley, A. C., Hajek, P., & Lycett, D. (2012). Interventions for preventing weight gain after smoking cessation. *The Cochrane Database of Systematic Reviews, 1*, CD006219. doi:10.1002/14651858.CD006219.pub3

FDA, U. S. Food and Drug Adminstration. (2009, July 1). FDA requires new boxed warnings for the smoking cessation drugs Chantix and Zyban. *Public Health Advisory*. Retrieved from www.fda.gov/Drugs/DrugSafety/PostmarketDrugSafetyInformationforPatientsandP.

FDA, U. S. Food and Drug Administration. (2010). *Guidance for Industry and FDA Staff: Use of "Light," "Mild," "Low," or Similar Descriptors in the Labeling or Advertising of Tobacco Products*. Rockville, Maryland: USFDA, Center for Tobacco Products. Retrieved January 17, 2018, from www.fda.gov/TobaccoProducts/GuidanceComplianceRegulatoryInformation/ucm214597.htm

FDA, U.S. Food and Drug Administration. (2012, March 6). *Press Announcements > FDA Issues Warning Letter to Makers of AeroShot "Caffeine Inhaler"*. Retrieved October 5, 2016, from FDA Press Statement: www.fda.gov/NewsEvents/Newsroom/PressAnnouncements/ucm294874.htm

FDA, U. S. Food and Drug Administration. (2016a, August 8). Extending authorities to all tobacco products, including e-cigarettes, cigars, and hookah. Retrieved July 16, 2017, from www.fda.gov/TobaccoProducts/Labeling/RulesRegulationsGuidance/ucm388395.htm

FDA, U.S. Food and Drug Administration. (2016b, December 16). *Chantix (varenicline) and Zyban (bupropion): Drug Safety Communication—Mental Health Side Effects Revised. Safety Alerts for Human Medical Products*) (pp. 1–12). Silver Spring, Maryland: U.S. Food and Drug Administration.

Fisone, G., Borgkvist, A., & Usiello, A. (2004, April). Caffeine as a psychomotor stimulant: Mechanism of action. *Cellular and Molecular Life Sciences, 61*(7–8), 857–872. doi:10.1007/s00018-003-3269-3

Fluharty, M., Taylor, A. E., & Grabski, M. (2017). The association of cigarette smoking with depression and anxiety: A systematic review. *Nicotine & Tobacco Research*, 3–13. doi: 10.1093/ntr/ntw40

Food Standards Agency. (2008, November 3). Foods Standards Agency publishes new caffeine advice for pregnant women. *Press Release*. Retrieved from tna.europarchive.org/20111116080332/www.food.gov.uk/news/pressreleases/2008/nov/caffeineadvice

Forray, A., Gotman, N., & Kershaw, T. (2014). Perinatal smoking and depression in women with concurrent substance use. *Addictive Behaviors, 39*(4), 749–756. doi:10.1016/j.addbeh.20123.12.008

Foulds, J., Veldheer, S., & Berg, A. (2011). Electronic cigarettes (e-cigs): Views of aficionados and clinical/public health perspectives. *International Journal of Clinical Practice, 65*(10), 1037–1042. doi:10.1111/j.1742-1241.2011.02751.x

Fox, M. (2017, May 15). Caffeine overdose killed South Carolina teen, coroner rules. *NBC News*.

Franklin, T. R., Ehrman, R., & Lynch, K. G. (2008). Menstrual cycle phase at quit date predicts smoking status in an NRT treatment trial: A retrospective analysis. *Journal of Women's Health, 17*(2), 287–292. doi:10.1089/jwh.2007.0423

Frishman, W. H. (2007). Smoking cessation pharmacotherapy—Nicotine and non-nicotine preparations. *Preventive Cardiology, 10*(2, Supplement 1), 10–22.

Frishman, W. H. (2009). Smoking cessation pharmacotherapy. *Therapeutic Advances in Cardiovascular Disease, 3*(4), 287–308.

Fuemmeler, B. F., Kollins, S. H., & McClernon, F. J. (2007, November–December). Attention deficit hyperactivity disorder symptoms predict nicotine dependence and progression to regular smoking from adolescence to young adulthood. *Journal of Pediatric Psychology, 32*(10), 1203–1213. doi:10.1093/jpepsy/jsm051

Fulgoni, V. L., Keast, D. R., & Lieberman, H. R. (2015). Trends in intake and sources of caffeine in the diets of US adults: 2001–2010. *American Journal of Clinical Nutrition, 101*(5), 1081–1087. doi:10.3945/ajcn.113.080077

Gallaway, M. S., Henley, S. J., & Steele, C. B. (2018, November 2). Surveillance for cancers associated with tobacco use —United States, 2010–2014. *MMWR, Morbidity and Mortality Weekly Report, 67*(12), 1–42.

Gamaleddin, I. H., Trigo, J. M., & Gueye, A. B. (2015). Role of endogenous cannabinoid system in nicotine addiction: Novel insights. *Frontiers in Psychiatry, 6*(Article 41), 1–2. doi:10.3389/psyt.2015.00041

Garrison, G. D., & Dugan, S. E. (2009). Varenicline: A first-line treatment option for smoking cessation. *Clinical Therapeutics, 31*(3), 463–491.

Generali, J. A. (1992). Nicotine transdermal patches. *Facts and Comparisons Drug Newsletter, 11*, 33–34.

Gentzke, A. S., Creamer, M., & Cullen, K. A. (2019, February 15). Vital signs: Tobacco product use among middle and high school students—United States, 2011–2018. *MMWR, Morbidity and Mortality Weekly Report, 68*(6), 157–164.

Ghose, T. (2014, November 16). Energy drinks can be deadly for young children. *Live Science*.

Gierach, G. L., Freedman, N. D., & Andaya, A. (2012). Coffee intake and breast cancer risk in the NIH-AARP diet and health study cohort. *International Journal of Cancer, 131*(2), 452–460. doi:10.1002/ijc.26372

Goldbach, J. T., Mereish, E. H., & Burgess, C. (2017). Sexual orientation disparities in the use of emerging drugs. *Substance Use & Misuse, 52*(2), 265–271. doi:10.1080/10826084.2016.1223691

Goniewicz, M., Gupta, L., & Lee, L. (2015). Electronic cigarettes are a source of thirdhand exposure to nicotine. *Nicotine & Tobacco Research, 17*(2), 256–258. doi:10.1093/ntr/ntu152

Gonzales, D., Rennard, S. I., & Nides, M. (2006). Varenicline: An alpha4beta2 nicotine acetylcholine receptor partial agonist vs. sustained-release bupropion and placebo for smoking cessation. *JAMA, the Journal of the American Medical Association, 296*(1), 47–55.

Goodwin, R. D., Cheslack-Postava, K., & Nelson, D. B. (2017, October 1). Smoking during pregnancy in the United States, 2005–2014: The role of depression. *Drug and Alcohol Dependence, 179*, 159–166. doi:10.1016/j.drugalcdep.2017.06.021

Goodwin, R. D., Keyes, K. M., & Hasin, D. S. (2009). Changes in cigarette use and nicotine dependence in the United States: Evidence from the 2001–2002 wave of the National Epidemiologic Survey of alcoholism and related conditions. *American Journal of Public Health, 99*(8), 1471–1477.

Gottlieb, S. (2018, November 15). Statement from FDA Commissioner Scott Gottlieb, M.D., on proposed new steps to protect youth by preventing access to flavored tobacco products and banning menthol in cigarettes. *FDA Statement*, 1–7. Department of Health and Human Services.

Graham, T. E. (2001). Caffeine and exercise: Metabolism, endurance and performance. *Sports Medicine, 31*(11), 785–807.

Grana, R., Benowitz, N., & Glantz, S. A. (2014, May 13). Contemporary reviews in cardiovascular medicine: E-Cigarettes: A scientific review. *CIRCULATION. 129*, pp. 1972–1986. Dallas, Texas: American Heart Association). doi:10.116/CIRCULATIONAHA.114007667, p.1978

Gray, K. M., McClure, E. A., & Baker, N. L. (2015). An exploratory short-term double-blind randomized trial of varenicline versus nicotine patch for smoking cessation in women. *Addiction, 110*(6), 1027–1034. doi:10.111/add.12895

Greenwood, D. C., Thatcher, N. J., & Ye, J. (2014). Caffeine intake during pregnancy and adverse birth outcomes: A systematic review and dose-response meta-analysis. *European Journal of Epidemiology, 29*(10), 725–734.

Grekin, E. R., & Ayna, D. (2012). Waterpipe smoking among college students in the United States: A review of the literature. *Journal of American College Health, 60*(3), 244–249. doi:10.1080/07448481.2011.589419

Grimshaw, G. M., & Stanton, A. (2006, October 18). Tobacco cessation intervention for young people. *Cochrane Database of Systematic Reviews, 4*, CD003289.

Guais, A., Brand, G., & Jacquot, L. (2011). Toxicity of carbon dioxide: A review. *Chemical Research in Toxicology, 24*(12), 2061–2070. doi:10.1021/tx200220r

Gunja, N., & Brown, J. A. (2012, January 16). Energy drinks: Health risks and toxicity. *MJA, 196*, 46–49. doi:10.5694/mja11.10838

Hackshaw, A., Morris, J. K., & Boniface, S. (2018). Low cigarette consumption and risk of coronary heart disease and stroke: Meta-analysis of 141 cohort studies in 55 study reports. *BMJ*, 1–15. doi:10.1136/bmj.j3984

Haddock, C. K., Lando, H., & Klesges, R. C. (1999). A study of the psychometric and predictive properties of the Fagerstrom Test for Nicotine Dependence in a population of young smokers. *Nicotine & Tobacco Research, 1*(1), 59–66.

Hahn, B. (2015). Nicotinic receptors and attention. *Current Topics in Behavioral Neurosciences, 23*, 103–135. doi:10.1007/978-3-319-13665-3_5

Hahn, K. A., Wise, L. A., & Rothman, K. J. (2015). Caffeine and caffeinated beverage consumption and risk of spontaneous abortion. *Human Reproduction (Journal), 30*(5), 1246–1255. doi:10.1093/humrep/dev063

Hammig, B., Daniel-Dobbs, P., & Blunt-Vinti, H. (2017). Electronic cigarette initiation among minority youth in the United States. *The American Journal of Drug and Alcohol Abuse, 43*(3), 306–310. doi:10.1080/00952990.2016.1203926

Harakeh, Z., Engels, R. C., & Monshouwer, K. (2010). Adolescent's weight concerns and the onset of smoking. *Substance Use/ Misuse, 45*(12), 1847–1860. doi:10.3109/10826081003682149

Harrell, P. T., Trenz, R. C., & Scherer, L. R. (2012). Cigarette smoking, illicit drug use, and routes of administration among heroin and cocaine users. *Addictive Behaviors, 37*(5), 678–681. doi:10.1016/j.addbeh.2012.01.011

Hartz, S. M., Short, S. E., & Saccone, N. L. (2012). Increased genetic vulnerability to smoking at CHRNA5 in early-onset smokers. *Archives of General Psychiatry, 69*(8), 854–860. doi:10.1001/archgenpsychiatry.2012.124

Hays, J. T. (2015, June 17). *Is Hookah Smoking Safer than Cigarette Smoking?* Retrieved April 13, 2016, from Mayo Clinic, pp.1–3: http://www.mayoclinic.org/healthy-lifestyle/quit-smoking/expert-answers/hookah/faq-20057920?p=1

Hays, J. T., Croghan, I. T., & Schroeder, D. R. (2010, October 12). Varenicline for tobacco dependence treatment in recovering alcohol-dependent smokers: An open-label pilot study. *Journal of Substance Abuse Treatment, 40*(1), 102–107.

Heatherton, T. F., Kozlowski, L. T., & Frecker, R. C. (1991). The Fagerstrom test for nicotine dependence: A revision of the Fagerstrom tolerance questionnaire. *British Journal of Addiction, 86*(9), 1119–1127.

Hecht, S. S. (2014). It is time to regulate carcinogenic tobacco-specific nitrosamines in cigarette tobacco. *Cancer Prevention Research*, 7(7), 639–647. doi:10.1158/1940-6207. CAPR-14-0095

Heeschen, C., Weis, M., & Aicher, A. (2002). A novel angiogenic pathway mediated by non-neuronal nicotinic acetylcholine receptors. *Journal of Clinical Investigation*, *110*(4), 527–536. doi:10.1172/JCI14676

Henley, S. J., Thomas, C. C., & Sharapova, S. R. (2016). Vital signs: Disparities in tobacco-related cancer incidence and mortality—United States, 2004–2013. *MMWR, Morbitity and Mortality Weekly Report*, *65*, 1212–1218. doi: http://dx.doi.org/10.15585/mmwr.mm6544a3

Herman, A. O. (2017, November 27). Coffee's numerous health benefits detailed in new analysis. *NEJM, New England Journal of Medicine*, *1*. Retrieved from www.jwatch.org/fw113569/2017/11/27/coffees-numerous-health-benefits-detailed-new-analysis?query=pfwTOC&jwd=000020000 2443&jspc=

Hindmarch, I., Rigney, U., & Stanley, N. (2000, April). A naturalistic investigation of the effects of day-long consumption of tea, coffee and water on alertness, sleep onset and sleep quality. *Psychopharmacology*, *149*(3), 203–216.

Ho, M. K., & Tyndale, R. F. (2007). Overview of the pharmacogenomics of cigarette smoking. *Pharmacogenomics Journal*, 7(2), 81–98.

Hoffmann, D., & Hoffmann, I. (1997). The changing cigarette, 1950–1995. *Journal of Toxicology and Environmental Health*, *50*(4), 307–364.

Holbrook, B. D. (2016, June). The effects of nicotine on human fetal development. *Birth Defects Research, Part C, Embryo Today*, *108*(2), 181–192. doi:10.1002/bdrc.21128

Horn, J. R., & Hansten, P. D. (2007, November 1). Get to know an enzyme: CYP1A2. *Pharmacy Times*.

Hoyt, A. T., Browne, M., & Richardson, S. (2014, August). Maternal caffeine consumption and small for gestational age births: Results from a population-based case-control study. *Maternal and Child Health Journal*, *18*(6), 1540–1551. doi:10.1007/s10995-013-1397-4

Huang, C. L., Lin, H. H., & Wang, H. H. (2006). Psychometric evaluation of the Chinese version of the Fagerstrom Tolerance Questionnaire as a measure of cigaretted dependence. *Journal of Advanced Nursing*, *55*(5), 596–603.

Huang, L. L., Kowitt, S. D., & Sutfin, E. L. (2016, August 4). Electronic cigarette use among high school students and its association with cigarette use and smoking cessation, North Carolina Youth Tobacco Surveys, 2011 and 2013. *Preventing Chronic Disease*, *13*, E103. doi:10.5888/pcd13.150564

Hukkanen, J., Jacob, P., & Benowitz, N. L. (2005, April). Metabolism and disposition kinetics of nicotine. *Pharmacological Reviews*, *57*(1), 79–115. doi:10.1124/pr.57.1.3

Huntley, E. D., & Juliano, L. M. (2012). Caffeine expectancy questionnaire (CaffEQ): Construction, psychometric properties, and associations with caffeine use, caffeine dependence, and other related variables. *Psychological Assessment*, *24*(3), 592–607. doi:10.1037/a0026417

Huttlin, E. A., Allen, A. M., & Tosun, N. L. (2015, November). Associations between adrenocortical activity and nicotine response in female smokers by menstrual phase. *Addictive Behaviors*, *50*, 135–139. doi:10.1016/j.addbeh.2015.06.026

Hyde, R. F., Paxton, R., & Carr, T. E. (1982, September 18). Nicotine chewing-gum. *British Medical Journal (Clinical Research Edition)*, *285*(6344), 811–812.

Hyland, A., Garten, S., & Giovino, G. A. (2002). Mentholated cigarettes and smoking cessation: Findings from COMMIT (Community Intervention Trial for Smoking Cessation). *Tobacco Control*, *11*(2), 135–139.

Jabber, S. B., & Hanly, M. G. (2013, December). Fatal caffeine overdose: A case report and review of literature. *The American Journal of Forensic Medicine and Pathology*, *34*(4), 321–324. doi:10.1097/PAF.0000000000000058

Jalonick, M. C. (2012, March 6). *FDA Issues Warning to Inhalable Caffeine Maker*. Retrieved October 6, 2016, from The San Diego Union-Tribune: www.sandiegouniontribune.com/sdut-fda-issues-warning-to-inhalable-caffeine-maker-2012mar06-story.html

Jaslow, R. (2012, March 7). FDA warns AeroShot caffeine inhaler's maker, saying supplements can't be inhaled. *CBS News*. Retrieved December 23, 2017, from www.cbsnews.com/news/fda-warns-aeroshot-caffeine-inhalers-maker-saying-supplements-cant-be-inhaled/

Johnson, J. L., Eaton, D. K., & Pederson, L. L. (2009). Associations of trying to lose weight, weight control behaviors, and current cigarette use among US high school students. *Journal of School Health*, *79*(8), 355–360.

Johnstone, E., Benowitz, N., & Cargill, A. (2006, October). Determinants of the rate of nicotine metabolism and effects on smoking behavior. *Clinical Pharmacology and Therapeutics*, *80*(4), 319–330. doi:10.1016/j.cjpt.2006.06.011

Jones, A. W. (2017, April 1). Review of caffeine-related fatalities along with postmortem blood concentrations in 51 poisoning deaths. *Journal of Analytical Toxicology*, *41*(3), 167–172. doi:10.1093/jat/bkx011

Jorenby, D. E., Hays, J. T., & Rigotti, N. A. (2006). Efficacy of varenicline, an alpha4beta2 nicotinic acetylcholine receptor partial agonist, vs. placebo or sustained-release bupropion for smoking cessation: A randomized controlled study. *JAMA, the Journal of the American Medical Association*, *296*(1), 56–63.

Juliano, L. M., Evatt, D. P., & Richards, P. D. (2012). Characterization of individuals seeking treatment for caffeine dependence. *Psychology of Addictive Behaviors*, *26*(4), 948–954. doi:10.1037/a0027246

Juliano, L. M., & Griffiths, R. R. (2004). A critical review of caffeine withdrawal: Empirical validation of symptoms and signs, incidence, severity, and associated features. *Psychopharmacology (Berlin), 176*, 1–29. doi:10.1007/s00213-004-2000-x

Kamat, A. D., & Van Dyke, A. L. (2017, February 1). Use of electronic nicotine delivery systems among adolescents: Status of the evidence and public health recommendations. *Pediatric Annals, 46*(2), e69–e77. doi:10.3928/19382359-20170111-01

Kamboj, A., Spiller, H. A., & Casavant, M. J. (2016). Pediatric exposure to e-cigarettes, nicotine, and tobacco products in the United States. *Pediatrics, 137*(6), e20160041. doi:10.1542/peds.2016-0041

Kassem, N. O., Kassem, N. O., & Liles, S. (2018, March 6). Acrolein exposure in hookah smokers and non-smokers exposed to hookah tobacco secondhand smoke: Implications for regulating hookah tobacco products. *Nicotine & Tobacco Research, 20*(4), 492–501. doi:10.1093/ntr/ntx133

Kasza, K. A., Ambrose, B. K., & Conway, K. P. (2017, January 26). Tobacco-product use by adults and youths in the United States in 2013 and 2014. *The New England Journal of Medicine, 376*, 342–353.

Kavuluru, R., Han, S., & Hahn, E. J. (2018, April 13). On the popularity of the USB flash drive-shaped electronic cigarette Juul. *Tobacco Control*. doi: 10.1136/tobaccocontrol-2018-054259.

Keisler, B. D., & Armsey, T. D. (2006). Caffeine as an ergogenic aid. *Current Sports Medicine Reports, 5*(4), 215–219.

Kenny, P. J., & Markou, A. (2001). Neurobiology of the nicotine withdrawal syndrome. *Pharmacology Biochemistry and Behavior, 70*(4), 531–549.

Keyes, K. M., Davey Smith, G., & Susser, E. (2014, March). Associations of prenatal maternal smoking with offspring hyperactivity: Causal or confounded? *Psychological Medicine, 44*(4), 857–867. doi:10.1017/S0033291713000986

Keyes, K. M., Hamilton, A., & Kandel, D. B. (2016). Birth cohorts analysis of adolescent cigarette smoking and subsequent marijuana and cocaine use. *American Journal of Public Health, 106*(6), 1143–1149. doi:10.2105/AJPH.2016.303128

Kim, S. S. (2017). Comparison of two nicotine dependence measures for use with Korean American women: The FTND and AUTOS. *Asian/Pacific Island Nursing Journal, 2*(2), 66–72.

Kimura, R., Ushiyama, N., & Fujii, T. (2003). Nicotine-induced Ca2+ signaling and down-regulation of nicotinic acetylcholine receptor subunit expression in the CEM human leukemic T-cell line. *Life Sciences, 72*(18–19), 2155–2158.

Kinugawa, T., Kurita, T., & Nohara, R. (2011). A case of atrial tachycardia sensitive to increased caffeine intake. *International Heart Journal, 52*(6), 398–400.

Klatsky, A. L., Hasan, A. S., & Armstrong, M. A. (2011, Summer). Coffee, caffeine, and risk of hospitalization for arrhythmias. *The Permanente Journal, 15*(3), 19–25.

Koch, G., Datta, A. N., & Jost, K. (2017, December). Caffeine citrate dosing adjustments to assure stable caffeine concentrations in preterm neonates. *The Journal of Pediatrics, 191*, 50–56. doi:10.10165/j.jpeds.2017.08.064

Kohut, S. J. (2017, March). Interactions between nicotine and drugs of abuse: A review of preclinical findings. *The American Journal of Drug and Alcohol Abuse, 43*(2), 155–170. doi:10.1080/00952990.2016.1209513

Korte, K. J., Capron, D. W., & Zvolensky, M. (2013). The Fragerstrom Test for Nicotine Dependence: Do revisions in the item scoring enhance the psychometric properties?. *Addictive Behaviors, 38*(3), 1757–1763. doi:10.1016/j.addbeh.2012.10.013

Kovess, V., Keyes, K. M., & Hamilton, A. (2015). Maternal smoking and offspring inattention and hyperactivity: Results from a cross-national European survey. *European Child & Adolescent Psychiatry, 24*(8), 919–929. doi:10.1007/s00787-014-0641-9

Krebs, N. M., Chen, A., & Zhu, J. (2016, July 1). Comparison of puff volume with cigarettes per day in predicting nicotine uptake among daily smokers. *American Journal of Epidemiology, 184*(1), 48–57. doi:10.1093/aje/kwv341

Krishnan-Sarin, S., Morean, M., & Kong, G. (2017). E-cigarettes and "dripping" among high-school youth. *Pediatrics, 139*(3), e201263224. doi:10.1542/peds.2016-3224

Kudlow, P. A., Naylor, K. T., & Xie, B. (2013). Cognitive enhancement in Canadian medical students. *Journal of Psychoactive Drugs, 45*(4), 360–365.

Kuper, H., Boffetta, P., & Adami, H. O. (2002). Tobacco use and cancer causation: Association by tumour type. *Journal of Internal Medicine, 252*(3), 206–224.

Laizure, S. C., Meibohm, B., & Nelson, K. (2017). Comparison of caffeine disposition following administration by oral solution (energy drink) and inspired powder (AeroShot) in human subjects. *British Journal of Clinical Pharmacology, 83*(12), 2687–2694. doi:10.1111/bcp.13389

Langley, K., Heron, J., & Smith, G. D. (2012, August 1). Maternal and paternal smoking during pregnancy and risk of ADHD symptoms in offspring: Testing for intrauterine effects. *American Journal of Epidemiology, 176*(3), 261–268. doi:10.1093/aje/kwr510

Laniado-Laborin, R. (2010). Smoking cessation intervention: An evidence-based approach. *Postgraduate Medicine, 122*(2), 74–82. doi:10.3810/pgm.2010.03.2124

Lanza, H. I., Grella, C. E., & Chung, P. J. (2014). Does adolescent weight status predict problematic substance use patterns?. *American Journal of Health Behavior, 38*(5), 708–716. doi:10.5993/ajhb.38.5.8

Lara, B., Gonzalez-Millan, C., & Salinero, J. J. (2014). Caffeine-containing energy drink improves physical performance in female soccer players. *Amino Acids, 46*(5), 1385–1392. doi:10.1007/s00726-014-1709-z

Lasser, K. E., Quintiliani, L. M., & Truong, V. (2017, October 30). Effect of patient navigation and financial incentives on smoking cessation among primary care patients at an urban safety-net hospital: A randomized clinical trial. *JAMA Internal Medicine* . doi: 10.1001/jamainternmed.2017.4372.

LaVito, A. (2018, November 8). CDC says smoking rates fall to record low in US. *CNBC TV*, 1–4. CNBC.

Leal, W. E., & Jackson, D. B. (2017, November 29). Energy drinks and escalation in drug use severity: An emergent hazard to adolescent health. *Preventive Medicine, 17*, 30475–30479. doi:10.1016/j.ypmed.2017.11.033

Leischow, S. J., Muramoto, M. L., & Matthews, E. (2016, May). Adolescent smoking cessation with bupropion: The role of adherence. *Nicotine & Tobacco Research, 18*(5), 1202–1205. doi:10.1093/ntr/ntv179

Lemke, R. P. (2002). Drug dosing for neonates. In L. A. Pagliaro & A. M. Pagliaro (Eds.), *Problems in Pediatric Drug Therapy* (4th ed. ed., pp. 531–554). Hamilton, Illinois: American Pharmaceutical Association.

Li, J., Zhao, H., & Song, J. M. (2015). A meta-analysis of risk of pregnancy loss and caffeine and coffee consumption during pregnancy. *International Journal of Gynaecology & Obstetrics, 130*(2), 116–122. doi:10.1016/j.ijgo.2015.03.033

Lieberman, H. R., Stavinoha, T., & McGraw, S. (2012). Caffeine use among active duty US Army soldiers. *Journal of the Academy of Nutrition and Dietetics, 112*(6), 902–912. doi:10.1016/j.jand.2012.02.001

Lindson-Hawley, N., Hartmann-Boyce, J., & Fanshawe, T. R. (2016, October 13). Interventions to reduce harm from continued tobacco use. *The Cochrane Database of Systematic Reviews, 10*, CD005231. doi:10.1002/14651858.CD005231.pub3

Linn, A. (2007, September 10). Starbucks rethinks stance on young customers. *msnbc.com*, 1–3. MSNBC.

Littleton, J., Barron, S., & Prendergast, M. (2007). May-June). Smoking kills (alcoholics)! Should we do something about it?. *Alcohol and Alcoholism, 42*(3), 167–173. doi:10.1093/alcalc/agm019

Lorist, M. M., & Tops, M. (2003). Caffeine, fatigue, and cognition. *Brain and Cognition, 53*(1), 82–94.

Ma, J. Z., Li, M. D., & Payne, T. J. (2012). Evaluation of the brief Wisconsin Inventory of smoking dependence motives in African-American and European-American heavy smokers. *Frontiers in Psychiatry, 3*(36). doi:10.3389/fpsyt.2012.00036

Mahoney, C. R., Giles, G. E., & Marriott, B. P. (2018). Intake of caffeine from all sources and reasons for use by college students. *Clinical Nutrition*, 1–8. doi:10.1016/j.clnu.2018.04.004

Malaiyandi, V., Sellers, E. M., & Tyndale, R. E. (2005, March). Implications of CYP2A6 genetic variation for smoking behaviors and nicotine dependence. *Clinical Pharmacology and Therapeutics*, 77(3), 145–158. doi:10.1016/j.clpt.2004.10.011

Malson, J. L., Sims, K., & Murty, R. (2001). Comparison of the nicotine content of tobacco used in bidis and conventional cigarettes. *Tobacco Control, 10*, 181–183.

Marczinski, C. A. (2015). Can energy drinks increase desire for more alcohol? *Advances in Nutrition, 6*(1), 96–101. doi:10.3945/an.114.007393

Marczinski, C. A., & Fillmore, M. T. (2014). Energy drinks mixed with alcohol: What are the risks?. *Nutrition Reviews, 72*(1), 98–107. doi:10.1111/nure.12127

Marczinski, C. A., Fillmore, M. T., & Bardgett, M. E. (2011). Effects of energy drinks mixed with alcohol on behavioral control: Risks for college students consuming trendy cocktails. *Alcoholism: Clinical and Experimental Research, 35* (7), 1282–1292. doi:10.1111/j.1530-0277..?

Marczinski, C. A., Fillmore, M. T., & Henges, A. L. (2012). Effects of energy drinks mixed with alcohol on information processing, motor coordination and subjective reports of intoxication. *Experimental and Clinical Psychopharmacology, 20*(2), 129–138. doi:10.1037/a0026136..?

Maritz, G. S. (2008). Nicotine and lung development. *Birth Defects Research Part C: Embryo Today: Reviews, 84*(1), 45–53. doi:10.1002/bdrc.20116

Maritz, G. S., & Harding, R. (2011). Life-long programming implications of exposure to tobacco smoking and nicotine before and soon after birth: Evidence for altered lung development. *International Journal of Environmental Research and Public Health, 8*(3), 875–898. doi:10.3390/ijerph8030875

Marmorstein, N. R. (2016). Energy drink and coffee consumption and psychopathology symptoms among early adolescents: Cross-sectional and logitudinal associations. *Journal of Caffeine Research, 6*(2), 1–10. doi:10.1089/jcr.2015.0018

Martinez-Ortega, J. M., Franco, S., & Rodriguez-Fernandez, J. M. (2017, April). Temporal sequencing of nicotine dependence and major depressive disorder: A U.S. national study. *Psychiatry Research, 250*, 264–269. doi:10.1016/j.psychres.2017.01.087

Martinez-Ortega, J. M., Goldstein, B. I., & Gutierrez-Rojas, L. (2013). Temporal sequencing of nicotine dependence and bipolar disorder in the National Epidemiologic Survey on Alcohol and Related Conditions (NESARC). *Journal of Psychiatric Research, 47*(7), 858–864. doi:10.1016/j.jpsychires.2013.03.012

Martyn, D., Lau, A., & Richardson, P. (2018, January). Temporal patterns of caffeine intake in the United States. *Food and Chemical Toxicology, 111*, 71–83. doi:10.1016/j.fct.2017.10.059

Martz, M. E., Patrick, M. E., & Schulenberg, J. E. (2015, May). Alcohol mixed with energy drink use among U.S. 12th-grade students: Prevalence, correlates, and associations with unsafe driving. *The Journal of Adolescent Health, 56*(5), 557–563. doi:10.1016/j.jadohealth.2015.01.019

Masadeh, M. M., Hussein, E. I., & Alzoubi, K. H. (2015). Identification, characterization and antibiotic resistance of bacterial isolates obtained from waterpipe device hoses. *International Journal of Environmental Research and Health, 12*(5), 5108–5115. doi:10.3390/ijerph120505108

Mathew, A. R., Wahlquist, A. E., & Garrett-Mayer, E. (2014, October). Affective motives for smoking among early-stage smokers. *Nicotine & Tobacco Research, 16*(10), 1387–1393. doi:10.1093/ntr/ntu093

Mathews, T. J. (2016, June 10). QuickStats: Smoking cessation during pregnancy—46 States and the District of Columbia. *MMWR, Morbidity and Mortality Weekly Report, 65*(22), 588. doi:10.15585/mmwr.mm6522a6

Mattson, M. E. (2013, January 10). *Update on Emergency Department Visits Involving Energy Drinks: A Continuing Public Health Concern.* Retrieved October 6, 2016, from www.ncbi.nlm.gov/pubmed/27606410

Maughan, R. J., & Griffin, J. (2003, December). Caffeine ingestion and fluid balance: A review. *Journal of Human Nutrition and Dietetics, 16*(6), 411–420.

Mayer, B. (2014). How much nicotine kills a human? Tracing back the generally accepted lethal dose to dubious self-experiments in the nineteenth century. *Archives of Toxicology, 88*(1), 5–7. doi:10.1007/s00204-013-1127-0

Maynard, C. (2015, April 3).Energy drinks the cause of many sudden cardiac deaths in young people, researchers find. *Consumer Affairs, 1*(278), 1–2

Mazure, C. M., Toll, B., & McKee, S. A. (2011, March). Menstrual cycle phase at quit date and smoking abstinence at 6 weeks in an open label trial of bupropion. *Drug and Alcohol Dependence, 114*, 68–72. doi: 10.1016/j.drugalcdep.2010.07.024

McConnell, R., Barrington-Trimis, J. L., & Wang, K. (2017, April 15). Electronic cigarette use and respiratory symptoms in adolescents. *American Journal of Respiratory and Critical Care Medicine, 195*(8), 1043–1049. doi:10.1164/rccm.2021604-087040C

McGinnis, J. (2018, May 28). Why are more teens, children drinking coffee?. *The Intelligencer*, 1–4.

McKetin, R., Coen, A., & Kaye, S. (2015, June 1). A comprehensive review of the effects of mixing caffeinated energy drinks with alcohol. *Drug and Alcohol Dependence, 151*, 15–30. doi:10.1016/j.drugalcdep.2015.01.047

McLaughlin, I., Dani, J. A., & De Biasi, M. (2015). Nicotine withdrawal. *Current Topics in Behavioral Neurosciences, 24*, 99–123. doi:10.1007/978-3-319-13482-6_4

McLellan, T. M., Caldwell, J. A., & Lieberman, H. R. (2016). A review of caffeine's effects on cognitive, physical and occupational performance. *Neuroscience and Biobehavioral Reviews, 71*, 294–312.

Mennella, J. A., & Beauchamp, G. K. (1998, November 19). Smoking and the flavor of breast milk. *The New England Journal of Medicine, 339*, 1559–1560. doi:10.1056/NEJM199811193392119

Mennella, J. A., Yourshaw, L. M., & Morgan, L. K. (2007, September). Breastfeeding and smoking: Short-term effects on infant feeding and sleep. *Pediatrics, 120*(3), 497–502.

Meredith, S. E., Juliano, J. L., & Hughes, J. R. (2013). Caffeine use disorder: A comprehensive review and research agenda. *Journal of Caffeine Research, 3*(3), 114–130. doi:10.1089/jcr.20123.0016

Merianos, A. L., Jandarov, R. A., & Mahabee-Gittens, M. (2018, September). Adolescent tobacco smoke exposure, respiratory symptoms, and emergeny department use. *Pediatrics, 142*(3), 1-11. doi: 10.1542/peds.2018-02666

Miech, R., Johnston, L., & O'Malley, P. M. (2018, December 17). Adolescent vaping and nicotine use in 2017–2018 — U.S. national estimates. *The New England Journal of Medicine*, 1–2. doi:10.1056/NEJMc1814130

Mikami, I., Akechi, T., & Kugaya, A. (1999). Screening for nicotine dependence among smoking-related cancer patients. *Japanese Journal of Cancer Research, 90*(10), 1071–1075.

Mineur, Y. S., & Picciotto, M. R. (2010). Nicotine receptors and depression: Revisiting and revising the cholinergic hypothesis. *Trends in Pharmacological Sciences, 31*(12), 580–586. doi:10.1016/j.tips.2010.09.004

Mishra, A., Chaturvedi, P., & Datta, S. (2015). Harmful effects of nicotine. *Indian Journal of Medical Paediatric Oncology, 36*(1, January-March), 24–31. doi:10.4103/0971-5851.151771.

Mitchell, D. C., Knight, C. A., & Hockenberry, J. (2014). Beverage caffeine intakes in the U. S. *Food and Clinical Toxicology, 63*, 136–142.

Mitchell, J. T., McIntyre, E. M., & McClernon, F. J. (2013). Smoking motivation in adults with attention-deficit/hyperactivity disorder using the Wisconsin Inventory of smoking dependence motives. *Nicotine & Tobacco Research*, 120–125. doi:10.1093/ntr/ntt144

Modesto-Lowe, V., Danforth, J. S., & Neering, C. (2010). Can we prevent smoking in children with ADHD: A review of the literature. *Connecticut Medicine, 74*(4), 229–236.

Moolchan, E. T., Radzius, A., & Epstein, D. H. (2002). The Fagerstrom test for nicotine dependence and the diagnostic interview schedule: Do they diagnose the same smokers? *Addictive Behaviors, 27*(1), 103–113.

Moon, K., Rule, A. M., & Magid, H. S. (2018, March). Biomarkers of secondhand smoke exposure in waterpipe tobacco venue employees in Istanbul, Moscow, and Cairo. *Nicotine & Tobacco Research, 20*(4), 482–491. doi:10.1093/ntr/ntx125

Moon, R. Y., Darnall, R. A., & Goodstein, M. H. (2011). SIDS and other sleep-related infant deaths: Expansion of recommendations for a safe infant sleeping environment. *Pediatrics, 128*(5), 1030–1039. doi:10.1542/peds.2011-2284

Moran-Santa Maria, M. M., Flanagan, J., & Brady, K. (2014). Ovarian hormones and drug abuse. *Current Psychiatry Reports, 16*(11), 511–522. doi:10.1007/s11920-014-0511-7

Mora-Rodriguez, R., & Pallares, J. G. (2014). Performance outcomes and unwanted side effects associated with energy drinks. *Nutrition Reviews, 72*(Supplement 1), 108–120. doi:10.1111/nure.12132

Moreno-Coutino, A., & Villalbos-Gallegos, L. (2017, January/March). Psychometric properties of the Fagerstrom Test for Nicotine Dependence in a sample of Mexican smokers. *Journal of Addictions Nursing, 28*(1), 27–33. doi:10.1097/JAN.0000000000000156

Morris, D. S., Fiala, S. C., & Pawlak, R. (2012). Opportunities for policy interventions to reduce youth hookah smoking in the United States. *Preventing Chronic Disease, 9*, E165. doi:10.5888/pcd9.120082

Mostofsky, E., Schlaug, G., & Mukamal, K. J. (2010). Coffee and acute ischemic stroke onset: The Stroke Onset Study. *Neurology, 75*(18), 1583–1588. doi:10.1212/WNL.0b013e3181fb443d

Muramoto, M. L., Leischow, S. J., & Sherrill, D. (2007). Randomized, double-blind, placebo-controlled trial of 2 dosages of sustained-release bupropion for adolescent smoking cessation. *Archives of Pediatric and Adolescent Medicine, 161*(11), 1068–1074.

Mwenifumbo, J. C., & Tyndale, R. F. (2007). Genetic variability in CYP2A6 and the pharmacokinetics of nicotine. *Pharmacogenomics, 8*(10), 1385–1402.

Nabi-Burza, E., Regan, S., & Drehmer, J. (2012). Parents smoking in their cars with children present. *Pediatrics, 130*, e1471–e1477. doi:10.1542/peds.2012-0334

Nakajima, M., al'Absi, M., & Dokam, A. (2012, November-December). An examinaion of the Fagerstrom test for nicotine dependence among concurrent tobacco and khat users. *J Psychoactive Drugs, 44*(5), 437–441. doi:10.1080/02791072.2012.737224

Nakajima, M., Kuroiwa, Y., & Yokoi, T. (2002, November). Interindividual differences in nicotine metabolism and genetic polymorphisms of human CYP2A6. *Drug Metabolism Reviews, 34*(4), 865–877. doi:10.1081/DMR-120015696

Nakajima, M., & Yokoi, T. (2005, August). Interindividual variability in nicotine metabolism: C-oxidation and glucuronidation. *Drug Metabolism and Pharmacokinetics, 20*(4), 227–235.

Nakazawa, A., Shigeta, M., & Ozasa, K. (2004). Smoking cigarettes of low nicotine yield does not reduce nicotine intake as expected: A study of nicotine dependency in Japanese males. *BMC Public Health, 4*, 28–36. doi:10.1186/1471-2458-4-28

National Academies of Sciences, Engineering, and Medicine. (2018). *Public Health Consequences of E-Cigarettes*. National Academies of Sciences, Engineering, and Medicine. Washington, DC: The National Academies Press. Retrieved from https://doi.org/10.17226/24952

Nawrot, P., Jordan, S., & Eastwood, J. (2003). Effects of caffeine on human health. *Food Additives and Contaminants, 20* (1), 1–30. doi:10.1080/0265203021000007840

Nehlig, A. (2010). Is caffeine a cognitive enhancer?. *Journal of Alzheimer's Disease, 20*, S85–S94. doi:10.3233/JAD-2010-091315

Nehlig, A. (1992). Caffeine and the central nervous system: Mechanisms of action, biochemical, metabolic and psychostimulant effects. *Brain Research Brain Research Review, 17*(2), 139–170.

Nehlig, A., & Debry, G. (1994, November-December). Potential teratogenic and neurodevelopmental consequences of coffee and caffeine exposure: A review on human and animal data. *Neurotoxicology and Teratology, 16*(6), 531–543.

NIDA, National Institute on Drug Abuse. (2016, May). *Drug Facts: Cigarettes and Other Tobacco Products*. Rockville, Maryland: U.S. Department of Health and Human Services. Retrieved September 8, 2016, from www.drugabuse.gov/publications/drugfacts/cigarettes-other-tobacco-products

Nides, M., Oncken, C., & Gonzales, D. (2006). Smoking cessation with varenicline, a selective alpha-4 beta-2 nicotinic receptor partial agonist: Results from a 7-week, randomized, placebo- and bupropion-controlled trial with 1-year follow-up. *Archives of Internal Medicine, 166*, 1561–1568.

Novotny, T. E., Hardin, S. N., & Hovda, L. R. (2011). Tobacco and cigarette butt consumption in humans and animals. *Tobacco Control, 20*(Supplement 1), i17–i20. doi:10.1136/tc.2011.043489

O'Brien, M. C., McCoy, T. P., & Rhodes, S. D. (2008). Caffeinated cocktails: Energy drink consumption, high-risk drinking, and alcohol-related consequences among college students. *Academic Emergency Medicine, 15*(5), 453–460. doi:10.1111/j.1553-2712.2008.00085.x

O'Cleirigh, C., Valentine, S. E., & Pinkston, M. (2015). The unique challenges facing HIV-positive patients who smoke cigarettes: HIV viremia, ART adherence, engagement in HIV care, and concurrent substance use. *AIDS and Behavior, 19*(1), 178–185. doi:10.1007/s10461-014-0762-7

Odani, S., Agaku, I. T., & Graffunder, C. M. (2018). Tobacco product use among military veterans—United States, 2010–2015. *MMWR, Morbidity and Mortality Weekly Report, 67*, 7–12. Retrieved from http://dx.doi.org/10.15585/mmwr.mm6701a2

Odani, S., Armour, B. S., & Agaku, I. T. (2018, August 31). Racial/ethnic disparities in tobacco product use among middle and high school students—United States, 2014–2017. *MMWR, Morbidity and Mortality Weekly Report, 67* (34), 952–957.

Oddy, W. H., & O'Sullivan, T. A. (2009, December 10). Energy drinks for children and adolescents. *BMJ, 339*, b5268.

Oh, A. Y., & Kacker, A. (2014). Do electronic cigarettes impart a lower potential disease burden than conventional tobacco cigarettes? Review on E-cigarette vapor versus tobacco smoke. *Laryngoscope, 124*(12), 2702–2706. doi:10.1002/lary.24750

Oh, J. K., Sandin, S., & Strom, P. (2015). Prospective study of breast cancer in relation to coffee, tea, and caffeine in Sweden. *International Journal of Cancer, 137*(8), 1979–1989. doi:10.1002/ijc.29569

Okuyemi, K. S., Pulvers, K. M., & Cox, L. S. (2007). Nicotine dependence among African American light smokers: A comparison of three scales. *Addictive Behaviors, 32*(10), 1989–2002.

Oo, C. Y., Burgio, D. E., & Kuhn, R. C. (1995). Pharmacokinetics of caffeine and its demethylated metabolites in lactation: Predictions of milk to serum concentration ratios. *Pharmaceutical Research, 12*, 313–316.

Ostroumov, A., Thomas, A. M., & Dani, J. A. (2015, October). Cigarettes and alcohol: The influence of nicotine on operant alcohol self-administration and the mesolimbic dopamine system. *Biochemical Pharmacology, 97*(4), 550–557. doi:10.1016/j.bcp.2015.07.038

Owens, J. A., Mindell, J., & Baylor, A. (2014). Effect of energy drink and caffeinated beverage consumption on sleep, mood, and performance in children and adolescents. *Nutrition Reviews, 72*(S1), 65–71. doi:10.1111/nure.12150

Pacifici, R., Pichini, S., & Graziano, S. (2015). Successful nicotine intake in medical assisted use of e-cigarettes: A pilot study. *International Journal of Environmental Research and Public Health, 12*(7), 7638–7646. doi:10.3390/ijerph120707638

Pagliaro, A. M., & Pagliaro, L. A. (Eds.). (1986). *Pharmacologic Aspects of Nursing*. St. Louis, Missouri: C.V. Mosby.

Pagliaro, A. M., & Pagliaro, L. A. (2018). *Women's Drug and Substance Abuse: A Comprehensive Analysis and Reflective Synthesis*. New York, New York: Routledge.

Pagliaro, L. A., & Pagliaro, A. M. (1999). *PNDR: Psychologists' Neuropsychotrophic Drug Reference*. Philadelphia, Pennsylvania: Brunner/Mazel.

Pagliaro, L. A., & Pagliaro, A. M. (Eds.). (2002). *Problems in Pediatric Drug Therapy* (4th ed. ed.). Washington, DC: American Pharmaceutical Association.

Pagliaro, L. A., & Pagliaro, A. M. (2004). *Pagliaros' Comprehensive Guide to Drugs and Substances of Abuse*. Washington, DC: American Pharmacists Association.

Pagliaro, L. A., & Pagliaro, A. M. (2009). *Pagliaros' Comprehensive Guide to Drugs and Substances of Abuse* (2nd ed.). Washington, DC: American Pharmacists Association.

Pagliaro, L. A., & Pagliaro, A. M. (2012). *Handbook of Child and Adolescent Drug and Substance Abuse: Pharmacological, Developmental, and Clinical Considerations*. Hoboken, New Jersey: John Wiley & Sons.

Palamar, J. J., Zhou, S., & Sherman, S. (2014, August). Hookah use among US high school seniors. *Pediatrics, 134*(2), 1–8. doi:10.101542/peds.2014-0538

Pancani, L., D'Addario, M., & Cappelletti, E. (2015). Smoking behavior: A cross-sectional study to assess the dimensionality of the Brief Wisconsin Inventory of Smoking Dependence Motives and identify different typologies among young daily smokers. *Nicotine & Tobacco Research*, 98–105. doi:10.1093/ntr/ntu143

Pang, R. D., Bello, M. S., & Stone, M. D. (2016). Premenstrual symptoms and smoking-related expectancies. *Addictive Behaviors, 57*, 38–41. doi:10.1016/j.addbeh.2016.01.015

Paolini, M., & De Biasi, M. (2011, October 15). Mechanistic insights into nicotine withdrawal. *Biochemical Pharmacology, 82*(8), 996–1007. doi:10.1016/j.bcp.2011.07.075

Parrott, C. E., Rathnataka, N., & Blalock, J. A. (2014). Examination of the Wisconsin Inventory of Smoking Dependence Motives (WISDM-68) factor structure in a sample of pregnant smokers. *Nicotine & Tobacco Research, 6*, 653–660. doi:10.1093/ntr/ntu238

Patnode, C. D., Henderson, J. T., & Thompson, J. H. (2015a). *Behavioral Counseling and Pharmacotherapy Interventions for Tobacco Cessation in Adults, Including Pregnant Women*. Rockville, MD: Agency for Healthcare Research and Quality.

Patnode, C. D., Henderson, J. T., & Thompson, J. H. (2015b, October 20). Behavioral counseling and pharmacotherapy interventions for tobacco cessation in adults, including pregnant women: A review of reviews for the U.S. Preventive Services Task Force. *Annals of Internal Medicine, 163*(8), 608–621. doi:10.7326/M15-0171

Patrick, M. E., Macuada, C., & Maggs, J. L. (2015). Who uses alcohol mixed with energy drinks? Characteristics of college student users. *Journal of American College Health, 64*(1), 74–79. doi:10.1080/07448481.2015.1042877

Paul, O. (1989, July). Background of the prevention of cardiovascular disease. II. Arteriosclerosis, hypertension, and selected risk factors. *Circulation, 80*(1), 206–214.

Peacock, A., Pennay, A., & Droste, N. (2014). "High" risk? A systematic review of the acute outcomes of mixing alcohol with energy drinks. *Addiction, 109*(10), 1612–1633. doi:10.1111/add.12622

Pelchovitz, D. J., & Goldberger, J. J. (2011). Caffeine and cardiac arrhythmias: A review of the evidence. *The American Journal of Medicine, 124*(4), 284–289. doi:10.1016/j.amjmed.2010.10.017

Perez-Rios, M., Santiago-Perez, M. I., & Alonso, B. (2009). Fagerstrom test for nicotine dependence vs heavy smoking index in a general population survey. *BMC Public Health, 9*, 493.

Perez-Stable, E. J., Herrera, B., & Jacob, P. (1998). Nicotine metabolism and intake in black and white smokers. *JAMA, Journal of the American Medical Association, 280*(2), 152.

Perkins, K. A., Karelitz, J. L., & Michael, V. C. (2017, August). Effects of nicotine versus placebo e-cigarette use on symptom relief during intitial tobacco abstinence. *Experimental and Clinical Pharmacology, 25*(4), 249–254. doi:10.1037/pha0000134

Pfeifer, G. P., Denissenko, M. F., & Olivier, M. (2002). Tobacco smoke carcinogens, DNA damage and p53 mutations in smoking-associated cancers. *Oncogene, 21*(48), 7435–7451.

Phelan, S. (2014). Smoking cessation in pregnancy. *Obstetrics and Gynecology Clinics of North America, 41*(2), 255–266. doi:10.1016/j.ogc.2014.02.007

Pinkerton, J. V., Guico-Pabia, C. J., & Taylor, H. S. (2010). Menstrual cycle-related exacerbation of disease. *American Journal of Obstetrics & Gynecology, 202*(3), 221–231. doi:10.1016/j.ajog.2009.07.061

Piper, M. E., Cook, J. W., & Schlam, T. R. (2010). Gender, race, and education differences in abstinence rates among participants in two randomized smoking cessation trials. *Nicotine & Tobacco Research, 12*(6), 647–657.

Piper, M. E., McCarthy, D. E., & Baker, T. B. (2008). Assessing dimensions of nicotine dependence. *Nicotine & Tobacco Research, 10*(6), 1009–1020. doi:10.1080/146222008020897563

Piper, M. E., McCarthy, D. E., & Bolt, D. M. (2008, June). Assessing dimensions of nicotine dependence: An evaluation of the Nicotine Dependence Scale (NDSS) and the Wisconsin Inventory of Smoking Dependence Motives (WISDM). *Nicotine & Tobacco Research, 10*(6), 1009–1020. doi:10.1080/14622200802097563

Piper, M. E., Piasecki, T. M., & Federman, E. B. (2004). A multiple motives approach to tobacco dependence: The Wisconsin Inventory of Smoking Dependence Motives (WISDM-68). *Journal of Consulting and Clinical Psychology, 72*(2), 139–154. doi:10.1037/0022-006X.72.2.139

Polak, K., Dillon, P., & Koch, J. R. (2016, June 29). Energy drink use is associated with alcohol and substance use in eighth, tenth, and twelfth graders. *Preventive Medicine Reports, 4*, 381–384. doi:10.1016/j.pmedr.2016.06.019

Pomerleau, C. S., Carton, S. M., & Lutzke, M. L. (1994). Reliability of the Fagerstrom Tolerance Questionnaire and the Fagerstrom Test for Nicotine Dependence. *Addictive Behaviors, 19*(1), 33–39.

Poulos, N. S., & Pasch, K. E. (2015, November). Energy drink consumption is associated with unhealthy dietary behaviours among college youth. *Perspectives in Public Health, 135*(6), 316–321. doi:10.1177/1757913914565388

Prochaska, J. J., & Hilton, J. F. (2012). Risk of cardiovascular serious adverse events associated with varenicline use for tobacco cessation: Systematic review and meta-analysis. *BMJ, 344*, e2856. doi:10.1136/bmj.e2856

Prokhorov, A. V., Koehly, L. M., & Pallonen, U. E. (1998). Adolescent nicotine dependence measured by the Modified Fagerstrom Tolerance Questionnaire at two time points. *Journal of Child & Adolescent Substance Abuse*, 7(4), 35–47.

Red Bull. (2018, October 8). RedBull.com website.

Reid, K. M., Forrest, J. R., & Porter, L. (2018, June 1). Tobacco product use among youths with and without lifetime asthma—Florida, 2016. *MMWR Morbidity and Mortality Weekly Reports, 67*(21), 599–601.

Reissig, C. J., Strain, E. C., & Griffiths, R. R. (2009). Caffeinated energy drinks—A growing problem. *Drug and Alcohol Dependence, 99*(1–3), 1–10. doi:10.1016/j.drugalcdep.2008.08.001

Reuters. (2015, February 25). Tobacco companies to settle smoking lawsuits for $100 million. *CNBC News*.

Rhee, J., Kim, R., & Kim, Y. (2015). Maternal caffeine consumption during pregnancy and risk of low birth weight: A dose-response meta-analysis of observational studies. *PLOS One, 10*(7), 1–2. doi:10.1371/journal.pone.0132334

Rhodes, J. D., Pelham, W. E., & Gnagy, E. M. (2016, August). Cigarette smoking and ADHD: An examination of prognostically-relevant smoking behaviors among adolescents and young adults. *Psychology of Addictive Behaviors, 30*(5), 588–600. doi:10.1037/adb0000188

Ribeiro, J. A., & Sebastiao, A. M. (2010). Caffeine and adenosine. *Journal of Alzheimers Disease*, 20(Suppl 1), S3–S15. doi: 10.3233/JAD-2010-1379

Richardson, C. C., & Ratner, P. A. (2005). A confirmatory factor analysis of the Fagerstrom Test for Nicotine Dependence. *Addictive Behaviors, 99*(1–3), 697–709.

Riggs, P. D. (2003). Treating adolescents for substance abuse and comorbid psychiatric diagnoses. *Science & Practice Perspectives, 2*(1), 18–29.

Robles, G. I., Singh-Franco, D., & Ghin, H. L. (2008). A review of the efficacy of smoking-cessation pharmacotherapies in nonwhite populations. *Clinical Therapeutics, 30*(5), 800–812. doi:10.1016/j.clinthera.2008.05.010

Roemer, A., & Stockwell, T. (2017, March). Alcohol mixed with energy drinks and risk of injury: A systematic review. *Journal of Studies on Alcohol and Drugs, 78*(2), 175–183.

Roger, J. M., Abayon, M., & Elad, S. (2016January 7). Oral tooth trauma and tooth avulsion following explosion of e-cigarette. *Journal of Oral and Maxillofacial Surgery*, 1–2. doi:10.1016/j.joms.2015.12.017

Rogers, A. J., Denk, L. D., & Wax, P. M. (2004). Catastrophic brain injury after nicotine insecticide ingestion. *Journal of Emergency Medicine, 26*(2), 169–172.

Rom, O., Pecorelli, A., & Valacchi, G. (2015, March). Are e-cigarettes a safe and good alternative to cigarette smoking?. *Annals of the New York Academy of Sciences, 1340*, 65–74. doi:10.1111/nyas.12609

Roosevelt, M. W. (2012, March 5). *Breathable Foods, Inc.—Warning Letter. Inspections, Compliance, Enforcement, and Criminal Investigations*. College Park, Maryland: U.S. Food and Drug Administration. Retrieved October 6, 2016, from. : . www.fda.gov/ICECI/EnforcementActions/WarningLetters/2012/ucm294774.htm

Rubin, R. (2008, January 20). New studies, different outcomes on caffeine, pregnancy. *News: Behavior & Health*. USA Today. Retrieved October 6, 2016, from http://usatoday30.usatoday.com/news/health/2008-01-20-caffeine_N.htm

Rubinstein, M. L., Shiffman, S., & Moscicki, A.-B. (2013, February). Nicotine metabolism and addiction among adolescent smokers. *Addiction, 108*(2), 406–412. doi:10.1111/j.1360-443.2012.4026.x

Ryu, J. E. (1985). Caffeine in human milk and in serum of breast-fed infants. *Developmental Pharmacology and Therapeutics, 8*, 329–337.

Saladin, M. E., McClure, E. A., & Baker, N. L. (2015). Increasing progesterone levels are associated with smoking abstinence among free-cycling women smokers who receive brief pharmacotherapy. *Nicotine & Tobacco Reasearch, 17*(4), 398–406. doi:10.1093/ntr/ntu262

Saladin, M. E., Wray, J. M., & Carpenter, M. J. (2015). Menstrual cycle phase effects in the gender dimorphic stress cue reactivity of smokers. *Nicotine & Tobacco Research, 17*, 607–611. doi: 10.1093/ntr/ntu203

SAMHSA, Substance Abuse and Mental Health Services Administration. (2011, November 22). *Emergency Department Visits Involving Energy Drinks. The DAWN Report*. Rockville, Maryland: Center for Behavioral Health Statistics and Quality.

SAMHSA, Substance Abuse and Mental Health Services Administration. (2014, March 13). 1 in 10 Energy Drink-related Emergency Department Visits Results in Hospitalization. *The DAWN Report*. Rockville, Maryland.

Sanchis-Gomar, F., Pareja-Galeano, H., & Cervellin, G. (2015, May). Energy drink overconsumption in adolescents: Implications for arrhythmias and other cardiovascular events. *Canadian Journal of Cardiology*, 31(5), 572–575. doi: 10.1016/j.cjca.2014.12.019

Sathya, C. (2014, July 7). *Hookah gains popularity: Nearly 1 in 5 teens have tried*. Retrieved April 13, 2016, from CNN. com: www.cnn.com/2014/07/07/health/hookah-teen-popularity/index.html

Sato, N., Sato, T., & Nozawa, A. (2012). Assessment scales for nicotine dependence. *Journal of Addiction Research & Therapy, S1*(008), 1–5. doi:10.4172/2155-6105.S1-008

Schaffer, S. D., Yoon, S., & Zadezensky, I. (2009, June). A review of smoking cessation: Potentially risky effects on prescribed medications. *Journal of Clinical Nursing, 18*(11), 1533–1540. doi:10.1111/j.1365-2702.20078.02724.x

Schoedel, K. A., Hoffmann, E. B., & Rao, Y. (2004). Ethnic variation in CYP2A6 and association of genetically slow nicotine metabolism and smoking in adult Caucasians. *Pharmacogenetics, 14*(9), 615–626.

Schroeder, M. J., & Hoffman, A. C. (2014, May 23). Electronic cigarettes and nicotine clinical pharmacology. *Tobacco Control*, Supplement 2 30–35. doi:10.1136/tobaccocontrol-2013-051469

Schwartz, L., Guais, A., & Chaumet-Riffaud, P. (2010). Carbon dioxide is largely responsible for the acute inflammatory effects of tobacco smoke. *Inhalation Toxicology, 22*(7), 543–551. doi:10.3109/08958370903555909

Seifert, S. M., Schaechter, J. L., & Hershorin, E. R. (2011, March). Health effects of energy drinks on children, adolescents, and young adults. *Pediatrics, 127*(3), 511–528. doi:10.1542/peds.2009-3592

Seifert, S. M., Seifert, S. A., & Schaechter, J. L. (2013). An analysis of energy-drink toxicity in the National Poison Data System. *Clinical Toxicology, 51*(7), 566–574. doi:10.3109/15563650.2012.820310

Seo, A. D., Kim, D. C., & Yu, H. J. (2016, December). Accidental ingestion of E-cigarette liquid nicotine in a 15-month-old child: An infant mortality case of nicotine intoxication. *Korean Journal of Pediatrics, 59*(12), 490–493. doi:10.3345/kjp.2016.59.12.490

Sharwood, L. N., Elkington, J., & Meuleners, L. (2013). Use of caffeinated substances and risk of crashes in long distance drivers of commercial vehicles: Case-control study. *BMJ, 346*. doi:10.1136/bmj.f1140

Shea, A. K., & Steiner, M. (2008). Cigarette smoking during pregnancy. *Nicotine & Tobacco Research, 10*(2), 267–278. doi:10.1080/14622200701825908

Sheen, S. J. (1988). Detection of nicotine in foods and plant materials. *Journal of Food Science, 53*(5), 1572–1573. doi:10.1111/j.1365-2621.1988.tb09328.x

Sherburne Hawkins, S., Bach, N., & Baum, C. F. (2018, February 15). Impact of tobacco control policies on adolescent smokeless tobacco and cigar use: A difference-in-defferences approach. *BMC Public Health*. https://doi.org/10.1186/s12889-018-5063-z

Shields, P. G., Berman, M., & Brasky, T. M. (2017, August). A review of pulmonary toxicity of electronic cigarettes in the context of smoking: A focus on inflammation. *Cancer Epidemiology, Biomarkers & Prevention, 26*(8), 1175–1191. doi:10.1158/1055-9965.EPI-17-0358

Shihadeh, A. (2003, January). Investigation of mainstream smoke aerosol of the argileh water pipe. *Food and Chemical Toxicology, 41*(1), 143–152.

Singh, S., Loke, Y. K., & Spangler, J. G. (2011). Risk of serious adverse cardiovascular events associated with varenicline: A systematic review and meta-analysis. *CMAJ, Canadian Medical Association Journal, 183*(12), 1359–1366. doi:10.1503/cmaj.110218

Siqueira, L. M. (2017, December 20). Nicotine and tobacco as substances of abuse in children and adolescents. *Pediatrics, 139*(1), e1–e13. doi:10.1542/peds.2016-3436

Smith, A. (2002). Effects of caffeine on human behavior. *Food and Chemical Toxicology, 40*(9), 1243–1255.

Smith, P. H., Kasza, K. A., & Hyland, A. (2015). Gender differences in medication use and cigarette smoking cessation: Results from the International Tobacco Control Four Country Survey. *Nicotine & Tobacco Research, 17*(4), 463–472. doi:10.1093/ntr/ntu212

Smith, S. S., Piper, M. E., & Bolt, D. M. (2010). Development of the Brief Wisconsin Inventory for Smoking Dependence Motives. *Nicotine & Tobacco Research, 12*(5), 489–499. doi:10.1093/ntr/ntq032

Sobkowiak, R., & Lesicki, A. (2013). Absorption, metabolism and excretion of nicotine in humans. *Postepy Biochemii, 59* (1), 33–44.

Solinas, M., Ferre, S., & You, Z.-B. (2002, August 1). Caffeine induces dopamine and glutamate release in the shell of the nucleus accumbens. *The Journal of Neuroscience, 22*(15), 6321–6324.

Somogyi, L. P. (2010). *Caffeine Intake by the U. S. Population (subcontract Number: 70000073494)*, pp. *1–85*. Oakridge National Laboratory. Kensington, California: The Food and Drug Administration.

Soneji, S., Barrington-Trimis, J. L., & Wills, T. A. (2017). Association between initial use of e-cigarettes and subsequent cigarette smoking among adolescents and young adults: A systematic review and meta-analysis. *JAMA Pediatrics, 171*(8), 788–797. doi:10.1001/jamapediatrics.2017.1488

St Helen, G., Dempsey, D., & Wilson, M. (2013, March). Racial differences in the relationship between tobacco dependence and nicotine and carcinogen exposure. *Addiction, 108*(3), 607–617. doi:10.1111/j.1360-0443.2012.04077.x

Stead, L. F., Koilpillai, P., & Fanshawe, T. R. (2016, March 24). Combined pharmacotherapy and behavioural interventions for smoking. *The Cochrane Database of Systematic Reviews, 24*(CD008286). doi:10.1002/14651858. CD008286.pub3

Steiner, M. (2000). Premenstrual syndrome and premenstrual dysphoric disorder: Guidleines for management. *Journal of Psychiatry and Neuroscience, 25*(5), 459–468.

Stokes, T., Fox, M., & Carroll, L. (2012, October 23). When caffeine kills: Energy drinks under the spotlight. *NBC News*, 1–2.

Streller, S., & Roth, K. (2014, November 4). The chemistry of tobacco—Part 2. *Chemistry Views Magazine*. Chemis in unserer, *47*, 248–268.

SurgeStix—Inhalable Caffeine Stix. (2012, March). Retrieved December 27, 2016, from ThinkGeek, pp. 1–2: www.thinkgreek.com/stuff/41/surgestix.shtml

Sutfin, E. L., McCoy, T. P., & Morrell, H. E. (2013). Electronic cigarette use by college students. *Drug and Alcohol Dependence, 131*(3), 214–221. doi:10.1016/j.drugalcdep.2013.05.001

Sutfin, E. L., McCoy, T. P., & Reboussin, B. A. (2011, May 1). Prevalence and correlates of waterpipe tobacco smoking by college students in North Carolina. *Drug and Alcohol Dependence, 115*(1–2), 131–136. doi:10.1016/j.drugalcdep.2011.01.018

Sutherland, M. T., Carroll, A. J., & Salmeron, B. J. (2013, October 1). Down-regulation of amygdala and insula functional circuits by varenicline and nicotine in abstinent cigarette smokers. *Biological Psychiatry, 74*(7), 538–546. doi:10.1016/j.biopsych.2013.01.035

Svikis, D. S., Berger, N., & Haug, N. A. (2005). Caffeine dependence in combination with a family history of alcoholism as a predictor of continued use of caffeine during pregnancy. *The American Journal of Psychiatry, 162* (12), 2344–2351.

Tanner, J. A., Chenoweth, M. J., & Tyndale, R. F. (2015). Pharmacogenetics of nicotine and associated smoking behaviors. *Current Topics in Behavioral Neurosciences, 23*, 37–86. doi:10.1007/978-3-319-13665-3_3

Tarnopolsky, M. A. (2008). Effect of caffeine on the neuromuscular system—Potential as an ergogenic aid. *Applied Physiology, Nutrition, and Metabolism, 33*(6), 1284–1289. doi:10.1139/H08-121

Tarnopolsky, M. A. (2010). Caffeine and creatine use in sport. *Annals of Nutrition & Metabolism, 57*(Supplement 2), 1–8. doi:10.1159/000322696

Temple, J. L. (2009). Caffeine use in children: What we know, what we have left to learn, and why we should worry. *Neurosciences and Biobehavioral Reviews, 33*, 793–806. doi:10.1016/j.neubiorev.2009.01.001

Temple, J. L., Bernard, C., & Lipshultz, S. E. (2017, May 26). The safety of ingested caffeine: A comprehensive review. *Frontiers in Psychiatry* . doi: 10.3389/fpsyt.2017.00080.

Temple, J. L., Dewey, A. M., & Briatico, L. N., (2010). Effects of acute caffeine administration on adolescents. *Experimental and Clinical Psychopharmacology, 18*(6), 510–520.doi: 10.1037/a002165.

Thorner-Bantug, E. W., Jaszyna-Gasior, M., & Schroeder, J. R. (2009). Weight gain, related concerns, and treatment outcomes among adolescent smokers enrolled in cessation treatment. *Journal of the National Medical Association, 101*(10), 1009–1014.

Thun, M. J., Henley, S. J., & Calle, E. E. (2002, October 21). Tobacco use and cancer: An epidemiologic perspective for geneticists. *Oncogene, 21*(48), 7307–7325. doi:10.1038/sj.onc.1205807

Tiesler, C. M., & Heinrich, J. (2014). Prenatal nicotine exposure and child behavioral problems. *European Child & Adolescent Psychiatry, 23*, 913–929. doi:10.1007/s00787-014-0615-y

TODAY. (2012, March 21). *Teen Girl Dies of "Caffeine Toxicity" after Downing 2 Energy Drinks*. Retrieved December 27, 2016, from Today.com, pp. 1–2: www.today.com/health/teen-girl-dies-caffeine-toxicity-after-downing-2-energy-drinks-506441

Tomizawa, M., & Casida, J. E. (2005). Neonicotinoid insecticide toxicology: Mechanisms of selective action. *Annual Review of Pharmacology and Toxicology, 45*, 247–268.

Tomizawa, M., & Casida, J. E. (2009). Molecular recognition of neonicotinoid insecticides: The determinants of life or death. *Accounts of Chemical Research, 42*(2), 260–269. doi:10.1021/ar800131p

Tonstad, S., Tonnesen, P., & Hajek, P. (2006). Effect of maintenance therapy with varenicline on smoking cessation: a randomized controlled trial. *JAMA, the Journal of the American Medical Association, 296*(1), 64–71.

Tran, N. L., Barraj, L. M., & Bi, X. (2016). Trends and patterns of caffeine consumption among US teenagers and young adults, NHANES 2003–2012. *Food and Chemical Toxicology, 94*, 227–242. doi:10.1016/j.fct.2016.06.007

Trehy, M. L., Ye, W., & Hadwiger, M. E. (2011). Analysis of electronic cigarette cartridges, refill solutions, and smoke for nicotine and nicotine related impurities. *Journal of Liquid Chromatography & Related Technologies, 34*(14), 1442–1458. doi:10.1080/10826076.2011.572213

Tsai, J., Walton, K., & Coleman, B. N. (2018, February 16). Reasons for electronic cigarette use among middle and high school students—National Youth Tobacco Survey, United States, 2016. *MMWR, Morbidity and Mortality Weekly Reports, 67*(6), 196–200.

Turnbull, D., Rodricks, J. V., & Mariano, G. F. (2017). Caffeine and cardiovascular health. *Regulatory Toxicology and Pharmacology, 89*, 165–185. doi:10.1016/j.yrtph.2017.07.025

Turner, C. (2018, May 2). What are NCAA athletes allowed to put in their bodies? *The Daily Universe*, 1–2. BYU School of Communications.

Upadhyaya, H. P., Brady, K. T., & Wang, W. (2004). Bupropion SR in adolescents with comorbid ADHD and nicotine dependence: A pilot study. *Journal of the American Academy of Child & Adolescent Psychiatry, 43*(2), 199–205. doi: https://doi.org/10.1097/00004583-200402000-00016

USDHHS, U. S. Department of Health and Human Services. (2010). *How Tobacco Smoke Causes Disease: The Biology and Behavioral Basis for Smoking-Attributable Disease.* Centers for Disease Control and Prevention, U. S. Department of Health and Human Services. Atlanta: Office on Smoking and Health, National Center for Chronic Disease Prevention and Health Promotion. Retrieved January 17, 2018, fromwww.cdc.gov/tobacco/data_statistics/sgr/2010/index.htm

USDHHS, U. S. Department of Health and Human Services. (2014). *The Health Consequences of Smoking—50 Years of Progess.* CDC, USDHHS. Atlanta, Georgia: Office on Smoking and Health, National Center for Chronic Disease Prevention and Health Promotion.

USDHHS, U.S. Department of Health and Human Services. (2016a). Deeming tobacco products to be subject to the Federal Food, Drug, and Cosmetic Act, as amended by the Family Smoking Prevention and Tobacco Control Act; Restrictions on the sale and distribution of tobacco products and required warning statements. *Federal Register, 81*(Fed. Reg. 28974).

USDHHS, U.S. Department of Health and Human Services. (2016b). *E-cigarette Use among Youth and Young Adults: A Report of the Surgeon General.* Public Health Service, Office of the Surgeon General. Rockville, Maryland: USDHHS.

Uysal, M. A., Kadakai, F., & Karsidag, C. (2004). Fagerstrom test for nicotine dependence: Reliability in a Turkish sample and factor analysis. *Tuberkuloz Ve Toraks, 52*(2), 115–121.

Uysal, M. A., Oztuna, D., & Bahadir, A. (2015). Psychometric properties of the Turkish version of the Fagerstrom test for nicotine dependence. *Tuberkuloz Ve Toraks, 63*(4), 250–256.

van Duinen, H., Lorist, M. M., & Zijdewind, I. (2005). The effect of caffeine on cognitive task performance and motor fatigue. *Psychopharmacology (Berlin), 180*(3), 539–547.

Varlet, V. (2016, December). Drug vaping: From the dangers of misuse to new therapeutic devices. *Toxics, 4*(4), 29–34. doi:10.3390/toxics4040029

Verplaetse, T. L., & McKee, S. A. (2017, March). An overview of alcohol and tobacco/nicotine interactons in the human laboratory. *The American Journal of Drug and Alcohol Abuse, 43*(2), 186–196. doi:10.1080/00952990.2016.1189927

Vetulani, J. (2001, May-June). Drug addiction: Part I. Psychoactive substances in the past and present. *Polish Journal of Pharmacology, 53*(3), 201–214.

Visram, S., Cheetham, M., & Riby, D. M. (2016). Consumption of energy drinks by children and young people: A rapid review examining evidence of physical effects and consumer attitudes. *BMJ Open, 6(e010380)*, 1–23. doi:10.1136/bmjopen-2015-010380

Vu, A. T., Taylor, K. M., & Holman, M. R. (2015). Polycyclic aromatic hydrocarbons in the mainstream smoke of popular U. S. cigarettes. *Chemical Research in Toxicology, 28*(8), 1616–1626. doi:10.1021/acs.chemrestox.5b00190

Wang, H., Li, X., & Guo, J. (2016, February 10). Distribution of toxic chemicals in particles of various sizes from mainstream cigarette smoke. *Inhalation Toxicology, 28*(2), 89–94.

Wang, T. S., Tynan, M. A., & Hallett, C. (2017, June 22). Smoke-free and tobacco-free policies in colleges and universities—United States and territories. *MMWR, Morbity and Mortality Weekly Report, 67*(24), 686–689.

Wang, T. W., Marynak, K. L., & Agaku, I. T. (2017, May). Secondhand exposure to electronic cigarette aerosol among US youths. *JAMA Pediatrics, 171*(5), 490–492.

Warner, K. E., & Pollack, H. A. (2014, November 13). The nicotine fix. *The Atlantic*, pp. 1–28. Retrieved October 8, 2016, from www.theatlantic.com/national/archive/2014/11/the-nicotine-fix/382666/

Watson, J., Deary, I., & Kerr, D. (2002). Central and peripheral effects of sustained caffeine use: Tolerance is incomplete. *British Journal of Clinical Pharmacology, 54*(4), 400–406.

Watson, T. D., Sweeney, J. F., & Louis, H. (2014). Neurocognitive, psychological and behavioral correlates of binge drinking and use of alcohol with caffeinated beverages in college-aged adults. *The American Journal of Alcohol Abuse, 40*(1), 58–66. doi:10.3109/009952990.2013.843005

Weinberger, A. H., Smith, P. H., & Allen, S. S. (2015). Systematic and meta-analytic review of research examining the impact of menstrual cycle phase and ovarian hormones on smoking and cessation. *Nicotine & Tobacco Research, 17* (4), 407–421. doi: 10.1093/ntr/ntu249

Weinberger, A. H., Reutenauer, E. L., & Allen, T. M. (2007). Reliability of the Fagerstrom Test for Nicotine Dependence, Minnesota Nicotine Withdrawal Scale, and Tiffany Questionnaire for Smoking Urges in smokers with and without schizophrenia. *Drug and Alcohol Dependence, 86*(2–3), 278–282.

Weiss, D., Tomasallo, C. D., & Meiman, J. G. (2016, December). Electronic cigarette exposure: Calls to Wisconsin poison control centers, 2010–2015. *Wisconsin Medical Journal, 115*(6), 306–310.

Wellman, R. J., DiFranza, J. R., & Morgenstern, M. (2012). Psychometric properties of the Autonomy Over Tobacco Scale in German. *European Addiction Research, 18*(2), 76–82. doi:10.1159/000334410

Wellman, R. J., DiFranza, J. R., & O'Loughlin, J. (2015, November). Confirmatory factor analysis of the Autonomy Over Tobacco Scale (AUTOS) in adults. *Addictive Behaviors, 50*, 217–221. doi:10.1016/j.addbeh.2015.06.033

Wellman, R. J., Edelen, M. O., & DiFranza, J. R. (2015, June). Item response theory analysis of the Autonomy Over Tobacco Scale (AUTOS). *Addictive Behaviors, 45*, 195–200. doi:10.1016/j.addbeh.2015.01.036

Westling, E., Rusby, J. C., & Crowley, R. (2017). Electronic cigarette use by youth: Prevalence, correlates, and use trajectories from middle to high school. *Journal of Adolescent Health, 60*(6), 660–666. doi:10.1016/j.jadohealth.2016.12.019

Wetherill, R. R., Franklin, T. R., & Allen, S. S. (2016, March 1). Ovarian hormones, menstrual cycle phase, and smoking: A review with recommendations for future studies. *Current Addiction Report, 3*(1), 1–8. doi:10.1007/s40429-016-0093-z

White, J. R., Padowski, J. M., & Zhong, Y. (2016). Pharmacokinetic analysis and comparison of caffeine administered rapidly or slowly in coffee chilled or hot versus energy drink in healthy young adults. *Clinical Toxicology, 54*(4), 308–312.

Whitten, L. (2009, November). Studies link family of genes to nicotine addiction. *NIDA Notes, 22*(6), 1, 10–14.

Wickham, R. J. (2015). How menthol alters tobacco-smoking behavior: A biological perspective. *Yale Journal of Biology and Medicine, 88*, 279–287.

Wikoff, D., Welsh, B. T., & Henderson, R. (2017, November). Systematic review of the potential adverse effects of caffeine consumption in healthy adults, pregnant women, adolescents, and children. *Food and Chemical Toxicology, 109*(pt1), 585–648. doi: 1016/j.fct.2017.04.002

WHO, World Health Organization. (2009). *WHO Study Group on Tobacco Product Regulation: Report on the Scientific Basis of Tobacco Product Regulation: Third Report of a WHO Study Group.* Geneva: World Health Organization. Retrieved October 7, 2016, from www.worldcat.org/title/who-study-group-on-tobacco-product-regulation-report-on-the-scientific-basis-of-tobacco-product-regulation-third-report-of-.

Willett, J. G., Bennett, M., & Hair, E. C. (2018, April 18). Recognition, use and perceptions of JUUL among youth and young adults. *Tobacco Control.* doi: 10.1136/tobaccocontrol-2018-054273

Williams, J. M., & Gandhi, K. K. (2008, June). Use of caffeine and nicotine in people with schizophrenia. *Current Drug Abuse Reviews, 1*(2), 155–161.

Wise, B. K., Cuffe, S. P., & Fischer, T. (2001, October). Dual diagnosis and successful participation of adolescents in substance abuse treatment. *Journal of Substance Abuse Treatment, 21*(3), 161–165.

Woolf, A., Burkhart, K., & Caraccio, T. (1997, May). Childhood poisoning involving transdermal nicotine patches. *Pediatrics, 99*(5), E4.

Wright, T. E., & Tam, E. (2010). Disparate rates of persistent smoking and drug use during pregnancy of women of Hawaiian ancestry. *Ethnicity & Disease, 20*(1 Supplement 1), S1-215–218.

Wu, W., Zhang, L., & Jain, R. B. (2005). Determination of carcinogenic tobacco-specific nitrosamines in mainstream smoke from U. S.-brand and non-U. S. brand cigarettes from 14 countries. *Nicotine & Tobacco Research*, 7(3), 443–451.

Yang, T. O., Crowe, B. J., & Cairns, B. J. (2015). Tea and coffee and risk of endometrial cancer: Cohort study and meta-analysis. *The American Journal of Clinical Nutrition, 101*(3), 570–578. doi:10.3945/ajcn.113.081836

Yardley, M. M., Mirbaba, M. M., & Ray, L. A. (2015). Pharmacological options for smoking cessation in heavy drinking smokers. *CNS Drugs, 29*(10), 833–845. doi:10.1007/s40263-015-0284-5

Zevin, S., & Benowitz, N. L. (1999). Drug interactions with tobacco smoking. An update. *Clinical Pharmacokinetics, 36* (6), 425–438. doi:10.2165/00003088-199936060-00004

Zhu, S.-H., Cummins, S. E., & Gamst, A. C. (2016, July). Quitting smoking before and after varenicline: A population study based on two representative samples of U.S. smokers. *Tobacco Control, 25*(4), 464–469. doi:10.1136/tobaccocontrol-2015-052332

Zhu, S.-H., Sun, J. Y., & Bonnevie, E. (2014). Four hundred and sixty brands of e-cigarettes and counting: Implications for product regulation. *Tobacco Control, 23*, iii43–4iii9. doi:10.1136/tobaccocontrol-2014-051670

Zickler, P. (2003, March). Nicotine's multiple effects on the brain's reward system drive addiction. *NIDA Notes, 17*(6), 1–3. Retrieved October 7, 2016, from www.ehd.org/health_tobacco_19.php

4
Cannabis and Other Psychodelics

The psychodelics encompass a major group of drugs and substances of abuse that was originally named, "psych**e**delics," by Osmond (1957) in order to differentiate them from "hallucinogens." As later explained by Cohen (1967), the term, "hallucinogen," was generally used to denote drugs and substances of abuse that produced a "temporary madness," whereas the term, "psychedelics," was used to denote drugs and substances of abuse that induced "valuable states of self-transcendence and mystical unity" (p. xv). Other names, such as "phantasticants" and "illusinogens" were also used to reflect the vivid sensory experiences and common visual illusions and misperceptions associated with the psychodelics. In addition, other names associated with, or reflecting, the specific professional stance of the person proposing the name (e.g., mystic; physician; psychiatrist; psychologist), were also used, such as: "psychotogens" (i.e., inducers of psychosis); "psychotomimetics" (i.e., mimickers of psychosis); "schizophrenomimetics" (i.e., mimickers of schizophrenia); "mysticomimetics" (i.e., mimickers of mystic states); and "psychotomystics" (i.e., mimickers of psychosis and mystic states).

The psychodelic group of the drugs and substance of abuse expanded with the more recent popularity of 3,4-methylenedioxymethamphetamine ("MDMA;" "Ecstasy") and other related drugs and substances of abuse that act as:

- "Empathogens" (i.e., drugs that produce feelings of "empathy" toward others);
- "Entactogens" (i.e., "touch," or "hug drugs" that produce feelings of "closeness," "belonging," and "love."

For clarity, and in keeping with the terms used to denote the other two major groups of abusable psychotropics discussed in this text (i.e., psych**o**depressants and psych**o**stimulants), we have selected to use the term, "psych**o**delics,"[1] to denote this major class of the abusable psychotropics.

Three major subclasses of psychodelics also were identified and comprise: (1) "amphetamine-like psychodelics;" (2) "d-lysergic-acid diethylamide (LSD)" and "LSD-like psychodelics;" and (3) "miscellaneous psychodelics" (see Table 4.1). This chapter focuses on four psychodelics that

1 We began using this term approximately 30 years ago following the development of our classification system, "abusable and nonabusable psychotropics," which was constructed to address and attempt to clarify the: (1) confusion we encountered in the published journal articles and textbooks; (2) miscommunication among health and social care professionals, including both undergraduate and graduate students; and (3) misunderstanding among patients and the general public regarding the identification and use of "abusable" and "nonabusable" psychotropic drugs. The system also simplified the categorization and organization of all of the abusable psychotropics—natural, synthetic, and semisynthetic—into three major classes along with their associated subclasses. Over the new millennium, we found this system consistent with our intent and simply designated the three major classes of the drugs and substances of abuse as: "psychodepressants," "psychostimulants," and "psychodelics." (See, for example, Pagliaro & Pagliaro, 1998, 1999a, 1999b, 2000, 2004, 2009, 2012, 2018). See also Figure P.1.

are the most commonly used by adolescents and young adults in the U.S. during the first two decades of the new millennium. These most commonly used psychodelics are:

1. Cannabis—principally its constituent, delta-9-tetrahydrocannabinol (THC);
2. Lysergic acid diethylamide (LSD);
3. Methylenedioxymethamphetamine (MDMA);
4. Phencyclidine (PCP).

Table 4.1 The Psychodelics

Subclassification *Generic Name*[2]	*Common Street Names*[3]
Amphetamine-Like Psychodelics—Phenethylamines	
4-Bromo-2,5-dimethoxyphenethylamine	"2-CB;" "Bromo;" "Nexus"
2,5 Dimethoxy-4-methylamphetamine	"DOM;" "STP"
Mescaline	"Buttons;" "Cactus;" *Peyote*
3,4-Methylenedioxyamphetamine	"Adam;" "Love Drug;" "MDA"
3,4-Methylenedioxyethylamphetamine	"Eve;" "MDE;" "MDEA"
3,4-Methylenedioxymethamphetamine	"Dancing Shoes;" "Ecstasy;" "MDMA;" "XTC"
N-Methyl-1-(3,4-methylenedioxyphenyl)-2-butanamine	"Eden;" "Fido-Dido;" "MBDB"
4-Methylthioamphetamine	"4-MTA;" "Flatliners;" "Golden Eagle"
Nutmeg	"Magic;" *Noz Moscada; Muskatbaum*
Paramethoxyamphetamine	"Death;" *Mitsubishi*; "PMA"
3,4,5-Trimethoxyamphetamine	"Mescalamphetamine;" "TMA"
LSD & LSD-Like Psychodelics	
Indoles	
Amanita Muscaria	"Flesh of the gods;" "Fly Agaric;" "Soma"

(*Continued*)

2 There are no brand/trade names for the psychodelics, other than those for the therapeutically approved and available cannabinoids—dronabinol (Marinol®) in the U.S., and nabilone (Cesamet®) in Canada.

3 Partial list. Examples of the most common street names are provided, when available. See Pagliaro and Pagliaro (2009) for a comprehensive listing of the drugs and substances of abuse and their common street names.

Table 4.1 (Cont.)

Subclassification *Generic Name*	*Common Street Names*
Harmala alkaloids	"Yage;" *Yaje*
Lysergic acid amide	"Blue Stars;" "LSA;" "Morning Glory"
Lysergic acid diethylamide	"Acid;" "LSD;" "25"
Tryptamines[4, 5]	
Alpha-Ethyltryptamine[6]	"Alpha-ET;" "ET;" "Love Pearls"
N,N-Diethyltryptamine	"DET"
N,N-Dipropyltryptamine	"DIPT"
5-Hydroxy-N,N-dimethyltryptamine[7]	"Bufo;" "5-0H-DMT;" "Toad"
5-Methoxy-N,N-dimethyltryptamine	"5-MeO-DMT"
Indole-Tryptamines	
Alpha-methyltryptamine	"3-IT;" "AMT;" "Spirals;"
N,N-Dimethyltryptamine	"45 Minute Trip;" "Businessman's Lunch;" "DMT"
5-Methoxy-N,N-diisopropyltryptamine	"Foxy;" "Foxy Methoxy;" "5-MeO-DIPT"
Psilocin	"Magic Mushrooms;" "Pizza Toppings;" "Shrooms"
Psilocybin	"Fungus;" "Sacred Mushrooms;" "Smurf Hats"
Miscellaneous Psychodelics	
Cannabis	*Ganja*; "Grass;" "Weed"

(*Continued*)

4 Virtually all of the tryptamines are classified as LSD-like psychodelics because of their observed psychotropic actions. However, they also are classified as "tryptamines" in this taxonomy because each has the amino acid, tryptamine, as its core chemical structure.

5 Psilocybin (i.e., O-phosphoryl-4-hydroxy-N,N-ethyltryptamine) and psilocin (i.e., 4-hydroxy-N,N-dimethyltryptamine) also can be added to this taxonomy.

6 Alpha-ethyltryptamine is not currently widely used and available data are extremely limited. Therefore, it is not discussed in this text.

7 Also known as "bufotenine." There is some question as to its psychodelic action, but the lack of psychodelic activity in human subjects may be simply due to its poor ability to cross the blood-brain barrier.

Table 4.1 (Cont.)

Subclassification Generic Name	*Common Street Names*
Ibogaine[8]	"Bocca;" "Iboga;" *Lebuga*
Ketamine	"Cat;" "K;" "Special K;" "Vitamin K"
Phencyclidine	"Angel Dust;" "PCP;" "Peace Pill"
Piperazine derivatives	"A2;" "Fly;" "Nemesis"
Salvia Divinorum[9]	"Big Sal;" "Diviner's Mint;" *Ska Maria Pastoral*

Common Misbelief: The use of psychodelics peaked during the 1960s and has steadily declined ever since.

Not true. Actually, adolescent and young adult psychodelic usage rates in the U.S., during the new millennium, are higher than at any other time in the history of the U.S., including during the "hippie subculture era" of the 1960s. Several factors are largely responsible for these observed high rates of psychodelic use, particularly the:

1. Adoption of more positive attitudes toward psychodelic use (e.g., Digitale, 2016; Motel, 2015; Samuels, 2015);
2. Decriminalization/legalization of cannabis in most states (e.g., Grucza, Vuolo, & Krauss, 2018; Williams & Bretteville-Jensen, 2014);
3. Relatively new and convenient sources of availability.

Contributing to the increasing sources of availability, and, consequently, increased use, is the widespread access of adolescents to the:

1. "Dark web;"
2. Numerous online, illicit drug marketplaces, such as the "Silk Road 3"(Barratt, Ferris, & Winstock, 2014; Pagliaro & Pagliaro, *Clinical Patient Data Files*; Pagliaro & Pagliaro, 2018; van Hout & Bingham, 2013).[10]

We begin with cannabis.

8 At lower dosages, ibogaine acts as a psychostimulant, primarily affecting the NMDA receptors. At higher dosages, it acts as a psychodelic, primarily involving the serotonin receptors.

9 Johnston, O'Malley, and Bachman (2011), in their 2010 in-school survey of adolescent use of the drugs and substances of abuse, found that 1.7% of 8th grade students, 3.7% of 10th grade students, and 5.5% of 12th grade students reported use of *Salvia Divinorum* during the previous year.

10 Cannabis is a "special case" because it is the only psychodelic commonly used by adolescents and young adults—at least currently, in most states—that can be legally purchased for medical and/or personal (i.e., "recreational") use (National Conference of State Legislatures, 2018).

Cannabis

> Cannabis is the most commonly used illicit drug worldwide.
>
> (Power, Verweij, & Zuhair, 2014, p. 1201)

It should not be surprising that, for adolescents and young adults, cannabis—primarily in the form of marijuana—is the most widely known and used psychodelic in the U.S. (Pagliaro & Pagliaro, 2009, 2012, 2018). As identified by Radhakrishnan, Wilkinson, and D'Souza (2014):

> Cannabis is the most commonly used illicit drug by adults, with 18.1 million current users in the U.S. and approximately 5 million daily cannabis users.
>
> (p. 1)

As similarly identified by Azofeifa, Mattson, and Schauer (2016):

> In the United States, marijuana is the most commonly used illicit drug. In 2013, 7.5% (19.8 million) of the U.S. population ... [12 years of age or older] ... reported using marijuana during the preceding month.
>
> (p. 1)

Finally, as noted by Murphy, Barry, and Vaughn (2013):

> Marijuana is by far the most commonly used illicit drug among adolescents.
>
> (p. 1)

With the legalization of medicinal marijuana, the resultant increased availability of high-percentage THC (delta-9-tetrahydrocannabinol) varieties in newly opened marijuana dispensaries and, more recently, recreational "herb," "pot," and "vapor" shops, which also offer electronic marijuana smoking devices—bongs, hookahs, and vaporizers; and candies and other edible cannabis "treats"—rates of marijuana use are rising in the U.S., as we previously predicted (Pagliaro & Pagliaro, 2012). We now predict that they will continue to rise into the foreseeable future. (See also the related discussion in the later cannabis section, "Adolescent and Young Adult Cannabis Use").

Not all researchers agree with our "prediction." For example, some researchers (e.g., Choo, Benz, & Zaller, 2014) have not found a significant increase in the incidence of adolescent marijuana use in relation to the legalization of medical marijuana. However, the preponderance of available research data (e.g. Hopfer, 2014; Miech, Johnston, & O'Malley, 2015; Salas-Wright, Vaughn, & Todic, 2015) support the theory that adolescent marijuana use significantly increases in jurisdictions in which its use has (at least for adults) been decriminalized or legalized. For example, Miech, Johnston, and O'Malley (2015), in their analysis of adolescent marijuana use in California prior to decriminalization in 2010, found that:

> In 2012 and afterwards California 12th graders as compared to their peers in other states became (a) 25% *more* likely to have used marijuana in the past 30 days, (b) 20% *less* likely to perceive regular marijuana use as a great health risk, (c) 20% *less* likely to strongly disapprove of regular marijuana use, and (d) about 60% *more* likely to expect to be using marijuana five years in the future.
>
> (p. 336)[11]

11 N.B. On January 1, 2018 the "recreational" use of marijuana became legal in California (Mikelionis, 2018).

Cannabis Pharmacognosy

Whereas "pharmacology" is the study of the origin, nature, chemistry, effects, and uses of drugs, a related science, "pharmacognosy,"[12] focuses specifically on the identification, recognition, extraction, and medicinal use of plants and other natural substances. For this reason, and because of the high rates of cannabis use in the U.S., we begin with an additional section on its pharmacognosy (including its botany). We then continue with the pharmacology of cannabis, a member of the miscellaneous subclass of psychodelics. Categorized as one of the three major products of cannabis (i.e., marijuana; hash [hashish]; and hashish oil), marijuana—commonly referred to as: "bud;" "dope;" "grass;" "Mary Jane;" "pot;" and "weed"—remains the most popular and, consequently, the most widely used form in the U.S.

Cannabis Botany

There are several species of cannabis,[13] including *Cannabis lativa* and *Cannabis sativa* (Indian hemp). *Cannabis sativa* is the principal variety from which marijuana, hashish, and hashish oil are prepared. Within the species of *Cannabis sativa*, there are several varieties including *Cannabis sativa indica, Cannabis sativa ruderalis,* and *Cannabis sativa sativa.* These varieties significantly differ in regard to their concentration of THC, the primary pharmacologically active cannabinoid found in the species,[14] with the *indica* variety having the highest concentration of THC.[15]

Within the cannabis plant, the highest concentration of THC is found in the bracts, or small leaves, at the base of the cannabis flowers, and their resin. The next highest concentration is found in the flowering tops, and then, in decreasing order, the upper leaves, large stems, and seeds, with the roots having the lowest concentration.[16] Additionally, the female plants tend to have a much higher THC concentration than the male plants. Thus, the reason for advertisements and sales of tools (e.g., ultraviolet lights) in drug-paraphernalia stores (i.e., headshops; hemp stores; hydroponic grow stores), the internet, and drug culture magazines (e.g., *High Times*) to "detect plant sex."

The desire for higher THC concentrations also accounts for the popularity of *sinsemilla*—unfertilized female cannabis plants that are cultivated specifically for their higher THC concentration. The cultivation of *sinsemilla* is generally accomplished by planting female seeds or by destroying the male plants before pollen is produced and the female plants are fertilized. These procedures allow the unfertilized female plants to flower more abundantly and, consequently, to produce more THC-containing resin.

12 "Pharmacognosy" is the study of bioactive natural products, particularly medicinals that are extracted or otherwise obtained (e.g., in natural dried state) from plants and other natural sources. It includes the recognition, extraction, and use of these natural products. In many taxonomies, pharmacognosy is considered to be an esoteric branch of pharmacology. Of note, pharmacognosy, as a distinct discipline, generally has not been a formal part of the academic curriculum of schools of medicine, nursing, or pharmacy, in the U.S., for over 50 years.

13 Cannabis is a genus of flowering plants found within the Cannabaceae family.

14 Over 100 different pharmacologically active cannabinoids have been identified in cannabis, including "cannabidiol" (CBD) and "cannabinol" (CBN). These other cannabinoids, particularly CBD, have been largely ignored over the past 75 years. However, with the legalization of marijuana for medical and/or recreational use in several states during the new millennium, interest in CBD containing edibles and drinks has proliferated (e.g., Lagerquist, 2019; Scipion, 2019).

15 N.B. Some botanical taxonomies classify *indica, ruderalis,* and *sativa* as belonging to different species of cannabis.

16 N.B. The roots, stalks, and stems, of the cannabis (marijuana) plant contain low concentrations of THC and are more fibrous than the rest of the plant leaves. Historically referred to as "hemp," these parts of the cannabis plant have been specifically cultivated and used to produce boat sails, canvas, clothing, fish nets, and paper for literally thousands of years (Pagliaro & Pagliaro, 2004). In December 2018, a bipartisan farm bill was signed into law that, as a component, formally legalized the industrial production of hemp in the U.S. (Angell, 2018; Kasana, 2018).

Cannabis is produced worldwide as illustrated by the names given to the many varieties that are distributed and sold across the U.S. These names include, for example: "Acapulco Gold;" "BC Bud;" "Cambodian Red;" "Hawaiian Buds;" "Indian Hash;" "Jamaican Ganja;" "Lebanese Hash;" "Moroccan Kif;" "New Mexico Sinse;" "Panama Gold;" "Thai Sticks;" and "Ukrainian Ditchweed." In addition to worldwide distribution and sale, several states (i.e., Alabama, California, Florida, Hawaii, Kentucky, North Carolina, Oregon, Tennessee, Washington, West Virginia, Wisconsin) produce cannabis to the extent that it is the state's most significant cash crop with the combined annual revenues reaching the tens of billions of dollars (Pagliaro & Pagliaro, 2009).

> The domestic marijuana crop is: larger than cotton in Alabama; larger than grapes, vegetables, and hay combined in California; larger than peanuts in Georgia; and larger than tobacco in both South Carolina and North Carolina.
>
> (Gettman, 2006, p. 1)

As individual states (e.g., California, Colorado, Washington) begin to re-legalize marijuana (i.e., marijuana was legal and unregulated in the U.S. prior to the early 20th Century), both for medicinal and personal use, hundreds of millions of dollars in tax revenue are being added to state tax coffers. For example, Colorado, which was the first state to legalize "recreational" marijuana use and retail sales in 2014, collected approximately $40 million in additional tax dollars in 2014 (La Corte, 2014; Smith, 2017). As reported by the Colorado Department of Revenue, for 2018:

> Total marijuana tax revenue includes the 2.9% retail and medical marijuana sales tax, 10% retail marijuana special sales tax, 15% marijuana excise tax, and retail/medical marijuana application and license fees.
>
> (2018, p. 1)

The combined "marijuana tax" for the calendar year 2017 was reported to be $247,368,473.00 (Colorado Department of Revenue, 2018).

In the state of Washington, legal marijuana sales yielded over $70 million in tax revenue during the 2014/2015 fiscal year (Williams, 2015). During the 2017/2018 fiscal year, the state of Washington increased its marijuana sales tax revenue to over $320 million (Kovacevich, 2018). It has been estimated that if marijuana sales were legalized in all 50 states, the associated tax revenue generated could exceed three billion dollars annually (Ferner, 2014).[17]

Despite its worldwide production and commerce—and production, to varying degrees, in every state—approximately 50% of the cannabis that is used in the U.S. is smuggled in from one specific country, Mexico, particularly along the U.S. southern border with Mexico (Hurley, West, & Ehleringer, 2010; Pagliaro & Pagliaro, 2012, 2018).[18] Additionally, increasing amounts of high grade marijuana are smuggled into the U.S. from Canada, particularly along the U.S. northern border with Canada (Hurley, West, & Ehleringer, 2010; Pagliaro & Pagliaro, 2012, 2018).

17 Based upon the consideration of more recent data, we believe that this prediction is an extremely conservative estimate and that the generated tax revenue could well exceed $30 billion annually by the end of the third decade of the new millennium.

18 Over the first decade of the new millennium, increasing amounts of high potency marijuana (i.e., 15% to 25% THC) began to enter the U.S. from Canada, produced predominantly from indoor growing operations (i.e., "grow-ops") in the Province of British Columbia (i.e., "BC Bud"). This trend is expected to significantly intensify through the end of the second decade of the new millennium, and well beyond, because the possession and use of both medical and recreational cannabis became legalized across all of Canada in 2018 (Paperny & Saminather, 2017; Reith, 2017).

During the second decade of the new millennium, a related trend began that has now become entrenched—state legalization of the "recreational" use of cannabis.[19] Associated with this trend was the rapid and increasing occurrence of the:

1. Illicit production and distribution of cannabis in states that had legalized recreational cannabis use;
2. Provision of the opportunity for transnational drug cartels to "set up shop" in these states and, consequently, facilitate the illicit distribution and sale of cannabis in states that had not legalized "recreational" use of cannabis.

(e.g., Cain, 2017; Romero, Gutierrez, & Blankstein, 2018; Shen, 2017)

The transnational, or foreign, drug cartels—primarily from China, Cuba, and Mexico—that are involved in producing cannabis within states where "recreational" use of cannabis has been legalized, operate by: (1) concealing production within a legal environment; and (2) facilitating distribution to other states—without having to smuggle the cannabis across international borders (i.e., into the U.S.). The methods adopted by these transnational "growers," who are operating within states where the "recreational" use of cannabis has been legalized, are actually quite simple to operationalize. They either purchase, or lease:

1. Farms and areas of rural land to grow large cannabis crops;
2. Hundreds of homes in which to established small hydroponic "grow-ops" of up to 50 plants.

Quite often, the transnational grow-ops are operated (i.e., maintained on a day-to-day basis) by illegal immigrants—often adolescents and often in the context of human trafficking (Pagliaro & Pagliaro, *Clinical Patient Data Files*).

Marijuana

"Marijuana" (i.e., "grass;" "pot;" "weed") is the dried, shredded plant form (generally, flowers and leaves) of cannabis.[20] Marijuana is generally grayish-green to greenish-brown in color and, when compared to hashish or hashish oil, contains significantly lower concentrations of THC. Marijuana is prepared for pulmonary inhalation (i.e., smoking, or "toking") using methods that are similar to those used for preparing tobacco leaves for smoking. However, marijuana preparation generally requires less time and involvement in regard to curing and drying.[21]

Hashish

"Hashish" (i.e., "Candy Bar;" "Hash;" "Lebanese") is prepared from the dried resin and compressed flowers of the cannabis plant and is generally light brown to black in color. Prepared and distributed for use in compressed blocks or cubes, it has a relatively high concentration of THC.

19 N.B. According to current U.S. federal laws (i.e., Schedule I of the Controlled Substances Act), cannabis possession, distribution, sale, and use are illegal.

20 Kif (i.e., "kaif;" "keef;" "kief"), an Arabic word meaning "well-being" or "pleasure," was originally the name given to a powder that was made from the dried flowers of the female cannabis plant. Indigenous to the Rif mountain area of northern Morocco, it was usually mixed with tobacco (i.e., one part to two parts) prior to smoking. Although the use of kif in the U.S. has been reported over the years, its use is relatively uncommon. The term is now more commonly used to denote marijuana or hashish that is from Morocco (Pagliaro & Pagliaro, 2004).

21 Whereas the rolled tobacco product prepared for smoking commonly is called a "cigarette," "cig," or "coffin nail," the rolled marijuana product prepared for smoking commonly is called a "doobie," "joint," "reefer," or "spliff."

Hashish Oil

"Hashish oil" is prepared from hashish by the means of extraction with an organic solvent, often isopropyl alcohol (i.e., "rubbing alcohol"). It is then filtered and concentrated. Hashish oil contains the highest concentration of THC and ranges in color from clear to almost black. Food coloring is often added for color enhancement.

Cannabis Concentrations

The concentration of THC in marijuana, hashish, and hashish oil can generally range from:

- 1% to 10% for "home grown" marijuana cigarettes;[22]
- 5% to 30% for "commercially grown" marijuana;
- 15% to 65% for hashish;
- 30% to 90% for hashish oil.

Whereas these concentrations vary depending on the specific part of the plant (e.g., buds, leaves, or stems) from which the THC was obtained, it also depends on the: (1) quality and source of the cannabis—the state, province, or country of origin (e.g., Hawaii, U.S.; British Columbia, Canada; Mexico); and (2) cultivation techniques (e.g., hydroponic cultivation). It is extremely important to recognize that, since the beginning of the new millennium, THC concentrations have significantly increased, on average, from 25% to 300% across the U.S. primarily depending upon: (1) pre-millennial comparison year; (2) form of cannabis; (3) type/variety of cannabis; and (4) location.

An average, a high potency marijuana joint during the 1960s and 1970s, contained only approximately ten mg of THC. However, during the beginning of the new millennium, the average, high potency, marijuana joint contained approximately 150 mg of THC (e.g., Ashton, 2001; Pagliaro & Pagliaro, 2004). As the third decade of the new millennium approaches, high potency marijuana joints contain up to 300 mg of THC (Pagliaro & Pagliaro, *Clinical Patient Dara Files*). However, regarding "apparent potency" in terms of pharmacological effects, it is important to keep in mind that the blood THC concentration achieved when smoking a marijuana joint varies significantly depending on the:

1. Amount of THC in the cannabis that is smoked;
2. Smoking technique used, including the rate, depth, and length of inhalation before exhaling (i.e., the "drag," "hit," or "toke");
3. Amount of THC that is destroyed by pyrolysis.[23]

Cannabis Pharmacology

Over 400 different chemicals are found in cannabis smoke, including: ammonia, benz[a]anthracene, benzene, benzo[a]pyrene, carbon monoxide, cresols, cyanogen, nitric oxide,

22 Also, the same for "blunts" (i.e., marijuana that is rolled in tobacco leaves) and "cigar wraps." (See related discussion in the later subsection, "Blunts").

23 N.B. Given the well-documented partial degradation of THC by pyrolysis and related undesired effects and toxicities related to "smoke," several researchers (e.g., Eisenberg, Ogintz, & Almog, 2014; Hartman, Brown, & Milavetz, 2015) studied potentially less harmful methods of use demonstrating that vaporization is an extremely effective form of THC delivery (see also the related discussion in the later cannabis subsections, "Vaping," and "Vaporizers.")

phenols, and tars.[24] Of these chemicals, approximately 100 different cannabinoids (e.g., cannabidiol [CBD]; cannabinol [CBN]; THC)—compounds that are only naturally found in cannabis plants and that function as exogenous ligands for the endocannabinoid system—have been identified (Weissman, 1981). (See also the related discussion in the following subsection.) Of these, the principal active cannabinoid, in terms of psychodelic actions, is THC.

A variety of clearly defined dose-related effects have been associated with the psychotropic actions of THC. "Lower" dosages may produce: decreased intraocular pressure; drowsiness; euphoria; hypertension; increased appetite; memory impairment; reddened eyes; relaxation; tachycardia; and temporal disintegration. "Moderate" dosages may produce: anxiety; decreased muscle strength and motor performance; decreased visual acuity; impaired coordination; and paranoia. "Higher" dosages may produce: confused thinking; delusions; hallucinations; synesthesia; and toxic psychosis.

> The interchanging of the senses ... the hashish eater knows what it is ... to smell colors, to see sounds, and, much more frequently, to see feelings.
>
> (Ludlow, 1857, p. 72)

Pharmacodynamics: Mechanism of Action

This section presents and discusses several important concepts regarding the mechanism of cannabis action, particularly those associated with the endocannabinoid system.

ENDOCANNABINOID SYSTEM

The mechanism by which THC produces its psychodelic and other effects is not yet fully understood. Undoubtedly, the greatest advancement has been the identification of the endocannabinoid system—the endogenous system of cannabinoid receptors and agonists, or ligands (Breivogel & Childers, 1998). Anandamide (N-archidonoyl ethanolamine), 2-arachidonoylglycerol, and 2-arachidonyl glycerol ether have been identified as the three major endogenous agonists, or ligands, of the endocannabinoid receptors.

Endocannabinoids typically are produced in response to increased intracellular calcium concentrations at postsynaptic sites—"in response to sustained synaptic activity" (Kendall & Yudowski, 2017, p. 3). The endocannabinoids elicit several of the pharmacologic actions, which have been associated with the use of THC (Maccarrone & Finazzi-Agro, 2002; Martin, Mechoulam, & Razdan, 1999; Pertwee & Ross, 2002; Singh & Budhiraja, 2006), including effects on learning, memory, mood, and pain perception.

Important strides have been made since the beginning of the new millennium in this regard. For example, a model of cannabinoid signaling was posited by Elphick and Egertova (2001), "in which anandamide is synthesized by postsynaptic cells and acts as a retrograde messenger molecule to modulate neurotransmitter release from presynamptic terminals" (p. 381). As identified by Wilson and Nicoll (2002):

> In contrast to classical neurotransmitters, endogenous cannabinoids can function as retrograde synaptic messengers: They are released from postsynaptic neurons and travel backward across synapses, activating CB_1 on presynaptic axons and suppressing neurotransmitter release.
>
> (p. 678)

24 N.B. Several of these chemicals are known human carcinogens (e.g., benzo[a]pyrene, a highly carcinogenic hydrocarbon found in coal tar; cresols; phenols; and tars). (See also the later cannabis pharmacology subsection, "Undesired, or Harmful, Effects and Toxicities.")

Thus, overall, the endocannabinoid system appears to primarily act as a neuromodulator of the CNS by affecting the release of several identified neurotransmitters, including: acetylcholine; dopamine; endorphins; gamma-aminobutyric acid (GABA); glutamate; noradrenaline; and serotonin (Lopez-Moreno, Gonzalez-Cuevas, & Moreno, 2008; Moreira & Lutz, 2008).

CB_1 AND CB_2 RECEPTORS. Two major cannabinoid G-protein coupled receptor subtypes exist—Subtype 1 (i.e., CB_1) receptors and Subtype 2 (i.e., CB_2) receptors (Pertwee, 2000). THC elicits its effects primarily by activating CB_1 receptors (Wilson & Nicoll, 2002), which are primarily present on central and peripheral neurons, predominantly within the CNS (Pertwee, 2000). These receptors appear to mediate the: (1) inhibition of adenylate cyclase and various calcium channels (i.e., opening of postsynaptic calcium channels followed by inhibition of presynaptic calcium influx); (2) stimulation of post-synaptic potassium channels facilitating potassium and neurotransmitter release; and (3) activation of mitogen-activated protein kinase (Ameri, 1999). The endocannabinoid activity of these receptors suggests a role in the modulation of neurotransmitter release and action (e.g., increasing dopaminergic neuronal activity in the ventral tegmental area-mesolimbic pathway) (Di Marzo, Melck, & Bisogno, 1998).

CB_1 RECEPTORS CB_1 receptors are one of the most abundant neuromodulatory receptors within the CNS with particularly high concentrations found in the basal ganglia, brainstem, cerebellum, cortex, hippocampus, and neocortex (Wilson & Nicoll, 2002). CB_1 receptors are "also found on peripheral nerve terminals and some extra-neural sites such as the testis, eye, vascular endothelium and spleen" (Kendall & Yudowski, 2017, p. 2). The majority of THC pleiotropic effects (i.e., the influence of one gene on two or more seemingly unrelated phenotypic traits simultaneously) are mediated by means of binding to the CB_1 receptor (Pagliaro & Pagliaro, 2009). For example, Cooper and Haney (2009) identified that:

> The rewarding and positive reinforcing effects of the primary psychoactive component of smoked cannabis, delta-9-tetrahydrocannabinol (THC), are mediated by the cannabinoid CB_1 receptor. The CB_1 receptor has also been shown to mediate cannabinoid dependence and expression of withdrawal upon cessation of drug administration.
>
> (p. 104)

CB_2 RECEPTORS CB_2 receptors are primarily present on immune cells, predominantly outside of the CNS (Klein, Lane, & Newton, 2000; Pertwee & Ross, 2002). These receptors appear to mediate the activation of mitogen-activated protein kinase and the inhibition of adenylate cyclase (Ameri, 1999). The endocannabinoid activity of these receptors (e.g., enhanced physiological response to cytokines) suggests a role in immuno-suppression and anti-inflammatory action (Nocerino, Amato, & Izzo, 2000). In addition, although not yet confirmed, these mechanisms may play an active role in the treatment of medical disorders such as chronic neuropathic pain, which is often refractory to standard pharmacotherapeutic interventions (Eisenberg, Ogintz & Almog, 2014; Wilsey, Marcotte, & Deutsch, 2013). CB_2 receptors also appear to be involved in "regulatory roles" in the context of "drug abuse" (Kendall & Yudowski, 2017, p. 2).

Pharmacokinetics: Absorption, Distribution, Metabolism, and Excretion

This section presents and discusses the absorption, distribution, metabolism, and excretion of THC.

ABSORPTION

Following ingestion, THC bioavailability is low (i.e., approximately 10%) because of extensive first-pass hepatic metabolism. Following pulmonary inhalation, THC bioavailability is much higher having a mean of 27% (range, 17% to 37%) due to its rapid absorption from the lungs and avoidance of first-pass hepatic metabolism. THC blood concentrations peak shortly after (i.e., ~ 10 minutes) the end of the pulmonary inhalation of cannabis (McGilveray, 2005). Once in the circulatory system, oxidative metabolism, primarily in the liver, produces both its active metabolite, 11-hydroxy-delta-9-tetrahydrocannabinol (11-OH-THC),[25] and its inactive metabolite, 11-nor-hydroxy-delta-9-tetrahydrocannabinol (THCCOOH). While the blood 11-OH-THC concentrations peak just after the end of the pulmonary inhalation of cannabis, the blood THCCOOH concentrations peak 1.5 to two hours after the pulmonary inhalation of cannabis.

DISTRIBUTION

THC is approximately 97% protein bound, while its active metabolite 11-OH-THC is slightly more protein bound (i.e., 99%). The apparent volume of distribution of THC is approximately 10 liters per kg, primarily because of its high lipid solubility (Hunt, Jones, & Herning, 1981). The long-term storage of THC in body fat helps to explain the poor correlation between THC blood concentrations and clinical effects, particularly during the initial period of establishing equilibrium, or a period of hysteresis (e.g., Cone & Huestis, 1993; Goulle & Guerbet, 2014; Heather, 2001).

METABOLISM

THC is primarily metabolized in the liver by the hepatic microsomal enzyme system (i.e., cytochrome P450 complex). Both P450 CYP2C9 and CYP3A4 are involved in the oxidative metabolism of THC.[26] Other body organs (e.g., brain; intestines; lungs) also contain CYP450 enzymes and also contribute, albeit to a significantly lesser extent, to the metabolism of THC. Cannabidiol is metabolized in a manner similar to THC and is also subject to significant first-pass hepatic metabolism (Anderson & Chan, 2016; Huestis, 2007; Yamaori, Kushihara, & Yamamoto, 2010).

EXCRETION

Some researchers report a mean initial "alpha" distribution half-life of elimination of approximately 30 hours for THC. However, the later "beta" phase elimination half-life is about 3.5 days because of its preferential concentration and storage in the spleen and body fat (range, one to seven days). In addition, it has long been recognized that cannabis smoke has the potential, like tobacco smoke, to induce hepatic microsomal isoenzymes. In this regard, regular, long-term cannabis users generally eliminate THC more rapidly (half-life of elimination, approximately 28 hours) than nonusers (half-life of elimination, approximately 57 hours).

Total body clearance of THC generally ranges from 750 to 1200 ml/minute with rates being, on average, approximately 10% lower in females compared to males. The elimination half-life of its inactive metabolite, THCCOOH, is two to six days. Both metabolites are

25 N.B. The pharmacological activity of 11-OH-THC is greater than that of the parent compound (i.e., THC).

26 CYP2C9 and CYP3A4 also are primarily involved in the metabolism of CBN while CYP2C19 and CYP3A4 are involved in the metabolism of CBD.

excreted in the urine. They are also secreted back into the gastrointestinal system by means of enterohepatic recirculation, where they are reabsorbed into the circulatory system or excreted in the feces. THC and its two major metabolites, 11-OH-THC and THCCOOH, are present in the urine as glucuronide conjugates. Low concentrations of both of the THC metabolites are often detected in the feces (primarily, 11-OH-THC) and urine (primarily, THCCOOH) for more than five weeks after cannabis—marijuana; hashish; or hash oil—was last used.

Tetrahydrocannabinol is subject to significant renal tubular reabsorption because of its high lipid solubility. Consequently, the renal excretion of unchanged THC is low (Sharma, Murthy, & Srinivas Bharath, 2012). Although, urinary concentrations of THC exceeding 1.5 ng/ml are suggestive of cannabis use during the previous eight hours, because of pharmacokinetic variance and extreme interindividual variability, a presumptive THC blood concentration cannot be reliably related to a specific measurable level of cognitive or behavior impairment. The blood to plasma concentration ratio for THC is 0.55.

URINE TESTING FOR CANNABIS USE/ABUSE

The urine tests currently used for identifying illicit cannabis use detect concentrations of THC and its major inactive metabolite, THCCOOH. The two general types of urinalysis involve either the use of immunoassay (IA) or Gas Chromatography/Mass Spectrometry (GC/MS). Immunoassay is less expensive and easier to perform and hence, it is usually the test of first choice—often in the context of a rapid "screening" test. Immunoassay utilizes a drug-enzyme complex to determine the presence of THC metabolites in the urine. Results are binary and are qualitative in nature—either positive or negative, as indicated by the color produced. For the immunoassay test, the standard cutoff threshold for cannabinoids in the urine is typically set at 50 ng/ml.

Gas Chromatography/Mass Spectrometry utilizes a more complex, or sophisticated method of analysis that is also more time consuming and expensive. Gas chromatography, which must be conducted in a suitably-equipped chemical laboratory, initially is used to separate the chemicals present in the urine sample. This is followed by the use of MS to ionize molecules present in the sample and to identify each by their specific molecular weights. The standard cutoff threshold for cannabinoids in the urine, when utilizing GC/MS, is typically set at 15 ng/ml. The major advantage of the GC/MS is that the results are quantitative. Thus, GC/MS is typically used in the context of a "confirmatory" test (i.e., following an initial, positive cannabis immunoassay test result).

The primary glucuronide conjugate of THC, THCCOOH, is predominantly detected in the urine. Levels of THCCOOH as low as one ng/ml of urine can be detected with good validity and reliability.[27] However, the validity of urine tests is not always accurate because false positive results can occur due to the:

1. Interference of certain other drugs or substances of abuse that may have been concurrently used (e.g., ibuprofen, Motrin®);
2. Inability of a test to differentiate between cannabis "smoke" or "vapor" that is deliberately, or directly, inhaled and that which is passively, or indirectly, inhaled (i.e., as "sidestream," or "second-hand," smoke/vapor).

27 N.B. In addition to assay sensitivity and specificity, individual factors (e.g., dosage; method of use [i.e., relative bioavailability]; state of hydration; rate of elimination) can significantly affect detection times (Goodwin, Darwin, & Chiang, 2008).

In addition, the ingestion of large quantities of products that contain hemp seed oil may produce "false positive" results if the cutoff values designated by the laboratory for the urine test are too low. Urine tests also can give "false negative" results. These false negative results are much more likely to occur when the urine test sample is deliberately adulterated with an in vitro adulterant that is added to the urine sample after collection (e.g., peroxidase and peroxide, which are found in Stealth®; pyridinium chlorochromate, which is found in Urine Luck®—products specifically developed to invalidate urine tests) (e.g., Dasgupta, 2015).

Gordon detailed how his college coaches at Baylor enabled his drug use:

> I've been enabled by coaches, teachers, professors, everybody, pretty much, gave me a second chance because of my ability. Not too long after I got arrested for possession of marijuana at Baylor, one of my coaches came by saying, "You are going to get drug tested by the compliance office. This how it's going to work, this is what they are going to do. If they do call you in, here goes these bottles of detox," Gordon said. "He showed me how to drink them, showed me how to take them. That was my first experience with getting over on the system and the authority not really being serious because it was being guided by someone who was employed by the university.
>
> (Masisak, 2017, p. 1)

<u>Related Professional Reminder:</u> Obtaining urine samples from adolescents for cannabis testing, unless court ordered, requires both: (1) consent of the parent(s) or other legal guardian(s)—if the adolescent is a minor; and (2) assent of the adolescent if the adolescent is mentally competent.[28]

Cannabis Drug–Drug Interactions

A surprising paucity of empirical data exist regarding drug–drug interactions involving THC. This lack of published research may be related to several variables that make quantification of potentially significant THC drug–drug interactions difficult to identify and study. These difficulties include differences in:

- THC and other cannabinoid concentrations among various natural sources (i.e., marijuana versus hashish versus hashish oil);
- THC and other cannabinoid concentrations among various *synthetic* sources (i.e., prescription THC formulations [i.e., dronabinol, Marinol®; nabilone, Cesamet®]);[29, 30]
- Methods of cannabis use (i.e., ingestion versus pulmonary inhalation);

28 N.B. Assent from the adolescent should also include permission, as might be required, to share test results with others. Federal Regulations, Part 2 (42 CFR Part 2) requires written permission from adolescent patients prior to the release or disclosure of related information that is not part of routine clinical care. Exceptions are noted in the context of: (1) law enforcement use (e.g., road-side checks); and (2) court-ordered mandates (e.g., used to maintain drug-free compliance for related probation, or child custody, orders).

29 Usually prescribed for the management of severe nausea and vomiting associated with cancer pharmacotherapy.

30 In addition, nabiximols (Sativex®), which was developed in the UK, is made from a cannabis extract. Sativex®, which is available in over 30 countries, including Canada, is pending FDA approval in the U.S. primarily for the treatment of neuropathic pain. It contains an equal ratio (i.e., 1:1) of THC and CBD, as well as a variety of other cannabinoids, flavonoids, and terpenes. Sativex® is administered as an oromucosal spray (Nurmikko, Serpell, & Hoggart, 2007; Russo, Guy, & Robson, 2007). Epidiolex® (CBD oral solution) received FDA approval in 2018 for the treatment of the Lennox-Gastaut syndrome and Dravet syndrome—both rare forms of childhood onset epilepsy that are difficult to treat (Devinsky, Cross, & Laux, 2017; FDA, 2018; Forster, 2018; Wirrell, 2016). (See also the related discussion in the later cannabis subsection, "Medical Cannabis Use.")

- Marijuana smoking techniques—such as number of "tokes" per joint; depth of inhalation; length of time that the marijuana smoke is inhaled and retained in the lungs;
- Effects of "polycyclic aromatic hydrocarbons" (PAHs) contained in marijuana smoke.

In addition, the federal illegal status of cannabis use, in the U.S., has significantly impeded related research. As states increasingly move to legalize cannabis use, this situation is expected to significantly change over the next decade.

Consequently, data concerning potentially significant THC drug–drug interactions generally are limited to theoretical questions involving the cytochrome P-450 enzymes. In this regard, the cannabinoids variably act as "inducers," "inhibitors," or "substrates" of the cytochrome P-450 enzymes (see related discussion in the earlier cannabis section, "Pharmacology, Pharmacokinetics—Metabolism") (e.g., Motycka, Glinton, & Brennan, 2016; Rong, Carmona, & Lee, 2018; Stout & Cimino, 2014). Each of these three mechanisms of cannabis drug–drug interactions are briefly discussed in the following list:

1. Inducers of CYP2C9 (e.g., barbiturates; carbamazepine [Tegretol®]; phenytoin [Dilantin®]) and CYP3A4 (e.g., carbamazepine; phenytoin; and rifampin [Rifadin®]) may increase the metabolism of THC and CBD and, consequently, reduce related plasma concentrations.
2. Inhibitors of CYP2C9 (e.g., amiodarone [Cordarone®]; cimetidine [Tagamet®]; fluoxetine [Prozac®]) and CYP3A4 (e.g., clarithromycin [Biaxin®]; ketoconazole [Nizoral®]; verapamil [Calan®]) may decrease the metabolism of THC and CBD and, consequently, increase related plasma concentrations.
3. Marijuana and tobacco smoke induce CYP1A2. Consequently, dosage adjustments may be required with drugs that are primarily metabolized by CYP1A (e.g., caffeine, clozapine [Clozaril®], theophylline [Theo-Dur®]), particularly when regular, or long-term, marijuana or tobacco smoking is initiated or discontinued.[31]
4. Polycyclic aromatic hydrocarbons (PAHs) contained in marijuana smoke (similar to those contained in tobacco smoke) can induce CYP450 enzymes and, consequently, increase the metabolism of certain drugs (e.g., chlorpromazine [Thorazine®]; theophylline [Theo-Dur®])(e.g., Anderson & Chan, 2016; Arellano, Papaseit, & Romaguera, 2017; Horn & Hansten, 2014; Melton, 2017; Yamaori, Koeda, & Kushihara, 2012).

Undesired, or Harmful, Effects and Toxicities

There are several characteristic signs and symptoms associated with acute cannabis use, primarily the: (1) pungent odor of cannabis smoke[32] that is often recognized on clothing and in closed areas where the cannabis has been smoked (e.g., in automobiles, bathrooms, bedrooms, and offices); and (2) reddened, or "blood shot," eyes. Whether or not users become "stoned," common toxicities that are associated with the use of cannabis can be readily divided into toxicities associated with: (1) occasional, or short-term use; and (2) regular, long-term use.

31 This effect is particularly significant among those who regularly smoke both marijuana and tobacco—a fairly common practice among adolescents and young adults.

32 Hence, the common names for cannabis—"skunk" and "skunk weed."

Common Misbelief: Cannabis is a relatively non-toxic, natural psychodelic that is associated with little harm.

OCCASIONAL OR SHORT-TERM USE

Short-term cannabis use has been generally associated with the following undesired, or harmful, effects and toxicities:

- Academic or work achievement decreased;
- Acute ischemic stroke (Rumalla, Reddy, & Mittal, 2016);
- Anxiety;
- Appetite increased (colloquially known as the "munchies");[33]
- Blood pressure increased;
- Burn injuries (Jehle, Nazir, & Bhavsar, 2015);
- Cognitive impairment;
- Executive functioning impaired;
- Confusion;
- Delusions;
- Depersonalization;
- Drowsiness;
- Hallucinations;
- Memory impairment, particularly episodic, short-term, verbal, and working memory (Colizzi & Bhattacharyya, 2017);
- Panic attacks;
- Paranoia;
- Psychomotor impairment;
- Psychotic disorder (for further discussion, see also the later section, "Cannabis-Induced Psychotic Disorder");
- Pulmonary irritation;
- Reddened eyes;
- Synesthesia;
- Tachycardia;
- Temporal disintegration;
- Toxic delirium;
- Visual acuity decreased.

REGULAR, LONG-TERM USE

Over the 1970s, 1980s, and 1990s, the potency of cannabis increased five-fold, from an average THC concentration of 2% to a THC concentration of 10% (Harrison, Backenheimer, & Inciardi, 1996).[34] The increase in potency reflected a preferential change among users from cannabis (sativa) sativa to cannabis (sativa) indica and the increased selective cultivation of sinsemilla varieties (see earlier discussion). Consequently, several undesired, or harmful, effects

33 This common effect, colloquially known as "the munchies," has been commercialized by the Jack in the Box® fast-food restaurant chain. In response to the 2018-legalization of the "recreational" use of marijuana in California, Jack in the Box® began marketing its "Merry [a reference to the common street name for cannabis, 'Mary Jane'] Munchie Meal" (Gant, 2017; Morris, 2017).

34 As briefly discussed earlier in this chapter, these "standard" THC concentrations have continued to steadily and significantly increase over the first two decades of the new millennium.

and toxicities have now been associated with the regular, long-term use of cannabis.[35] These effects and toxicities include:[36, 37]

- Academic or work achievement decreased;
- Cannabinoid hyperemesis syndrome (CHS) (Beech, Sterrett, & Babiuk, 2015);[38]
- Cannabis withdrawal syndrome (relatively mild);
- Cognitive impairment;[39]
- Decreased sperm count;
- Developmental or maturational delay or arrest;
- Disruption of normal ovulation;
- Gynecomastia;
- Immunosuppression;
- Lethargy;
- Mental depression;
- Physical dependence;

35 It may seem logical to conclude, based upon these observations, that potential cannabis users, being aware of the significant increases in the THC concentrations of current cannabis products, would take appropriate precautions (e.g., avoidance of cannabis use or reduction of dosage, or amount consumed or inhaled). However, new millennial trends—in terms of medicalization, decriminalization, and legalization of cannabis use in many cities and states across the U.S.—have significantly affected people's related attitudes (e.g., Cerda, Wall, & Keyes, 2012; Samuels, 2015).

For example, a decreased perception of the significant risk associated with cannabis use has been positively associated with: (1) younger age; (2) high school graduation; (3) annual family income over $75k; and (4) current cannabis use (Pacek, Mauro, & Martins, 2015). In addition, Cerda, Wall, and Keyes (2012) noted two related and potentially problematic, but expected, trends that: (1) residents of states, which have enacted laws decriminalizing cannabis use, have higher odds of cannabis use; and (2) states with legalized cannabis use have higher rates of cannabis use.

36 The intensity and clinical significance of these toxicities depend, to a significant degree, upon the: (1) amount of THC absorbed; (2) environmental setting or circumstances of use; and (3) physical, mental, and social characteristics of the user.

37 A better understanding of cannabis pharmacology (see earlier cannabis pharmacology subsection, "Mechanism of Action") provides possible explanations for many of these observed undesired, or harmful, effects and toxicities. For example, the undesired effects involving human immune response are likely mediated by interactions involving THC, or other cannabinoids, with the CB_2 receptor. The mental depression and psychosis are likely mediated by effects of the endocannabinoid system on the neurotransmitters, dopamine and serotonin. In addition, a genetic expression of various harmful effects (e.g., development of schizophrenia), as noted by Power, Verweij, and Zuhair (2014), likely plays a significant mediating role.

38 The CHS was first identified by Allen, de Moore, and Heddle (2004). It is characterized by: (1) regular, long-term cannabis use; (2) cyclic, intractable nausea and vomiting; and (3) compulsive hot water bathing (Andrews & Bracero, 2015; Nicolson, Denysenko, & Mulcare, 2012).

The hyperemesis phase of the CHS is self-limiting with a usual duration of one to two days. However, continued or resumed cannabis use will generally exacerbate the signs and symptoms. Although the use of standard antiemetic pharmacotherapy is ineffective for most CHS patients, a hot bath or shower, as reported by patients, provides effective, although only temporary relief. Hospitalization may be required in cases of severe volume depletion or other acute medical contexts (Galli, Andari Sawaya, & Friedenberg, 2011).

39 As identified by van Holst and Schilt (2011), the neuropsychological dysfunction (e.g., cognitive impairment; memory impairment), which is associated with the occasional, or short-term, use of cannabis, does not persist following a period of abstinence from its use (i.e., does not appear to be permanent—in contrast to the neurotoxicity associated with regular, long-term amphetamine use). (For further related discussion, see Chapter 2, "Amphetamines and Cocaine".) However, this conclusion remains open to debate and warrants further research, particularly in the context of the regular, long-term use of higher-dosages/potencies of cannabis that is attendant with the legalization of cannabis for "recreational use" in several states.

For example, Camchong, Lim, and Kumra (2017) conducted a longitudinal study of the effects of high-dosage cannabis use among adolescents (mean age of 17 years) and determined that, "repeated exposure to cannabis during adolescence may have detrimental effects on brain resting functional connectivity, intelligence, and cognitive function" (p. 1922).

- Prenatal developmental interference (see later cannabis subsection, "Pregnancy and Lactation");
- Psychosis (see additional related discussion in later section, "Cannabis-Induced Psychotic Disorder");
- Pulmonary irritation (e.g., cough and colds, with the eventual development of related COPD [i.e., asthma; bronchitis]);[40]
- Suicidality (i.e., suicide ideation, suicide planning, suicide attempt, and suicide completion);[41]
- Xerostomia.

<u>Related Professional Reminder:</u> Because of the similarities of the CHS to both the cyclic vomiting syndrome and hyperemesis gravidarum, its clinical diagnosis is often missed among adolescent girls and young women who are pregnant. A differential diagnosis of CHS should always be considered when patients present with cyclic intractable vomiting, particular that which is temporarily relieved by compulsive hot water bathing.

Although these and other toxicities associated with regular, long-term use have been extensively documented in the published literature, relatively few serious (i.e., incapacitating or life threatening) toxicities have been directly associated with cannabis use. The available evidence, from controlled clinical studies and common sense (i.e., logical conclusions based on knowledge of cannabis pharmacology), point to four relatively major toxicities that are directly linked to the regular, long-term use of cannabis: (1) amotivational syndrome; (2) motor vehicle and other crashes, including airplane, train, and truck crashes; (3) psychosis; and (4) pulmonary toxicity. (Also see later subsections, "Physical and Mental Dependence" and "Pregnancy and Lactation.")

AMOTIVATIONAL SYNDROME

Amotivational syndrome, or burn out, is identified among regular, long-term cannabis users.[42] Generally, after several months to years of using cannabis to "mellow-out" or to forget their problems, these individuals tend to lose interest in their homes, work and social environments and the challenges of life. They typically content themselves, alone, each day, doing little else

40 Although not listed because of a paucity of available reliable published data, lung cancer would be an expected chronic toxicity associated with regular, long-term cannabis smoking. This toxic effect would be expected because of: (1) the presence of known human carcinogens in cannabis smoke in concentrations significantly higher than those found in tobacco cigarette smoke (e.g., Ashton, 2001); and (2) the method of smoking cannabis (i.e., inhaling the cannabis smoke deeply into the lungs and holding it in the lungs as long as possible) (e.g., Pagliaro, 1983). This smoking technique is thought to maximize the contact of the smoke with the alveoli and, hence, increase the amount of THC absorbed by the capillaries for distribution through the circulatory system. Vaporized THC significantly decreases or eliminates this risk (see also the related discussion in the later cannabis subsections, "Pulmonary Toxicities" and "Vaping").

41 The relationship between regular, long-term cannabis use and suicide is reportedly positive, but modest (e.g., Borges, Bagge, & Orozco, 2016; Delforterie, Lynskey, & Huizink, 2015). However, we tend to question these findings and suggest that other underlying variables (e.g., mental depression), or other concomitant cofactors, likely play a major—if not determining—role in this reported relationship between cannabis use and suicidality. Interestingly, in comparison to states in which cannabis use was not legalized, its legal use among middle-aged men has been associated with a reduction in suicides (Anderson, Rees, & Sabia, 2014).

42 This syndrome, which has been generally recognized since the 1970s, is supported by evidence that is largely anecdotal and is derived from case reports and uncontrolled studies. Several researchers (e.g., Johns, 2001; Pagliaro & Pagliaro, *Clinical Patient Data Files*) question the validity of this syndrome and suggest that what is observed is simply the expected behavior associated with "chronic," long-term cannabis intoxication. In this context, it may be more pronounced among some cannabis users because of their related: (1) age and developmental level; (2) pattern of use; (3) personality characteristics; and (4) social factors.

than looking through favorite magazines, listening to music, watching their favorite television programs, and playing android or iPhone games on their cell phones while they smoke cannabis. As noted by Castle (2013):

> An "amotivational syndrome" has been described in chronic, heavy cannabis users. The syndrome resembles the negative symptoms of schizophrenia and is characterized by apathy, amotivation, social withdrawal, narrowing of interests, lethargy, impaired memory, impaired concentrations, disturbed judgment, and impaired occupational achievement.
>
> (p. 2)

Whether the use of cannabis causes this syndrome, or whether it merely brings out the latent personality characteristics of an individual adolescent or young adult, has not yet been clearly determined.

MOTOR VEHICLE AND OTHER CRASHES

Motor vehicle and other crashes are a major concern in regard to adolescents and young adults who use/abuse any form of cannabis.

Common Misbelief: It is relatively safe to smoke marijuana while driving a car.

Several large meta-analyses have found that acute cannabis intoxication results in a significant increase in the odds ratios of being involved in a motor vehicle crash (motor vehicle collision, MVC). For example, Li, Brady, and DiMaggio (2012) reported that:

> The results of this meta-analysis suggest that marijuana use by drivers is associated with a significantly increased risk of being involved in motor vehicle crashes.
>
> (p. 65)

As found by Asbridge, Hayden, and Cartwright (2012):

> Acute cannabis consumption is associated with an increased risk of a motor vehicle crash, especially for fatal collisions.
>
> (p. 1)

Regular, long-term cannabis users, are at greatest risk for motor vehicle and other crashes, particularly if they: (1) use high potency cannabis; (2) are drivers who concomitantly abuse both cannabis and alcohol, which can result in deleterious, synergistic effects—associated with different mechanisms of action—on driving ability; and (3) are younger, or inexperienced, drivers (Pagliaro & Pagliaro, 2009; Stein, Caviness, & Anderson, 2014).[43]

43 N.B. It is particularly important to recognize that the incidence of cannabis-related MVCs is increasing (e.g., Christophersen, Morland, & Stewart, 2016) and we fully expect it to continue to do so over the next decade as increasing numbers of states legalize marijuana use or decriminalize its possession and use. For example, Couper and Peterson (2014), in their comprehensive study of drug use and motor vehicle accidents, or MVAs—pre- and post-legalization in Washington state, found that while other drug use remained constant, marijuana use significantly increased (i.e., from 25% to over 50%).

While most cannabis researchers generally agree that there is a direct relationship between cannabis intoxication and decreased driving performance, others (e.g., Sewell, Poling, & Sofuoglu, 2009) continue to argue the contrary, positing the following rationale in support of their position:

1. That alcohol, which is legal and, generally, socially acceptable, impairs driving performance to a significantly greater extent than does cannabis;
2. That cannabis users are less likely to smoke and drive than to drink and drive;
3. That cannabis users, because cognition is significantly less compromised than with alcohol use, are consciously aware of the "impairment" associated with their cannabis use, and, therefore, take conscious precautions (e.g., driving more slowly) in order to compensate and prevent associated motor vehicle crashes.[44]

We believe, however, that it is socially irresponsible (as well as illogical) to disregard the significance of cannabis use in relation to motor vehicle crashes by simply stating that the statistics are not as bad as those associated with alcohol use. The fact is that drivers, who are under the influence of cannabis, cannot drive as well as they can when they are not under the influence of cannabis. The driving impairment—which is directly related to the acute toxicities associate with cannabis use—becomes increasingly severe in direct relation to increasingly high cannabis dosages (i.e., using larger amounts of cannabis or using cannabis that is more potent in terms of relative blood THC concentration) (e.g., Ramaekers, Berghaus, & van Laar, 2004; Sewell, Poling, & Sofuoglu, 2009).

The association between marijuana use and motor vehicle crashes has been supported by the analysis of related data from states where marijuana use has been legalized for "recreational" use (among adults). As identified by Hagler (2017), citing data from the 2015 report entitled, *The Legalization of Marijuana in Colorado: The Impact*:

> The statistics reveal that between 2013 and 2014 there was a 45% increase in marijuana-associated impaired driving, a 32% increase in marijuana-related motor vehicle deaths (with a 92% increase from 2010 to 2014), as well as 29% and 38% increases in emergency room visits and hospital admissions secondary to marijuana use.
>
> (p. 11)

As cannabis use has significantly increased among drivers—coincident with its legalization—law enforcement officers now require a rapid detection quick-screen test for detecting cannabis use. The Draeger Drug Test 5000®, which is produced in Europe, is a mobile drug screening system that can be used to determine cannabis use with a simply obtained roadside sample of the driver's saliva (Platt, 2018). The system is portable, easy to use, and provides immediate results.[45]

In addition, as previously noted, when cannabis is used in combination with alcohol—a fairly common practice, particularly among adolescents and young adults—the research is abundantly clear that the degree of driving impairment is significantly greater (i.e., in comparison to that caused by the use of either cannabis or alcohol alone) (e.g., Ramaekers, Berghaus, & van Laar, 2004; Sewell, Poling, & Sofuoglu, 2009).

44 Sewell, Poling, and Sofuoglu (2009) do point out that, regarding the third posit, it is negated when both cannabis and alcohol are used concomitantly.

45 The Draeger Drug Test 5000® also can be used to determine the use of: amphetamines; benzodiazepines; cocaine; and methadone.

Related Professional Recommendation: ***Without exception, drivers should not smoke or vape cannabis and drive.***[46]

CANNABIS-INDUCED PSYCHOTIC DISORDER—SCHIZOPHRENIA

While severe mental health problems are not generally associated with cannabis use among most cannabis users, it is currently widely recognized that, for some cannabis users, cannabis use can be associated with a wide variety of schizophrenic-like effects, both "positive" and "negative," and negative cognitive effects.[47]

POSITIVE SCHIZOPHRENIA-LIKE EFFECTS. Positive schizophrenia-like effects include:

- Abnormalities in time perception;
- Catatonic behaviors;
- Conceptual disorganization;
- Delusions, usually grandiose;
- Depersonalization;
- Derealization;
- Disorganized speech;
- Fragmented thinking;
- Grossly disorganized behavior;
- Hallucinations;
- Paranoid thoughts;
- Racing thoughts;
- Thought alienation.

NEGATIVE SCHIZOPHRENIA-LIKE EFFECTS. Negative schizophrenia-like effects include:

- Affective flattening;
- Alogia;
- Anhedonia;
- Apathy;

46 Despite this admonition, and its strong support in the published professional and scientific literature (e.g., Hartman & Huestis, 2013), the effects of cannabis use on driving performance have not as yet been ingrained into the public psyche in the U.S. To illustrate this lack of awareness, which is commonly observed among various members of the general public regarding the deleterious effects of cannabis use on motor vehicle driving performance, we share the following two anecdotal cases that we personally recently observed. In the first case, a middle-aged woman, whose driver's license was revoked because of an alcohol-related impaired driving conviction, requested that her adolescent daughter—a daily recreational user of marijuana—be her designated driver.

In another case, an older man—who required a designated driver because his eyes were being dilated as part of his examination—was accompanied by his son in the ophthalmologist's waiting room. After a while, the son told his father that he needed to "go out for a smoke" and to "stretch a bit" to relieve his "back pain." As he left the waiting room, another patient shared that he had recently lost his wife to lung cancer and that, perhaps the man's son should stop smoking. The father quickly clarified that it was "okay." His son was not going out to smoke a tobacco cigarette, but was going out to smoke his medical marijuana, which he used to manage his chronic back pain (Pagliaro & Pagliaro, *Clinical Patient Data Files*.)

47 This has not always been the case in the U.S., nor in the related published western clinical and scientific literature. For example, we were among the first to formally identify this relationship in presentations and publications during the 1970s and 1980s (e.g., Pagliaro, 1983; Pagliaro, 1988) based upon both our clinical experience (i.e., Pagliaro & Pagliaro, *Clinical Patient Data Files*) and review of 100 years of related published East Indian literature from the mid-19th to the mid-20th centuries. However, we commonly received "push back" that either this observation was: (1) inaccurate; or (2) accurate and applicable in India, but not in the U.S.—because of the significant differences in patterns of cannabis use.

- Avolition;
- Decreased rage response;
- Lack of spontaneity;
- Poverty of thought;
- Psychomotor retardation;
- Reduced rapport;
- Social withdrawal.

NEGATIVE COGNITIVE EFFECTS. Negative "cognitive" effects include:

- Decreased attention;
- Impaired executive functioning;
- Reduced ability for abstract thought;
- Reduced problem-solving ability;
- Short-term memory deficits;
- Verbal memory deficits;
- Working memory deficits.

Depending upon the personal characteristics of the adolescent or young adult (e.g., age; genetics, including gender and continental descent) and the patterns of cannabis use (e.g., THC concentration; amount used; frequency of use), these cognitive effects can range in (1) severity (i.e., from mild to severe); and (2) duration (i.e., from transient to "permanent"). Thus, the various effects, which are observed among cannabis users, are not uniform. The etiological relationship between cannabis use and psychosis (i.e., schizophrenia-like effects) also appears to be largely mediated by a shared mechanism involving the endogenous "cannabinoid" receptor, CB_1 (Cohen, Solowij, & Carr, 2008; D'Souza, 2007; Leweke & Koethe, 2008). (Also see earlier cannabis pharmacology subsection, "Pharmacodynamics—Mechanism of Action.")

It is also important to recognize that adolescents and young adults, who are diagnosed with schizophrenia, often use cannabis in an effort to self-medicate related undesired positive, negative, and cognitive effects, as listed earlier (Castle, 2013). Among other adolescents and young adults, for whom schizophrenia is directly induced by the use of cannabis, the effects can be either:

1. Transient, in which case, they may be considered to be undesired, or harmful, effects or toxicities associated with cannabis use;
2. Long-term or "permanent," in which case, the use of cannabis likely elicited or exacerbated the onset, or display, of schizophrenia—particularly in susceptible "pre-schizophrenics" (i.e., those with pre-dispositions to schizophrenia) (Castle, 2013; Radhakrishnan, Wilkinson, & D'Souza, 2014).[48]

It also should be recognized that adolescents and young adults, who have been diagnosed with schizophrenia and who are also in remission, may relapse—with full-blown symptomatology—when cannabis use is resumed (Pagliaro & Pagliaro, *Clinical Patient Data Files*).

PULMONARY TOXICITIES

Cannabis smoking, particularly among adolescents and young adults who also smoke tobacco cigarettes or have chronic obstructive pulmonary disease (COPD), is associated with a further compromise of pulmonary function due to additive or synergic irritation and damage to lung

48 Adolescents and young adults, who have polymorphisms of COMT and AKT1 genes, may be at increased risk for psychotic disorders in association with the use of cannabinoids (Radhakrishnan, Wilkinson, & D'Souza, 2014).

tissue (e.g., Hancox, Poulton, & Ely, 2010; Lee & Hancox, 2011; Pagliaro & Pagliaro, 2009; Taylor, Fergusson, & Milne 2002).

The pulmonary toxicity identified among regular, long-term, or heavy, cannabis smokers is primarily related to the components (e.g., ammonia, hydrogen cyanide, and nitric oxide) in cannabis smoke other than THC (Pagliaro, 1983, 1988, 2012, 2018).[49] Therefore, the severity of these pulmonary effects depends more on the:

1. Amount of cannabis smoked;
2. Smoking techniques employed;
3. Combustion properties of the materials used in the production of cannabis products, including the "joint" wrapping paper (Pagliaro & Pagliaro, 2009).[50]

For example, regarding effects on airway obstruction, Aldington, Williams, and Nowitz (2007)—utilizing high-resolution computed tomography (HRCT) scanning, pulmonary function tests, and a smoking questionnaire—found that "one cannabis joint had a similar effect to 2.5–five tobacco cigarettes" (p. 1058). Although replication studies and confirmatory data are currently lacking, we have long warned of the risk of cannabis smoking as a carcinogen or co-carcinogen contributing to lung cancer in genetically susceptible individuals. Joshi, Joshi and Bartter (2014), in their review of the effects of marijuana smoke on the respiratory system, noted that:

> The immuno-histopathologic and epidemiologic evidence in marijuana users suggest biological plausibility of marijuana smoking as a risk for the development of lung cancer. (p. 173)

Tashkin (2013), as well as other researchers, suggest that the association between cannabis smoking and lung cancer is only evident with "heavy, long-term use" and not with "light or moderate [occasional or regular, short-term] use" (p. 239).

In addition, the respiratory toxicity associated with smoking cannabis can, on occasion, be due to a contaminant, or additive, to the cannabis. For example, Gilbert, Baram, and Cavarocchi (2013) reported two cases of "respiratory failure soon after they had smoked 'wet' marijuana cigarettes" (p. 64). "Wet" marijuana cigarettes, or joints, are typically dipped, prior to smoking, in either "formaldehyde"—known on the street as "embalming fluid"—or phencyclidine (PCP). (See also the discussion in the later psychodelic section, "Phencyclidine.")

PHYSICAL AND PSYCHOLOGICAL DEPENDENCE

The question as to whether the regular, long-term use of cannabis results in physical dependence has been extensively argued over the previous century. However, the new

49 Consequently, although empirical data currently are lacking, we would expect that "vaping" THC would result in a significant reduction of the significant respiratory toxicity that is associated with "smoking a joint."

50 Over 400 chemicals—primarily formed as a result of pyrolysis—can be found in marijuana smoke, including many of the same chemicals that are found in tobacco smoke. When marijuana is smoked, it yields more tar than tobacco. In addition, the tar from marijuana smoke has higher concentrations of certain carcinogens (e.g., benzo(a)pyrene) than are found in the tar from tobacco smoke. Thus, it is probable that marijuana smoking will produce more lung cancer when compared to tobacco smoking, which currently is the leading cause of lung cancer in the world.

Based upon the chemical constituents found in the pyrolysis products of marijuana smoke versus the pyrolysis products of tobacco smoke, and comparative differences in smoking techniques for marijuana versus tobacco (i.e., smoking the entire joint and inhaling the marijuana smoke more deeply into the lungs where it is held in the lower respiratory tract for a longer period of time), we have, for several decades (e.g., Pagliaro, 1974, 1983, 1988; Pagliaro & Pagliaro 1996, 2004, 2009) estimated that smoking one joint of marijuana subjects smokers to as much irritation and associated damage to the respiratory system, along with subsequent risk for lung cancer, as smoking one package (i.e., 20) filter-tipped tobacco cigarettes.

millennial consensus is that it does.[51] The regular, long-term, high-dosage use of cannabis is clearly recognized as being associated with the development of physical dependence (e.g., Khalsa, Genser, & Francis, 2002; Maldonado & Rodriguez de Fonseca, 2002). Reflecting the classic definition of physical dependence, regular, long-term cannabis use is associated with both tolerance and withdrawal. Winstock, Ford, and Witton (2010) noted that approximately 10% of regular cannabis users develop dependence.[52]

For adolescent girls and young women, the length of time from the initiation of cannabis use to the development of cannabis dependence or use disorder, as well as, "time to entrance into treatment"—is generally significantly shorter than that for adolescent boys and young men (Ehlers, Gizer, & Vieten, 2010; Hernandez-Avilla, Rounsaville, & Kranzler, 2004; Khan, Secades-Villa, & Okuda, 2013). This phenomenon is referred to as "telescoping." In addition, young women of African continental descent, particularly those whose marijuana use preceded their alcohol use, are significantly more likely to experience telescoping than are young women of European continental descent (Sartor, Agrawal, & Lynskey, 2013).

CANNABIS TOLERANCE. The development of tolerance to cannabis, as related to its regular, long-term use, has been associated with the interaction of CB_1 receptors with cannabis agonists, particularly THC. This prolonged interaction results in the:

1. Desensitization of the receptors (i.e., a decrease in their ability to activate effector pathways);
2. Corresponding reduction in the number of related receptors.

(Kendall & Yudowski, 2017)

Since the 1960s, the higher average potency of cannabis in the U.S. (as noted in earlier cannabis subsections), has been tremendous (i.e., a five- to ten-fold plus increase in THC concentration). This higher potency appears to have significantly increased the probability for developing cannabis physical dependence or CUD—and the associated recognition of the: (1) clinically significant development of tolerance, or the need to use increasing amounts of cannabis in an effort to achieve initial desired effects; and (2) occurrence of the cannabis withdrawal syndrome when regular, long-term use is abruptly discontinued.

CANNABIS WITHDRAWAL SYNDROME. Following the abrupt discontinuation of regular, long-term cannabis use, the cannabis withdrawal syndrome is commonly experienced. In fact,

51 For example, since its 4th edition in 1994, the *Diagnostic and Statistical Manual of Mental Disorders* (DSM-IV) (APA, 2000) has listed cannabis dependence in its taxonomy based largely upon noted tolerance and a well-recognized withdrawal syndrome. However, until the last decade of the 20th century, it was generally thought that only psychological dependence, not physical dependence, was likely to develop with the regular, long-term use of cannabis. Currently, the DSM-5 (APA, 2013) subsumes these related conditions under the classification of "cannabis use disorder" (CUD)—the continued use of cannabis regardless of significant impairment ranging from mild to severe. (See also the related discussion in the later cannabis subsections, "Assessment and Diagnosis of Adolescent and Young Adult Cannabis Dependence or Use Disorder" and "Treating Adolescent and Young Adult Cannabis Dependence or Use Disorder.")

52 In comparison, Hasin, Kerridge, and Saha (2016), in their analysis of data from the *National Epidemiologic Survey on Alcohol and Related Conditions-III* (NESARC-III), found that adults, 18 years-of-age and older, had a lifetime prevalence of CUD to be 6.3%. This number appears to be consistent with that reported by Winstock, Ford, and Witton (2010)—given that adolescents were largely excluded from the analysis and that the young adult cohort (i.e., 18 to 29 years-of-age) reportedly had the highest rate of lifetime CUD among adults.

Budney, Hughes, and Moore (2004) identified that up to 85% of cannabis users experience withdrawal.[53] The occurrence of the cannabis withdrawal syndrome is supported by two major pieces of evidence:

1. Pharmacological characterization of the endocannabinoid system (see the discussion in the earlier cannabis subsection, "Pharmacology, Pharmacodynamics—Mechanism of Action");
2. Acute demonstration of characteristic signs and symptoms when a CB_1 cannabinoid receptor antagonist is administered to an active cannabis user as part of a controlled research study.

(e.g., Budney & Hughes, 2006; Cooper & Haney, 2009)

The characteristic signs and symptoms, which are generally considered to be relatively mild, or non-life threatening, include:

- Aggression;
- Anger;
- Anorexia;
- Anxiety;
- Chills;
- Cramping;
- Craving for cannabis;
- Diaphoresis;
- Dreaming increased;
- Headaches;
- Hypersomnia;
- Hyperthermia;
- Insomnia;
- Irritability;
- Mental depression;
- Nausea;
- Nervousness;
- Nightmares;
- Restlessness;
- Rebound increase in rapid eye movement (REM) sleep;
- Tremor;
- Weakness;
- Weight loss.

(Bonnet & Preuss, 2017; Budney, Hughes, & Moore, 2004; Cornelius, Chung, & Martin, 2008; Pagliaro & Pagliaro, 2004)

Lasting for up to five days, the signs and symptoms associated with the cannabis withdrawal syndrome generally peak on day one (Pagliaro & Pagliaro, 2009; Preuss, Watzke, & Zimmermann, 2010).

Most adolescents and young adults, who experience the cannabis withdrawal syndrome, report a wide variance in the severity of the characteristic signs and symptoms of the cannabis

53 N.B. The self-medication of this withdrawal syndrome, whether performed consciously or unconsciously, has been determined to be a major factor contributing to recidivism following discontinuation of cannabis use (Pagliaro & Pagliaro, *Clinical Patient Data Files*; Winstock, Ford, & Witton, 2010).

withdrawal syndrome. This variance appears to be associated with several factors, including the:

1. Amount and potency of the cannabis used;
2. Concurrent use of other drugs and substances of abuse;
3. Duration of regular, long-term use;
4. Genetic predisposition;
5. History of childhood physical or sexual abuse (Sartor, Agrawal, & Grant, 2015; Sartor, Waldron, & Duncan, 2013; Simpson & Miller, 2002);
6. Major depressive or psychotic disorder—the factor that appears to account for most of the observed variance.

(Arendt, Rosenberg, & Foldager, 2007; Khan, Secades-Villa, & Okuda, 2013; Preuss, Watzke, & Zimmermann, 2010)

Cannabis Overdosage/Unintentional Poisoning

Surprisingly, given the historical record of 5,000-plus years of human cannabis use (Pagliaro & Pagliaro, 2004), the toxicities associated with its use have not yet been fully evaluated. However, it appears that fatal overdosages are relatively rare. In fact, during the last two centuries, the general medical consensus has been that the occasional use of cannabis is not particularly harmful and that the intermittent use of low potency cannabis is not generally associated with obvious signs and symptoms of toxicity (ARF/WHO, 1981).

However, cannabis exposure and unintentional poisoning involving infants and young children increased during the first two decades of the new millennium. Of concern, it is expected to continue to increase as additional states legalize the medical and recreational use of cannabis (Pagliaro & Pagliaro, *Clinical Patient Data Files*). When such exposure occurs, recommended medical treatment is largely supportive and guided by the presenting signs and symptoms.

There is no available antidote for cannabis overdosage/unintentional poisoning. Additionally, although several authors (e.g., Crippa, Derenusson, & Chagas, 2017) have recommended various pharmacotherapeutic approaches for the management of cannabis overdosage/unintentional poisoning (e.g., antagonists of CB_1; antipsychotics; beta-adrenergic blockers; cannabidiol), none of these approaches have consistently demonstrated clinical efficacy and none have received specific FDA approval for these indications. Consequently, pharmacotherapy is primarily individually selected on the basis of presenting signs and symptoms and applied, as needed, on a case by case basis. (See also the related discussion in the later cannabis subsection, treating adolescent and young adult cannabis dependence or use disorder—"Pharmacotherapy").[54]

During the new millennium, in the U.S., increasing numbers of states passed laws to:

1. Decriminalize cannabis use;
2. Legalize medical cannabis use;
3. Legalize recreational cannabis use.

Within this context, Wang, Roosevelt, and Le Lait (2014) identified an associated increase in "unintentional pediatric exposures." As found by Hagler (2017), in a report on behalf of the American College of Pediatricians:

54 N.B. Gastric decontamination with activated charcoal is generally ineffective and may place infants at risk of aspiration associated with possible vomiting.

> There is evidence legalization of marijuana limited to medical dispensaries and/or adult recreational use has led to increased unintended exposure to marijuana among young children. By 2011, rates of poison center calls for accidental pediatric marijuana ingestion more than tripled in states that decriminalized marijuana before 2005. In states which passed legislation between 2005 and 2011 call rates increased nearly 11.5% per year. There was no similar increase in states that had not decriminalized marijuana as of December 31, 2011. Additionally, exposures in decriminalized states where marijuana use was legalized were more likely than those in non-legal states to present with moderate to severe symptoms requiring admission to a pediatric intensive care unit. The median age of children involved was 18–24 months.
>
> (p. 1–2)

A subsequent related study by Onders, Casavant, and Spiller (2016) confirmed these general findings. In their analyses of cannabis exposure among children younger than six years-of-age, utilizing data obtained from the National Poison Data System for the years 2000 through 2013, they found that:

> The rate of marijuana exposure was significantly (2.82 times) higher in states where its use was legalized prior to 2000 compared with states where its use is *not* legal.
>
> (p. 428)

In addition, they reported that the:

1. Mean age of exposure was two years-of-age;
2. Majority of exposures (i.e., 75%) were by means of ingestion;
3. Approximately, one in five exposures required admission to a health care facility.

In another related study, Cao, Srisuma, and Bronstein (2016) analyzed data from the National Poison Data System for the years 2013 through 2015—specifically in regard to human exposure calls involving edible marijuana products (i.e., beverages, brownies, candies, and cookies). The majority of cases occurred among children, younger than six years-of-age, followed by adolescents, 13 to 19 years-of-age. In addition, over 90% of related calls, which were reported to the National Poison Data System, were from states in which marijuana use for medical and/or recreational use was decriminalized/legalized.

> A young girl got sick after eating cannabis-infused gummy bears ... the child was reported to have been in the back seat of her parents' vehicle when she discovered some discarded candies and then ate an unknown number of them.
>
> (Wood, 2018, p. 1)

<u>Related Professional Reminder:</u> Cases of cannabis poisoning involving children, whether intentional or unintentional, should be reported to Child Protective Services.

Pregnancy and Lactation

Although THC crosses the placenta, a number of studies of infrequent or moderate use by adolescent girls and young women during pregnancy have not been significantly associated with teratogenic effects. However, some studies and reports (e.g., Bryant, 2015; Fried & Smith, 2001; Richardson, Ryan, & Willford, 2002) suggest that higher order cognitive functioning among children, such as attentional processes and analysis/hypothesis testing, is negatively correlated with in utero exposure to cannabis. We also note concerns regarding possible long-term negative effects of in utero exposure upon subsequent memory processes (e.g., encoding and retrieval mechanisms) (Pagliaro & Pagliaro, 1996, 2009). THC also is excreted into breast milk and expected effects (e.g., drowsiness) can be observed among breastfed neonates and infants.

In addition, because the endocannabinoid system appears to be involved in brain development—cell proliferation and differentiation—several authors (e.g., Crane, Schuster, & Gonzalez, 2013; Schneider, 2008; Trezza, Cuomo, & Vanderschuren, 2008) have expressed concerns that there is a significant risk for cannabis toxicity during periods of high neuronal plasticity (e.g., prenatal period, late adolescence, and early adulthood) and, consequently, its potential effects on executive functioning, including problem solving and other higher cognitive functions.

These potential effects are cause for particular concern during the new millennium because of the recognition that the use of cannabis has become the primary reason for seeking inpatient treatment for SUDs among pregnant adolescent girls and young women. For example, in 2007, 45.9% of the admissions of pregnant adolescent girls and young women for inpatient treatment, across the U.S., were primarily related to cannabis use (Substance Abuse and Mental Health Services Administration, 2011). This statistic reflects a significant change from the statistics reported 15 years earlier, in 1992, when admission for pregnant adolescent girls and young women for treatment of SUDs were primarily related to alcohol use—with marijuana use accounting for only 19.3 % of other admissions at that time.

Another noted change among pregnant adolescent girls and young women during the new millennium in the U.S. is the finding that they are usually more likely to concurrently use two or more drugs or substances of abuse while pregnant. Buchi, Suarez, and Varner (2013), in their analysis of data obtained from women in labor and delivery units across Utah, found that the most frequently detected abusable psychotropic drugs were:

- Alcohol;
- Cocaine;
- Marijuana;
- Methamphetamine;
- Opiate analgesics.

These findings appear to be generally consistent among pregnant women, including adolescent girls and young women, across the U.S. However, regional differences—primarily in relation to age, drug availability, and sociocultural/ethnic factors, as well as, continental and other descent—affect the choice of drugs and substances of abuse used by pregnant adolescent girls and young women.

In response to the increasing use of cannabis by adolescent girls and young women during pregnancy—particularly at a time of growing social acceptance of its use—Gunn, Rosales, and Center (2016) sought to assess maternal and fetal outcomes regarding the effects of cannabis use during pregnancy. Retrospective meta-analysis of 24 studies from seven electronic databases was conducted. Major findings included a significantly increased odds ratio of: (1) anemia among women who used cannabis during pregnancy; (2) decreased birth weights among neonates exposed to cannabis in utero; and (3) increased need for placement of neonates, who were born to mothers who used cannabis during pregnancy, in neonatal intensive care units (NICUs).

> "Teen Mom" Jenelle Evans reveals drug use while pregnant with daughter ... I tested positive for THC ...
>
> (Evans, 2018, p.1)

Applying an approach which favors the utilization of an "abundance of caution," it has been recommended that adolescent girls and young women should *not* smoke or otherwise use cannabis because of the potential risks to their offspring (O'Mara & Nahata, 2002; Pagliaro, 1995; Pagliaro & Pagliaro, 2002, 2018). In addition to the concerns already stipulated, the NIH reported that the risk for stillbirth increases up to 2.3-fold in association with maternal marijuana use. Cannabis use by young mothers of infants and young children may also negatively affect their mothering/parenting (Pagliaro & Pagliaro, *Clinical Patient Data Files*). It also has been associated with a higher incidence of marijuana use by offspring later in life. For these reasons, several professional organizations (e.g., *The American Congress of Obstetricians and Gynecologists* [ACOG]) have made formal recommendations that the use of marijuana be totally avoided by all pregnant adolescent girls and young women and by those who are breastfeeding (ACOG, 2015a, 2015b). However, others (e.g., *American Academy of Pediatrics*)—noting "the lack of definitive research"—urge discussion with pregnant cannabis users regarding possible risks (Ryan, Ammerman, & O'Connor, 2018, p. 10).

We now turn to child, adolescent, and young adult cannabis exposure and use during the new millennium.

New Millennial Trends in Cannabis Use

This section presents and discusses new trends in cannabis use during the new millennium, in the U.S., with attention both to the medical use of cannabis and to exposure for children, adolescents, and young adults. Also presented and discussed are trends in adolescent and young adult illicit/recreational use of cannabis including methods of use and drug involvement.

Child Medical Cannabis Use

"Medical marijuana" has been prescribed for children, adolescents, and young adults for the treatment of ADHD—as a non-FDA approved indication—since 2009. "Medicinal marijuana" also has been advocated and used for children in the U.S. for the treatment of a wide variety of other conditions, including:

- Anorexia;
- Autism;
- Chemotherapy-induced nausea and vomiting;
- Chronic pain;
- Developmental disorders;
- Neuroblastoma;
- Seizure disorders[55](e.g., Campbell, Shaw Phillips, & Manasco, 2017; Rieder, 2016; Shucheng Wong & Wilens, 2017).

We do not generally recommend the medical use of marijuana for children[56] because of the:

1. Inadequate quantity and quality of supportive published research;

55 In June 2018, the FDA approved the use of CBD oral solution (Epidiolex®) for the treatment of two rare and severe seizure disorders for patients two years-of-age and older: (1) Lennox-Gastaut Syndrome; and (2) Dravet Syndrome (FDA, 2018).

56 The only exception that we have endorsed for several decades is the use of cannabis, in its various forms, for the attempted medical management of seizure disorders among children who have been refractory to traditional anticonvulsant pharmacotherapy (Pagliaro & Pagliaro, *Clinical Patient Data Files*).

2. Inconsistent therapeutic results, based virtually exclusively, on uncontrolled published case studies and reports—or animal and in vitro research studies;
3. Lack of formal FDA approval.

Adolescent and Young Adult Medical Cannabis Use

Cannabis, in the form of its chemical surrogates dronabinol [Marinol®; Syndros®]),[57] and nabilone (Cesamet®),[58] are approved by the FDA for the medical management of:

1. Anorexia with weight loss among patients with AIDS;
2. Mild to moderate nausea and vomiting associated with cancer chemotherapy.

However, contrary to existing U.S. federal law (e.g., Mead, 2017), a majority of states have individually legalized the medicinal use of cannabis in a variety of formulations (e.g., foods, beverages, pharmaceuticals) for the treatment of many physical and mental conditions including:

- Acquired immune deficiency syndrome (AIDS);
- Anorexia;
- Arthritis;
- Cachexia;
- Chronic pain;
- Glaucoma;
- Migraine headaches;
- Nausea (severe);
- Persistent muscle spasms (e.g., as related to multiple sclerosis);[59]
- Seizure disorders;
- Any other chronic or persistent medical signs or symptoms that either: (1) limit the patient's ability to conduct a major life activity as defined in the *Americans With Disabilities Act* of 1990, Public Law 101–3336; or (2) if not alleviated, may cause serious harm to the patient's safety or physical and/or mental health (e.g., medical marijuana has been prescribed, as noted earlier, for children and adolescents for the treatment of ADHD since 2009).[60]

Supporting evidence regarding claims of efficacy for these and other conditions has been largely anecdotal, but is summarized in Table 4.2.

In states in which cannabis is legalized, adults, including young adults, who have a medical prescription—including prescriptions for their children—can legally purchase, possess, and use various prescribed forms and amounts of cannabis, particularly marijuana.

57 Dronabinol is a synthetic form of THC.

58 Nabilone is a synthetic cannabinoid.

59 In Canada, a formulation of equal parts of CBD and THC was approved in 2015 for the symptomatic relief of spasticity in adults with multiple sclerosis. The combination is referred to as "nabiximols" and is available under the trade name, "Sativex®." Sativex® is administered as a buccal (i.e., oromucosal) spray (Russo, Calabro, & Naro, 2015).

60 Given the growing attention to the devastating opiate analgesic epidemic in the U.S. (see related discussion in Chapter 5, "Prescription Opiate Analgesics and Heroin"), several "cannabis proponents"—including legislators (e.g., Senator Elizabeth Warren [Granowicz, 2016]) and lay proponents (e.g., Herman, 2018; Kaplan, 2018; Lieber, 2018) —have touted the beneficial role of medical cannabis use in the context of reducing opioid overdosage deaths. However, related empirical evidence has been characterized as being "very weak" (Swift Yasgur, 2018).

Table 4.2 Evidence Supporting Claims of Medicinal Cannabis/Cannabinoid Efficacy for Selected Indications

Indication	*Evidence of Cannabis/Cannabinoid Efficacy*[61]
Acute Pain	Subjective reports of pain relief among users have not been generally supported by human, placebo-controlled studies. Animal studies have suggested an effect on the natural analgesic system
AIDS-Related Cachexia	Approved by the FDA to treat AIDS-related anorexia and associated weight loss
Alzheimer's Disease	Preliminary results from animal and in vitro studies, as well as the study of human post-mortem brain samples, suggest possible benefits
Anxiety	May reduce anxiety among some users
Antineoplastic-Related Nausea and Vomiting	Synthetic cannabinoids (i.e., dronabinol [Marinol; Syndros®]; nabilone [Cesamet®; Canemes®]) have been approved by the FDA for this indication
Glaucoma	Some studies have demonstrated that cannabis use can decrease intraocular pressure. However, results are generally short-lived, lasting for only a few hours
Neuropathic Pain, Multiple Sclerosis, and Related Spasticity	Cannabis use may reduce the intensity of chronic neuropathic pain in a minority of users. Reduction in motor dysfunction and pain may be related to anti-inflammatory and neuroprotective endocannabinoid actions in the CNS. Cannabis use may reduce associated muscle stiffness or spasms
Traumatic Brain Injury (TBI)	Animal models and limited human clinical data suggest that the endocannabinoid system is involved in the response to TBI and that agonists (both endogenous and exogenous) can decrease brain inflammation and related edema

Sources: Canadian Pharmacists Association (2018); Maida & Daeninck (2016); Kendall & Yudowski (2017); Mayo Clinic Staff (2017); Pagliaro & Pagliaro (2004, 2009, 2018).

Marijuana also can be grown for personal, or recreational, use.[62] However, it is more commonly purchased from specialized marijuana dispensaries. Currently, 41 states have some form of an active, voter-approved medical marijuana program.

61 N.B. Particularly regarding cannabis use, reported efficacy also includes the contribution of any related "placebo effect," which has also been reported in relation to the use of edible cannabis products (Loflin, Earleywine, & Farmer, 2017).

62 N.B. Several states (i.e., Alaska, California, Colorado, Illinois, Michigan, Nevada, Oregon, and Washington), as well as the District of Columbia, have legalized the non-medical, recreational/social use of marijuana (Berke, 2018; Miller, 2016). However, even in these states and district, an individual must be 21 years of age to legally buy, possess, or use "retail" marijuana (Robinson, 2018; Sanchez, 2014).

Embryo/Fetus, Neonate/Infant, and Child Cannabis Exposure

Infant and young child exposure to cannabis, usually marijuana, is related to: (1) in utero exposure; (2) breastfeeding exposure; and (3) accidental/unintentional exposure or poisoning. Fortunately, none of these exposures are typically associated with significant clinical sequelae. (See related discussion in the earlier cannabis pharmacology subsections, "Pregnancy and Lactation" and "Cannabis Overdosage.") Children also may be (4) medically exposed to cannabis for a variety of indications. (See the previous subsection, "Child Medical Cannabis Use.")

Adolescent and Young Adult Illicit/Recreational Marijuana Use

"Marijuana is the most frequently used illicit substance in the U.S." (Cerda, Wall, & Keyes, 2012, p. 22). It also "is the most commonly used illicit drug among adolescents" (Murphy, Barry, & Vaughn, 2013). For example, Murphy, Barry, and Vaughn (2013), citing data from the *Monitoring the Future Survey*, report that lifetime prevalence of marijuana use among U.S. high school seniors was approximately 50%. Johnson, Fairman, and Gilreath (2015), utilizing data from the *National Youth Risk Behavior Survey* of 9th to 12th grade students in the U.S., found that:

> The prevalence of past 30-day use from 1999–2013 for all groups and both sexes was 22.5%, and it was lowest among Asians and highest among American Indian/Alaska Natives. Although boys have historically had a higher prevalence of marijuana use, results indicate that male-female differences in marijuana use decreased over time.
>
> (p. 8)

The Office of Adolescent Health (2017) reported that lifetime marijuana use among U.S. high school students (i.e., grades nine to 12) was approximately 40% for 2013 and 2015 with adolescent boys and girls reporting relatively equal use rates.

During the new millennium, adolescent use of marijuana has been increasingly guided by related changing trends in public attitudes toward marijuana use. For example, as found by Motel (2015, pp. 1–3), the changing trends supporting marijuana legalization are rapidly outpacing opposition:

- 68% of Americans say marijuana should be legalized in the U.S.
- 70% of Americans say alcohol is more harmful to a person's health than marijuana.
- 57% of Americans would not be bothered if a store or business selling legal marijuana opened-up in their neighborhood.
- 50% of Americans say they have tried marijuana.
- Several states (i.e., Alaska; California; Colorado; Illinois; Michigan; Oregon; Washington) and the District of Columbia have legalized the "recreational" use of marijuana.

As identified by Azofeifa, Mattson, and Schauer (2016)—and previously discussed earlier in this chapter:

> A decrease in the perception of great risk from smoking marijuana combined with increases in the perception of availability (i.e., fairly easy or very easy to obtain marijuana) and fewer punitive legal penalties (e.g., no penalty) for the possession of marijuana for personal use might play a role in increased use among adults.
>
> (p. 1)

Several other authors (e.g., Berg, Stratton, & Schauer, 2015; Hanby Hudgens, 2017; Newman, 2017) have noted similar findings among adolescents and young adults in the U.S.

> Teen marijuana use increased 24% after Colorado allowed medical marijuana in 2010. That number increased another 8 percent after the passing of recreational marijuana in 2013.
>
> (Ballinger, 2018, p. 1)

According to a 2016 Gallup poll of over 1,000 adults in all 50 states and the District of Columbia:

> The percentage of American adults who say they currently smoke marijuana has nearly doubled since 2013. Thirteen percent of adults in the U.S. now say they currently smoke pot—up from 7 percent in 2013.
>
> (Miller, 2016, p. 3)[63]

As identified by Frobe, Leeman, and Patock-Peckham (2018):

> Cannabis is the most commonly used illicit substance in the United States and is increasing among young adults (18- to 25-year-olds).
>
> (p. 32)

Additionally, Schulenberg, Johnston, and O'Malley (2017) reported that daily use of cannabis among 18 to 23 year-olds was approximately 8%—the highest it has been in 40 years.

COMMON METHODS OF MARIJUANA USE

Generally, adolescents use two common methods of marijuana self-administration: (1) ingestion; and (2) pulmonary inhalation (i.e., smoking; vaporizing). The more recent legalization of medicinal marijuana in many states (see previous bullet list) has resulted in the development of a wide variety of edible marijuana products (e.g., brownies; butters; cakes; caramels; chocolates; granola bars; "gummy bears;" and lollipops).[64] These edible products can be purchased at local marijuana dispensaries along with, or as alternatives to, the extensive varieties of marijuana buds and leaves that are also legally sold in these dispensaries.

However, because the bioavailability of ingested marijuana products is low (i.e., ~ 10%), in order to achieve equivalent actions, the required dosage of ingested products must be generally five times higher than that of inhaled marijuana products.[65] This difference in

63 Given the consistent and growing movement toward decriminalization, medical use, and legalized "recreational" use of cannabis across the U.S. during the second decade of the new millennium, we fully expect, as previously noted, that, over the next several decades, the: (1) percentage of both adolescents and adults, who use cannabis, will continue to increase; and (2) usage discrepancies between the genders, which have been decreasing over the new millennium, will totally "disappear" (Pagliaro & Pagliaro, *Clinical Patient Data Files*). These trends in adolescent marijuana use statistics are supported by the signaling hypothesis, "which posits [that] decriminalization is a [significant] risk factor for future increases in youth marijuana prevalence and acceptance" (Miech, Johnston, & O'Malley, 2015, p. 340). Additionally, the concomitant use of both cannabis and nicotine (i.e., smoking both marijuana "joints" and tobacco cigarettes over the past 30 days) has significantly increased in states where medical marijuana is legal compared to illegal (Wang, Ramo, & Lisha, 2016).

64 During the 19th century, cannabis was also ingested as candy bonbons or baked into foods, such as cookies and brownies. The ingestion of cannabis in its various forms continued through the 1950s, 1960s, and 1970—often utilizing a classic "brownie hashish fudge" recipe that was developed and popularized by Alice B. Toklas (1954).

65 Although hashish oil may be injected intravenously, this method of use is relatively rare because of the associated severe pain and inflammation that occurs at the injection site secondarily to the injection of an oil. This pain and inflammation also are the reasons why, whenever possible, injectable drugs are mostly prepared as aqueous solutions or suspensions. Therefore, like other types of cannabis, hashish oil is more often ingested in edible products or inhaled by "toking"—generally in combination with cannabis or tobacco—or "vaping."

dosage is required because pulmonary absorption is much greater than that achieved from the GI tract (see the related discussion in the earlier cannabis pharmacology subsection, "Pharmacokinetics—Absorption"). Thus, smoking ("toking" and hookah smoking), including the use of "blunts;" inhaling vaporized cannabis (i.e., "vaping"); and, more recently, "dabbing" are the most common methods of use among adolescents and young adults for all three forms of cannabis—marijuana, hashish, hashish oil. See the related discussion in the following subsections, "Blunt Smoking," "Dabbing," "Hookah Smoking," and "Vaping."

BLUNT SMOKING. A blunt is a tobacco cigar that is split with a razor, the tobacco emptied and replaced with marijuana, and re-rolled either with the original tobacco wrap or a more exotic, and expensive, wrap.[66] Blunts, also referred to as "Dutch," "El-P," "L," "LPs," and "White Owl," are particularly used by adolescents and young adults of Hispanic descent. The respective street names for these blunts refer to the "Dutch Masters®," "El Producto®," and "White Owl®" brands of American machine-made cigars. In addition, cigar wraps, or blunt wraps, can be separately purchased and used to roll the marijuana.[66]

Blunts got their name during the early 1980s when Jamaican/Rastafarians, who were living in New York City, began using Phillies Blunt® cigars in which they substituted the tobacco filler with marijuana. Smoking blunts increased in popularity among marijuana smokers, particularly young males from ethnic minority groups, because of several perceived advantages when compared to smoking "joints," including:

- Blunts, being larger in size, hold more marijuana and, consequently, can: (1) be smoked, extinguished, and relit at a later time; and (2) enable "tokers" to obtain a very large hit (i.e., a "mondo");
- Blunts burn more slowly than "joints" and, consequently, offer an extended period of time to "toke up" or share with friends;
- Blunts, compared to a hand-rolled "joint," resemble a legal product (i.e., cigar) and, consequently, are less likely to be recognized by parents, police, and teachers as an illicit substance of abuse;[67]
- Blunts, particularly among adolescent boys, display a characteristic, distinctive appearance when smoked that gives them a perception of being "cool," "tough," or "macho"—similar to the perceptual difference often associated with smoking a cigar versus smoking a cigarette;
- Blunts, because of their tobacco wrap, contain and deliver nicotine, as well as THC, and, consequently, reportedly provide a more pleasurable experience;
- Blunt preparation and use rituals significantly contribute to their popularity and use.

(e.g., Pagliaro & Pagliaro, *Clinical Patient Data Files*;
Sifaneck, Johnson, & Dunlap, 2006)

Blunt use among adolescents in the U.S. is highest among boys of African or Asian continental and Hispanic descents (Delnevo, Bover-Manderski, & Hrywna, 2100; Dunlap, Benoit, & Sifaneck, 2006; Lee, Battle, & Lipton, 2010; Soller & Lee, 2010). This blunt use is currently largely due to its active promotion among the "hip-hop" culture that these adolescents are actively engaged in (Foster, 2016; Ketchum, 2017). These blunt users,

66 Included among the other more exotic and expensive wraps that can be purchased for making blunts include Shine Papers®, which are 24k edible/smokable gold foil wraps that are designed specifically for rolling "blunts" or "joints."

67 As cannabis is decriminalized/legalized for medical/recreational use, this particular perceived advantage is expected to correspondingly decrease.

generally, have a lower perception of harm associated with cannabis use (Sinclair, Foushee, & Scarinci, 2013).

Utilizing data from the 2013 National Survey on Drug Use and Health (NSDUH), Montgomery and Bagot (2016) studied a group of 935 current (i.e., within the past 30 days) marijuana or hashish using subjects (12 years-of-age and older) of African continental descent within the U.S. They found that:

1. 73.2% were blunt users;
2. Blunt users initiated their blunt use at an earlier age (i.e., 15.9 years) than other marijuana/hashish users, who initiated their use at a later age (i.e., 17.3 years);
3. Blunt users reported more days of marijuana use in the past month (i.e., 16 days versus eight days) than other marijuana/hashish users;
4. 25% of blunt users reported a higher incidence of past year marijuana abuse or dependence than other marijuana/hashish users.

Dabbing. A more recent method of cannabis use, particularly among adolescents and young adults, is referred to as "dabbing." Dabbing involves passing pressurized butane gas over dried marijuana to extract a concentrated gummy resin of THC and its related cannabinoids and terpenes. The end product is often referred to as, "butane hash oil," or "BHO," because of its method of preparation.[68] It also is referred to as "dabs," which can typically have a THC concentration as high as 60% to 90%. The dabs, which are also referred to as "amber," "budder," "earwax," or "honey/honey oil," are then pressed through a filter for use in bongs, water pipes, or vaporizers (including e-cigarettes and e-hookahs). The product is also commonly used by simply "dabbing" it onto a heated surface (commonly referred to as a "nail") and inhaling the vapor that is produced.[69]

The use of this high-concentration THC product steadily increased during the second decade of the new millennium. The major concerns associated with dabbing—in addition to the toxic outcomes associated with the higher concentration of THC—is the significant danger of explosions and fires associated with the dabbing production process (Miller, Stogner, & Miller, 2016; Pagliaro & Pagliaro, *Clinical Patient Data Files*). The production process is commonly associated with explosions, fires, and related burn injuries because dabs are produced using highly volatile pressurized butane as a solvent.[70] Third degree burns are common and associated deaths have been reported (e.g., Romanowski, Barsun, & Kwan, 2017).

A review of the related published literature indicates that the burn injuries can be significant with a median 25% total-body-surface-area burn size. Demographically, the overwhelming majority of these burn injuries occurred among young adult men with a mean age of 26 years (Bell, Slim, & Flaten, 2015; Jensen, Bertelotti, & Greenhaigh, 2015; Romanowski, Barsun, & Kwan, 2017). It is expected that the demographics of the "dab-preparation" burn injuries reflect the general demographic characteristics of the population of "butane hash oil" users.

In addition, as found by Chan, Hall, and Freeman (2017), in their 20-country anonymous online survey of cannabis users, those who used "butane hash oil" were significantly more likely than other cannabis users to report:

68 The end product, "shatter," more closely resembles a sheet of toffee or maple syrup candy. The name is derived from its hard glass-like texture that—much like peanut brittle—shatters when it is broken up to be used.

69 Additionally, in states where cannabis use has been legalized, BHO is often used to make "edibles" (Pagliaro & Pagliaro, *Clinical Patient Data Files*).

70 These injuries are reminiscent of the burn injuries suffered during the early 1980s due to the flammability of the ether used to produce "freebase" cocaine (for related discussion, see Chapter 2, "Amphetamines and Cocaine").

1. Having been diagnosed with mental depression;
2. Using a greater number of different drugs and substances of abuse.

HOOKAH SMOKING.[71] In addition to rolling the cannabis into a cigarette paper to form a "reefer," or "joint," to "toke," cannabis users may also use a traditional conical pipe, small-bowled pipe, or water pipe—also referred to as a "bong," "chillim," "galyan," "goza," "hookah," "narghile," or "shisha"—to inhale cannabis smoke (Chaouachi, 2009).

Hookah smoking has become increasingly popular among adolescents and young adults, over the new millennium, as evidenced by the growing number of hookah bars, or "Shisha Bars," that are appearing across the U.S. Favorable attitudes regarding hookah use have been reported in up to 90% of research participants (Krauss, Sowles, & Moreno, 2015). In the U.S., approximately 15% to 20% of high school seniors and 20% to 40% of U.S. college/university students have reported hookah use during the past year (CDC, 2015a).[72] Factors identified by Morris, Fiala, and Pawlak (2012) that tend to support high levels of hookah smoking, include:

1. Social acceptance;
2. Having friends and family members who smoke hookahs;
3. Believing that hookah smoking is less harmful than smoking a "joint."

"Smokers" are increasingly recognizing that, when they inhale cannabis smoke deeply into their lungs to enhance THC absorption and achieve resultant high blood THC concentrations, they are also inhaling other chemicals and constituents along with the THC—including carcinogens (see also the following subsection, "Vaping").

Hookah smoking is also associated with several other undesired, or harmful, effects and toxicities. For example, in addition to the potential for physical and psychological dependence, cannabis or tobacco warmed by the charcoal heat source in the hookah, can produce high levels of carbon monoxide, heavy metals, and cancer-causing chemicals that, when inhaled, increase the risk for pulmonary toxicities. In addition, when users pass the same mouthpiece from one to another during smoking sessions, they can spread several communicable diseases, including: acute bronchitis; gonorrhea; herpes; syphilis; and tuberculosis (e.g., American Lung Association, 2016, p. 1; CDC, 2015a, 2015b; Pagliaro & Pagliaro, *Clinical Patient Data Files*). As a result, many adolescents and young adults are increasingly turning to the use of an "electronic hookah," or "e-hookah," an increasingly popular product available for vaporizing cannabis that is much like the e-cigarette (see related discussion in Chapter 3, "Caffeine and Nicotine").

VAPING. Several terms are used, often interchangeably, to describe the pulmonary inhalation of a drug or substance of abuse that has been vaporized by the heat produced by an electronic device, such as a vaporizer (e.g., for nicotine, this device is usually, an electric coil in an e-cigarette or e-pen). (See the related discussion in Chapter 3, "Caffeine and Nicotine", "E-Cigarettes"). Various types of vaporizers also are commonly used by cannabis users, who also have developed related argot, or slang, including:

1. "Vaper." A noun that is commonly used to describe someone who vapes;

71 See also related discussion in the subsection, "Hookahs" in Chapter 3, "Caffeine and Nicotine."

72 Schulenberg, Johnston, and O'Malley (2017) identified that hookah use among college/university students and their non-college/university peers, 19 to 23 years-of-age, significantly decreased from 2011 to 2016 (i.e., from ~ 30% to ~ 20%). We, too, have observed this significant decline in hookah use among adolescents. However, it appears to be related to a significant and corresponding concomitant increase, for both adolescents and young adults, in electronic hookah use (see the related discussion in the later subsection, "Electronic Hookahs").

2. "Vapes." An intransitive verb used to denote the process of vaping;
3. "Vaping." A present participle of the verb "vapes."

"Vapes" and "vaping" are often used interchangeably, much like "smoke" and "smoking." These terms originated in the argot of the cannabis subculture during the 1980s and were widely adopted and used in conjunction with the introduction from China of the first commercial e-cigarette to the U.S. during the first decade of the new millennium. They have since become mainstream with "vape" being chosen, in 2014, as "the word of the year" and formally added to the Oxford Dictionary. By 2017, the director of the NIDA identified that "nearly 1 in 3 students in 12th grade report past year use of some kind of vaping device" (Volkow, 2017, p. 1).

For efficient pulmonary absorption, a drug or substance of abuse must be vaporized into an aerosolized or gaseous form to facilitate the process of inhaling: (1) volatile solvents (e.g., "sniffing" gasoline or glue); (2) smoking (e.g., smoking opium from an opium pipe; smoking a tobacco cigarette); and (3) vaporizing (e.g., inhaling crack cocaine from a crack pipe). Although "volatile inhalants" are generally "ready for use," in each of the examples, the volatile solvent drug or substance of abuse—prior to inhalation—must be changed from a solid, or liquid, form to a gas form. The major difference in their transformation into a gas (i.e., how much heat is required) is determined by the boiling point of the drug or substance of abuse (i.e., the temperature at which its liquid form boils and turns into a vapor).

The combustion of organic material, such as cannabis or tobacco, produces an aerosol (i.e., smoke) that contains active ingredients in the form of fine particles or liquid droplets suspended in air—that can be inhaled. The temperature involved in smoking can reach close to 900° C during a puff (i.e., as drawn-in oxygen "fuels the fire" at the burning end of the cigarette/joint). Consequently, many chemicals, in addition to the "desired" drug or substance of abuse, are aerosolized, as well as formed de novo by the processes of combustion, distillation, pyrolysis, and pyrosynthesis (Dubie & Green, 1982; Streller & Roth, 2015).

Smoking can provide high enough temperatures to aerosolize drugs and chemicals found in organic matter (e.g., marijuana; tobacco). Whereas vaporizing produces lower heat, which can vaporize drugs and substances of abuse (e.g., nicotine; THC) that have lower boiling points and, consequently, avoids the chemical processes of combustion, distillation, pyrolysis, and pyrosynthesis.

Vaporizing cannabis involves using a commercial vaporizer to heat the cannabis and evaporate the THC into a gas that, when inhaled, delivers up to 95% of the evaporated THC. In comparison to smoking, the gas has significantly less carbon monoxide and other toxins (e.g., tars found in cannabis smoke). Because the required temperature for vaporizing is significantly lower than that needed for smoking, the cannabis is not burned, diminishing associated cancer risk because related carcinogens are not produced.

VAPORIZERS Vaporizers are generally available in two forms: (1) quasi-stationary desktop models; and (2) portable devices. The desk-top models (e.g., subHERBan Art®; Volcano® forced air vaporizer) are powered by electricity provided by a standard electrical outlet. The most recent major innovation in relation to desktop vaporizers are the availability of vaporizer pods (e.g., Canna Cloud®; Wisp®). The vaporizer pods are similar in form and appearance to coffee pods and are used in much the same way as for pod coffee machines (e.g., Keurig®). Similar to the variety of available coffee pods, the vaporizer pods allow users to conveniently purchase and use sealed, prefilled single-use pods that are available in a variety of CBD and THC strengths and aromas.

Portable devices (i.e., "portable vapes;" "vape pens" such as "Cloud Pen®," "Executive®," "Links®," "PuffCo®," and "Puff Fog Pen®") are battery operated and, by far, more widely used than desktop vaporizers (Pagliaro & Pagliaro, *Clinical Patient Data Files*). As shared by a typical electronic pen user:

> You know, it's convenient for something to take to, like, a movie theater, or a concert—where you're not necessarily supposed to be smoking a joint or having a pipe.
>
> (Bryan & Simon, 2014, p. 1)

ELECTRONIC HOOKAHS Electronic hookahs are commonly referred to as "E-Heads," "E-Hookahs," "E-Pens" (an abbreviation for "electronic shisha pens"), and "Vape Pens." They typically consist of three major components: (1) a rechargeable lithium battery to generate the heat necessary for vaporizing the e-liquid; (2) a delivery device about the size and general shape as a Sharpie® marking pen or an insulin pen; and (3) the "e-liquid" cartridge/tank that contains the product to be vaporized—THC. Inhalation[73] through the end of the automizer results in the automatic and virtually instantaneous heating and vaporization of the THC-containing e-liquid which is, subsequently, rapidly absorbed into the circulatory system.[74]

The noted benefits of e-hookah use, according to many users, include:

- Its smaller size when compared to traditional hookahs, which makes it more convenient to carry from place to place (and conceal);
- Use of a battery as a heat source that produces cleaner and less toxic smoke rather than the burning charcoal, which is required with the traditional hookahs;
- Fewer associated restrictions, laws, and regulations—resulting in both more private and public use;
- Lower production of hazardous "sidestream smoke."

Consequently, the use of vaporizers and e-hookahs for delivering various types of available cannabis (e.g., marijuana, hashish, or hashish oil) to get "high" increased geometrically during the last few years with over one in 10 U.S. high school seniors reporting use in 2017 (Newman, 2018).

Adolescent Illicit Drug Involvement

Adolescent involvement in the illicit distribution and sale of cannabis exceeds related involvement with all of the other drugs and substances of abuse—combined (Pagliaro & Pagliaro, *Clinical Patient Data Files*). Involvement runs the entire gamut of illicit activities including:

- "Runner" for dial-a-dope cellular phone-based marijuana sales;
- Grower of marijuana plants;
- Harvester and dryer of marijuana "buds;"
- Preparer of hashish, hashish oil, and "dabs;"
- Preparer of edible marijuana products (e.g., hashish brownies);
- Seller of marijuana products from home;
- Seller of marijuana products at school;
- Seller of marijuana products on-the-street;
- Smuggler of cannabis across either the Canadian or Mexican borders into the U.S.;
- Smuggler of cannabis from "legal" jurisdictions in the U.S. to other jurisdictions where possession and use are "illegal."

73 In some models, a button must be pressed while simultaneously inhaling in order to activate the electronic hookah.

74 Generally, the e-liquid also contains four other ingredients that function as a "vehicle" for facilitating the vaporization of the product to be vaporized and as a flavor, fragrance, or taste enhancer. These ingredients are: (1) fruit flavoring; (2) propylene glycol; (3) vegetable glycerine; and (4) water.

For example, in regard to related adolescent involvement in drug dealing:

> Task force Cmdr. John Burke has called [18-year-old] Pagenstecher a "little czar" in the [marijuana] drug ring and said most were students at Mason High and Kings High, two highly ranked public schools.
>
> (Associated Press, 2012a, p. 1)

> A teenager convicted of selling up to $20,000 worth of high-grade marijuana a month to high school students in southwestern Ohio was sentenced Monday to serve six months to three years in a juvenile prison by a judge who called him "a pretty fine young person that went down a bad trail."
>
> (Associated Press, 2012b, p. 1)

> Gordon told Sports Illustrated that he made upwards of $10,000 per month selling marijuana while playing football at Baylor [University].
>
> (Masisak, 2017, p. 1)

> An underage girl called police to report someone had stolen her drugs ... Around 8 p.m. Tuesday, the girl called police and said two boys came to her home, put a gun to her head, and stole the marijuana she had planned to sell them. Police said the incident involved a total of five teenagers, all between 14 and 16 years old. Officers found drug paraphernalia "all over the house" including marijuana, smoking pipes, a digital scale, and a grinder, according to police.
>
> (Tribune Media Wire, 2017, p. 1)

> A 15-year-old Massachusetts high school freshman was arrested after she was accused by police of running a drug pickup business—using her bedroom window as a service hub. Haverhill police believe she was selling the drugs with the consent of her mother, who also was taken into custody, FOX25 reported, citing court documents.
>
> (Norman, 2018, p. 1)

> There was no deep undercover operation, no long-term surveillance, no wiretaps that led authorities to Josue Lomeli and his drug-smuggling work. It was as simple and as obvious as the poorly concealed bulge in the clothes of the teenager who approached the Customs and Border Protection officer assigned to Lane 59 at the San Ysidro Port of Entry. Drug gangs target youths who can legally cross the border because they are U.S. citizens who may live in Tijuana and go to school in the United States or have a Border Crossing Card.
>
> (Moran, 2016, p. 2)

Or, as presented in another seemingly "common story"—based on our years of related experience:

> In Eagle Pass, Texas, where poverty and dirt roads outnumber jobs and opportunities, Mexico's drug cartels prey on kids—offering them thousands of dollars to smuggle hundreds of pounds of drugs each week ... The summer after sixth grade, 12-year-old Cesar was at a party with Leo when he was introduced to another boy, Alejandro. Two days later, Leo called Cesar to pass on a message from Alejandro: Do you want to work for Los Zetas?[75] ... The work started that night,

75 Los Zetas is a major Mexican criminal sydicate that is primarily involved in drug trafficking.

> with Cesar ordered to drive a truck 20 miles to a ranch where it was stripped packed with cash and reassembled for Cesar to drive back to Eagle Pass. For that he was paid $15,000 in cash . . .
>
> There were other boys in Eagle Pass working for Los Zetas, including Eduardo, who was about 15 and had been smuggled from Mexico to work for the gang . . . His main role was to pick up vehicles packed with cocaine and marijuana that had been smuggled into the United States and drive them with other youths three hours away to San Antonio.
>
> (Contreras, 2015, pp. 1–10)

Adolescents, who are involved in drug dealing and other drug involvement, generally "work" alone or as members of low-level, unorganized, street-level gangs or high-level, formally organized gangs. As rhetorically asked and answered by McElroy (2016, p. 1):

> Why would a 22-year-old want to do the dial-a-dope street operations and put a target on his back if he has 13, 14-year-old cousins that are willing to make a couple of thousand dollars a week? Why would he take that risk? "For the money."

Many adolescents and young adults become involved in drug dealing and other illicit activities to support their own cannabis use,[76] while others may become more intensely involved as a means for obtaining their primary source of income (see earlier exemplar scenarios). Given this situation, it is both surprising and disappointing that only a limited amount of published research is available regarding this widespread and perennial problem. Regardless of the paucity of published research, it is clear to us—based on several decades of professional clinical and forensic work with adolescents and young adults, who have been part of the cannabis or marijuana drug trade and other drug dealing—that the primary and virtually exclusive motivation for their involvement is "financial." Over the years the most common responses to our question, "Why are you involved in this activity?" are words to the effect that it is easy and pays better than a "mc-job" (i.e., working hard for a minimum wage at McDonalds®). In addition, "it's more prestigious," particularly within their own social group of friends, gang members, or other acquaintances.

These observations have been noted for some time in the U.S.—although originally in the context of street gang involvement during the 1990s by adolescent boys of African continental descent, who lived in low income, urban areas (e.g., Altschuler & Brounstein, 1991; Li, Stanton, & Feigelman, 1999). As identified, at that time, by Stanton and Galbraith (1994):

> Existing data indicate that approximately 10% of male, urban, African-American early adolescents report having engaged in drug trafficking, with a higher percent of youths reporting having been asked to sell drugs and/or indicating that they expect to become involved in drug trafficking.
>
> (p. 1039)

Adolescents in the U.S. of Hispanic descent also were quick to adopt participation in street-level, drug-dealing gangs (e.g., Walker, 1990). Much more recently (i.e., particularly during the second decade of the new millennium), a similar disturbing phenomenon appears to have expanded among adolescents of Hispanic descent, particularly those living in proximity to the Mexican border (e.g., Contreras, 2015; Moran, 2016).

76 For example, in their analysis of data from the *National Survey of Drug Use and Health*, which sampled 13,706 adolescents 12 to 17 years-of-age, Floyd, Alexandre, and Hedden (2010) found that marijuana use was a major risk factor for engaging in the sale of marijuana by these youth. In this context, high school students have frequently shared with us that they would purchase marijuana (for example, one ounce), divide and sell ¾ to friends and fellow students to "recoup" the original purchase price, and be left with ¼ for their own use—"free of charge" (Pagliaro & Pagliaro, *Clinical Patient Data Files*).

Related Professional Reminder: ***Adolescents, who are involved in the trafficking of marijuana are significantly more likely, than other adolescents, to use marijuana.***[77]

Additionally, mental health care professionals should be cognizant of the "not unusual" occurrence, among parents who use cannabis, of providing cannabis to their children—sometimes for self-diagnosed "medical" reasons (e.g., promote sleep; relieve anxiety) and sometimes for "recreational" reasons. For example, as reported by the Associated Press (2018):

> A Virginia mom who gave her 3 kids (ages 7, 11, and 14) marijuana gets 10 days in jail. (p. 1)

We have previously reported (e.g., Pagliaro & Pagliaro, 2012; Pagliaro & Pagliaro, *Clinical Patient Data Files*) several cases of mothers, fathers, and older siblings giving a "puff" of their joint to a toddler or young child in order to "observe the effects"—which, reportedly, commonly include: "blood shot eyes;" "looking stoned;" and "jumping around." These effects are often recorded and shared on social media (e.g., Facebook®).

Assessment and Diagnosis of Adolescent and Young Adult Cannabis Dependence or Use Disorder

The assessment and diagnosis of cannabis dependence or use disorder (CUD) is generally achieved by means of an initial clinical interview with the adolescent or young adult during which: (1) cannabis use is established; and, if established, (2) answers are obtained to questions concerning both the qualitative and quantitative nature of the reported cannabis use.

This section presents and discusses DSM-5 criteria for CUD and quick-screen psychometric tests for detecting cannabis dependence among adolescents and young adults, who use cannabis. For a comprehensive overview, also see the related discussion of assessment and diagnosis in the context of adolescent and young adult AUD and SUDs in Chapter 1, "Alcohol."

DSM-5 Criteria for Detecting CUD

Typically, answers to the following 11 behaviors, which are based on DSM-5 criteria for CUD (e.g., APA, 2013; Hasin, O'Brien, & Auriacombe, 2013) are sought. In addition, an indication of both the severity and duration of cannabis use and associated harmful effects is also sought. In this context, adolescents and young adults are asked to identify their experiences (i.e., endorse or not endorse the following behaviors):

1. Continuing to use cannabis despite physical or psychological problems related to use;
2. Continuing to use cannabis despite relationship or social problems related to use;
3. Craving for cannabis (i.e., have a longing for, or strong desire to use, cannabis);
4. Have difficulty controlling, cutting down, or discontinuing cannabis use (e.g., repeated unsuccessful attempts to quit cannabis use);
5. Giving up, or significantly reducing, other activities—particularly, occupational, recreational, or social activities—in favor of cannabis use;
6. Having problems at home, school, or work as a result of cannabis use;
7. Spending a lot of time on cannabis use, including: obtaining cannabis or recovering from effects associated with its use;
8. Displaying tolerance to cannabis;

77 In one of the few published studies on adolescent "drug dealing" in the U.S., Shook, Vaughn, and Salas-Wright (2013) found that "the vast majority of [adolescent] dealers use alcohol, tobacco, and marijuana" (p. 365).

9. Using cannabis in hazardous situations (e.g., while driving a motor vehicle);
10. Using more cannabis than intended, more frequently than intended, or for longer periods than intended;
11. Experiencing withdrawal when unable to obtain cannabis or when discontinuing cannabis use.

Positive endorsement of two, or more, of the listed behaviors generally signifies CUD. In addition, the number of items endorsed provides an indication of the severity of the CUD (i.e., "mild," two or three endorsements; "moderate," four or five endorsements; and "severe," six or more endorsements).[78]

Selected Cannabis Quick-Screen Psychometric Tests[79]

Several quick-screen psychometric tests have been developed, including the: "Cannabis Experiences Questionnaire," or CEQ (Stirling, Barkus, & Nabosi, 2008); "Cannabis Use Problem Identification Test," or CUPIT (Bashford, Flett, & Copeland, 2010); "Marijuana Adolescent Problem Inventory," or MAPI (Knapp, Babbin, & Budney, 2018); "Marijuana Craving Questionnaire," or MCQ (Heishman, Singleton, & Liguori, 2001); and "Rutgers Marijuana Problem Index," or RMPI (White, Labouvie, & Papadaratsakis, 2005). However, for virtually all of these tests: (1) the availability of published test statistics is severely limited, particularly for adolescents; and (2) no single test is currently identified as being the "standard" for detecting cannabis dependence or use disorder (CUD) for this age group.

Three quick-screen psychometric tests [i.e., the: (1) "Cannabis Abuse Screening Test," or CAST; (2) "Cannabis Use Disorder Identification Test," or CUDIT; and (3) "Cannabis Use Disorder Identification Test-Revised," or CUDIT-R] have been specifically developed to detect cannabis dependence or use disorder among adolescents and have more available published test statistics than do other associated tests. A discussion of the use of each of these tests, and their available psychometric properties, are presented in the following subsections.[80]

<u>Related Professional Reminder:</u> As with the use of all quick-screen psychometric tests, but particularly with the tests for CUD—because of the absence of a clinical "gold" standard diagnostic test, or best available benchmark—suggestive positive findings must be carefully supported by appropriate clinical assessment and interview.

CANNABIS ABUSE SCREENING TEST (CAST)

The CAST (Table 4.3) is a self-administered six-item quick-screen psychometric test that was developed by Legleye, Karila, and Beck (2007) to detect cannabis abuse, particularly among adolescents and young adults. The CAST was developed at the University of Paris, Paris, France. Thus, psychometric values, or test statistics, reflect sampled populations of adolescents and young adults of European continental descent—particularly representing those from

78 We (e.g., Pagliaro & Pagliaro, *Clinical Patient Data Files*) and others (e.g., Mewton, Slade, & Teesson, 2013) have noted concerns related to the DSM-5 criteria for CUD—particularly in regard to the: (1) lack of distinction between social, habitual, abusive, and compulsive cannabis use; and (2) accepted discriminating, or cutoff score, of 2 that has the potential to make the diagnosis for CUD over-inclusive, or significantly overestimated.

79 See also the related discussion and overview of quick-screen psychometric test statistics, selection, use, and interpretation in Chapter 1, "Alcohol," and the description and discussion of additional nonspecific (i.e., generic) tests for the detection of SUDs in Chapter 2, "Amphetamines and Cocaine."

80 Additionally, some general tests for detecting various SUDs have been used to detect CUD (e.g., "Severity Dependence Scales" [SDS]). A brief discussion and review of these quick-screen psychometric tests are presented in Chapter 2, "Amphetamines and Cocaine."

Table 4.3 The CAST

Item/question	*Scoring Criteria [Point Allocation]*
1. Have you ever smoked cannabis before midday?	Never, [0]; rarely, [1]; from time to time, [2]; fairly often, [3]; very often, [4]
2. Have you ever smoked cannabis when you were alone?	Never, [0]; rarely, [1]; from time to time, [2]; fairly often, [3]; very often, [4]
3. Have you ever had memory problems when you smoked cannabis?	Never, [0]; rarely, [1]; from time to time, [2]; fairly often, [3]; very often, [4]
4. Have friends or members of your family ever told you that you ought to reduce your cannabis use?	Never, [0]; rarely, [1]; from time to time, [2]; fairly often, [3]; very often, [4]
5. Have you ever tried to reduce or stop your cannabis use without succeeding?	Never, [0]; rarely, [1]; from time to time, [2]; fairly often, [3]; very often, [4]
6. Have you ever had problems because of your use of cannabis (argument, fight, accident, bad result at school, etc.)?	Never, [0]; rarely, [1]; from time to time, [2]; fairly often, [3]; very often, [4]

Source: Legleye, Karila, & Beck (2007).

France, Hungary, Italy, and Spain. Equivalent psychometric values, which represent adolescents and young adults in the U.S., are not available.

Using different forms of factor analysis, some researchers found the CAST to be one-dimensional (e.g., Bastiani, Siciliano, & Curzio, 2013), while others found the CAST to be two-dimensional (e.g., Legleye, 2017). However, the two dimensional, or two-factor model, appears to be the more satisfactory representation with: factor one, representing "frequency of use/problems;" and factor two, representing "non-recreational use/dependency symptoms" (Legleye, Eslami, & Bougeard, 2017).[81]

SCORING OF THE CAST. Responses to each item of the CAST are scored on a five-point Likert scale (see Table 4.3). Scores are then summed for a possible maximal score of 24. A discriminating, or cutoff, score of six is generally considered indicative of cannabis abuse (Legleye, Karila, & Beck, 2007; Legleye, Kraus, & Piontek, 2012; Legleye & Rouquette, 2018; Stoner, 2016).

AVAILABLE TEST STATISTICS AND RECOMMENDATIONS. Data are available regarding the specificity, sensitivity, validity, and reliability of the CAST. These data are discussed in the following subsections.

81 Sznitman (2017), in an analysis of the CAST using three age groups (i.e., 18 to 24 years-of-age; 25 to 29 years-of-age; 30 to 40 years-of-age) of cannabis users in Israel, also found the CAST to be two-dimensional across all age groups studied. However, the factors were descriptively identified in a slightly different manner as "cannabis use problems" and "deviation from a common standard of use."

SPECIFICITY AND SENSITIVITY In a general population sample, the specificity and sensitivity for the CAST is reported to be 81.4% and 92.9%, respectively, when using a criterion value, or cutoff score, of 4. In addition, the positive predictive value is 45.8% and the negative predictive value is 96.5% (Legleye, Karila, & Beck, 2007; Piontek, Kraus, & Klempova, 2008).

Legleye, Karila, and Beck (2007), using a cutoff score of 4 in their CAST study of 123 French school students, reported a sensitivity of 92.9% and a specificity 81.4%. In another study, using a cutoff score of 5, Legleye (2017) found a sensitivity of 78.2% and a specificity of 79.6%. With a cutoff score of 6, a sensitivity of 93.0% and a specificity of 66.7% were reported (Legleye, Kraus, & Piontek, 2012). In a later study, using a cut-off score of 8, Legleye (2017) found a sensitivity of 86% and a specificity of 86.7%. Bastiani, Siciliano, and Curzio (2013), using a cutoff score of 7 with a sample of 5,787 Italian adolescent cannabis users, found that the CAST significantly overestimated the DSM-IV referenced diagnosis of cannabis dependence.

VALIDITY AND RELIABILITY In terms of construct validity, the factor loadings of the CAST items are moderate. In addition, as a measure of convergent validity, the CAST correlates well with the related dimensions of the POSIT when using a cutoff score of 4 (Legleye, Karila, and Beck, 2007).

When used with a general population sample, the reliability of the CAST, in terms of internal consistency (i.e., inter-item consistency), is relatively high with a Cronbach's alpha coefficient of 0.81. However, reliability is lower (i.e., 0.74) when used with French cannabis users, 16 to 62 years-of-age (Legleye, Karila, & Beck, 2007; Legleye, Guignard, & Richard, 2015). Similar values were reported for Cronbach's alpha coefficient when the CAST was tested among: Italian adolescents, 15 to 19 years-of-age (i.e., 0.78) (Bastiani, Siciliano, & Curzio, 2013); Spanish young adult cannabis users (i.e., 0.71) (Cuenca-Royo, Sanchez-Niubo, & Forero, 2012); Hungarian high school students (i.e., 0.71) (Gyepesi, Urban, & Farkas, 2014); and French young adult cannabis users, 15 to 26 years-of-age (i.e., 0.73) (Legleye, Kraus, & Piontek, 2012).

Test-retest reliability has been calculated at greater than 0.80 (Cuenca-Royo, Sanchez-Niubo, & Forero, 2012). This value for the reliability coefficient is acceptable, but relatively low.

RECOMMENDATIONS Although the overall statistics for the CAST are acceptable, the low positive predictive value (i.e., less than 50%) indicates that: (1) the cutoff score needs to be lowered; or (2) the test items need to be modified (e.g., by the addition of valid and reliable items). We generally do not recommend the use of the CAST because of its low positive predictive value and the lack of sampling among U.S. adolescents and young adults.

CANNABIS USE DISORDER IDENTIFICATION TEST (CUDIT)

The CUDIT is a 10-item quick-screen psychometric test (Table 4.4, CUDIT) based on the "Alcohol Use Disorder Identification Test" (AUDIT) (for a discussion of the AUDIT, see Chapter 1, "Alcohol"). Developed by Adamson and Sellman (2003) to detect CUD, the development and testing of the CUDIT was predicated on diagnostic criteria obtained from the DSM-IV.

SCORING OF THE CUDIT. Responses to each item of the CUDIT are given a score of 0 to 4 (see Table 4.4 for scoring criteria). The maximal score possible is 40. A discriminating cutoff score of 8 is generally considered to be equivalent to the DSM-IV diagnosis for CUD, or cannabis dependence (Adamson & Sellman, 2003).[82]

82 Annaheim, Rehm, and Gmel (2008), using a community sample of Swiss adolescents and young adults, identified that "7" was the "ideal" cutoff score. They also noted that two items (i.e., "injuries" and "hours being stoned") "had loadings below 0.5 on the unidimensional construct and correlated lower than 0.4 with the total CUDIT score" (p. 190)—prompting them to recommend the revision of these items.

Table 4.4 The CUDIT

Item/question	*Scoring Criteria [Point Allocation]*
Over the past six months...	
1. How often did you use cannabis?	Never, [0]; monthly or less, [1]; two to four times a month, [2]; two to three times a week, [3]; four or more times a week, [4]
2. How many hours were you stoned on a typical day when you had been using cannabis?	One or two, [0]; three or four, [1]; five or six, [2]; seven to nine, [3]; 10 or more, [4]
3. How often were you stoned for six or more hours?	Never, [0]; less than monthly, [1]; monthly, [2]; weekly, [3]; daily or almost daily, [4]
4. How often did you find that you were not able to stop using cannabis once you had started?	Never, [0]; less than monthly, [1]; monthly, [2]; weekly, [3]; daily or almost daily, [4]
5. How often did you fail to do what was normally expected from you because of using cannabis?	Never, [0]; less than monthly, [1]; monthly, [2]; weekly, [3]; daily or almost daily, [4]
6. How often did you need to use cannabis in the morning to get yourself going after a heavy session of using cannabis?	Never, [0]; less than monthly, [1]; monthly, [2]; weekly, [3]; daily or almost daily, [4]
7. How often did you have a feeling of guilt or remorse after using cannabis?	Never, [0]; less than monthly, [1]; monthly, [2]; weekly, [3]; daily or almost daily, [4]
8. How often have you had a problem with your memory or concentration after using cannabis?	Never, [0]; less than monthly, [1]; monthly, [2]; weekly, [3]; daily or almost daily, [4]
9. Have you or someone else been injured as a result of your use of cannabis?	No, [0]; Yes, [4]
10. Has a relative, friend or doctor or other health worker been concerned about your use of cannabis or suggested you cutdown?	No, [0]; Yes, [4]

Source: Adamson & Sellman (2003).

The original CUDIT has been revised several times to facilitate its use and to improve its test statistics—as illustrated by a few of its revised titles and associated test developers:

- "Cannabis Use Disorder Identification Test-Revised" (CUDIT-R) (Adamson, Kay-Lambkin, & Baker, 2010);
- "Cannabis Use Disorder Identification Test-Modified" (CUDIT-M) (Annaheim, Scotto, & Gmel, 2010);

- "Cannabis Use Disorder Identification Test-Short Form" (CUDIT-SF) (Bonn-Miller, Heinz, & Smith, 2016).[83]

Of these tests, only the CUDIT-R has received broad attention and use. Consequently, it is discussed separately in its own subsection. See "Cannabis Use Disorder Identification Test-Revised (CUDIT-R)."

AVAILABLE TEST STATISTICS AND RECOMMENDATIONS. CUDIT test statistics are available for specificity, sensitivity, and positive and negative predictive values, as well as validity. We conclude with our recommendations for the use of the CUDIT for adolescents.

SPECIFICITY, SENSITIVITY, AND POSITIVE AND NEGATIVE PREDICTIVE VALUES The following values were found when using a discrimination, or cutoff, score of 8 for a convenience sample of 53 New Zealand alcohol dependent cannabis users: specificity, 94.7%; sensitivity, 73.3%; positive predictive value, 84.6%; and negative predictive value, 90.0% (Adamson & Sellman, 2003). Annaheim, Rehm, and Gmel (2008), using a cutoff score of 7 for a sample of 593 adolescent cannabis users, found, in relation to "cannabis use at school," a sensitivity of 71.1%, a specificity of 64.2%, a positive predictive value of 14.1%, and a negative predictive value of 96.4%.

VALIDITY AND RELIABILITY In terms of construct validity, factor loadings of items were moderate for all items except item nine, "injured." A very weak factor loading was obtained for this item, indicating that it probably should not have been included in this quick-screen psychometric test. The reliability of the CUDIT is low to moderate as indicated by the reported ranges for item total correlation for general and alcohol dependent population samples. For the general population sample, the reported range was 0.07 to 0.55 (Annaheim, Rehm, & Gmel, 2008). For the alcohol dependent sample, the reported range was 0.44 to 0.77 (Adamson & Sellman, 2003). Overall, internal consistency for the CUDIT is moderate as indicated by reported Cronbach's alpha coefficients in the mid-0.70s range (Adamson & Sellman, 2003; Annaheim, Rehm, & Gmel, 2008). Two items (i.e., item two, "hours stoned," and item nine, "injured") are reported to have lower correlation (i.e., below 0.4) with the total CUDIT score (Annaheim, Rehm, & Gmel, 2008). Thus, the validity and reliability of the CUDIT is expected to increase if these two items are appropriately modified or deleted.

RECOMMENDATIONS Given the problems associated with CUDIT test items, particularly item nine ("injured"), the moderate overall psychometric evaluation, and the relative paucity of published test statistics that utilize samples of U.S. adolescents and young adults, we recommend that, until additional valid and reliable supportive data become available, the use of the CUDIT be avoided.

83 The CUDIT-SF is comprised of three items (i.e., Item three; Item five, and Item six), which were taken directly from the CUDIT-R. Scored in the same manner as the CUDIT-R, the CUDIT-SF uses a recommended cutoff score of 2 or higher to obtain a positive quick-screen test result. Using two samples (i.e., sample one, adults from a medical cannabis facility in the U.S.; and sample two, adults from a community sample of regular "recreational" marijuana users in Australia), Bonn-Miller, Heinz, and Smith (2016) found: (1) moderate test reliability based on Cronbach alpha coefficients of 0.66 in sample one and 0.80 in sample two; (2) agreement with the CUDIT-R (using a cutoff score of 13) of 95%; (3) specificity of 77%; and (4) positive prediction values for subjects who met DSM-5 criteria for CUD of 78% (using a cutoff score of 2). (For additional related discussion, see the CUDIT-R in the following subsection.)

CANNABIS USE DISORDER IDENTIFICATION TEST-REVISED (CUDIT-R)

The CUDIT-R is an eight-item, self-administered quick-screen psychometric test (Table 4.5 CUDIT-R). It was derived from the CUDIT by Adamson, Kay-Lambkin, and Baker (2010) to detect CUD among users, who have used marijuana within the past six months. The CUDIT-R is comprised of four items from the original test and four new items. It contains two items from each of the domains: "consumption;" "cannabis problems/abuse;" "dependence;" and "psychological features."

Table 4.5 The CUDIT-R

Item	*Question*	*Scoring [Point allocation]*
If you have used marijuana [cannabis] in the past six months, please answer the following questions about your cannabis use. Select the responses that are most correct for you in relation to your cannabis use over the past six months.		
1.	How often do you use cannabis?	Never, [0]; monthly or less, [1]; two to four times a month, [2]; Two to three times a week, [3]; four or more times a week, [4]
2.	How many hours were you "stoned" on a typical day when you had been using cannabis?	Less than one, [0]; one or two, [1]; three or four, [2]; five or six, [3]; seven or more, [4]
3.	How often during the last six months did you find that you were not able to stop using cannabis once you had started?	Never, [0]; less than monthly, [1]; monthly, [2]; weekly, [3]; daily or almost daily, [4]
4.	How often during the past six months did you fail to do what was normally expected from you because of using cannabis?	Never, [0]; less than monthly, [1]; monthly, [2]; weekly, [3]; daily or almost daily, [4]
5.	How often in the past six months have you devoted a great deal of your time to getting, using, or recovering from cannabis?	Never, [0]; less than monthly, [1]; monthly, [2]; weekly, [3]; daily or almost daily, [4]
6.	How often in the past six months have you had a problem with your memory or concentration after using cannabis?	Never, [0]; less than monthly, [1]; monthly, [2]; weekly, [3]; daily or almost daily, [4]
7.	How often do you use cannabis in situations that could be physically hazardous, such as driving, operating machinery, or caring for children?	Never, [0]; less than monthly, [1]; monthly, [2]; weekly, [3]; daily or almost daily, [4]
8.	Have you ever thought about cutting down, or stopping, your use of cannabis?	Never, [0]; Yes, but not in the past 6 months, [2]; Yes, during the past 6 months, [4]

Source: Adamson, Kay-Lambkin, & Baker (2010).

SCORING OF THE CUDIT-R. Items one to seven of the CUDIT-R are scored on a five-point Likert scale (see Table 4.5). Item eight is scored as 0, 2, or 4. The item scores are summed to give a total score of 0 to 32. A cutoff score of 8 is indicative of hazardous cannabis use, while a cutoff score of 12 is indicative of CUD.[84]

AVAILABLE TEST STATISTICS AND RECOMMENDATIONS. Data are available regarding the specificity, sensitivity, validity, and reliability of the CUDIT-R. These statistics are presented and discussed in the following subsections.

SPECIFICITY AND SENSITIVITY Using a cut-off score of 13 for 144 Australians with concurrent major depressive disorder (MDD) and SUDs, Adamson, Kay-Lambkin, and Baker (2010) obtained a specificity of 0.90 and sensitivity of 0.91. Using this cut-off score, they also obtained a positive predictive value of 0.96 and a negative predictive value of 0.80.

VALIDITY AND RELIABILITY Looking at the eight items that comprise the CUDIT-R, it is obvious that the test has good *face* validity. In terms of *predictive* validity, Adamson, Kay-Lambkin, and Baker (2010) found that the:

> CUDIT-R score, which reflects the level of cannabis use problems over the preceding six months, was highly correlated with recent cannabis use frequency as measured by the OTI Q-Score (Spearman's rho = 0.705, p < 0.001).
>
> (p. 140)

The validity of the CUDIT-R, in terms of internal consistency, is acceptable, but moderate with a Cronbach's alpha coefficient of 0.73 (Loflin, Babson, & Browne, 2017).

RECOMMENDATIONS CUDIT-R is the best quick-screen psychometric test for detecting CUD that is currently available. However, we recommend cautious use because the: (1) test statistics of the CUDIT-R have not been replicated by researchers other than the innovators; and (2) norming was performed primarily with Australian samples (i.e., there is a paucity of test statistics obtained for adolescents in the U.S.).

Treating Adolescent or Young Adult Cannabis Dependence or Use Disorder

Given the extent of cannabis use among adolescents and young adults in the U.S.—as well as the occurrence of cannabis dependence or use disorder in these age groups—it is both surprising and disappointing that so little published research regarding treatment are currently available.[85]

> No intervention to date has proved consistently effective for the majority of those with dependence on cannabis.
>
> (Winstock, Ford, & Witton, 2010, p. 803)

> There is no unique treatment modality for the treatment of dependence on cannabis.
>
> (Banys & Cermak, 2016, p. 1)

84 Australian researchers, Marshal (2013) and Bruno, Marshall, and Adamson (2013), used a cut-off score of 13 to detect DSM-IV dependence and DSM-5 moderate to severe CUD.

85 This may be due, at least in part, to the observation that, while cannabis dependence or use disorder is likely the most common drug or substance of abuse disorder in the U.S., only a minority of adolescents and young adults with this disorder (i.e., ~ 10%) seek formal professional assistance for its treatment (Gates, Sabioni, & Copeland, 2016; Sherman, & McRae-Clark, 2016).

Pharmacotherapy and Psychotherapy/Counseling Approaches

Optimal treatment for drug or substance of abuse disorders, as frequently noted throughout this text, generally involves a selected combination of both efficacious pharmacotherapy and efficacious psychotherapy/counseling. Unfortunately, as noted in the following sections, there is currently a dearth of empirical data to support the consistent effectiveness of any form of therapy for the treatment of CUD for adolescents and young adults.

PHARMACOTHERAPY

Unfortunately, to date, no specific pharmacotherapy has been determined to provide consistent beneficial effects in regard to the treatment of cannabis dependence or use disorder (Copeland & Swift, 2009; Sherman & McRae-Clark, 2016).

> Although pharmacologic treatments have shown promise, none have emerged as clearly efficacious.
>
> (Sherman & McRae-Clark, 2016, p. 511)

As recognized by the NIDA (2018b):

> Currently, the FDA has not approved any medications for the treatment of marijuana use disorder.
>
> (p. 40)[86]

PSYCHOTHERAPY/COUNSELING

To date, psychotherapy/counseling has been the mainstay of treatment for cannabis dependence or use disorder. The major identified approaches have included:

- Abstinence-based voucher incentives;
- Cognitive-behavioral therapy (CBT);
- Contingency management (CM);
- Multidimensional family therapy (MFT);
- Motivational enhancement therapy (MET);
- 12-Step Programs;
- Combination therapy with two or more approaches, as listed above
  (e.g., Budney, Moore, & Rocha, 2006; Dennis, Godley, & Diamond, 2004; NIDA, 2018b; Sherman & McRae-Clark, 2016).[87]

Each of the listed psychotherapy/counseling approaches have demonstrated some limited success in the treatment of cannabis dependence or use disorder. CBT—particularly that involving nine or more, individual sessions—appears to be the most likely successful approach for reducing cannabis use among adolescents and young adults (e.g., Copeland, Swift, & Roffman, 2001; Denis, Lavie, & Fatseas, 2006; Gates, Sabioni, &

86 N.B. We would add that we are not aware of any current related "off-label" use of pharmacotherapy that we would recommend, with a significant degree of confidence, for the treatment of adolescents or young adults with cannabis dependence or use disorder.

87 For a discussion of each of these approaches, see the alcohol treatment approaches subsection, "Psychotherapy/Counseling," in Chapter 1, "Alcohol."

Copeland, 2016). However, the following major concerns must be noted and made explicit in regard to the related supportive, published empirical research findings:

1. Abstinence rates post-treatment were low and unstable;
2. Sample sizes were relatively small;
3. The majority of subjects were adults.

Consequently, although we personally favor and have used CBT with success in the treatment of adolescents and young adults, who have been diagnosed with cannabis dependence or use disorder, the available empirical data preclude—at least at this time—our full endorsement and recommendation of this therapeutic approach for the treatment of cannabis dependence or use disorder for other mental health care professionals.

Contemporaneous Diagnoses Involving Cannabis Dependence or Use Disorder[88]

Adolescents and young adults, who develop cannabis dependence or use disorder, generally have higher rates of:

- Anxiety Disorders, including panic attacks (e.g., Buckner, Heimberg, & Schneier, 2012; Hasin, Kerridge, & Saha, 2016; Karolina Kedzior & Tabata Laeber, 2014);
- Alcohol dependence or use disorder (NIDA, 2018c);
- Bipolar Disorder (e.g., Kvitland, Melle, & Aminoff, 2016; Kazour, Awaida, & Souaiby, 2018; Taub, Feingold, & Rehm, 2018);
- MDD (e.g., Karolina Kedzior & Martin-Iverson, 2010);[89]
- Nicotine dependence or use disorder (e.g., Dierker, Braymiller, & Rose, 2018; Hasin, Kerridge, & Saha, 2016; NIDA, 2018c; Richter, Pugh, & Smith, 2017);
- Personality Disorders (e.g., Gillespie, Aggen, & Neale, 2018; Hasin, Kerridge, & Saha, 2016);
- PTSD (e.g., Gentes, Schry, & Hicks, 2016; Hasin, Kerridge, & Saha, 2016 Kevorkian, Bonn-Miller, & Belendiuk, 2015);
- Psychotic Disorders (e.g., DeRosse, Kaplan, & Burdick, 2010; Koskinen, Lohonen, & Koponen, 2010).

In addition, for adolescent and young adults of African continental descent or North American-Puerto Rican descent, initiating marijuana use at an early age and its regular long-term use was associated with anger, depression, and other mental disturbances (Pahl, Brook, & Koppel, 2011).

Lysergic Acid Diethylamide (LSD)

> LSD is just a tool to turn us into what we are supposed to be.
>
> Albert Hofmann, 1906–2008

This major section of Chapter 4 presents and discusses adolescent and young adult use and abuse of *lysergic acid diethylamide* (LSD). Commonly known as "acid," "blotter," "dots," "kool-

88 See also the related discussion in the following lysergic acid diethylamide subsection, "LSD-Induced Disorders."

89 N.B. Feingold, Rehm, and Lev-Ran (2017) posited that the association between cannabis dependence or use disorder and MDD is not direct, but rather related to "associated sociodemographic and clinical factors" (p. 225).

aid," "trips," "window panes," and a myriad of other names, LSD is generally used to obtain such psychodelic actions as:

- Micropsia, seeing things much smaller than they are;
- Macropsia, seeing things much larger than they are;
- Synesthesia, blending of sensory input—such as, hearing colors and seeing sounds;
- Temporal disintegration, perceiving time as passing extremely slowly—such as, watching "grass grow" or "paint dry;"
- Visual, or optical, illusions;[90]
- Vivid thoughts and memories—including "flashbacks."

These psychodelic actions have been particularly attractive to adolescents and young adults for over seven decades. The pharmacology of LSD and its use/abuse by adolescents and young adults, during the new millennium in the U.S., are presented and discussed in the following subsections.

LSD Pharmacology

LSD is the most widely used "indole" psychodelic in the U.S. A semi-synthetic derivative of an ergot alkaloid, it was first synthesized in 1938 by Albert Hoffman from lysergic acid, a substance that occurs naturally in the parasitic ergot fungus (*Claviceps purpurea*) that grows on the grain-bearing tip, or ear, of stem cereal plants (e.g., barley, wheat, and rye). 25th in a series of ergot derivatives, LSD was initially named "LSD-25." However, because of its failure to yield significant results in preliminary animal studies, interest in LSD-25 rapidly diminished. In fact, little was done with the compound until April 16, 1943, when Hofmann prepared a fresh supply. Inadvertently absorbing a small amount on his fingertips (due to poor laboratory technique), he quickly and pleasantly became overcome by both an intense stimulation of the imagination and altered state of awareness of the world (i.e., resultant illusions and hallucinations). Three days later, he deliberately ingested 250 mcg of the compound (under controlled, experimental conditions), to confirm his first experience (Hofmann, 1970, 1980a, 1980b; Pagliaro & Pagliaro, 2004). The rest of the story, as they say, is "history."

Pharmacodynamics: Mechanism of Action

Although vast amounts of published research have now accumulated regarding the general pharmacology of LSD, its exact mechanism of action remains largely unknown (Passie, Halpern, & Stichtenoth, 2008). However, it has long been suggested that binding to 5-HT2 receptors is the primary mechanism responsible for the "hallucinogenic" activity of LSD (e.g., Glennon, Titeler, & McKenney, 1984). LSD interacts as a partial agonist with the serotonin 5-HT(2A) and 5-HT(2B) receptors (Chen & Tesmer, 2017; De Gregorio, Comai, & Posa, 2016; Wacker, Wang, & McCorvy, 2017), particularly those on neocortical pyramidal cells (Nichols, 2004). As identified by Passie, Halpern, and Stichtenoth (2008), LSD also appears to act as an agonist at the 5-HT(1A) receptors in the cortex, locus coeruleus, and raphe nuclei.

90 In the obituary for Albert Hofmann, which was written for the *Scientific American*, Biello (2008, p. 1) cited Albert Hoffman's report following his initial investigative self-administration of LSD, during which he:

> Perceived an uninterrupted stream of fantastic pictures, extraordinary shapes with intense, kaleidoscopic play of colors . . .

Consequently, they suggest that "LSD is probably best referred to as a mixed 5-HT2/HT1 receptor partial agonist" (p. 305).

Other published data suggest that:

> LSD reduces connectivity within brain networks and reduces the extent to which separate networks remain distinct in their patterns of firing.
>
> (*American College of Neuropsychopharmacology*, 2015, p. 1)

The resultant "more chaotic" brain state, suggested by this proposed mechanism of LSD action, is consistent with both the:

1. Prodromal phase of psychosis/schizophrenia;
2. Characterization/nomenclature that refers to the psychodelics as "psychotogens" or "schizophrenomimetics" (as described in the introduction of this chapter).

Pharmacokinetics: Absorption, Distribution, Metabolism, and Excretion

When ingested, LSD is readily absorbed from the GI tract on an empty stomach. Its onset of action generally begins within 30 to 60 minutes. Maximal plasma concentrations are achieved in approximately 90 minutes (Passie, Halpern, & Stichtenoth, 2008). The intensity of expected LSD-related psychodelic effects (e.g., experience of perceptual changes) depends on the classical determining factors of "drug, set, and setting" (Zinberg, 1986):

1. "Drug." Amount of LSD that is used (i.e., LSD effects are dose-dependent);
2. "Set." Personality traits, predisposition, or tendencies of an adolescent or young adult to react in a particular way;
3. "Setting." Context of use (e.g., alone or with others, who may be coaching or who may be also using LSD; initial use versus repeated regular use).

The psychodelic effects produced by LSD generally peak within one to six hours and usually dissipate within eight to 12 hours. Approximately 1% of LSD is excreted in unchanged form in the urine within 24 hours. Approximately 15% is excreted as the metabolite, 2-oxo-3-hydroxy-lysergic acid diethylamide. The half-life of elimination for LSD is two to five hours (Dolder, Schmid, & Haschke, 2015; Dolder, Schmid, & Steuer, 2017; Pagliaro & Pagliaro, 2009). Additional pharmacokinetic data are not available.

LSD Drug–Drug Interactions

LSD, as an agonist of the serotonin 5-HT receptors (see earlier LSD subsection, "Pharmacology, Pharmacodynamics: Mechanism of Action") can theoretically interact with a wide range of psychodelic indolealkylamines, including:

- LSD-like psychodelics (e.g., lysergic acid amide [LSA]);
- Tryptamines (e.g., N,N-dimethyltryptamine [DMT]; psilocybin [magic mushrooms]);
- Beta-carbolines (e.g., harmaline).

Depending upon the dosages of the concurrently used psychodelic(s), as well as the context of use, intensified associated psychodelic effects or the occurrence of the serotonin syndrome, may result (Yu, 2008). To date, these concerns, which are very likely valid, have not been empirically supported with human studies.[91]

Undesired, or Harmful, Effects and Toxicities

The use/abuse of LSD has been associated with several physical toxicities. It also has been associated with other long recognized, and generally much more serious, mental toxicities, which have been generally related to "drug, set, and setting." The "physical" toxicities associated with LSD use, include: anorexia; blurred vision; diaphoresis; dizziness; headache; heart palpitations; hypertension; incoordination; insomnia; mydriasis; nausea; tachycardia; and xerostomia.

The "mental" toxicities include: anxiety; difficulty locating the source of a sound; distortions of body image; dysphoria; fear of fragmentation, or disintegration, of the self; mood swings from happiness to sadness; and prolonged visual afterimages. While troublesome, these mental toxicities are generally short-lived. However, they can be extremely frightening when experienced in the context of a "bad trip" or "flashback." (See the later related discussion in this subsection.)

LSD-INDUCED DISORDERS

The relatively common, and generally more serious, mental toxicities associated with LSD use are well-recognized, and include: mental depression; severe panic reactions or "bad trips;" paranoia; and prolonged psychosis, particularly among adolescents and young adults who use LSD and have a predisposition for these toxicities (i.e., have a positive family history of schizophrenia). These common, and generally more serious, toxicities have been classified into four LSD-induced disorders according to the American Psychiatric Association's DSM taxonomy:

1. LSD-induced anxiety disorder;
2. LSD-induced hallucinogen persisting perception disorder;
3. LSD-induced mood disorder;
4. LSD-induced psychotic disorder.

These more serious LSD-induced disorders are managed in various ways, as follows.

LSD-INDUCED ANXIETY DISORDER. LSD-induced anxiety disorder is characterized by nervous behavior or panic that occurs during or following LSD use. It is often managed with sedative-hypnotic pharmacotherapy (e.g., diazepam, Valium®).

LSD-INDUCED HALLUCINOGEN-PERSISTING PERCEPTION DISORDER (FLASHBACKS). Hallucinogen-persisting perception disorder is the transient recurrence of perceptual disturbances associated with previous LSD use that can occur days, months, or even years after the last use of LSD. Due, particularly, to their unexpected occurrence, the transient recurrence of perceptual disturbances can result in significant clinical, or social, mental stress and impairment—determined, to a large degree, by the context in which they occur.

Hallucinogen-persisting perception disorder, or "flashbacks," typically involve visual hallucinations, but can also involve olfactory, tactile, or other sensory hallucinations that can last for

91 N.B. A number of additional LSD drug–drug interactions have been listed on the internet—primarily by LSD users. These unsubstantiated, anecdotal reports are considered to be generally unreliable and cannot be evaluated further until appropriate research investigation and support (i.e., empirical research data) become available.

minutes to hours. Although they are encountered more commonly with the frequent use of LSD, flashbacks can also occur following the initial use of LSD.[92] Flashbacks may be triggered by any type of environmental stimuli but, are commonly associated with the people, places, and things related to the initial use of LSD.[93] In addition, flashbacks have been related to physical or mental stress (Pagliaro & Pagliaro, *Clinical Patient Data Files*). When they do occur, they should be treated in the same way as LSD-induced psychotic disorder (see the following brief discussion in this subsection). Unplanned and unexpected, virtually all flashbacks have the potential to be unpleasant.

LSD-INDUCED MOOD DISORDER. LSD-induced mood disorder is associated with the regular, long-term use of LSD. Much like major depressive disorder (MDD), LSD-induced mood disorder is characterized by mental depression and associated risk for suicide attempts or completions. Occurring during or following LSD use, LSD-induced mood disorder generally persists for 24 hours or longer.

The MDD associated with LSD-induced mood disorder generally occurs among adolescents and young adults who have:

1. A predisposing, or genetic, tendency for MDD;
2. Concomitant use of other drugs and substances of abuse, particularly the psychodepressants (e.g., alcohol);
3. Other significant environmental risk factors (e.g., chronic debilitating medical conditions or disorders).

In the absence of these factors, lifetime LSD use generally has not been associated with an increased likelihood of: suicide attempt or completion related to LSD-induced mood disorder; serious psychological distress associated with other mental disorders; or history of mental health treatment (Hendricks, Thorne, & Clark, 2015; Johansen & Krebs, 2015; Krebs & Johansen, 2013; Pagliaro & Pagliaro, *Clinical Patient Data Files*).

LSD-INDUCED PSYCHOTIC DISORDER. LSD-induced psychotic disorder is characterized by disordered thinking, extreme alterations in emotions, and hallucinations that occur during LSD use. Generally resolving within hours, this psychotic disorder can progress to a long-term schizophreniform disorder. LSD-induced psychotic disorder, which is similar to "amphetamine-induced psychotic disorder" (see Chapter 2, "Amphetamines and Cocaine"), is more likely to occur with the repeated use of LSD. Adolescents and young adults, who use/abuse LSD and develop associated signs and symptoms of psychosis/schizophrenia, usually have a pre-existing, positive family history of schizophrenia.

LSD-induced psychotic disorder generally resolves with the discontinuation of LSD use. If necessary, it also responds well to appropriate antipsychotic pharmacotherapy. However, the psychosis may last for several days or several months—even with treatment. Less severe "bad trips" are usually temporary, lasting for approximately 24 hours (see also the related discussion in the earlier LSD subsection, "LSD-Induced Hallucinogen-Persisting Perception Disorder"). They generally can be successfully managed by providing reassurance and other psychological support in a familiar environment. Antipsychotic pharmacotherapy

92 During the new millennium, particularly with the generally lower dose of LSD that is being used (i.e., approximately half the dose used during the 1960s and 1970s), the incidence of flashbacks has been significantly reduced to the point that they are becoming a relatively uncommon phenomenon (Pagliaro & Pagliaro, *Clinical Patient Data Files*).

93 We have suggested that, for example, flashbacks, like the déjà vu experience, may be related, at least in some cases, to olfactory memory (Pagliaro, 1991).

(e.g., chlorpromazine, Thorazine®), which antagonizes most of the pharmacologic actions of LSD, usually is not required.

Physical and Psychological Dependence

The regular, long-term use of LSD has not been associated with physical dependence characterized by a classic withdrawal syndrome that: (1) occurs when regular, long-term use is abruptly discontinued; and (2) is immediately relieved when use is resumed. However, the use of LSD has been associated with the development of tolerance, cross tolerance, and reverse tolerance.

LSD TOLERANCE, CROSS TOLERANCE, AND REVERSE TOLERANCE

The regular use of LSD produces tolerance, cross tolerance, and reverse tolerance to LSD. "Tolerance," a reduced sensitivity to both the physical and psychological effects of LSD, often occurs among adolescents and young adults who are regular LSD users. Becoming insensitive to the LSD effects they desire, adolescents and young adults often unsuccessfully use increasingly higher doses of LSD in their efforts to achieve desired results. Heightened sensitivity to LSD can be rapidly returned, however, by discontinuing LSD use for three or four days (Pagliaro & Pagliaro, *Clinical Patient Data Files*; Passie, Halpern, & Stichtenoth, 2008; Scholey, Parrott, & Buchanan, 2004). The extent of physical and psychological tolerance to LSD can be significant—to the same degree as that observed for alcohol, prescription sedative-hypnotics (e.g., benzodiazepines; z-drugs); and phencyclidine ("PCP;" "Angel Dust"). Tolerance to the cardiovascular effects of LSD also occurs, but to a lesser degree.

"Cross tolerance" is the ability of a drug or substance of abuse to produce tolerance to the effects of other certain pharmacologically similar drugs and substances of abuse. The use of LSD is associated with cross tolerance to:

- Mescaline ("Cactus Buttons;" Peyote);
- Methylenedioxymethamphetamine ("Ecstasy;" "MDMA");
- Psilocybin ("Magic Mushrooms;" "Psychodelic Mushrooms;" "Schrooms").

The occurrence of LSD cross tolerance with these other drugs and substances of abuse suggests a common cellular/molecular mechanism of action.

"Reverse tolerance," or increased sensitivity to the effects of LSD, also has been rarely reported (Pagliaro & Pagliaro, *Clinical Patient Data Files*).

LSD WITHDRAWAL SYNDROME

There is no available evidence, anecdotal or otherwise, that supports the occurrence of a classic LSD withdrawal syndrome when regular, long-term use is abruptly discontinued.

LSD Overdosage

LSD has a high LD_{50} and, thus, is relatively safe to use. Although LSD has not been directly associated with overdosage fatalities, it has been indirectly associated with several accidental deaths and completed suicides. These fatalities have occurred among adolescents and young adults, who were under the influence of its psychodelic actions (e.g., an adolescent girl, believing she can "fly like a bird," fatally jumps off the roof of a building to her death; a young man, believing he is being chased by an illusionary figure, races across a street in terror and is fatally struck by a passing motor vehicle).

Procedures that are commonly used to facilitate the elimination of other drugs and substances of abuse overdosages (e.g., administration of activated charcoal; gastric lavage; hemodialysis; manipulation of urinary pH), have minimal efficacy in cases of LSD overdosage and, thus, are not recommended.

There is no known antidote for LSD overdosage and medical management is largely supportive. Based on presenting signs and symptoms, interventions may include the use of appropriate sedative-hypnotics (e.g., diazepam [Diazepam®]), for the treatment of associated anxiety/panic reactions, and antipsychotics (e.g., haloperidol [Haldol®]; chlorpromazine [Thorazine®]).[94] Fortunately, most related frightening experiences (i.e., "bad trips;" or panic reactions) can be managed by a safe environment and appropriate reassurance, or "talking down" the adolescent or young adult.[95]

Pregnancy and Lactation

Although LSD was commonly considered to be a human teratogen, particularly during the 1960s and 1970s, no empirical data have been published that support a clear link between the maternal use of LSD during pregnancy and teratogenesis (i.e., congenital malformations, including chromosomal damage among offspring).[96] In addition, the excretion of LSD into the breastmilk of mothers who use LSD and are breastfeeding, has not been demonstrated (Pagliaro & Pagliaro, 2000, 2009, 2012, 2018).

New Millennial Trends in LSD Use

The medical use of LSD is presented and discussed with attention to children, adolescents, and young adults. Embryo/fetal, infant, and child exposure also are presented and discussed. The section concludes with new millennial trends in adolescent and young adult LSD use.

Medical LSD Use

LSD never received FDA approval for the management of specific medical indications. However, it was evaluated in a number of clinical trials between 1947 and 1967,[97] when it

94 N.B. As emphasized by Passie, Halpern, and Stichtenoth, (2008), antipsychotics (e.g., chlorpromazine [Thorazine®]) are not antidotes for LSD overdosage. They are incomplete antagonists of LSD. Thus, although they may reduce or eliminate some LSD-induced effects, such as: anxiety; dizziness; nausea; and vomiting; they generally do not alter the production of delusions and hallucinations.

95 Adolescents and young adults often present to emergency departments with a possible LSD toxicity/overdosage. Routine toxicology tests and the comprehensive clinical assessment of these adolescents and young adults is indicated to identify all possible presenting toxicities. This assessment approach is required because many adolescents and young adults, who use LSD, also concurrently use other drugs and substances of abuse—all of which, in addition, may have been "cut" with other psychodelics (e.g., MMDA; PCP) or other unknown adulterants. Conscientious follow-up, based on test results and medical and other professional intervention, are also indicated.

96 Teratogenic effects have long been believed to be associated with the maternal use of LSD. However, this belief was mainly based on individual case reports in which severe physical abnormalities were identified among neonates whose mothers used LSD and other drugs and substances of abuse during the 1960s and 1970s. This erroneous conclusion was also supported by laboratory reports and studies by several researchers, who found human chromosomal damage (i.e., breakage) after in vitro exposure to LSD (e.g., Cohen, Marinello, & Back, 1967; Dishotsky, Loughman, & Mogar, 1971; Robinson, Chitham, & Greenwood, 1974).

97 During this time, LSD was experimentally evaluated in a variety of therapeutic contexts, including the treatment of schizophrenia (e.g., Abramson, Waxenberg, & Levine, 1955; Aronson & Waterman, 1962; Savage, 1955; Sloane & Lovett Doust, 1954; Wapner & Krus, 1960). Additionally, LSD was used: (1) to create a model of psychosis for the development and evaluation of antipsychotic pharmacotherapies; and (2) as an adjunct to psychotherapy for the treatment of refractory patients, such as violent sexual offenders (e.g., Bonson, 2017; Pagliaro & Pagliaro, *Clinical Patient Data Files*).

was placed on Schedule I of the U.N. Convention on Drugs (Pagliaro & Pagliaro, 2004; Pagliaro & Pagliaro, *Clinical Patient Data Files*; Rucker, Iliff, & Nutt, 2017). LSD is not currently approved for any medical indications in the U.S., although requests for the reconsideration of the use of LSD as an adjunct to psychotherapy is perennially expressed by various mental health professionals and researchers (e.g., Das, Barnwal, & Ramasamy, 2016; Gasser, Holstein, & Michel, 2014; Passie, Halpern, & Stichtenoth, 2008).

Given both the growing acceptance of cannabis, as discussed in the first major section of this chapter, and the relatively low to moderate risk of significant toxicity associated with the use of low-dosage LSD among carefully selected patients (e.g., nonpregnant and nonpsychotic adults), we expect that its medical use will eventually be approved. However, because of the possible various subjective and unpredictable reactions associated with LSD use, we recommend that the medical use of LSD be rigorously supervised in carefully controlled medical psychotherapeutic contexts with particular attention to the characteristics of individual LSD users, their environments, and their responses.

Embryo/Fetus, Neonate/Infant, and Child LSD Exposure

Although children rarely use LSD, they are often exposed to LSD primarily in the context of: (1) in utero exposure; (2) exposure through breastfeeding; and (3) accidental/unintentional poisoning. Fortunately, clinical sequelae associated with these exposures are not severe. See related discussion in the earlier LSD subsections, "Overdosage/Unintentional Poisoning" and "Pregnancy and Lactation."

Adolescent and Young Adult Illicit/Recreational LSD Use

Embodied by the "hippies" as a "Turn on, Tune-in, Dropout," and "antiestablishment" drug, which was musically eternalized in song lyrics by Bob Dylan, "The Beatles," and "The Rolling Stones," adolescent and young adult use of LSD flourished during the 1960s. However, during the late 1970s and 1980s, its use gradually declined. During the 1990s, LSD and other psychodelic drugs—at significantly lower dosages than those typically used during the 1960s—underwent renewed popularity as their use exploded among adolescents and young adults in the U.S., who were increasingly drawn to dance clubs and raves where they extensively used LSD and other psychodelics by every method of administration possible. Nevertheless, during the first two decades of the new millennium, the use of LSD has stabilized, if not declined.

As found by *Partnerships for a Drug-Free America* (2006), in their national survey: 6% of adolescents, in grades seven through 12, reported "having ever tried" LSD. This finding was 50% lower than the 12% that was reported for their 2000 survey and followed the decline in adolescent LSD use that was observed through 2004—at which time, LSD use appeared to stabilize at 6%. Wu, Schlenger, and Galvin (2006), in their review of data from the NSDUH, reported that, among their participants—16 to 23 year-old, noninstitutionalized household Americans—13.2% reported lifetime prevalence of LSD use and 2.3% reported use "within the past year."

In another study, Johnston, O'Malley, and Bachman (2008) found—in their 2007 nationwide survey (MTFS)—that, of 50,000 8th, 10th, and 12th graders, 1.1% of 8th graders, 1.9% of 10th graders, and 2.1% of 12th graders reported LSD use within the 12 months prior to the survey. They also found that 0.5% of 8th graders, 0.7% of 10th graders, and 0.6 % of 12th graders reported using LSD within the previous month (i.e., 30 days prior to the survey). In a later survey, Johnston, O'Malley, and Bachman (2011) found essentially the same level of reported LSD use—0.6%, 0.7%, and 0.8%, respectively. While reported lifetime use slightly increased among respondents from 8th grade through 12th grade over the past several years, recent use reportedly remained low (i.e., less than 1%) and relatively unchanged.

However, a change that was noted, during the second decade of the new millennium in the U.S, was the increase in LSD use by college/university students. As identified by Kruzman (2017), citing data from the NSDUH:

> The proportion of 18- to 25-year-olds who reported using LSD in the past year grew by 40% between 2013 and 2015.
>
> (p. 1)

In addition, Lipari and Ahrnsbrak (2017), in their presentation of the results from the 2016 NSDUH, found that: (1) new users ranged in age from 12 to 49 years-of-age (mean 20.6 years-of-age); (2) 160,000 adolescents, 12 to 17 years-of-age, used LSD for the first time in 2016; and (3) 567,000 young adults, 18 to 25 years-of-age, used LSD for the first time in 2016. Presenting highlights for the *2017 Monitoring the Future* annual report, the NIDA Press Office (2018a) reported that, "Past year use of LSD among 12th graders is at 3.3 percent" (p. 1).

A possible major contributing factor for the relatively low LSD use rates compared to other psychodelics (e.g., cannabis) is "perception of risk." As identified by Lipari and Ahrnsbrak (2017), regarding the results of the 2016 NSDUH, about 50% of adolescents and young adults "perceive great risk of harm from trying LSD once or twice." They also identified that about 75% of adolescents and young adults, "perceive great risk of harm from weekly LSD use" (p. 5).

Finally, when considering the statistics for LSD use, it is extremely important—as long identified by us and others—to give appropriate attention to the specific characteristics of the populations being sampled (e.g., high school students). For example, Swaim, Beauvais, and Chavez (1997) examined differences in self-reported LSD use statistics among: (1) adolescents, who were from three different ethnic groups; and (2) adolescents, who were currently enrolled in high school, versus adolescents, who dropped out of school. They found significant differences in reported use rates of LSD among the different groups of adolescents. For example, regarding "lifetime use of LSD," the highest rate was reported for adolescent high school students of European continental descent (i.e., 18%). In addition, the rate of use among matched age-controlled adolescents, who had dropped out of high school, was significantly higher (i.e., 47%).

Related Professional Reminder: ***Extreme care must be used by clinicians when using research generated statistics, particularly in regard to over-generalization from a limited or partial population sample—such as a non-random, non-stratified convenience sample.***

METHODS OF LSD USE

Most adolescents and young adults ingest a tiny LSD microdot tablet or place it under the tongue for sublingual absorption. Others ingest a sugar cube, gelatin square (or other shaped "window pane"), or small piece of blotter paper, upon which a drop of LSD solution is carefully placed. Additionally, a newer trend in LSD use developed—"microdosing." Microdosing is the ingestion of a very small dose of LSD (i.e., generally one-tenth of a usual dose) to, reportedly, increase creativity and everyday experiences—without the usual LSD-related undesired, or harmful, effects, and toxicities, such as, hallucinations and extreme sensory distortions, or illusions. To date, all available data regarding LSD microdosing is based on anecdotal reports (Boseley, 2018; Brodwin, 2017; Pagliaro & Pagliaro, *Clinical Patient Data Files*).

Assessment and Diagnosis of Psychodelic Dependence or Use Disorder—LSD, MDMA, and PCP

The assessment and diagnosis of psychodelic dependence or use disorders—particularly, LSD, MDMA, and PCP—among adolescents and young adults are presented and discussed in this subsection as a group because of their similarities.[98] As previously presented specifically for cannabis, attention also is given to the clinical professional's initial interview with an adolescent and use of relevant DSM-criteria and available quick-screen psychometric tests.

The assessment and diagnosis of LSD, MDMA, or PCP use disorder generally begins with the initial clinical interview with the adolescent or young adult during which: (1) the use of LSD, MDMA, or PCP is established; and, if established, (2) answers to questions concerning both the qualitative and quantitative nature of the adolescent's or young adult's use of the psychodelic of focus (i.e., LSD, MDMA, or PCP) are obtained. Commonly used questions, which can facilitate this process, include:

- How often do you use LSD/MDMA/PCP?
- When you use LSD/MDMA/PCP, how much do you usually use?
- Have you continued to use LSD/MDMA/PCP despite physical or psychological problems related to use?
- Have you continued to use LSD/MDMA/PCP despite relationship or social problems related to use?
- Have you experienced difficulties controlling, cutting down, or stopping LSD/MDMA/PCP use?
- Have you given up, or significantly reduced, other activities—particularly occupational, recreational, or social activities in favor of LSD/MDMA/PCP use?
- Have you experienced problems at home, school, or work as a result of LSD/MDMA/PCP use?
- Have you used more LSD/MDMA/PCP than intended, more frequently than intended, or for longer periods than intended?
- Have you spent a lot of time on LSD/MDMA/PCP use—including obtaining LSD/MDMA/PCP or recovering from effects associated with use?
- Have you used LSD/MDMA/PCP in potentially hazardous situations (e.g., while driving a motor vehicle)?

No specific validated psychometric screening tests have been developed to assist in the assessment and diagnoses of LSD, MDMA, or PCP dependence or use disorders. However, several generic psychometric screening tests for SUDS have been developed and are available for use to detect LSD, MDMA, or PCP dependence or use disorder(s). For a presentation and further discussion of these generic tests, see the amphetamine subsection in Chapter 2, "Amphetamines and Cocaine," "Selected Quick-Screen Psychometric Tests."

Methylenedioxymethamphetamine (MDMA)

Commonly known "on-the-street" as: "Ecstasy;" "E;" "Eve;" "Hug Drug;" "Love Drug;" "Molly;"[99] "X;" "XTC;" and a variety of other common names, MDMA is primarily used by adolescents and young adults to achieve such desired empathogenic/entactogenic actions as:

1. Emotional closeness;
2. Empathy—affection, compassion, identification, love, responsiveness, sympathy, understanding, warm-heartedness;
3. Euphoria—ecstasy, elation, joy, jubilation, rapture;

98 N.B. Although these psychodelics are discussed together here because of their similarities, DSM-5 addresses PCP use disorder as a separate distinct mental disorder.

99 The popular street name, "Molly," is derived from the word, "molecule."

4. Extroversion—friendliness, outgoingness, self-confidence, sociability, socialness;
5. Happiness—cheerfulness, contentment, gladness, joy, pleasure;
6. Sensory pleasure.

As identified by Hysek, Schmid, and Simmler (2014), MDMA increases and intensifies, "explicit and implicit emotional empathy," particularly among females (p. 1645). The use of MDMA also is associated with mild hallucinations that can last for four to eight hours without the anxiety, dissociation, perceptual distortion, or other undesired effects that are commonly associated with the use of other psychodelics (e.g., LSD). Desired psychostimulant effects associated with MDMA use include: alleviation of fatigue; heightened perceptions; stress relief; and wakefulness. All of these desired pharmacological effects, particularly the feelings of calmness, euphoria, understanding, and closeness to others (i.e., "pro-social effects"), have made MDMA especially appealing to adolescents and young adults, particularly adolescent girls and young women (Kirkpatrick & de Wit, 2015; Pagliaro & Pagliaro, 2009, 2012, 2018; Piper, 2007; Wardle, Kirkpatrick, & de Wit, 2014).

Interestingly, Thomasius, Petersen, and Zapletalova (2005) identified that, for both current and former MDMA users:

> The motivation for ecstasy use is not likely to be self-medication of pre-existing depressive or anxiety disorders as these did *not* occur more frequently in the ecstasy users than in control groups or in the general population.
>
> (p. 1310)

MDMA Pharmacology

MDMA is a synthetic psychodelic that is chemically related to the amphetamines, which explains its psychostimulant actions. The attachment of a methylenedioxy group to the aromatic ring also makes MDMA structurally similar to the natural psychodelic, "mescaline." MDMA was originally known as "methylsafrylaminc" and originally synthesized in 1912 by the German pharmaceutical company, Merck and Company—in an attempt to develop drugs to "control bleeding" (NIDA, 2017). However, there was little interest in MDMA for the next 50 years, at which time it was rediscovered and popularized by the "Hippies" during the counter-culture movement.

The majority of MDMA, which is currently used in the U.S., is synthesized in Canada. A significant amount is also illicitly imported from the Netherlands (NIDA, 2017).

Pharmacodynamics: Mechanism of Action

The feelings of elation, emotional closeness, and sensory pleasure, which are associated with the use of MDMA, are thought to be caused by the:

1. Release of neurotransmitters, primarily serotonin (i.e., 5-hydroxytryptamine, 5-HT), but also—to a lesser extent—dopamine and norepinephrine;
2. Prevention of their reuptake (i.e., MDMA acts as an indirect biogenic amine agonist).

This mechanism of action involves the interaction of MDMA with 5-HT membrane transporters (SERTS) as substrates—consequently, affecting neurotransmitter membrane reuptake and vesicular storage systems (de la Torre, Farre, & Roset, 2004; Pagliaro & Pagliaro, 2004; Schmid, Rickli, & Schaffner, 2015).

Several researchers (e.g., Meyer, 2013; Parrott, Lock, & Conner, 2008) also argue that the MDMA-associated neuro-hormonal release—particularly, the release of cortisol and oxytocin—may be a key underlying factor in producing the observed effects that are typically associated with MDMA use. Parrott, Lock, and Conner (2008) identified that cortisol release is increased by such stimulatory factors as physical activity, thermal stress, and psychostimulant drugs. Parrott (2009), citing data from a previous study that found that cortisol levels increased significantly (i.e., by 800%) among participants on MDMA when "dance clubbing," concluded that:

> In MDMA-using dance clubbers, the cortisol levels are ... possibly due to the combined factors of stimulant drug, physical exertion and psychosocial stimulation.
>
> (p. 148)

As found by Hysek, Schmid, and Simmler (2014), in their "placebo-controlled, double-blind, random-order, cross-over design" study of "32 healthy volunteers:"

> MDMA increased plasma levels of cortisol and prolactin, which are markers of serotonergic and noradrenergic activity, and of oxytocin, which has been associated with prosocial behavior.
>
> (p. 1645)

The identified situational, or contextual, factors, as well as the MDMA dosage ingested, probably explain, or at least help to account for, the majority of the observed variance in individual response to MDMA use.

In addition, McGregor, Callaghan, and Hunt (2008) advanced the theory that the neuropeptide, oxytocin, may play an integral and significant role in the action of MDMA.[100] As noted by the researchers, oxytocin often has been referred to as the "social" neuropeptide because of its "prosocial" and "pro-sexual" effects (i.e., as have been associated with MDMA use). This action appears to be mediated by oxytocin-dopamine interactions that occur in the mesolimbic region of the brain. However, the purported mechanism of action for MDMA, as for many other psychodelics, involves several different mechanisms. In addition, these mechanisms also can vary in their extent of contribution to the action of MDMA based upon several variables (e.g., age, gender, genetics).

Pharmacokinetics: Absorption, Distribution, Metabolism, and Excretion

MDMA is readily absorbed from the GI tract following ingestion and has an onset of action of approximately 30 minutes. Peak serum MDMA concentrations are achieved within one to three hours. The half-life of elimination for MDMA is approximately seven hours. Effects generally last for three to six hours (NIDA, 2016).

MDMA is metabolized in the liver to an active metabolite, "methylenedioxyamphetamine" (e.g., "MDA;" "Adam"), primarily by the hepatic microsomal enzyme cytochrome P450-2D6 (i.e., CYP2D6).[101] As emphasized by de la Torre, Farre, and Roset (2004):

100 Although oxytocin is probably best known for its physiological effects, such as increasing contractions during parturition and increasing breast milk ejection during lactation and breastfeeding, it also is known for several significant psychological effects. For example, oxytocin has been specifically associated with: (1) increased ability to cope with stress, elevated mood, sociability, and trust; and (2) decreased feelings of anxiety, aggression, and irritability.

101 Consequently, enzyme inducers and inhibitors of cytochrome P450-2D6 can significantly increase or decrease, respectively, the half-life of elimination of MDMA. (See also the related discussion in the later MDMA subsection, "MDMA Drug–Drug Interactions").

> MDMA metabolism is rather complex and includes 2 main metabolic pathways: (1) O-demethylation followed by catechol-O-methyltransferase (COMT)-catalyzed methylation and/or glucuronide/sulfate conjugation; and (2) N-dealkylation, deamination, and oxidation to the corresponding benzoic acid derivatives conjugated with glycine.
>
> (p. 137)

The half-life of MDA (i.e., 12 to 36 hours) is longer than that of its active parent drug, MDMA, and is associated with more neurotoxicity (Pagliaro & Pagliaro, 2009). Other human pharmacokinetic data are not available.

MDMA Drug–Drug Interactions

Typically, adolescents and young adults, who use MDMA, concomitantly use other drugs and substances of abuse, including alcohol and cannabis (Pagliaro & Pagliaro, 2009), that may result in significant drug–drug interactions that are often of an additive or synergistic nature (Parrott, 2006). They also may use a variety of non-abusable psychotropics (e.g., antidepressants). However, published research and related data concerning drug–drug interactions involving MDMA are primarily based on theoretical concerns. Although limited, available published data concerning MDMA interactions involving alcohol, bupropion, monoamine oxidase inhibitors, and the serotonin reuptake inhibitor, paroxetine, are presented and discussed in the following subsections.

ALCOHOL AND MDMA

Alcohol and MDMA are commonly concurrently used by adolescents and young adults in the U.S. (Pagliaro & Pagliaro, 2009, 2012; Pagliaro & Pagliaro, *Clinical Patient Data Files*). However, the majority of studies of a possible interaction between the two abusable psychotropics have been performed with laboratory animal models (e.g., Upreti, Eddington, & Moon, 2009). A significant contributory factor to this situation is the illegal status of the use of MDMA in the U.S. and, consequently, the associated difficulty associated with obtaining ethical approval for related research involving humans.

A Spanish research group (i.e., Hernandez-Lopez, Farre, & Roset, 2002) found, in their study of a group of human research participants, that concurrent use of alcohol and MDMA resulted in:

1. Decreased blood alcohol concentrations (approximately 12%);
2. Increased blood MDMA concentrations (approximately 13%);
3. Decreased subjective feelings associated with alcohol intoxication;
4. No objective effects on the alcohol-induced impairment of psychomotor skills;
5. Longer-lasting MDMA-induced feelings of euphoria than that induced by the use of either alcohol or MDMA alone.

Although not replicated, these laboratory findings suggest a very real potential for increased impaired hazardous motor vehicle driving among adolescents and young adults, who concurrently use alcohol and MDMA and drive. In addition, based on the consideration of both related case reports and data from MDMA-related ED visits, SAMHSA (2013b, p. 1) concluded that:

> When Ecstasy is mixed with alcohol, the stimulating effects of Ecstasy cause the user to be *less* aware of alcohol intoxication. This mixture can lead to poor decision making and bodily harm. The Ecstasy-alcohol mixture also causes a longer lasting euphoria than Ecstasy or alcohol alone, which could *increase* the potential for abuse.

See also the related discussion in the later subsection, "MDMA Overdosage."

BUPROPION (WELLBUTRIN®, ZYBAN®) AND MDMA

Bupropion is an antidepressant that is also used to facilitate smoking cessation (see related discussion in Chapter 3, "Caffeine and Nicotine"). Because of its action as a dopamine-norepinephrine reuptake inhibitor, bupropion has been anticipated to interact with MDMA, which facilitates the release and inhibits the reuptake of the biogenic amines (i.e., dopamine, norepinephrine, and serotonin). Swiss researchers (i.e., Schmid, Rickli, & Schaffner, 2015), in their study of this interaction involving human subjects, found that:

1. Bupropion reduced MDMA-induced elevations in plasma norepinephrine concentrations;
2. Bupropion reduced the cardiostimulant effects of MDMA;
3. Bupropion increased MDMA concentrations and prolonged its subjective mood effects;
4. MDMA reduced the plasma concentrations of bupropion.

MONOAMINE OXIDASE INHIBITORS (MAOIs) AND MDMA

MAOIs, such as moclobemide (Manerix®), phenelzine (Nardil®), and tranylcypromine (Parnate®), have been postulated to interact with MDMA producing the serotonin syndrome that can be potentially fatal. Although no related empirical studies are available, several cases of this interaction involving MAOIs and MDMA have been reported. For example, both Pilgrim, Gerostamoulos, and Woodford (2012) and Vuori, Henry, and Ojanpera (2003) each reported an independent series of four cases of fatal serotonin toxicity caused by the combination of a MAOI and MDMA. All eight individual cases involved moclobemide, a reversible MAOI-A inhibitor. Signs and symptoms included: diaphoresis; hyperkalemia; hyperthermia; shaking; and twitching (see also the related discussion in the following MDMA subsection, "Pharmacology, Undesired, or Harmful Effects and Toxicities").

PAROXETINE (PAXIL®) AND MDMA

Paroxetine is a selective serotonin reuptake inhibitor (SSRI). It is both a substrate for and a potent inhibitor of CYP2D6. Deficiency, or impairment, of CYP2D6 places MDMA users at significantly increased risk of acute toxicity at moderate dosages (Pagliaro & Pagliaro, 2009). It is estimated that approximately 10% of U.S. adolescents and young adults of European continental descent are genetically deficient in regard to this hepatic microsomal isoenzyme (Pagliaro & Pagliaro, 2009) (See the earlier related discussion in the subsection, "Pharmacology, Pharmacokinetics"). Consequently, drugs, such as paroxetine, which may reduce CYP2D6, can be expected, at least theoretically, to increase MDMA blood concentrations—and related toxicity.

In order to formally investigate the interaction of paroxetine and MDMA in humans, Spanish researchers (i.e., Farre, Abanades, & Roset, 2007) pretreated their volunteer human subjects with paroxetine and then administered a single dose of MDMA. They found that pretreatment with paroxetine resulted in:

1. A 30% increase in MDMA plasma concentrations—presumably due to decreased metabolism by CYP2D6;
2. Marked decreases in both the objective physiological effects (e.g., cardiovascular effects; pupil diameter; temperature); and subjective psychological effects (e.g., euphoria) associated with MDMA use—presumably due to decreased serotonin reuptake.

Consequently, they posited that a:

> Marked *decrease* in the effects of MDMA could lead users to take *higher* doses of MDMA and to produce potential life-threatening toxic effects.
>
> (p. 954)

Undesired, or Harmful, Effects and Toxicities.

The use of MDMA is associated with both acute and chronic toxicities. These and other undesired, or harmful, effects and toxicities are presented in the following MDMA subsections. Interestingly, several researchers (e.g., Allott & Redman, 2007; Ogeil, Rajaratnam, & Broadbear, 2013; Wu, Grady, & Rosales, 2011) have reported that, when compared to adolescent boys and young men, adolescent girls and young women, who use MDMA, have a higher incidence of toxicity and/or a greater severity of toxicity. For example, as reported by Rosenson, Smollin, and Sporer (2007):

> Female sex was associated with increased odds of hyponatremia and increased odds of hyponatremia-associated coma among persons with ecstasy intoxication.
>
> (p. 164)

Moritz, Kalantar-Zadeh, and Ayus (2013) suggested that the noted higher incidence of MDMA-related symptomatic hyponatremia among adolescent girls and young women is due to: (1) estrogen-mediated impairment of brain cell volume; and (2) the more pronounced vasocontrictive effects of arginine vasopressin (AVP) noted in the female brain.

Also see the related discussion in the later MDMA subsection, "Overdosage/Unintentional Poisoning."

ACUTE AND CHRONIC TOXICITIES

The use of MDMA is associated with several acute mental and physical toxicities, including: agitation; anxiety; blurred vision; bruxism; cardiac dysrhythmias; diaphoresis; dissociative signs and symptoms;[102] dizziness; fatigue; fear; hallucinations (mild); headache; hepatitis (MDMA-induced); hyperkinesia; hypertension; hyperthermia;[103] hyponatremia;[104] impulsive behavior; mental confusion; mental depression; mydriasis; nausea; panic attacks; perceptual disturbances (mild); restless legs; seizures; tachycardia; thirst; urinary retention; vomiting; and xerostomia

102 Dissociative signs and symptoms (e.g., elevated feelings of depersonalization and derealization) are not usually reported, particularly when MDMA is used alone. However, these signs and symptoms have been induced in controlled laboratory studies (e.g., Puxty, Ramaekers, & de la Torre, 2017; van Heugten-Van der Kloet, Giesbrecht, & van Wel, 2015) following typical single doses to volunteer subjects. These MDMA-associated signs and symptoms generally exceed those observed among patients with schizophrenia.

Puxty, Ramaekers, and de la Torre (2017), in a human laboratory experiment conducted in the Netherlands in which subjects were pretreated with the 5-HT_{2A} receptor antagonist, ketanserin (Sufrexal®), the dissociative symptoms (as measured by the responses to the "Clinician-Administered Dissociative States Scale" [CADSS]) were not significantly modified (i.e., the dissociative symptoms do not appear to be mediated by receptor MDMA interaction with the 5-HT_{2A} receptor).

103 The increase in body temperature is usually minimal (i.e., 0.5° to 1.0° C) with low to moderate dosages (Parrott, 2012). However, increases in body temperature can be significant with higher dosages and can result in hyperthermia (see related discussion in later subsection, "Overdosage/Unintentional Poisoning").

104 Generally mild, except in cases of overdosage (see related discussion in later subsection, "Overdosage.") In a related study, van Dijken, Blom, and Hene (2013) noted that "most cases of hyponatremia occurred in females" (p. 2277). Also see earlier related observations by Rosenson, Smollin, and Sporer (2007).

(Baylen & Rosenberg, 2006; Pagliaro & Pagliaro, *Clinical Patient Data Files*; Pagliaro & Pagliaro, 2009; Smith, Larive, & Romanelli, 2002).

Regarding chronic toxicities, the regular, long-term use of MDMA is associated with: anorexia; dehydration related to hyperkinesia and hyperthermia; insomnia; irritability; neurogenic bladder; renal failure; soreness of the jaw muscles related to bruxism and trismus; and weight loss related to nausea and vomiting. In addition, neurological/neuropsychiatric impairments (e.g., attention problems; memory deficits) have been associated with the regular, long-term use of MDMA (e.g., Morgan, 2000; Thomasius, Zapletalova, & Petersen, 2006).

The regular, long-term use of MDMA is also directly associated with the loss of serotonergic axons in the corpus striatum and other areas associated with higher-level brain functioning, including that involving the frontal cortex (Quednow, Jessen, & Kuhn, 2006). Adolescents may be at particular risk for these MDMA-related neurotoxicities, including neuropsychiatric impairment (Montoya, Sorrentino, & Lukas, 2002). Of increasing concern, are findings that some neurotoxic effects do not appear to abate, even after several years following the discontinuation of MDMA use. Consequently, these neurotoxic effects may be permanent (Gouzoulis-Mayfrank & Daumann, 2006, 2009; Pagliaro & Pagliaro, 2009).

Several researchers support this contention regarding more serious neurotoxic effects affecting attention and memory, particularly, verbal memory[105] (Parrott, 2006; Piper, 2007). For example, as identified by Parrott (2006):

> Most heavy (ecstasy/MDMA) users report memory or other psychobiological problems ... confirmed by objective deficits in working memory, attention, frontal-executive memory tasks, and episodic memory tasks.
>
> (p. 147)

As found by Quednow, Jessen, and Kuhn (2006):

> Abstinent MDMA users have memory deficits ... users revealed impairments in learning, consolidation, recall and recognition.
>
> (p. 373)

In another example, as reported by Roberts, Nestor, and Garavan (2009):

> Ecstasy users performed significantly worse in learning and memory compared to controls and cannabis users.
>
> (p. 71)

In addition, mental depression (i.e., "mid-week blues") has been reported by both occasional and regular, long-term MDMA users. Usually occurring two to five days following the last use of MDMA, it is unclear as to whether the depressive symptomatology is related to: (1) the specific pharmacological mechanisms associated with MDMA; or (2) a negative placebo effect,

105 Memory and other neurological impairments associated with regular, long-term use of MDMA is not always experienced by all users (Gouzoulis-Mayfrank & Daumann, 2006; Gouzoulis-Mayfrank, Fischermann, & Rezk, 2005). The reason for this apparent variation in response to MDMA is unknown. However, it is most likely associated with the: (1) concomitant use of other neurotoxic drugs and substances of abuse (e.g., alcohol; methamphetamine)—for example, over 90% of MDMA users also report use of cannabis (Parrott, 2006); (2) dosage of MDMA used; and (3) genetic predisposition. In addition, several researchers (e.g., Parrott, 2006, p. 147) suggest the venues in which MDMA is typically used (i.e., "hot and crowded dance clubs and raves") may significantly raise the body temperature of users and, consequently, contribute to the observed neuropsychobiological effects (including noted deficits in learning and memory).

such as an adolescent girl wishing that she was back in the MDMA-clubbing scene again. In any event, severe MDMA-midweek blues is more often reported by girls than boys, who similarly use MDMA (Falck, Wang, & Carlson, 2006; Meyer, 2013). (Also see related discussion in the following MDMA subsection, "Physical and Psychological Dependence—MDMA Withdrawal Syndrome.")

PHYSICAL AND PSYCHOLOGICAL DEPENDENCE OR USE DISORDER

Whereas the regular, long-term use of most psychodelics (e.g., LSD; PCP) has not been associated with "classic" physical and psychological dependence, the regular, long-term use of MDMA has been increasingly associated with physical dependence—albeit, reportedly significantly less severe in nature than that associated with alcohol, methamphetamine, nicotine, or opiate analgesics (Degenhardt, Bruno, & Topp, 2010; Meyer, 2013). MDMA physical dependence is characterized by acute tolerance and a MDMA withdrawal syndrome. MDMA psychological dependence is characterized by craving for MDMA (e.g., Cottler, Womack, & Compton, 2001; Leung & Cottler, 2008; Wu, Ringwalt, & Weiss, 2009).

ACUTE TOLERANCE. Acute tolerance to MDMA has been identified and appears to be associated with the use of repeated doses of MDMA over two to four hours (Cottler, Womack, & Compton, 2001). The short-term reduction or absence of desired MDMA effects (e.g., euphoria)—as well as undesired, or harmful, effects (e.g., tachycardia)—are believed to be due to the inhibition of serotonin synthesis and/or the depletion of serotonin stores (Farre, Tomillero; & Perez-Mana, 2015; Gallagher, Hadjiefthyvoulou, & Fisk, 2014; Hysek, Simmler, & Schillinger, 2014; Peiro, Farre, & Roset, 2013).

MDMA WITHDRAWAL SYNDROME. A MDMA withdrawal syndrome has been identified (e.g., Cottler, Womack, & Compton, 2001) and generally occurs three to five days following the abrupt discontinuation of regular, long-term MDMA use. It is primarily characterized by feelings of dysphoria and emotional withdrawal. The relationship of the MDMA withdrawal syndrome to "mid-week blues" (see earlier discussion) has been suggested, but has not been formally established (Pagliaro & Pagliaro, 2009).

CRAVING. Craving for MDMA is commonly reported by adolescents and young adults who are MDMA users (Pagliaro & Pagliaro, *Clinical Patient Data Files*). To better understand this construct, Davis and Rosenberg (2014) developed an eight-item "Ecstasy" craving questionnaire with a seven-point Likert response scale. Among their sample of 240 "MDMA/Ecstasy" users, the questionnaire was found to have high reliability in terms of internal consistency (i.e., Cronbach's alpha = 0.95). They also found:

> Frequency counts for six of the eight statements revealed that one-third to one-half of the recreational users in our sample agreed with statements indicative of craving.
>
> (p. 160)

MDMA Overdosage/Unintentional Poisoning

Although relatively rare, during the first decade of the new millennium, over 300 overdose fatalities were associated with MDMA in the U.S. (Pagliaro & Pagliaro, 2009). Primarily involving adolescent boys and men, 15 to 40 years-of-age, most of these deaths were accidental (i.e., unintentional) and were related to dehydration and hyperthermia (Gill, Hayes, & deSousa, 2002). Suicides involving MDMA use—such as that involving a 15 year-old adolescent girl—are also considered to be relatively rare events (Fernando, Gilbert, & Carroll, 2012).

> According to the Drug Abuse Warning Network (DAWN), the estimated number of emergency department (ED) visits involving Ecstasy in patients younger than 21 years old increased 128 percent, from 4,460 visits in 2005 to 10,176 visits in 2011.
>
> (SAMHSA, 2013a, p. 1)

In many of these cases, uncharacteristic behavior and vomiting are initially observed, followed by seizures, disorientation, coma, and death. Death is usually associated with acute renal failure, cardiac dysrhythmias, cerebrovascular accident, disseminated intravascular coagulation, hyperkalemia, hyperthermia, hyponatremic encephalopathy, renal toxicity, and rhabdomyolysis (Pagliaro & Pagliaro, 2009; Patel, Belson, & Longwater, 2005).

MDMA-induced hyperthermia commonly occurs among adolescents and young adults, who have experienced a significant acute overdosage, and significantly contributes to associated morbidity and mortality. The major factors that appear to contribute to the severity of MDMA-induced hyperthermia, include the: (1) dose of MDMA ingested; (2) temperature of the immediate surroundings (e.g., dance club; rave); and (3) amount of physical exertion—often related to continuous dancing throughout the night (Armenian, Mamantov, & Tsutaoka, 2013; Pagliaro & Pagliaro, 2009).

MDMA-induced renal toxicity is most often related to: (1) acute renal injury (e.g., nontraumatic rhabdomyolysis); or (2) severe hyponatremia (Campbell & Rosner, 2008; Ghatol & Kazory, 2012). As identified by Campbell and Rosner (2008), the factors contributing to MDMA-associated hyponatremia, include:

- Absorption of hypotonic solutions from the GI tract;
- Misdirected, usually by "friends," to drink lots of fluids at dance clubs or raves;
- MDMA-induced secretion of arginine vasopressin (AVP), or antidiuretic hormone (ADH);
- MDMA-induced thirst;
- Ready availability of fluids.

The severe MDMA-induced hyponatremia is most often observed among adolescent girls and young women (Campbell & Rosner, 2008; Rosenson, Smollin, & Sporer, 2007; van Dijken, Blom, & Hene, 2013). It is commonly medically managed with infusions of hypertonic saline solution (Pagliaro & Pagliaro, 2009). Malignant hypotension, secondary to volume depletion, also may significantly contribute to the acute renal injury (Campbell & Rosner, 2008).

A clear picture as to the cause and sequelae of MDMA overdosage is difficult to obtain because the overwhelming majority of MDMA users (i.e., 80% to 90%) are known to be users of several other drugs and substances of abuse, which commonly include the concurrent use of alcohol, cannabis, and LSD (e.g., Ho, Karimi-Tabesh, & Koren, 2001; Pagliaro & Pagliaro, 2009). For example, alcohol is frequently used concurrently with MDMA by adolescents and young adults in the U.S. (Pagliaro & Pagliaro, 2004, 2009, 2012) and is involved as a co-intoxicant in approximately one-third of reported ED visits of patients under 21 years-of-age for evaluation and treatment of MDMA overdosage (SAMHSA, 2013b). (See also the related discussion in the earlier MDMA subsection, "MDMA Drug–Drug Interactions—Alcohol and MDMA.")

It also should be noted that street samples of MDMA are commonly misrepresented, adulterated, and/or deliberately "cut" with other drugs—drugs that can contribute to, or exacerbate, the signs and symptoms of MDMA overdosage. As identified by the NIDA (2016):

> Much of the Molly seized by the police contains additives such as cocaine, ketamine, methamphetamine, over-the-counter cough medicine, or synthetic cathinones (i.e., "bath salts").
>
> (p. 3)

As further reported by the National Highway Traffic Safety Administration (2016):

> Potency of street samples is highly variable, and tablets sold as "ecstasy" may in fact contain little or no MDMA, but may contain caffeine, ephedrine, phenylpropanolamine, paramethoxyamphetamine (PMA), methylenedioxyamphetamine (MDA), dextromethorphan, amphetamine, methamphetamine, and ketamine.
>
> (p. 1)

It also has been suggested that, what is often identified as MDMA overdosage, may, in many cases, actually be an expression of the "serotonin syndrome." The serotonin syndrome may occur as a result of the interaction of MDMA with a selective serotonin reuptake inhibitor (SSRI), such as the antidepressant, fluoxetine (Prozac®), or other interacting drugs (Pilgrim, Gerostamoulos, & Drummer, 2011; Schifano, 2004). (See also the earlier MDMA subsection, "MDMA Drug–Drug Interactions.") In addition, many of the signs and symptoms of fatal MDMA overdosage (e.g., hyponatremic encephalopathy) can be related to several other risk factors, including the concurrent ingestion of an excessive amount of beer or water.[106]

The serious and potentially fatal consequences of MDMA overdosage require emergency medical evaluation and support of body systems (e.g., IV fluids and cooling baths, pads, or compresses, as indicated). In addition, dantrolene (Dantrium®) has been recommended by some poison control centers to aid in the treatment of MDMA overdosages characterized by hyperthermia and rigidity (Grunau, Wiens, & Brubacher, 2010; Grunau, Wiens, & Greidanus, 2010). There is no known antidote for MDMA overdosage. (See also, the later subsection, "New Millennial Trends in MDMA Use—Embryo/Fetal, Neonate/Infant, and Child Exposure to MDMA")

Pregnancy and Lactation

The use of MDMA by adolescent girls and young women during pregnancy does not appear to present a significant risk for teratogenesis (Pagliaro & Pagliaro, 2009).[107] However, some researchers (Singer, Moore, & Fulton, 2012; Singer, Moore, & Min, 2012) found, in their sample of 96 women (28 MDMA users, and 68 non-MDMA users), that prenatally exposed infants displayed poorer mental and motor development at four and 12 months of age. They also noted that these observed effects were consistent with those observed in some animal species (i.e., chicks; rats) that were experimentally exposed to MDMA neonatally. Parrott, Moore, and Turner (2014) posited that these neuro-psychobiological deficits may be related to the high levels of cortisol associated with MDMA use (see related discussion in the earlier MDMA pharmacology subsection, "Pharmacodynamics: Mechanism of Action").

No data are readily available on the excretion of MDMA in breast milk (Pagliaro & Pagliaro, 2009). In the absence of these data, it is strongly recommended that adolescent girls and young women, who use MDMA, avoid breastfeeding. The caution is predicated upon: (1) the mechanism of action of MDMA; (2) reports of neurotoxicity among MDMA users; and (3) the potential for toxicity to the developing CNS of breast-fed neonates and infants.

106 MDMA use, even in healthy volunteers has resulted in an increase in vasopressin secretion with consequent reduced sodium concentrations and polydipsia because of its effects on the serotonergic system. When excess fluids (e.g., beer, water) have been ingested, resultant hyponatremia and/or hypervolemia may—as previously noted—occur (Campbell & Rosner, 2008; Traub, Hoffman, & Nelson, 2002).

107 N.B. This conclusion is based primarily on the *absence* of related published data (i.e., case reports or clinical studies identifying the presence of teratogenic effects)—particularly, when considering that adolescents and young adults have been the primary users of MDMA in the U.S. for the past 40 years.

New Millennial Trends in MDMA Use

The medical use of MDMA is presented and discussed followed by the presentation and discussion of embryo/fetal, neonate/infant, and child exposure to MDMA. The section concludes with new millennial trends in adolescent and young adult illicit/recreational MDMA use.

Medical MDMA Use

Following its synthesis in 1912, interest in the use of MDMA quickly waned. It was briefly used—off-label—as a possible adjunct to psychotherapy, particularly for the treatment of post-traumatic stress disorder (PTSD) during the late 1970s and early 1980s, (Jerome, Schuster, & Yazar-Klosinski, 2013; Meyer, 2013). In 1985, the FDA placed MDMA on the list of Schedule I drugs (NIDA, 2017). MDMA currently has no FDA-approved therapeutic medical indication for use in the U.S. However, interest in such use remains high (e.g., Nutt, 2012; Scharff, 2014) and we expect that, as with the other psychodelics, FDA approval for research purposes and medical use will be received within the next two decades.

Infant and Child MDMA Exposure

MDMA has been associated with a number of pediatric overdosages, worldwide (e.g., England, Germany, Spain, Taiwan, and the U.S.), which generally occur in the context of accidental, unintentional poisonings that involve infants and toddlers, usually two years-of-age or younger. Although reports of these poisonings are relatively rare (e.g., Chang, Lai, & Kong, 2005; Duffy & Swart, 2006; Feldman & Mazor, 2007; Kung, Chan, & Tse, 2008; Melian, Burillo-Poutze, & Campo, 2004), they exceed the total number of unintentional poisonings reported for all of the other psychodelics combined.

Adolescent and Young Adult Illicit/Recreational MDMA Use

The use of MDMA by adolescents and young adults has an interesting history. After a relatively slow start, the use of MDMA among adolescents and young adults virtually exploded worldwide, particularly in response to two trends that began in the 1980s: (1) "raving;" and (2) "clubbing." As described by the CDC (2010):

> A rave is an all-night dance party with electronic music. When raves first emerged in the late 1980s, they were underground parties usually held at abandoned warehouses and outdoor sites. Since then, raves have become organized commercial events staged by promoters at established venues, often with high ticket prices and elaborate laser light effects.
>
> (p. 677)

Clubbing, or club culture, is related to raving with a focus on social gathering at nightclubs (e.g., discotheques; festivals; and techno clubs), where adolescents (usually with false identification cards, or accompanied by an adult) and young adults: listen to music, particularly electronic dance music; dance; drink alcohol; and use "recreational" drugs, including MDMA.

Whereas MDMA capsules and tablets are usually ingested, often with a "swig of beer," some adolescents and young adults empty the powder from a capsule or crush a tablet into a fine powder and intranasally insufflate, or "snort," their MDMA. Rarely, the MDMA powder is dissolved and intravenously injected (Pagliaro & Pagliaro, *Clinical Patient Data Files*).

During the first decade of the new millennium, widespread use of MDMA continued throughout the U.S., particularly, among middle class adolescent girls and young women of

European continental descent (Parsons, Grov, & Kelly, 2009; Wu, Liu, & Hoang Pham, 2010). This trend continued into the second decade of the new millennium with both sellers and users having little difficulty obtaining illicitly produced MDMA capsules and tablets from supplies, primarily produced in Western Europe—particularly Belgium, Luxembourg, and the Netherlands and often transported through Canada and Mexico for distribution and sale across the U.S. (Shukla, Crump, & Chrisco, 2012). A small number of laboratories also illicitly produce MDMA in Canada and the U.S. (NIDA, 2017).

In their review of data from the NSDUH, which used a sample of non-institutionalized household members 16 years-of-age to 23 years-of-age, Wu, Schlenger, and Galvin (2006) identified that: (1) 13.6% of participants reported "lifetime prevalence of MDMA use;" and (2) 6% of participants reported "past year use." In a later study, Murphy, Barry, and Vaughn (2013) found that 5% of both 10th and 12th graders reported "ecstasy use in the past year" (p. 4). In comparison, Palamar, Mauro, and Han (2017), in their secondary analysis of data from the 2007–2014 *National Survey on Drug Use and Health* (NSDUH), found among participants, 12 to 34 years-of-age, that past-year prevalence of MDMA use was stable across years at 2%. However, the proportion of MDMA users with a college degree increased from 11.5% to 24.5%

Bearing in mind these results, it is critical to consider the findings of Palamar, Keyes, and Cleland (2016), who analyzed data from a nationally representative survey of 6,250 U.S. high school seniors, with specific attention to the use of "MDMA" or "Ecstasy" versus the use of "Molly" in the wording of questionnaire forms aimed at detecting MDMA use:

> The form including "Molly" in the definition had significantly higher prevalence than the two (combined) forms that did not. Lifetime use (8.0% vs. 5.5%) and 12-month use (5.1% vs. 3.6%) were significantly higher with "Molly" in the definition.
>
> (p. 279)[108]

<u>Related Professional Reminder:</u> Adolescents and young adults are often not as well-informed regarding issues of drug and substance abuse as their health care professional may assume. Verify your assumptions, beliefs, and hunches with open-ended questioning and other appropriate techniques (e.g., parental and other validation).

Several factors highly correlate with MDMA use among adolescents and young adults during the new millennium, including:

- A high sensation-seeking personality;
- A history of childhood physical abuse;
- Childhood use of drugs and/or substances of abuse;
- Concurrent use of other drugs and substances of abuse;[109]
- Low academic achievement;
- Multiple continental or other descent, or ethnicity;
- Parental use of drugs and substances of abuse;
- Peer use of drugs and substances of abuse (e.g., Martins & Alexandre, 2009; Martins, Storr, & Alexandre, 2008; Pagliaro & Pagliaro, *Clinical Patient Data Files*; Wu, Liu, & Hoang Pham, 2010).

108 Obviously, the high school seniors in this survey recognized MDMA and "Ecstasy" as the same drug but did *not* also recognize "Molly" as the same drug.

109 MDMA is often used concurrently with alcohol and/or cannabis (NIDA, 2016). It also is used with cocaine, methamphetamine, and opiate analgesics (Meyer, 2013). See the related discussion in the earlier MDMA subsection, "MDMA Drug–Drug Interactions."

In addition, several researchers (e.g., Hopfer, Mendelson, & Van Leeuwen, 2006, 2010; NIDA, 2017; Santos, Rapues, & Wilson, 2014; Van Leeuwen, Hopfer, & Hooks, 2004) have identified that the use of MDMA is highest among adolescents and young adults, who are:

1. Bisexual, gay, lesbian, or transgendered (see the related discussion in the following subsection);
2. Homeless or "living-on-the-street;"
3. Regular attendees of dance clubs and rave events;
4. Enrollees in treatment programs aimed at quitting the use of drugs and substances of abuse.

BISEXUAL, GAY, AND LESBIAN ADOLESCENTS AND YOUNG ADULTS

Bisexual, gay, and lesbian adolescents and young adults, including those who are college/university students (e.g., medical students), reportedly use significantly larger amounts of MDMA than do their heterosexual counterparts (Horowitz, Galanter, & Dermatis, 2008; McCabe, Boyd, & Hughes, 2003; NIDA, 2017; Parsons, Kelly, & Wells, 2006). In fact, bisexual, gay, and lesbian college/university students are twice as likely as their heterosexual cohorts to have used MDMA in the past year (Boyd, McCabe, & d'Arcy, 2003). This difference also was found to be more pronounced during adolescence (i.e., 12 to 17 years-of-age) than during young adulthood (i.e., 18 to 23 years-of-age) by Corliss, Rosario, and Wypji (2010) in their study of U.S. adolescents and young adults.

In addition, several researchers (e.g., Eiserman, Diamond, & Schensul, 2005; Ramo, Grov, & Delucchi, 2010) have identified significant correlations between MDMA use and recent history of unprotected anal intercourse among bisexual and gay adolescent boys and young men. Other researchers also have reported that, particularly during "circuit party" weekends, MDMA use by bisexual and gay adolescent boys and young men has been highly correlated with unprotected sex with multiple partners, as well as, with partners who knowingly are HIV positive (e.g., Klitzman, Pope, & Hudson, 2000; Pagliaro & Pagliaro, *Clinical Patient Data Files*).

ADOLESCENTS AND YOUNG ADULTS OF AFRICAN CONTINENTAL DESCENT

Another trend during the new millennium in relation to MDMA use is the significant increase in use among adolescents and young adults of African continental descent. This trend has been specifically related to the perceived influence of hip-hop/rap music lyrics that endorse MDMA use "as a way to have fun or get women 'loose'" (Rigg & Estreet, 2018, p. 1). As noted by Linden (cited by Diamond, Bermudez, & Schensul, 2006, p. 274):

> What is new is that Ecstasy, once an almost exclusive plaything of White subcultures, is being increasingly embraced by young African Americans. And heading up the X appreciation society are chart-topping platinum artists who have found in the drug a new lyrical obsession and de facto status symbol.

Diamond, Bermudez, and Schensul (2006), in their content analysis of 69 rap songs that mention MDMA, portrayed these songs as describing "men and women using ecstasy for sex:"

> The women in these songs are generally referred to as "hoes," "freaks," or "bitches." Graphic and crude sexual lyrics are a feature of "booty rap" songs ... In booty rap songs, which celebrate male machismo and hedonistic party culture, ecstasy use is frequently associated with kinky and promiscuous sex and money.
>
> (p. 283)

ADOLESCENTS AND YOUNG ADULTS OF HISPANIC DESCENT

Another noted trend during the new millennium in relation to MDMA use has been the proportionate increase in MDMA use by Hispanic adolescents, particularly those adolescents from low-income families (Wu, Liu, & Hoang Pham, 2010). In their study of injection drug users in New York City that involved 715 participants (62.4% of Hispanic descent and 27.3% of African continental descent), Ompad, Galea, and Fuller (2005) found that "lifetime ecstasy use" was reported by 26% of those of Hispanic descent and 16% of those of African continental descent. In addition, Schinke, Schwinn, and Hopkins (2016), citing data from the CDC, noted that "Relative to their non-Hispanic Black and White classmates, 9th grade Hispanic youths have higher use rates of ecstasy" (p. 185).

Lack of acculturation, speaking Spanish at home, lack of high school diploma, and gang membership have consistently been shown to be factors associated with increased risk for drug abuse, including MDMA use among Hispanic youth in the U.S. (e.g., Pagliaro & Pagliaro, *Clinical Patient Data Files*; Schinke, Schwinn, & Hopkins, 2016). As the numbers of unaccompanied, undocumented adolescents increase in the U.S., the occurrence of the identified risk factors also increases, and, unless appropriate corrective interventions are initiated, we can expect a continuing and increase in the use of MDMA among adolescents in the U.S. of Hispanic descent.

Access to the Dark Net

Another major factor contributing to increased use of MDMA, among adolescents and young adults during the new millennium in the U.S., is access to the Dark Net (darknet) from which MDMA, as well as virtually any other drug or substance of abuse, can be readily obtained. In this regard, Winstock (2016), reviewing related data from the 2015 *Global Drug Survey* of 23 different countries, found that the purchase of drugs and substances of abuse from the darknet was significant—ranging from a high of 18% of respondents from Sweden to a low of 0.4% of respondents from Greece. The average percentage of purchases, by country, was reported at 4.5%. The U.S. reported 8% (p. 21).

Typically, adolescents and young adults, who want to purchase a particular drug or substance of abuse:

1. Sign on to a service (e.g., TOR) that masks the purchaser's identity;
2. Proceed to a digital black-market site (e.g., Silk Road 3);
3. Complete the purchase using "bitcoins."

The drug or substance of abuse is then sent directly to the adolescent or young adult purchaser by postal service or courier delivery.

Based upon other responses obtained from study participants regarding the benefits and issues related to a darknet drug purchase versus a conventional drug purchase, Winstock (2016, p. 20) identified several "clear benefits" associated with darknet purchases:

- Reduced rates of exposure to violence;
- Fewer adulterated drugs;
- Greater confidence in product quality;
- Removal from the street dealing environment.

Assessment and Diagnoses of MDMA Dependence or Use Disorder

See the earlier related discussion in the LSD subsection, "Assessment, Diagnosis, and Treatment of LSD, MDMA, or PCP Dependence or Use Disorder."

Treating MDMA Dependence or Use Disorder

There is a dearth of published clinical research available regarding the treatment of MDMA dependence or use disorder for adolescents and young adults. As noted by the NIDA (2017):

> There are currently no FDA-approved medications to treat MDMA use disorder . . .The most effective current treatments for patients with MDMA use disorder are cognitive behavioral interventions.
>
> (p. 24)

Unfortunately, the evidence available to support the use of "cognitive-behavioral" interventions is largely anecdotal. There are no published research studies concerning the treatment of adolescents and young adults diagnosed with MDMA dependence or use disorder.[110]

Phencyclidine (PCP)

Phencyclidine (PCP),[111] commonly known as "Angel Dust," "Elephant," "Hog," "Horse Tranquilizer," "PeaCe Pill," "Rocket Fuel," "Tranq," and many other street names,[112] became a "controlled substance" in the U.S. in 1978 when it was designated a Schedule II drug by the DEA. PCP had already gained popularity among many groups of users (e.g., members of organized motorcycle gangs [OMGs]) and, when no longer able to obtain legal pharmaceutical grade PCP for their use, these groups soon found that PCP could be illegally produced and sold on the street in various forms for intravenous or subcutaneous injection, intranasal insufflation, oral ingestion, or pulmonary inhalation (e.g., smoking a "Sherman"). The Hell's Angels OMG was extremely successful in producing tremendous profits in relation to the production, distribution, and sale of PCP across the U.S. during the early 1970s. It was during this time, and as a result of their "marketing campaign," that PCP received its most popular street names (i.e., "Angel Dust" and "Hog"), which continue to be commonly used today.

Since the 1980s, adolescents and young adults have used low dosages of PCP to:

- Achieve a "buzz," or an "alcohol-like" disinhibitory euphoria;
- Elevate mood;
- Promote relaxation;
- Relieve pain;
- Reduce sexual inhibitions.

They also used PCP to achieve such desired psychodelic effects as:

- Feelings of "unreality" (detachment from reality);
- Distortions in the perception of time, space, and body image.

110 For a related overview and discussion of cognitive-behavioral interventions, see the alcohol subsection in Chapter 1, "Alcohol," "Treating Alcohol Dependence or Use Disorder—Psychotherapy/Counseling."

111 The popular and commonly used acronym, "PCP," for phencyclidine is derived from its organic chemical name, 1-(1-**p**henyl**c**yclohexyl) **p**iperidine.

112 For example, when PCP powder is sprinkled on dried marijuana or tobacco, or when marijuana joints or tobacco cigarettes are dipped into PCP solution ("Embalming Fluid"), the resulting combination product is commonly referred to as: "Crystal Weed;" "*Frios;*" "Fry;" "Illies;" "Macho Weed," "Wet;" and "*Yerba Mala.*"

Approximately 30 years ago, Carrol (1990) analyzed available published retrospective studies that examined the effects associated with PCP use and identified two different categories of "dose-related" effects:

1. "Subjective effects," which appear to vary dramatically in relation to personality characteristics, or predisposition, of the user;
2. "Secondary effects," which appear to vary dramatically during different episodes of PCP use by the same user.

In addition to desired effects, the use of low dosages of PCP was associated with cognitive impairment in most cases. As described by Domino[113] and Luby (2012):

> It was astounding to us that phencyclidine became a major street drug of abuse . . . Few of our volunteer subjects were ever willing to take the drug a second time. One former resident still recalls her PCP experience as intensely psychologically painful.
>
> (p. 916)

However, perhaps as expected, it has been suggested that PCP users, who experience a positive subjective experience, are more likely to develop a pattern of regular, long-term use than PCP users who initially experienced dysphoria, or other undesired effects. Other researchers, who have surveyed PCP users, have generally found that the desired effects of PCP are experienced only about half of the time, while undesired, or harmful, effects are experienced during the other half of the time.[114] As reported by many regular, long-term PCP users, in addition to the desired effects, it is the unpredictable effects that make it—seemingly contrary to common sense—"attractive" (Pagliaro & Pagliaro, *Clinical Patient Data Files*).

PCP Chemistry

PCP, 1-(1-phenocyclohexyl) piperidine, is produced by illicit chemical laboratories across the U.S., but primarily located in Southern California. It is generally produced as a white crystalline powder from readily available chemical precursors. The crystalline PCP powder, which is readily soluble in water or alcohol, has a distinctive, bitter chemical taste. It is prepared in a variety of dosage formulations, including: capsules; solutions; and tablets, for ingestion, or when crushed or diluted as needed—nasal insufflation, or "snorting," pulmonary inhalation, and both subcutaneous and intravenous injection. Rarely, PCP is prepared in a solution for ophthalmic instillation (Pagliaro & Pagliaro, *Clinical Patient Data Files*). The most common methods of PCP use are ingestion and pulmonary inhalation.

PCP Pharmacology

This subsection provides a brief overview of the proposed pharmacodynamics, or mechanism of action, of PCP and its pharmacokinetics—absorption, distribution, metabolism, and excretion. It also presents and discusses the undesired, or harmful, effects and relatively serious

113 Edward F. Domino was one of the original PCP researchers.

114 This response may be, at least in part, due to drug–drug interactions. As noted by West, Helman, and McKeown (2015):

> Of PCP-related ED visits in 2011, 72% involved PCP combined with other drugs. (p.1)

toxicities associated with PCP use, including PCP-induced: (1) aggressive and violent behavior ("bad trips"); (2) anterograde amnesia; (3) delusional and mood disorders; and (4) psychosis. Also presented and discussed are indirect fatalities, physical and psychological dependence or use disorder, and PCP overdosage.[115]

Pharmacodynamics: Mechanism of Action

The exact mechanism, by which PCP exerts its psychodelic actions in humans, has not been determined.[116] However, noncompetitive antagonism of the N-methyl-D-aspartate (NMDA) receptor channel complexes, located in the basal ganglia, cortex, hippocampus, and limbic regions of the brain, has been postulated. This antagonism is thought to block the action of the excitatory amino acids—aspartate and glutamate (Morris, Cochran, & Pratt, 2005). PCP also inhibits GABA and increases dopamine and norepinephrine concentrations by: (1) increasing synthesis; and (2) inhibiting presynaptic reuptake. PCP possesses significant anticholinergic activity. These actions of PCP and the associated medically desired clinical effects of amnesia, analgesia, immobility, and sedation initially led to its development as an intravenous surgical anesthetic for human use (Pagliaro & Pagliaro, 2004).

Pharmacokinetics: Absorption, Distribution, Metabolism, and Excretion

PCP is relatively well-absorbed (i.e., 50% to 100%) from all routes of administration (e.g., ingestion; intranasal insufflation; intravenous and subcutaneous injection; pulmonary inhalation). Once absorbed into the circulatory system, PCP reaches the CNS, where it becomes ionized within the acidic environment of the cerebrospinal fluid (CSF). The ionization causes "ion trapping" that results in spinal fluid PCP concentrations that are several times higher than plasma PCP concentrations. However, following pulmonary inhalation (e.g., smoking a tobacco cigarette or a marijuana joint that has been dipped into PCP solution), 50% of the PCP is degraded, or lost, because of heating and the pyrolysis associated with smoking tobacco and cannabis cigarettes.

The onset of action, when smoked, is generally within five minutes. However, when a PCP tablet is ingested or when PCP powder is intranasally insufflated (i.e., "sniffed" or "snorted"), the onset of action can be delayed for up to 60 minutes. Effects generally last for four to six hours, but may persist for up to 24 hours.

PCP is both lipid and water soluble and has a volume of distribution of approximately six liters/kg. A weak base, PCP is significantly secreted into the acidic environment of the stomach and, subsequently, cyclically reabsorbed in the small intestine. Regardless of the method of use, PCP is extensively metabolized to inactive metabolites in the liver primarily by the hepatic microsomal isoenzyme P450 CYP3A and undergoes extensive first-pass hepatic metabolism (i.e., oxidative hydroxylation)—with large interindividual differences (Laurenzana & Owens, 1997). PCP and its metabolites are excreted primarily in the urine (Cook, Perez-Reyes, & Jeffcoat, 1983). Approximately 10% of PCP is excreted in

115 Because of the difficulties associated with the "street synthesis" of PCP—which ranges from a lack of needed precursor chemicals to a lack of needed laboratory facilities and "cooks" who are familiar with related recipes and techniques—street samples are often contaminated with precursors and byproducts, each of which increase the toxicity of the PCP product in unique and often unexpected and harmful ways (e.g., unintentional production of "PCC," a PCP precursor that releases cyanide) (Shulgin & MacLean, 1976; Soine, Vincek, & Agee, 1979).

116 Several laboratory researchers (e.g., Freed, Weinberger, & Bing, 1980; Hardin, Wessinger, & Wenger, 2002) have identified additional details involving the mechanism of action of PCP, such as binding to a PCP receptor. However, most of these studies used the brains of mice or rats and, consequently, are not generalizable to humans.

unchanged form in the urine. The half-life of elimination is approximately 17 hours (Bey & Patel, 2007; Cook, Perez-Reyes, & Jeffcoat, 1983; Pagliaro & Pagliaro, 2009; West, Helman, & McKeown, 2015).

PCP is commonly included with other drugs and substances of abuse in urine drug-screening tests requested for adolescents and young adults, who are admitted to emergency departments (EDs) in unconscious, or unresponsive, states. These tests generally involve an immunoassay (e.g., Siemens Syva EMIT II Immunoassay®) that may be subject to false-positive results for PCP resulting from the use of several medications including Venlafaxine (Effexor®), tramadol (Ultram®) or dextromethorphan (Benylin DM®) (Ly, Thornton, Buono, 2012; Rengarajan & Mullins, 2013). To assure the accuracy of urinary PCP analysis, gas chromatography/mass spectrophotometry (GC/MS) must be used.

Undesired, or Harmful, Effects and Toxicities

Several common toxicities associated with PCP use appear to be dose-related (see Table 4.6). In addition, certain PCP toxicities may be fatal, including:

1. Cardiac arrest;
2. Intracranial hemorrhage secondary to hypertension;
3. Hyperkalemia secondary to rhabdomyolysis.[117]

Table 4.6 PCP Dose-Related Toxicities

Toxicities Associated with Low PCP Dosage	*Toxicities Associated with High PCP Dosage*	*Toxicities Associated with Low or High PCP Dosages*
Ataxia	Abnormal breathing	Agitation
Diaphoresis	"Blank stare"	Analgesia
Edema	Blurred vision	Anxiety
Flushing	Bradycardia	Belligerence
Impaired judgment	Cardiac arrest	Dissociative anesthetic action
Incoordination	Catatonia	"Flashbacks"
Muscle rigidity	Coma	Hallucinations
Numbness of extremities	Compulsive and repetitive movements	Hypertension
Polydipsia with polyuria	Confusion	Illusions

(*Continued*)

117 The rhabdomyolysis is itself secondary to PCP-induced seizures.

Table 4.6 (Cont.)

Toxicities Associated with Low PCP Dosage	*Toxicities Associated with High PCP Dosage*	*Toxicities Associated with Low or High PCP Dosages*
Rapid mood swings	Difficulty concentrating	Irritability
Restlessness	Disorientation	Nystagmus (both vertical and horizontal)
Speech disturbances (e.g., slowed or slurred speech)	Dizziness	Paranoia
Tachycardia	Drooling	PCP-induced aggressive and violent behavior ("bad trips")
Xerostomia	Incoherent speech	PCP-induced anterograde amnesia
	Nausea	PCP-induced delusional and mood disorders
	Proprioceptive balance disorder	PCP-induced psychotic disorder
	Punding	
	Seizures	
	Vomiting	

Sources: Bey & Patel 2007; Hendricks, Daugherty, & Dang 2017; NIDA (2009); Peters, Kelder, & Meshack (2005); Pagliaro & Pagliaro (2009); Pradhan (1984).

Several other undesired, or harmful, effects and toxicities are directly related to the use of PCP. Although available data do not provide strong evidence implicating the regular, long-term use of PCP with major body organ (e.g., cardiac, hepatic, renal) or cellular damage, they do provide evidence for the occurrence of several major mental toxicities. These toxic effects are presented and briefly discussed in the following subsections, PCP-induced: aggressive and violent behavior; anterograde amnesia; delusional and mood disorders; and psychotic disorder.

PCP-INDUCED AGGRESSIVE AND VIOLENT BEHAVIOR

One of the most troublesome toxicities associated with the regular, long-term use of PCP is its tendency to precipitate, or aggravate, aggressive and violent behavior—behavior that is often bizarre, sudden, and unexpected.[118] Three contexts of aggressive and violent behavior have been observed:

118 When compared to adults, PCP-induced aggression and violent behavior is less frequently encountered in children. However, apnea, respiratory depression, and seizures appear to occur more frequently in children than adolescents and young adults (Bey & Patel, 2007).

1. Toxic organic brain disorders (i.e., psychosis);
2. Primitive sadistic criminal behaviors (e.g., brutal murders; extreme self-mutilation);
3. "Bad trips."

The bad trips associated with PCP use occur suddenly and unexpectedly among users and are characterized by sudden and severe acts of violence against themselves and others. Generally, users, who experience a bad trip, have previously used PCP and experienced expected desirable effects (e.g., alcohol-like euphoria). For these reasons, it has been suggested that the bad trips may be due to the adulteration/contamination of street supplies of PCP with formaldehyde or other impurities that could cause these effects (Marceaux, Dilks, & Hixson, 2008).

The use of PCP also has been associated with intimate partner violence (IPV) (e.g., Crane, Easton, & Devine, 2013; Spindel & Brody, 2016). (See also the "Intimate Partner Violence" subsection in Chapter 2, "Amphetamines and Cocaine.") Whereas the disinhibition caused by PCP may explain uncharacteristic behavior, the PCP-induced aggressive and violent behavior is most likely related to the underlying, or latent, psychological characteristics of the user (e.g., angry; depressed; fearful; hostile). The "superhuman" strength that has been observed among PCP users during episodes of aggressive and violent behavior is primarily due to the analgesic and dissociative anesthetic effects. These PCP effects, which decrease or eliminate the pain experienced by users, consequently, enables them to perform aggressive and violent acts—acts that they would otherwise not be able to complete because of the associated self-injuries inflicted on their body tissues and the resultant pain. As such, PCP users do not become superhuman, they only think, or feel, that they are.[119]

PCP-INDUCED ANTEROGRADE AMNESIA

Following the absorption of PCP into the systemic circulation, amnesia begins and lasts until the effects of PCP wear off as PCP blood concentrations diminish.[120] During this time, users may behave uncharacteristically in ways that, while not generally harmful, may be later identified as being bizarre (e.g., removing their clothing and running around naked). Usually, users "black-out" and later report no conscious memory of the events that occurred during the amnestic episode (Pagliaro & Pagliaro, 2009).

Although potentially "embarrassing" acts may occur while "high" on PCP, its amnestic effects probably contribute to continued use (i.e., the potentially aversive behaviors are not remembered by the user and, thus, do not serve as a deterrent to future use). The PCP-induced memory impairment has resulted in the use of the amnesia defense in some criminal trials to establish diminished capacity (e.g., Berman & Coccaro, 1998; Pagliaro & Pagliaro, *Clinical Patient Data Files*). (Also see previous PCP subsection, "PCP-Induced Aggressive and Violent Behavior.")

119 The unpredictable toxicities associated with PCP have contributed to its street folk lore and to its increased popularity of use among certain groups of users. For example, adolescent boys and young men of Hispanic descent, particularly those who are involved in criminal youth gangs (Pagliaro & Pagliaro, *Clinical Patient Data Files*), are attracted to PCP and other drugs and substances of abuse that have unpredictable, and possibly horrific consequences associated with their use (i.e., their willingness to use such "dangerous" drugs denotes that they are "macho").

120 This anterograde amnesia is similar to that associated with the use of alcohol or benzodiazepine sedative-hypnotics (see the related discussion in Chapter 1, "Alcohol," and Chapter 6, "Prescription Sedative-Hypnotics").

PCP-INDUCED DELUSIONAL AND MOOD DISORDERS

PCP-induced delusional disorder may appear up to one week following a PCP overdosage and is characterized by: (1) disheveled or eccentric appearance; (2) dysphoria; (3) mild cognitive impairment; (4) rambling, garbled, and incoherent speech; and (5) ritualistic stereotypic behavior. (See also the later subsection, "PCP Overdosage"). The PCP-induced mood disorders—primarily anxiety disorder, as well as bipolar disorder and major depressive disorder—may appear within one- or two-weeks following PCP use.

These delusional and mood disorders are characterized by a prominent, and persistently depressed, elevated, or expansive mood, with anxiety, delusions, hallucinations, irritability, panic attacks, and somatization. Although the association of these disorders with PCP use is relatively uncommon, resultant effects may be long-lasting and have been associated with suicidal behaviors.

PCP-INDUCED PSYCHOTIC DISORDER

PCP-induced psychotic disorder is similar, in many regards to amphetamine-induced psychosis (Murray, 2002), and can occur after a single use of PCP—whether or not the user has a prior positive history of mental illness. However, it is more likely to occur among users who have previously used PCP or who have a genetic predisposition for schizophrenia. The psychosis may last for several days or months, even with appropriate medical management (e.g., antipsychotic pharmacotherapy, such as haloperidol [Haldol®]). PCP-induced psychotic disorder also may recur spontaneously, even with the use of lower dosages of PCP.

PCP is pharmacologically recognized as a "psychotomimetic." In this regard, it has been used to study psychosis, particularly that which is associated with catatonic or negative features (Pagliaro & Pagliaro, 2009). Common related signs and symptoms that occur to a moderate to high degree among adolescent and young adult PCP users—as well as among patients diagnosed with schizophrenia—include: ambivalence; attention disorder; disordered thinking or loosening of associations; delusions; depersonalization; hallucinations; mood disorders; over inclusive thoughts; and paranoia (Domino & Luby, 2012; NIDA, 2009; Pagliaro & Pagliaro, 2009).

Physical and Psychological Dependence

In response to the epidemic use of PCP reported during the late 1960s and 1970s, a considerable amount of research was undertaken in an effort to identify its abuse potential and addiction liability. The general consensus derived from this research included that:

1. PCP is not associated with the development of physical dependence[121] (i.e., abrupt discontinuation of regular, long-term use of PCP is not associated with a classic PCP withdrawal syndrome);
2. Tolerance—the need to increase the amount of PCP used in an attempt to achieve desired pharmacologic actions—develops with continued, regular use;
3. Cross-tolerance between PCP and other drugs and substances of abuse has not been reported;

121 However, using animal laboratory models, several researchers (e.g., Balster & Woolverton, 1980; Noda & Nabeshima, 2006) found that the regular, long-term use of PCP is associated with physical dependence.

4. Abrupt discontinuation of regular, long-term use of PCP is associated with various degrees of *psychological* dependence[122] characterized by various degrees of mental depression, lack of energy, and physical distress.

PCP Overdosage/Unintentional Poisoning

The signs and symptoms of PCP overdosage, include: aggression; agitation; ataxia; catatonia; coma; hallucinations; hypertension; hyperthermia; incoordination; nystagmus; psychosis; rhabdomyolysis; seizures; and tachycardia. Similar to LSD overdosage, the associated fatalities are most often indirectly caused and are related to accidental injuries, drownings, and physical trauma—including self-inflicted trauma (i.e., most overdosage fatalities involve homicides and suicides).

> Overall, the estimated number of phencyclidine (PCP)-related emergency department (ED) visits increased more than 400 percent between 2005 and 2011 (from 14,825 to 75,538 visits); more recently, the number of these visits doubled between 2009 and 2011 (from 36,719 to 75,538).
>
> (SAMHSA, 2013a, p.1)

Most PCP overdosage victims, who present to the ED, usually only require medical observation and supportive care (D'Onofrio, McCausland, & Tarabar, 2006). Chemical restraint, if necessary, is preferred over physical restraint because the latter may exacerbate the risk of rhabdomyolysis. Benzodiazepine (e.g., diazepam, Valium®) pharmacotherapy may be used to manage associated anxiety and fear.[123] An antipsychotic, which does not have high anticholinergic actions (e.g., haloperidol [Haldol®]; olanzapine [Zyprexa®]; risperidone [Risperdal®]), may be of benefit for the management of the behavioral toxicities (e.g., agitation; psychosis) associated with PCP overdosage (MacNeal, Cone, & Sinha, 2012; Pagliaro & Pagliaro, 2009).[124] PCP overdosages, particularly those involving infants, children, and adolescents, require hospitalization to ensure appropriate assessment, management (including cardiac monitoring), and follow-up. There is no known antidote for PCP overdosage.

Urinary acidification may increase PCP elimination (Domino & Wilson, 1977; Peres-Reyes, Di Guiseppi, & Brine, 1982). However, efficacy is limited and related acidification has been associated with acute tubular necrosis. Gastric lavage with repeated dosages of activated charcoal (one gm/kg) have been used—with prior consideration of respiratory function and the initiation of measures to prevent aspiration. Hyperthermia (in excess of 40°C) should be treated with mechanical cooling measures. As reported by SAMSHSA (2013a, p. 1):

> Other illicit drugs, such as marijuana, cocaine, and heroin, were involved in approximately half (48%) of PCP-related ED visits in 2011.

Consequently, clinicians, who treat PCP overdosage, should always request a full toxicology screen and be prepared to treat concurrent overdosages involving several drugs and substances of abuse.

122 Regarding psychological dependence, the abrupt discontinuation of PCP use has been associated with significant "craving." In addition, compulsive, PCP-seeking behavior has been observed among PCP users despite risks for severe adverse consequences that are related to use (Pagliaro & Pagliaro, *Clinical Patient Data Files*).

123 Intravenous diazepam (Valium®) is also used to treat associated status epilepticus.

124 Antipsychotics that have high anticholinergic actions (e.g., phenothiazines) may exacerbate PCP-induced hyperthermia.

Pregnancy and Lactation

This section discusses maternal use of PCP during pregnancy and lactation.

PREGNANCY[125]

The maternal use of PCP during pregnancy has been associated with certain birth defects, including neonatal dysmorphogenesis, characterized by distorted facial features, low birth weight, and a small head circumference (Tabor, Smith-Wallace, & Yonekura, 1990; Wachsman, Schuertz, & Chan, 1989). However, these reported teratogenic effects are poorly documented and generally have been deemed to be clinically insignificant (i.e., if they do occur, then they are extremely rare).[126] However, acute, short-term abnormal neurological findings associated with PCP use (e.g., decreased attention; decreased neonatal reflexes; hyperactive deep tendon ankle reflexes) have been identified among neonates who were prenatally exposed to PCP (e.g., Golden, Kuhnert, & Sokol, 1987). In addition, the long-term effects of prenatal PCP exposure on the later development of infants and children, including effects on learning, have been raised, but remain inconclusive (Pagliaro & Pagliaro, 1996, 2002, 2009).

LACTATION

The safety of PCP use by adolescent girls and young women, who are breastfeeding, has not been established. However, PCP is excreted in breast milk and has been associated with behavioral problems, coma, irritability, and lethargy among breastfed infants whose mothers use PCP (Pagliaro & Pagliaro, 2009). Adolescent girls and young women, who breastfeed, should not use PCP (Pagliaro & Pagliaro, 2002).

New Millennial Trends in PCP Use

The medical use of PCP is presented and discussed with attention to children, adolescents, and young adults. Embryo/fetal, infant, and child exposure also are presented and discussed. The section concludes with new millennial trends in adolescent and young adult illicit/recreational PCP use.

Medical PCP Use

First synthesized in 1926, PCP was not introduced until 1958 as an intravenous surgical dissociative anesthetic (i.e., Sernyl®; Sernylan®). When a low to moderate dosage of PCP was intravenously administered according to recommended dosing schedules, it was physically well-tolerated during surgery and produced few undesired physical effects (e.g., excessive changes in blood pressure, depth and rate of respirations, or heart rate). However, during the immediate recovery period following surgery, several troublesome psychological effects were observed among patients, including agitation, hallucinations, post-operative delirium, and violent behavior. As a result, PCP was withdrawn from medical use and was replaced with a

125 The overwhelming majority of available related published data are from laboratory animal studies that cannot be extrapolated to humans.

126 In addition, the noted "birth defects" ascribed to the use of PCP during pregnancy could be caused by the concurrent maternal use/abuse of other drugs and substances of abuse such as alcohol, cannabis, or tobacco.

derivative—the dissociative anesthetic, ketamine.[127] By 1967, because of its undesired, or harmful, mental effects and toxicities,[128] the use of PCP was restricted by the FDA for "veterinary use only."

Child PCP Exposure

Child exposure to PCP primarily involves one of three contexts: (1) in utero exposure; (2) exposure during breastfeeding; and (3) accidental/unintentional poisoning. See related discussion in the earlier subsections, "Pregnancy and Lactation" and "PCP Overdosage/Unintentional Poisoning."

Adolescent and Young Adult Illicit/Recreational PCP Use

> PCP is predominately abused by young adults and high school students.
>
> (DEA, 2013, p. 1)

In 2011, over six million Americans, 12 years-of-age and older, reported lifetime PCP use, including over 1% of high school seniors (DEA, 2013). However, these estimates are probably low because national and other surveys generally miss large numbers of adolescents and young adults who are not represented in major collection sites (e.g., colleges/universities; high schools). For example, many PCP users:

1. Do not attend high school or college/university (e.g., prior to graduation, they "drop-out" of high school or college/university in order to, for example, join the military or obtain needed part- or full-time jobs);
2. Are not detected with usual emergency department blood and urine screening tests because PCP, for economic reasons, is not always included in these and other screens (e.g., emergency admissions; sports testing; and police arrest).

127 Ketamine (Ketalar®), which is a mixture of two enantiomers, is similar to PCP. It is a dissociative anesthetic that minimally suppresses breathing. It has a relatively rapid onset of action (i.e., less than five minutes by IM or IV injection and less than 30 minutes when ingested). Ketamine is metabolized by the hepatic microsomal enzyme system, CYP3A4, with greater than 90% excreted in the urine—both in its unchanged form and as its major metabolite, norketamine. The duration of action is approximately one hour, and the half-life of elimination is approximately three hours. The primary mechanism of action of ketamine is as a non-competitive antagonist of the NMDA receptor (Pagliaro & Pagliaro, 2009).

The acute undesired, or harmful, effects associated with ketamine include amnesia and cognitive impairment, particularly of executive functioning. Ketamine, commonly known on the street as "Cat", "K" "Kit-Kat", or "Special K," is abused for its psychodelic effects at dance clubs and raves. With high dosages or regular, long term use, some users describe the experience of going into the "K-hole"—a negative or terrifying state of extreme dissociation with both auditory and visual hallucinations. Of interest, a young woman, who received ketamine as part of her obstetric care during labor and delivery, reported her experience to us with attention to each detail of the "unusual" experience—which we clearly recognized as a "K-hole" experience (Pagliaro & Pagliaro, *Clinical Patient Data Files*).

Of particular interest—and in keeping with the significant interest, particularly among health and social care professionals, to attempt to use the various psychodelics therapeutically—in 2019 the FDA approved the use of esketamine (Spravato®), in conjunction with an oral antidepressant, for the treatment of refractory depression among adults. Esketamine, the s-enantiomer of ketamine, is intranasally self-administered by the patient. A required "black box" warning cautions that the use of esketamine is associated with several mental risks including: abuse and misuse; impaired attention, judgement, and thinking; and suicidal thoughts and behaviors (FDA, 2019; Kelley, 2019).

128 For example, while post-operatively recovering from the anesthetic effects of PCP, patients often became agitated, delusional, and irrational.

In one of the few available national drug surveys of psychodelic use, the NIDA (2016) reported that, in 2014, approximately 3% of adults in the U.S. (26 years-of-age and older) reported lifetime use of PCP. Contributing to the ability of PCP to "fly under the radar" is its changing pattern of adolescent and young adult use over the last decade, including its use:

1. In combination with other drugs and substances of abuse, particularly alcohol and marijuana;
2. In lower dosages;
3. By increasingly diverse ethnic groups.

For example, by the end of the first decade of the new millennium, data suggested an increase in PCP use among adolescents and young adults of Hispanic descent, living in the southwestern U.S., including, the large metropolitan areas of Houston, Texas, and Los Angeles, California (DEA, 2013). As the second decade of the new millennium comes to an end, the highest principle groups of PCP-users in the U.S. are now consistently found to be adolescent boys and young adults of African continental or Hispanic descent.

Assessment, Diagnosis, and Treatment of PCP Dependence or Use Disorder

Although specifically identified in DSM-5, PCP use disorder shares many similarities with other psychodelic dependence or use disorders. Consequently, PCP also shares various assessment, diagnosis, and treatment approaches with LSD and MDMA (see the earlier related discussion in the LSD subsection, "Assessment, Diagnosis, and Treatment of LSD, MDMA, and PCP Dependence or Use Disorders").

Adolescents and young adults with PCP dependence or use disorder generally do not self-refer or actively seek professional treatment. More often, they are referred by family, law enforcement, school counselors, or others (e.g., courts) for assessment, diagnosis, and therapeutic intervention following:

1. PCP overdosage/Unintentional poisoning;
2. Injury sustained while intoxicated with PCP;
3. Arrest for bizarre or violent behavior/crimes associated with PCP use;
4. Medical complications (e.g., rhabdomyolysis; seizures) related to PCP use.

References

Abramson, H. A., Waxenberg, S. E., & Levine, A. (1955). Lysergic acid diethylamide (LSD-25): XIII Effect on Bender-Gestalt test performance. *Journal of Psychology, 40*, 341–349.

ACOG, The American Congress of Obstetricians and Gynecologists. (2015a, July). *Marijuana Use during Pregnancy and Lactation (committee Opinion, No. 637)*. Retrieved from ACOG.org, pp. 1–5: www.acog.org/Resources-And-Publications/Committee-Opinions/Committee-on-Ob..

ACOG, The American Congress of Obstetricians and Gynecologists. (2015b, June 22). *Ob-gyns Warn against Marijuana Use for Pregnant Women*. Retrieved from ACOG.org, ppp. 1–2: http://www.acog.org/About-ACOG/News-Room/News-Releases/2015/Ob-gyns-Warn-Aga..

Adamson, S. J., Kay-Lambkin, F. J., & Baker, A. L. (2010). An improved brief measure of cannabis misuse: The Cannabis Use Disorders Identification Test-Revised (CUDIT-R). *Drug and Alcohol Dependence, 110*, 137–143. doi:10.1016/j.drugalcvdfep.2010.02.017

Adamson, S. J., & Sellman, J. D. (2003). A prototype screening instrument for cannabis use disorder: The Cannabis Use Disorders Identification Test (CUDIT) in an alcohol-dependent clinical sample. *Drug and Alcohol Review, 22*(3), 309–315.

Aldington, S., Williams, M., & Nowitz, M. (2007). Effects of cannabis on pulmonary structure, function and symptoms. *Thorax, 62*(12), 1058–1063.

Allen, J. H., de Moore, G. M., & Heddle, R. (2004). Cannabinoid hyperemesis: Cyclical hyperemesis in association with chronic cannabis use. *Gut, 53*, 1566–1570.

Allott, K., & Redman, J. (2007). Are there sex differences associated with the effects of ecstasy/3,4-methylenedioxymethamphetamine (MDMA)? *Neuroscience and Behavioral Reviews, 31*(3), 327–347.

Altschuler, D. M., & Brounstein, P. J. (1991, November). Patterns of drug use, drug trafficking, and other delinquency among inner-city adolescent males in Washington, DC. *Criminology, 29*(4), 589–622.

Ameri, A. (1999). The effects of cannabinoids on the brain. *Progress in Neurobiology, 58*(4), 315–348.

American College of Neuropsychopharmacology. (2015, December 10). *LSD changes consciousness by reorganizing human brain networks*. Retrieved February 1, 2016, from ScienceDaily, pp. 1–6: www.sciencedaily.com/releases/2015/12/151210144910.htm

American Lung Association. (2016). *Hookah Smoking: A Growing Threat to Public Health*. Washington, DC: American Lung Association. Retrieved June 6, 2016

Anderson, D. M., Rees, D. I., & Sabia, J. J. (2014). Medical marijuana laws and suicides by gender and age. *American Journal of Public Health, 104*(12), 2369–2376. doi:10.2105/AJPH.2013.301612

Anderson, G. D., & Chan, L. N. (2016). Pharmacokinetic drug interactions with tobacco, cannabinoids and smoking cessation products. *Clinical Pharmacokinetics, 55*(11), 1353–1368. doi:10.1007/s40262-016-0400-9

Andrews, K. H., & Bracero, L. A. (2015). Canabinoid hyperemesis syndrome during pregnancy: A case report. *The Journal of Reproductive Medicine, 60*(9-10), 430–432.

Angell, T. (2018, June 28). U.S. senate votes to legalize hemp after decades-long ban under marijuana prohibition. *Forbes*, 1–2. Washington, DC.

Annaheim, B., Rehm, J., & Gmel, G. (2008). How to screen for problematic cannabis use in population surveys? An evaluation of the Cannabis Use Disorders Identification Test (CUDIT) in a Swiss sample of adolescents and young adults. *European Addiction Research, 14*(4), 190–197.

Annaheim, B., Scotto, T. J., & Gmel, G. (2010, September). Revising the Cannabis Use Disorders Identification Test (CUDIT) by means of Item Response Theory. *International Journal of Methods in Psychiatric Research, 19*(3), 142–155. doi:10.1002/mpr.308

APA, American Psychiatric Association. (2000). *DSM-IV, Diagnostic and Statistical Manual of Mental Disorders* (4th ed.). Washington, DC: American Psychiatric Association.

APA, American Psychiatric Association. (2013). *DSM-5, Diagnostic and Statistical Manual of Mental Disorders* (5th ed.). Washington, DC: American Psychiatric Association.

Arellano, A. L., Papaseit, E., & Romaguera, A. (2017). Neuropsychiatric and general interactions of natural and synthetic cannabinoids with drugs of abuse and medicines. *CNS & Neurological Disorders - Drug Targets, 16*(5), 554–566. doi:10.2174/1871527316666170413104516

Arendt, M., Rosenberg, R., & Foldager, L. (2007). Withdrawal symptoms do not predict relapse among subjects treated for cannabis dependence. *American Journal on Addictions, 16*(6), 461–467.

ARF/WHO, Addiction Research Foundation/World Health Organization. (1981). *Report of an ARF/WHO Scientific (6) Meeting on the Adverse Health and Behavioral Consequences of Cannabis Use*. Toronto: Addiction Research Foundation.

Armenian, P., Mamantov, T. M., & Tsutaoka, B. T. (2013). Multiple MDMA (Ecstasy) overdoses at a rave event: A case series. *Journal of Intensive Care Medicine, 28*(4), 252–258. doi:10.1177/0885066612445982

Aronson, H., & Waterman, C. E. (1962). The effect of D-lysergic acid diethylamide (LDS-25) on learning and retention. *Journal of Clinical and Experimental Psychopathology, 23*, 17–23.

Asbridge, M., Hayden, J. A., & Cartwright, J. L. (2012, February 9). Acute cannabis consumption and motor vehicle collison risk: Systematic review of observational studies and meta-analysis. *BMJ*, 344. doi:10.1136/bmj.e536

Ashton, C. B. (2001). Pharmacology and effects of cannabis: A brief review. *The British Journal of Psychiatry, 178*(2), 101–106. doi:10.1192/bjp.178.2.101

Associated Press. (2012a, October 22). Ohio teen dealer to be sentenced in drug trafficking. *FoxNews.com*. Lebanon, OH: Fox News. Retrieved from http://foxnews.com/us/2012/10/22/ohio-teen-dealer-to-be-sentenced-in-drug-trafficking-case.html

Associated Press. (2012b, October 22). Prolific teenage drug dealer who sold $20K in marijuana per month could spend three years in prison. *National Post*. Lebanon, OH: National Post. Retrieved from http://nationalpost.com/news/prolific-teenage-drug-dealer-who-sold-23k-in-marijuana-per-month-could-spend-three-years-in-prison

Associated Press. (2018, November 7). Virginia mom who gave 3 kids marijuana gets 10 days in jail. *AP News*, 1. Staunton, VA: Associated Press.

Azofeifa, A., Mattson, M. E., & Schauer, G. (2016, September 2). National estimates of marijuana use and related indicators–National survey on drug use and health, United States, 2002-2014. *MMWR, Morbidity and Mortality Weekly Report, 65*(11), pp. 1–25.

Ballinger, D. (2018, March 11). Teen drug use in Denver metro becoming public concern. *9News.com*. Denver, CO: 9News.com. Retrieved from www.9news.com/article/news/health/teen-drug-use-in-denver-metro-becoming-public-problem/234216948

Balster, R. L., & Woolverton, W. L. (1980, September). Continuous-access phencyclidine self-administration by rhesus monkeys leading to physical dependence. *Psychopharmacology, 70*(1), 5–10.

Banys, P., & Cermak, T. (2016, July 22). Clinical treatment of cannabis use disorders in adolescents. *Marijuana Legalization and Youth: Briefings for California Policy Makers*, 1–18. California Society of Addiction Medicine.

Barratt, M. J., Ferris, J. A., & Winstock, A. R. (2014). Use of Silk Road, the online drug marketplace, in the United Kingdom, Australia and the United States. *Addiction, 109*(5), 774–783. doi:10.1111/add.12470

Bashford, J., Flett, R., & Copeland, J. (2010). The Cannabis Use Problems Identification Test (CUPIT): Development, reliability, concurrent and predictive validity among adolescents and adults. *Addiction, 105*(4), 615–625. doi:10.1111/j.1360-0443.2009.02859.x

Bastiani, L., Siciliano, V., & Curzio, O. (2013). Optimal scaling of the CAST and of SDS Scale in a national sample of adolescents. *Journal of Addictive Behaviors, 38*(4), 2060–2067. doi:10.1016/j.addbeh.2012.12.016

Baylen, C. A., & Rosenberg, H. (2006). A review of the acute subjective effects of MDMA/ecstasy. *Addiction, 101*(7), 933–947.

Beech, R. A., Sterrett, D. R., & Babiuk, J. (2015). Cannabinoid hyperemesis syndrome: A case report and literature review. *Journal of Oral Maxillofacial Surgery, 73*(10), 1907–1910. doi:10.1016/joms.2015.03.059

Bell, C., Slim, J., & Flaten, H. K. (2015, December). Butane hash oil burns associated with marijuana liberalization in Colorado. *Journal of Medical Toxicology, 11*(4), 422–425. doi:10.1007/s13181-015-0501-0

Berg, C. J., Stratton, E., & Schauer, G. L. (2015). Perceived harm, addictiveness, and social acceptability of tobacco products and marijuana among young adults: Marijuana, hookah, and electronic cigarettes win. *Substance Use & Misuse, 50*(1), 79–89. doi:10.3109/10826084.2014.958857

Berke, J. (2018, November 7). Here's where you can legally consume marijuana in the US in 2018. *Business Insider*, 1-3.

Berman, M. E., & Coccaro, E. F. (1998). Neurobiologic correlates of violence: Relevance to criminal responsibility. *Behavioral Sciences and the Law, 16*(3), 303–318. doi: 10.1002/(SICI)1099-0798(199822)16:3<285::AID-BSL308>3.0.C0;2-4

Bey, T., & Patel, A. (2007, February). Phencyclidine intoxication and adverse effects: A clinical and pharmacological review of an illicit drug. *California Journal of Emergency Medicine, 8*(1), 9–14.

Biello, D. (2008, April 30). Albert Hofmann, inventor of LSD, embarks on final trip. *Science American*, 1.

Bonnet, U., & Preuss, U. W. (2017). The cannabis withdrawal syndrome: Current insights. *Substance Abuse and Rehabilitation, 8*, 9–37.

Bonn-Miller, M. O., Heinz, A. J., & Smith, E. V. (2016). Preliminary development of a brief cannabis use disorder screening tool: The Cannabis Use Disorder Identification Test Short Form. *Cannabis and Cannabinoid Research, 1* (1), 252–261. doi:10.1089/can.2016.0022

Bonson, K. R. (2017, November 17). Regulation of human research with LSD in the United States (1949-1987). *Psychopharmacology*. doi:10.1007/s00213-017-4777-4

Borges, G., Bagge, C. L., & Orozco, R. (2016, May). A literature review and meta-analyses of cannabis use and suicidality. *Journal of Affective Disorders, 195*, 63–74. doi:10.1016/j.jad.2016.02.007

Boseley, S. (2018, September 1). First ever trials on the effects of microdosing LSD set to begin. *The Guardian*, 1–3.

Boyd, C. J., McCabe, S. E., & d'Arcy, H. (2003). Ecstasy use among college undergraduates: Gender, race and sexual identity. *Journal of Substance Abuse Treatment, 24*(3), 209–215.

Breivogel, C. S., & Childers, S. R. (1998). The functional neuroanatomy of brain cannabinoid receptors. *Neurobiology Disease, 5*(6 Pt B), 417–431.

Brodwin, E. (2017, January 30). The truth about 'microdosing,' which involves taking tiny amounts of psychedelics like LSD. *Business Insider*, 1–10.

Bruno, R., Marshall, S., & Adamson, S. (2013). Screening for DSM-5 cannabis dependence using the Cannabis Use Identification Test-Revised. *NIDA Abstract Database*. NIH, National Institute on Drug Abuse. Retrieved March 7, 2018, from www.drugabuse.gov/international/abstracts/screening-dsm-5-cannabis-dependence-usingcanna bis-use-identification-test-revised

Bryan, M., & Simon, S. (2014, May 24). Pot vape pens, the crack cocaine of marijuana. *NPR Now*. NPR.

Bryant, A. (2015, June 22). Marijuana: ACOG encourages abstinence while pregnant or breast-feeding. *Obstetrics & Gynecology*, ACOG Committee on Obstetric Practice. (Committee opinion no. 637). Retrieved April 18, 2016, from NEJM Journal Watch, p. 1: 10.1097/AOG.0000000000000993

Buchi, K. F., Suarez, C., & Varner, M. W. (2013). The prevalence of prenatal opioid and other drug use in Utah. *American Journal of Perinatology, 30*(3), 241–244. doi:10.1055/s-0032-1323586

Buckner, J. D., Heimberg, R. G., & Schneier, F. R. (2012). The relationship between cannabis use disorders and social anxiety disorder in the National Epidemiological study of Alcohol and Related Conditions (NESARC). *Drug and Acohol Dependence, 124*(1-2), 128–134.

Budney, A. J., & Hughes, J. R. (2006, May). The cannabis withdrawal syndrome. *Current Opinion in Psychiatry, 19*(3), 233–238.

Budney, A. J., Hughes, J. R., & Moore, B. A. (2004). Review of the validity and significance of cannabis withdrawal syndrome. *The American Journal of Psychiatry, 161*(11), 1967–1977.

Budney, A. J., Moore, B. A., & Rocha, H. L. (2006, April). Clinical trial of abstinence-based vouchers and cognitive-behavioral therapy for cannabis dependence. *Journal of Consulting and Clinical Psychology, 24*(2), 307–316.

Cain, P. (2017, September 22). Non-Americans barred from U.S. for smoking pot – Even in states where it's legal. *Global News Online*. Global News.

Camchong, J., Lim, K. O., & Kumra, S. (2017). Adverse effects of cannabis on adolescent brain development: A longitudinal study. *Cerebral Cortex*, *27*(3), 1922–1930. doi:10.1093/cercor/bhw015

Campbell, C. T., Shaw Phillips, M., & Manasco, K. (2017, May-June). Cannabinoids in pediatrics. *The Journal of Pediatric Pharmacology and Therapeutics*, *22*(3), 176–185. doi:10.5863/1551-6776-22.3.176

Campbell, G. A., & Rosner, M. H. (2008). The agony of ecstasy: MDMA (3,4-methylenedioxymethamphetamine) and the kidney. *Clinical Journal of the American Society of Neprhology*, *3*(6), 1852–1860. doi:10.2215/CJN.02080508

Canadian Pharmacists Association. (2018, January 25). Cannabis for medical purposes evidence guide: Information for pharmacists and other health care professionals. *Medical Cannabis*, 1–11. Canadian Pharmacists Association.

Cao, D., Srisuma, S., & Bronstein, A. C. (2016, November). Characterization of edible marijuana product exposures reported to United States poison centers. *Clinical Toxicology*, *54*(9), 840–846. doi:10.1080/15563650.2016.12099761

Carroll, M. E. (1990, September). PCP and hallucinations. *Advances in Alcohol and Substance Abuse*, *9*(1-2), 167–185.

Castle, D. J. (2013). Cannabis and psychosis: What causes what? *Faculty of 1000 Medicine Reports*, *5*(1), 1–4. doi:10.3410/M5-1

CDC, Center for Disease Control and Prevention. (2015b, November 9). *Dangers of Hookah Smoking*. Retrieved June 25, 2016, from http:www.cdc.gov/chronicdisease/

CDC, Centers for Disease Control and Prevention. (2015a, September 14). *Hookahs*. Retrieved June 25, 2016, from Office on Smoking and Health: www.cdc.gov/chronicdisease/

Cerda, M., Wall, M., & Keyes, K. M. (2012). Medical marijuana laws in 50 states: Investigating the relationship between state legalization of medical marijuana and marijuana use, abuse and dependence. *Drug and Alcohol Dependence*, *120*(1-3), 22–27. doi:10.1016/j.drugalcdep.2011.06.011

Cermak, T. L., & Banys, P. (2016). Prevention of youthful marijuana use. *Journal of Psychoactive Drugs*, *48*(1), 21–23. doi:10.1080/02791072.2015.1117689

Chan, G. C., Hall, W., & Freeman, T. P. (2017, September 1). User characteristics and effect profile of Butane Hash Oil: An extremely high-potency cannabis concentrate. *Drug and Alcohol Dependence*, *178*, 32–38. doi:10.1016/j.drugalcdep.2017.04.014

Chang, Y. J., Lai, M. W., & Kong, M. S. (2005). Accidental ingestion of ecstasy in a toddler. *Journal of the Formosan Medical Association*, *104*(12), 946–947.

Chaouachi, K. (2009). Hookah (shisha, narghile) smoking and environmental tobacco smoke (ETS). A critical review of the relevant literature and the public health consequences. *International Journal of Environmental Research and Public Health*, *6*(2), 798–843. doi:10.3390/ijerph6020798

Chen, Q., & Tesmer, J. J. (2017, January 26). A receptor on acid. *Cell*, *168*(3), 339–341. doi:10.1016/j.cell.2017.01.012

Choo, E. K., Benz, M., & Zaller, N. (2014, August). The impact of state medical marijuana legislation on adolescent marijuana use. *Journal of Adolescent Health*, *55*(2), 160–166.

Christophersen, A. S., Morland, J., & Stewart, K. (2016). International trends in alcohol and drug use among vehicle drivers. *Forensic Science Review*, *28*(1), 37–66.

Cohen, M., Solowij, N., & Carr, V. (2008). Cannabis, cannabinoids and schizophrenia: Integration of the evidence. *Australian & New Zealand Journal of Psychiatry*, *42*(5), 357–368. doi:10.1080/00048670801961156

Cohen, M. M., Marinello, M. J., & Back, N. (1967). Chromosomal damage in human leukocytes induced by lysergic acid diethylamide. *Science*, *155*, 1417–1419.

Cohen, S. (1967). Psychotomimetic agents. *Annual Review of Pharmacology*, 7, 301–318. doi:10.1146/annurev.pa.07.040167.001505

Colizzi, M., & Bhattacharyya, S. (2017). Does cannabis composition matter? Differential effects of delta-9-tetrahydrocannabinol and cannabidiol on human cognition. *Current Addiction Reports*, *4*, 62–74. doi:10.1007/s40429-017-0142-2

Colorado Department of Revenue. (2018). *Colorado marijuana tax data*. Retrieved March 13, 2018, from Department of Revenue, pp. 1–2: www.colorado.gov/pacific/revenue/colorado-marijuana-tax-data

Cone, E. J., & Huestis, M. A. (1993, December). Relating blood concentrations of tetrahydrocannabinol and metabolites to pharmacologic effects and time of marijuana use. *Therapeutic Drug Monitoring*, *15*(6), 527–532.

Contreras, E. (2015, August 13). Inside the life of a drug-trafficking teen. *CNN.com*, 1. Eagle Pass, TX: CNN. Retrieved from www.cnn.com/2015/08/12/us/inside-the-life-of-a-drug-trafficking-teen/index.html

Cook, C. E., Perez-Reyes, M., & Jeffcoat, A. R. (1983, July). Phencyclidine disposition in humans after small doses of radiolabeled drug. *Federation Proceedings*, *42*(9), 2566–2569.

Cooper, Z. D., & Haney, M. (2009, April). Actions of delta-9-tetrahydrocannabinol in cannabis: Relation to use, abuse, dependence. *International Review of Psychiatry*, *21*(2), 104–112. doi:10.1080/09540260902782752

Copeland, J., & Swift, W. (2009). Cannabis use disorder: Epidemiology and management. *International Review of Psychiatry*, *21*(2). doi:10.1080/09540260902782745

Copeland, J., Swift, W., & Roffman, R. (2001). A randomized controlled trial of brief cognitive-behavioral interventions for cannabis use disorder. *Journal of Substance Abuse Treatment*, *21*, 55–64.

Corliss, H. L., Rosario, M., & Wypji, D. (2010). Sexual orientation and drug use in a longitudinal cohort study of US adolescents. *Addictive Behaviors, 35*(5), 517–521. doi:10.1016/j.addbeh.2009.12.019

Cornelius, J. R., Chung, T., & Martin, C. (2008). Cannabis withdrawal is common among treatment-seeking adolescents with cannabis dependence and major depression, and is associated with rapid relapse to dependence. *Addictive Behaviors, 33*(11), 1500–1505.

Cottler, L. B., Womack, S. B., & Compton, W. M. (2001, December). Ecstasy abuse and dependence among adolescents and young adults: Applicability and reliability of DSM-IV criteria. *Human Psychopharmacology, 16* (8), 599–606.

Couper, F. J., & Peterson, B. L. (2014). The prevalence of marijuana in suspected impaired driving cases in Washington state. *Journal of Analytical Toxicology, 38*(8), 569–574. doi:10.1093/jat/bku090

Crane, A., Easton, C. J., & Devine, S. (2013). Between phencyclidine use and partner violence: An initial examination. *Journal of Addictive Diseases, 32*(2), 150–157. doi: 10.1080/10550887.2013.797279

Crane, N. A., Schuster, R. M., & Gonzalez, R. (2013). Preliminary evidence for a sex-specific relationship between amount of cannabis use and neurocognitive performance in young adult cannabis users. *Journal of International Psychology and Sociology, 19*(9), 1009–1015. doi:10.1017/S135561771300088X

Crippa, J., Derenusson, G. N., & Chagas, M. (2017). Pharmacological interventions in the treament of the acute effects of cannabis: A systematic review of literature. *Harm Reduction Journal, 9*, 7–13.

Cuenca-Royo, A. M., Sanchez-Niubo, A., & Forero, C. G. (2012). Psychometric properties of the CAST and SDS scales in young adult cannabis users. *Journal of Addictive Behaviors, 37*(6), 709–715. doi:10.1016/j.addbeh.2012.02.012

D'Onofrio, G., McCausland, J. B., & Tarabar, A. F. (2006). Illy: Clinical and public health implications of a street drug. *Substance Abuse, 27*(4), 45–51.

D'Souza, D. C. (2007). Cannabinoids and psychosis. *International Review of Neurobiology, 78*, 289–326. doi:10.1016/S0074-7742(06)78010-2

Das, S., Barnwal, P., & Ramasamy, A. (2016). Lysergic acid diethylamide: A drug of 'use'? *Therapeutic Advances in Psychopharmacology, 6*(3), 214–228. doi:10.1177/2045125316640440

Dasgupta, A. (2015, February 1). How people try to beat drug testing: Issues with urinary adulterants and their detection. *Clinical Laboratory News*, 1–5.

Davis, A. K., & Rosenberg, H. (2014). The prevalence, intensity, and assessment of craving for MDMA/ecstasy in recreational users. *Journal of Psychoactive Drugs, 46*(2), 154–161. doi:10.1080/02791072.2014.901586

De Gregorio, D., Comai, S., & Posa, L. (2016). D-lysergic acid diethylamide (LSD) as a model of psychosis: Mechanism of action and pharmacology. *International Journal of Molecular Sciences, 17*, 1–20. doi:10.3390/ijms17111953

de la Torre, R., Farre, M., & Roset, P. N. (2004, April). Human pharmacology of MDMA: Pharmacokinetics, metabolism, and disposition. *Therapeutic Drug Monitoring, 26*(2), 137–144.

DEA, Drug Enforcement Administration. (2013, January). *Phencyclidine*. Arlington, VA: Drug Enforcement Administration.

Degenhardt, L., Bruno, R., & Topp, L. (2010, February 1). Is ecstasy a drug of dependence? *Drug and Alcohol Dependence, 107*(1), 1–10. doi:10.1016/j.drugalcdep.2009.09.009

Delforterie, M. J., Lynskey, M. T., & Huizink, A. C. (2015, May 1). The relationship between cannabis involvement and suicidal thoughts and behaviors. *Drug and Alcohol Dependence, 150*, 98–104. doi:10.1016/j.drugalcdep.2015.02.01

Denis, C., Lavie, E., & Fatseas, M. (2006, July 19). Psychotherapeutic interventions for cannabis abuse and/or dependence in outpatient settings. *The Cochrane Database of Systematic Reviews, 3*, CD005336.

Dennis, M., Godley, S. H., & Diamond, G. (2004, October). The Cannabis Youth Treatment (CYT) Study: Main findings from two randomized trials. *Journal of Substance Abuse Treatment, 27*(3), 197–213.

DeRosse, P., Kaplan, A., & Burdick, K. E. (2010, July). Cannabis use disorders in schizophrenia: Effects on cognition and symptoms. *Schizophrenia Research, 120*(1-3), 95–100. doi:10.1016/j.schres.2010.04.007

Devinsky, O., Cross, J. H., & Laux, L. (2017, May 25). Trial of cannabidiol for drug-resistant seizures in the Dravet syndrome. *The New England Journal of Medicine, 376*(21), 2011–2020. doi:10.1056/NEJMoa1611618

Di Marzo, V., Melck, D., & Bisogno, T. (1998). Endocannabinoids: Endogenous cannabinoid receptor ligands with neuromodulatory action. *Trends in Neurosciences, 21*(12), 521–528.

Diamond, S., Bermudez, R., & Schensul, J. (2006, May). What's the rap about ecstasy? Popular music lyrics and drug trends among American youth. *Journal of Adolescent Research, 21*(3), 269–298. doi:10.1177/0743558406287398

Dierker, L., Braymiller, J., & Rose, J. (2018, June 1). Nicotine dependence predicts cannabis use disorder symptoms among adolescents and young adults. *Drug and Alcohol Dependence, 187*, 212–220. doi:10.1016/j.drugalcdep.2018.02.037

Digitale, E. (2016, October 31). Teens' beliefs about marijuana documented in new Stanford study. *Scope*. Stanford Medicine.

Dishotsky, N. I., Loughman, W. D., & Mogar, R. E. (1971, April 30). LSD and genetic damage. *Science, 172*(3982), 431–440.

Dolder, P. C., Schmid, Y., & Haschke, M. (2015, June 24). Pharmacokinetics and concentration-effect relationship of oral LSD in humans. *International Journal of Neuropsychopharmacology*, *19*(1), pii: pyv072. doi:10.1093/injp/pyv072

Dolder, P. C., Schmid, Y., & Steuer, A. E. (2017). Pharmacokinetics and pharmacodynamics of lysergic acid diethylamide in healthy subjects. *Clinical Pharmacokinetics*, *56*(10), 1219–1230. doi:10.1007/s40262-017-0513-9

Domino, E. F., & Luby, E. D. (2012). Phencyclidine/Schizophrenia: One view toward the past, the other to the future. *Schizophrenia Bulletin*, *38*(5), 914–919. doi:10.1093/schbul/sbs011

Domino, E. F., & Wilson, A. E. (1977). Effects of urine acidification on plasma and urine phencyclidine levels in overdosage. *Clinical Pharmacology and Therapeutics*, *22*(4), 421–424.

Dubie, M. F., & Green, C. R. (1982). Methods of collection of smoke for analytical purposes. *Recent Advances in Tobacco Science*, *8*(42), 102.

Duffy, M. R., & Swart, M. (2006). Severe ecstasy poisoning in a toddler. *Anaesthesia*, *61*(5). doi:10.1111/j.1365-2044.2006.04620.x

Dunlap, E., Benoit, E., & Sifaneck, S. J. (2006, June). Social constructions of dependency by blunts smokers: Qualitative reports. *The International Journal on Drug Policy*, *17*(3), 171–182. doi:10.1016/j.drugpo.2006.01.004

Ehlers, C. L., Gizer, I. R., & Vieten, C. (2010). Cannabis dependence in the San Francisco Family Study: Age of onset of use, DSM-IV symptoms, withdrawal, and heritability. *Addictive Behaviors*, *35*(2), 102–110. doi:10.1016/j.addbeh.2009.09.009

Eisenberg, E., Ogintz, M., & Almog, S. (2014). The pharmacokinetics, efficacy, safety, and ease of use of a novel portable metered-dose cannabis inhaler in patients with chronic neuropathic pain: A phase 1a study. *Journal of Pain and Palliative Care Pharmacotherapy*, *28*(3), 216–225. doi:10.3109/15360288.2014.941130

Eiserman, J. M., Diamond, S., & Schensul, J. J. (2005). Rollin' on E. *Journal of Ethnicity in Substance Abuse*, *4*(2), 9–38. doi:10.1300/j233v04n02_02

Elphick, M. R., & Egertova, M. (2001, March 29). The neurobiology and evolution of cannabinoid signaling. *Philosophical Transactions of the Royal Society of London B Biological Sciences*, *356*(1407), 381–408. doi:10.1098/rstb.2000.0787

Evans, M. M. (2018, February 20). 'Teen Mom' Jenelle Evans reveals drug use while pregnant with daughter. *FoxNews.com*. Fox News.

Falck, R. S., Wang, J., & Carlson, R. G. (2006). Prevalence and correlates of current depressive symptomatology among a community sample of MDMA users in Ohio. *Addictive Behaviors*, *31*(1), 90–101. doi:10.1016/j.addbeh.2005.04.017

Farre, M., Abanades, S., & Roset, P. N. (2007, December). Pharmacological interaction between 3,4-methylenedioxymethamphetamine (ecstasy) and paroxetime: Pharmacological effects and pharmacokinetics. *Journal of Pharmacology and Experimental Therapeutics*, *323*(3), 954–962.

Farre, M., Tomillero, A., & Perez-Mana, C. (2015). Human pharmacology of 3,4-methylenedioxymethamphetamine (MDMA, ecstasy) after repeated doses taken 4 h apart. *European Neuropsychopharmacology*, *25*(10), 1637–1649. doi:10.1016/j.euroneuro.2015.05.007

FDA. (2019, March 5). FDA approves new nasal spray medication for treatment-resistant depression; available only at a certified doctor's office or clinic. *FDA News Release*.

Feingold, D., Rehm, J., & Lev-Ran, S. (2017, May). Cannabis use and the course and outcome of major depressive disorder: A population based longitudinal study. *Psychiatry Research*, *251*, 225–234. doi:10.1016/j.psychres.2017.02.027

Feldman, K. W., & Mazor, S. (2007). Ecstasy ingestion causing heatstroke-like multiorgan injury in a toddler. *Pediatric Emergency Care*, *23*(10), 725–726.

Fernando, T., Gilbert, J. D., & Carroll, C. M. (2012). Ecstasy and suicide. *Journal of Forensic Sciences*, *57*(4), 1137–1139. doi:10.1111/j.1556-4029.2012.02107.x

Ferner, M. (2014, September 22). *Marijuana Tax Revenue May Top $3 Billion a Year with Legalization*. Retrieved April 13, 2016, from HOFFPOST POLITICS: www.huffingtonpost.com/2014/09/22/legal-marijuana-taxes_n_5863860.html

Floyd, L. J., Alexandre, P. K., & Hedden, S. L. (2010, March). Adolescent drug dealing and race/ethnicity: A population-based study of the differential impact of substance use on involvement in drug trade. *The American Journal of Drug and Alcohol Abuse*, *36*(2), 87–91. doi:10.3109/00952991003587469

Forster, V. (2018, June 25). FDA approves first-ever drug directly purified from cannabis. *Forbes*, 1–2.

Foster, D. (2016, April 19). How blunts came to define hip-hop's golden age in New York city. *Elite Daily*.

Freed, W. J., Weinberger, D. R., & Bing, L. A. (1980, December). Neuropharmacological studies of phencyclidine (PCP)-induced behavioral stimulation in mice. *Psychopharmacology*, *71*(3), 291–297.

Fried, P. A., & Smith, A. M. (2001). A literature review of the consequences of prenatal marihuana exposure. An emerging theme of a deficiency in aspects of executive function. *Neurotoxicology and Teratology*, *23*(1), 1–11.

Frobe, T., Leeman, R. F., & Patock-Peckham, J. (2018). Correlates of cannabis vape-pen use and knowledge among U.S. college students. *Addictive Behaviors Reports*, 7, 32–39.

Gallagher, D. T., Hadjiefthyvoulou, F., & Fisk, J. E. (2014). Prospective memory deficits in illicit polydrug users are associated with the average long-term typical dose of ecstasy typically consumed in a single session. *Neuropsychology, 28*(1), 43–54. doi:10.1037/neu0000004

Galli, J. A., Andari Sawaya, R., & Friedenberg, F. K. (2011, December). Cannabinoid hyperemesis syndrome. *Current Drug Abuse Reviews, 4*(4), 241–249.

Gant, M. (2017, December 29). Jack in the Box launching weed-themed Merry Munchie Meal in California. *Fox News*. FoxNews.com.

Gasser, P., Holstein, D., & Michel, Y. (2014). Safety and efficacy of lysergic acid diethylamide-assisted psychotherapy for anxiety associated with life-threatening diseases. *The Journal of Nervous and Mental Disease, 202*(7), 513–520. doi:10.1097/NMD.0000000000000113

Gates, P. J., Sabioni, P., & Copeland, J. (2016, May 5). Psychosocial interventions for cannabis use disorder. *The Cochrane Database of Systematic Reviews, 5*, CD005336. doi:10.1002/14651858.CD005336.pub4

Gentes, E. L., Schry, A. R., & Hicks, T. A. (2016, May). Treatment and correlates of cannabis use in an outpatient VA posttraumatic stress disorder clinic. *Psychology of Addictive Behaviors, 30*(3), 415–421. doi:10.1037/adb0000154

Gettman, J. (2006, December). *Marijuana Production in the United States (2006)*. Retrieved August 1, 2015, from The Bulletin of Cannabis Reform, pp. 1–28: www.drugscience.org/bcr/index.html

Ghatol, A., & Kazory, A. (2012). Ecstasy-associated acute severe hypnonatremia and cerebral edema: A role for osmotic diuresis? *The Journal of Emergency Medicine, 42*(6), e137–e140. doi:10.1016/j.jemermed.2009.05.001

Gilbert, C. R., Baram, M., & Cavarocchi, N. C. (2013). "Smoking wet": Respiratory failure related to smoking tainted marijuana cigarettes. *Texas Heart Institute Journal, 40*(1), 64–67.

Gill, J. R., Hayes, J. A., & deSousa, I. S. (2002). Ecstasy (MDMA) deaths in New York City: A case series and review of the literature. *Journal of Forensic Sciences, 47*, 121–126.

Gillespie, N. A., Aggen, S. H., & Neale, M. C. (2018). Associations between personality disorders and cannabis use and cannabis use disorders: A population-based twin study. *Addiction, 113*(8), 1488–1498. doi:10.1111/add.14209

Glennon, R. A., Titeler, M., & McKenney, J. D. (1984, December 17). Evidence for 5-HT2 involvement in the mechanism of action of hallucinogenic agents. *Life Sciences, 35*(25), 2505–2511. doi:10.210126/0024-3205(84)90436-3

Golden, N. L., Kuhnert, B. R., & Sokol, R. J. (1987). Neonatal manifestations of maternal phencyclidine exposure. *Journal of Perinatal Medicine, 15*, 185–191.

Goodwin, R. S., Darwin, W. D., & Chiang, C. N. (2008). Urinary elimination of 11-nor-9-carboxy-9-tetrahydrcannabinol in cannabis users during continuously monitored abstinence. *Journal of Analytical Toxicology, 32*(8), 562–569.

Goulle, J. P., & Guerbet, M. (2014). Tetrahydrocannabinol pharmacokinetics; new synthetic cannabinoids; road safety and cannabis. *Bulletin De l'Academie Nationale De Medecine, 198*(3), 541–556.

Gouzoulis-Mayfrank, E., & Daumann, J. (2006). Neurotoxicity of methylenedioxymethamphetamines (MDMA; ecstasy) in humans: How strong is the evidence for persistent brain damage? *Addiction, 101*(3), 348–361. doi:10.1111/j.1360-0443.2006.01314.x

Gouzoulis-Mayfrank, E., & Daumann, J. (2009). Neurotoxicity of drugs of abuse–The case of methylenedioxymethamphetamines (MDMA, ecstasy), and amphetamines. *Dialogues in Clinical Neuroscience, 11*(3), 305–317.

Gouzoulis-Mayfrank, E., Fischermann, T., & Rezk, M. (2005). Memory performance in polyvalent MDMA (ecstasy) users who continue or discontinue MDMA use. *Drug and Alcohol Dependence, 78*(3), 317–323. doi:10.1016/j.drugalcdep.2004.12.002

Granowicz, J. (2016). Senator Elizabeth Warren asks the CDC to study marijuana as opiate alternative. *The Marijuana Times*, 1.

Grucza, R. A., Vuolo, M., & Krauss, M. J. (2018, September). Cannabis decriminalization: A study of recent policy change in five U.S. states. *The International Journal on Drug Policy, 59*, 67–75. doi:10.1016/j.drugpo.2018.06.016

Grunau, B. E., Wiens, M. O., & Brubacher, J. R. (2010, September). Dantrolene in the treatment of MDMA-related hyperpyrexia: A systematic review. *CJEM, 12*(5), 435–442.

Grunau, B. E., Wiens, M. O., & Greidanus, M. (2010, September). Dantrolene for the treatment of MDMA toxicity. *CJEM, 12*(5), 457–459.

Gunn, J. K., Rosales, C. B., & Center, K. E. (2016). Prenatal exposure to cannabis and maternal and child health outcomes: A systematic review and meta-analysis. *BMJ Open, 6*, 1–7. doi:10.1136/bmjopen-2015-009986

Gyepesi, A., Urban, R., & Farkas, J. (2014). Psychometric properties of the Cannabis Abuse Screening Test in Hungarian samples of adolescents and young adults. *European Addiction Research, 20*(3), 119–128. doi:10.1159/000353238

Hagler, D. (2017, April). Marijuana use: Detrimental to youth. *Position Statement*, 1–14. American College of Pediatricians.

Hanby Hudgens, L. (2017, April 20). Teens tend to think marijuana use is no big deal, but they're wrong. *The Washington Post*. The Washigton Post. Retrieved from www.washingtonpost.com/news/parenting/wp/2017/04/20/teens-tend-to-think-marijuana-use-is-no-big-deal-but-theyre-wrong/?utm_term=c7dc749a5b6e

Hancox, R. J., Poulton, R., & Ely, M. (2010). Effects of cannabis on lung function: A population-based cohort study. *European Respiratory Journal, 35*(1), 42–47. doi:10.1183/09031936.00065009

Hardin, J. S., Wessinger, W. D., & Wenger, G. R. (2002, July). A single dose of monoclonal anti-phencyclidine IgG offers long-term reductions in phencyclidine behavioral effects in rats. *Journal of Pharmacology and Experimental Therapeutics, 202*(1), 119–126. doi:10.1124/jpet.302.1.119

Harrison, L. D., Backenheimer, M., & Inciardi, J. A. (1996). Cannabis use in the United States: Implications for policy. In P. Cohen & A. Sas, *Cannabisbeleid in Duitsland, Frankrijk En De Verenigde Staten* (pp. 179–276). Amsterdam: Centrum voor Drugsonderzoek.

Hartman, R. L., Brown, T. L., & Milavetz, G. (2015). Controlled cannabis vaporizer admininstration: Blood and plasma cannabinoids with and without alcohol. *Clinical Chemistry, 61*(6), 850–869. doi:10.1373/clinchem.2015.238287

Hartman, R. L., & Huestis, M. A. (2013). Cannabis effects on driving skills. *Clinical Chemistry, 59*(3), 478–492. doi:10.1373/clinchem.2012.194381

Hasin, D. S., Kerridge, B. T., & Saha, T. D. (2016). Prevalence and correlates of DSM-5 cannabis use disorder, 2012-2013: Findings from the National Epidemiologic Survey on Alcohol and Related Conditions-III. *The American Journal of Psychiatry, 173*(6), 588–599.

Hasin, D. S., O'Brien, C. P., & Auriacombe, M. (2013). DSM-5 criteria for substance use disorders: Recommendations and rationale. *American Journal of Psychiatry, 170*(8), 834–851. doi:10.1176/appi.ajp.2013.12060782

Heather, A. C. (2001, February). Pharmacology and effects of cannabis: A brief review. *The British Journal of Psychiatry, 178*, 101–106.

Heishman, S. J., Singleton, E. G., & Liguori, A. (2001). Marijuana craving questionnaire: Development and initial validation of a self-report instrument. *Addiction, 96*(7), 1023–1034.

Hendricks, L.-V., Daugherty, J. L., & Dang, Q. (2017). Phencyclidine ("PCP"): A dangerous drug impacting youth. *Journal of Substance Abuse & Alcoholism, 5*(4), 1065.

Hendricks, P. S., Thorne, C. B., & Clark, C. B. (2015). Classic psychedelic use is associated with reduced psychological distress and suicidality in the United States adult population. *Journal of Psychopharmacology, 29*(3), 280–288. doi:10.1177/0269881114565653

Herman, B. (2018, February 28). This scientist is testing a marijuana ingredient as a way to prevent relapse. *STAT*, 1–5.

Hernandez-Avilla, C. A., Rounsaville, B. J., & Kranzler, H. R. (2004). Opioid-, cannabis- and alcohol-dependent women show more rapid progression to substance abuse treatment. *Drug and Alcohol Dependence, 74*(3), 265–272.

Hernandez-Lopez, C., Farre, M., & Roset, P. N. (2002). 3,4-methylenedioxymethamphetamine (ecstasy) and alcohol interactions in humans: Psychomotor performance, subjective effects, and pharmacokinetics. *The Journal of Pharmacology and Experimental Therapeutics, 300*(1), 236–244.

Ho, E., Karimi-Tabesh, L., & Koren, G. (2001). Characteristics of pregnant women who use ecstasy (3, 4-methylene-dioxymethamphetamine). *Neurotoxicology and Teratology, 23*(6), 561–567.

Hofmann, A. (1970). Notes and documents concerning the discovery of LSD. *Agents and Actions, 1*(3), 148–150.

Hofmann, A. (1980a). *LSD - My Problem Child.* New York, NY: McGraw Hill.

Hofmann, A. (1980b). How LSD originated. *Journal of Psychedelic Drugs, 11*(1-2), 53–60.

Hopfer, C. (2014). Implications of marijuana legalization for adolescent substance use. *Substance Abuse, 35*(4), 331–335. doi:10.1080/08897077.2014.943386

Hopfer, C., Mendelson, B., & Van Leeuwen, J. M. (2010). Club drug use among youths in treatment for substance abuse. *The American Journal on Addictions, 15*(1). doi:10.1080/10550490500419144

Horn, J. R., & Hansten, P. D. (2014, December 9). Drug interactions with marijuana. *Pharmacy Times.*

Horowitz, A., Galanter, M., & Dermatis, H. (2008). Use of and attitudes toward club drugs by medical students. *Journal of Addictive Disease, 27*(4), 35–42. doi:10.1080/10550880802324705

Huestis, M. A. (2007). Human cannabinoid pharmacokinetics. *Chemistry & Biodiversity, 4*(8), 1770–1804.

Hunt, C. A., Jones, R. T., & Herning, R. I. (1981, June). Evidence that cannabidiol does not significantly alter the pharmacokinetics of tetrahydrocannabinol in man. *Journal of Pharmacokinetics and Biopharmaceutics, 9*(3), 245–260.

Hurley, J. M., West, J. B., & Ehleringer, J. R. (2010). Tracing retail cannabis in the United States: Geographic origin and cultivation patterns. *International Journal of Drug Policy, 21*, 222–228. doi:10.1016/j.drugpo.2009.08.001

Hysek, C. M., Schmid, Y., & Simmler, L. D. (2014). MDMA enhances emotional empathy and prosocial behavior. *Social Cognitive & Affective Neuroscience, 9*(11), 1645–1652. doi:10.1093/scan/nst161

Hysek, C. M., Simmler, L. D., & Schillinger, N. (2014). Pharmacokinetic and pharmacodynamic effects of methylphenidate and MDMA administered alone or in combination. *International Journal of Neuropsychopharmacology, 17*(3), 371–381. doi:10,1017/S1461145713001132

Jehle, J. C. C., Nazir, N., & Bhavsar, D. (2015). The rapidly increasing trend of cannabis use in burn injury. *Journal of Burn Care & Research, 36*(1), e12-e17. doi:10.1097/BCR.0000000000000192

Jensen, G., Bertelotti, R., & Greenhaigh, D. (2015, March-April). Honey oil burns: A growing problem. *Journal of Burn Care & Research, 36*(2), e34-e37. doi:10.1097/BCR.0000000000000067

Jerome, L., Schuster, S., & Yazar-Klosinski, B. B. (2013). Can MDMA play a role in the treatment of substance abuse? *Current Drug Abuse Reviews, 6*(1), 54–62.

Johansen, P. O., & Krebs, T. S. (2015). Psychedelics not linked to mental health problems or suicidal behavior; A population study. *Journal of Psychopharmacology, 29*(3), 270–279. doi:10.1177/0269881114568039
Johns, A. (2001). Psychiatric effects of cannabis. *The British Journal of Psychiatry, 178*, 116–122.
Johnson, R. M., Fairman, B., & Gilreath, T. (2015, October 1). Past 15-year trends in adolescent marijuana use: Differences by race/ethnicity and sex. *Drug and Alcohol Dependence, 155*, 8–15. doi:10.1016/j.drugalcdep.
Johnston, L. D., O'Malley, P. M., & Bachman, J. G. (2011). *Monitoring the Future national results on adolescent drug use: Overview of key findings*. Ann Arbor, Michigan: Institute for Social Research, The University of Michigan.
Joshi, M., Joshi, A., & Bartter, T. (2014). Marijuana and lung diseases. *Current Opinion in Pulmonary Medicine, 20*(2), 173–179. doi:10.1097/MCP.0000000000000026
Kaplan, M. (2018, March 5). Weed is helping me quit opioids. *New York Post*, 1.
Karolina Kedzior, K., & Martin-Iverson, M. (2010). Association between severity of cannabis dependence and depression. *Psychology, 1*, 233–237. doi:10.4236/psych.2010.14031
Karolina Kedzior, K., & Tabata Laeber, L. (2014). A positive association between anxiety disorders and cannabis use or cannabis use disorders in the general population: A meta analysis of 31 studies. *BMC Psychiatry, 14*, 136. doi:10.1186/1471-244X-14-136
Kasana, M. (2018, December 21). Hemp is legal in the US now – Here's what that actually means. *Bustle*, 1–2.
Kazour, F., Awaida, C., & Souaiby, L. (2018, February). A study on a sample of patients hospitalized for bipolar disorder. *L'Encephale, 44*(1), 14–21. doi:10.1016/j.encep.2016.08.005
Kelley, K. J. (2019, March 7). FDA approves intranasal esketamine as adjunctive treatment for depression. *NEJM Journal Watch*, 1.
Kendall, D. A., & Yudowski, G. A. (2017, January). Cannabinoid receptors in the central nervous system: Their signaling and roles in disease. *Frontiers in Cellular Neuroscience, 10*, 1–10. doi:10.3389/fncel.2016.00294
Ketchum, W. E. (2017, January 19). 25 iconic rap lyrics about weed. *Billboard Magazine*, 1-3.
Kevorkian, S., Bonn-Miller, M. O., & Belendiuk, K. (2015, September). Associations among trauma, posttraumatic stress disorder, cannabis use, and cannabis use disorder in a nationally representative epidemiologic sample. *Psychology of Addictive Behaviors, 29*(3), 633–638. doi:10.1037/adb0000110
Khalsa, J. H., Genser, S., & Francis, H. (2002). Clinical consequences of marijuana. *Journal of Clinical Pharmacology, 42* (Supplement 11), 7S-10S.
Khan, S. S., Secades-Villa, R., & Okuda, M. (2013). Gender differences in cannabis use disorders: Results from the National Epidemiologic Survey of Alcohol and Related Conditions. *Drug and Alcohol Dependence, 130*(1-3), 101–108. doi:10.1016/j.drugalcdep.2012.10.015
Kirkpatrick, M. G., & de Wit, H. (2015). MDMA: A social drug in a social context. *Psychopharmacology (Berlin), 232*(6), 1155–1163. doi:10.1007/s00213-014-3752-6
Klein, T. W., Lane, B., & Newton, C. A. (2000). The cannabinoid system and cytokine network. *Proceedings of the Society for Experimental Biology and Medicine, 225*(1), 1–8.
Klitzman, R. L., Pope, H. G., & Hudson, J. I. (2000). MDMA ("Ecstasy") abuse and high-risk sexual behaviors among 169 gay and bisexual men. *American Journal of Psychiatry, 157*(7), 1162–1164.
Knapp, A. A., Babbin, S. F., & Budney, A. J. (2018). Psychometric assessment of the Marijuana Adolescent Problem Inventory. *Addictive Behaviors, 79*, 113–119. doi:10.1016/j.addbeh.2017.12.013
Koskinen, J., Lohonen, J., & Koponen, H. (2010, November 1). Rate of cannabis use disorders in clinical samples of patients with schizophrenia: A meta-analysis. *Schizophrenia Bulletin, 36*(6), 1115–1130. doi:10.1093/schbul/sbp031
Kovacevich, N. (2018, December 5). Cannabis is a tax bonanza for states. *Forbes*, 1–2.
Krauss, M. J., Sowles, S. J., & Moreno, M. (2015, July 30). Hookah-related twitter chatter: A content analysis. *Preventing Chronic Disease, 12*(e121), 1–9. doi:10.5888/pcd12.150140
Krebs, T. S., & Johansen, P. O. (2013, August 19). Psychedelics and mental health: A population study. *PLoS One, 8*(8), e63972. doi:10/1371/journal.pone.0063972
Kruzman, D. (2017, July 26). You're not tripping: LSD is making a comeback. *USA Today*, 1.
Kung, S. W., Chan, Y. C., & Tse, M. L. (2008). Accidental ecstasy poisoning in a five-year-old boy. *Hong Kong Journal of Emergency Medicine, 15*, 111–114.
Kvitland, L. R., Melle, I., & Aminoff, S. R. (2016, February). Cannabis use in first-treatment bipolar I disorder: Relations to clinical characteristics. *Early Intervention in Psychiatry, 10*(1), 36–44. doi:10.1111/eip.12138
La Corte, R. (2014). Legal pot bringing in even more tax revenue than predicted. Retrieved from: www.huffingtonpost.com/2014/11/20
Lagerquist, J. (2019, February 25). Starbucks could be the first big chain to launch cannabis drinks. *Yahoo Finance*.
Laurenzana, E. M., & Owens, S. M. (1997). Metabolism of phencyclidine by human liver microsomes. *Drug Metabolism and Disposition, 25*(5), 557–563.
Lee, J. P., Battle, R. S., & Lipton, R. (2010, February). 'Smoking': Use of cigarettes, cigars and blunts among Southeast Asian American youth and young adults. *Health Education Research, 25*(1), 83–96. doi:10.1093/her/cyp066
Lee, M. H., & Hancox, R. J. (2011). Effects of smoking cannabis on lung function. *Expert Review of Respiratory Medicine, 5*(4), 537–546. doi:10.1586/ers.11.40

Legleye, S. (2017, November 10). The Cannabis Abuse Screening Test and the DSM-5 in the general population: Optimal thresholds and underlying common structure using multiple factor analysis. *International Journal of Methods in Psychiatric Research*. doi:10.1002/mpr.1597

Legleye, S., Eslami, A., & Bougeard, S. (2017, March). Assessing the structure of the CAST (Canabis Abuse Screening Test) in 13 European countries using multigroup analyses. *International Journal of Methods in Psychiatric Research, 26* (1). doi:10.1002/mpr.1552

Legleye, S., Guignard, R., & Richard, J. B. (2015, June). Properties of the Cannabis Abuse Screening Test (CAST) in the general population. *International Journal of Methods in Psychiatric Research, 24*(2), 170–183. doi:10.1002/mpr.1465

Legleye, S., Karila, L., & Beck, F. (2007). Validation of the CAST, a general population cannabis abuse screening test. *Journal of Substance Use, 12*(4), 233–242.

Legleye, S., Kraus, L., & Piontek, D. (2012). Validation of the Cannabis Abuse Screening Test in a sample of cannabis inpatients. *European Addiction Research, 18*(4), 193–200. doi:10.1159/000336553

Legleye, S., & Rouquette, A. (2018, March 1). Age invariance of the Cannabis Abuse Screening Test in a probabilistic sample of cannabis users. *European Addiction Research, 24*(1), 37–42. doi:10.1159/000487480

Leung, K. S., & Cottler, L. B. (2008). Ecstasy and other club drugs: A review of recent epidemiologic studies. *Current Opinion in Psychiatry, 21*(3), 234–241. doi:10.1097/YCO.0b013e3282f9b1f1

Leweke, F. M., & Koethe, D. (2008). Cannabis and psychiatric disorders: It is not only addiction. *Addiction Biology, 13* (2), 264–275. doi:10.1111/j.1369-1600.2008.00106.x

Li, M. C., Brady, J. E., & DiMaggio, C. J. (2012). Marijuana use and motor vehicle crashes. *Epidemiologic Reviews, 34*, 65–72. doi:10.1093/epirev/mxr017

Li, X., Stanton, B., & Feigelman, S. (1999, February). Exposure to drug trafficking among urban, low-income African American children and adolescents. *Archives of Pediatrics & Adolescent Medicine, 153*, 161–168.

Lieber, M. (2018, April 26). Marijuana legalization could help offset opioid epidemic, studies find. *CNN*, 1.

Lipari, R. N., & Ahrnsbrak, R. D. (2017, September). Risk and protective factors and estimates of substance use initiation: Results from the 2016 National Survey on Drug Use and Health. *SAMHSA NSDUH Data Review*, 1–30. SDMHSA.

Loflin, M., Babson, K., & Browne, K. (2017). Assessment of the validity of the CUDIT-R in a subpopulation of cannabis users. *The American Journal of Drug and Alcohol Abuse, 44*(1), 19–23. doi:10.1080/00952990.2017.1376677

Loflin, M. J., Earleywine, M., & Farmer, S. (2017, August 3). Placebo effects of edible cannabis: Reported intoxicaiton effects at a 30-minute delay. *Journal of Psychoactive Drugs*, 1–5. doi:10.1080/02791072.2017.1354409

Lopez-Moreno, J. A., Gonzalez-Cuevas, G., & Moreno, G. (2008). The pharmacology of the endocannabinoid system: Functional and structural interactions with other neurotransmitter systems and their repercussions in behavioral addiction. *Addiction Biology, 13*(2), 160–187. doi:10.1111/j.1369-1600.2008.00105.x

Ludlow, F. H. (1857). *The Hashish Eater: Being Passages from the Life of Pythagorean*. New York, NY: S. G. Rains.

Ly, B. T., Thornton, S. L., & Buono, C. (2012). False-positive urine phencyclidine immunoassay screen caused by interferrence by tramadol and its metabolites. *Annals of Emergency Medicine, 59*(6), 545–547. doi:10.1016/j.annemergmed.2011.08.013

Maccarrone, M., & Finazzi-Agro, A. (2002). Endocannabinoids and their actions. *Vitamins and Hormones, 65*, 225–255.

MacNeal, J. J., Cone, D. C., & Sinha, V. (2012). Use of haloperidol in PCP-intoxicated individuals. *Clinical Toxicology (Philadelphia, PA), 59*(9), 851–853. doi:10.3109/15563650.2012.722222

Maida, V., & Daeninck, P. J. (2016, December). A user's guide to cannabinoid therapies in oncology. *Current Oncology, 23*(6), 398–406.

Maldonado, R., & Rodriguez de Fonseca, F. (2002, May 1). Cannabinoid addiction: Behavioral models and neural correlates. *Journal of Neuroscience, 22*(9), 3326–3331.

Marceaux, J. C., Dilks, L. S., & Hixson, S. (2008). Neuropsychological effects of formaldehyde use. *Journal of Psychoactive Drugs, 40*(2), 207–210. doi:10.1080/02791072.2008.10400632

Marshal, S. E. (2013). *The Cannabis Use Disorder Identification Test - Revised (CUDIT-R): Categorisation and Interpretation*. Australia: University of Tasmania. Retrieved March 5, 2018.

Martin, B. R., Mechoulam, R., & Razdan, R. K. (1999). Discovery and characterization of endogenous cannabinoids. *Life Sciences, 65*(6-7), 573–595.

Martins, S. S., & Alexandre, P. K. (2009). The association of Ecstasy use and academic achievement among adolescents in two U.S. national surveys. *Addictive Behaviors, 34*(1), 9–16. doi:10.1016/j.addbeh.2008.07.022

Martins, S. S., Storr, C. L., & Alexandre, P. K. (2008). Adolescent Ecstasy and other drug use in the National Survey of Parents and Youth: The role of sensation-seeking, parental monitoring and peer's drug use. *Addictive Behaviors, 33*(7), 919–933. doi:10.1016/j.addbeh.2008.02.010

Masisak, C. (2017, November 29). Troubled NFL star Josh Gordon reveals his past as a gun toting, drug selling gangster. *NY Post*, 1–2.

Mayo Clinic Staff. (2017). *Marijuana*. Mayo Clinic. Retrieved March 6 2018

McCabe, S. E., Boyd, C., & Hughes, T. L. (2003, June). Sexual identity and substance use among undergraduate students. *Substance Abuse, 24*(2), 77–91.

McElroy, J. (2016, July 13). Why children as young as 12 are joining the Surrey drug trade. *Global News*, 1. Surrey, BC: Global News. Retrieved from https://globalnews.ca/news/2822741/why-children-as-young-as-12-are-joining-the-surrey-drug-trade/

McGilveray, I. J. (2005, Autumn). Pharmacokinetics of cannabinoids. *Pain Research & Management, 10*(Supplement A), 15A-22A.

McGregor, I. S., Callaghan, P. D., & Hunt, G. E. (2008). From ultrasocial to antisocial: A role for oxytocin in the acute reinforcing effects and long-term adverse consequences of drug use? *British Journal of Pharmacology, 154*(2), 358–368. doi: 10.1038/bjp.2008.132

Mead, A. (2017, May). The legal status of cannabis (marijuana) and cannabidiol (CBD) under U.S. law. *Epilepsy & Behavior, 70*(Part B), 288–291. doi:10.1016/j.yebeh.2016.11.021

Melian, A. M., Burillo-Poutze, G., & Campo, C. G. (2004). Accidental ecstasy poisoning in a toddler. *Pediatric Emergency Care, 20*(8), 534–535.

Melton, S. T. (2017, June 8). Stirring the pot: Potential drug interactions with marijuana. *MedScape.*

Meyer, J. S. (2013, November 21). 3,4-methylenedioxymethamphetamine (MDMA): Current perspectives. *Substance Abuse and Rehabilitation, 4*, 83–99. doi:10.2147/SAR.S37258

Miech, R. A., Johnston, L., & O'Malley, P. M. (2015). Trends in use of and attitudes toward marijuana among youth before and after decriminalization: The case of California 2007-2013. *The International Journal on Drug Policy, 26* (4), 336–344. doi:10.1016/j.drugpo.2015.01.009

Mikelionis, L. (2018, January 1). With new year, California's recreational pot laws take effect. *Fox News*. FoxNews.com.

Miller, S. G. (2016, August 8). High numbers? 1 in 8 US adults smokes pot. *Live Science*, 1–10.

Montgomery, L., & Bagot, K. (2016). Let's be blunt: Consumption methods matter among black marijuana smokers. *Journal of Studies on Alcohol and Drugs, 77*, 451–456.

Montoya, A. G., Sorrentino, R., & Lukas, S. E. (2002). Long-term neuropsychiatric consequences of "ecstasy" (MDMA): A review. *Harvard Review of Psychiatry, 10*(4), 212–220.

Moran, G. (2016, June 20). There has been some progress, but youth drug smuggling persists at the U.S.-Mexico border. *LA Times*, 1–5. San Diego, CA: LA Times. Retrieved from www.latimes.com/local/lanow/la-me-youths-drug-smuggling-20160620-snap-story.html

Moreira, F. A., & Lutz, B. (2008). The endocannabinoid system: Emotion, learning and addiction. *Addictive Behaviors, 13* (2), 196–212. doi:10.1111/j.1369-1600.2008.00104.x

Morgan, M. J. (2000, October). Ecstasy (MDMA): A review of its possible persistent psychological effects. *Psychopharmacology, 152*(3), 230–248.

Moritz, M. L., Kalantar-Zadeh, K., & Ayus, J. C. (2013). Ecstasy-associated hyponatremia: Why are women at risk? *Nephrology, Dialysis, Transplantation, 28*(9), 2206–2209. doi:10.1093/ndt/gft192

Morris, B. J., Cochran, S. M., & Pratt, J. A. (2005). PCP: From pharmacology to modelling schizophrenia. *Current Opinion in Pharmacology, 5*(1), 101–106.

Morris, D. S., Fiala, S. C., & Pawlak, R. (2012, November 15). Opportunities for policy interventions to reduce youth hookah smoking in the United States. *Preventing Chronic Disease, 9*, 1–4. doi:10.5888/pcd9.120082

Morris, D. Z. (2017, December 26). Jack in the Box is launching a 'Munchie Meal' for stoners. *Fortune.*

Motel, S. (2015, April 14). *6 Facts about Marijuana*. Retrieved April 14, 2016, from PewResearchCenter: www.pewresearch.org/author/smotel/

Motycka, C., Glinton, M., & Brennan, C. (2016). Side effects and drug interactions with marijuana. *International Archives of Nursing and Health Care, 2*(1), 1–2.

Murphy, D., Barry, M., & Vaughn, B. (2013, September). Adolescent health highlight: Use of illicit drugs. *Child Trends: Adolescent Health Highlight(#2013-11)*, 1–8. (H. J. Scarupa, Ed.) Child Trends.

Murray, J. B. (2002). Phencyclidine (PCP): A dangerous drug, but useful in schizophrenia research. *The Journal of Psychology, 136*(3), 319–327.

National Conference of State Legislatures. (2018, November 8). State medical marijuana laws. *Summary Report*, 1–10. National Conference of State Legislatures.

National Highway Traffic Safety Administration (NHTSA). (n.d.). *Drugs and Human Performance FACT SHEETS*. Retrieved April 10, 2016, from Methylyenedioxymethamphetamine (MDMA, Ecstasy), pp. 1–5: www.nhtsa.gov/people/injury/research/job185drugs/methylenedioxymethamphetamine.htm

Newman, K. (2017, December 14). NIH survey: Students vaping, using marijuana more in 2017. *U.S. News & World Report*, 1–4. Retrieved from www.usnews.com/news/national-news/articles/2017-12-14/nih-survey-alcohol-and-marijuana-and-vaping-top-students-2017-drug-use

Nichols, D. E. (2004). Hallucinogens, *Pharmacology & Therapeutics, 101*(2), 131–181.

Nicolson, S. E., Denysenko, L., & Mulcare, J. L. (2012, May-June). Cannabinoid hyperemesis syndrome: A case series and review of previous reports. *Journal of Psychosomatics, 53*(3), 212–219. doi:10.1016/j.psym.2012.01.003

NIDA, National Institute on Drug Abuse. (2009, June). Hallucinogens: LSD, peyote, psilocybin, and PCPP. 1-7. U.S. Department of Health and Human Services.

NIDA, National Institute on Drug Abuse. (2016, January). *Hallucinogens*. Retrieved April 10, 2016, from National Institute on Drug Abuse (NIDA), pp. 1–4: www.drugabuse.gov/drugs-abuse/hallucinogens

NIDA, National Institute on Drug Abuse. (2017). *MDMA (ecstasy) Abuse*. Bethesda, MA: National Institutes on Drug Abuse.

NIDA, National Institute on Drug Abuse. (2018a). Highlights from the 2017 survey. *Press Release*, 1–3. NIDA.

NIDA, National Institute on Drug Abuse. (2018b, June). *Marijuana*. Bethesda, MD: NIH.

NIDA, National Institute on Drug Abuse. (2018c, February). *Common Comorbidities with Substance Use Disorders*. Bethesda, MD: NIH.

Nocerino, E., Amato, M., & Izzo, A. A. (2000). Cannabis and cannabinoid receptors. *Fitoterapia*, *71*(Supplement 1), S6-S12.

Noda, Y., & Nabeshima, T. (2006, January 12). Involvement of signal transduction cascade via dopamine-D1 receptors in phencyclidine dependence. *Annals of the New York Academy of Sciences*. doi:10.1196/annals.1316.008

Norman, G. (2018, January 10). Massachusetts teen, 15, accused of running drug pickup operation out of bedroom window. *FoxNews.com*, 1. FoxNews.com. Retrieved from www.foxnews.com/us/2018/01/10/massachusetts-teen-15-accused-running-drug-pickup-operation-out-bedroom-window.html

Nurmikko, T. J., Serpell, M. G., & Hoggart, B. (2007, August). Sativex successfully treats neuropathic pain characterised by allodynia: A randomised, double-blind, placebo-controlled clinical trial. *Pain*, 1–11. doi:10.1016/j.pain.2007.08.028

Nutt, D. (2012, July 18). Scientists' agony over ecstasy. *The Guardian*, 1–2.

O'Mara, N. B., & Nahata, M. C. (2002). Drugs excreted in human breast milk. In L. A. Pagliaro & A. M. Pagliaro (Eds.), *Problems in Pediatric Drug Therapy* (4th ed., pp. 201–244). Washington, DC: American Pharmaceutical Association.

Office of Adolescent Health. (2017). *United States Adolescent Substance Abuse Facts*. Washington, DC: U.S. Deparmtent of Health & Human Services.

Ogeil, R. P., Rajaratnam, S. M., & Broadbear, J. H. (2013). Male and female ecstasy users: Differences in patterns of use, sleep quality and mental health outcomes. *Drug and Alcohol Dependence*, *132*(1-2), 223–230. doi:10.1016/j.drugalcdep.2013.02.002

Ompad, D. C., Galea, S., & Fuller, C. M. (2005). Ecstasy use among Hispanic and black substance users in New York city. *Substance Use & Misuse*, *40*, 1399–1407. doi:10.1081/JA-200066960

Onders, B., Casavant, M. J., & Spiller, H. A. (2016, May). Marijuana exposure among children younger than six years in the United States. *Clinical Pediatrics*, *55*(5), 428–436. doi:10.1177/0009922815589912

Osmond, H. (1957). A review of the clinical effects of psychotomimetic agents. *Annals of the New York Academy of Sciences*, *66*(3), 418–434.

Pacek, L. R., Mauro, P. M., & Martins, S. S. (2015). Perceived risk of regular cannabis use in the United States from 2002 to 2012: Differences by sex, age, and race/ethnicity. *Drug and Alcohol Dependence*, *149*, 232–244. doi:10.1016/j.drugalcdep.2015.02.009

Pagliaro, A. M., & Pagliaro, L. A. (1996). *Substance Use among Children and Adolescents: Its Nature, Extent, and Effects from Conception to Adulthood*. New York, NY: John Wiley & Sons.

Pagliaro, A. M., & Pagliaro, L. A. (2000). *Substance Use among Women: A Reference and Research Guide*. Philadelphia, PA: Brunner/Mazel.

Pagliaro, A. M., & Pagliaro, L. A. (2018). *Women's Drug and Substance Abuse: A Comprehensive Analysis and Reflective Synthesis*. New York, NY: Routledge.

Pagliaro, L. A. (1983). Up in smoke? A brief overview of marijuana toxicity. *Kergma*, *41*, 1–4.

Pagliaro, L. A. (1988, June). Marijuana and hashish: What are the risks? *Let's Talk*, *13*, 12–14.

Pagliaro, L. A. (1991). The deja vu phenomena (letter). *American Journal of Psychiatry*, *148*, 1418.

Pagliaro, L. A. (1995). Psychopharmacology updates: Marijuana reconsidered. *Psymposium*, *5*(2), 12–13.

Pagliaro, L. A., & Pagliaro, A. M. (1998). *The Pharmacological Basis of Psychotherapeutcs: An Introduction for Psychologists*. Washington, DC: Brunner/Mazel.

Pagliaro, L. A., & Pagliaro, A. M. (1999a). *PPDR: Psychologists' Psychotropic Drug Reference*. Philadelphia, PA: Brunner/Mazel.

Pagliaro, L. A., & Pagliaro, A. M. (1999b). *PNDR: Psychologists' Neuropsychotropic Drug Reference*. Philadelphia, PA: Brunner/Mazel.

Pagliaro, L. A., & Pagliaro, A. M. (Eds.). (2002). *Problems in Pediatric Drug Therapy* (4th ed.). Washington, DC: American Pharmaceutical Association.

Pagliaro, L. A., & Pagliaro, A. M. (2004). *Pagliaros' Comprehensive Guide to Drugs and Substances of Abuse* (1st ed.). Washington, DC: American Pharmacists Association.

Pagliaro, L. A., & Pagliaro, A. M. (2009). *Pagliaros' Comprehensive Guide to Drugs and Substances of Abuse* (2nd ed.). Washington, DC: American Pharmacists Association.

Pagliaro, L. A., & Pagliaro, A. M. (2012). *Handbook of Child and Adolescent Drug and Substance Abuse*. Hoboken, NJ: Wiley & Sons.

Pahl, K., Brook, J. S., & Koppel, J. (2011). Trajectories of marijuana use and psychological adjustment among urban African American and Puerto Rican women. *Psychological Medicine, 41*(8), 1775–1783. doi:10.1017/S0033291710002345

Palamar, J. J., Keyes, K., & Cleland, C. M. (2016, August). Underreporting of ecstasy use among high school seniors in the US. *Drug and Alcohol Dependence, 165*, 279–282. doi:10.1016/j.drugalcdep.2016.06.001

Palamar, J. J., Mauro, P. M., & Han, B. H. (2017). Shifting characteristcs of ecstasy users ages 12-34 in the United States, 2007-2014. *Drug and Alcohol Dependence, 181*, 20–24. doi:10.1016/j.drugalcdep.2017.09.011

Paperny, A. M., & Saminather, N. (2017, November 17). Just months away, here's how pot legalization is shaping up in Canada. (C. Reese, Ed.) Global News. Retrieved from https://globalnews.ca/news/3867467/marijuana-legalization-canada-progress/

Parrott, A. C. (2006). MDMA in humans: Factors which affect the neuropsychobiological profiles of recreational ecstasy users, the integrative role of bioenergetic stress. *Journal of Psychopharmacology, 20*(2), 147–163. doi:10.1177/0269881106063268

Parrott, A. C. (2009). Cortisol and 3,4-methylenedioxymethamphetamine: Neurohormonal aspects of bioenergetic stress in ecstasy users. *Neuropsychobiology, 60*(3-4), 148–158. doi:10.1159/000253551

Parrott, A. C. (2012). MDMA and temperature: A review of the thermal effects of 'Ecstasy' in humans. *Drug and Alcohol Dependence, 121*(1-2), 1–9. doi:10.1016/j.drugalcdep.2011.08.012

Parrott, A. C., Lock, J., & Conner, A. C. (2008). Dance clubbing on MDMA and during abtinence from Ecstasy/MDMA: Prospective neuroendocrine and psychobiological changes. *Neuropsychobiology, 57*(4), 165–180. doi:10.1159/000147470

Parrott, A. C., Moore, D. G., & Turner, J. (2014). MDMA and heightened cortisol: A neurohormonal perspective on the pregnancy outcomes of mothers who used Ecstasy during pregnancy. *Human Psychopharmacology: Clinical and Experimental, 29*(1), 1–7.

Parsons, J. T., Grov, C., & Kelly, B. C. (2009). Club drug use and dependence among young adults recruited through time-space sampling. *Public Health Reports, 124*(2), 246–254.

Parsons, J. T., Kelly, B. C., & Wells, B. E. (2006). Differences in club drug use between heterosexual and lesbian/bisexual females. *Addictive Behaviors, 31*(12), 2344–2349.

Partnership for a Drug-Free America. (2006, May 17). Key findings of: 18th annual Partnership Attitude Tracking Study on Teen Drug Abuse 2005. *Press Release*, 1–2. Partnership for a Drug-Free America.

Passie, T., Halpern, J. H., & Stichtenoth, D. O. (2008, Winter). The pharmacology of lysergic acid diethylamide: A review. *CNS Neurosciences & Therapeutics, 14*(4), 295–314. doi:10.1111/j.1755-5949.2008.00059.x

Patel, M. M., Belson, M. G., & Longwater, A. B. (2005). Methylenedioxymethamphetamine (ecstasy)-related hyperthermia. *The Journal of Emergency Medicine, 29*(4), 451–454.

Peiro, A. M., Farre, M., & Roset, P. N. (2013). Human pharmacology of 3,4-methylenedioxymethamphetamine (MDMA, ecstasy) after repeated doses taken 2 h apart. *Psychopharmacology (Berlin), 225*(4), 883–893. doi:10.1007/s00213-012-2894-7

Peres-Reyes, M., Di Guiseppi, S., & Brine, D. R. (1982). Urine pH and phencyclidine excretion. *Clinical Pharmacology and Therapeutics, 32*, 635–641. doi:10.1038/clpt.1982.214

Pertwee, R. G. (2000). Cannabinoid receptor ligands: Clinical and neuropharmacological considerations, relevant to future drug discovery and development. *Expert Opinion on Investigative Drugs, 9*(7), 1553–1571.

Pertwee, R. G., & Ross, R. A. (2002). Cannabinoid receptors and their ligands. *Prostaglandins, Leukotrienes, and Essential Fatty Acids, 66*(2-3), 101–121.

Peters, Jr., R. J., Kelder, S. H., & Meshack, A. (2005). Beliefs and social norms about cigarettes or marijuana sticks laced with embalming fluid and phencyclidine (PCP): Why youth use "fry". *Substance Use & Misuse, 40*(4), 563–571.

Pilgrim, J. L., Gerostamoulos, D., & Drummer, O. H. (2011). Deaths involving MDMA and the concomitant use of pharmaceutical drugs. *Journal of Analytical Toxicology, 35*(4), 219–226.

Pilgrim, J. L., Gerostamoulos, D., & Woodford, N. (2012, February 10). Serotonin toxicity involving MDMA (ecstasy) and moclobemide. *Forensic Science International, 215*(1-3), 184–188. doi:10.1016/j.forsciint.2011.04.008

Piontek, D., Kraus, L., & Klempova, D. (2008). Short scales to assess cannabis-related problems: A review of psychometric properties. *Substance Abuse Treatment, Prevention, and Policy, 3*, 25–35.

Piper, B. J. (2007). A developmental comparison of the neurobehavioral effects of ecstasy (MDMA). *Neurotoxicology and Teratology, 29*(2), 288–300. doi:10.1016/j.ntt.2006.10.002

Platt, B. (2018, July 30). Federal government set to approve first device for testing drivers' saliva for cannabis. *National Post.* Ottawa: National Post.

Power, R. A., Verweij, K. J., & Zuhair, M. (2014). Genetic predisposition to schizophrenia associated with increaed use of cannabis. *Molecular Psychiatry, 19*(11), 1201–1204. doi:10.1038/mp.2014.51

Pradhan, S. N. (1984, Winter). Phencyclidine (PCP): Some human studies. *Neuroscience & Biobehavioral Reviews, 8*(4), 493–501.

Preuss, U. W., Watzke, A. B., & Zimmermann, J. (2010). Cannabis withdrawal severity and short-term course among cannabis-dependent adolescent and young adult inpatients. *Drug and Alcohol Dependence, 106*(2-3), 133–141.

Puxty, D., Ramaekers, J. G., & de la Torre, R. (2017, July). MDMA-induced dissociative state not mediated by the 5-HT2A receptor. *Frontiers in Pharmacology*, *8*(Article 455), 1–9. doi:10.3389/fphar.2017.00455

Quednow, B. B., Jessen, F., & Kuhn, K. U. (2006, May). *Memory Deficits in Abstinent MDMA (ecstasy) Users: Neuropsychological Evidence of Frontal Dysfunction*. Retrieved March 30, 2016, from PubMed - NCBI, pp. 1–2: www.ncbi.nim.gov/pubmed/16574711

Radhakrishnan, R., Wilkinson, S. T., & D'Souza, D. C. (2014). Gone to pot - A review of the association between cannabis and psychosis. *Frontiers in Psychiatry*, *5*(Article 54), 1–24. doi:10.3389/psyt.2014.00054

Ramaekers, J. G., Berghaus, G., & van Laar, M. (2004). Dose related risk of motor vehicle crashes after cannabis use. *Drug and Alcohol Dependence*, *73*(2), 109–119.

Ramo, D. E., Grov, C., & Delucchi, K. (2010). Typology of club drug use among young adults recruited using time-space sampling. *Drug and Alcohol Dependence*, *107*(2-3), 119–127.

Reith, T. (2017, November 3). Legalized marijuana presents opportunity of a lifetime for Canadian entrepreneurs. *CBC News*.

Rengarajan, A., & Mullins, M. E. (2013). How often do false-positive phencyclidine urine screens occur with use of common medications? *Clinical Toxicology (Philadelphia, PA)*, *51*(6), 493–496. doi:10.3109/15563650.2013.801982

Richardson, G. A., Ryan, C., & Willford, J. (2002). Prenatal alcohol and marijuana exposure: Effects on neuropsychological outcomes at 10 years. *Neuotoxicology and Teratology*, *24*(3), 309–320.

Richter, L., Pugh, B. S., & Smith, P. H. (2017). The co-occurrence of nicotine and other substance use and addiction among youth and adults in the United States: Implications for research, practice, and policy. *The American Journal of Drug and Alcohol Abuse*, *43*(2), 132–145. doi:10.1080/00952990.2016.1193511

Rieder, M. J. (2016). Is the medical use of cannabis a therapeutic option for children? *Paediatric and Child Health*, *21*(1), 31–34.

Rigg, K. K., & Estreet, A. T. (2018). MDMA (ecstasy/molly) use among African Americans: The perceived influence of hip-hop/rap music. *Journal of Ethnicity in Substance Abuse*, *53*(7), 1. doi:10.1080/15332640.2018.1430646

Roberts, G. M., Nestor, L., & Garavan, H. (2009, October 6). Learning and memory deficits in ecstasy users and their neural correlates during a face-learning task. *Brain Research*, 71–81. doi:10.1016/j.brainres.2009.07.040

Robinson, J. T., Chitham, R. G., & Greenwood, R. M. (1974). Chromosome aberrations and LSD. *British Journal of Psychiatry*, *125*, 238–244.

Robinson, M. (2018, January 1). Here's where you can legally smoke weed in 2018. *Business Insider*, 1-2.

Romanowski, K. S., Barsun, A., & Kwan, P. (2017, January/February). Butane hash oil burns: A 7-year perspective on a growing problem. *Journal of Burn Care & Research*, *38*(1), e165-e171. doi:10.1097/BCR.0000000000000334

Romero, D., Gutierrez, G., & Blankstein, A. (2018, May 29). Foreign cartels embrace home-grown marijuana in pot-legal states. *NBC News*. Los Angeles.

Rong, C., Carmona, N. E., & Lee, Y. L. (2018). Drug-drug interactions as a result of co-administering delta9-THC and CBD with other psychotropic agents. *Expert Opinion on Drug Safety*, *17*(1), 51–54. doi:10.1080/14740338.2017.1397128

Rosenson, J., Smollin, C., & Sporer, K. A. (2007). Patterns of ecstasy-associated hyponatremia in California. *Annals of Emergency Medicine*, *49*(2), 164–171. doi:10.1016/j.annemergmed.2006.09.018

Rucker, J. J., Iliff, J., & Nutt, D. J. (2017, December 25). Psychiatry & the psychedelic drugs. Past, present & future. *Neuropharmacology*. doi:10.1016/j.neuropharm.2017.12.040

Rumalla, K., Reddy, A. Y., & Mittal, M. K. (2016, May 15). Recreational marijuana use and acute ischemic stroke: A population-based analysis of hospitalized patients in the United States. *Journal of the Neurological Sciences*, *304*, 191–196. doi:10.1016/j.jns.2016.01.066

Russo, E. B., Guy, G. W., & Robson, P. J. (2007). Cannabis, pain, and sleep: Lessons from therapeutic clinical trials of Sativex, a cannabis-based medicine. *Chemistry & Biodiversity*, *4*, 1729–1743.

Russo, M., Calabro, R., & Naro, A. (2015, January 29). Sativex in the management of multiple sclerosis-related spasticity: Role of the corticospinal modulation. *Neural Plasticity*, 1–6. doi:10.1155/2015/656582

Ryan, S. A., Ammerman, S. D., & O'Connor, M. E. (2018, September). Marijuana use during pregnancy and breastfeeding: Implications for neonatal and childhood outcomes. *Pediatrics*, *142*(3), e20181889.

Salas-Wright, C. P., Vaughn, M. G., & Todic, J. (2015). Trends in the disapproval and use of marijuana among adolescents and young adults in the United States: 2002-2013. *The American Journal of Drug and Alcohol Abuse*, *41*(5), 392–404. doi:10.3109/00952990.2015.1049493

SAMHSA, Substance Abuse and Mental Health Services Administration. (2011). *Results from the 2010 National Survey on Drug Use and Health: Summary of National Findings, NSDUH Series H-41, HHS Publication No. (SMA) 11-4658.* Rockville, MD.

SAMHSA. (2013b). *Ecstasy-related Emergency Department Visits by Young People Increased between 2005 and 2011: Alcohol Involvement Remains a Concern.* Washington, DC: Substance Abuse and Mental Health Services Administration.

SAMHSA, Substance Abuse And Mental Health Services Administration. (2013a, November 12). Emergency department visits involving phencyclidine (PCP). *The DAWN Report*, 1–5. Rockville, MD: U.S. Department of Health & Human Services.

Samuels, A. (2015, July 16). Study: Marijuana disapproval rate down among millennials. *USA Today College News*. Retrieved from USA Today College News.

Sanchez, R. (2014, January 1). 10 things you can and can't do under Colorado's new cannabis law. *Telegraph*. Washington: Telegraph Media Group.

Santos, G. M., Rapues, J., & Wilson, E. C. (2014). Alcohol and substance use among transgender women in San Francisco: Prevalence and association with human immunodeficiency virus infection. *Drug and Alcohol Review, 33*(3), 287–295. doi:10.1111/dar.12116

Sartor, C. E., Agrawal, A., & Grant, J. D. (2015). Differences between African-American and European-American women in the association of childhood sexual abuse with initiation of marijuana use and progression to problem use. *Journal of Studies on Alcohol and Drugs, 76*(4), 569–577.

Sartor, C. E., Agrawal, A., & Lynskey, M. T. (2013). Cannabis or alcohol first? Differences by ethnicity and in risk for rapid progression to cannabis-related problems among women. *Psychological Medicine, 43*(4), 813–823. doi:10.1017/S0033291712001493

Sartor, C. E., Waldron, M., & Duncan, A. E. (2013). Childhood sexual abuse and early substance use in adolescent girls: The role of familial influences. *Addiction*, 993–1000. doi:10.1111/add.12115

Savage, C. (1955). Variations in ego feeling induced by D-lysergic acid diethylamide (LDS-25). *Psychoanalytic Review, 1*, 1–16.

Scharff, C. (2014, September 16). Does MDMA have psychotherapeutic potential? *Psychology Today*, 1–2.

Schifano, F. (2004). A bitter pill. Overview of ecstasy (MDMA, MDA) related fatalities. *Psychopharmacology (Berlin), 173* (3-4), 242–248. doi:10.1007/s00213-003-1730-5

Schinke, S., Schwinn, T., & Hopkins, J. (2016). Drug abuse risk and protective factors among Hispanic adolescents. *Preventive Medicine Reports, 3*, 185–188. doi:10.1016/j.pmedr.2016.01.012

Schmid, Y., Rickli, A., & Schaffner, A. (2015, April). Interactions between bupropion and 3,4-methylenedioxy-methamphetamine in healthy subjects. *The Journal of Pharmacology and Experimental Therapeutics, 353*(1), 102–111. doi:10.1124/jpet.114.222356

Schneider, M. (2008). Puberty as a highly vulnerable developmental period for the consequences of cannabis exposure. *Addiction Biology, 13*(2), 253–263.

Scholey, A. B., Parrott, A. C., & Buchanan, T. (2004). Increased intensity of ecstasy and polydrug usage in the more experienced recreational ecstasy/MDMA users: A WWW study. *Addictive Behaviors, 29*(4), 743–752. doi:10.1016/j.addbeh.2004.02.022

Schulenberg, J. E., Johnston, L. D., & O'Malley, P. M. (2017). *Monitoring the Future National Survey Results on Drug Use, 1975-2016: Volume 2, College Students and Adults Ages 19-55*. The University of Michigan, Institute for Social Research. Ann Arbor: The University of Michigan.

Scipion, J. (2019, February 28). Martha Stewart partners with pot company to develop CBD products. *Fox Business News*.

Sewell, R. A., Poling, J., & Sofuoglu, M. (2009). The effect of cannabis compared with alcohol driving. *The American Journal on Addictions, 18*(3), 185–193. doi:10.1080/105504909027869..

Sharma, P., Murthy, P., & Srinivas Bharath, M. M. (2012, Fall). Chemistry, metabolism, and toxicology of cannabis: Clinical implications. *Iranian Journal of Psychiatry*, 7(4), 149–156.

Shen, A. (2017, December 7). US police arrest 50 Chinese in raid on US$80m illegal marijuana growing operation. *South China Morning Post*. Inkstone.

Sherman, B. J., & McRae-Clark, A. L. (2016). Treatment of cannabis use disorder: Current science and future outlook. *Pharmacotherapy, 36*(5), 511–535. doi:10.1002/phar.1747

Shook, J. J., Vaughn, M. G., & Salas-Wright, C. P. (2013). Expoloring the variation in drug selling among adolescents in the United States. *Journal of Criminal Justice, 41*(6), November-December, 365–374.

Shucheng Wong, S., & Wilens, T. E. (2017). Medical cannabinoids in children and adolescents: A systematic review. *American Academy of Pediatrics, 140*(5), e20171818. doi: 10.1542/peds.2017-2018

Shukla, R. K., Crump, J. L., & Chrisco, E. S. (2012). An evolving problem: Methamphetamine production and trafficking in the United States. *International Journal of Drug Policy, 23*(6), 426–435. doi:10.1016/j.drugpo.2012.07.004

Shulgin, A. T., & MacLean, D. E. (1976). Illicit synthesis of phencyclidine (PCP) and several of its analogs. *Clinical Toxicology, 9*(4), 553–560.

Sifaneck, S. J., Johnson, B. D., & Dunlap, E. (2006). Cigars-for-blunts: Choice of tobacco products by blunt smokers. *Journal of Ethnicity in Substance Abuse, 4*(3-4), 23–42.

Simpson, T. L., & Miller, W. R. (2002). Concomitance between childhood sexual and physical abuse and substance use problems: A review. *Clinical Psychology Review, 22*(1), 27–77.

Sinclair, C. F., Foushee, H. R., & Scarinci, I. (2013). Perceptions of harm to health from cigarettes, blunts, and marijuana among young adult African-American men. *Journal of Health Care for the Poor and Underserved, 24*, 1266–1275. doi:10.1353/hpu.2013.0126

Singer, L. T., Moore, D. G., & Fulton, S. (2012). Neurobehavioral outcomes of infants exposed to MDMA (Ecstasy) and other recreational drugs during pregnancy. *Neurotoxicology and Teratology, 34*, 303–310.

Singer, L. T., Moore, D. G., & Min, M. O. (2012, September). One-year outcomes of prenatal exposure to MDMA and other recreational drugs. *Pediatrics, 130*(3), 407–413. doi:10.1542/peds.2012-0666

Singh, J., & Budhiraja, S. (2006, April). Therapeutic potential of cannabinoid receptor ligands: Current status. *Methods and Findings in Experimental and Clinical Pharmacology, 28*(3), 177–183.

Sloane, B., & Lovett Doust, J. W. (1954). Psychophysiological investigations in experimental psychoses: Results of the exhibition of d-lysergic acid diethylamide to psychiatric patients. *The Journal of Mental Science, 100*, 129–144.

Smith, A. (2017, July 19). Colorado passes a milestone for pc. *CNN.com*. CNN. Retrieved January 17, 2018, from http://money.cnn.com/2017/07/19/news/colorado-marijuana-tax-revenue/index.html

Smith, K. M., Larive, L. L., & Romanelli, F. (2002). Club drugs: Methylenedioxymethamphetamine, flunitrazepam, ketamine hydrochloride, and gamma-hydroxybutyrate. *American Journal of Health-System Pharmacy: AJHP, 59* (11), 1067–1076.

Soine, W. H., Vincek, W. C., & Agee, D. T. (1979). Phencyclidine contaminant generates cyanide. *New England Journal of Medicine, 301*(8), 438.

Soller, B., & Lee, J. P. (2010, September 8). Drug-intake methods and social identity: The use of marijuana in blunts among southeast Asian adolescents and emerging adults. *Journal of Adolescent Research, 25*(6), 783–806.

Spindel, M., & Brody, J. (2016). *Risks Associated with Parental Use of Phencyclidine (PCP)*. Washington, DC: DC Vounteer Lawyers Project.

Stanton, B., & Galbraith, J. (1994, June). Drug trafficking among African-American early adolescents: Prevalence, consequences, and associated behaviors and beliefs. *Pediatrics, 93*(6, part 2), 1039–1043.

Stein, M. D., Caviness, C. M., & Anderson, B. J. (2014). Alcohol use potentiates marijuana problem severity in young adult women. *Womens Health Issues, 24*(1), e77-e82. doi:10.1016/j.whi.2013.10.005

Stirling, J., Barkus, E. J., & Nabosi, L. (2008). Cannabis-induced psychotic-like experiences are predicted by high schizotypy. *Psychopathology, 41*(6), 371–378.

Stoner, S. A. (2016). *Screening and Assessment for Cannabis Use Disorder*. University of Washington, Alcohol & Drug Abuse Institute. Seattle: University of Washington. Retrieved from http://adai.uw.edu/pubs/pdf/2016marijuanascreeningassess.pdf

Stout, S. M., & Cimino, N. M. (2014, February). Exogenous cannabinoids as substrates, inhibitors, and inducers of human drug metabolizing enzymes: A systematic review. *Drug Metabolism Reviews, 46*(1), 86–95. doi:10.3109/03602532.2013.849268

Streller, S., & Roth, K. (2015, January 6). The chemistry of tobacco – Part 4. *ChemViews*, 1–10. doi:10.1002/chemv.2014.400135

Swaim, R. C., Beauvais, F., & Chavez, E. L. (1997). The effects of school dropout rates on estimates of adolescent substance use among three racial/ethnic groups. *American Journal of Public Health, 87*(1), 51–55.

Swift Yasgur, B. (2018, March 2). Legalized marijuana: Fewer risks, fewer benefits. *Medscape*, 1.

Sznitman, S. R. (2017, December). The Cannabis Abuse Screening Test (CAST) revisisted: Examining measurement invariance by age. *International Journal of Methods in Psychiatric Research, 26*(4), 1. doi:10.1002/mpr.1529

Tabor, B. L., Smith-Wallace, T., & Yonekura, M. L. (1990). Perinatal outcome associated with PCP versus cocaine use. *The American Journal of Drug and Alcohol Abuse, 16*(3-4), 337–348.

Tashkin, D. P. (2013). Effects of marijuana smoking on the lung. *Annals of the American Thoracic Society, 10*(3), 239–247. doi:10.1513/AnnalsATS.201212-127FR

Taub, S., Feingold, D., & Rehm, J. (2018, January). Patterns of cannabis use and clinical correlates among individuals with major depressive disorder and bipolar disorder. *Comprehensive Psychiatry, 80*, 89–96. doi:10.1016/j.comppsych.2017.09.004

Taylor, D. R., Fergusson, D. M., & Milne, B. J. (2002). A longitudinal study of the effects of tobacco and cannabis exposure on lung function in young adults. *Addiction, 97*(8), 1055–1061.

Thomasius, R., Petersen, K. U., & Zapletalova, P. (2005). Mental disorders in current and former heavy ecstasy (MDMA) users. *Addiction, 100*(9), 1310–1319.

Thomasius, R., Zapletalova, P., & Petersen, K. (2006, March). Mood, cognition and serotonin transporter availability in current and former ecstasy (MDMA) users: The longitudinal perspective. *Journal of Psychopharmacology, 20*(2), 211–225.

Toklas, A. B. (1954). *The Alice B. Toklas Cookbook*. New York, NY: Harper Collins.

Traub, S. J., Hoffman, R. S., & Nelson, L. S. (2002). The "ecstasy" hangover: Hyponatremia due to 3,4-methylenedioxymethamphetamine. *Journal of Urban Health, 79*(4), 549–555.

Trezza, V., Cuomo, V., & Vanderschuren, L. J. (2008). Cannabis and the developing brain: Insights from behavior. *European Journal of Pharmacology, 585*(2-3), 441–452.

Tribune Media Wire. (2017, September 21). Teen drug dealer calls Indiana police to report someone stole her drugs. *WREG News Channel 3*. Greenwood, IN: WREG News Channel 3. Retrieved from http://wreg.com/2017/09/21/teen-drug-dealer-calls-indiana-police-to-report-someone-stole-her-drugs/

Upreti, V. V., Eddington, N. D., & Moon, K. H. (2009, July 24). Drug interactons between ethanol and 3,4-methylenedioxymethamphetamine ("ecstasy"). *Toxicology Newsletters, 188*(2), 167–172. doi:10.1016/j.toxlet.2009.03.023

van Dijken, G. D., Blom, R. E., & Hene, R. J. (2013). High incidence of mild hyponatremia in females using ecstasy at a rave party. *Nephrology Dialysis Transplantation, 28*(9), 2277–2283. doi:10.1093/ndt/gft023

van Heugten-Van der Kloet, D., Giesbrecht, T., & van Wel, J. (2015). MDMA, cannabis, and cocaine produce acute dissociative symptoms. *Psychiatry Research, 228*(3), 907–912. doi:10.1016/j.psychres.2015.04.028

van Holst, R. J., & Schilt, T. (2011). Drug-related decrease in neuropsychological functions of abstinent drug users. *Current Drug Abuse Reviews, 4*(1), 42–56.

van Hout, M. C., & Bingham, T. (2013). 'Surfing the Silk Road': A study of users' experiences. *International Journal of Drug Policy, 24*(6), 524–529. doi:10.1016/j.drugpo.2013.08.011

Van Leeuwen, J. M., Hopfer, C., & Hooks, S. (2004, June). A snapshot of substance abuse among homeless and runaway youth in Denver, Colorado. *Journal of Community Health, 29*(3), 217–229.

Volkow, N. (2017, December 14). Vaping popular among teens; opioid misuse at historic lows. *National Institute on Drug Abuse Report.* National Institutes of Health.

Vuori, E., Henry, J. A., & Ojanpera, I. (2003). Death following ingestion of MDMA (ecstasy) and moclobemide. *Addiction, 98*(3), 365–368.

Wachsman, L., Schuertz, S., & Chan, L. S. (1989). What happens to babies exposed to phencyclidine (PCP) in utero? *The American Journal of Drug and Alcohol Abuse, 15*(1), 31–39.

Wacker, D., Wang, S., & McCorvy, J. D. (2017, January 26). Crystal structure of an LSD-bound human serotonin receptor. *Cell, 168*(3), 377–389. doi:10.1016/j.cell.2016.12.033

Walker, J. (1990, May 29). Surge of hispanic gangs seen in Los Angeles. *The Washington Post*, 1. Los Angeles, CA: The Washington Post.

Wang, G. S., Roosevelt, G., & Le Lait, M. C. (2014, February 3). Association of unintentional pediatric exposures with decriminalization of marijuana in the United States. *Annals of Emergency Medicine, 63*(6), 684–689.

Wang, J. B., Ramo, D. E., & Lisha, N. E. (2016, September 1). Medical marijuana legalization and cigarette and mairjuana co-use in adolescents and adults. *Drug and Alcohol Dependence, 166*, 32–38. doi:10.1016/j.drugalcdep.2016.06.016

Wapner, S., & Krus, D. M. (1960, November/December). Effects of lysergic acid diethylamide and differences between normals and schizophrenics on the Stroop Color-Word Test. *Journal of Neuropsychiatry, 2*, 76–81.

Wardle, M. C., Kirkpatrick, M. G., & de Wit, H. (2014). "Ecstasy' as a social drug: MDMA preferentially affects responses to emotional stimuli with social content. *Social Cognitive & Affective Neuroscience, 9*(8), 1076–1081. doi:10.1093/scan/nsu035

Weissman, A. (1981). On the definition of cannabinoids: Botanical? Chemical? Pharmacological? *Journal of Clinical Pharmacology, 21*(8-9 Supplement), 159S-165S.

West, P. L., Helman, R. S., & McKeown, N. J. (2015, April 20). *Phencyclidine Toxicity.* Retrieved from Medscape, pp. 1–3: http://emedicine.medscape.com/article/816348-overview

White, H. R., Labouvie, E. W., & Papadaratsakis, V. (2005). Changes in substance use during the transition to adulthood: A comparison of college students and their noncollege age peers. *Journal of Drug Issues, 35*(2), 281–306.

Williams, J., & Bretteville-Jensen, A. L. (2014, July). Does liberalizing cannabis laws increase cannabis use? *Journal of Health Economics, 36*, 20–32. doi:10.1016/j.healeco.2014.03.006

Williams, S. (2015, July 12). *Washington's marijuana tax revenue tops estimates, but big problems still exist.* Retrieved April 13, 2016, from The Motely Fool, pp. 1–8: www.fool.com/investing/general/2015/07/12/washingtons-marijuana-tax-revenue-tops-estimates-b.aspx

Wilsey, B., Marcotte, T., & Deutsch, R. (2013). Low-dose vaporized cannabis significantly improves neuropathic pain. *The Journal of Pain, 14*(2), 136–148. doi:10.1016/j.pain.2012.10.009

Wilson, R. I., & Nicoll, R. A. (2002, April 26). Endocannabinoid signaling in the brain. *Science, 296*(5568), 678–682. doi:10.1136/science.1063545

Winstock, A. (2016). *What Did We Learn from GDS2015? an Overview of Our Key Findings.* Retrieved January 12, 2016, from The Global Drug Survey 2015 findings, pp. 1–27: www.globaldrugsurvey.com/the-global-drug-survey-2015-findings/

Winstock, A. R., Ford, C., & Witton, J. (2010, April 10). Assessment and management of cannabis use disorders in primary care. *BMJ, 340*, 800–804. doi:10.1136/bmj.c1571

Wirrell, E. C. (2016, June). Treatment of Dravet syndrome. *The Canadian Journal of Neurological Sciences, 43*(Supplement 3), S13-S18. doi:10.1017/cjn.2016.249

Wood, J. (2018, October 5). Comox valley RCMP investigating after child sent to hospital by weed gummy bears. *My Comox Valley Now*, 1. Courtenay.

Wu, L. T., Ringwalt, C. L., & Weiss, R. D. (2009). Hallucinogen-related disorders in a national sample of adolescents: The influence of ecstasy/MDMA use. *Drug and Alcohol Dependence, 104*(1-2), 156–166.

Wu, L. T., Schlenger, W. E., & Galvin, D. M. (2006). Concurrent use of methamphetamine, MDMA, LSD, ketamine, GHB, and flunitrazepam among American youths. *Drug and Alcohol Dependence, 84*(1), 102–113.

Wu, P., Liu, X., & Hoang Pham, T. (2010, November). Ecstasy use among U.S. adolescents from 1999 to 2008. *Drug and Alcohol Dependence, 112*(1-2), 33–38. doi:10.1016/j.drugalcdep.2010.05.006

Wu, Z. H., Grady, J. J., & Rosales, S. (2011). Ecstasy use and its correlates among young, low-income womem. *Substance Use & Misuse, 46*(4), 404–410. doi: 10.3109/10826084.2010.501680

Yamaori, S., Koeda, K., & Kushihara, M. (2012). Comparison in the in vitro inhibitory effects of major phytocannabinoids and polycyclic aromatic hydrocarbonbs contained in marijuana smoke on cytochrome P450 2C9 activity. *Drug Metabolism and Pharmacokinetics, 27*(3), 294–300.

Yamaori, S., Kushihara, M., & Yamamoto, I. (2010, June 1). Characterization of major phytocannabinoids, cannabidiol and cannabinol, as isoform-selective and potent inhibitors of human CYP1 enzymes. *Biochemical Pharmacology, 79* (11), 1691–1698. doi:10.1016/j.bcp.2010.01.028

Yu, A. M. (2008, June). Indoealkylamines: Biotransformations and potential drug-drug interactions. *The AAPS Journal, 10*(2), 242–253. doi:10.1208/s12248-008-9028-5

Zinberg, N. (1986). *Drug, Set, and Setting: The Basis for Congtrolled Intoxicant Use.* New Haven, CT: Yale University Press

5
Prescription Opiate Analgesics and Heroin

Since the beginning of the new millennium, the nonmedical use of prescription opiate analgesics increased significantly among adolescents and young adults across the US., particularly:

- Buprenorphine;
- Fentanyl;
- Hydrocodone;
- Hydromorphone;
- Methadone;
- Morphine;
- Oxycodone.[1]

Primarily medically prescribed for the relief of moderate to severe pain, adolescents and young adults now use, and continue to use, prescription opiate analgesics to achieve:

1. An intense feeling of euphoria;
2. An overall warm and pleasant feeling, or "rush;"
3. A sleepy, dream-like state, commonly known as "being on-the-nod;"

They also use perscription opiate analgesics to:

4. Self-manage physical pain, often related to sports injuries;
5. Prevent, or self-manage, the opiate analgesic withdrawal syndrome.

Interestingly, Young, Esteban McCabe, and Cranford (2012), in their web-based, self-administered survey of 2,597 7th through 12th grade students, found that:

> Approximately 14% (n = 373) of the sample reported medical use of prescription opioids in the past 12 months, while 5% (n = 148) of the sample reported nonmedical use of prescription opioids in the past 12 months. The most common reason for nonmedical use was "to relieve pain" (n = 91, 62.8%) followed by "to get high" (n = 23, 15.9%) and to "experiment" (n = 16, 11.0%).
>
> (p. 336)

1 Over the new millennium, several other prescription opiate analgesics (e.g., codeine, loperamide [Imodium®], and tramadol [Ultram®]) also were used by adolescents and young adults in the U.S. However, these opiate analgesics are not discussed in detail in this text because they were less frequently used. (Readers, who require additional information that may be specific to each of these other drugs, are referred to Pagliaro and Pagliaro (2009).

In addition to the prescription opiate analgesics, the use of heroin increased significantly particularly among adolescents and young adults for whom prescription opiate analgesics became more difficult to obtain.

We begin with an overview and discussion of the basic pharmacognosy/botany, chemistry, and pharmacology of the prescription opiate analgesics and heroin with attention to their similarities and differences regarding:

1. Pharmacodynamics, or mechanisms of action;
2. Pharmacokinetics—absorption, distribution, metabolism, and excretion; and dosage formulations and methods of use;
3. Drug–Drug interactions;
4. Undesired, or harmful, effects and toxicities;
5. Overdosage, including unintentional poisonings;
6. Use during pregnancy and lactation.

We then present and discuss new millennial trends in prescription opiate analgesic and heroin use, including: medical use; embryo/fetus, neonate, infant, and child exposure; and adolescent and young adult illicit/recreational use.[2]

Opiate Analgesic Pharmacognosy/Botany, Chemistry, and Pharmacology

Pharmacognosy/Botany

Opium is prepared from the dried resin of the unripe seed pod of the poppy plant *(Papaver somniferum)*—the poppy that causes sleep.[3] The crude resin is often called "poppy tears" (*lachryma papaveris*). The opium alkaloids[4] are then extracted from the resin by various methods. Raw opium contains approximately 10% morphine by weight. Morphine is considered the standard against which all other opiate analgesics are compared regarding potency and efficacy. The relative potencies of the various opiate analgesics—the average dosages that are required to generally provide equivalent pain relief, or equal efficacy—are listed in Table 5.1.

Chemistry

The opiate analgesics comprise three subgroups, or "families:" (1) natural pure agonists; (2) synthetic pure agonists; and (3) synthetic mixed agonist/antagonists (see Table 5.2). The first,

2 Due to the paucity of published research regarding the abuse of opiate analgesics among children, one to 10 years-of-age, during the new millennium, we are unable to extract, interpret, and discuss associated valid and reliable trends for this age group.

3 As soon as the petals have fallen from the pod of the opium flower, it is lanced in order to obtain the raw opium resin.

4 In addition to the opiate analgesic alkaloids of morphine (10% to 15%) and codeine (1% to 3%), opium alkaloids also contain noscapine (i.e., narcotine; 4% to 8%), papaverine (1% to 3%), and thebaine (1% to 2%) depending on the country of origin and techniques used to lance the opium seed pod so that the opium resin, or latex, can run out (e.g., the number of times that a pod is lanced), and the amount and type of nitrogen-based fertilizers used to cultivate the opium plants (Annett, 1920).

Table 5.1 Relative Potencies of the Opiate Analgesics[5]

Opiate Analgesic *Generic and Trade/Brand Names*®[6]	*Average Dosage (mg)* *Intramuscular (IM)/Oral Ingestion (PO)*	
	IM (mg)	*PO (mg)*
Butorphanol (Stadol®)	2	—
Codeine (Ratio-Codeine®)	120	200
Fentanyl (Actiq®)	0.1	—
Hydrocodone	—	45
Hydromorphone (Dilaudid®)	1.5	7.5
Levorphanol (Levo-Dromoran®)	2	4
Meperidine (Demerol®)	75	300
Methadone (Dolophine®)	10	20
Morphine (MS Contin®)	10	30
Nalbuphine (Nubain®)	10	—
Oxycodone (OxyContin®)	15	20
Oxymorphone (Numorphan®)	1	10
Pentazocine (Talwin®)	60	180

and original family, includes opium and its pure natural derivatives—codeine and morphine. The second family includes several synthetic modifications of morphine, such as fentanyl, heroin (diacetylmorphine), methadone, and oxycodone. These synthetic modifications have chemical structures and pharmacologic actions that resemble their natural parent drug,

Table 5.2 Subgroups of the Opiate Analgesics

Category *Generic Name*	*Brand/Trade Names®*	*Common Street Names*[7]
PURE AGONISTS—Natural		
Opium		"Big O;" "Chinese Molasses;" "Poppy"

(Continued)

5 N.B. These are single, average dosage equivalents. Consequently, for adolescents and young adults who use/abuse opiate analgesics, variability may be significant.

6 Brand/trade names are denoted by the symbol, "®." They are included primarily for "illustrative purposes (i.e., to facilitate clinical practice application for readers who comprise a wide range of mental health care professionals). The inclusion of a brand/trade name is not meant to endorse an opiate analgesic, nor is it meant to suggest—unless explicitly stated otherwise—that the pharmacology and other data presented are preferentially associated with that particular brand/trade name. It should be noted that some of these brand trade names have been discontinued by the original manufacturer, but are still available by this name over the internet.

7 Partial list. When available, examples of three to five of the most common street names are provided. See Pagliaro and Pagliaro (2009) for a comprehensive listing of the drugs and substances of abuse, and their common street names.

Table 5.2 (Cont.)

Category Generic Name	*Brand/Trade Names®*	*Common Street Names*[7]
Opium derivatives:		
Codeine[8]	Codeine Contin®; Ratio-Codeine®	"Codies;" "Cough Syrup;" "School Boy;" "T3;" "T4"
Morphine	Duramorph®; M.O.S.®; MS Contin®	"Drug Store;" "Good Ole M;" "Hospital Heroin;" "Morph;" "MS"
PURE AGONISTS—SYNTHETIC		
Fentanyl	Actiq®; Duragesic®	"Fen;" "Murder 8;" "Perc-O-Pop"
Heroin		"Black Tar;" "Brown Sugar;" "Capital H;" "Charley;" "Horse;" "Junk;" "Smack"
Hydrocodone[9]		"Hydros;" "Hyke;" "Tuss;" "Vikes"
Hydromorphone	Dilaudid®	"Delaud;" "Dillies"
Levorphanol	Levo-Dromoran®	
Meperidine	Demerol®	"Demmies;" "Dems;" "Mep"
Methadone	Dolophine®	"Adolph;" "Dollies;" "Done;" "Wafer"
Oxycodone	OxyContin®	"Cotton;" "Hillbilly Heroin;" "Oxy;" "Oxycotton;" "Poor Boy's Heroin;" "Percs"
Oxymorphone	Numorphan®; Opana®	"Blue Heaven;" "Mrs. O"
Propoxyphene[10]	Darvon®	"Footballs;" "Pinks"
Tramadol	Ultram®	"Trammies;" "Ultras"
MIXED AGONIST/ANTAGONISTS—SYNTHETIC		
Buprenorphine	Buprenex®; Suboxone®	"Oranges;" "Tems"
Butorphanol	Stadol®	
Nalbuphine	Nubain®	"Nubian"
Pentazocine	Talwin®	"Big T;" "Ts"

8 Usually available as one of the ingredients in a multi-ingredient product (e.g., Empirin #4; Tylenol #4).

9 Usually available as one of the ingredients in a multi-ingredient product (e.g., Loratab®; Vicodin®).

10 In December 2010, the FDA removed propoxyphene from licit production and use within the U.S. This action followed a similar move in Europe and was in response to related risk for developing potentially serious, or even fatal, cardiac dysrhythmias associated with propoxyphene use (Gandey, 2010).

morphine. The third family includes the synthetic, mixed agonist/antagonists—buprenorphine, nalbuphine, and pentazocine.

Pharmacology

Pharmacologically, the opiate analgesics—for over a century—have been traditionally referred to as narcotic analgesics reflecting their major therapeutic indication—to relieve pain.[11] They also have been simply called, "narcotics." Derived from the Greek word, "narke," narcotic means a lack of feeling or sensation—a feeling of numbness. However, the general use of the term narcotic has caused much confusion because of its "legal" meaning.

Legally, the term, narcotic, is used to denote all the various drugs and substances of abuse that are listed under the U.S. and international narcotic acts and laws. One of the first such laws in the U.S. was the Harrison Narcotics Tax Act (Ch.1, 38 Stat. 785) that was approved on December 17, 1914 and took effect March 1, 1915. This federal tax law regulated and taxed, for the first time in the U.S., the production, importation, and distribution of opiate analgesics and coca products (e.g., Coca-Cola® and Van Mariani®—both of which, at that time, legally contained cocaine). Under these laws, cannabis, cocaine, heroin, and lysergic acid diethylamide (LSD), for example, are all legally classified as narcotics. However, of the four drugs and substances of abuse listed in this example, only heroin is pharmacologically classified as a narcotic based upon its chemical structure and pharmacological action.

Adding to the confusion, the opiate analgesics are most often referred to as "opioids"—a term that is also used to denote the: (1) opiate analgesic antagonist, naloxone (Narcan®); and (2) opiate analgesic-like substances that are naturally found in the body (i.e., endogenous opioid peptides). Consequently, in order to minimize any potential confusion associated with the use of these various terms, we selected to use the term, "opiate analgesic," throughout this book, for any natural (e.g., codeine) or synthetic (e.g., heroin) drug that exerts morphine-like actions on the human brain and spinal cord.

Pharmacodynamics: Mechanism of Action

The opiate analgesics have an interesting mechanism of action. Rather than raising the pain threshold to achieve analgesia—as happens, for example, with most sedative-hypnotics and general anesthetics—they modify the brain's interpretation of painful stimuli by depressing CNS activity. Thus, the sensation of pain is still experienced, but, subjectively, it does not seem to "hurt as much."

The endogenous opioid peptides are short sequences of amino acids that were identified in the brain during the 1970s and were named "endomorphins," "dynorphins," "endorphins," and "enkephalins." Various opiate analgesic receptors also were discovered within the body and were extensively studied. Although the receptor classification system that evolved from this research remains incomplete, three major groups of opiate analgesic receptors were pharmacologically characterized and named, delta, kappa, and mu.[12] The highest concentrations of these cell surface

11 Opiate analgesics have been used therapeutically over the millennia to treat moderate to severe pain, both acute and chronic (Pagliaro & Pagliaro, 1986, 1999, 2004). They are, however, generally ineffective for the management of either chronic idiopathic pain (e.g., fibromyalgia) or neuropathic pain (e.g., pain associated with diabetic peripheral neuropathy) (Arner & Meyerson, 1988; Malleson, Connell, & Bennett, 2001; Schreiber, Nones, & Reis, 2015)—except for the associated pain relief potentially provided by the placebo effect.

12 Three other receptors (i.e., sigma [σ], epsilon [ε], and nociceptive receptors) also have been identified and studied. However, their full role in regard to the mechanisms of opiate analgesic action in humans remains controversial. Nociceptive receptors, or "nociceptors," are found in the brain and spinal cord—as well as other body organs and tissues (e.g., gastrointestinal, integumentary, and muscular systems). In the context of opiate analgesic use, these receptors appear to be primarily associated with anxiety, mental depression, and the development of tolerance.

receptors are found in the: limbic system; midbrain, which also includes the ventral tegmental area (VTA); and spinal cord (see Figure 5.1). These G-protein-coupled inhibitory receptors (i.e., delta, kappa, and mu), which mediate the inhibition of adenylyl cyclase, are essential to the analgesic actions of the opiate analgesics (Traynor, 2012; Zhang, Ferguson, & Barak, 1998).

Agonist-dependent processes, including receptor phosphorylation, desensitization, internalization, and down regulation, are responsible for the regulation of the opiate analgesic receptors (Zhang, Ferguson, & Barak, 1998). The conformational changes induced in the receptors, as a consequence of their binding to opiate analgesics, causes "downstream signaling events" that result in associated expressed actions, including analgesia, constipation, euphoria, and respiratory depression. "Continuing activation of these signaling pathways leads to homeostatic changes that result in [the development of] tolerance and the opiate-dependent state" (Traynor, 2012, p. 173).

The similarities and differences in the pharmacology and toxicology (i.e., undesired, or harmful, effects and toxicities) of the opiate analgesics is due primarily to their similarities and differences in selectivity for, and binding to, the delta, kappa, and mu opiate analgesic receptors (Gharagozlou, Demirci, & Clark, 2002; Inturrisi, 2002; Okada, Tsuda, & Bryant, 2002; Zuurmond, Meert, & Noorduin, 2002).

"Pure" opiate analgesics (e.g., morphine) appear to exert their analgesic action primarily at the mu receptors found in the brain, spinal cord, and intestinal tract. These receptors are associated with analgesia and euphoria. Mu receptors are also associated with: constipation;

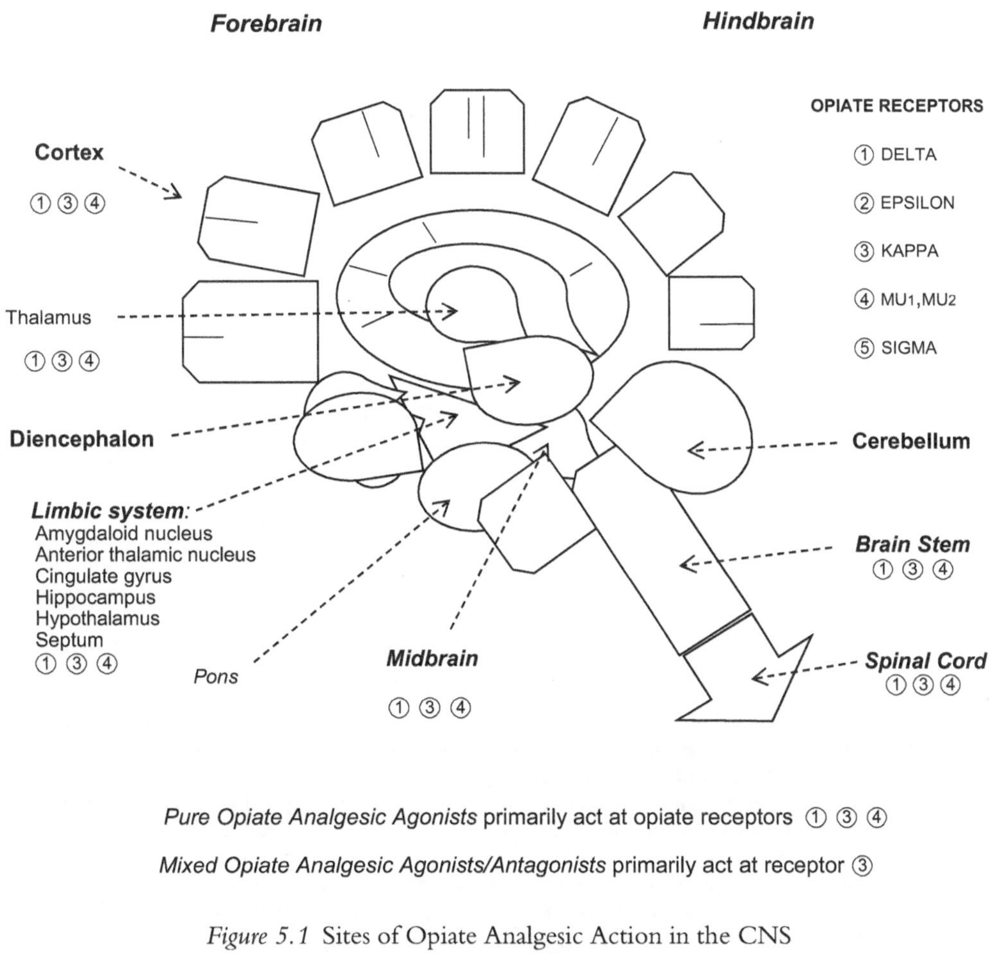

Figure 5.1 Sites of Opiate Analgesic Action in the CNS

miosis; respiratory depression; and the development of physical dependence. "Synthetic" opiate analgesics, including meperidine (Demerol®), appear to act at the delta receptors, which are located primarily in the limbic system of the brain. Delta receptors are associated with an exaggerated feeling of mental depression or unhappiness (i.e., dysphoria), hallucinations, and other "psychotomimetic" effects. "Mixed" opiate analgesics (e.g., butorphanol [Stadol®]) act primarily at the kappa receptors, which are associated with sedation and spinal analgesia, as well as miosis.

Pharmacologically, drugs that stimulate any of the opiate analgesic receptors (i.e., delta, kappa, or mu receptors) have been designated as "agonists." Those that block the opiate analgesic receptors have been designated as "antagonists" (i.e., naloxone [Narcan®]; naltrexone [Trexan®]). Opiate analgesics that stimulate one receptor and block another have been designated as "mixed agonist/antagonists" (i.e., buprenorphine [Buprenex®]) (see Table 5.1).

The mechanism of action of the opiate analgesic antagonist, naloxone [Narcan®], is particularly important regarding opiate analgesic overdosage. Naloxone can bind to and block all opiate analgesic receptors and, thus, prevent opiate analgesics from attaching to the receptors and eliciting their analgesic and other effects. Naloxone is particularly attracted to mu receptors to which it readily binds reversing the respiratory depression associated with opiate analgesic overdosage. Naloxone's affinity for mu receptors is at least tenfold higher than its affinity for kappa receptors. This greater affinity for mu receptors may explain why naloxone readily reverses the respiratory depression that occurs with opiate analgesic overdosage involving the mixed agonist/antagonists (e.g., butorphanol [Stadol®]), but only minimally reverses the analgesia that occurs with the stimulation of the kappa receptors in the spinal cord.

Pharmacokinetics: Absorption, Distribution, Metabolism, and Excretion

Opiate analgesics can be ingested as capsules (e.g., propoxyphene, Darvon®), liquids (e.g., methadone, Dolophine®), or tablets (e.g., codeine).[13] In addition, opiate analgesics can be: vaporized and inhaled into the pulmonary system by "chasing the dragon" (e.g., heroin; opium); intranasally insufflated or "snorted," as a powder (e.g., heroin; hydrocodone); transbucally absorbed by sucking on a lozenge (e.g., fentanyl, Actiq®);[14] or sublingually absorbed by placing a sublingual tablet under the tongue (e.g., buprenorphine, Buprenex®; sufentanil, Dsuvia®).[15] They can be intravenously (IV) injected (i.e., "mainlined") as an aqueous solution (e.g., heroin; pentazocine, Talwin®) or they can be subcutaneously injected

13 Another method of ingestion for the opiate analgesics involves the traditional preparation and use of poppy tea, or "doda." The dried opium poppy seed pods, which generally are crushed and finely ground, are brewed as an "herbal tea." The tea is used traditionally in many parts of the world, particularly in South Asian countries and in the U.S. where Asian grocery and convenience specialty stores often stock and sell dried poppy seed pods. Increasingly, U.S. high school students and young adults have been experimenting with "doda," sometimes with lethal results (Homebrewed, 2017; Pagliaro & Pagliaro, *Clinical Patient Data Files*; Powers, Erickson, & Swortwood, 2017; Sam Houston, 2017).

14 Actiq®, the fentanyl "lollipop," is a solid drug matrix of fentanyl on a plastic stick. It was designed to facilitate easy removal from the mouth, where it is buccally (i.e. transmucosally) absorbed, in the event of early signs of fentanyl overdosage (i.e., respiratory depression) during medical use.

15 Dsuvia®—which is five to 10 times more potent than its parent drug, fentanyl—delivers a sublingual dose of sufentanil by means of a disposable, prefilled single dose applicator. It was specifically designed for patients who cannot swallow oral dosage formulations or who require rapid analgesic intervention when IV access is extremely difficult or hazardous (e.g., treatment of wounded soldiers in active combat situations). In 2018, the FDA restricted approved use to certified, medically supervised health care settings. Data regarding diversion and illicit use are not currently available (FDA, 2018a).

(SC), or "popped" under the skin (e.g., heroin).[16] They can also be absorbed through the various skin layers (e.g., epidermis; dermis) by the application of a transdermal delivery system or "patch" (e.g., fentanyl, Duragesic®). These different formulations and methods of use, or administration, can affect opiate analgesic pharmacokinetics—absorption, distribution, metabolism, and excretion—in several ways, as discussed in the following subsections.

ABSORPTION

The absorption of the various opiate analgesics depends on their:

1. Dosage formulation (e.g., oral tablet or transdermal delivery system);
2. Method of use/route of administration (e.g., ingestion; IV injection; pulmonary inhalation);[17]
3. Purity, presence of adulterants, and method of production (e.g., a tablet that is too tightly compressed, or otherwise incorrectly formulated, may not break-up or dissolve in the stomach, or intestines, when ingested—thus, reducing, or preventing, the absorption of its active ingredients from the GI tract into the systemic circulation).

Following ingestion, opiate analgesics are mainly absorbed from the intestines, where absorption can be more erratic and unpredictable when compared to that associated with other methods of use. Absorption also is slowed and less complete from the GI tract because of first-pass hepatic metabolism. For example, only approximately 40% of the morphine that is ingested is delivered to the systemic circulation—and mu receptor sites—because of pre-systemic clearance (i.e., significant first-pass hepatic metabolism). Consequently, opiate analgesic blood concentrations that are achieved after ingestion are often half, or less than half, of those achieved when the same dose of the opiate analgesic is injected IV—a method that insures immediate and complete absorption and effects.

It is important to note that, when compared to IV injection, absorption following SC injection into the fatty tissues under the skin layers or intramuscular (IM) injection into muscle tissues is also more variable and produces less rapid rise in blood concentrations than does IV injection. These and other basic pharmacological differences often affect the selection of an opiate analgesic and its dose and method of use (see, for example, Table 5.1).

In addition to IV injection, other methods of opiate analgesic use that may largely avoid first-pass hepatic metabolism, include:

- Intranasal instillation (e.g., heroin "nose drops") and intranasal insufflation (e.g., crushing hydrocodone tablets and snorting the powder);[18]
- Pulmonary inhalation (e.g., "chasing the dragon");
- SC injection (e.g., "chipping");
- Sublingual absorption from under the tongue (e.g., buprenorphine, Subutex®);

16 The SC injection of heroin has been referred to as "chipping" (Pagliaro & Pagliaro, *Clinical Patient Data Files*). The term "chipping" also has been used to refer to occasional (e.g., once per week) heroin use (e.g., Bass, Brown, & DuPont, 1972).

17 This factor accounts, to a significant extent, for the differences in potencies noted for the same opiate analgesic when administered by different routes (see, for example, Table 5.1).

18 Transmucosal absorption also is the mechanism used for intranasal drug delivery (e.g., nasal drops; nasal sprays). Increasingly, intranasal administration of opiate analgesics (e.g., butorphanol [Stadol NS®]; fentanyl [Lazanda®]) have been advocated and used to manage breakthrough cancer pain (Dietrich & Gums, 2012; Grassin-Delyle, Buenestado, & Naline, 2012; Vellucci, Mediati, & Gasperoni, 2017). It is also used as a route of administration of the opiate analgesic antagonist, naloxone (Narcan®). (See also the discussion in the later subsection, "Opiate Analgesic Overdosage/Unintentional Poisoning").

- Transdermal absorption (e.g., applying a fentanyl, Duragesic®, transdermal delivery system); or the use of an iontophoretic transdermal system, such as Ionsys®, for the delivery of fentanyl;
- Transmucosal buccal absorption (e.g., buprenorphine, Belbuca® film; fentanyl [Actiq®] "lollipop" or "lozenge on-a-stick").

DISTRIBUTION

Different opiate analgesics, once absorbed into the systemic circulation, have different distribution characteristics. These differences may help to explain why some users prefer one opiate analgesic over another. For example, morphine, which is not as lipophilic as heroin, does not cross the blood-brain barrier as readily and, thus, does not achieve its onset of opiate analgesic action as rapidly. This distribution characteristic may explain why adolescents and young adults, who abuse opiate analgesics, typically prefer heroin over morphine (Pagliaro & Pagliaro, *Clinical Patient Data Files*) (For further discussion, see the following section, "Metabolism and Excretion").

METABOLISM AND EXCRETION

Morphine and other opiate analgesics are largely metabolized into several inactive products by the liver before being excreted by the kidneys. Some opiate analgesics, such as small amounts of codeine and most of a dose of heroin (i.e., diacetylmorphine), are first metabolized into morphine before they are further metabolized into inactive metabolites and excreted by the kidneys. The metabolism of most opiate analgesics is relatively rapid. Thus, their duration of action, on average, is four to five hours.

Consequently, children, adolescents, and young adults, who require an opiate analgesic for the management of moderate to severe pain following an injury or a surgical procedure, generally require additional dosing every four to five hours to maintain adequate pain relief. This time frame for metabolism and excretion also helps to explain why adolescents and young adults, who are physically dependent on opiate analgesics, must use them daily, at intervals as short as every three to five hours,[19] to prevent the onset of the opiate analgesic withdrawal syndrome (for further discussion, see the later pharmacology subsection, "Undesired, or Harmful, Effects and Toxicities—Physical and Psychological Dependence").

The opiate analgesics undergo metabolism predominantly by Phase I and Phase II metabolic reactions (Overholser & Foster, 2011).[20] Whereas most opiate analgesics undergo both phases: (1) hydromorphone, morphine, and oxymorphone, do not undergo Phase I metabolism; and (2) fentanyl, hydrocodone, and tramadol do not undergo Phase II metabolism (DePriest, Puet, & Holt, 2015; Feng, Zhu, & Zhou, 2017; Gudin, 2012). (See also the related discussion in the later section, "Opiate Analgesic Drug–Drug Interactions.")

Urine screening for opiate analgesic use detects codeine and morphine (either as "free" drug or conjugated metabolite), as well as, the active metabolites dihydrocodeine, dihydromorphine, and hydromorphone.

19 For example, when heroin is available, adolescents and young adults, who "mainline," generally "shoot up," on average, four times per day (Pagliaro & Pagliaro, *Clinical Patient Data Files*).

20 Phase I metabolic reactions include hydrolysis and oxidation (e.g., N-demethylation; O-dealkylation; O-demethylation). These metabolic reactions are predominately mediated by the hepatic cytochrome P450 isoenzyme system with the most important isoenzymes being CYP3A4 and CYP2D6 (Lotsch, 2005). Phase II metabolic reactions are conjugation reactions that primarily involve glucuronidation to more water-soluble metabolites. These reactions are predominantly catalyzed by glucuronosyltransferase (e.g., UGT1A3; UGT1A9; UGT2B7).

Common Misbelief: Finding morphine and codeine in the results of a urine drug test for an adolescent or young adult indicates recent use of both opiate analgesics.

Not true. In fact, heroin use may be suspected when both morphine and codeine are found in the urine screen results because heroin is metabolized into morphine. However, a small amount of codeine also is metabolized to morphine. Therefore, rapid screening assays cannot be used to differentially determine whether codeine, heroin, or morphine has been used.[21, 22]

Heroin has a rapid onset of action after IV injection (i.e., within 10 seconds) and is a potent inducer of histamine release that dilates the blood vessels of the skin and, through this mechanism, increases feelings of body warmth, or "rush." Heroin crosses the blood-brain barrier more rapidly than morphine and produces greater euphoric effects when used in equivalent amounts. However, once in the brain, heroin is rapidly hydrolyzed back into morphine.

Heroin functions essentially as a "pro-drug" with a short half-life of elimination (i.e., two to six minutes) because it is rapidly metabolized from diacetylmorphine to 6-acetylmorphine and morphine—both of which are pharmacologically active (Clarification, 2016). Consequently, heroin does not produce a significantly superior analgesic response in comparison to morphine—thus, the subjective reports of user preference for heroin over morphine, may be largely confounded by expected placebo effects—as well as the noted "rush" (Pagliaro & Pagliaro, *Clinical Patient Data Files*).

Opiate Analgesic Drug–Drug Interactions

Opiate analgesic drug–drug interactions are relatively common (e.g., Mauer & Bartkowski, 1993; Megarbane, Gueye, & Baud, 2003; Overholser & Foster, 2011; Pergolizzi, 2011). For example, Pergolizzi, Labhsetwar, and Puenpatom (2011), in their study of patients who were receiving long-term opiate analgesic pharmacotherapy for chronic low back pain, found that the potential for drug–drug interactions involving opiate analgesics was 27%. Additionally, Pergolizzi, Ma, and Foster (2014)—utilizing data obtained from over 57,000 patients who had chronic, non-cancer pain and who were receiving a long-acting opiate analgesic for at least 30 days—found that approximately 6% were exposed to a "potentially major drug–drug interaction" (p. 467).

21 To precisely determine that a certain opiate analgesic has been used, a more specific chemical assay using gas chromatography with mass spectroscopy (GC/MS) or high-pressure liquid chromatography (HPLC) must be used. These methods of chemical analysis are significantly more complex, time consuming, and costly to perform than are the rapid immunoassay screenings test. However, they are more specific and accurate.

22 Urine screening for illicit or problematic patterns of opiate analgesic use can produce both "false positive" and "false negative" results. (For additional discussion of the concepts of "false positive" and "false negative" test results see Chapter 1, "Alcohol.") For example, codeine is widely available in cough and cold products and combination analgesic products. Poppy seeds also contain small amounts of morphine. If any of these products, or if enough poppy seeds are consumed, morphine can be detected in the urine for two to four days and yield positive urine screens for morphine and codeine—false positive results regarding opiate analgesic use (Farzan, 2018; Pagliaro & Pagliaro, 2009).

False negative tests also occur. For example, increasingly, specific adulterants (e.g., Absolute Detox®; Stealth®) are being used by illicit opiate analgesic users, including those in treatment programs, to produce false negative urine test results to avoid detection of their illicit opiate analgesic use (Cody, Valtier, & Kuhlman, 2001; Dasgupta, 2015; Stolberg & Gerth, 2000). These products are widely advertised and are easily obtained by means of purchase from vendors over the internet (Hoyle, 2002; Pagliaro & Pagliaro, *Clinical Patient Data Files*).

All drug–drug interactions, including those involving opiate analgesics, may be classified as occurring by means of either pharmacodynamic or pharmacokinetic mechanisms (Hansten, 1986, 2002).

PHARMACODYNAMIC DRUG–DRUG INTERACTIONS

Virtually all major clinically significant opiate analgesic opiate analgesic pharmacodynamic interactions involve: (1) non-opiate analgesic psychodepressants; (2) psychostimulants; or (3) serotonin reuptake inhibitors.

NON-OPIATE ANALGESIC PSYCHODEPRESSANT AND OPIATE ANALGESIC DRUG–DRUG INTERACTIONS. Interactions involving non-opiate analgesic psychodepressants and opiate analgesics may produce additive, and potentially synergistic, CNS depressant effects that can result in a significant reduction in respiratory rate and the promotion of sedation, which, ultimately, can be fatal (e.g., Kumar, 2017; Pagliaro & Pagliaro, 2009). Given this demonstrated and well-documented concern, the FDA, for example, added a mandatory "boxed warning" on August 31, 2016 (FDA, 2016a) for related drug monographs in an effort to decrease the concurrent use of opiate analgesics and benzodiazepines (see also the related discussion in Chapter 6, "Prescription Sedative-Hypnotics").[23]

PSYCHOSTIMULANT AND OPIATE ANALGESIC DRUG–DRUG INTERACTIONS. Contrary to most drug–drug interactions, psychostimulant (e.g., amphetamines; cocaine) and opiate analgesic interactions are often consciously pursued—albeit in the illicit context of "recreational" opiate analgesic use—to: (1) achieve desired psychodepressant and psychostimulant effects; and (2) modulate the contributory effects of each drug. For example, the IV injection of a "speedball," traditionally defined as a mixture of cocaine and heroin, reportedly results in a simultaneous and extreme "rush" and intense euphoric "high." The combined IV injection of a psychodepressant and a psychostimulant first became popular in the 1970s (Pagliaro & Pagliaro, *Clinical Patient Data Files*). A resurgence in this pattern of use was identified during the second decade of the new millennium with reported prevalence rates "during the past six months—among IV drug users—ranging from 20% to 50% (e.g. Al-Tayyib, Koester, & Langegger, 2017; Meacham, Strathdee, & Rangel, 2016).

SELECTIVE SEROTONIN REUPTAKE INHIBITOR AND OPIATE ANALGESIC DRUG–DRUG INTERACTIONS. A potentially significant, but decidedly less common, and less well-defined, drug–drug interaction involves the interaction between selective serotonin reuptake inhibitors (e.g., duloxetine, Cymbalta®; fluoxetine, Prozac®; fluvoxamine, Luvox®; paroxetine, Paxil®; sertraline, Zoloft®) and opiate analgesics, which can result in the serotonin syndrome (e.g., Gnanadesigan, Espinoza, & Smith, 2005; Houlihan, 2004; Nelson & Philbrick, 2012; Rastogi, Swarm, & Patel, 2011; Solhaug & Molden, 2017).

PHARMACOKINETIC DRUG–DRUG INTERACTIONS

Virtually all major opiate analgesic pharmacokinetic drug–drug interactions involve drugs—including various opiate analgesics themselves—that induce or inhibit the production of cytochrome P450 isoenzymes, particularly CYP3A4 and CYP2D6, which predominantly

23 On September 20, 2017, the FDA issued a related update and addendum advising that drugs used to treat opiate analgesic dependence or "addiction" (e.g. buprenorphine; methadone) "should not be withheld from patients taking benzodiazepines" because "the harm caused by untreated opioid addiction can outweigh" the related risks (FDA, 2017a, p. 1).

affect opiate analgesic metabolism (Feng, Zhu, & Zhou, 2017; Overholser & Foster, 2011; Pagliaro & Pagliaro, 2009). (See Table 5.3) (See also the related discussion of opiate analgesic metabolism in the previous pharmacology section, "Pharmacokinetics—Metabolism.") Consequently, drugs that induce or inhibit the production of P450 isoenzymes, can result in clinically significant drug interactions when used with opiate analgesics, particularly those that have a lower therapeutic index and/or are used at high dosages.

Inducers of either CYP3A4 or CYP2D6 stimulate the production of these enzymes and, consequently, cause an increased metabolism and, correspondingly, a lower serum concentration of the opiate analgesics. Based on patient response and, if applicable, opiate analgesic serum levels, the dosage of the opiate analgesic may need to be increased. Conversely, inhibitors of either CYP3A4 or CYP2D6 will have the exact opposite effects.

<u>Related Professional Reminder:</u> The clinical significance of all opiate analgesic drug–drug interactions, including those involving other opiate analgesics, is dependent upon several factors associated with each interacting drug: (1) dosage; (2) route of administration; (3) frequency of administration; (4) half-life of elimination; and (5) therapeutic index. Clinical significance is also dependent upon several factors associated with each recipient or user: (6) age; (7) gender; (8) concomitant medical

Table 5.3 Major Inducers and Inhibitors of CYP3A4 and CYP2D6

CYP3A4		*CYP2D6*	
Inducers	*Inhibitors*	*Inducers*	*Inhibitors*
Carbamazepine	Amiodarone	Dexamethasone	Amiodarone
Fentanyl	Clarithromycin	Rifampin	Bupropion
Griseofulvin	Clotrimazole		Chlorpromazine
Methadone	Dexamethasone		Cimetidine
Modafinil	Diazepam		Citalopram
Oxycodone	Diltiazem		Clomipramine
Pentobarbital	Erythromycin		Codeine
Phenobarbital	Fluconazole		Fluoxetine
Phenytoin	Fluoxetine		Fluvoxamine
Primidone	Fluvoxamine		Haloperidol
Rifampin	Indinavir		Methadone
Ziprasidone	Itraconazole		Moclobemide
	Ketoconazole		Paroxetine
	Nefazodone		Quinidine
	Ritonavir		Ritonavir
	Valproic Acid		Sertraline
	Verapamil		Thioridazine
	Voriconazole		Valproic Acid
			Venlafaxine

Sources: FDA (2017b); Feng, Zhu, & Zhou (2017); Gudin (2012); Holmquist (2009); McCance-Katz, Sullivan, & Nallani (2010); Pagliaro & Pagliaro (2009); Pergolizzi, Ma, & Foster (2014).

conditions, including pregnancy; (9) overall health status, including hepatic and renal function; and (10) genetic variability, including polymorphisms for the hepatic microsomal isoenzymes.

Undesired, or Harmful, Effects and Toxicities

The opiate analgesics are associated with many undesired, or harmful, effects and toxicities that can affect virtualy every body system. The occurrence and significance of these opiate analgesic-related undesired, or harmful, effects and toxicities are generally associated with their patterns of use—irregular, short-term use or regular, long-term use—and dosage.[24] The toxicities associated with the opiate analgesics can be immediate (i.e., acute) or can develop over time (i.e., chronic) (see Table 5.4). Acute toxicities occur more commonly and can be quite severe, while chronic toxicities occur less commonly and are usually relatively mild.[25] Consequently, the risk of

Table 5.4 Signs and Symptoms of Acute and Chronic Opiate Analgesic Toxicities

BODY SYSTEM	*SIGNS & SYMPTOMS*	
	Acute	*Chronic*
CNS	Cognitive impairment; headache; syncope	Physical dependence; psychological dependence
CV	Bradycardia; cardiac arrest; circulatory depression; orthostatic, or postural, hypotension; sedation; shock; with intravenous injection, local pain or phlebitis at injection site	Anemia
Cutaneous	Diaphoresis; dilation of superficial blood vessels with resultant warming of the skin ("flushing"); erythema; pain at injection site with subcutaneous injection; pruritus; urticaria	
GI	Constipation; nausea; vomiting	Constipation
Genitourinary	Impotence (boys and young men); reduced sexual desire; urinary retention	Menstrual irregularities (girls and young women); reduced sexual desire
Muscular-Skeletal	With intramuscular injection, pain at injection site	
Ophthalmic	Miosis	
Respiratory	Bronchospasm; laryngospasm; respiratory arrest; respiratory depression	

24 The difference between a "desired" pharmacological effect that is associated with the use of an opiate analgesic and an "undesired," "harmful," or "toxic" effect often is related to the context of use. For example, the development of an undesired effect, such as "constipation," for an adolescent who is being successfully treated with an opiate analgesic for the pain associated with a broken leg compared to an adolescent, who is being treated for severe diarrhea with an opiate analgesic, or a derivative anti-diarrheal product, for its desired constipating effects.

25 In fact, chronic toxicities associated with the opiate analgesics are generally considered to be lower than for any other psychodepressant as well as for most of the other drugs and substances of abuse.

morbidity and mortality for adolescents and young adults, who use the opiate analgesics, is primarily associated with acute toxicity. Generally, there is little direct residual physiological damage associated with the regular, long-term use of the opiate analgesics.[26]

Opiate analgesics have long been known to cause the release of histamine from mast cells[27] likely by means of the direct activation of G-proteins (Barke & Hough, 1993; Moss & Roscow, 1983; Stellato, Cirillo, & de Paulis, 1992; Withington, Patrick, & Reynolds, 1993). This histamine release has been related to the "rush" experienced with the IV injection of heroin (e.g., vasodilation of most blood vessels; warming of the skin), as well as several other expected signs and symptoms, including: bronchospasm; erythema; hypotension; pruritus; tachycardia; and urticaria (e.g., Flacke, Flacke, & Bloor, 1987; Mauer, Kager, & Fellinger, 2014). In addition, Cygan, Trunsky, and Corbridge (2000) reported a series of five young adults with asthma who developed status asthmaticus after "snorting" heroin. Others have also noted that the intranasal insufflation, IV injection, or pulmonary inhalation of heroin, by users who have asthma, has been associated with acute exacerbation of related nasal and respiratory signs and symptoms (Underner, Perriot, & Peiffer, 2017; Weeks, Clark, & Mycyk, 2016).

Persistent constipation commonly occurs with regular, long-term opiate analgesic use, particularly when ingested. As the opiate analgesic management of non-cancer pain significantly increased during the new millennium, the incidence of constipation related to opiate analgesic use (i.e., "opioid-induced constipation," or OIC) correspondingly increased (Weber, 2016).[28]

Significant recent pharmacotherapeutic advances in the treatment of OIC/OIBD have primarily focused on peripheral-acting mu opiate analgesic receptor antagonists (PAMORAs) (Holder & Rhee, 2016; Jones, Prommer, & Backstedt, 2016; Leppert, 2016). For example, naloxegol (Movantik®) prevents opiate analgesics from binding to mu opiate analgesic receptors in the GI tract (Garnock-Jones, 2015). It was approved for adult oral ingestion by the FDA in September 2014 (FDA, 2014a). As such, it became the first drug in this new pharmacological classification of drugs developed for the treatment of OIC (Anantharamu, Sharma, & Gupta, 2015; Corsetti & Tack, 2015).

PAMORAs are "PEGylated" derivatives of naloxone that, when ingested, are specifically developed to have negligible penetration of the CNS. Consequently, they block the constipating effects associated with the use of the opiate analgesics, but not the associated analgesic effects. Their clinical use in patients with advanced/severe OIC/OIBD symptoms, who do not respond well to traditional oral laxatives, has resulted in significant relief of adverse GI symptoms without compromising related opiate analgesia. As such, their use is particularly indicated for adults with chronic, severe pain who require opiate analgesic pharmacotherapy.[29]

Common undesired, or harmful, effects associated with naloxegol, include: abdominal pain, diarrhea, and excessive gas and flatulence (FDA, 2014). Additionally, the use of

26 For example, although deficits in executive cognitive functioning may occur with periods of opiate analgesic use, residual impairment among former opiate analgesic users has not been reported. This observation is in stark contrast to former amphetamine users who, although abstinent, continue to display deficits in executive cognitive functioning related to their former regular, long-term amphetamine use (Ersche, Clark, & London, 2006; Pagliaro & Pagliaro, *Clinical Patient Data Files*). (Also see the related discussion in Chapter 2, "Amphetamines and Cocaine").

27 The mast cells display significantly different histamine release responses that depend upon: (1) specific opiate analgesic used (e.g., buprenorphine versus morphine); (2) dose; (3) frequency of use; (4) method of use, or administration (e.g., ingestion versus IV injection); and (5) tissue type/location (e.g., lung versus skin).

28 When additional opiate analgesic-related GI signs and symptoms (e.g., abdominal pain; bloating; gastric stasis; nausea; vomiting; and xerostomia) are combined with OIC, the resultant spectrum/syndrome of GI complaints is commonly referred to as "opioid-induced bowel dysfunction" (OIBD) (Leppert, 2015).

29 PAMORAs have also demonstrated significant therapeutic efficacy as a prophylactic against severe OIC among adolescents and young adults who occasionally require an opiate analgesic for the treatment of acute pain (e.g., painful dental or medical procedure)—particularly, among those who have previously experienced severe OIC (Pagliaro & Pagliaro, *Clinical Patient Data Files*).

PAMORAs are associated with several undesired, or harmful, effects, which are not dose-related, including: fecal impaction; bowel obstruction; and bowel perforation. Tolerance to these undesired, or harmful, effects does not develop (Jones, Prommer, & Backstedt, 2015).

TOXICITIES ASSOCIATED WITH OPIATE ANALGESIC INTRAVENOUS INJECTION

In addition to direct toxicities associated with the use of opiate analgesics, there are several significant undesired, or harmful, effects and toxicities that are specifically associated with their method of use, particularly, IV injection (Bangsberg, Rosen, & Aragon, 2002; Ciccarone & Bourgois, 2003; Pieper & Templin, 2001; Schoener, Hopper, & Pierre, 2002).[30] These undesired effects, which specifically involve IV injection sites, include: abscesses; scarring of the skin (i.e., "needle tracks" or "railroad tracks"); soft-tissue infection or inflammation (e.g., cellulitis; cutaneous venous ulcer; necrotizing fasciitis); and thrombophlebitis. Other asssociated undesired, or harmful, effects, include:

- Aneurysms;
- Blood infections (e.g., bacteremia; sepsis; septicemia);
- Brain and spinal cord infections;
- Endocarditis;[31]
- Gangrene;
- Muscular infection (e.g., myonecrosis; myositis; pyomyositis);
- Pulmonary abnormalities (e.g., talc granulomas);
- Systemic viral infections (e.g., hepatitis B virus [HBV]; hepatitis C virus [HCV];[32, 33] HIV[34]);
- Tetanus;
- Wound botulism.

Not directly caused by the opiate analgesics, themselves, these infections and other undesired effects are caused by: (1) the adulterants used by dealers to "cut" the opiate analgesic to increase its weight and street value; (2) crushing and injecting drugs intended for ingestion together with related excipients; (3) infection caused by using unsterile, shared needles and syringes; and (4) improper injection techniques and resultant local tissue damage.

Obviously, these serious complications do not occur when opiate analgesics are swallowed, smoked, or "snorted." However, these other methods of use may be associated with their

30 Commonly used anatomic sites for illicit IV injection of the opiate analgesics, in decreasing order of frequency of use, include the: antecubital fossa, or forearm at the bend of the elbow; foot, generally between the toes; leg; breast; groin (e.g., femoral vein); and neck (e.g., jugular vein)—which, when used is commonly referred to as a "pocket shot" (Pagliaro & Pagliaro, *Clinical Patient Data Files*).

31 Infective endocarditis related to intravenous injection has increased significantly during the new millennium, with the highest rates reported for young adult men and women of European continental descent, who live in rural areas (e.g., Fleischauer, Ruhl, & Rhea, 2017). In a related study of injection and non-injection drug use and infectious disease, Keen, Khan, and Clifford (2014) found that approximately 70% of their Baltimore, Maryland sample of injection drug users were of European continental descent.

32 Often a precursor to cirrhosis of the liver or hepatocellular carcinoma—either of which may be fatal or require liver transplantation. The most common cause of hepatitis C in the U.S. is the sharing of contaminated needles and syringes among IV users of drugs and substances of abuse.

33 In 2016, the CDC announced that hepatitis C virus (HCV) infection had its most significant increase among women of childbearing age and cautioned about an increased risk in the U.S. for mother-to-child transmission. The increased rates of HCV were identified as being directly related to increased intravenous drug use (IVDU) (Koneru, Nelson, & Hariri, 2016). In addition, Akyar, Seneca, and Akyar (2016) identified that over 40% of their sample of heroin using adolescents and young adults tested positive for HCV.

34 In this context, Cedarbaum and Banta-Green (2016), in their study of IV heroin users, found that "young adults were significantly more likely to re-use syringes two to four times" (p. 102).

own undesired, or harmful, effects. For example, during the past decade, the intranasal use (i.e., "snorting") of the opiate analgesics, particularly crushed hydrocodone-acetaminophen combination tablets (e.g., Lortab®; Vicodin®), has been associated with:

- Bacterial infection of the nasal surfaces with a resultant rhinorrhea containing a mixture of mucopurulent exudate;
- Erosion of the lateral nasal walls, nasopharynx, and soft palate;
- Fungal invasion of the nasal surfaces;
- Inflammation of the nasal passages and sinuses;
- Perforation of the nasal septum.

(Alexander, Alexander, & Valentino, 2012; Sloan & Klimkina, 2009; Yewell, Haydon, & Archer, 2002)

In addition, severe, life-threatening asthmatic attacks have been associated with the intranasal insufflation, or "snorting," of heroin by users who have pre-existing asthma (Krantz, Hershow, & Prachand, 2003; Pagliaro & Pagliaro, *Clinical Patient Data Files*).

PHYSICAL AND PSYCHOLOGICAL DEPENDENCE

Throughout the 20th century, several of the opiate analgesics, including heroin, methadone (Dolophine®), and propoxyphene (Darvon®), were specifically developed, and originally marketed, to provide analgesia without causing physical or psychological dependence. However, it is now generally known that the regular, long-term use of any opiate analgesic, including the synthetic derivatives, is associated with the development of both physical and psychological dependence, characterized by: (1) tolerance; (2) an opiate analgesic withdrawal syndrome; and (3) craving. As identified by the National Institute on Drug Abuse:

> An estimated 2.1 million people in the United States suffer from substance use disorders related to prescription opioid pain relievers in 2012 and an estimated 467,000 [are] addicted to heroin.
>
> (Volkow, 2014, p. 1)

***Related Professional Reminder:* Opiate analgesics that are capable of relieving pain, also are capable of causing both physical and psychological dependence.**

OPIATE ANALGESIC TOLERANCE. "Tolerance" is the need to use increasingly higher doses of an opiate analgesic, or at more frequent intervals, in an effort to achieve the desired effects that were experienced with initial use. Tolerance develops within a few months of regular, long-term opiate analgesic use. Replacing the usual opiate analgesic with a different opiate analgesic generally does not help to achieve desired effects (e.g., analgesia; euphoria) due to the common occurrence of "cross-tolerance" (i.e., when tolerance occurs to one of the opiate analgesics, such as heroin, tolerance to the other opiate analgesics, such as morphine, also occurs). In addition, for many of the opiate analgesics, including heroin and methadone, the higher the dosage of the opiate analgesic used, the more severe the physical dependence and the associated opiate analgesic withdrawal syndrome when regular, long-term use is abruptly discontinued.

Common Misbelief: If adolescents and young adults use their opiate analgesics exactly as medically prescribed, they can avoid the development of tolerance.

Not true. As noted by Volkow and McLellan (2016) from the NIDA:

> There is lingering *misunderstanding* among some physicians about the important differences between physical dependence and addiction. The repeated administration of any opioid almost inevitably results in the development of tolerance and physical dependence.
>
> (p. 1)

The euphorigenic action that opiate analgesics produce among non-tolerant people is generally reduced, or eliminated, as tolerance develops. It is important to note that whereas tolerance and opiate analgesic withdrawal are two components of physical dependence, "craving" is a characteristic of psychological dependence.

To once again achieve the desired euphorigenic actions, tolerant adolescents and young adults, who regularly use opiate analgesics, may significantly increase the amount of the opiate analgesic they use—and, consequently, place themselves at higher risk for overdosage and death associated with severe respiratory depression. In addition, among adolescents and young adults, who are regular, long-term opiate analgesic users, the higher the dosage of the opiate analgesic used, the more severe the physical dependence, and, thus, the more severe the associated opiate analgesic withdrawal syndrome. Consequently, an increased desire to avoid the opiate analgesic withdrawal syndrome develops and this desire becomes a powerful, and very often persuasive, motive for continued opiate analgesic use. (See the following section for additional discussion of the opiate analgesic withdrawal syndrome.)

Opiate Analgesic Withdrawal Syndrome.[35] The opiate analgesic withdrawal syndrome occurs when regular, long-term opiate analgesic use is abruptly discontinued and is immediately relieved when opiate analgesic use is resumed. Signs and symptoms[36] of the opiate analgesic withdrawal syndrome generally include:

- Abdominal cramps and pain;
- Anorexia;
- Anxiety;
- Asthenia;
- Backache;
- Chills with goose flesh (i.e., "going cold turkey");
- Diaphoresis;
- Diarrhea;
- Dysphoria;
- Fever of unknown origin;
- Hyperalgesia;
- Hypertension;
- Hyperthermia;
- Hyperventilation;
- Insomnia;
- Irritability
- Muscle aches and jerks (i.e., "kicking the habit");
- Nausea;
- Nervousness;

35 See also the related discussion in the later subsection, "Pharmacotherapy: Opiate Analgesic Withdrawal Syndrome."

36 These signs and symptoms, often resembling those associated with a severe case of the "flu," are not generally life-threatening (Pagliaro & Pagliaro, *Clinical Patient Data Files*).

- Piloerection;
- Restlessness;
- Rhinitis;
- Rhinorrhea;
- Shivering;
- Sneezing;
- Tachycardia;
- Tremors;
- Vomiting;
- Watery eyes;
- Worrying;
- Yawning.

Additionally, in severe cases, terrifying hallucinations, convulsions, and coma may occur.

The signs and symptoms of opiate analgesic withdrawal usually begin within eight to 16 hours following the last time that an opiate analgesic was used and resolve after two to 12 days. The occurrence and severity largely depend on the: (1) specific opiate analgesic used;[37] (2) the length of time that the opiate analgesic was regularly used; (3) dosage used (higher compared to lower); and (4) the method of use (ingestion versus IV injection). Although many users, who have undergone opiate analgesic withdrawal, report the experience as being extremely difficult and painful, most cases are relatively mild in terms of the pain and physical stress that is experienced.[38] (See also the later pharmacology subsection, "Opiate Analgesic Overdosage/Unintentional Poisoning—Opiate Analgesic Overdosage."

In addition, the opiate analgesic withdrawal syndrome is not usually fatal, even when nonmedically managed (i.e., quitting "cold turkey"). Fatalities related to opiate analgesic withdrawal are generally rare. However, when they do occur, they are usually the result of such complicating factors as concurrent use of other drugs or substances of abuse, heart disease, or mental depression leading to suicide attempts or completions.[39] Both buprenorphine (see also the related discussion in the later opiate analgesic "Pharmacology" subsection, "Neonatal Opiate Analgesic Abstinence Syndrome") and clonidine have been used to ameliorate the signs and symptoms associated with the opiate analgesic withdrawal syndrome.

37 Reportedly, the abrupt discontinuation of methadone (Dolophine®) has been identified as resulting in the most severe withdrawal syndrome when compared to other opiate analgesics at equivalent dosages and length of use (Hiltunen & Eklund, 2002; Pagliaro & Pagliaro, 2009; Pagliaro & Pagliaro, *Clinical Patient Data Files*).

38 Despite the objective documentation of the relatively mild, undesired effects associated with the opiate analgesic withdrawal syndrome, the conscious attempt to avoid or diminish these effects is, reportedly, one of the major reasons—following, "to achieve feelings of euphoria"—for the continued regular, long-term use of opiate analgesics (Pagliaro & Pagliaro, *Clinical Patient Data Files*). As such, when their favorite opiate analgesic is not available, adolescent and young adult "opiate addicts" will use whatever opiate analgesic is available to them to avoid or diminish the undesired effects even if they would not generally otherwise use that opiate analgesic (e.g., codeine) because they "don't like it" or think it is "junk."

Loperamide (Imodium®) is one-such opiate analgesic. It was developed and approved by the FDA as an antidiarrheal. Because it acts primarily at the intestinal opiate analgesic mu-receptor in the myenteric plexus of the GIT, its potential for abuse is officially labeled as "low." Consequently, it is widely available "over-the-counter," without a prescription. However, at higher dosages, it can readily cross the blood-brain barrier resulting in central systemic effects, including euphoria and respiratory depression–and relieve the opiate analgesic withdrawal syndrome. The abuse of loperamide has been associated with physical and psychological dependence, respiratory depression, and life-threating ventricular dysrhythmias (MacDonald, Heiner, & Villarreal, 2015; Marraffa, Holland, & Sullivan, 2014; Spinner, Lonardo, & Mulamalla, 2015).

39 Except in cases of opiate analgesic withdrawal involving: (1) high dosages; or (2) methadone use—which are often reported to be significantly more severe than the withdrawal syndromes associated with other opiate analgesics (Pagliaro & Pagliaro, 2009).

OPIATE ANALGESIC CRAVING. Craving—the memory of, and the desire for, the feeling of euphoria initially experienced—appears to be one of the major factors of psychological dependence underlying the high potential for recidivism among regular, long-term opiate analgesic users who attempt to quit their use of opiate analgesics.

***Related Professional Reminder:* Intervention for the opiate analgesic withdrawal syndrome should always be used as an opportunity to initiate appropriate treatment aimed at the cessation of opiate analgesic use and the prevention of recidivism.**

Opiate Analgesic Overdosage/Unintentional Poisoning

This section presents and discusses published new millennial research statistics regarding opiate analgesic overdosage and unintentional poisoning involving infants, children, adolescents, and young adults.

OPIATE ANALGESIC OVERDOSAGE

Between 1997 and 2009, the rate of hospitalizations in the U.S., related to opiate analgesic overdosage, increased sharply and significantly from two hospitalizations per 100,000 U.S. population to 15 hospitalizations per 100,000 population (Unick, Rosenblum, & Mars, 2013).[40]

Analyzing data from the *National Survey on Drug Use and the Health* and *National Vital Statistics System*, the CDC and FDA found that:

> During 2002–2013, heroin overdose death rates nearly quadrupled in the United States, from 0.7 deaths to 2.7 deaths per 100,000 population, with a near doubling of the rates from 2011–2013.
>
> (Jones, Logan, & Gladden, 2015, p. 719)

In some of these cases, death is often a rapid event in which the needle and syringe may be found still attached to the adolescent's or young adult's injection site (e.g., antecubital fossa; dorsum of the hand) (Pagliaro & Pagliaro, *Clinical Patient Data Files*). However, the highest number of annual overdosage deaths—as well as the highest rate of increase in overdosage death in the U.S. during the first decade of the new millennium (i.e., 2000 to 2011) involved the prescription opiate analgesics, particularly oxycodone (OxyContin®) (Brown, 2011; Girion, Glover, & Smith, 2011; Rudd, 2014).

The CDC identified that "prescription opioid-related overdose deaths increased sharply during 1999–2010 in the United States in parallel with increased opioid prescribing" (Guy, Zhang, & Bohm, 2017, p. 697). As noted by Nora Volkow, Director of the National Institute on Drug Abuse:

> We are seeing an increase in the number of people who are dying from overdoses, predominantly after abuse of prescribed opioid analgesics. This disturbing trend appears to be associated with a growing number of prescriptions in and diversion from the legal market.
>
> (Volkow & McLellan, 2016, p. 8)

Several others have reported similar findings. For example, as reported by Frieden and Houry (2016): "Death from prescription-opioid overdose has dramatically increased in the United States, quadrupling in the past 15 years" (p. 10).

40 It is important for health and social care professionals to keep in mind that approximately 20% of these hospitalizations—and related deaths—involve the concomitant use of alcohol (CDC, 2018; Jones, Paulozzi, & Mack, 2014). (For additional related discussion, see Chapter 1, "Alcohol.")

Most adolescent and young adult heroin users also concurrently use other drugs and substances of abuse (see also the related discussion in the earlier section, "Opiate Analgesic Drug–Drug Interactions"). Thus, these overdosages, as previously discussed, may also display serious synergistic effects[41] related to the use of: (1) heroin and another psychodepressant (e.g., alcohol; benzodiazepine); or (2) heroin and a psychostimulant (e.g., cocaine; methamphetamine), which may have been used concurrently by the same, or by a different, method of use (Jones, Paulozzi, & Mack, 2014; Pagliaro & Pagliaro, 2009; Sharp & Melnik, 2015; Sporer, 1999).

> Kyle Belitto, a lawyer and her husband, Glenn Belitto, 59, a finance professional—both with Harvard degrees—of the leafy Bronxville, a Westchester suburb in New York where the median household income is $200,000 a year, learned the hard way when their 19-year-old Ivy League son died in December of a suspected opioid overdose, The New York Post reported . . .
>
> "Cocaine was really big for him," Will Rabsey, 19, who went to all 12 years of elementary, middle and high school with Gage, told The Post. "I remember a few times he'd put a line out and I'd say, 'Damn, Gage, that's a lot.' He'd say, 'No I've done this before. I can handle it.'" . . .
>
> According to the Post, Gage lied to his psychiatrist to up his prescription of Klonopin, anti-anxiety pill. He'd also been prescribed Vyvanse, a stimulant, and methylphenidate—commonly known as Ritalin—to treat attention deficit disorder.
>
> (Miles, 2018, p. 1)

Seth, Scholl, and Rudd (2018) noted that:

> Drug overdose deaths in the United States increased 11.4% from 2014 to 2015 resulting in 52,404 deaths in 2015, including 33,091 (63.1%) that involved an opioid. The largest rate increases from 2014 to 2015 occurred among deaths involving synthetic opioids other than methadone (72.2%) . . . The largest absolute rate increases of opioid-involved deaths, and deaths involving synthetic opioids occurred among males aged 25–44 years and persons aged 25–34 years. However, deaths involving synthetic opioids increased in every subgroup examined.
>
> (p. 349)

Unfortunately, the rates of opiate analgesic-related hospitalizations and deaths have not abated during the second decade of the new millennium (e.g., Fleischauer, Ruhl, & Rhea, 2017). As identified by Williams and Bisaga (2016, p. 813):

> The United States is facing a vast epidemic of opioid-related deaths. More than 2.4 million Americans have a severe opioid-use disorder (OUD)[42] involving dependence on pain medications, heroin, or both, and rates of drug-overdose deaths in this country have outpaced mortality from motor vehicle accidents since 2013.

Additionally, as identified by Vivolo-Kantor, Seth, and Gladden (2018)—on behalf of the CDC:

41 Synergistic drug effects occur when two or more drugs, including the drugs and substances of abuse, work together to produce, either: (1) an effect that neither drug can produce on its own; or (2) an effect size that is significantly greater than the sum of the individual drug effects when added together. For example, fatal overdosages involving either alcohol, alone, or a benzodiazepine, alone, are relatively rare. However, when both alcohol and benzodiazepines are ingested together, overdosages are much, more common—including fatal overdosages (see the related discussion in Chapters 1, "Alcohol", and 6, "Prescription Sedative Hypnotics").

42 This term is used in the 5th addition of the DSM taxonomy (APA, 2013).

> During July 2016-September 2017, ED visits among those aged ≥ 11 years for opioid overdoses in the United States increased 29.7% overall and 34.5% in 16 states with high prevalence of overdose mortality. Significant rate increases were found in five Midwest region states (largest in Wisconsin [109%]) and three Northeast region states (largest in Delaware [105%]).
>
> (p. 279)

Particularly tragic, in this context, is the observation by Doctor, Nguyen, and Lev (2018) that:

> Most opioid prescription deaths occur among people with common conditions for which prescribing risks outweigh benefits.
>
> (p. 588)

In 2005, it was noted that approximately 16,000 people in the U.S. die annually because of a prescription opiate-analgesic overdosage and an additional number of approximately 8,000 people die annually because of heroin-related overdosages (i.e., approximately 65 people daily) (NIDA, 2015b). By 2017, this number had significantly increased. As noted by Soelberg, Brown, and Du Vivier (2017):

> The United States is in the midst of a devastating opioid misuse epidemic leading to over 33,000 deaths per year [i.e., approximately 100 people daily] for both prescription and illegal opioids. Roughly, half of these deaths are attributable to prescription opioids.
>
> (p. 1675)

In 2018, the director of the National Institutes of Health reiterated this observation:

> Every day, more than 115 Americans die after overdosing on opioids, that is a fourfold increase since 2000, and the numbers continue to climb.
>
> (NIH, 2018, p. 1)

Deaths associated with opiate analgesic overdosage, in the U.S., have increased significantly during the new millennium. For example, by over 200% from 2000 to 2014 (Rudd, Aleshire, & Zibbell, 2016).[43] We expect that these numbers of opiate analgesic overdosage deaths will continue to increase significantly over the next 20 years, as increasing numbers of baby boomers reach age 65+ (Colliver, Compton, & Gfroerer, 2006; Gossop & Moos, 2008; Han, Gfroerer, & Colliver, 2009a, 2009b; Nordrum, 2016).

Related Professional Reminder: ***Opiate analgesic overdosage is a life-threatening medical emergency that generally requires: (1) immediate administration of naloxone; (2) monitoring of respirations and provision of any required respiratory support; and (3) detection and treatment of any other suspected concurrent overdosage involving other drugs and substances of abuse (e.g., alcohol; benzodiazepines; cocaine; methamphetamine).***

The signs and symptoms of acute opiate analgesic overdosage are listed in Table 5.5. As shown, several major organ systems may be involved.

43 Geographically, the highest reported increases in these opiate analgesic overdosage deaths occurred in the Appalachian and Southwestern states (Park & Bloch, 2016).

Table 5.5 Signs and Symptoms of Acute Opiate Analgesic Overdosage

Body System	*Acute Opiate Analgesic Overdosage Signs & Symptoms*
Cardiovascular	Hypotension; shock
Central Nervous	Stupor or coma. Seizures may occur with meperidine (Demerol®) or propoxyphene (Darvon®). Seizures also may occur with hypoxemia
Gastrointestinal	Diminished or absent bowel sounds; constipation
Peripheral Nervous	Reflex arc effects, including diminished or absent reflexes (e.g., abdominal reflex; ankle jerk reflex; quadriceps knee jerk reflex; and radial brachialis reflex)
Ophthalmic	Miosis. Mydriasis may occur with meperidine (Demerol®) and with extreme hypoxia
Pulmonary	Apnea; hypopnea; hypoxia
Thermoregulatory	Hypothermia

TREATMENT OF OPIATE ANALGESIC OVERDOSAGE: NALOXONE PHARMACOTHERAPY. The opiate analgesic antagonist, naloxone (Narcan®),[44] can literally bring an adolescent or young adult, who has overdosed on an opiate analgesic, back from death's doorstep.[45] Naloxone, which is not well absorbed from the GI tract, is therapeutically administered by a variety of other routes, including: IM injection; intranasal insufflation; endotracheal (ET) instillation; IV injection or infusion; and SC injection. Absorption following IV and ET administration is generally rapid. However, absorption may be slow, and the related onset of action delayed, with IM or SC injection. Consequently, we generally recommend that naloxone be administered by IV injection, whenever possible.[46]

The generally recommended dosage of naloxone is 0.1 mg/kg. The dosage can be repeated, if needed, within a couple of minutes. Thereafter, dosages are repeated at hourly intervals commensurate with the half-life of elimination of naloxone. A constant IV infusion of naloxone, although generally not required, may also be initiated (Kauffman, Banner, &

44 Naloxone (Narcan®) is a relatively inert drug that has no significant actions—other than to competitively bind to endogenous opiate analgesic receptor sties, and, subsequently, prevent the opiate analgesic from binding to the sites and eliciting their expected therapeutic and undesired, or toxic, effects. (See also the related discussion in the earlier pharmacology section, "Pharmacodynamics: Mechanism of Action.")

45 N.B. It is extremely important to be mindful that, naloxone only reverses the actions of the opiate analgesics. Naloxone does not reverse the actions of any other drug, including any other drug and substance of abuse that may also be involved in the overdosage. Other drugs and substances of abuse that are suspected to be involved in the overdosage must be appropriately identified and individually dealt with accordingly—for example, with activated charcoal, gastric lavage, or a specific antidote as per established clinical protocols. As noted in an analysis of related data by the CDC and FDA:

> Overall, 96% of past-year heroin users reported use of at least one other drug during the past year, and 61% reported using at least three different drugs.
>
> (Jones, Logan, & Gladden, 2015, p. 721)

46 N.B. Administration into a large vein is the most efficient method. The use of peripheral veins can be problematic in cases of opiate analgesic overdosage because of, for example, collapsed veins, hypotension, trauma, and vasoconstriction. In these cases, when a central vein is not easily accessible, the IN or ET routes are generally recommended. See also the related use of intranasal naloxone as discussed in the following subsection, "Unintentional Poisoning."

Blumer, 1990; Pagliaro & Pagliaro, 1999, 2002). (See also the related discussion in the later subsection, "Unintentional Poisoning").

Although naloxone has generally become more widely available, death due to acute heroin overdosage is a relatively common event that has been increasing since the early 1990's—from less than 1,000 deaths per year to more than 30,000 deaths per year (NIDA, 2015b; Ochoa, Hahn, & Seal, 2001; Rudd, 2014). As identified by Jones, Logan, and Gladden (2015, p.1), "Heroin use and overdose deaths have increased significantly in the United States"—quadrupling from 2002 to 2013 (Nordrum, 2015) and more than tripling from 2010 to 2014 (Rudd, Aleshire, & Zibbell, 2016). (See related discussion in the previous section.)

As part of the response to this horrific situation, the FDA approved the use of a hand-held naloxone auto-injector (Evzio®) in 2014 (FDA, 2014b). The single dose naloxone autoinjector (Evzio®) is available by prescription for use by family members, or caregivers, for the emergency treatment of known or suspected cases of opiate analgesic overdosage. A single two mg IM[47] or SC dose of naloxone is injected with a 0.4 ml pre-filled, hand-held auto-injector. Use is facilitated by verbal instructions provided to the user by an electronic voice instruction system—once the unit has been turned on—similar to the verbal instructions provided by some automated defibrillators. Additional doses can be administered, utilizing a new autoinjector, at two- to three- minute intervals as indicated by patient response (i.e., failure to respond to the initial dose or response to the initial dose followed by relapse into respiratory depression).

Over the last 30 years, increasingly pure supplies of heroin (i.e., higher relative concentrations of heroin in actual street samples) became generally available in the U.S. These supplies of heroin were associated with literally thousands of deaths as noted earlier.[48] From 2012 to 2015, heroin was the most frequently mentioned drug associated with overdosage deaths in the U.S. (Hedegaard, Bastian, & Trinidad, 2018, p. 1). In many of these cases, the deaths were the result of users not making allowances for the increasingly pure supplies of heroin that they were obtaining (i.e., they failed to reduce their usual dosages).

Additionally, while a significant increase in overdosage deaths was identified among IV heroin users in the U.S. during the second decade of the new millennium, the chemical analyses—which were conducted by both the CDC and DEA—determined that fentanyl and its analogs, which were added to the street heroin, were the most frequent cause for the significant increase in overdosage deaths (Gladden, Martinez, & Seth, 2016; Peterson, Gladden, & Delcher, 2016).[49]

In 2016, fentanyl was the most frequently mentioned drug that was involved with overdosage deaths in the U.S. (Hedegaard, Bastian, & Trinidad, 2018). The NIH (2018, p. 1), based upon an analysis of data from their searchable internal database, *CDC Wonder*, found that:

> Among the more than 72,000 drug overdose deaths estimated in 2017, the sharpest increase occurred among deaths related to fentanyl and fentanyl analogs (synthetic opioids) with nearly 30,000 overdose deaths.

47 It is recommended that the IM injection of naloxone be made into the anterolateral aspect of the thigh (i.e., quadriceps femoris or vastus lateralis muscles), through clothing if necessary, for children, adolescents, and young adults.

48 N.B. Not only has the number of heroin-related overdosage deaths increased significantly in the U.S., but also has the rate of heroin-related ED visits.

49 Generally, in national statistical reports, overdosage deaths are not identified separately for individual opiate analgesics (e.g., fentanyl overdosages are not distinguished from those involving oxycodone; heroin overdosages are not distinguished from those involving all combined prescription opiate analgesic overdosages).

The highest increase in these fentanyl-related, overdosage deaths occurred in eight "high burden" states—Florida, Kentucky, Maine, Maryland, Massachusetts, New Hampshire, North Carolina, and Ohio. Overall, the number of fentanyl-related overdosage deaths in the U.S. increased significantly from approximately 3,000 deaths, in 2010, to approximately 6,000 deaths, in 2014. (Also see the related discussion in the later section, "Fentanyl.")

As part of the concerted action of the government to combat the growing epidemic of opiate analgesic deaths, HHS recommended, in December 2018, that clinicians consider the routine prescription of naloxone for patients who are considered to be at high risk for overdosage. Specifically, the HHS recommended that:

> In order to reduce the risk of overdose deaths, clinicians should strongly consider prescribing or co-prescribing naloxone, and providing education about its use for the following patients who are at risk of opioid overdose:
>
> - Patients prescribed opioids who:
>   - Are receiving opioids at a dosage of 50 morphine milligram equivalents (MME) per day or greater;
>   - Have respiratory conditions such as chronic obstructive pulmonary disease (COPD) or obstructive sleep apnea (regardless of opioid dose);
>   - Have been prescribed benzodiazepines (regardless of opioid dose);
>   - Have a non-opioid substance use disorder, report excessive alcohol use, or have a mental health disorder (regardless of opioid dose).
>
> - Patients at high risk for experiencing or responding to an opioid overdose, including individuals:
>   - Using heroin, illicit synthetic opioids or misusing prescription opioids;
>   - Using other illicit drugs such as stimulants, including methamphetamine and cocaine, which could potentially be contaminated with illicit synthetic opioids like fentanyl;
>   - Receiving treatment for opioid use disorder, including medication-assisted treatment with methadone, buprenorphine, or naltrexone;
>   - With a history of opioid misuse that were recently released from incarceration or other controlled settings where tolerance to opioids has been lost.
>
> (HHS, 2018, p. 5)

OPIATE ANALGESIC UNINTENTIONAL POISONING

Along with the growing opiate analgesic epidemic in the U.S. during the new millennium, childhood poisonings involving the opiate analgesics likewise increased significantly. As found by Allen, Casavant, and Spiller (2017), in their analysis of data from the *National Poison Data System*:

> Poison control centers received reports of 188,468 prescription opioid exposures among children [and adolescents] under 20 years of age from 2000 through 2015.[50]
>
> (p. e20163382)

50 Of the reported exposures, 60% involved children five years-of-age or younger; 55% were referred to a health care facility; and 12% required hospitalization.

In a SAMHAS report, Crane (2017) identified that:

> The number of ED visits involving accidental ingestion of opioid pain relievers among children aged 1 to 5 tripled between 2004 and 2011. About one quarter of these ED visits were serious enough to have ended with hospitalization or transfer to another health facility.
>
> (p. 4)

Glenza (2016) similarly reported that:

> The incidence of American children overdosing on opioids increased dramatically between 1997 and 2012, including a two-fold increase among toddlers.
>
> (p. 1)

> A toddler in Michigan died after ingesting an "extraordinary level" of fentanyl ... Ava Floyd, 18 months old, died on Christmas Day. The prosecutor's office in the Detroit suburb of Macomb County said the child's parents had been producing and packing fentanyl in their home and she ingested the narcotic.
>
> (Phillips, 2019, p. 1)

***Related Professional Reminder:* In cases of opiate analgesic poisoning, a toxicology screen is indicated to confirm the exact suspected intoxicant and any co-intoxicants.**

The signs and symptoms of opiate analgesic poisoning among children include:

- Constipation;
- Hypotension;
- Lethargy;
- Miosis;
- Nausea;
- Pruritus;
- Respiratory depression;
- Vomiting.

The treatment and management for pediatric opiate analgesic poisoning involves: (1) immediate assessment and diagnosis; (2) as medically indicated, either ET or IV administration of naloxone (Narcan®)—the antidote for opiate analgesic poisoning;[51] (3) careful monitoring; and (4) supportive medical care. The usual dosage of naloxone is 0.1 mg/kg and is repeated at hourly intervals, as needed (Pagliaro & Pagliaro, 2002).

***Related Professional Reminder:* Child and adolescent opiate analgesic overdosage/unintentional poisoning requires immediate emergency intervention. Once stabilized, children (and**

51 Although associated with a slower onset of action, the IM or SC injection of naloxone also can be used. In addition, the intranasal route of administration has been increasingly used by family members, "lay bystanders," needle exchange patients, paramedics, patients, and police in emergency situations. Approved for use by the FDA, intranasal naloxone is available in a single, four-mg dose intranasal device. The efficacy of this intranasal naloxone delivery device is reportedly almost identical to that associated with IV injection (e.g., Barton, Colwell, & Wolfe, 2005; Doe-Simkins, Walley & Epstein, 2009; Robinson & Wermeling, 2014). (See also the related use of the naloxone auto-injector in the later section, "Pharmacotherapy: Naloxone.")

adolescents), who are diagnosed with opiate analgesic overdosage/unintentional poisoning should be assessed for suicide risk. If confirmed, or even strongly suspected, referral for appropriate psychiatric/psychotherapeutic intervention and follow-up are indicated.[52] Additionally, the precise related circumstances must be identified to prevent re-occurrence. As indicated, referral to child protective (or family) services and/or law enforcement is usually required.

Pregnancy and Lactation

Adolescent girls and young women, who use opiate analgesics during pregnancy, expose their embryos and fetuses to opiate analgesics. Additionally, adolescent girls and young women, who use opiate analgesics and breastfeed, expose their nursing neonates and infants to opiate analgesics. This section presents and discusses medical and nonmedical prescription opiate analgesic use during pregnancy and lactation with attention to the potential for maternal and fetal/neonatal dependence or use disorder, including the opiate analgesic-induced neonatal abstinence syndrome (NAS) and its management.

PREGNANCY

Although opiate analgesics readily cross the placental barrier, their maternal use during pregnancy has not been directly associated with teratogenesis, or congenital malformations. In fact, the intermittent use of low dosages of opiate analgesics by adolescent girls and young women, who are pregnant, is relatively safe for themselves and their fetuses. Opiate analgesics are also medically used to provide maternal pain relief just prior to, and during labor and delivery—which may result in drowsiness, lethargy, or other expected pharmacologic actions (e.g., constipation; respiratory depression) among neonates.

However, caution is required with regular, long-term maternal use of moderate to high dosages of opiate analgesics during pregnancy because of the risk for: (1) maternal and fetal physical dependence; and—following birth—(2) signs and symptoms of maternal opiate analgesic withdrawal syndrome and opiate analgesic induced-neonatal abstinence syndrome (NAS), which occur as opiate analgesic blood concentrations decrease. For further discussion, see the following subsection discussion, "Opiate Analgesic-Induced Neonatal Abstinence Syndrome."

STATISTICS. Of concern over the new millennium are troubling statistics related to opiate analgesic use by adolescent girls and young women during pregnancy. For example, Heil, Jones, and Arria (2011) found, in their study of a large sample of women who abused opiate analgesics, that 90% had a history of drug abuse treatment admission episodes, and 86% reported having had an "unintended" pregnancy.

In their study of adolescent girls and women of reproductive-age, who were enrolled in Medicaid in selected states in the U.S. during 2008–2012, Ailes, Dawson, and Lind (2015) found that approximately 40% of the women received a prescription for an opiate analgesic from their prescribers. In a similar study of adolescent girls and women of reproductive age (i.e., 15 to 45 years-of-age), who were enrolled in Medicaid during 2008–2013 in New York state, approximately 20% filled a prescription for an opiate analgesic at their neighborhood pharmacy (Gallagher, Shin, & Roohan, 2016).

In another example, Bateman, Hernandez-Diaz, and Rathmell (2014, p. 1216), in a review of data from 534,500 women in the U.S., who completed their pregnancies while enrolled in a commercial insurance plan, found that "76,742 (14.4 %) were dispensed an opiate analgesic (primarily codeine, hydrocodone, and oxycodone) at some point during their pregnancies."

52 The abuse of other psychodepressants (e.g., alcohol; heroin)—as well as the presence of mental depression—has been associated with increased risk for suicide attempts and completions among adolescents (Wong, Zhou, & Goebert, 2013).

As reported by Patrick and Schiff (2017)—on behalf of the American College of Obstetricians and Gynecologists:

> The use of opioids during pregnancy has grown rapidly in the past decade.
>
> (p. e20164070)

And, as noted by Jumah (2016), "opioids are now the most common reason for seeking treatment for illicit substances during pregnancy" (p. 35).

OPIATE ANALGESIC-INDUCED NEONATAL ABSTINENCE SYNDROME (NAS).[53]

> In his first three weeks of life, Brayden suffered through a form of new-born drug dependency called Neonatal Abstinence Syndrome. He trembled and wailed inconsolably, clenching his muscles and sometimes gasping for breath as he went through withdrawal.
>
> (Wilson & Shiffman, 2015, p. 2)

In their two-year study (2010 to 2011) of 242 neonates confirmed as having NAS, Lind, Petersen, and Lederer (2015) found that over 235 of the neonates (i.e., over 97%) required admission to an NICU for an average of 26 days. Fortunately, all the neonates in this study survived.[54]

The occurrence of NAS is significantly increased among neonates whose mothers: (1) regularly abused opiate analgesics during pregnancy; or (2) abused opiate analgesics during the last trimester (Desai, Huybrechts, & Hernandez-Diaz, 2015).[55] As reported by Lind, Petersen, and Lederer (2015), the mothers, who participated in their study of maternal opiate analgesic use during pregnancy, provided the following reasons for their use of opiate analgesics, listed in descending order:[56]

1. Illicit personal use (133 mothers, or 55%);
2. Drug abuse treatment (100 mothers, or 41%);
3. Chronic pain (52 mothers, or 22%);
4. Unknown or unspecified (25 mothers, or 10%).

Of related concern is the consistent observation that the incidence of NAS in the U.S. has increased significantly during the new millennium. For example: Ko, Patrick, and Tong (2016) noted that:

53 Also referred to in the published literature as the "neonatal opioid withdrawal syndrome" (NOWS).

54 However, as in Brayden's case, survival is not equivalent to "happily and safely ever after." As noted in the related NBC/Reuters report:

> Reuters identified 110 cases since 2010 that are similar to Brayden's: Babies and toddlers whose mothers used opioids during pregnancy and who later died preventable deaths.
>
> Being born drug-dependent didn't kill these children. Each recovered enough to be discharged from the hospital. What sealed their fates was being sent home to families ill-equipped to care for them.
>
> Like Brayden, more than 40 of the children suffocated. Thirteen died after swallowing toxic doses of methadone, heroin, oxycodone or other opioids.
>
> (Wilson & Shiffman, 2015, p. 3)

55 Other major health risks for women, who are physically dependent on opiate analgesics, and who are pregnant or breastfeeding—as well as for their developing fetuses or breastfed neonates—are related to the use of illicit opiate analgesics that: (1) contain adulterants; or (2) are self-injected (see the related discussion in the earlier pharmacology subsection, "Undesired, or Harmful, Effects and Toxicities").

56 The total percentage exceeds 100% because some of the mothers provided more than one reason for their opiate analgesic use during pregnancy.

> The overall NAS incidence increased 400% from 1.5 per 1,000 hospital births in 1999, to 6.0 per 1,000 hospital births in 2013.
>
> (p. 799)

Similarly, Sessions Cole, Wegner, and Davis (2017) reported an increasing trend in the number of NAS cases in the U.S. from seven cases/1,000 neonatal intensive care unit admissions in 2004 to 27 cases/1,000 in 2013. The associated reported rates of NAS per 1,000 hospital live births were highest in the states of Vermont (i.e., 33.3 cases) and West Virginia (i.e., 33.4 cases).[57]

In association with the increasing rate of opiate analgesic abuse among adolescent girls and young women in the U.S. during the new millennium, rates of NAS also have significantly increased—as foreseen or expected (Davies, Gilbert, & Johnson, 2016; Pagliaro & Pagliaro, 2000, 2004; Pagliaro & Pagliaro, *Clinical Patient Data Files*).

MAT AND THE PREVENTION OF NAS[58] Various opiate analgesics (e.g., methadone [Dolophine®]) have been used to maintain maternal opiate analgesic dependence (i.e., "medication-assisted treatment" [MAT]) during pregnancy and to decrease the risk for neonatal opiate analgesic physical dependence and associated NAS (e.g., Brown, Hayes, & Thornton, 2015; Logan, Brown, & Hayes, 2013; Osborn, Jeffery, & Cole, 2010a). Currently, it appears that the use of sublingual buprenorphine (Buprenex®), a mixed opiate agonist/antagonist (see earlier discussion), is preferred because it is associated with a significantly:

1. Milder form of the NAS, such as lower incidents of preterm labor and neonatal respiratory distress (Jansson & Velez, 2012; Thomas, Fullerton, & Kim, 2014; Unger, Jagsch, & Jones, 2011; Wilder & Winhusen, 2015);
2. Less severe maternal opiate analgesic physical dependence that is relatively easier to manage than that associated with methadone use (Gaalema, Heil, & Badger, 2013);
3. Longer mean gestational age, larger head circumference, longer body length, and heavier body weight at birth for neonates whose mothers received buprenorphine maintenance

57 These reported increases in the rates of NAS in the U.S. are also consistent with an earlier report by Patrick, Schumacher, and Benneyworth (2012). In their retrospective analysis of a nationally representative sample of newborns with NAS, they found that the rate of incidence increased from 1.20 per 1,000 hospital births in 2000 to 3.39 per 1,000 hospital births in 2009 (p. 1934).

58 N.B. In 2016, the FDA added a "boxed warning" for buprenorphine and methadone products regarding the potential danger of NAS associated with buprenorphine or methadone pharmacotherapy among pregnant adolescent girls and women:

> Since NOWS [(i.e., NAS] can result from in utero exposure to opioids—whether medically authorized or illicit—the risk of NOWS from MAT [medication-assisted treatment] must be balanced against the risk of untreated opioid addiction during pregnancy; an independent advisory committee and numerous reproductive health experts agree this balance is important. If left untreated, illicit opioid use is associated with poor pregnancy outcomes such as low birth weight, preterm birth, or fetal death.
>
> (FDA, 2016b, p. 1)

They go on to note that:

> The FDA's action requiring safety labeling changes for MAT-only methadone and buprenorphine products is intended to appropriately inform prescribers about the risks of NOWS without inadvertently discouraging treatment for pregnant women with opioid addiction.
>
> (FDA, 2016b, p. 1)

pharmacotherapy when compared to neonates whose mothers received methadone maintenance pharmacotherapy during pregnancy (Brogly, Saia, & Walley, 2014);

4. Fewer hospital days for neonates born to mothers who received buprenorphine maintenance pharmacotherapy when compared to mothers who received methadone maintenance pharmacotherapy (Pritham, Paul, & Hayes, 2012).

SIGNS AND SYMPTOMS OF NAS Signs and symptoms of the NAS include: body temperature instability; body weight loss or lower than expected weight gain; dehydration; diaphoresis; diarrhea; disruption of maternal-infant attachment or bonding;[59] exaggerated Moro reflex; excessive crying, usually high-pitched; feeding difficulties (i.e., poor feeding behaviors); hyperreflexia; hyperthermia; increased muscle tone; increased number of stools; irritability; mottling; nasal stuffiness and flaring; piloerection; poor sleep; respiratory distress; seizures; sneezing; tachypnea; tremors; vomiting; and yawning (Hudak & Tan, 2012; Ko, Patrick, & Tong, 2016; Osborn, Jeffery, & Cole, 2010a, 2010b).

MANAGEMENT OF NAS The onset of the NAS is variable, dependent on the half-life of elimination of the opiate analgesic involved (e.g., for heroin, within 24 hours following birth; for methadone, within two to six days following birth). (See the earlier related discussion in the pharmacology subsection, "Pharmacokinetics—Metabolism.")

The intensity of these signs and symptoms does not always reflect the amount or duration of maternal opiate analgesic use during pregnancy. Several researchers (e.g., Cole, Wegner, & Davis, 2017) suggest that neonatal genomic variants—particularly in regard to genes that encode catechol-O-methyltransferase, the mu-opiate analgesic receptor, and prepronociceptin—are associated with significant differences in NAS outcomes (i.e., intensity/ severity; length of hospitalization; and response to pharmacotherapy). Unfortunately, although several genes have been implicated, consensus regarding their significance has not yet been achieved.[60]

The opiate analgesics, methadone and morphine, are widely used for the medical management of neonates experiencing the NAS (e.g., Cramton & Gruchala, 2013; Johnson, Gerada, & Greenough, 2003). However, there is no consensus as to the best approach for its medical management (Pagliaro & Pagliaro, 2002). In addition to methadone and morphine, buprenorphine is also used in the management of the NAS. Recommended dosage schedules, which should be individually adjusted based on the: (1) severity of the NAS; (2) characteristics of the neonate; and (3) clinical response, are presented in Table 5.6.

If a neonate requires additional pharmacotherapy for the medical management of NAS, a sedative-hypnotic may be added to reduce withdrawal severity. In related systematic reviews performed for the Cochrane Database, Osborn, Jeffery, and Cole (2005, 2010a, 2010b) found that the use of a barbiturate (i.e., phenobarbital)—generally using a loading dose of 20 mg/kg

59 Also, see the related discussion in the later subsection, "New Millennial Trends of Adolescent and Young Adult Opiate Analgesic Use—Mothering."

60 Interestingly, Oei, Xu, and Abdel-Latif (2012, p. F193), in their study of the characteristics of dopamine D2 receptor gene (DRD2) polymorphisms in heroin- or methadone-exposed and drug-free control neonates and the relationship to NAS, found that the:

1. A2A2 allele is more common in drug-exposed neonates;
2. 141ins allele is significantly more common in drug-exposed neonates and in drug-free control neonates with less severe postnatal withdrawal.

These findings help to further our understanding of the NAS and its characteristic signs and symptoms as well as its potential mechanisms of action.

Table 5.6 Pharmacotherapy for Managing NAS[61]

Opiate Analgesic	*Initial Dose*	*Maintenance Dose*	*Discontinuing NAS Pharmacotherapy*
Buprenorphine	5 mcg/kg, delivered sublingually with oral dosing syringe placed under the neonate's tongue	As indicated, increase by 1.25 mcg/kg/dose to a maximum of 60 mcg/kg/day	Following three days of stabilization, decrease maintenance dosage by 10% per day and discontinue when dosage has been reduced to 10% of the maintenance dosage
Methadone	0.1 mg/kg/dose orally every 12 hours	As indicated, increase to a maximal dose of 0.5 mg/kg (i.e., 1 mg/kg/day)	Decrease maintenance dosage by 10% every week and discontinue when dosage has been reduced to 0.05 mg/kg/dose
Morphine	0.1 mg/kg/dose orally every four hours	As indicated, increase by 0.025 mg/kg/dose to a maximum of 1.25 mg/kg/day	Decrease maintenance dosage by 10% per day and discontinue when dosage has been reduced to 0.15 mg/kg/dose

Sources: Cramton & Gruchala (2013); Kocherlakota (2014); Kraft, Adeniyi-Jones, & Chervoneva (2017); Kraft, Dysart, & Greenspan (2011).

and a maintenance dose of 2.5 mg/kg every 12 hours, as indicated by clinical response—provided superior results when compared to a benzodiazepine (i.e., diazepam) in terms of the "reduction in treatment failure." We, too, have endorsed this approach in the context of managing seizures associated with NAS (see, for example, Lemke, 2002). Additionally, clonidine (i.e., 0.5–1 mcg/kg/dose orally ingested every four to six hours) has been used as an adjunct to the selected pharmacotherapy for NAS (e.g., Agthe, Kim, & Mathias, 2009; Broome & So, 2011; Cramton & Gruchala, 2013).[62]

Related Professional Reminder: ***Clearly, health and social care professionals require accurate knowledge about opiate analgesic use by pregnant adolescent girls and young women and the potential effects on their developing embryos/fetuses. They also require accurate knowledge regarding the related postnatal effects on these adolescent girls and young women and their neonates and infants. In this context, health and social care professionals would be well-advised to heed the cautionary advice of Krans and Patrick (2016) and others (e.g., Pagliaro & Pagliaro, 2018) to be sensitive to and cognizant of the fears of pregnant adolescent girls and young women, that disclosing their use of opiate analgesics, or other drugs and substances of abuse, may place them at risk for related negative consequences, including criminal charges, the***

61 Naloxone should always be readily available for use in case of opiate analgesic overdosage.

62 In the U.S., the mean hospital stay for infants with NAS is 17 days, usually in a NICU (Ko, Wolicki, & Barfield, 2017).

need to surrender their infant to social care authorities, and other consequences that can prevent them from seeking beneficial prenatal and postnatal health care services as needed.

LACTATION

Intermittent use of low dosages of opiate analgesics is relatively safe for mothers who are breastfeeding their neonates and infants. However, opiate analgesics have been detected in breast milk in amounts that can cause expected pharmacologic actions in neonates and infants (e.g., CNS depression; constipation; hypoventilation). Neonates and infants may also develop opiate analgesic physical dependence and are at risk for experiencing the opiate analgesic withdrawal syndrome if maternal use of opiate analgesics, or breastfeeding, is abruptly discontinued.

Generally, we recommend that adolescent girls and young women, who are breastfeeding, should not use opiate analgesics, or, alternatively, should discontinue breastfeeding (Pagliaro & Pagliaro, 2012; 2018). However, there are other perspectives on this topic.

For example, Welle-Strand, Skurtveit, and Jansson (2013, p. 1060), in a national cohort study of 124 Norwegian women treated with either methadone of buprenorphine maintenance pharmacotherapy during pregnancy, found that "breast fed neonates exposed to methadone prenatally had significantly lower incidence of NAS requiring pharmacotherapy (53% vs. 80%)."[63]

New Millennial Trends

During the new millennium, the use of "prescription" (e.g., oxycodone) and "non-prescription" (e.g., heroin) opiate analgesics increased significantly among adolescents and young adults with the licit use of prescription drugs often preceding the illicit use of heroin. This section presents and discusses: (1) commonly used prescription opiate analgesics and trends in their use, including their medical and nonmedical, or illicit/recreational, use; and (2) heroin and trends in its use, including adolescent and young adult illicit drug involvement. We begin with the prescription opiate analgesics.

Commonly Used Prescription Opiate Analgesics

The four prescription opiate analgesics that are most commonly abused during the new millennium by adolescents and young adults—from highest to lowest—are:

1. Oxycodone;
2. Hydrocodone;
3. Buprenorphine;
4. Fentanyl.

Each of these prescription opiate analgesics are presented and discussed in the following sections along with trends in their use.

Oxycodone

Oxycodone (OxyContin®) is one of the most widely abused prescription opiate analgesics in the U.S. (Cicero, Inciardi, & Munoz, 2005). Illicitly used to primarily achieve euphoric

63 The confounding variable in this study and conclusions drawn regarding NAS, are the potential residual effects of prenatal methadone exposure—in the absence of subsequent breastfeeding (i.e., the slow reduction in neonatal methadone blood concentrations). In addition, several researchers (e.g., Cramton & Gruchala, 2013; Hudak & Tan, 2012) have found that breastfeeding alone—as an alternative nonpharmacological treatment intervention—may have an ameliorating effect on the severity of NAS.

effects, or a "rush," and to prevent or manage the opiate analgesic withdrawal syndrome, use and associated toxicities "skyrocketed" during the 1990s and have remained high ever since. It has been estimated that, during the new millennium, 99% of the world's production of oxycodone, as well as hydrocodone, was consumed in the U.S. (Winstock, 2016).

The extended-release formulation of oxycodone, "OxyContin®," was approved by the FDA in 1995. Although initially considered to have a lower abuse potential because of its slow-release properties—and marketed as such—its widespread use began in 2000 and continued throughout the first decade of the new millennium. Almost immediately, users discovered that crushing and "snorting" the extended-release tablets enabled them to achieve a rapid release of the OxyContin® and resultant high blood oxycodone concentrations (Aquina, Marques-Baptista, & Bridgeman, 2009; Cicero, Inciardi, & Munoz, 2005; Pagliaro & Pagliaro, 2009). In 2010, the most potent strength tablet of OxyContin® (i.e., 160 mg) was discontinued and a new formulation was introduced that made crushing and dissolving the extended-release tablets more difficult (MacLaren, 2015). These changes resulted in only a temporary and moderate degree of success in terms of decreasing OxyContin® abuse.[64]

During the first decade of the new millennium, the use of oxycodone was highest in rural and suburban regions of the Western U.S. (Cicero, Surratt, & Inciardi, 2007). In an earlier study, Carise, Dugosh, and McLellan (2007) analyzed data obtained from approximately 28,000 participants, who were admitted to 157 addiction treatment programs in the U.S., from 2001 to 2004. The researchers found that approximately 5% used OxyContin® predominantly obtained from nonmedical sources. In a later study comparing past-year Oxy-Contin® users to past-year users of other opiate analgesic, Martins, Storr, and Zhu (2009) found that OxyContin® users were more likely to be 18 to 25 years-of-age and to have a concurrent mental health problem.

More recently, in an analysis of trends in the nonmedical use of Oxy Contin® in the U.S. —from 2000 to 2013—Jones, Muhuri, and Lurie (2017) found that:

> In 2013, the percentage of past-year nonmedical use of OxyContin® among people 12 years of age and older in the United States was 0.5%.
>
> (p. 452)

Johnston, Miech, and O'Malley (2018) found that past-year oxycodone use among high school students, based on self-reports, was 2.7% in 2017.

Hydrocodone

Hydrocodone (e.g., Hycodan®; Hysingla ER®; Vicodin®), like oxycodone, is another prescription opiate analgesic that is widely used in the U.S. (Cicero, Inciardi, & Munoz, 2005). It is a semisynthetic opiate analgesic that can be derived from a number of precursors, including: codeine, morphine, and thebaine. Hydrocodone is extensively metabolized in the liver, primarily by CYP3A4, to several metabolites, including the active metabolite, hydromorphone.

Hydrocodone is most commonly used by young adults of European descent, 20 to 40 years-of-age (Pagliaro & Pagliaro, 2009). In their analysis of data from the Researched Abuse Diversion and Addiction-Related Surveillance (RADARS®) System, Zosel, Bucher Bartelson, and Bailey (2013) found that the most frequently abused prescription drug was hydrocodone. Of the over 16,000 intentional exposures of adolescents (i.e., 13 to 19 years-of-age) to the various prescription drugs and substances of abuse, 32% involved hydrocodone.

64 In August of 2015, the FDA approved the use of extended-release oxycodone for adolescents, 11 to 16 years of age, who experienced "pain severe enough to require daily, around-the-clock, long-term opioid treatment for which alternative treatment options are inadequate" (Yang, Chen, & Bennett, 2016, p. 1).

Between 2014 and 2015, the FDA approved two "extended-release" formulations of hydrocodone—Hysingla ER® and Zohydro ER®—for the medical management of chronic, severe pain (Extended-Release, 2014, 2015). To address the potential risk for the abuse of these products, they were formulated with several "abuse-deterrent" properties. For example, whether the tablets were coarsely or finely ground, the resultant powder was formulated to fall out of the nostrils when intranasally insufflated, or "snorted." In addition, when attempts were made to dissolve the tablets for IV injection, a viscous gel is formed that is difficult to inject. As part of a *Risk Evaluation and Mitigation Strategy* (REMS) program, the FDA also mandated that pharmaceutical manufacturers make training programs for the optimal use of these formulations available to prescribers. However, despite these efforts, Johnston, Miech, and O'Malley (2018) found that 2% of high school seniors self-reported past year use of Vicodin® (i.e., combination hydrocodone and acetaminophen) for 2017.

Buprenorphine

Buprenorphine (Buprenex®) is a synthetic opiate analgesic that was synthesized in the late 1970s for the medical management of moderate to severe pain. Acting primarily as an agonist, it has a high affinity to bind to, and slowly separate from, mu receptors. Consequently, buprenorphine produces expected opiate analgesic agonist effects, particularly at low to moderate dosages. However, at higher dosages, it can reach a ceiling effect and, subsequently, acts as an opiate analgesic antagonist (Buprenorphine, 2016).

Buprenorphine also acts as an antagonist at kappa receptors. Because of its mixed agonist/antagonist actions, it is FDA approved for the medical management of acute opiate analgesic detoxification, stabilization, and long-term maintenance of resumed nonuse of opiate analgesics (Connery, 2015; Greenwald, Comer, & Fiellin, 2014; Hard, 2014; Soyka, 2015)—including among adolescents and young adults (e.g., Chang, Klimas, & Wood, 2018; Hadland), Wharam, & Schuster, 2017; Saloner, Feder, & Krawczyk, 2017; Subramaniam, Warden, & Minhajuddin, 2011) (see the related discussion in the later "Pharmacotherapy" section). Naloxone (see the related discussion in the earlier pharmacology section, "Undesired, or Harmful, Effects and Toxicities—Opiate Analgesic Overdosage/Unintentional Poisoning") is often combined with a sublingual formulation of buprenorphine (e.g., Suboxone®, sublingual film; Zubsolv®, sublingual tablet) to minimize the risk for buprenorphine diversion or abuse (Smith, Bailey, & Woody, 2007)—in particular, that associated with IV use.

However, combination buprenorphine and naloxone is used in the U.S.—primarily to self-manage the signs and symptoms of the opiate analgesic withdrawal syndrome (Schuman-Oilivier, Albanese, & Nelson, 2010; Yokell, Zaller, & Green, 2011). Those, who use buprenorphine, tend to be younger and of European descent (Pagliaro & Pagliaro, *Clinical Patient Data Files*). Among buprenorphine users, who seek drug and substance abuse treatment in the U.S., 6% reported injecting buprenorphine to get "high" (Cicero, Surratt, & Inciardi, 2007). Interestingly, as might be expected, buprenorphine users are more likely to be "injection drug users," while those who use the buprenorphine/naloxone combination product are more likely to be "non-injection drug users" (Bazazi, Yokell, & Fu, 2011; Pagliaro & Pagliaro, *Clinical Patient Data Files*). Dart (2011) found that 45.5% of "intravenous" buprenorphine users and 16.3 % of combination buprenorphine/naloxone users reported use within the previous month.

The abuse of buprenorphine, particularly, combination buprenorphine/naloxone, is significantly limited in the U.S. by the ready availability—"on-the-street"—of high-quality heroin. As found by Cicero, Ellis, and Surratt (2014b):

> Buprenorphine is rarely preferred for its inherent euphorigenic properties, but rather serves as a substitute for other drugs, particularly heroin, or as a drug used, preferable to methadone, to self-medicate withdrawal sickness or wean off opioids.
>
> (p. 98)

Fentanyl

Fentanyl is an extremely potent prescription opiate analgesic that is 50 to 100 times more potent than morphine (see Table 5.1). It is currently approved by the FDA for the management of surgical/postoperative pain, severe pain, and breakthrough cancer pain.

Fentanyl is licitly available in eight different formulations in various dosages that are produced by pharmaceutical manufacturers and dispensed by pharmacists:

1. Soluble buccal film (Onsolis®);
2. Effervescent buccal tablet (Fentora®), that uses the OraVescent® drug delivery system;
3. Injectable formulation for intramuscular or intravenous use (Sublimaze®);
4. Intranasal spray (Lazanda®), available in both aqueous solution and pectin-based mucus-adhesive system;
5. Sublingual spray (Subsys®);
6. Sublingual tablet (Abstral®; Vellofent®);
7. Transdermal delivery system (Duragesic®), designed to continuously deliver a specific dosage of fentanyl over a period of 72 hours (i.e., "fentanyl patch"), as well as, a relatively newer "iontophoretic transdermal" system (Ionsys®);
8. Transmucosal lozenge for buccal absorption (Actiq®), a solid drug matrix on a handle (i.e., "fentanyl lollipop"), that, in the event of signs and symptoms of overdosage, facilitates removal of the lozenge from the mouth.

Fentanyl is less often prescribed for non-hospitalized, or outpatients, because of its high potency and associated risk for overdosage. However, illicitly manufactured fentanyl is readily available and easily obtained "on the street" in the U.S.—the current primary source for this "prescription" opiate analgesic. In this context of use, illicitly produced fentanyl is:

1. Generally produced in China—or in the U.S. from precursor chemicals that are predominantly manufactured in, and imported from, China;
2. Almost always clandestinely mixed with street heroin by opiate analgesic dealers prior to its sale—without the consent, or knowledge, of the buyer/user (Gladden, Martinez, & Seth, 2016; Pagliaro & Pagliaro, *Clinical Patient Data Files*; Peterson, Gladden, & Delcher, 2016);
3. Also produced in Mexico, it is usually transported—often by mail—across the U.S./ Mexican border, where it is distributed throughout the U.S. by Mexican transnational drug cartels (e.g., the Sinaloa Cartel);
4. Bought and sold, at the "wholesale" level, in 10-gram units that are vernacularly referred to as "fingers."

Fentanyl, because of its potency and variety of available formulations, has been widely abused in the U.S. It also is often: (1) added to heroin to increase the potency and "kick" of heroin; and (2) falsely represented and sold as alprazolam, hydrocodone, oxycodone, and other drugs and substances of abuse. As noted by the NIDA, "The fake pills are much cheaper than the real versions" (NIDA, 2016, p. 1).

More importantly, because buyers are generally unaware of what they are purchasing, "hundreds of people have overdosed on fentanyl across the nation since 2013, often because of using heroin that has been 'laced' with the much stronger substance [i.e., fentanyl]" (NIDA, 2015b, p. 1). Consequently, drug-related overdosages have significantly increased during the second decade of the new millennium (see related discussion in the earlier subsection, "Opiate Analgesic Overdosage"). As reported by Seth, Scholl, and Rudd (2018), the fentanyl-related deaths increased 100% in the U.S. from 2015 to 2016. O'Donnell, Halpin, and Mattson (2017), in their analysis for the CDC of "5,152 opioid-overdosage deaths in 10 states during July-December 2016," found that over 50% involved fentanyl (p. 1197).[65]

A warning shared by a current heroin user in regard to fentanyl use:

> Be careful. It's got a lotta bodies on it [i.e., it's so strong its killing people].
>
> (Carroll, Marshall, & Rich, 2017, pp. 136–137)

We now turn to heroin.

Heroin—Sources, Distribution, and Use

Sources and Distribution of Opium and Heroin

Opium cultivation and heroin production are higher than ever. Transshipped from Asia to Colombia and, finally, to the U.S. for distribution at specified geographical locations, heroin is readily available in both higher concentrations and purity than at any other time in history (Ciccarone, 2009).[66] In addition, over the new millennium, opium has been increasingly grown and heroin has been increasingly produced in South America (e.g., Republic of Colombia) for use in the U.S. Its distribution and commerce in the U.S. is largely controlled by ethnically defined criminal gangs.[67]

Thus, across the U.S., during the new millennium, the ready availability of purer, powdered heroin, rather than the more commonly available, and less pure black-tar heroin, resulted in:

1. Increased accessibility to heroin;
2. Lower street cost per dose;

65 N.B. Because of its physical characteristics, it is much easier to add fentanyl to powdered heroin (e.g., "china white") than to "black tar heroin"—which is a significantly less refined "tarry, opium-like substance." Consequently, fentanyl overdosages are much more likely to occur in areas of the U.S. where powdered heroin is predominantly available (e.g., east coast) and less common in areas of the U.S. where "black tar heroin" is predominantly available (e.g., southwest). As found by a young adult heroin user who wanted to avoid fentanyl use because of its associated increased risk for fatal overdosage:

> Black tar heroin I feel safer doing. It's harder to cut. It's not powder. Powder you can add anything to . . . Black tar heroin, in order to cut it, you have to do all this stuff to it, cook it, and it's a lot harder to cut, so I feel safer doing that.
>
> (Carroll, Marshall, & Rich, 2017, p. 140)

66 The average concentration of injectable forms of heroin at street level, is approximately 10% to 27%–in comparison to approximately 7% during the 1980s. The purity of street-level Colombian heroin typically ranges from 25% to 80% pure, while Mexican black tar heroin typically ranges from 14% to 60% pure with the highest purity found in cities along the U.S./Mexico border (e.g., El Paso, Texas) (Pagliaro & Pagliaro, 2012). Heroin purity, at street level, varies significantly in the U.S. from city to city and from time to time—depending upon availability and demand (Pagliaro & Pagliaro, *Clinical Patient Data Files*). For example, in 2008 heroin street level purity in San Francisco was reported as 8.5% while in Philadelphia it was reported as 60% (Mars, Bourgois, & Karandinos, 2014).

67 For example: the importation and distribution of heroin in Seattle Washington is mostly controlled by Chinese gangs; a significant amount of the retail-level heroin distribution and sales along the northeastern coast is controlled by Dominican gangs, based primarily in New York City; most of the importation and distribution of heroin from Mexico into the Southwestern U.S. is controlled by Mexican gangs (e.g., "Sinaloa Cowboys"); much of the smuggling of heroin into the U.S. from southeastern Asia is by Nigerian gangs, based primarily in Chicago; and much of the distribution of Asian heroin that is transshipped through the Port of Los Angeles is controlled by Thai gangs (National Drug Intelligence Center, 2001; Pagliaro & Pagliaro, 2009, 2012; Pagliaro & Pagliaro, *Clinical Patient Data Files*).

3. Increased intranasal use (i.e., "sniffing;" "snorting");
4. Increased use among adolescents and young adults.

(e.g., Pagliaro & Pagliaro, 2004; Pagliaro & Pagliaro, *Clinical Patient Data Files*; Tarabar & Nelson, 2003)

In a related study, using 55,940 young adults, 18 to 25 years-of-age—from the 2011–2013 *National Survey on Drug use and Health*—Ihongbe and Masho (2016, p. 74) found that: (1) approximately 20% self-reported lifetime heroin use; and (2) the single most common method of heroin use was "sniffing."

A re-emerging trend from the 1970s is the more casual, non-intravenous, non-daily, social use of heroin. During the 1970s, this pattern of use was often referred to as "chipping." Rather than intravenously injecting, or "mainlining," the heroin, it was injected SC, in much the same way as insulin is injected by people with diabetes. However, adolescents and young adults, who are "casual" heroin users, are still more likely to "chase the dragon" (i.e., smoke their heroin).

They also are more likely to intranasally insufflate, or "snort," their heroin (Katz, Dart, & Bailey, 2011; Pagliaro & Pagliaro, 2009, 2012; Stern, 2011). Adolescents and young adults may also use transmucosal opiate analgesic nasal sprays, or what is known on the street as, "heroin nose drops." Consequently, during the new millennium, approximately 60% of users administered their heroin by non-IV routes (e.g., Pagliaro & Pagliaro, 2004, 2012).

Particularly troubling is the noted change, during the new millennium, in the attitudes of adolescents and young adults toward the use of opiate analgesics, including heroin and its non-oral routes of administration—for which there is an apparent increasingly tacit acceptance that now ranks with "snorting a line of coke" or "smoking a joint" (Pagliaro & Pagliaro, *Clinical Patient Data Files*). The use of illicit prescription opiate analgesics, and their prelude to illicit heroin use significantly intensified during the new millennium, particularly among adolescents and young adults (e.g., Pagliaro & Pagliaro, *Clinical Patient Data Files*; Sharma, Bruner, & Barnett, 2016). In their study of subjects, who had used heroin within the previous four months, Peavy, Banta-Green, and Kingston (2012) found that "39% reported being 'hooked on' prescription-type opioids first" (p. 259). Additionally, as noted by Novak, Bluthenthal, and Wenger (2016):

> Individuals born after 1980 were more likely than were individuals born before 1980 to initiate opioids through nonmedical use of prescription opioids than heroin.
>
> (p. 298)

In their study of nonmedical prescription "opioid" (NMPO) use and heroin use among adolescents and young adults, 12 to 34 years-of-age, Martins, Segura, and Santaella-Tenoria (2017) found that, between 2002 and 2014:

> There was a four-fold and nine-fold increase over time in the odds of heroin use among emerging adults and young adults who were NMPO users, respectively.
>
> (p. 236)

Common Misbelief: The typical opiate analgesic "addict" in the U.S. is a young man of non-European descent, with a criminal history, and who is often "on welfare" or "living on the street."

This belief is simply not true. As identified by Cicero, Ellis, and Surratt (2014a):

> The abuse of heroin has migrated from low-income urban areas with large minority populations to more affluent suburban and rural areas with primarily white populations. (p. 821)

During the new millennium, adolescents and young adults, generally used opiate analgesics to achieve such desired psychodepressant effects as:

1. Extreme euphoria;
2. Warm "rush;"
3. Sleepy, dream-like state ("being on-the-nod").

Less commonly, they also used heroin for, (4) pain relief (see related discussion in the later subsection regarding opiate analgesic use among adolescent athletes [i.e., "Medical/Non-medical Use in the Contexts of Sports Injuries"]). Many adolescents and young adults also abuse heroin and other illicit prescription opiate analgesics to, (5) prevent, or self-manage, the undesired effects associated with the opiate analgesic withdrawal syndrome (see the previous section in this chapter, "Pharmacology, Undesired, or Harmful, Effects and Toxicities: Physical and Psychological Dependence—Opiate Analgesic Withdrawal Syndrome").

During the second decade of the new millennium, it was commonly recognized—by both government agencies and drug and substance abuse professionals—that a growing heroin epidemic was impacting states across the U.S. with rates of heroin addiction and overdosage increasing at alarming rates, particularly in Indiana, Kentucky and New Jersey (Whitman, 2015).

Amidst this growing epidemic of heroin use, a new phenomenon—the general increasing acceptance of adolescent and young adult heroin use, be it intranasal insufflation (i.e., "snorting"), pulmonary inhalation (i.e., "smoking"), or IV injection (i.e., "mainlining"). In this context, adolescents and young adults found themselves in a unique situation, in which:

1. Heroin is readily available;
2. Heroin use is not generally "frowned upon" (i.e., commonly viewed in a pejorative manner)—as it had been during the decades preceding the new millennium.

Additionally, the rapid rise in heroin use, in the U.S. during the new millennium, has been largely due to the "unanticipated consequences" of government interventions[68] set in the context of a "perfect storm" (i.e., the convergence of several individual factors that, together, strongly encouraged and supported increases in heroin use). As reported by the National Institute on Drug Abuse (NIDA, 2014):

> For a few years, NIDA and other Federal partners have been sounding the alarm over the rise in heroin use, particularly among people with addictions to prescription opioids who switch to heroin because it is cheaper and easier to obtain. Half a million Americans are

68 Specifically, responding to an epidemic of opiate analgesic use, the FDA issued several rules, and Congress passed several laws, intended to limit the illicit production, and often inappropriate over-prescription, of opiate analgesics, particularly oxycodone (OxyContin®). (See the related discussion in the earlier section, "Commonly Used Prescription Opiate Analgesics–Oxycodone").

> now addicted to heroin, and four out of five recent heroin initiates had previously used prescription opioids non-medically.
>
> (p. 1)

Similarly, Case and Deaton (2015) noted that:

> Tighter controls on opioid prescription brought some substitution into heroin and, in this period, the U.S. saw falling prices and rising quality of heroin, as well as availability in areas where heroin had been previously largely unknown.
>
> (p. 15081)

As shared by Mars, Bourgois, and Karandinos (2014), in their ethnographic study of transitions from "opioid pills to heroin injecting" in Philadelphia and San Francisco:

> From accounts of younger/recent heroin injectors in this study, it is evident that since the rise of the opioid pill epidemic, the barriers to heroin use and to injection have been reduced by the normalized pervasiveness of these pharmaceuticals. The widespread availability of opioid analgesics outside sanctioned channels and, paradoxically, medical and regulatory attempts to curb this through monitoring and limiting prescribing, appear to be drawing a new generation into higher risk heroin injecting. Unlike those substances previously labeled "gateway drugs," opioid pills seem to have a direct relationship with progression to heroin initiation.
>
> (p. 264)

The consequence is significantly increased opiate analgesic use, particularly heroin use—both IN and IV. For example, several researchers found that approximately 1.5% of U.S. high school seniors, currently enrolled in and attending school, reported "lifetime heroin use" (Boyd, Young, & McCabe, 2014; Martins, Segura, & Santaella-Tenoria, 2017; Palamar, Shearston, & Dawson, 2016; Wu & Howard, 2007). (See also the related discussion of opiate analgesic use by high school athletes in the later subsection, "Medical/Nonmedical Use in the Context of Sports Injuries.")

During the new millennium, several characteristic behaviors were identified that favor injectable heroin use. For example, Wu and Howard (2007), in a National survey of U.S. adolescents, 12 to 17 years-of-age, found that:

> Adolescent drug users who were females, school dropouts, whites, or delinquents had significantly increased odds of heroin use.
>
> (p. 265)

In addition, it was identified that adolescent girls and young women, who have used heroin, are more likely than adolescent boys and young men to:

- Have a current sexual partner who injects heroin intravenously;
- Have received their first intravenous injection of heroin from their sexual partner;
- Have their heroin intravenously injected by their sexual partner;
- Be influenced to intravenously self-inject their own heroin by encouragement/pressure exerted from their sexual partner;
- Inject their heroin, or other opiate analgesics, first thing in the morning.

(Back, Lawson, & Singleton, 2011; Pagliaro & Pagliaro, *Clinical Patient Data Files*; Pagliaro, Pagliaro, & Thauberger, 1993)

A decade into the new millennium, Holscher, Reissner, and Di Furia (2010) identified that there was no gender difference between men and women in the U.S. regarding the age of onset of regular, long-term heroin use.[69] Attracted to the opiate analgesics when offered by a sexual partner, friend, or acquaintance, many adolescent girls and young women become "hooked" and continue to seek and use opiate analgesics in an effort to obtain their desired effects.

> KB is a 16 yo WF [white female] from a suburban area. She was raised by her grandmother after her mother died of a heroin overdose. Her 21 yo brother is in a methadone treatment program . . . Last year she started seeing a 23 yo man who introduced her to heroin, first nasal then injection . . . EMS was called to her school because she was unresponsive; she was resuscitated with naloxone. She spent the night in an emergency room and was transferred to inpatient substance treatment. She reported daily injection heroin use.
>
> (Sharma, Bruner, & Barnett, 2016, p. 485)

Pooling data from the annual *National Survey on Drug Use and Health* (NSDUH) for 2002 through 2011, Muhuri, Gfroerer, and Davies (2013) found that the:

> Heroin incidence rate was 19 times higher among those who reported prior nonmedical pain reliever [i.e., prescription opiate analgesic] use than those who did not.
>
> (p. 1)

Heroin is often used in place of prescription opiate analgesics, particularly by adolescents and young adults of European continental descent[70] residing in suburban and rural areas because it is "more readily accessible and much less expensive" (Cicero, Ellis, & Surratt, 2014a, p. 821). This finding has been reaffirmed by several others (e.g., Jones, Logan, & Gladden, 2015; Martins, Sarvet, & Sanaella-Tenorio, 2017).

> Sean O'Conner [a teenager of European continental descent from a working middle class family] had what he considers an enjoyable, average childhood, but this did not stop him from becoming a heroin addict in high school.
>
> (Calefati, 2008, p. 1)

Medical Use of Prescription Opiate Analgesics

Prescription opiate analgesics are medically prescribed for children, adolescents, and young adults for various reasons:[71]

69 Research in this area often presents seemingly contradictory results (i.e., that men still significantly outnumber women in terms of heroin use in the U.S.). However, these apparent discrepancies are largely related to study design and sampling procedures (e.g., sampling within specific ethnic communities or specific age groups; variable definitions of heroin use from daily use to lifetime use).

70 A noted exception are young adults of Hispanic descent (Pagliaro & Pagliaro, *Clinical Patient Data Files*; Park & Bloch, 2016). As noted by Park and Bloch (2016):

> Heroin addiction has been "passed down from generation to generation in small cities around New Mexico" by "grandparents who have been heroin users for years, and it is passed down to younger generations; its almost like a way of life."
>
> (p. 7)

(See also the related discussion in the following subsection, "Adolescents and Young Adults of Hispanic Descent.")

71 Although opiate analgesics are capable of inducing sleep, they are not generally used for this indication because of their high potential for physical and psychological dependence and the availability of the safer and more effective sedative-hypnotic drugs (see Chapter 6, "Prescription Sedative-Hypnotics").

1. Treatment of severe, nonproductive cough;
2. Management of diarrhea;
3. Preoperative sedation;
4. Relief of moderate to severe pain due to, for example, injury, surgery, or cancer.

The medical prescription of opiate analgesics grew exponentially over the first two decades of the new millennium. As reported by Manchikanti (2007, p. 399):

> Opioid pill prescribing grew 533% from 1997–2005 with hydrocodone becoming the leading prescribed medication and oxycodone the top retailed opioid by weight in the United States.

Regarding the prescription of opiate analgesics for adolescents, 12 to 17 years-of-age, and young adults, the American Society of Addiction Medicine reported that:

> The prescribing rates for prescription opioids among adolescents and young adults nearly doubled from 1994 to 2007.
>
> (ASAM, 2016, p. 2)

> From 2002 to 2004, the prevalence of prescription opioid use disorder significantly increased among emerging adults aged 18–25 (11.98% to 15.11%), and likewise from 2002 to 2014 among young adults aged 26–34 (11.27% to 23.52%).
>
> (Martins, Segura, & Santaella-Tenoria, 2017, p. 238)

While much of this growth was due to the medical management of moderate to severe cancer pain, it also was due to the largely inappropriate management of chronic, nonmalignant pain.

> Americans, constituting only 4.6% of the world's population, have been consuming 80% of the global opioid supply, and 99% of the global hydrocodone supply.
>
> (Manchikanti & Singh, 2008, p. 563)

The pharmaceutical industry, specifically the "$13 billion-a-year opioid industry" has been not only complicit, but has played a major, direct, contributing role in initiating and sustaining the new millennial opiate analgesic epidemic in the U.S. (e.g., AP, 2018; Hadland, Cerda, & Li, 2018; Haffajee & Mello, 2017; Pagliaro & Pagliaro, *Clinical Patient Data Files*). The manufacturers of prescription opiate analgesics (e.g., Purdue Pharma L. P.—the manufacturer of OxyContin®) used several specific advertising techniques to increase the demand for and sustain the use of opiate analgesics in the U.S. starting in the mid-1990s and continuing throughout the new millennium (e.g., Lyapustina & Alexander, 2015; Pagliaro & Pagliaro, *Clinical Patient Data Files*). These techniques included:

1. Advocacy for increased prescribing of opiate analgesics for chronic pain management;
2. Advertising that deliberately minimized/omitted concerns regarding physical and psychological dependence;
3. Aggressive marketing (promotion campaigns), including the use of: free patient samples; gifts for prescribers; and all-expense paid CE programs/symposia;
4. An unprecedented increase in production—that far exceeded the amounts required to fill legitimate prescription needs in the U.S.

In partial response to the continuing and escalating epidemic of prescribed opiate analgesic use, the CDC released new guidelines for the prescription of opiate analgesics (Dowell, Haegerich, & Chou, 2016). In a follow-up investigation of "long-term opioid use"—which was based on the *CDC Guideline for Prescribing Opioids for Chronic Pain*—Shah, Hayes, and Martin (2017) found that:

> In a representative sample of opioid naïve, cancer-free adults who received a prescription for opioid pain relievers, the likelihood of chronic opioid use increased with each additional day of medication supplied starting with the third day ... The highest probability of continued opioid use at 1 and 3 years was observed among patients who started on a long-acting opioid ...
>
> (p. 265)

In a large international study, Winstock (2016) found that prescription opiate analgesic use was highest in the U.S. He also reported a somewhat unexpected finding for which he provided a related recommendation:

> Our study showed that less than 50% of patients in receipt of prescription opioids had ever been warned about the risks of addiction, so [as a request to his medical colleagues], please have that conversation upfront when you start prescribing. Informed patients are safer patients.
>
> (p. 19)

Nonmedical Use of Prescription Opiate Analgesics

As reported by the SAMHSA (2009), based on national data:

> Nearly 2 million individuals in the U.S. have opioid abuse or dependence, with the majority reporting abuse of prescription opioids.
>
> (p. 1)

Generally, most adolescents and young adults appropriately use opiate analgesics as prescribed by their physicians for the management of acute pain and other indications (e.g., diarrhea; nonproductive cough) and do not develop harmful patterns of use. However, other adolescents and young adults inappropriately use prescribed opiate analgesics by using them more frequently and in larger amounts than prescribed (e.g., Zosel, Bucher Bartelson, & Bailey, 2013). Additionally, still others illicitly obtain and nonmedically use prescription opiate analgesics. As identified by McCabe, Boyd, and Cranford (2009), in their representative national sample of 12,441 high school seniors:

> More than 1 in every 10 high school seniors reported nonmedical use of prescription opioids and 45% of past-year nonmedical users reported "to relieve physical pain" as an important motivation.
>
> (p. 739)

These adolescents and young adults often progress to a pattern of compulsive use—a particularly harmful pattern of use (see related discussion in Chapter 1, "Alcohol") that is associated with physical and psychological dependence or use disorder. As emphasized by Sharma, Bruner, and Barnett (2016):

> Opiate use has devastating consequences for youth and their families, including: progression to full addiction, severe psychosocial impairment, HCV and HIV transmission with injection use, exacerbation of co-occurring psychiatric disorders, overdose, and death.
>
> (p. 487)

Similarly, Jordan, Blackburn, and Des Jarlais (2017) noted that:

> Misuse of prescription opioids has played an important role in national increases of fatal and non-fatal overdose, heroin use and injection, and HIV and HCV infection among young people.
>
> (p. 31)

During the new millennium, the medical prescription of opiate analgesics significantly increased among every demographic in the U.S. (Brady, McCauley, & Back, 2016; Pagliaro & Pagliaro, 2009; Pagliaro & Pagliaro, *Clinical Patient Data Files*). Specific patient factors related to the medical prescription, and subsequent abuse of prescription opiate analgesics, include:

- Chronic, noncancer pain, including arthritis and back pain;
- Concurrent affective disorders (e.g., depression);
- Current, acute moderate to severe pain;
- History of alcohol abuse;
- Inability to fall and/or stay asleep;
- Increased severity of pain;
- Parental nonmedical opiate analgesic use.[72]

(e.g., Barth, Moran-Santa Maria, & Lawson, 2013; Jamison, Ross, & Michna, 2010; Shah, Hayes, & Martin, 2017; Tsui, Herman, & Kettavong, 2010)

In the U.S., young adults, particularly those who have several of these factors, are significantly more likely to engage in the practice of "double-doctoring," or "physician shopping." This practice is commonly used by young adults to obtain multiple opiate analgesic prescriptions from several different prescribers for the same medical condition (e.g., back pain—real or feigned). In a comprehensive study of data obtained from over 146 million opioid prescriptions dispensed by 76% of U.S. retail pharmacies during 2008, McDonald and Carlson (2013) found that "doctor shoppers:"

- Comprised approximately 1% of all prescription purchases;
- On average, obtained 32 prescriptions for opiate analgesics;
- On average, filled their prescriptions for opiate analgesics at 10 different pharmacies;
- Bought approximately 2% of all opiate analgesic prescriptions (4% of "weighed amounts;")
- Often paid for their prescriptions in cash to avoid detection.

In addition, as identified by Stanos, Bruckenthal, and Barkin (2012):

> A study of prescription opioid abusers in a drug rehabilitation program found that 80% tampered with opioid tablets to accelerate drug release by chewing the tablet or by administering the drug intranasally or intravenously.
>
> (p. 683)

72 Griesler, Hu, and Wall (2019), in their analysis of data from 35,000 parent-adolescent (12 to 17 years-of-age) dyads in the U.S., found that, after controlling for other factors, "parental nonmedical prescription opioid use was associated with adolescent nonmedical prescription opioid use" (p. e20182354). Interestingly, this effect was particularly significant in relation to "mothers" use—in comparison to "fathers" use.

Medical/Nonmedical Use in the Context of Sports Injuries

A related and tragic senario observed among adolescents and young adults, which has become acutely exacerbated during the new millennium, is the prescription of opiate analgesics to help manage both acute and chronic pain related to sports injuries and othopedic surgeries.[73] The regular, long-term use of these prescribed opiate analgesics results, as expected, in both physical and psychological dependence. "Dependent" on the opiate analgesics when continued prescription refills are eventually refused, the adolescent or young adult frequently turns to readily available illicit prescription and other opiate analgesics (e.g., heroin), that can be easily obtained on-the-street or from dark web sites—often tragically culminating with a fatal overdosage.

> Oates says her son was not the kind of teen one would expect to become a drug addict. He was a captain of his football and wrestling teams at Burlington High School and popular among his teammates. He got good grades and didn't have behavior problems ...
>
> But by his junior year, Christopher was experimenting with Percocet, another opioid pain killer. It had been prescribed to him for a football injury. By his senior year, he and some friends were using OxyContin; they got hooked. Soon after he graduated, he started using heroin, too.
>
> Two months ago, her 19-year-old son, Christopher, died of a heroin overdose.
>
> (Arnold, 2005, p. 7)

Adolescent and young adult athletes, who appear to be at particularly significant risk for this pattern of use, commonly share the following characteristics:

- Are male;
- Are highly motivated to succeed;
- Continue sport participation despite sustaining significant physical injuries;
- Participate in organized high school sports at a varsity level;
- Tend to be "star" players;
- Usually participate in high-contact sports (e.g., football; ice-hockey; soccer).

(e.g., Cook, 2016; Ford, Pomykacz, & Veliz, 2018; Pagliaro & Pagliaro, *Clinical Patient Data Files*; Veliz, Boyd, & Esteban McCabe, 2017; Veliz, Epstein-Ngo, & Meier, 2014)

> SM is a 17yo white male who lives with his parents and two younger siblings in a rural town. He was an A/B student in high school where he played on the varsity team... During his junior year he broke his ankle, requiring surgery and internal fixation. He was prescribed opioid analgesics peri-operatively, continued to have pain, and was given repeated prescriptions. Two months post-op, he started escalating his use, taking higher doses at shorter frequencies. He started crushing the pills and snorting them. As he ran out of his prescriptions, he took opioids he found at home in the medicine cabinet and then started stealing supplies from friends and neighbors. He progressed to sniffing or smoking heroin when it was difficult to get pills, stealing money from his parents.
>
> (Sharma, Bruner, & Barnett, 2016, p. 485)

> Rachel Staples and Brock Eurchuk say their son's drug use started after he was prescribed opioids for four surgical procedures last year, though they had requested alternative treatments. Two surgeries treated his fractured jaw, which he broke on a soccer field, and two others were

73 In a related context, Boyd, Young, and McCabe (2014), in their web-based *Secondary Student Life Survey* of 2,627 high school students, found that 3.5% "used someone else's" prescribed opiate analgesics "for pain relief only" (p. 284).

> for shoulder reconstructions from another sports injury… Stables and Eurchuk believe their son started buying street drugs, which were marketed as pharmaceutical-grade pills, in the five-month period between two surgeries, when he experienced chronic and acute pain.[74]
>
> (Smart, 2018, pp. 1–2)

In a related story published in *Sports Illustrated*, a mother of a star high school athlete, who died from an opiate analgesic overdosage, poignantly shared:

> You know what really breaks my heart? My son knew he was meant to be an athlete. Sports was his first addiction. He just ran into another addiction that was so much more powerful.
>
> (Wertheim & Rodriguez, 2015, p. 1)

Related Professional Reminder: ***It should be kept in mind that coaches, parents, physicians, teachers, and trainers need to better attend to, and monitor, the use of prescription opiate analgesics among young athletes—even when appropriately, initially medically prescribed for pain relief.***

Although opiate analgesic use, in the context of "sports," primarily involves adolescent boys and young men, the use of opiate analgesics by adolescent girls and young women is also of increasing concern.

Mothering and Heroin Use

The use of opiate analgesics by young mothers has been associated with extremely distressing consequences, including poor maternal-infant and child bonding and severe neglect and abuse of infants and children. As found by Nair, Black, and Schuler (1997), in their randomized, longitudinal cohort study of 152 mother/infant dyads for evidence of disruption of primary caregiving or neglect during the first 28 months of life, maternal heroin use during pregnancy was the most significant factor associated with disruption of the provision of maternal care. This trend has continued in the U.S. through the first two decades of the new millennium.

Extremely deleterious effects upon "mothering"—from neglect to active physical abuse of infants, children, and adolescents—have been associated with the use of opiate analgesics by mothers (Pagliaro & Pagliaro, *Clinical Patient Data Files*). The following related case reports serve as examples:

> On November 15, 2015, Child Protective Services investigators removed a 6-year-old boy, a 4-year-old girl and a 2-year-old girl from Hutt and McIver's home because there was heroin in the house, as well as needles and rat droppings. CPS employees noticed marks, bruising and cuts on the younger girl's body, indicative of heroin injection. The oldest child was interviewed a month later and described being choked by McIver and then injected with "feel good medicine." … The 2-year-old girl tested positive for heroin through a hair follicle test two months later.
>
> (Ocker, 2016, pp. 1–2)

> Mom whose 5-month-old baby died from drinking formula laced with heroin gets up to eight-year prison term
>
> (AP, 2016, p. 1)

> A woman from Ohio was sentenced to 51 years in prison for the "horrific" crime of allowing her drug dealer to have sex with her 11-year-old daughter to obtain heroin to feed her addiction … Prosecutors said the girl was raped, sodomized, and forced to

74 16-year-old Elliot Eurchuk died of an opiate analgesic overdosage on April 20, 2018.

> perform oral sex with the encounters sometimes videotaped ... The girl's grandmother told the courtroom she doesn't know if the young girl will ever recover form the ordeal.
>
> (Russell, 2016, p. 1)

> Police arrested a pregnant mother in Evansville after they found her passed out on heroin behind the wheel at a stoplight with her young child in the backseat.
>
> (Onay, 2017, p. 1)

> An infant in Michigan who was reportedly "being fussy," overdosed after her mother allegedly gave her methadone.[75] Jennifer Pickerd ... gave her six-week-old girl 20 mg of the drug because she believed the baby was going through withdrawal after she quit breastfeeding ... Authorities ... responded to a 911 call regarding an infant who was not breathing. The infant was revived with Narcan.
>
> (Darrah, 2018, p.1)[76]

Adolescents and Young Adults of Hispanic Descent

In the U.S., a unique category of adolescents and young adults, who use heroin, is known as the "tecato" ("tecata"). These youth typically adhere to the "Cholo"[77] culture—a Mexican-American/Chicano gang subculture. Similar to homeless and transient families that are generally largely "hidden" from mainstream society, they, consequently, are often overlooked by mainstream researchers. Adolescents and young adults of this subculture typically:

1. Are socioeconomically disadvantaged;
2. Have not graduated from high school;
3. Predominantly speak Spanish at home

(Pagliaro & Pagliaro, *Clinical Patient Data Files*; Ramos, 1995; Valdez, Kaplan, & Cepeda, 2000; Valdez, Neaigus & Kaplan, 2011).

Heroin ("carga;" "chiva;" "la heroina") use (often as a "speedball") is an integral part of this culture, which commonly extends back three, or more, generations. Consequently, normalizing the use of heroin in this unique subculture (Ramos, 1995; Valdez, Neaigus, & Kaplan, 2011).

75 We have noted, and previously reported (e.g., Pagliaro & Pagliaro, 2004, 2012), that mothers and grandmothers have administered opium derivatives to infants and young children to manage perceived problem behaviors, including: excessive crying; inability to fall asleep; and painful teething. One particularly interesting example involved the rather common cultural practice in one Ukrainian-American community for "babas" (i.e., grandmothers) to use the opium poppies that they raised it their gardens—grown primarily to harvest the seeds to use in baking (e.g., poppy seed bread and cakes)—packaged in a sachet and utilized as a pacifier to settle neonates and to help them to sleep and, primarily among infants, to manage their teething pain (Pagliaro & Pagliaro, *Clinical Patient Data Files*). Disturbingly, in the context of our forensic consulting, we have also encountered the administration of heroin, and other psychodepressants, to infants and young children by their mothers, their mother's boyfriends/fiancés, or others responsible for their care, to facilitate sexual assault (Pagliaro & Pagliaro, *Clinical Patient Data Files*).

76 At the time of her arrest, Pickerd was on probation for stealing a cellphone at a Denny's Restarurant in Kentwood and skipping out on her bill. She had been enrolled in a local methadone clinic ... (Hogan, 2018, p. 1)

77 The term, "Cholos," was originally used for Latin Americans with Indian blood; American Spanish, or mestizos, who originated from Cholollán, or what is now known as Cholula, in Mexico. Currently, in the U.S., the term is typically used to identify a specific Mexican-American gang subculture. Typically, they self-identify by having shaved heads and wearing baggy pants, a tank top, and a flannel shirt that is only buttoned at the top. They also typically wear gang-colored bandanas folded as a headband, sport numerous tattoos, and frequently flash gang hand signals. "Cholas" generally have long-permed black hair, use dark lipstick, and have a teardrop tattooed under their eye. Cholo/chola children (e.g., toddlers) often have shaved heads and are dressed in typical "cholo" garb.

In addition, selling and using a wide variety of other drugs and substances of abuse (e.g., alcohol; cannabis) is a characteristic of the majority of these families. A majority of family members also are involved in several additional illicit income-generating activities, including:

- Armed robbery;
- Break and entry;
- Drug smuggling/transportation;
- Extortion;
- Fencing;
- Forgery;
- Fraud;
- Prostitution;
- Shoplifting.

(e.g., Pagliario & Pagliaro, *Clinical Patient Data Files*; Ramos, 1995; Valdez, Kaplan, & Cepeda, 2000)

The mean age of initial heroin use for these adolescents and young adults is 18 years-of-age. Transition from the non-injection of heroin to the injection of heroin occurs at a high rate (Valdez, Neaigus, & Kaplan, 2011). Within this Mexican-American subculture it has been identified that "dropping out of school" and "cohabiting" are associated with high rates of heroin use, while, perhaps surprisingly, "early-nest leaving" and "teenage parenthood" appear to be protective factors against heroin use (Cepeda, Nowotny, & Frankeberger, 2016).

Assessment and Diagnosis of Adolescent and Young Adult Opiate Analgesic Dependence or Use Disorder[78]

Opioid use disorder (OUD) is a creation of DSM-5 (APA, 2013). It combines the previous DSM-IV diagnoses of "opioid dependence" and opioid abuse—with the deletion of the single item, "legal problems" (Compton, Dawson, & Goldstein, 2013; Hasin, O'Brien, & Auriacombe, 2013).[79]

The assessment and diagnosis of opiate analgesic dependence or use disorder (OUD) involves an initial clinical interview with the adolescent or young adult during which: (1) opiate analgesic use is established; and, if established, (2) questions are asked that obtain answers concerning both the qualitative and quantitative nature of reported opiate analgesic use (e.g., particular opiate analgesic used; history or pattern of use; attempts to quit; previous treatment approaches). The DSM-5 criteria and detection scoring for OUD are presented in Table 5.7.

The 11 criteria listed in Table 5.7 represent/measure four factors: (1) impaired control (criteria 1 through 4); (2) social impairment (criteria 5 through 7); (3) risky use (criteria 8 and 9); and (4) pharmacological properties (criteria 10 and 11). A contextual predicate of the DSM-5 diagnosis of OUD is that "legitimate medical use" of the opiate analgesics invalidates

78 For an overview of the general principles of assessment and diagnosis including the use of quick-screen psychometric tests—see the related discussion in Chapter 1, "Alcohol." See also Chapter 2, "Amphetamines and Cocaine," for examples of quick-screen psychotropic tests that can be used to detect SUDs, including opiate analgesic (opioid) use disorder, among adolescents and young adults.

79 N.B. The concordance between DSM-IV "opioid dependence" and DSM-5 "opioid use disorder" is high. For example, Boscarino, Rukstalis, and Hoffman (2011) reported an associated kappa value of 0.87.

Table 5.7 DSM-5 Criteria and Scoring for Opioid Use Disorder

Item #	*DSM-5 Criteria*
1.	Opioids are often taken in larger amounts or over a longer period than was intended
2.	There is a persistent desire or unsuccessful efforts to cutdown or control opioid use
3.	A great deal of time is spent in activities necessary to obtain the opioid, use the opioid, or recover from its effects
4.	Craving or a strong desire to use opioids
5.	Recurrent opioid use resulting in a failure to fulfill major role obligations at work, school, or home
6.	Continued use despite having a persistent or recurrent social or interpersonal problems caused or exacerbated by the effects of opioids
7.	Important social, occupational, or recreational activities are given up or reduced because of opioid use
8.	Recurrent opioid use in situations in which it is physically hazardous
9.	Continued use despite knowledge of having a persistent or recurrent physical or psychological problem that is likely to have been caused or exacerbated by opioids
10.	Tolerance,[80] as defined by either of the following: a Need for markedly increased amounts of opioids to achieve intoxication or desired effect b Markedly diminished effect with continued use of the same amount of opioid
11.	Withdrawal,[81] as manifested by either of the following: a Characteristic opioid withdrawal syndrome b Same (or a closely related) substance is taken to relieve or avoid withdrawal symptoms
SCORING	According to DSM-Criteria: The presence of at least two of these symptoms indicates an opioid use disorder (OUD). Additionally, the severity of the OUD is defined as: "Mild," the presence of two or three symptoms; "Moderate," the presence of four or five symptoms; or "Severe," the presence of six or more symptoms.

Source: APA (2013)

80 Patients who are prescribed opioid medications for analgesia may exhibit these two criteria (withdrawal and tolerance) but would not necessarily be considered to have a substance use disorder.

81 Please see comment in previous footnote.

the diagnosis (APA, 2013). We take extreme umbrage with this biased, dated, and profoundly unscientific view of opiate analgesic dependence.[82] Consequently, when we use the DSM-5 criteria for OUD, we simply ignore this aspect—for example, in regard to the DSM footnotes for criteria 10, tolerance, and criteria 11, withdrawal (Pagliaro & Pagliaro, *Clinical Patient Data Files*).

Screening, brief intervention, and referral to treatment (SBIRT) is widely endorsed by many groups, including the American Academy of Pediatrics. Unfortunately, the use of SBIRT, particularly to screen adolescents and young adults for heroin and other opiate analgesic abuse, has not been widely adopted (Harris, 2016; Harris, Shaw, & Sherman, 2016). This lack of adoption may be partly due to the lack of available, generic quick-screen psychometric tests. However, clinicians can use one of the several available "generic" quick-screen psychometric tests that are discussed in Chapter 2, "Amphetamines and Cocaine."

Treating Adolescent and Young Adult Opiate Analgesic Dependence or Use Disorder

The treatment of opiate analgesic physical and psychological dependence or use disorder among adolescents and young adults involves both pharmacotherapy and psychotherapy/counseling. As noted by Sharma, Bruner, and Barnett (2016):

> Although there is a limited evidence base for youth specific treatment, emerging consensus supports the incorporation of relapse prevention medications such as buprenorphine and extended release naltrexone into comprehensive psychosocial treatment including counseling and family involvement.
>
> (p. 487)

Pharmacotherapy[83]

Advances in the pharmacological treatment of opiate analgesic dependence or use disorder are quite diverse. For example, the use of methadone (Dolophine®) for opiate analgesic maintenance (i.e., methadone maintenance) (Fareed, Casarella, & Amar, 2010); buprenorphine (Buprenex®) as an aid for opiate analgesic detoxification (Flassing, 2010; Kovas, McFarland, & McCarty, 2007); and naloxone (Narcan®) for the treatment of opiate analgesic overdosage.

Related pharmaceutical and pharmacotherapeutic approaches are presented and discussed in the following sections:

1. Opiate analgesic abuse-deterrent technologies;
2. Opiate analgesic overdosage (acute);
3. Opiate analgesic maintenance, replacement, or substitution;
4. Opiate analgesic withdrawal syndrome;
5. Opiate analgesic relapse prevention.

82 N.B. Physical dependence, or OUD, is a clinical pharmacological, physiological process that is completely unrelated to the reasons for use (i.e., has no inherent moral or psychological basis—it has no conscious component). It is, consequently unrelated to whether use is for a medical indication or for "recreational" purposes.

83 The clinical efficacy of selected pharmacotherapies is significantly enhanced by concurrent psychotherapy/counseling. Consequently, to achieve optimal outcomes, we also consistently recommend the coordinated application of both approaches (see the related discussion in the later section, "Psychotherapy/Counseling").

Opiate Analgesic Abuse-Deterrent Technologies

An area of active pharmaceutical research and development over the new millennium has involved the pharmaceutical alteration of: (1) dosage formulations;[84] and (2) drug delivery systems. These efforts are aimed at both discouraging the use of a particular drug or substance of abuse, or its method of use, and to avoid or reduce associated harm. As noted by the FDA:

> Most abuse deterrent technologies developed to date are intended to make manipulation more difficult or to make abuse of the manipulated product less attractive or less rewarding. (USDHHS, 2015, p. 3)

Common Misbelief: Newer altered drug formulations totally prevent the abuse of opiate analgesics while maintaining desired pain-relieving effects.

Actually, the FDA-approved pharmaceutical formulations, which have been developed and implemented for use in the U.S., are designed to *deter* abuse. They are not designed to make use impossible. Thus, they do not fully prevent abuse. However, there is growing evidence that supports their efficacy in terms of deterring, or reducing, some opiate analgesic abuse.

As a result of the "steep increase in abuse, misuse, and both fatal and non-fatal overdoses involving prescription opioids" in the U.S., over the new millennium (see the earlier related discussion in this chapter), the focus of developmental research within the area of "abuse-deterrent formulations" has been primarily directed at opiate analgesic abuse, including the preparation of "tamper resistant formulations."[85] Several examples of abuse-deterrent technologies and formulations are presented and discussed in the following sections. We begin with a highly successful approach that involved the development of combination buprenorphine/naloxone sublingual tablets (Bunavail®; Suboxone®) to prevent the illicit intravenous use of buprenorphine. Other examples of this approach include EMBEDA®, as well as oxycodone, in controlled-release/extended release (CR/ER) formulations (e.g., OxyContin® CR/ER).

BUPRENORPHINE/NALOXONE SUBLINGUAL TABLETS

Illicit IV use of buprenorphine has been significantly reduced in the U.S. with an abuse-deterrent pharmacological/pharmaceutical strategy. The addition of naloxone to the buprenorphine sublingual tablet formulation prevents illicit intravenous use of buprenorphine by an interesting, and rather simple, mechanism.

When used sublingually, the naloxone is poorly absorbed and, thus, has virtually no effect on the analgesic action of buprenorphine—as clinically intended. However, if the combination

84 These formulations, which differ significantly, are often referred to as abuse-deterrent formulations, or ADFs (Schaeffer, 2012).

85 As noted by Passik, Hays, and Eisner (2006), in their study sample of adults who abused prescription drugs and who were entering drug rehabilitation, 80% reported tampering with prescription opiate analgesic tablets by chewing them or administering them by intranasal or intravenous routes. Interestingly, in another laboratory observational study of adults—who abused prescription opiate analgesics and were tasked with attempting to modify "crush-resistant" opiate analgesic prescription formulations to enable self-administration by either the intranasal or intravenous routes—Vosburg, Jones, and Manubay (2012, p. 206) found that:

> No particularly unique tools were requested for tampering purposes. Intranasal abusers worked primarily with a hammer, razor, and wax paper; while intravenous abusers primarily employed a razor, spoon, lighter, hammer, syringe and cotton, cookers, and water.

tablet is illicitly crushed, dissolved, and injected IV, the naloxone is immediately and completely absorbed blocking the desired action of the buprenorphine at the endogenous CNS opiate analgesic receptors (Connery, 2015; Hard, 2014). (See also the related discussion in the later subsection, "Opiate Analgesic Maintenance, Replacement, or Substitution—Buprenorphine/ Naloxone Combination.")

EMBEDA®

EMBEDA® is an extended-release combination of morphine and naltrexone in capsular form. Within the capsule are morphine pellets that contain a core of sequestered naltrexone. The analysis of post-marketing data regarding undesired, or harmful, effects and toxicities associated with approximately 97,000 prescriptions for EMBEDA®, indicated a significant reduction in abuse (Badalamenti, Buckley, & Smith, 2012).

This finding was consistent with the results of a related naltrexone bioavailability study by Johnson and Setnik (2011), who found that when the capsules are crushed, the naltrexone is immediately released "mitigating morphine-induced effects," including related "drug liking" scores (p. 391). However, as emphasized by Smith (2011), in a related review: "No product is likely to be abuse-proof in the hands of clever and determined abusers" (p. 1111).

OXYCODONE CR/ER

In August 2010, oxycodone CR/ER—including OxyContin®—tablets were reformulated in the U.S. with a polymer coating to reduce non-oral methods of use. When the tablets are crushed and, subsequently, attempted to be dissolved in water for intranasal or IV use, the polymer coating turns into a gel that deters intranasal and IV use.

As identified by Butler, Cassidy, and Chilcoat (2013, p. 351), preliminary analysis of "a sentinel surveillance sample of 140,496 individuals assessed for substance abuse treatment at 357 U.S. centers" indicated that the reformulated product was associated with a significant reduction (i.e., 41%) in abuse when compared to the original oxycodone product. However, the same research group—in a subsequent study involving "232,874 adults, at 437 facilities"—failed to detect a significant reduction in the abuse of the oxycodone CR/ER product (Cassidy, DasMahapatra, & Black, 2014, p. 440).

In another study, Havens, Leukefeld, and DeVeaugh-Geiss (2014), utilizing structured interviews of 189 adults with histories of opiate analgesic abuse, reported "mixed" results regarding the abuse of the OxyContin® CR/ER formulations (i.e., significant amounts of abuse, but significantly lower amounts than reported for the original, immediate-release [IR] formulations). Others (e.g., Michna, Kirson, & Shei, 2014; Sellers, Perrino, & Colucci, 2013) have reported similar findings.

Opiate Analgesic Overdosage, Acute[86]

Specific pharmacologic antagonists are available for the management of opiate analgesic overdosage. These antagonists include naloxone (Narcan®) and naltrexone (Trexan®), both of which reverse to a significant degree—if not completely—acute toxicities and other effects (e.g., pain relief) associated with the use of opiate analgesics. Naloxone is the preferred opiate analgesic antagonist for use in all cases of acute opiate analgesic overdosage because of its ability to be quickly and effectively administered from a variety of routes, including: IM and

86 See also the detailed related discussion in the earlier pharmacology section, "Treatment of Opiate Analgesic Overdosage: Naloxone Pharmacotherapy."

IV injection; intranasal instillation; and pulmonary inhalation (Orciari Herman, 2017b; Pagliaro & Pagliaro, 2004, 2009).

NALOXONE (NARCAN®)

Naloxone is the only essentially pure opiate analgesic antagonist currently available for the treatment of opiate analgesic overdosage. In response to the significant increase in opiate analgesic overdosage deaths in the U.S. during the new millennium, the FDA approved the use of a single dose naloxone auto-injector (Evzio®) (FDA, 2014b). Formulated for IM or SC use, it is indicated for the management of opiate analgesic overdosage for children, adolescents, and young adults, as well as older adults (A naloxone, 2014). Naloxone has: (1) a usual duration of action of one to two hours; (2) no other pharmacologic action other than its antagonism of the opiate analgesic agonists; (3) not been associated with overdosage toxicity; and (4) virtually no contraindications for its use. However, cautious use is indicated because, along with its rapid reversal of the respiratory depression associated with opiate analgesic overdosage, it also can precipitate the acute opiate analgesic withdrawal syndrome when administered to those who are physically dependent on opiate analgesics.

Naloxone is poorly absorbed following ingestion. Thus, it has been traditionally administered by IV, IM, or SC injection. However, because opiate analgesic users comprise a high-risk population for HIV, hepatitis, and other serious infections, concern was raised regarding possible needle-stick injuries among medical staff members, who injected naloxone to opiate analgesic users, who had overdosed. As a result of this concern, researchers explored other methods of naloxone administration that would be both expedient and safe.

The result of this research was the development of a "needleless," intranasal method of naloxone administration that appears to be effective in approximately 75% of pre-hospital treatment cases (Robinson & Wermeling, 2014; Weber, Tataris, & Hoffman, 2012). In November 2015, the FDA approved this route of administration and made it available to care givers, family members, and first responders under the formulation and product name of, "Narcan Nasal Spray®" (FDA, 2015; NIDA, 2015a). Narcan Nasal Spray® is dispensed in a box containing two individual doses of naloxone (four mg each in 0.1 ml of nasal spray solution) in self-contained, single use disposable nasal spray units (Nordrum, 2016).

Opiate Analgesic Maintenance, Replacement, or Substitution

Maintenance, replacement, or substitution (MRS) pharmacotherapy[87] for opiate analgesic dependence, or use disorder, is based on the principle of harm reduction—an integral component of tertiary prevention (see earlier related discussion). As such, MRS pharmacotherapy involves replacing an opiate analgesic, and/or its method of use, with another opiate analgesic or method of use that is, in comparison, less harmful. This section focuses on two such opiate analgesics: (1) buprenorphine, which is used alone or in combination with naloxone; and (2) methadone, which is most often used for young adults who use heroin.

BUPRENORPHINE

Buprenorphine has been found effective for both the: (1) management of acute opiate analgesic detoxification; and (2) long-term opiate analgesic maintenance pharmacotherapy (e.g., Kovas, McFarland, & McCarty, 2007; Pagliaro & Pagliaro, 2009). In a double-blind,

87 MRS pharmacotherapy is also referred to by the FDA as "medication-assisted treatment" (MAT).

placebo-controlled multicenter random-controlled study of "opioid-dependent" adolescents and young adults, 16 to 24 years-of-age, Marsch, Moore, and Ducat (2016) found that:

> Participants who received a 56-day buprenorphine taper in were retained in treatment significantly longer than participants who received a 28-day buprenorphine taper.
>
> (p. 1406)

In late 2017, the FDA approved the use of an injectable, extended-release form of buprenorphine (BUP-XR) for the treatment of OUD. BUP-XR is available under the trade name of Sublocade® and is administered once monthly as an IM injection. In early 2019, results of a randomized, double-blind study indicated that:

> Both BUP-XR regimens led to substantial proportions of participants achieving abstinence from opioids, relief of withdrawal symptoms, and control of craving without the need for daily medication adherence or supplemental buprenorphine.
>
> (NIDA, 2019, p. 1)

Buprenorphine also has been found to be safer than methadone in cases of overdosage and is associated with a less severe opiate analgesic withdrawal syndrome when regular, long-term use is abruptly discontinued (Raisch, Fye, & Boardman, 2002). In addition, in clinical circumstances in which opiate analgesic maintenance is required for adolescent girls and young women,[88] who are heroin-dependent and pregnant, we recommend the use of buprenorphine during their pregnancy.

Buprenorphine is equally efficacious as methadone and also offers three unique benefits for their embryos/fetuses and neonates:

1. Reduced embryo/fetal cardiac suppression;
2. Reduced fetal movement suppression;
3. Less severe opiate analgesic neonatal abstinence syndrome (NAS).[89]

(Jones, Finnegan, & Kaltenbach, 2012; Minozzi, Amato, & Bellisario, 2013; Pagliaro & Pagliaro, 2012; Sutter, Leeman, & Hsi, 2014)

In addition, as related to the latter benefit, Pritham (2013) found that both buprenorphine and methadone are excreted in breast milk and, consequently, for young mothers maintained on either buprenorphine or methadone, the severity of the neonatal abstinence syndrome among their neonates can be decreased by breastfeeding.

BUPRENORPHINE/NALOXONE COMBINATION

In an effort to curtail the widespread use of buprenorphine associated with the increasing opiate analgesic epidemic across the U.S. during the new millennium, the FDA endorsed the marketing of combination drug products that contained both buprenorphine (two mg) and naloxone (five mg) (e.g., Suboxone®).

Buprenorphine, a mixed opiate analgesic agonist/antagonist (i.e., partial mu-receptor agonist and full kappa-receptor antagonist), is preferentially administered sublingually

88 N.B. In this context, we tend to clearly differentiate between adolescent girls, for whom we do not recommend the use of methadone maintenance (see earlier related discussion), and young women, for whom we have recommended methadone maintenance pharmacotherapy—when clinically appropriate.

89 See related discussion in earlier section, "Opiate Analgesic-Induced Neonatal Abstinence Syndrome."

(absorption F = 0.5; half-life of elimination, approximately 30 hours). Naloxone, an opiate analgesic antagonist, also can be administered sublingually (absorption F = 0.1; half-life of elimination, approximately one hour) (Chiang & Hawks, 2003; Pagliaro & Pagliaro, 2009; Robinson, 2006). Thus, the pharmacokinetics of these two drugs, particularly their difference in "F," allows their combination as a mixed opiate analgesic agonist/antagonist in different buccal or sublingual formulations that can be dosed once daily:

- Buccal film (Bunavail®);
- Sublingual film (Suboxone® Film);
- Sublingual tablet (Suboxone®; SubSolv®).

When the combined product is administered by IV injection, absorption is 100% for both buprenorphine and naloxone (i.e., F=1) resulting in the desired euphoric and analgesic effects of buprenorphine being totally blocked by the naloxone. In addition to the expected undesired effects and toxicities associated with the use of buprenorphine, the buccal/sub-lingual formulations have been associated with numbness and redness of the mouth and tongue pain. In the U.S. since 2000, physicians are required to:

1. Undergo a training course;
2. Apply for a license to prescribe combination buprenorphine/naloxone opiate analgesic MRS pharmacotherapy on an outpatient basis.

However, as noted by Williams and Bisaga (2016), in their editorial regarding the "vast epidemic of opioid-related deaths" facing the U.S.:

> In 40% of U.S. counties there is currently no physician authorized to prescribe buprenorphine, and the majority of authorized providers actually treat few or no patients.
>
> (p. 814)

For adolescents (> 12 years-of-age) and young adults, the initial "induction" dose of buprenorphine/naloxone is 2 mg/0.5 mg SL on day one with incremental dose increases of 2mg/0.5 mg SL until achievement of the suppression of the signs and symptoms associated with the opiate analgesic withdrawal syndrome. The generally recommended target dosage is 16 mg/4 mg once daily with a maximum dose of 24 mg/6 mg per day. Subramaniam, Warden, and Minhajuddin (2011) found that their sample of 152 "opioid-dependent youth" (15 to 21 years-of-age) responded to 12 weeks of extended buprenorphine/naloxone pharmacotherapy.

METHADONE

Methadone (Dolophine®), a long-acting opiate analgesic, has been used in the U.S. as a legal form of pharmacotherapy for opiate analgesic maintenance for over 50 years for patients, who are "addicted" to heroin and who have been unable to successfully complete opiate analgesic detoxification. In this context of use, methadone has long been considered to be the "gold standard" of opiate analgesic maintenance therapy. However, we do not recommend the use of methadone maintenance therapy for adolescents. Instead, we have always attempted to facilitate the discontinuation of opiate analgesic use among adolescents (Pagliaro & Pagliaro, *Clinical Patient Data Files*).

Consequently, we recommend that other methods, including psychotherapy/counseling (see following section, "Psychotherapy/Counseling"), be used to achieve the cessation of opiate analgesic use in this age group. This recommendation is based on the:

1. Extremely long-term duration of methadone maintenance pharmacotherapy that would be required for adolescents (i.e., through adulthood);
2. Difficulties associated with the eventual discontinuation of methadone maintenance (i.e., a more severe withdrawal syndrome);
3. Risk for methadone diversion—or illicit use/sale—by adolescents;
4. Risk for methadone overdosage;
5. Greater likelihood of successful discontinuation of opiate analgesic use (i.e., in comparison to that experienced by adults).

Over the last decade, methadone maintenance has been associated with a disproportionate number of deaths related to prescription opiate analgesic overdosages. As noted by Faul, Bohm, and Alexander (2017):

> Methadone accounted for approximately 1% of all opioids prescribed for pain but accounted for approximately 23% of all prescription opioid deaths in 2014.
>
> (p. 320)

These overdosages have been reported particularly among patients who have been prescribed methadone in lieu of oxycodone for the management of chronic pain (Faul, Bohm, & Alexander, 2017; Pagliaro & Pagliaro, *Clinical Patient Data Files*). As reported by Collins (2010), many of these deaths, appear to be iatrogenic, specifically involving the:

1. Inappropriate use of conversion tables for dosing methadone;
2. Prescription of too high a dosage of methadone for initiating methadone maintenance (i.e., 80 mg/day as opposed to 30 mg/day).

Prescribed in dosages that generally do not produce euphoria or other desired psychotropic effects, methadone maintenance holds off, or keeps at bay, the signs and symptoms of the opiate analgesic withdrawal syndrome. Despite its associated limitations and problems, methadone—at least for adults, including some young adults—remains the "gold standard" for opiate analgesic maintenance pharmacotherapy (Connery, 2015, p. 63).

Methadone maintenance pharmacotherapy for young adults, who are dependent on heroin, is guided by the following goals:

- Cessation of the illicit use of heroin;
- Enhancement of the abilities of young adults to lead a more normal and, consequently, less harmful and more productive life than that generally associated with heroin use.

Methadone maintenance pharmacotherapy offers several benefits:

1. Ingested once daily[90] (i.e., an easier and more convenient administration schedule than that associated with the need to obtain illegal heroin, which is generally injected at least four times a day);
2. Prevents the harmful effects associated with heroin IV injection (e.g., HIV infection; overdosage) (See also the earlier related section, "Pharmacology, Undesired, or

90 Oral pharmacotherapy, for young adults, begins with 10 to 20 mg/day and increases by 10 mg every week until a maintenance dosage of 60 to 120 mg/day is achieved.

Harmful, Effects and Toxicities—Toxicities Associated with Intravenous Injection of Opiate Analgesics");
3. Decreases craving for heroin;
4. Is legally available at a relatively low-cost;
5. Is more conveniently and safely obtained at licensed neighborhood pharmacies;
6. Minimizes the occurrence of euphoria and excessive sedation.

Additionally, methadone maintenance has been associated with a significant reduction in "hustling" and other related behaviors (e.g., breaks and entries; child neglect; imprisonment; overdosage death; prostitution) that are commonly associated with young adult heroin use. It also has been associated with increased abilities to participate in psychotherapy and other tertiary prevention approaches and maintain effective parenting, work, school, and other social responsibilities (e.g., Farrell, Ward, & Mattick, 1994; Joseph, Stancliff, & Langrod, 2000).

Although methadone pharmacotherapy for opiate analgesic maintenance has many advantages, it also has some disadvantages. For example, the withdrawal syndrome associated with methadone use is much more severe than that associated with heroin use.[91] Thus, many young adults, who enroll in methadone maintenance programs, remain in these programs for several years. During this time, they often begin, or continue, to use other drugs and substances of abuse, such as alcohol and cocaine—drugs and substances of abuse whose use is not directly dissuaded by the use of methadone (Pagliaro & Pagliaro, 2009; Pagliaro & Pagliaro, *Clinical Patient Data Files*). Unfortunately, young adults, who decide to discontinue their methadone maintenance program, often resume their heroin use.[92]

Opiate Analgesic Withdrawal Syndrome[93]

The regular, long-term use of pure opiate analgesic agonists (e.g., morphine) or mixed opiate analgesic agonist/antagonists (e.g., pentazocine, Talwin®) are associated with the development of physical (and psychological) dependence. Thus, among adolescents and young adults, who are physically dependent on the opiate analgesics, abrupt discontinuation of regular, long-term use, or the use of an opiate analgesic antagonist (e.g., naloxone, Narcan®), may result in the opiate analgesic withdrawal syndrome.

Although the opiate analgesic withdrawal syndrome is not usually life threatening, the appropriate use of selected pharmacotherapeutic approaches for the management of opiate analgesic withdrawal and the monitoring of therapeutic response are generally indicated. Gradual discontinuation of the regular, long-term use of the opiate analgesic will prevent or minimize related signs and symptoms of withdrawal. A major reason to attempt to ameliorate the signs and symptoms of opiate analgesic withdrawal pharmacotherapeutically is that a relapse to resumed opiate analgesic use commonly occurs during unmedicated and unsupervised opiate analgesic withdrawal.

Naltrexone pharmacotherapy has been available and has been used for some time in "rapid and ultra-rapid opioid detoxification" treatment centers, which promise quick, painless, same-day detoxification for people who are physically dependent on opiate analgesics (e.g., O'Connor & Kosten, 1998; Singh & Basu, 2004). However, the procedures involved in this

91 This problem is often related to unidentified or untreated contemporaneous diagnoses (Wu & Blazer, 2014). (See also the related discussion in the subsection, "Contemporaneous Diagnoses.")

92 In addition, some simply "overcome" the methadone blockage of the opiate mu receptors by using "massive" dosages of other desired opiate analgesics (usually heroin)—often with fatal results (Pagliaro & Pagliaro, *Clinical Patient Data Files*).

93 See also the related discussion in the earlier subsection, "Opiate Analgesic Withdrawal Syndrome."

treatment approach (e.g., administration of a general anesthetic followed by a high-dose of opiate analgesic antagonists that induce severe withdrawal with the patient having no conscious experience of it) generally pose significant risks for patients, including several documented fatalities (Hamilton, Olmedo, & Shah, 2002). We do not recommend this form of opiate analgesic detoxification treatment.

Additionally, we generally do not recommend the use of specific pharmacological adjuncts for the management of the heroin withdrawal syndrome because it is generally relatively mild and can usually be handled "cold turkey" (i.e., signs and symptoms of the heroin withdrawal syndrome typically resemble those of a bad case of influenza—dependent, of course, on both the amount of heroin used daily and the length of time it has been used).[94]

In contrast, the methadone withdrawal syndrome may be quite severe with convulsions and other physiological effects that require appropriate treatment under direct medical supervision, generally in the context of inpatient treatment. Even when not required medically, we strongly recommend that patients undergo methadone withdrawal in an inpatient setting, particularly patients with concomitant histories of long-standing or high-dose use of alcohol or another drug or substance of abuse, in order to provide appropriate psychological support and significantly improve compliance (i.e., ensure that the patient successfully completes the withdrawal process). The average stay for people in detoxification units or centers in these situations typically is approximately three to seven days (Pagliaro & Pagliaro, *Clinical Patient Data Files*).

Opiate Analgesic Relapse Prevention[95]

Several pharmacological approaches involving opiate analgesic antagonists have been developed in an effort to ensure continued abstinence (i.e., relapse prevention) among opiate analgesic-dependent adolescents and young adults (and other adults), who have discontinued opiate analgesic use—generally for a minimum of seven days. In this context, relapse prevention pharmacotherapy generally attempts to ensure abstinence by means of blocking associated "rewarding" stimuli when opiate analgesics are used.

Naltrexone, a long-acting oral opiate antagonist, was originally developed and marketed in the U.S. in 1984 under the brand name, Trexan®, for the treatment of opiate analgesic dependence, or "addiction"—particularly among practicing physicians and other health care professionals (e.g., Greenstein, Arndt, & McLellan, 1984; Kirchmayer, Davoli, & Verster, 2000; Pagliaro & Pagliaro, Clinical Patient Data Files).[96]

The oral dosage form of naltrexone can be administered once daily without regard to meals or the ingestion of other foods and beverages. However, compliance has been problematic (Pagliaro & Pagliaro, *Clinical Patient Data Files*). In an effort to improve compliance and therapeutic outcomes, an injectable form of naltrexone was made available (Garbutt, Kranzler, & O'Malley,

94 N.B. This does not mean, nor in any way imply, that patients should be "left on their own." They should be closely monitored and appropriate therapeutic interventions—medical, pharmacological, and psychological—should always be applied as individually required in order to optimize clinical outcomes.

95 See also the earlier discussion in the related section, "Opiate Analgesic Maintenance, Replacement, or Substitution."

96 We have found that naltrexone is particularly beneficial for maintaining opiate analgesic nonuse among recovering health and social care professionals (e.g., nurses; pharmacists; physicians) and professional health and social care students who otherwise would be "at risk for relapsed use," particularly because of their accessibility to opiate analgesics in their clinical areas of practice.

In the context of professional rehabilitation/return to practice (i.e., after their misuse of the opiate analgesics has been identified and their professional regulatory body has formally ordered treatment prior to their re-registration/return to work in the clinical environment), we have had very good success with well-motivated subjects—particularly when combined, with: (1) effective psychotherapy/counseling (see following sections); and (2) appropriate and diligent monitoring /"follow-up."

2005; Gastfriend, 2014). The injectable form of naltrexone (Vivitrol®) is an extended-release suspension formulation that can be injected IM,[97] once monthly, by a health care professional. While found to significantly improve compliance for some patients, for others, poor patient compliance and low treatment retention rates continue (e.g., Minozzi, Amato, & Vecchi, 2011). For example, in a sample of over 300 community-living, ex-prisoners, who had limited use of heroin within the 30 days prior to the commencement of the research study, Lee, Friedmann, & Kinlock (2016) found that—when extended-release naltrexone (Vivitrol®)[98] was used in combination with relapse-prevention counseling and community support—monthly injections of naltrexone demonstrated significant efficacy only during the first six months of therapy. Several studies (e.g., NIDA, 2017; Orciari Herman, 2017a; Tanum, Solli, & Latif, 2017), compared the naltrexone injection formulation with the oral buprenorphine and naloxone combination formulation with the general finding that the two approaches were therapeutically equivalent.

The most common undesired effect associated with the use of naltrexone is nausea. However, its long-term safety and efficacy have not yet been clearly established and the FDA has added a "Boxed Warning" to its official monograph stating that:

> Naltrexone may cause liver damage when taken in large doses" [i.e., several times the normal recommended daily dose for an extended period].
>
> (Naltrexone, 2009, p. 1)

In addition, as previously noted, naltrexone—being an opiate analgesic antagonist—can precipitate the opiate analgesic withdrawal syndrome among regular, long-term users of opiate analgesics, including those who are being medically managed for moderate to severe chronic pain (e.g., chronic cancer pain). Thus, caution must be exercised when naltrexone pharmacotherapy is initiated for opiate analgesic relapse prevention for these patients, who would also require alternative pain relief measures (e.g., acupuncture/acupressure; non-opiate analgesics, such as acetaminophen [Tylenol®]; NSAIDs [e.g., aspirin, ibuprofen]; local anesthetic, such as topical lidocaine; regional nerve block) (Pagliaro & Pagliaro, 1999; Pagliaro & Pagliaro, *Clinical Patient Data Files*; Volpicelli, Clay, & Watson, 1995).

Psychotherapy/Counseling

Although virtually every form of psychotherapy/counseling has been used to treat adolescents and young adults who have opiate analgesic dependence or use disorder, cognitive-behavioral therapy (CBT) is the generally accepted mainstay of this therapeutic approach (Pagliaro & Pagliaro, *Clinical Patient Data Files*). (See also the related discussion in the "Psychotherapy/ Counseling" section of Chapter 1, "Alcohol").

In December 2018, the FDA approved the use of a CBT-related mobile "app" to be used in conjunction with a formal treatment program for OUD.

> The reSET-O app is a prescription cognitive behavioral therapy intended to be used in addition to outpatient treatment under the care of a health care professional, in conjunction with treatment that includes buprenorphine and contingency management …

97 Intramuscular injection of naltrexone has been associated with injection site reactions, including: dark scabbing; erythema; induration; intense pain; lumps; open wounds; pruritus; swelling; and tenderness. On occasion, these reactions can be severe enough to warrant surgical or other therapeutic intervention. Thus, naltrexone IM injection pharmacotherapy requires appropriate, routine monitoring of injection sites.

98 Vivitrol® is also approved for the treatment of alcohol dependence or use disorder. For further discussion, see Chapter 1, "Alcohol."

The reSET-O is an app that can be downloaded directly to a patient's mobile device after they receive a prescription to do so from their doctor. It is intended to be used while participating in an outpatient OUD treatment program.

(FDA, 2018b, p. 1)[99]

Safe Injection Facilities (SIFs)

For adolescents and young adults, who use opiate analgesics by IV injection, a somewhat related approach to harm reduction are "supervised injection facilities," or "safe injection sites." Although used for adults, who IV inject opiate analgesics and other drugs and substances of abuse in several countries[100] since the beginning of the new millennium, SIFs are not currently legally sanctioned in the U.S. (Kerr, Mitra, & Clare-Kennedy, 2017). However, there has been increased related interest and discussion regarding their use in several states because of the current opiate analgesic crisis. For example, Bouvier, Elston, and Hadland (2017) sampled 54 adolescents and young adults (median age 26 years), who reported recent "non-medical prescription opioid use" as part of the *Rhode Island Young Adult Prescription Drug Study*, found that almost two-thirds (i.e., 63%) said they would use a SIF. Additionally, several cities (e.g., Boston, Denver, New York, San Francisco, and Seattle) have endorsed, and are officially pursuing, the implementation of SIFs (Gorden, 2018; Sawyer, 2018).[101]

We do *not* recommend the use of SIFs for adolescents or young adults because we view SIFs as an enabling behavior that offers little in terms of long-term positive benefits for these young IV opiate analgesic users. Both professional and public opinion in this area have waxed and waned over the decades and we have quite often found ourselves in a "minority position." However, given our related long experience and clinical professional observations, we strongly believe that endorsement of the use of SIFs is simply tantamount to "kicking the can down the road"—eventually, to a time when the "piper must be paid." A time when the associated problems for adolescent and young adult IV opiate analgesic users, based on current trajectories and knowledge of the usual progression of OUD, will have significantly worsened and the potential for the implementation of successful positive interventions will have been significantly decreased—or lost.

Contemporaneous Diagnoses Involving Opiate Analgesics

Several common contemporaneous diagnoses have been identified among adolescents and young adults who use opiate analgesics. These diagnoses include: alcohol and other drug and substance of abuse dependence or use disorders, particularly, nicotine dependence or use disorder; other mental disorders; numerous PMDs; and "somatic symptom disorder" (SSD).

The concurrent use of other drugs and substances of abuse with opiate analgesics also depends largely on availability, reason for use, and context of use. For example, adolescents and young adults who use heroin typically drink alcohol and smoke or vape cannabis and/or tobacco.

99 The use of the reSET-O program has been demonstrated to increase program retention, but not efficacy in comparison to buprenorphine pharmacotherapy and contingency management alone (FDA, 2018, p. 2). For a further discussion of contingency management, see the treatment subsection, "Psychotherapy/Counseling" in Chapter 1, "Alcohol."

100 A number of countries—including Australia, Canada, France, Germany, Netherlands, Norway, and Switzerland—legally allow the use of SIFs.

101 States and cities in the U.S. have the authority to approve SIFs, but—as is the case for cannabis (see Chapter 4, "Cannabis and Other Psychodelics")—they cannot nullify related federal laws (Beletsky, Davis, & Anderson, 2008).

"Homeless" adolescents or young adults use opiate analgesics, when available—along with virtually any and all other available drugs and substances of abuse. In another example, high school and college athletes, may restrict use to prescription opiate analgesics to control acute, and later, chronic pain associated with sports-related injuries[102]—at least until their availability ceases, at which time they may increase their alcohol consumption and/or switch to heroin.

Several contemporaneous diagnoses involving opiate analgesic dependence or use disorder, as would be expected, include various PMDs, particularly pain disorders—both acute and chronic (i.e., the reason why opiate analgesics are initially prescribed for the vast majority of adolescents and young adults). However, as noted by Katz, Rosenbloom, and Fashler (2015):

> For the first time in more than 30 years, the most recent edition of the DSM no longer includes a pain-specific mental disorder. DSM-5 SSD with predominant pain replaces DSM-IV pain disorder but it is *not* recommended for people with chronic pain, because it lacks validity, and is overly inclusive and stigmatizing. Instead, *adjustment disorder* remains the most appropriate, accurate, and acceptable diagnosis for people who are overly concerned about their pain.
>
> (p. 165)

Managing Contemporaneous Diagnoses[103]

Appropriate pharmacotherapy for the management of contemporaneous diagnoses involving opiate analgesic dependence or use disorder is a common and integral component of the medical, psychological, and other health and social care services required by adolescents and young adults. In addition, as noted by several researchers (e.g., McCarthy, Tomlinson, & Anderson, 2005; Pagliaro & Pagliaro, *Clinical Patient Data Files*), failure to adequately treat other involved mental disorders may significantly contribute to—following initially successful treatment outcomes for opiate analgesic dependence or use disorder—relapsed opiate analgesic use.

Three major approaches are commonly used in the treatment of adolescents and young adults with contemporaneous diagnoses. These approaches have been categorized by Smith and Randall (2012) as:

1. Sequential;
2. Parallel;
3. Integrated.

The "sequential" approach, based largely on the hypotheses that a single clinician can optimally focus on, or address, a single dependence or use disorder, addresses only one selected dependence or use disorder.[104] This selected dependence or use disorder is treated

102 As discussed earlier in this chapter, among adolescents and young adults, sports injuries often lead to regular, long-term opiate analgesic use particularly when injuries are not given sufficient time to heal. "Acute pain" frequently converts to "chronic pain," often along with an anxiety disorder or major depressive disorder that requires additional pharmacotherapy, such as antidepressants and sedative-hypnotics, including antianxiety drugs (e.g., benzodiazepines, Ativan®; diazepam, Valium®). (See also Chapter 6, "Prescription Sedative Hypnotics"). The increasing complexity of pharmacotherapy also increases the risk for drug-drug interactions and other dependence or use disorders.

103 For a general overview of contemporaneous diagnoses and their general management, see the related discussion in Chapter 1, "Alcohol."

104 Unfortunately, in this situation, the order of treatment is almost always chosen on an "ad hoc" basis predicated primarily on the background, knowledge, and clinical strengths of the clinician as opposed to the individual needs of the specific patient, who is seeking treatment, and the relationship between, or among, the presenting concurrent disorders.

first while largely ignoring—or delaying—the treatment of the concurrent dependence or use disorder(s) or other mental or physical medical disorders. A related corollary is that once the single selected dependence or use disorder is treated and is in "control/remission," another dependence or use disorder (or other mental or physical medical disorder) can be successfully treated (i.e., is more amenable to intervention).

In the "parallel" approach, specific treatment approaches are delivered separately, but simultaneously. The treatments (e.g., for opiate analgesic or other dependence or use disorder; mental disorder; physical medical disorder) are usually delivered by different clinicians in different facilities. Coordination and communication among the patient and the clinicians involved in this approach are of critical importance for optimal therapeutic success—given that significant deficits in coordination and communication are the major reasons for the failures associated with the parallel approach. For example, when one clinician says one thing to a patient and the other clinician(s) says something else in terms of the cause of the condition, the preferred therapeutic approach, and the necessary length of treatment. Inadequate coordination and communication between and among the treating clinicians, as is particularly apt to occur when they are not part of the same clinic or treatment unit/site (e.g., university hospitals), is another major area of concern that can lead to therapeutic failures.

In the "integrated" approach, treatment is delivered in a similar way to the parallel approach, but by a single health care professional. This is our preferred approach for the treatment of contemporaneous diagnoses. We have consistently used this approach with great success over the decades as well as recommending its use to others. However, it is the most difficult approach to successfully employ because of the absolute requirements for a skilled, knowledgeable, and clinically experienced clinician or therapist. It also is important to note that, when needed, appropriate consultation, collaboration, and referral are extremely beneficial to the treatment outcomes. In the majority of "difficult" or previously "failed" cases that have been referred to us over the years, the most common problem has been the use of non-professionally educated para-professional therapists, usually recovering from their own drug or substance abuse, who have experience and strengths in group therapy and other related skills, but are ill-prepared to plan and deliver complex therapeutic treatment that tends to be far beyond their abilities when confronted with contemporaneous disorders involving opiate analgesic dependence, SUDs, and often multiple OMDs (Pagliaro & Pagliaro, *Clinical Patient Data Files*).

Additionally, we have frequently observed, particularly among patients who are extremely socially-economically (i.e., financially) or educationally successful, that therapeutic success is significantly hindered when the patient thinks that he or she is "superior" to the individual providing the therapeutic intervention. For example, in our clinical experience, adolescents and young adults, such as class presidents, varsity team captains, medical students, honors students, and graduate students, respond best to a therapist who they both respect and implicitly trust. Consequently, therapeutic success with the adolescents and young adults, who have opiate analgesic or other dependence or use disorder(s), and/or mental disorder(s), and/or physical medical disorder(s) is generally minimal when the therapist is, for example, a recovering alcoholic or heroin addict with little or no formal advanced education/clinical experience.[105]

105 This observation can also be related to differences in IQ—i.e., potential for successful therapeutic intervention is minimized when the IQ of the adolescent or young adult who has been diagnosed with opiate analgesic dependence or use disorder is significantly higher than that of the therapist.

References

Afghanistan, opium and the Taliban. (2001, February 15). Opioids.com, 1–5. Retrieved from http://opioids.com/afghanistan/index.html

Afghanistan opium survey 2008: Executive summary. (2008, August). 1–32. United Nations: Office on Drugs and Crime.

Agthe, A. G., Kim, G. R., & Mathias, K. B. (2009, May). Clonidine as an adjunct therapy to opioids for neonatal abstinence syndrome: A randomized, controlled trial. *Pediatrics, 123*(5), e849–e856. doi:10.1542/peds.2008-0978.

Ailes, E. C., Dawson, A. L., & Lind, J. N. (2015). Opioid prescription claims among women of reproductive age–United States, 2008-2012. *MMWR, Morbidity & Mortality Weekly Report, 64*, 37–41. Retrieved from www.ncbi.nlm.nih.gov/pubmed/25611168

Akyar, E., Seneca, K. H., & Akyar, S. (2016). Linkage to care for suburban heroin users with hepatitis C virus infection, New Jersey, USA. *Emerging Infectious Diseases, 22*(5), 907–909. doi:10.3201/eid2205.151980

Alexander, D., Alexander, K., & Valentino, J. (2012). Intranasal hydrocodone-acetaminophen abuse induced necrosis of the nasal cavity and pharynx. *Laryngoscope, 122*(11), 2378–2381. doi:10.1002/lary.23542

Allen, J. D., Casavant, M. J., & Spiller, H. A. (2017). Prescription opioid exposures among children and adolescents in the United States: 2000-2015. *Pediatrics, 139*(4), pii: e20163382. doi:10.1542/peds.2016-3382

Al-Tayyib, A., Koester, S., & Langegger, S. (2017, July 3). Heroin and methamphetamine injection: An emerging drug use pattern. *Substance Use & Misuse, 52*(8), 1051–1058. doi:10.1080/10826084.2016.1271432.

Anantharamu, T., Sharma, S., & Gupta, A. K. (2015). Naloxegol: First oral peripherally acting mu opioid receptor antagonists for opioid-induced constipation. *Journal of Pharmacology and Pharmacotherapeutics, 6*(3), 188–192. doi:10.4103/0976-500X.162015

Annett, H. E. (1920). Factors influencing alkaloidal content and yield of latex in the opium poppy (Papaver somniferum). *Biochemical Journal, 14*(5), 618–636.

AP, Associated Press. (2016, September 8). Mom whose baby drank formula laced with heroin gets prison. *Fox News*. Plymouth, Massachussetts, USA: Fox News.

AP, Associated Press. (2018, February 10). OxyContin maker will stop marketing opioids to doctors, company says. *The Guardian*, 1.

APA, American Psychiatric Association. (2013). *DMS-5, Diagnostic and Statistical Manual of Mental Disorders* (5th ed.). Washington, D.C.: American Psychiatric Association.

Aquina, C. T., Marques-Baptista, A., & Bridgeman, P. (2009). OxyContin abuse and overdose. *Postgraduate Medicine, 121*(2), 163–167. doi:10.3810/pgm.2009.03.1988

Arner, S., & Meyerson, B. A. (1988, April). Lack of analgesic effect of opioids on neuropathic and idiopathic forms of pain. *Pain, 33*(1), 11–23.

Arnold, C. (2005, December 19). Teen abuse of painkiller OxyContin on the rise. *NPR*, 1–8.

ASAM, American Society of Addiction Medicine. (2016). *Opioid Addiction 2016: Facts & Figures*. American Society of Addiction Medicine.

Back, S. E., Lawson, K. M., & Singleton, L. M. (2011). Characteristics and correlates of men and women with prescription opioid dependence. *Addictive Behaviors, 36*(8), 829–834. doi:10.1016/j.addbeh.2011.03.013

Badalamenti, V. C., Buckley, J. W., & Smith, E. T. (2012). Safety of EMBEda (morphine sulfate and naltrexone hydrochloride) extended-release capsules: Reveiw of postmarketing adverse events during the first year. *Journal of Opioid Management, 8*(2), 115–125.

Bangsberg, D. R., Rosen, J. I., & Aragon, T. (2002). Clostridial myonecrosis cluster among injection drug users: A molecular epidemiology investigation. *Archives of Internal Medicine, 162*(5), 517–522.

Barke, K. E., & Hough, L. B. (1993). Opiates, mast cells and histamine release. *Life Sciences, 53*(18), 1391–1399.

Barth, K. S., Moran-Santa Maria, M., & Lawson, K. (2013). Pain and motives for use among non-treatment seeking individuals with prescription opioid dependence. *The American Journal on Addictions, 22*(5), 486–491. doi:10.1111/j.1521-0391.2013.12038.x

Barton, E. D., Colwell, C. B., & Wolfe, T. (2005). Efficacy of intranasal naloxone as a needleless alternative for treatment of opioid overdose in the prehospital setting. *The Journal of Emergency Medicine, 29*(3), 265–271. doi:10.1016/j.jemermed.2005.03.007

Bass, U. F., Brown, B. S., & DuPont, R. L. (1972). The use of heroin by an offender population: A report over time. *Corrective Psychiatry & Journal of Social Therapy, 18*(4), 24–30.

Bateman, B. T., Hernandez-Diaz, S., & Rathmell, J. P. (2014). Patterns of opioid utilization in pregnancy in a large cohort of commercial insurance beneficiaries in the United States. *Anesthesiology, 120*(5), 1216–1224. doi:10.1097/ALN.0000000000000172

Bazazi, A. R., Yokell, M., & Fu, J. (2011). Illicit use of buprenorphine/naloxone among injecting and non-injecting opioid users. *Journal of Addiction Medicine, 5*, 175–180.

Beletsky, L., Davis, C. S., & Anderson, E. (2008). The law (and politics) of safe injection facilities in the United States. *American Journal of Public Health, 98*(2), 231–237.

Boscarino, J. A., Rukstalis, M. R., & Hoffman, S. N. (2011). Prevalence of prescription opioid-use disorder among chronic pain patients: Comparison of the DSM-5 vs. DSM-4 diagnostic criteria. *Journal of Addictive Diseases, 30* (3), 185–194.

Bouvier, B. A., Elston, B., & Hadland, S. E. (2017). Willingness to use a supervised injection facility among young adults who use prescription opioids non-medically: A cross-sectional study. *Harm Reduction Journal, 14*(13), 1–9. doi:10.1186/s12954-017-01139-0

Boyd, C. J., Young, A., & McCabe, S. E. (2014). Psychological and drug abuse symptoms associated with non-medical use of opioid analgesics among adolescents. *Substance Abuse, 35*(3), 284–289. doi:10.1080/08897077.2014.928660

Brady, K. T., McCauley, J. L., & Back, S. E. (2016). Prescription opioid misuse, abuse, and treatment in the United States: An update. *The American Journal of Psychiatry, 173*(1), 18–26. doi:10.1176/appi.ajp.2015.15020262

Brogly, S. B., Saia, K. A., & Walley, A. Y. (2014). Prenatal buprenorphine versus methadone exposure and neonatal outcomes: Systemic review and meta-analysis. *American Journal of Epidemiology, 180*(7), 673–686. doi:10.1093/aje/kwu190

Broome, L., & So, T.-Y. (2011). Neonatal abstinence syndrome: The use of clonidine as a treatment option. *NeoReviews, 12*(10), e575–e584. doi:10.1542/neo.12-10-e575

Brown, E. (2011, November 1). *Prescription Painkillers Outpace Heroin, Cocaine in OD Deaths. Los Angeles Times*, 1–2. Retrieved from http://articles.latimes.com/2011/nov01/news/la-heb-prescription-drug-overdose-deaths-2…

Brown, M. S., Hayes, M. J., & Thornton, L. M. (2015). Methadone versus morphine for treatment of neonatal abstinence syndrome: A prospective randomized clinical trial. *Journal of Perinatology, 35*(4), 278–283. doi:10.1038/jp.2014.194

Buprenorphine buccal film (Belbuca) for chronic pain. (2016). *The Medical Letter, 58*(1492), 47–48.

Butler, S. F., Cassidy, T. A., & Chilcoat, H. (2013). Abuse rates and routes of administration of reformulated extended-release oxycodone: Initial findings from a sentinel surveillance sample of individuals assessed for substance abuse treatment. *The Journal of Pain, 14*(4), 351–358. doi:10.1016/j.jpain.2012.08.008

Calefati, J. (2008, December 5). The teenage face of heroin abuse: Sean O'Connor, 19. *U.S. News & World Report*, 1.

Carise, D., Dugosh, K. L., & McLellan, A. T. (2007). Prescription OxyContin abuse among patients entering addiction treatment. *American Journal of Psychiatry, 164*(11), 1750–1756.

Carroll, J. J., Marshall, B., & Rich, J. D. (2017). Exposure to fentanyl-contaminated heroin and overdose risk among illicit opioid users in Rhode Island: A mixed methods study. *International Journal of Drug Policy, 46*, 136–145. doi:10.1016/j.drugpo.2017.05.023

Case, A., & Deaton, A. (2015, December 8). Rising morbidity and mortality in midlife among White non-Hispanic Americans in the 21st Century. *Proceedings of the National Academy of Science, 112*(49), 15078–15083. Retrieved from www.pnas.org/cgi/doi/10.1073/pnas.1518393112

Cassidy, T. A., DasMahapatra, P., & Black, R. A. (2014). Changes in prevalence of prescription opioid abuse after introduction of an abuse-deterrent opioid formulation. *Pain Medicine, 15*(3), 440–451. doi:10.1111/pme.12295

CDC, Centers for Disease Control and Prevention. (2018, February 21). *Alcohol Screening and Brief Intervention for People Who Consume Alcohol and Use Opioids*. Atlanta, Georgia: National Center for Injury Prevention and Control.

Cedarbaum, E. R., & Banta-Green, C. J. (2016, January 1). Health behaviors of young adult heroin injectors in the Seattle area. *Drug and Alcohol Dependence, 158*, 102–109. doi:10.1016/j.drugalcdep.2015.11.011

Cepeda, A., Nowotny, K. M., & Frankeberger, J. (2016, September). Precocious transitions and long-term heroin use outcomes: A longitudinal study of gang-affiliated Mexican-American males. *Addictive Behaviors, 60*, 48–52. doi:10.1016/j.addbeh.2016.03.023

Chang, D. C., Klimas, J., & Wood, E. (2018). Medication-assisted treatment for youth with opioid use disorder: Current dilemmas and remaining questions. *The American Journal of Drug and Alcohol Abuse, 44*(2), 143–146. doi:10.1080/00952990.2017.1399403

Chiang, C. N., & Hawks, R. L. (2003). Pharmacokinetics of the combination tablet of buprenorphine and naloxone. *Drug and Alcohol Dependence, 70*(2 Supplement), S39–S47.

Ciccarone, D. (2009). Heroin in brown, black and white: Structural factors and medical consequences in the US heroin market. *International Journal of Drug Policy, 20*(3), 277–282.

Ciccarone, D., & Bourgois, P. (2003). Explaining the geographical variation of HIV among injection drug users in the United States. *Drug and Substance Misuse, 38*(14), 2049–2063.

Cicero, T. J., Ellis, M. S., & Surratt, H. L. (2014a). The changing face of heroin use in the United States: A retrospective analysis of the past 50 years. *JAMA Psychiatry, 71*(7), 821–826. doi:10.1001/jamapsychiatry.2014.366

Cicero, T. J., Ellis, M. S., & Surratt, H. L. (2014b, September 1). Factors contributing to the rise of buprenorphine misuse: 2008-2013. *Drug and Alcohol Dependence, 142*, 98–104. doi:10.1016/j.drugalcdep.2014.06.005

Cicero, T. J., Inciardi, J. A., & Munoz, A. (2005). Trends in abuse of oxycontin and other opioid analgesics in the United States: 2002-2004. *The Journal of Pain*, 662–672.

Cicero, T. J., Surratt, H. L., & Inciardi, J. (2007). Use and misuse of buprenorphine in the management of opioid addiction. *Journal of Opioid Management, 3*, 302–308.

Clarification: Half-life of heroin. (2016). *The Medical Letter, 58*(1489), 32.

Cody, J. T., Valtier, S., & Kuhlman, J. (2001). Analysis of morphine and codeine in samples adulterated with Stealth. *Journal of Analytical Toxicology, 25*(7), 572–575.

Cole, F. S., Wegner, D. J., & Davis, J. M. (2017, August). The genomics of neonatal abstinence syndrome. *Frontiers in Pediatrics, 5*(176), 1–4. doi:10.3389/fped.2017.00176.

Collins, T. R. (2010, February 8). Deaths from methadone overdose disproportionate to number of prescriptions. *Medscape Medical News*. Retrieved from www.medscape.com/viewarticle/716603_print

Colliver, J. D., Compton, W. M., & Gfroerer, J. C. (2006). Projecting drug use among aging baby boomers in 2020. *Annals of Epidemiology, 16*, 257–265.

Compton, W. M., Dawson, D. A., & Goldstein, R. B. (2013, September). Crosswalk between DSM-IV dependence and DSM-5 substance use disorders for opioids, cannabis, cocaine and alcohol. *Drug and Alcohol Dependence, 132* (0), 387–390. doi:10.1016/j.drugalcdep.2013.02.036.

Connery, H. S. (2015). Medication-assisted treatment of opioid use disorder: Review of the evidence and future directions. *Harvard Review of Psychiatry, 23*(2), 63–75. doi:10.1097/HRP.0000000000000075

Cook, B. (2016, August 3). What is the risk of youth sports injuries leading to opioid, heroin abuse? *Forbes*, 1–4.

Corsetti, M., & Tack, J. (2015). Naloxegol: The first orally administered, peripherally acting, mu opioid receptor antagonist, approved for the treatment of opioid-induced consitpation. *Drugs of Today (barcelona), 51*(8), 474–489. doi:10.1358/dot.2015.51.8.2364896

Cramton, R. E., & Gruchala, N. E. (2013). Babies breaking bad: Neonatal and iatrogenic withdrawal syndromes. *Current Opinion in Pediatrics, 25*, 532–542. doi:10.1097/MOP.0b013e328362cd0d

Crane, E. H. (2017). *Emergency Department Visits Involving the Accidental Ingestion of Opioid Pain Relievers by Children Aged 1 to 5*. Rockville, Maryland: Center for Behavioral Health Statisitics and Quality, SAMHSA.

Cygan, J., Trunsky, M., & Corbridge, T. (2000). Inhaled heroin-induced status asthmaticus. *Chest, 117*(1), 272–275.

Darrah, N. (2018, November 14). Michigan mother gave infant methadone because she was being fussy:' Report. *Fox News*. Fox News.

Dart, R. C. (2011). 5th Annual Scientifica Meeting Presentation. *Evaluation of ADFs using RADARS system data*. Retrieved from www.radars.org/Home2/AnnualMeeting/RADARSSystem2011AnnualMeeting.aspx

Dasgupta, A. (2015, February 1). *How People Try to Beat Drug Testing - Issues with Urinary Adulterants Andn Their Detection*. 1–4. Clinical Laboratoty News. Retrieved from www.aacc.org/publications/cln/articles/2015/february/drug-testing.aspx

Davies, H., Gilbert, R., & Johnson, K. (2016). Neonatal drug withdrawal syndrome: Cross-country comparison using hospital administrative data in England, the USA, Western Australia and Ontario, Canada. *Archives of Disease in Childhood. Fetal and Neonatal Edition, 101*(1), F26–F30. doi:10.1136/archdischild-2015-308948

DePriest, A. Z., Puet, B. L., & Holt, A. C. (2015, July). Metabolism and dispositon of prescription opioids: A review. *Forensic Science Review, 27*(2), 115–145.

Desai, R. J., Huybrechts, K. F., & Hernandez-Diaz, S. (2015). Exposure to prescription opioid analgesics in utero and risk of neonatal abstinence syndrome: Population based cohort study. *BMJ, British Medical Journal*, h2102. doi:10.1136/bmj.h2102

Dietrich, E., & Gums, J. G. (2012). Intranasal fentanyl spray: A novel dosage form for the treatment of breakthrough cancer pain. *Annals of Pharmacotherapy, 46*(10), 1382–1391. doi:10.1345/aph.1R069

Doctor, J. N., Nguyen, A., & Lev, R. (2018, August 10). Opioid prescribing decreases after learning of a patient's fatal overdose. *Science, 361*, 588–590.

Doe-Simkins, M., Walley, A. Y., & Epstein, A. (2009). Saved by the nose: Bystander-administered intranasal naloxone hydrochloride for opioid overdose. *American Journal of Public Health, 99*(5), 788–791. doi:10.2105/AJPH.2008.146647

Dowell, D., Haegerich, T. M., & Chou, R. (2016, March 18). CDC guideline for prescribing opioids for chronic pain–United States, 2016. *MMWR, Morbidity and Mortality Recommendations and Reports, 65*(1), 1–49. doi:10.15585/mmwr.rr6501e1.

Ersche, K. D., Clark, L., & London, M. (2006). Profile of executive and memory function associated with amphetamine and opiate dependence. *Neuropsychopharmacology, 31*(5), 1036–1047. doi:10.1038/sj.np.1300889

Extended-Release hydrocodone (Hysingla ER) for pain. (2015). *The Medical Letter, 57*(1468), 71–72.

Extended-Release hydrocodone (Zohydro ER) for pain. (2014). *The Medical Letter, 56*(1444), 45–46.

Fareed, A., Casarella, J., & Amar, R. (2010). Methadone maintenance dosing guideline for opioid dependence: A literature review. *Journal of Addictive Diseases, 29*(1), 1–14.

Farrell, M., Ward, J., & Mattick, R. (1994, October 15). Methadone mainentance treatment in opiate dependence: A review. *BMJ, 309*, 997–1001.

Farzan, A. (2018, August 8). Yes, you can fail a drug test by eating a poppy seed bagel, as a Maryland mother learned. *The Star*. The Washington Post.

Faul, M., Bohm, M., & Alexander, C. (2017, March 31). Methadone prescribing and overdose and the association with Medicaid preferred drug list policies – United States 2007-2014. *MMWR, Morbidity and Mortality Weekly Report, 66*(12), 320–323.

FDA, U.S. Food and Drug Administration. (2014a, September 16). *Press Announcements > FDA Approves Movantik for Opioid-induced Constipation. FDA.gov.* Retrieved October 3, 2016, from www.fda.gov/NewEvents/Newsroom/PressAnnouncements/ucm414620.htm

FDA, U.S. Food and Drug Administration. (2014b, April 3). FDA approves new hand-held auto-injector to reverse opioid overdose. *FDA News Release.*

FDA, U.S. Food and Drug Administration. (2015, November 18). FDA News Release. *FDA moves quickly to approve easy-to-use nasal spray to treat opioid overdose.* Retrieved from www.fda.gov/NewsEvents/Newsroom/PressAnnouncements/ucm473505.htm

FDA, U.S. Food and Drug Administration. (2016a, August 31). FDA drug safety communication: FDA warns about serious risks and death when combining opioid pain or cough medicines with benzodiazepines: Requires its strongest warning. *Safety Announcement.*

FDA, U.S. Food and Drug Administration. (2016b, May 26). Neonatal opioid withdrawal syndrome and medication-assisted treatment with methadone and buprenorphine. *FDA News Release.*

FDA, U.S. Food and Drug Administration. (2017a, September 20). FDA drug safety communication: FDA urges caution about withholding opioid addiction medications from patients taking benzodiazepines or CNS depressants: Careful medication management can reduce risks. *Safety Announcement.*

FDA, U.S. Food and Drug Administration. (2017b, November 14). *Drug Development and Drug Interactions: Table of Substrates, Inhibitors and Inducers.* Maryland: Silver Springs.

FDA, U.S. Food and Drug Administration. (2018a, November 2). Statement from FDA commissioner Scott Gottlieb, M.D., on agency's approval of Dsuvia and the FDA's future consideration of new opioids. *Statement.*

FDA, U.S. Food and Drug Administration. (2018b, December 10). FDA clears mobile medical app to help those with opioid use disorder stay in recovery programs. *FDA News Release.*

Feng, X., Zhu, L., & Zhou, Q. (2017). Opioid analgesics-related pharmacokinetic drug interactions: From the perspectives of evidence based on randomized controlled trials and clinical risk management. *Journal of Pain Management, 10,* 1225–1239.

Flacke, J. W., Flacke, W. E., & Bloor, B. C. (1987). Histamine release by four narcotics: A double-blind study in humans. *Anesthesia and Analgesia, 66*(8), 723–730.

Flassing, J. (2010). Buprenorphine: A more accessible treatment for opioid dependence. *Journal of the American Academy of Physician Assistants, 23*(9), 40–43.

Fleischauer, A. T., Ruhl, L., & Rhea, S. (2017, June 9). Hospitalizations for endocarditis and associated health care costs among persons with diagnosed drug dependence – North Carolina, 2010-2015. *Morbidity and Mortality Weekly Report, 66*(22), 569–573.

Ford, J. A., Pomykacz, C., & Veliz, P. (2018). Sports involvement, injury history, and non-medical use of prescription opioids among college students: An analysis with a national sample. *The American Journal on Addictions, 27*(1), 15–22. doi:10.1111/ajad.12657

Frieden, T. R., & Houry, D. (2016, March 15). *Reducing the Risks of Relief - the CDC Opioid-Prescribing Guideline [epub Ahead of Print].* PubMed – NCBI. Retrieved April 7, 2016, from www.gov.nih.gov/pubmed/?term=frieden+houry

Gaalema, D. E., Heil, S. H., & Badger, G. J. (2013, November 1). Time to initiation of treatment for neonatal abstinence syndrome in neonates exposed in utero to buprenorphine or methadone. *Drug and Alcohol Dependence, 133*(1), 266–269. doi:10.1016/jdrugalcdep.2013.06.004.

Gallagher, B. K., Shin, Y., & Roohan, P. (2016, April 29). Opioid prescriptions among women of reproductive age enrolled in Medicaid–New York, 2008-2013. *MMWR, Morbidity and Mortality Weekly Report, 65*(16), 415–417. doi:10.15585/mmwr.mm6516a2.

Garbutt, J. C., Kranzler, H. R., & O'Malley, S. S. (2005). Efficacy and tolerability of long-acting injectable naltrexone for alcohol dependence: A randomized controlled study. *JAMA, the Journal of the American Medical Association, 293,* 1617–1625.

Garnock-Jones, K. P. (2015). Naloxegol: A review of its use in patients with opioid-induced constipation. *Drugs, 75*(4), 419–425. doi:10.1007/s40265-015-0357-2

Gastfriend, D. R. (2014). A pharmaceutical industry perspective on the economics of treatments for alcohol and opioid use disorders. *Annals of the New York Academy of Sciences, 1327,* 112–130. doi:10.1111/nyas.12538

Gharagozlou, P., Demirci, H., & Clark, J. D. (2002). Activation profiles of opioid ligands in HEK cells expressing delta opioid receptors. *BMC Neuroscience, 3*(1), 19.

Girion, L., Glover, S., & Smith, D. (2011, September 17). *Drug Deaths Now Outnumber Traffic Fatalities in U.S., Data Show. Los Angeles Times,* 1–3. Retrieved from http://articles.latimes.com/2011/sep/17/local/la-me-drugs-epidemic-20110918

Gladden, R. M., Martinez, P., & Seth, P. (2016, August 26). Fentanyl law enforcement submissions and increases in synthetic opioid-involved overdose deaths – 27 states, 2013-2014. *MMWR, Morbidity & Mortality Weekly Report, 65*(33), 837–843. doi:10.15585/mmwr.mm6533a2.

Glenza, J. (2016, October 31). US child opioid overdoses increased over past two decades, research finds. *The Guardian,* 1–5.

Gnanadesigan, N., Espinoza, R. T., & Smith, R. (2005, July-August). Interaction of serotonergic antidepressants and opioid analgesics: Is serotonin syndrome going undetected? *Journal of the American Medical Directors Association, 6* (4), 265–269.

Gorden, E. (2018, September 7). What's the evidence that supervised drug injection sites save lives? Boston: NPR.

Gossop, M., & Moos, R. (2008). Substance misuse among older adults: A neglected but treatable problem. *Addiction, 103*, 347–348.

Grassin-Delyle, S., Buenestado, A., & Naline, E. (2012). Intranasal drug delivery: An efficient and non-invasive route for systemic administration: Focus on opioids. *Pharmacology & Therapeutics, 134*(3), 366–379. doi:10.1016/j.pharmthera.2012.03.003

Greenstein, R. A., Arndt, I. C., & McLellan, A. T. (1984). Naltrexone: A clinical perspective. *The Journal of Clinical Psychiatry, 45*(9, part 2), 25–28.

Greenwald, M. K., Comer, S. D., & Fiellin, D. A. (2014, November 1). Buprenorphine maintenance and mu-opioid receptor availability in the treatment of opioid use disorder: Implications for clinical use and policy. *Drug and Alcohol Dependence, 144*, 1–11. doi:10.1016/j.drugalcdep.2014.07.035

Griesler, P. C., Hu, M.-C., & Wall, M. M. (2019, February). Nonmedical prescription opioid use by parents and adolescents in the US. *Pediatrics*, e20182354. doi:10.1542/peds.2018-2354

Gudin, J. (2012, December). Opioid therapies and cyctochrome P450 interactions. *Journal of Pain and Symptom Management, 44*(6S), S4–S14. doi:10.1016/j.jpainsymman.2012.08.013.

Guy, G. P., Zhang, K., & Bohm, M. K. (2017, July 7). Vital signs: Changes in opioid prescribing in the United States. 2006-2015. *MMWR, Morbidity and Mortality Weekly Report, 66*(26), 697–704.

Hadland, S. E., Cerda, M., & Li, Y. (2018). Association of pharmaceutical industry marketing of opioid products to physicians with subsequent opioid prescribing. *JAMA Internal Medicine, 178*(6), 861–863.

Hadland, S. E., Wharam, J. F., & Schuster, M. A. (2017). Trends in receipt of buprenorphine and naltrexone for opioid use disorder among adolescents and young adults, 2001-2014. *JAMA Pediatrics, 171*(8), 747–755. doi:10.1001/jamapediatrics.2017.0745

Haffajee, R. L., & Mello, M. M. (2017, December 14). Drug companies' liability for the opioid epidemic. *The New England Journal of Medicine, 377*, 2301–2305.

Hamilton, R. J., Olmedo, R. E., & Shah, S. (2002). Complications of ultrarapid opioid detoxification with subcutaneous naltrexone pellets. *Academic Emergency Medicine, 9*(1), 63–68.

Han, B., Gfroerer, J. C., & Colliver, J. D. (2009a). *An Examination of Trends in Illicit Drug Use among Adults Aged 50 to 59 in the United States*. Rockville, Maryland: Substance Abuse and Mental Health Services Administration, Office of Applied Studies.

Han, B., Gfroerer, J. C., & Colliver, J. D. (2009b). Substance use disorder among older adults in the United States in 2020. *Addiction, 104*(1), 88–96.

Hansten, P. D. (1986). Drug interactions. In A. M. Pagliaro & L. A. Pagliaro (Eds.), *Pharmacologic Aspects of Nursing* (pp. 170–179). St. Louis, Missouri: C. V. Mosby.

Hansten, P. D. (2002). Pediatric drug interactions. In L. A. Pagliaro & A. M. Pagliaro (Eds.), *Problems in Pediatric Drug Therapy* (4th ed., pp. 315–346). Washington, D. C.: American Pharmaceutical Association.

Hard, B. (2014, November 28). Management of opioid painkiller dependence in primary care: Ongoing recovery with buprenorphine/naloxone. *BMJ Case Reports*, 207308. doi:10.1136/bcr-2014-207308

Harris, B. R. (2016, October). Talking about screening, brief intervention, and referral to treatment for adolescents: An upstream intervention to address the heroin and prescription opioid epidemic. *Preventive Medicine, 91*, 397–399. doi:10.1016/j.ypmed.2016.08.022

Harris, B. R., Shaw, B. A., & Sherman, B. R. (2016). Screening, brief intervention, and referral to treatment for adolescents: Attitudes, perceptions and practice of New York school-based health center providers. *Journal of Substance Abuse, 37*(1), 161–167. doi:10.1080/08897077.2015.1015703

Hasin, D. S., O'Brien, C. P., & Auriacombe, M. (2013). DSM-5 criteria for substance use disorders: Recommendations and rationale. *The American Journal of Psychiatry, 170*(8), 834–851. doi:10.1176/appi.ajp.2013.12060782

Havens, J. R., Leukefeld, C. G., & DeVeaugh-Geiss, A. M. (2014, June 1). The impact of a reformulation of extended-release oxycodone designed to deter abuse in a sample of prescription opioid abusers. *Drug and Alcohol Dependence, 139*, 9–17. doi:10.1016/j.drugalcdep.2014.02.018

Hedegaard, H., Bastian, B. A., & Trinidad, J. P. (2018, December 12). Drugs most frequently involved in drug overdose deaths: United States, 2011-2016. *National Vital Statistics Reports, 67*(9), 1–14.

Heil, S. H., Jones, H. E., & Arria, A. (2011). Unintended pregnancy I opioid-abusing women. *Journal of Substance Abuse Treatment, 40*(2), 199–202.

HHS, Health and Human Services. (2018, December 19). HHS recommends prescribing or co-prescribing naloxone to those at high risk for an opioid overdose. *HHS Press Release*, 1–5.

Hiltunen, A. J., & Eklund, C. (2002). Withdrawal from methadone maintenance treatment. Reasons for not trying to quit methadone. *European Addiction Research, 8*(1), 38–44.

Hogan, J. (2018, November 13). Mother charged with giving infant methadone 'because she was fussy'. *ABC 13*, 1. Grand Rapids, Michigan: ABC News.

Holder, R. M., & Rhee, D. (2016, March 6). Novel oral therapies for opioid-induced bowel dysfuntion in patients with chronic noncancer pain [Epub ahead of print]. *Pharmacotherapy*. doi:10.1002/phar.1711.

Holmquist, G. L. (2009). Opioid metabolism and effects of cytochrome P450. *Pain Medicine, 10*(S1), S20–S29. doi:10.1111/j.1526-4637.2009.00596.x

Holscher, F., Reissner, V., & Di Furia, L. (2010). Differences between men and women in the course of opiate dependence: Is there a telescoping effect? *260*(3), 235–241. doi:10.1007/s00406-009-0053-x

Houlihan, D. J. (2004). Serotonin syndrome resulting from coadministration of tramadol, venlafaxine, and mirtazapine. *The Annals of Pharmacotherapy, 38*(3), 411–413.

Hoyle, J. (2002). Stealth advertising on the Internet: Scumware. *Journal of the American Dental Association, 133*(4), 427.

Hudak, M. L., & Tan, R. C. (2012). Neonatal drug withdrawal. *Pediatrics, 129*, e540–e560. doi:10.1542/peds.2011-3212

Ihongbe, T. O., & Masho, S. W. (2016, December). Prevalence, correlates and patterns of heroin use among young adults in the United States. *Addictive Behaviors, 63*, 74–81. doi:10.1016/j.addbeh.2016.07.003

Inturrisi, C. E. (2002). Clinical pharmacology of opioids for pain. *The Clinical Journal of Pain, 18*(4 Suppl), S3–S13.

Jamison, R. N., Ross, E. L., & Michna, E. (2010). Substance misuse treatment for high risk chronic pain patients on opioid therapy: A randomized trial. *Pain, 150*(3), 390–400. doi:10.1016/j.pain.2010.02.033

Jansson, L. M., & Velez, M. (2012). Neonatal abstinence syndrome. *Current Opinion in Pediatrics, 24*(2), 252–258. doi:10.1097/MOP.0b013e32834fdc.3a

Johnson, F., & Setnik, B. (2011). Morphine sulfate and naltrexone hydrochloride extended-release capsules: Naltrexone release, pharmacodynamics, and tolerability. *Pain Physician, 14*(4), 391–406.

Johnson, K., Gerada, C., & Greenough, A. (2003). Treatment of neonatal abstinence syndrome. *Archives of Disease in Childhood, 88*, F2–F5.

Johnston, L. D., Miech, R. A., & O'Malley, P. M. (2018). *Monitoring the Future National Survey Results on Drug Use, 1975-2017: Overview, Key Findings on Adolescent Drug Use*. Ann Arbor: Institute for Social Research, The University of Michigan.

Jones, C. M., Logan, J., & Gladden, R. M. (2015, July 10). Vital signs: Demographic and substance use trends among heroin users – United States, 2002-2013. *MMWR, Morbidity and Mortality Weekly Report, 64*, 719–725.

Jones, C. M., Muhuri, P. K., & Lurie, P. G. (2017). Trends in the nonmedical use of OxyContin, United States, 2006 to 2013. *The Clinical Journal of Pain, 33*(5), 452–461. doi:10.1097/AJP.0000000000000426

Jones, C. M., Paulozzi, L. J., & Mack, K. A. (2014). Alcohol involvement in opioid pain reliever and benzodiazepine drug abuse–Related emergency department visits and drug-related deaths – United States, 2010. *Morbidity and Mortality Weekly Report (MMWR), 63*(40), 881–885.

Jones, H. E., Finnegan, L. P., & Kaltenbach, K. (2012). Methadone and buprenorphine for the management of opioid dependence in pregnancy. *Drugs, 72*(6), 747–757. doi:10.2165/11632820-000000000-00000

Jones, R., Prommer, E., & Backstedt, D. (2015, July 6). Naloxegol: A novel therapy in the management of opioid-induced constipation. *American Journal of Hospice and Palliative Care*, Epub ahead of print. Retrieved March 12, 2016, from www.ncbi.nim.nih.gov/pubmed/26150678

Jordan, A. E., Blackburn, N. A., & Des Jarlais, D. C. (2017, June). Past-year prevalence of prescription opioid misuse among those 11 to 30 years of age in the United States: A systematic review and meta-analysis. *Journal of Substance Abuse Treatment*, 77, 31–37. doi:10.1016/j.jsat.2017.03.007

Joseph, H., Stancliff, S., & Langrod, J. (2000, October-November). Methadone maintenance treatment (MMT): A review of historical and clinical issues. *The Mount Sinai Journal of Medicine, New York, 67*(5–6), 347–364.

Jumah, N. A. (2016). Rural, pregnant, and opioid dependent: A systematic review. *Substance Abuse Research and Treatment, 10*(S1), 35–41. doi:10.4137/SART.s34547

Katz, J., Rosenbloom, B. N., & Fashler, S. (2015). Chronic pain, psychopathology, and DSM-5 somatic symptom disorder. *Canadian Journal of Psychiatry, 60*(4), 160–167. doi:10.1177/070674371506000402

Katz, N., Dart, R. C., & Bailey, E. (2011). Tampering with prescription opioids: Nature and extent of the problem, health consequences, and solutions. *The American Journal of Drug and Alcohol Abuse, 37*(4), 205–217. doi:10.3109/00952990.2011.569623

Kauffman, R. E., Banner, W., & Blumer, J. L. (1990, September). Naloxone dosage and route of administration for infants and children: Addendum to emergency drug doses for infants and children. *Pediatrics, 86*(3), 484–485.

Keen, L., Khan, M., & Clifford, L. (2014, September). Injection and non-injection drug use and infectious disease in Baltimore city: Diferences by race. *Addictive Behaviors, 39*(9), 1325–1328. doi:10.1016/j.addbeh.2014.04.020.

Kerr, T., Mitra, S., & Clare-Kennedy, M. (2017). Supervised injection facilities in Canada: Past, present, and future. *Harm Reduction Journal, 14*(28), 1–9. doi:10.1186/s12954-017-0154-1

Kirchmayer, U., Davoli, M., & Verster, A. (2000). Naltrexone maintenance treatment for opioid dependence. *Cochrane Database of Systematic Reviews, 2*, CD001333.

Ko, J. Y., Patrick, S. W., & Tong, V. T. (2016, August 12). Incidence of neonatal abstinence syndrome – 28 states, 1999-2013. *MMWR, Morbidity and Mortality Weekly Report, 65*(31), 799–802.

Ko, J. Y., Wolicki, S., & Barfield, W. D. (2017, March 10). CDC Grand Rounds: Public health strategies to prevent neonatal abstinence syndrome. *MMWR, Morbidity and Mortality Weekly Report, 66*(9), 242–245.

Kocherlakota, P. (2014, July 28). Neonatal abstinence syndrome. *Pediatrics, 134,* e547–e561. doi:10.1542/peds.2013-3524

Koneru, A., Nelson, N., & Hariri, S. (2016, July 22). Increased hepatitis C virus (HCV) detection in women of childbearing age and potential risk for vertical transmission–United States and Kentucky, 2011-2014. *MMWR, Mobidity and Mortality Weekly Report, 65*(28), 705–710. doi:10.15585/mmwr.mm6528a2(http://dx//doi.org/10.15585/mmwr.mm6528a2.

Kovas, A. E., McFarland, B. H., & McCarty, D. J. (2007). Buprenorphine for acute heroin detoxification: Diffusion of research into practice. *Journal of Substance Abuse Treatment, 32*(2), 199–206.

Kraft, W. K., Adeniyi-Jones, S. C., & Chervoneva, I. (2017, June 15). Buprenorphine for the treatment of the neonatal abstinence syndrome. *The New England Journal of Medicine, 376*(24), 2341–2348. doi:10.1056/NEJMoa1614835.

Kraft, W. K., Dysart, K., & Greenspan, J. S. (2011, March). Revised dose schema of sublingual buprenorphine in the treatment of the neonatal opioid abstinence syndrome. *Addiction, 106*(3), 574–580. doi:10.1111/j.1360-0443.2010.03170.x.

Krans, E. E., & Patrick, S. W. (2016). Opioid use disorder in pregnancy: Health policy and practice in the midst of an epidemic. *Obstetrics & Gynecology, 128*(1), 4–10. doi:10.1097/AOG.0000000000001446

Krantz, A. J., Hershow, R. C., & Prachand, N. (2003). Heroin insufflation as a trigger for patients with life-threatening asthma. *Chest, 123*(2), 510–517.

Kumar, R. (2017). Association between concurrent use of prescription opioids and benzodiazepines and overdose: Retrospective analysis. *BMJ, 356,* 760.

Lee, J. D., Friedmann, P. D., & Kinlock, T. W. (2016). Extended-release naltrexone to prevent opioid relapse in criminal justice offenders. *New England Journal of Medicine, 374*(13), 1232–1242. doi:10.1056/NEJMoa1505409

Lemke, R. P. (2002). Drug dosing for neonates. In L. A. Pagliaro & A. M. Pagliaro (Eds.), *Problems in Pediatric Drug Therapy* (4th ed., pp. 531–554). Washington, DC: American Pharmaceutical Association.

Leppert, W. (2015, April 16). Emerging therapies for patients with symptoms of opioid-induced bowel dysfunction. *Drug Design, Development and Therapy, 9,* 2215–2231. doi:10.2147/DDDT.S32684

Lind, J. N., Petersen, E. E., & Lederer, P. A. (2015). Infant and maternal characteristics in neonatal abstinence syndrome–Selected hospitals in Florida, 2010-2011. *MMWR, Morbidity and Mortality Weekly Report, 64*(8), 213–216.

Logan, B. A., Brown, M. S., & Hayes, M. J. (2013, March). Neonatal abstinence syndrome: Treatment and pediatric outcomes. *Clinical Obstetrics and Gynecology, 56*(1), 186–192. doi:10.1097/GFR.0b013e31827feea4.

Lotsch, J. (2005, May). Opioid metabolites. *Journal of Pain and Symptom Management, 29*(5S), S10–S24. doi:10.1016/j.jpainsymman.2005.01.004.

Lyapustina, T., & Alexander, G. C. (2015, June 13). The prescription opioid addiction and abuse epidemic: How it happened and what we can do about it. *The Pharmaceutical Journal, 294*(7866). doi:10.1211/PJ.2015.20068579

MacDonald, R., Heiner, J., & Villarreal, J. (2015). Loperamide dependence and abuse. *BMJ Case Reports, pii,* brc2015209705. doi:10.1136/bcr-2015-209705

MacLaren, E. (2015). *Oxycodone History and Statistics. Drugabuse.com,* 1–23. Retrieved March 12, 2016, from http://drugabuse.com/library/oxycodone-history-and-statistics/

Malleson, P. N., Connell, H., & Bennett, S. M. (2001). Chronic musculoskeletal and other idiopathic pain syndromes. *Archives of Disease in Childhood, 84,* 189–192.

Manchikanti, L. (2007). National drug control policy and prescription drug abuse. *Pain Physician, 10,* 399–424.

Manchikanti, L., & Singh, A. (2008). Therapeutic opioids: A ten-year perspective on the complexities and complications of the escalating use, abuse, and nonmedical use of opioids. *Pain Physician, 11*(2 Supplement), S63–S88.

Marraffa, J. M., Holland, M. G., & Sullivan, R. W. (2014). Cardiac conduction disturbance after loperamide abuse. *Clinical Toxicology (Philadelphia), 52*(9), 952–957. doi:10.3109/15563650.2014.969371

Mars, S. G., Bourgois, P., & Karandinos, G. (2014, March). "Every 'never' I ever said came true:" Transitions from opioid pills to heroin injecting. *International Journal on Drug Policy, 25*(2), 257–266. doi:10.1016/j.drugpo.2013.10.004.

Marsch, L. A., Moore, S. K., & Ducat, E. (2016). A randomized controlled trial of buprenorphine taper duration among opioid-dependent adolescents and young adults. *Addiction, 111*(8), 1406–1415. doi:10.1111/add.13363

Martins, S. S., Sarvet, A., & Sanaella-Tenorio, J. (2017). Changes in US lifetime heroin use and heroin use disorder: Prevalence from the 2001-2002 to 2012-2013 National Epidemiologic Survey on Alcohol and Related Conditions. *JAMA Psychiatry, 74*(5), 445–455. doi:10.1001/jamapsychiatry.2017.0113

Martins, S. S., Segura, L. E., & Santaella-Tenoria, J. (2017, February). Prescription opioid use disorder and heroin use among youth nonmedical prescription opioid users from 2002 to 2014. *Addictive Behaviors, 65,* 236–241. doi:10.1016/j.addbeh.2016.08.033

Martins, S. S., Storr, C. L., & Zhu, H. (2009). Correlates of extramedical use of OxyContin versus other analgesic opioids among the US general population. *Drug and Alcohol Dependence, 99*(1–3), 58–67. doi:10.1016/j.drugalcdep.2008.06.013

Mauer, P. M., & Bartkowski, R. R. (1993). Drug interactions of clinical significance with opioid analgesics. *Drug Safety, 8*(1), 30–48.

Mauer, U., Kager, C., & Fellinger, C. (2014, February 27). Risk of anaphylaxis in opioid dependent persons: Effects of heroin versus substitution substances. *Substance Abuse Treatment, Prevention, and Policy, 9*, 12. doi:10.1186/1747-597X-9-12

McCabe, S. E., Boyd, C. J., & Cranford, J. A. (2009). Motives for nonmedical use of prescription opioids among high school seniors in the United States: Self-treatment and beyond. *Archives of Pediatric & Adolescent Medicine, 163*(8), 739–744. doi:10.1001/archpediatrics.2009.120

McCance-Katz, E. F., Sullivan, L., & Nallani, S. (2010). Drug interactions of clinical importance among the opioids, methadone and buprenorphine, and other frequently prescribed medications: A review. *The American Journal on Addictions, 19*(1), 4–16. doi:10.1111/j.1521-0391.2009.00005.x

McCarthy, D. M., Tomlinson, K. L., & Anderson, K. G. (2005). Relapse in alcohol and drug disordered adolescents with comorbid psychopathology. *Psychology of Addictive Behaviors, 19*(1), 28–34.

McDonald, D. C., & Carlson, K. E. (2013, July 17). Estimating the prevalence of opioid diversion by "Doctor Shoppers" in the United States. *PLoS ONE, 8*(7), 1–25, e69241. doi:10.1371/journal.pone.0069241.

Meacham, M. C., Strathdee, S. A., & Rangel, G. (2016). Prevalence and correlates of heroin-methamphetamine co-injection among persons who inject drugs in San Diego, California, and Tijuana, Baja California, Mexico. *Journal of Studies on Alcohol and Drugs*, 77, 774–781.

Megarbane, B., Gueye, P., & Baud, F. (2003, November). Interactions between benzodiazepines and opioids. *Annales De Medicine Interne, 154*(Spec No 2), S64–S72.

Michna, E., Kirson, N. Y., & Shei, A. (2014). Use of prescription opioids with abuse-deterrent technology to address opioid abuse. *Current Medical Research and Opinion, 30*(8), 1589–1598. doi:10.1185/03007995.2014.915803

Miles, F. (2018, February 18). Promising Ivy League student, 19, killed in opioid crisis. *Fox News*, 1. FoxNews.com.

Minozzi, S., Amato, L., & Bellisario, C. (2013, December 23). Maintenance agonist treatments for opiate-dependent pregnant women. *Cochrane Database of Systematic Reviews, 12*, CD006318. doi:10.1002/14651858.CD006318.pub3

Minozzi, S., Amato, L., & Vecchi, S. (2011). Oral naltrexone maintenance treatment for opioid dependence. *Cochrane Database of Systematic Reviews, 4*, CD001333. doi:10,1002/14651858.CD001333.pub4

Moss, J., & Roscow, C. E. (1983, October). Histamine release by narcotics and muscle relaxants in humans. *Anesthesiology, 59*(4), 330–339.

Muhuri, P. K., Gfroerer, J. C., & Davies, M. C. (2013, August). *Associations of Nonmedical Pain Reliever Use and Initiation of Heroin Use in the United States.* CBHSQ (Center for Behavioral Health Statistics and Quality) Data Review. Retrieved March 3, 2016, from http://archive.samhsa.gov/data/2k13/DataReview/DR006/nonmedical-pain-reliever-use-2013.htm

Nair, P., Black, M. M., & Schuler, M. (1997, November). Risk factors for disruption in primary caregiving among infants of substance abusing women. *Child Abuse and Neglect, 21*(11), 1039–1051.

A naloxone. (2014, June 9). A naloxone auto-injector (Evzio). *The Medical Letter, 56*(1444), 45–46.

Naltrexone. (2009, February 1). *Medline Plus.* 1–4. Retrieved from www.nlm.nih.gov/medlineplus/druginfo/meds/a685041.html

National Drug Intelligence Center. (2001, May). *Heroin. California Central District Dug Threat Assessment.* 1–8. National Drug Intelligence Center. Retrieved from www.justice.gov/ndic/pubs0/668/heroin.htm

Nelson, E. M., & Philbrick, A. M. (2012, December 12). Avoiding serotonin syndrome: The nature of the interaction between tramadol and selective serotonin reuptake inhibitors. *Annals of Pharmacotherapy.*

NIDA, National Institute on Drug Abuse. (2014, June 24). What can we do about the heroin overdose epidemic? 1–6. Retrieved June 26, 2014, from www.drugabuse.gov/about-nida/noras-blog/2014/06/what-can-we-do-about-heroin-o...

NIDA, National Institute on Drug Abuse. (2015a, November 18). FDA approves naloxone nasal spray to reverse opioid overdose. 1–4. Retrieved January 12, 2016, from www.drugabuse.gov/news-events/news-releases/2015/11/fda-approves-naloxone-nas...

NIDA, National Institute on Drug Abuse. (2015b, December). Overdose Death Rates. Retrieved February 21, 2016, from www.drugabuse.gov/related-topics/trends-statistics/overdose-death-rates

NIDA, National Institute on Drug Abuse. (2016, May 5). *Fake Prescription Drugs Laced with Fentanyl.* 1–2. National Institute on Drug Abuse (NIDA). Retrieved May 5, 2016, from www.drugabuse.gov/emerging-trends/fake-prescription-drugs-laced-fentanyl?utm_source=NIDA+Emerging+Trends&utm_campaign=abd868b77...

NIDA, National Institute on Drug Abuse. (2017, November 14). *Opioid Treament Drugs Have Similar Outcomes once Patients Initiate Treatment. Press release.* Bethesda, Maryland: National Institutes of Health.

NIDA, National Institute on Drug Abuse. (2019, February 19). Monthly buprenorphine injections effective for opioid use disorders. *News Release.* National Institutes of Health.

NIH, National Institute on Drug Abuse. (2018, August). Overdose death rates. *Advancing Addiction Science*, 1–4. NIH.

Nordrum, A. (2015, July 7). *Deaths from Heroin Overdoses Have Quadrupled over past Decade in US*, CDC *Says.* IBTimes. Retrieved March 19, 2016, from www.ibtimes.com/deaths-heroin-overdoses-have-quadrupled-over-past-decade-us-cdc-says-1998702?rel=rel2

Nordrum, A. (2016, January 21). *Addiction 2016: As Heroin Use Escalates, a New Drug to Reverse Overdoses Hits US Drugstores*. IBTimes.com. Retrieved from http://www.ibtimes.com/addiction-2016-heroin-use-escalates-new-drug-reverse-overdoses-hits-us-drugstores-2271924

Novak, S. P., Bluthenthal, R., & Wenger, L. (2016). Initiation of heroin and prescription opioid pain relievers by birth cohort. *American Journal of Public Health, 106*, 298–300. doi:10.2105/AJPH.2015.302972

O'Connor, P. G., & Kosten, T. R. (1998). Rapid and ultrarapid opioid detoxification techniques. *JAMA, 279*(3), 229–234. doi:10.1001/jama.279.3.229

O'Donnell, J. K., Halpin, J., & Mattson, C. L. (2017, November 3). Deaths involving fentanyl, fentanyl analogs, and U-47700-10 states, July-December 2016. *MMWR, Morbidity and Mortality Weekly Report, 66*(43), 1197–1202.

Ochoa, K. C., Hahn, J. A., & Seal, K. H. (2001). Overdosing among young injection drug users in San Francisco. *Addictive Behaviors, 26*(3), 453–460.

Ocker, K. (2016, October 31). Mom gave kids heroin as 'feel-good medicine,' charges say. *The News Tribune*, 1–2. Parkland, Washington. Retrieved November 1, 2016

Oei, J. L., Xu, H. X., & Abdel-Latif, M. E. (2012). Dopamine D2 receptor gene polymorphisms in newborn infants of drug-using women. *Archives of Disease in Childhood. Fetal and Neonatal Edition, 97*(3), F193–F198. doi:10.1136/archdischild-2011-300235

Okada, Y., Tsuda, Y., & Bryant, S. D. (2002). Endomorphins and related opioid peptides. *Vitamins and Hormones, 65*, 257–279.

Onay, N. (2017, December 13). Police: Pregnant mother in southern Indiana pases out behind wheel with child in backseat. *FOX59 web*. Evansville, Indiana: FOX59 TV.

Orciari Herman, A. (2017a, October 19). Extended-release naltrexone seems as effective as standard treatment for opioid dependence. *NEJM Journal Watch*. NEJM.

Orciari Herman, A. (2017b, November 28). Out-of-hospital naloxone for opioid overdose: What's the optimal strategy? *NEJM Journal Watch*. NEJM.

Osborn, D. A., Jeffery, H. E., & Cole, M. J. (2005, July 20). Sedatives for opiate withdrawal in newborn infants. *Cochrane Database of Systematic Reviews, 3*, CD002053. doi:10.1002/14651858.CD002053.pub2

Osborn, D. A., Jeffery, H. E., & Cole, M. J. (2010a, October 6). Opiate treatment for opiate withdrawal in newborn infants. *Cochrane Database of Systematic Reviews, 10*, CD002059. doi:10.1002/14651858.CD002059.pub3

Osborn, D. A., Jeffery, H. E., & Cole, M. J. (2010b, October 6). Sedatives for opiate withdrawal in newborn infants. *Cochrane Database of Systematic Reviews, 10*, CD002053. doi:10.1002/14651858.CD002053.pub3

Overholser, B. R., & Foster, D. R. (2011). Opioid pharmacokinetic drug-drug interactions. *The American Journal of Managed Care, 17*, S276–S287.

Pagliaro, A. M., & Pagliaro, L. A. (Eds.). (1986). *Pharmacologic Aspects of Nursing*. St. Louis: C. V. Mosby.

Pagliaro, A. M., & Pagliaro, L. A. (2000). *Substance Use among Women: A Reference and Resource Guide*. Philadelphia, PA: Brunner/Mazel.

Pagliaro, A. M., & Pagliaro, L. A. (2018). *Women's Drug and Substance Abuse: A Comprehensive Analysis and Reflective Synthesis*. New York, New York: Routledge.

Pagliaro, A. M., Pagliaro, L. A., & Thauberger, P. C. (1993). Knowledge, behaviours, and risk perception of intravenous drug users in relation to HIV infection and AIDS: The PIARG Projects. *Advances in Medical Psychotherapy, 6*, 1–28.

Pagliaro, L. A., & Pagliaro, A. M. (1999). *PNDR: Psychologists' Neuropsychotropic Drug Reference*. Philadelphia, PA: Brunner/Mazel.

Pagliaro, L. A., & Pagliaro, A. M. (Eds.). (2002). *Problems in Pediatric Drug Therapy* (4th ed.). Washington, DC: American Pharmaceutical Association.

Pagliaro, L. A., & Pagliaro, A. M. (2004). *Pagliaros' Comprehensive Guide to Drugs and Substances of Abuse*. Washington, D. C.: American Pharmacists Association.

Pagliaro, L. A., & Pagliaro, A. M. (2009). *Pagliaros' Comprehensive Guide to the Drugs and Substances of Abuse* (2nd ed.). Washington, DC: American Pharmacists Association.

Pagliaro, L. A., & Pagliaro, A. M. (2012). *Handbook of Child and Adolescent Drug and Substance Abuse*. Hoboken, New Jersey: Wiley & Sons.

Palamar, J. J., Shearston, J. A., & Dawson, E. W. (2016, January 1). Nonmedical opioid use and heroin use in a nationally representative sample of US high school seniors. *Drug and Alcohol Dependence, 158*, 132–138. doi:10.1016/j.drugalcdep.2015.11.005

Park, H., & Bloch, M. (2016, January 19). *How the Epidemic of Drug Overdose Deaths Ripples across America. The New York Times*. Retrieved July 16, 2016, from www.nytimes.com/interactive/2016/01/07/us/drug-overdose-deaths-in-the-us.html

Passik, S. D., Hays, L., & Eisner, N. (2006). Psychiatric and pain characteristics of prescription drug abusers entering drug rehabilitation. *Journal of Pain and Palliative Care Pharmacotherapy, 20*(2), 5–13.

Patrick, S. W., & Schiff, D. M. (2017). A public health response to opioid use in pregnancy. *Pediatrics, 39*(3), pii: e20164070. doi:10.1542/peds.2016-4070

Patrick, S. W., Schumacher, R. E., & Benneyworth, B. D. (2012). Neonatal abstinence syndrome and associated health care expenditures: United States, 2000-2009. *JAMA: Journal of the American Medical Association, 307*(18), 1934–1940. doi:10.1001/jama.2012.3951

Peavy, K. M., Banta-Green, C. J., & Kingston, S. (2012, July-August). "Hooked on" prescription-type opiates prior to using heroin: Results from a survey of syringe exchange clients. *Journal of Psychoactive Drugs, 44*(3), 259–265. doi:10.1080/02791072.2012.704591.

Pergolizzi, J. V. (2011, September 20). Quantifying the impact of drug-drug interactions associated with opioids. *The American Journal of Managed Care, 17*, S288–S292.

Pergolizzi, J. V., Labhsetwar, S. A., & Puenpatom, R. A. (2011). Prevalence of exposure to potential CYP450 pharmacokinetc drug-drug interactions among patients with chronic low back pain taking opioids. *Pain Practice, 11*(3), 230–239.

Pergolizzi, J. V., Ma, L., & Foster, D. R. (2014). The prevalence of opioid-related major potential drug-drug interations and their impact on health care costs in chronic pain patients. *Journal of Manged Care & Specialty Pharmacy, 20*(5), 467–476.

Peterson, A. B., Gladden, R. M., & Delcher, C. (2016, August 26). Increases in fentanyl-related overdose deaths – Florida and Ohio, 2013-2015. *MMWR, Morbidity and Mortality Weekly Report, 65*(33), 844–849. doi:10.15585/mmwr.mm6533a3.

Phillips, K. (2019, January 15). An overdose victim had more fentanyl in her than officials had ever seen: She was 18 months old. *The Washington Post*, 1.

Pieper, B., & Templin, T. (2001). Chronic venous insufficiency in persons with a history of injection drug use. *Research in Nursing & Health, 24*(5), 423–432.

Powers, D., Erickson, S., & Swortwood, M. J. (2017, October). Quantification of morphine, codeine, and thebaine in home-brewed poppy seed tea by LC-MS/MS. *Journal of Forensic Sciences, 63*(4). doi:10.1111/1556-4029.13664

Pritham, U. A. (2013). Breastfeeding promotion for management of neonatal abstinence. *Journal of Obstetric, Gynecologic, & Neonatal Nursing, 42*(5), 517–526. doi:10.1111/1552-6909.12242

Pritham, U. A., Paul, J. A., & Hayes, M. J. (2012). Opioid dependency in pregnancy and length of stay for neonatal abstinence syndrome. *Journal of Obstetric, Gynecologic, & Neonatal Nursing, 41*(2), 180–190. doi:10.1111/j.1552-6909.2011.01330.x

Raisch, D. W., Fye, C. L., & Boardman, K. D. (2002). Opioid dependence treatment, including buprenorphine/naloxone. *Annals of Pharmacotherapy, 36*(2), 312–321.

Ramos, R. (1995). *An Ethnographic Study of Heroin Abuse by Mexican Americans in San Antonio, Texas*. Austin, Texas: Texas Commission on Alcohol and Drug Abuse.

Rastogi, R., Swarm, M. D., & Patel, T. A. (2011, December). Case scenario: Opioid association with serotonin syndrome: Implications to the practitioners. *Anesthesiology, 15*(6), 1291–1298.

Robinson, A., & Wermeling, D. P. (2014, December 15). Intranasal naloxone administration for treatment of opioid overdose. *American Journal of Health-Systems Pharmacy, 71*(24), 2129–2135. doi:10.2146/ajhp130798.

Robinson, S. E. (2006). Buprenorphine-containing treatments: Place in the management of opioid addiction. *CNS Drugs, 20*(9), 697–712.

Rudd, R. A. (2014, October 3). Increases in heroin overdose deaths–28 States, 2010 to 2012. *MMWR, Morbidity and Mortality Weekly Report, 63*(39), 849–854.

Rudd, R. A., Aleshire, N., & Zibbell, J. E. (2016). Increases in drug and opioid overdose deaths–United States, 2000-2014. *MMWR, Morbidity and Mortality Weekly Report, 64*(50), 1378–1382.

Russell, A. (2016, July 20). *Ohio Woman Sentenced to 51 Years for Letting Drug Dealer Rape Her 11-year-old Daughter for Heroin. National | Globalnews.ca.* Retrieved July 16, 2016, from http://globalnews.ca/news/2836699/ohio-woman-sentenced-to-51-years-for-letting-drug-dealer-rape-her-11-year-old-daughter-for-heroin/?utm_source=...

Saloner, B., Feder, K. A., & Krawczyk, N. (2017). Closing the medication-assisted treatment gap for youth with opioid use disorder. *JAMA Pediatrics, 171*(8), 729–731.

Sam Houston State University. (2017, October 10). Home-brewed poppy seed tea can be lethal. *ScienceDaily*. ScienceDaily.

SAMHSA, Substance Abuse and Mental Health Services Administration, Office of Applied Studies. (2009). Results from the 2008 National Survey on Drug Use and Health: National Findings (HHNSDUH Series H-36, HHS Publication No. SMA 09-4434). Rockville, Maryland.

Sawyer, N. (2018, April 25). S.F. pins down its needle problem. *SF Weekly*, 1–2.

Schaeffer, T. (2012). Abuse-deterrent formulations, an evolving technology against the abuse and misuse of opioid analgesics. *Journal of Medical Toxicology, 8*, 400–407. doi:10.1007/s13181-012-0270-y

Schoener, E. P., Hopper, J. A., & Pierre, J. D. (2002). Injection drug use in North America. *Infectious Disease Clinics of North America, 16*(3), 535–551.

Schreiber, A. K., Nones, C., & Reis, R. C. (2015, April 15). Diabetic neuropathic pain: Physiopathology and treatment. *World Journal of Diabetes, 6*(3), 432–444. doi:10.4239/wjd.v6.i3.432.

Schuman-Oilivier, Z., Albanese, M., & Nelson, S. E. (2010). Self treatment: Illicit buprenorphine use by opioid-dependent treatment seekers. *Journal of Substance Abuse Treatment, 39*(1), 41–50.

Sellers, E. M., Perrino, P. J., & Colucci, S. V. (2013). Attractiveness of reformulated OxyContin(R) tablets: Assessing comparative preferences and tampering potential. *Journal of Psychopharmacology, 27*(9), 808–816. doi:10.1177/0269881113493364

Sessions Cole, F., Wegner, D. J., & Davis, J. M. (2017). The genomics of neonatal abstinence syndrome. *Frontiers in Pediatrics, 5*, 176. doi:10.3389/fped.2017.00176

Seth, P., Scholl, L., & Rudd, R. A. (2018, March 30). Overdose deaths involving opioids, cocaine, and psychostimulants – United States, 2015-2016. *MMWR, Morbidity and Mortality Weekly Report, 67*(12), 349–358.

Shah, A., Hayes, C. J., & Martin, B. C. (2017, March 17). Characteristics of initial prescription episodes and likelihood of long-term opioid use – United States, 2006-2013. *MMWR, Morbidity and Mortality Weekly Report, 66*(10), 265–269.

Sharma, B., Bruner, A., & Barnett, G. (2016, July). Opioid use disorders. *Child and Adolescent Psychiatric Clinics of North America, 25*(3), 473–487. doi:10.1016/j.chc.2016.03.002.

Sharp, M. J., & Melnik, T. A. (2015). Poisoning deaths involving opioid analgesics - New York State, 2003-2012. *MMWR Morbidity and Mortality Weekly Report, 64*(14), 377–380.

Singh, J., & Basu, D. (2004). Ultra-rapid opioid detoxification: Current status and controversies. *Journal of Postgraduate Medicine, 50*(3), 227–232.

Sloan, P. A., & Klimkina, O. (2009). Intranasal abuse of prescription hydrocodone/acetaminophen results in oronasal fistula: A case report. *Journal of Opioid Management, 5*(6), 383–385.

Smart, A. (2018, April 22). Victoria teen's accidental overdose started with prescription drugs, parents say. *The Canadian Press*, 1–4. CBC.

Smith, H. S. (2011). Morphine sulfate and naltrexone hydrochloride extended release capsules for the management of chronic, moderate-to-severe pain, while reducing morphine-induced subjective effects upon tampering by crushing. *Expert Opinion on Pharmacotherapy, 12*(7), 1111–1125. doi:10.1517/14656566.2011.571205

Smith, J. P., & Randall, C. L. (2012). Anxiety and alcohol use disorders: Comorbidity and treatment considerations. *Alcohol Research, 34*(4), 414–431.

Smith, M. Y., Bailey, J. E., & Woody, G. E. (2007). Abuse of buprenorphine in the United States: 2003-2005. *Journal of Addictive Diseases, 26*(3), 107–111.

Soelberg, C. D., Brown, R. E., & Du Vivier, D. (2017, November). The US opioid crisis: Current federal and state legal issues. *Anesthesia and Analgesia, 125*(5), 1675–1681. doi:10.1213/ANE.0000000000002403.

Solhaug, V., & Molden, E. (2017, October). Individual variability in clinical effect and tolerability of opioid analgesics-Importance of drug interactions and pharmacogenetics. *Scandinavian Journal of Pain, 17*, 193–200. doi:10.1016/j.sjpain.2017.09.009

Soyka, M. (2015). Buprenorphine-naloxone buccal soluble film for the treatment of opioid dependence: Current Update. *Expert Opinion on Drug Delivery, 12*(2), 339–347. doi:10.1517/17425247.2014.953479

Spinner, H. L., Lonardo, N. W., & Mulamalla, R. (2015). Ventricular tachycardia associated with high-dose chronic loperamide use. *Pharmacotherapy, 35*(2), 234–238. doi:10.1002/phar.1540

Sporer, K. A. (1999). Acute heroin overdose. *Annals of Internal Medicine, 130*(7), 584–590.

Stanos, S. P., Bruckenthal, P., & Barkin, R. L. (2012). Strategies to reduce the tampering and subsequent abuse of long-acting opioids: Potential risks and benefits of formulations with physical or pharmacologic deterrents to tampering. *Mayo Clinic Proceedings, 87*(7), 683–694.

Stellato, C., Cirillo, R., & de Paulis, A. (1992, November). Human basophil/mast cell releasability. IX. Heterogeneity of the effects of opioids on mediator release. *Anesthesiology*, 77(5), 932–940.

Stern, A. (2011, November 17). *Afghan Heroin Traffic Thrives in War: Russia. Reuters.com*, 1. Retrieved from www.reuters.com/assets/print?aid=USTRE7AG2LM20111117

Stolberg, S. G., & Gerth, J. (2000, November 16). High-tech stealth being used to sway doctor prescriptions. *New York Times*, A1, A22.

Subramaniam, G. A., Warden, D., & Minhajuddin, A. (2011). Predictors of abstinence: National Institute of Drug Abuse multisite buprenorphine/naloxone treatment trial in opioid-dependent youth. *Journal of the American Academy of Child & Adolescent Psychiatry, 50*(11), 1120–1128.

Sutter, M. B., Leeman, L., & Hsi, A. (2014). Neonatal opioid withdrawal syndrome. *Obstetrics and Gynecology Clinics of North America, 41*(2), 317–334. doi:10.1016/j.ogc.2014.02.010

Tanum, L., Solli, K. K., & Latif, Z. E. (2017, October 18). The effectiveness of injectable extended-release naltrexone vs daily buprenorphine-naloxone for opioid dependence: A randomized clinical noninferiority trial. *JAMA Psychiatry*. doi:10.1001/jamapsychiatry.2017.3206.

Tarabar, A. F., & Nelson, L. S. (2003, April). The resurgence and abuse of heroin by children in the United States. *Current Opinion in Pediatrics, 15*(2), 210–215.

Thomas, C. P., Fullerton, C. A., & Kim, M. (2014). Medication-assisted treatment with buprenorphine: Assessing the evidence. *Psychiatric Services, 65*(2), 158–170. doi:10.1176/appi.ps.201300256

Traynor, J. (2012). Mu-opioid receptors and regulators of G protein signaling (RGS) proteins: From a symposium on new concepts in mu-opioid pharmacology. *Drug and Alcohol Dependence, 121*(3), 173–180. doi:10.1016/j.drugalcdep.2011.10.027

Tsui, J. I., Herman, D. S., & Kettavong, M. (2010). Physician introduction to opioids for pain among patients with opioid dependence and depressive symptoms. *Journal of Substance Abuse Treatment, 39*(4), 378–383. doi:10.1016/j.jsat.2010.06.012

Underner, M., Perriot, J., & Peiffer, G. (2017, July-August). Asthma and heroin use. *La Presse Medicale, 46*(7–8 (Part 1)), 660–675. doi:10.1016/j.lpm.2017.06.002.

Unger, A., Jagsch, R., & Jones, H. (2011). Randomized controlled trials in pregnancy: Scientific and ethical aspects. Exposure to different opioid medications during pregnancy in an intra-individual comparison. *Addiction, 106*(7), 1355–1362.

Unick, G. J., Rosenblum, D., & Mars, S. G. (2013). Intertwined epidemics: National demographic trends in hospitalizations for heroin- and opioid-related overdoses, 1993–2009. *PloS One, 8*, e54496.

USDHHS, U.S. Department of Health and Human Services. (2015). *Abuse-Deterrent Opioids – Evaluation and Labeling: Guidance for Industry. USDHHS, Division of Drug Information.* Silver Springs: Food and Drug Administration.

Valdez, A., Kaplan, C. D., & Cepeda, A. (2000). The process of paradoxical automomy and survival in the heroin careers of Mexican American women. *Contemporary Drug Problems, 27*, 189–200.

Valdez, A., Neaigus, A., & Kaplan, C. (2011, April 1). High rates of transitions to injecting drug use among Mexican American non-injecting heroin users in San Antonio, Texas. *Drug and Alcohol Dependence, 114*(2–3), 233–236. doi:10.1016/j.drugalcdep.2010.09.014.

Veliz, P., Boyd, C. J., & Esteban McCabe, S. (2017). Nonmedical use of prescription opioids and heroin use among adolescents involved in competitive sports. *The Journal of Adolescent Health, 60*(3), 346–349. doi:10.1016/j.jadohealth.2016.09.021

Veliz, P., Epstein-Ngo, Q. M., & Meier, E. (2014). Painfully obvious: A longitudinal examination of medical use and misuse of opioid medication among adolescent sports participants. *The Journal of Adolescent Health, 54*(3), 333–340. doi:10.1016/j.jadohealth.2013.09.002

Vellucci, R., Mediati, R. D., & Gasperoni, S. (2017). Assessment and treatment of breakthrough cancer pain: From theory to clinical practice. *Journal of Pain Research, 10*, 2147–2155. doi:10.2147/JPR.S135807

Vivolo-Kantor, A. M., Seth, P., & Gladden, R. M. (2018, March 9). Vital signs: Trends in emergency department visits for suspected opioid overdoses – United States, July 2016 - September 2017. *MMWR, Morbidity and Mortality Weekly Report, 67*(9), 279–285.

Volkow, N. D. (2014, May 14). *America's Addiction to Opioids: Heroin and Prescription Drug Abuse*. National Institute on Drug Abuse (NIDA). Retrieved March 12, 2016, from www.drugabuse.gov/about-nida/legislative-activities/testimony-to-congress/2016/americas-addiction-to-opioids-heroin-prescription-drug-abuse

Volkow, N. D., & McLellan, A. T. (2016, March 31). *Opioid Abuse in Chronic Pain*. NEJM Resident E-Bulletin. Retrieved March 30, 2016, from resebulletin@nejm.org

Volpicelli, J. R., Clay, K. L., & Watson, N. T. (1995). Naltrexone in the treatment of alcoholism: Predicting response to naltrexone. *The Journal of Clinical Psychiatry, 56*(Supplement 7), 39–44.

Vosburg, S. K., Jones, J. D., & Manubay, J. M. (2012). Assessment of a formulation designed to be crush-resistant in prescription opioid abusers. *Drug and Alcohol Dependence, 126*(0), 206–215. doi:10.1016/j.drugalcdep.2012.05.013

Weber, H. C. (2016). Opioid-induced constipation in chronic noncancer pain. *Current Opinion in Endocrinology, Diabetes and Obesity, 23*(1), 11–17. doi:10.1097/MED.0000000000000220

Weber, J. M., Tataris, K. L., & Hoffman, J. D. (2012). Can nebulized naloxone be used safely and effectively by emergency medical services for suspected opioid overdose? *Prehospital Emergency Care, 16*(2), 289–292. doi:10.3109/10903127.2011.640763

Weeks, M. A., Clark, E. P., & Mycyk, M. B. (2016). Characteristics of heroin-dependent patients seeking asthma care in the ED. *The American Journal of Emergency Medicine, 34*(5), 896–898. doi:10.1016/j.ajem.2016.02.005

Welle-Strand, G. K., Skurtveit, S., & Jansson, L. M. (2013). Breastfeeding reduces the need for withdrawal treatment in opioid-exposed infants. *Acta Paediatrica, 102*(11), 1060–1066. doi:10.1111/apa.12378

Wertheim, L. J., & Rodriguez, K. (2015, June 18). How painkillers are turning young athletes into heroin addicts. *Sports Illustrated*, 1–8.

Whitman, E. (2015, April 10). *US heroin epidemic growing rates of addiction and overdose reported in New* Jersey, *Kentucky, Indiana. IBTimes.com*. Retrieved April 19, 2016, from www.ibtimes.com/us-heroin-epidemic-growing-rates-addiction-overdose-reported-new-jersey-kentucky-1877064?rel=rel2

Wilder, C. M., & Winhusen, T. (2015). Pharmacological management of opioid use disorder in pregnant women. *CNS Drugs, 29*(8), 625–636. doi:10.1007/s40263-015-0273-8

Williams, A. R., & Bisaga, A. (2016). From AIDS to opioids – How to combat an epidemic. *The New England Journal of Medicine, 375*(9), 813–815.

Wilson, D., & Shiffman, J. (2015, December 7). U. S. NewS. *Newborns Die after Going Home with Moms Fighting Drug Addiction*. Lehighton, Pennsylvania: NBC News. Retrieved from www.nbcnews.com/news/us-news/newborns-die-after-going-home-moms-fighting-drug-addiction-n475531

Winstock, A. R. (2016, January 12). *The Global Drug Survey 2015 Findings – What Did We Learn from GDS2015?* 1–27. Global Drug Survey. Retrieved from www.globaldrugsurvey.com/the-global-drug-survey-2015-findings/

Withington, D. E., Patrick, J. A., & Reynolds, F. (1993). Histamine release by morphine and diamorphine in man. *Anaesthesia, 48*(1), 26–29.

Wong, S. S., Zhou, B., & Goebert, D. (2013). The risk of adolescent suicide across patterns of drug use: A nationally representative study of high school students in the United States from 1999 to 2009. *Social Psychiatry and Psychiatric Epidemiology, 48*(10), 1611–1620. doi:10.1007/s00127-013-0721-z

Wu, L.-T., & Blazer, D. G. (2014, April). Substance use disorders and psychiatric comorbidity in mid and later life: A review. *International Journal of Epidemiology, 43*(2), 304–317. doi:10.1093/ije/dyt173.

Wu, L.-T., & Howard, M. O. (2007). Is inhalant use a risk factor for heroin and injection drug use among adolescents in the United States? *Addictive Behaviors, 32*(2), 265–281.

Yang, Y. T., Chen, B., & Bennett, C. L. (2016). FDA approval of extended-release oxycodone for children with severe pain. *Pediatrics, 137*(5), 1–3. doi:10.1542/peds.2016-0205

Yewell, J., Haydon, R., & Archer, S. (2002). Complications of intranasal prescription narcotic abuse. *The Annals of Otology, Rhinology, and Laryngology, 111*(2), 174–177.

Yokell, M. A., Zaller, N. D., & Green, T. C. (2011). Buprenorphine and buprenorphine/naloxone diversion, misuse, and illicit use: An international review. *Current Drug Abuse Reviews, 4*(1), 28–41.

Young, A., Esteban McCabe, S., & Cranford, J. A. (2012, October). Nonmedical use of prescription opioids among adolescents: Subtypes based on motivation for use. *Journal of Addictive Diseases, 31*(4), 332–341. doi:10.1080/10550887.2012.735564.

Zhang, J., Ferguson, S., & Barak, L. S. (1998, June). Role for G protein-coupled receptor kinase in agonist-specific regulation of mu-opioid receptor responsiveness. *Proceedings of the National Academy of Sciences of the United States of America, 95*, 7157–7162.

Zuurmond, W. W., Meert, T. F., & Noorduin, H. (2002). Partial versus full agonists for opioid-mediated analgesia—Focus on fentanyl and buprenorphine. *Acta Anaesthesiologica Belgica, 53*(3), 193–201.

6
Prescription Sedative-Hypnotics

A "sedative" drug reduces response to all sensory input by mildly depressing the central nervous system (CNS). A "hypnotic" drug causes a state of natural sleep by moderately depressing the CNS. A "sedative-hypnotic" drug causes dose-dependent drowsiness, sleep, or coma, depending on its dosage, respectively, and corresponding blood concentration. Pharmacologically, all the drugs discussed in this chapter are classified as "sedative-hypnotics" (Table 6.1).[1, 2] Some of these drugs, because of their pharmaceutical company development and marketing, as well as FDA approval, may also be classified according to their "approved" indication for use (e.g. "anxiolytics;" "anticonvulsants;" or "muscle relaxants"). To avoid confusion, these sedative-hypnotics are clearly identified whenever they are discussed in this chapter.

Three subclasses of the prescription sedative-hypnotics—"benzodiazepines," "z-drugs," and "miscellaneous sedative-hypnotics" (i.e., suvorexant [Belsomra®] and gamma-hydroxybutyrate [GHB])—are the primary focus of this chapter because of their common use by adolescents and young adults in the U.S. during the new millennium.

We first present and discuss the benzodiazepines, followed by the z-drugs, and conclude with two miscellaneous sedative-hypnotics—suvorexant and gamma-hydroxybutyrate. For each of these subclasses of prescription sedative-hypnotics, we give special attention to their basic pharmacology—"pharmacodynamics," or mechanism of action; "pharmacokinetics," or absorption, distribution, metabolism, and excretion; "drug–drug interactions;" and "undesired, or harmful, effects and toxicities," including physical and psychological dependence. Also presented and discussed are "overdosage/ unintentional poisoning" and "pregnancy and lactation." We conclude the chapter with an overview and discussion of new millennial trends in embryo/fetus, neonate/infant, and child exposure to prescription sedative-hypnotics and both their medical and nonmedical use by adolescents and young adults.

1 Other prescription sedative-hypnotics, including the "barbiturates" (e.g., pentobarbital [Nembutal®]; phenobarbital [Luminal®]; secobarbital [Seconal®]) and "miscellaneous sedative-hypnotics" (e.g., chloral hydrate [Noctec®]), which were more commonly used in the U.S. during the last century, are not discussed in this chapter. For related detailed information and discussion, see Pagliaro and Pagliaro (2004, 2009).

2 For an overview and discussion of the "non-prescription" sedative-hypnotic most commonly used by adolescents and young adults, see Chapter 1, "Alcohol."

Table 6.1 Prescription Sedative-Hypnotics

Category *Generic Name*	*Brand/Trade Names*[3]	*Common Street Names*[4]
BARBITURATES		
Amobarbital	Amytal®	
Butabarbital	Butisol®	
Butalbital[5]		
Pentobarbital	Nembutal®	"Abbots;" "Nembs;" "Yellows"
Phenobarbital	Luminal®	"Pheno;" "Sleepers"
Secobarbital	Seconal®	"Lillys;" "Pinks;" "Reds"
Thiopental	Pentothal®	
BENZODIAZEPINES		
Alprazolam	Xanax®	"Bars;" "Footballs;" "Xan;" "Zannies"
Bromazepam	Lectopam®	
Chlordiazepoxide	Librium®	"Libs;" "Libbies"
Clobazam	Onfi®	
Clonazepam	Klonopin®; Rivotril®	"Clo;" "Klonnies;" "K-Pin"
Clorazepate	Tranxene®	
Diazepam	Valium®	"Blues;" "Mother's Little Helper;" "Vs"
Estazolam	ProSom®	
Flunitrazepam[6]	Rohypnol®	"Forget Me Pill;" "La Roche;" "Mexican Valium;" "Papas;" "Roofies"
Flurazepam	Dalmane®	
Halazepam	Paxipam®	
Lorazepam	Ativan®	"Zzz"
Midazolam	Versed®	
Nitrazepam	Mogadon®	"Dons;" "Moggies"
Oxazepam	Serax®	

(*Continued*)

3 When available, examples of common brand/trade names are provided.
4 Partial list. Examples of three to five of the most common street names are provided, when available.
5 Butalbital is only available in combination products (e.g., Fiorinal®).
6 Although not legally produced in the U.S., flunitrazepam is widely available worldwide under the brand/trade name, "Rohypnol®." It is commonly known and used as a date-rape drug.

Table 6.1 (Cont.)

Category Generic Name	*Brand/Trade Names*	*Common Street Names*
Prazepam	Centrax®	
Quazepam	Doral®	
Temazepam	Restoril®	"Green Devils;" "Temmies"
Triazolam	Halcion®	"Halcyon;" "Halcyon Daze"
Z-DRUGS		
Eszopiclone	Lunesta®	
Zaleplon	Sonata®	
Zolpidem	Ambien®; Edluar®; Intermezzo®; Lunata®; Zolpimist®	"A-minus;" "Nappien;" "No-Go;" "Tic-Tacs;" "ZIM"
Zopiclone	Imovane®; Zimovane®	"Zim-Zims"
MISCELLANEOUS SEDATIVE-HYPNOTICS		
Gamma-Hydroxybutyrate	Xyrem®	"Easy Lay;" "Georgia Home Boy;" "GHB;" "Grievous Bodily Harm"
Suvorexant	Belsomra®	

Benzodiazepines

The benzodiazepine molecule[7] was synthesized in the 1950s as a pharmacotherapeutic alternative to the barbiturates (i.e., derivatives of barbituric acid) that had dominated the sedative-hypnotic market for the previous 100 years. Over the last 70 years more than 2,000 different benzodiazepine derivatives have been developed. The benzodiazepines were widely advertised and marketed as being the safest drugs available for managing anxiety and insomnia because, in comparison to the barbiturates, they possess a significantly higher therapeutic index. For this reason, and because the benzodiazepines were found to be relatively safe and effective for use in clinical practice—they became the most widely medically-prescribed and abused sedative-hypnotics in the U.S., as well as the rest of the world. Although the benzodiazepines continue to be widely used for their desired sedative and hypnotic actions, their use is now being increasingly replaced by the more recently developed z-drugs. In fact, the z-drugs have now become the most medically-prescribed and abused sedative-hypnotics in the U.S. (see the later subsection, "Z-Drugs").[8]

7 The core chemical structure of the benzodiazepines consists of a seven-member heterocyclic diazepine ring fused to a benzene ring.

8 N.B. Although the use of the z-drugs has significantly increased in popularity during the new millennium (see later discussion), currently there are insufficient data to fully support their significant superiority in terms of clinical efficacy and safety over the benzodiazepines.

Benzodiazepine Pharmacology

The benzodiazepines and their active metabolites share similar sedative and hypnotic actions with no one benzodiazepine being significantly superior to the others.[9] However, some children, adolescents, and young adults may react differently to various benzodiazepines, particularly regarding associated undesired, or harmful, effects and toxicities (see the later related discussion; see also the later benzodiazepine subsection, "Pharmacology, Pharmacokinetics—Metabolism"). These effects and toxicities are discussed in the following sections, along with other related basic pharmacological principles and concepts. It is important to note that the variability in individual response may, in large part, be due to a "placebo effect."[10] We begin with the pharmacodynamics of the benzodiazepines—their mechanism of psychodepressant action.

Pharmacodynamics: Mechanism of Action

Although the benzodiazepines have been commercially available since the late 1950s, the precise sites and specific mechanisms of their sedative and hypnotic actions, even now, are not fully understood. It is thought that the benzodiazepines act in the CNS, in concert with gamma-aminobutyric acid (GABA),[11] to inhibit neurotransmission, particularly in the cerebral cortex and the limbic system, including the amygdala and the thalamus (Bergman, 1986). A GABA receptor complex has been identified, at which, the benzodiazepines appear to enhance GABA-mediated chloride influx through chloride ion channels (see Figure 6.1).

Over 50 years ago, three GABA receptors were identified and designated as "$GABA_A$," "$GABA_B$," and "$GABA_C$."[12] Approximately 16 years later, their importance was realized. The $GABA_A$ receptor is the most important and the most studied. More appropriately conceptualized as a receptor complex, $GABA_A$ is comprised of five protein subunits that are arranged in a specific pentameric order/structure of subunits surrounding a central trans-cell membrane ion pore, or channel, that is permeable to chloride and other anions (Nutt & Malizia, 2001; Pagliaro & Pagliaro, 2004; Sieghart, 1994).[13] Consequently, the $GABA_A$ receptor is considered to be an ionotropic receptor that functions in concert with a ligand-gated ion channel. The endogenous ligand for the $GABA_A$ receptor, as indicated by its name, is "GABA." Thirty different isoforms of the $GABA_A$ receptor have been identified that contain the alpha (α), beta (β), and gamma (γ) subunits in different combinations that are arranged in a unique pentameric order. The biological complexity of the $GABA_A$ receptors is largely accounted for by the numerous diverse

9 However, the benzodiazepines do significantly differ regarding their anticonvulsant actions. Generally, only clonazepam (Rivotril®), clorazepate (Tranxene®), diazepam (Valium®), and lorazepam (Ativan®) are used to pharmacologically manage seizure disorders. Clonazepam is probably more appropriately classified primarily as an anticonvulsant rather than as a sedative-hypnotic because of its pharmacologic actions and primary medical use.

10 The placebo effect is a psychological mechanism of drug action that applies to all drugs, whether pharmacologically active (e.g., opiate analgesic) or not (e.g., sugar tablet; normal saline injection). Placebo and other drug actions are not mutually exclusive. In fact, they generally occur together with the use of most drugs (e.g., the headache relief that is often obtained within seconds after swallowing an aspirin tablet with a glassful of water—prior to complete absorption and achievement of therapeutic serum concentrations). Only the percentage of response due to the placebo effect differs from individual to individual and drug to drug based largely on several variables that are related to the patient, prescriber, drug, and clinical context of use.

11 GABA is the major inhibitory neurotransmitter in the CNS and is found, in particularly high concentrations, in the cerebral cortex and the limbic system.

12 The $GABA_C$ receptor is often alternatively considered not to be a separate receptor, but rather an isoform of the $GABA_A$ receptor (Sigel & Steinmann, 2012).

13 The $GABA_A$ receptor complex is similar in form and function to other Cys loop ligand-gated ion channel receptors, such as, the nicotinic acetylcholine receptor (See Chapter 3, "Caffeine and Nicotine").

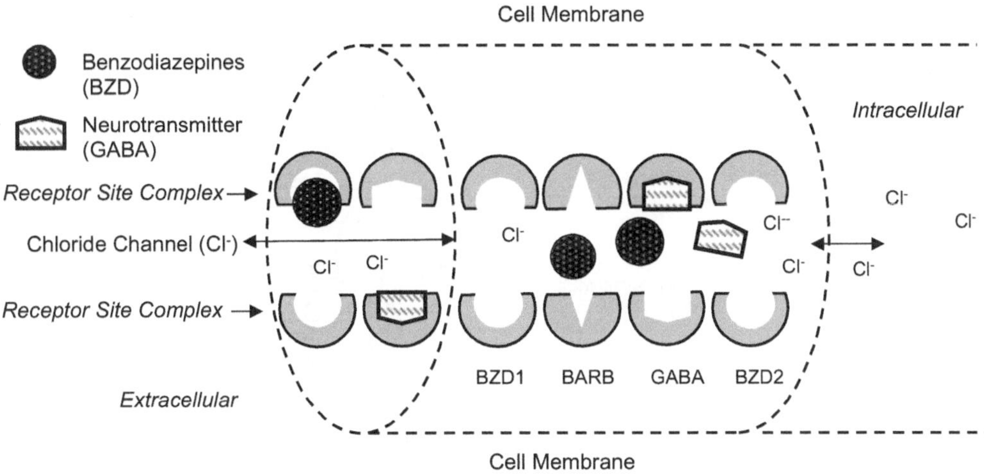

Figure 6.1 The GABA Benzodiazepine Receptor

combinations of the receptor subunits. The most common isoform for the $GABA_A$ receptor contains the α, β, and γ subunits arranged in the following pentameric order—"α_1, β_2, α_1, β_2, and γ_2" (see Figures 6.2 and 6.3).

Several exogenous chemicals (e.g., bicuculline;[14] muscimol[15]) have been developed, primarily for laboratory research purposes, which can bind directly to the $GABA_A$ receptor. Additionally, the $GABA_A$ receptor protein complex contains a number of allosteric binding sites that can modulate the activity of the $GABA_A$ receptor. Examples of sedative-hypnotics that bind to these allosteric sites include: alcohol; barbiturates; benzodiazepines; and z-drugs.

BENZODIAZEPINE RECEPTORS

The benzodiazepines bind primarily, in a nonspecific manner, to two receptors that have been commonly referred to as the benzodiazepine 1 (BZD1) and benzodiazepine 2 (BZD2) receptors.[16] BZD1 receptors, which are concentrated in the cerebral cortex, thalamus, and cerebellum, contain α_1, β_1, β_2, β_3, and γ_2 subunits. BZD2 receptors, which are concentrated in the limbic system, motor neurons, and the dorsal horn of the spinal cord, contain α_2, α_3, α_5, β_1, β_2, β_3, and γ_2 subunits (Atack, 2005; Crestani, Low, & Keist, 2001; Griffin, Kaye, & Rivera Bueno, 2013; Sieghart, 1994).

14 Bicuculline is a synthetic antagonist of the $GABA_A$ receptor. It was originally identified as a pharmacologically active plant alkaloid found naturally in the family *Papaveraceae*, subfamily *Fumarioideae*.

15 Muscimol is one of the principal active components found naturally in the psychodelic mushroom, *Amanita muscaria*. It is a potent agonist of the $GABA_A$ receptor.

16 To be more precise, it is generally agreed that the benzodiazepines do not bind to specific "benzodiazepine receptors," but rather to allosteric modulatory regions near the GABA receptor complex (i.e., between the alpha and gamma subunits). The reasoning for the conclusion that the benzodiazepine binding sites are not considered to be true receptors is based primarily upon the observation that—in the absence of GABA—benzodiazepines do not elicit their associated psychodepressant effects (Bergman, 1986; Sieghart, 1994). Consequently, the "benzodiazepine receptors" are, more appropriately, currently referred to as "benzodiazepine binding sites."

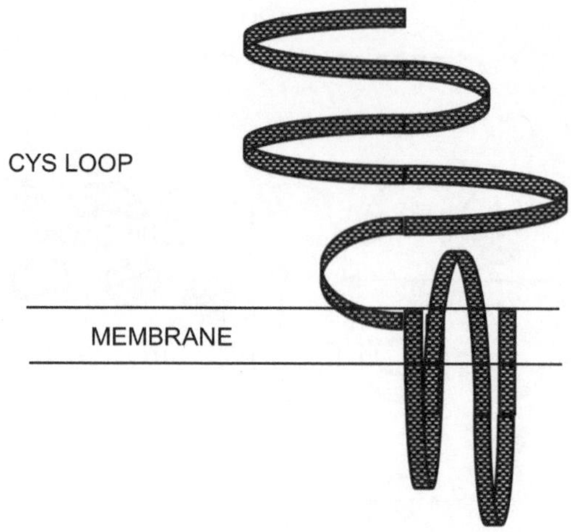

Figure 6.2 Typology of the Cys Loop $GABA_A$ Receptor

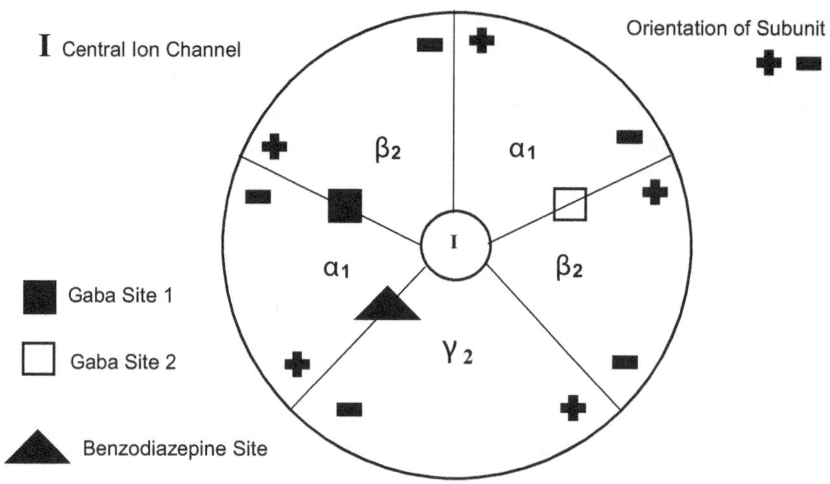

Figure 6.3 Major Isoform of $GABA_A$ Receptors $\alpha 1$, $\beta 2$, $\gamma 2$: A Transverse Perspective

The α_1 subunit is the most commonly distributed subunit in the CNS. Agonistic action involving the α_1 subunit is primarily related to the production of sedation and anterograde amnesia. The α_2 and α_3 subunits are more closely related to the effects of anxiolysis, muscle relaxation, and sleep regulation (Gunja, 2013b).

Although it has been clearly demonstrated that the benzodiazepines have a high affinity for binding at the GABA receptor complex,[17] it has not yet been proved that this action is directly, and solely, responsible for their observed pharmacologic actions in humans. For example, it has also been suggested that, following the onset of menarche, progesterone may have some direct agonistic action at the $GABA_A$ receptor that may enhance the actions of the benzodiazepines and contribute to their abuse by adolescent girls and young women (Babalonis, Lile, & Martin, 2011a, 2011b). More generally, and for both genders, these effects may be related to the direct modulatory actions of endogenous neurosteroids (e.g., allopregnanolone and tetrahydrodeoxycorticosterone) at the $GABA_A$ receptor (Belelli & Lambert, 2005; Hosie, Wilkins, & Da Silva, 2006).

Pharmacokinetics: Absorption, Distribution, Metabolism, and Excretion

The basic pharmacokinetics of the benzodiazepines—the processes of absorption, distribution, metabolism, and excretion—are described and discussed. We begin with "absorption."

ABSORPTION

The benzodiazepines are generally well-absorbed after ingestion. Although the ingestion of food can sometimes delay the rate of absorption, it does not generally affect the extent of absorption. However, the route of administration can affect the absorption of the benzodiazepines. For example, diazepam (Valium®) is virtually completely absorbed after ingestion and can achieve peak blood concentrations within one to two hours. Following IV injection,[18] peak blood concentrations are achieved within 15 minutes. After IM injection,[19] peak blood concentrations usually occur within two hours. The administration of sublingual formulations of diazepam (e.g., alprazolam; triazolam) generally results in a more rapid and complete absorption in comparison to ingestion (Garzone & Kroboth, 1989).

DISTRIBUTION

The benzodiazepines are highly bound (i.e., > 96%) to plasma proteins (e.g., albumin) and are widely distributed throughout body tissues. However, because they are highly lipophilic, the benzodiazepines and their metabolites readily cross the blood-brain and placental "barriers." They also are excreted in breast milk. (See also the related discussion in the later subsection, "Pregnacy and Lactation").

METABOLISM AND EXCRETION

Most of the benzodiazepines are metabolized mainly in the liver by the hepatic microsomal enzyme system, primarily by CYP3A4.[20] Therefore, hepatic disease or dysfunction (e.g.,

17 Endogenous ligands for the benzodiazepine-binding site (i.e., the "brain's Valium") are known as "endozepines" and consist of a group, or family, of neuropeptides. The major identified ligands in this family include: (1) nonpeptidic endozepines; (2) oleamides; and (3) diazepam-binding inhibitor (Farzampour, Reimer, & Huguenard, 2015).

18 Absorption is immediate and, by definition, 100% following IV injection (i.e., F = 1.0—for all IV-injected drugs).

19 Absorption may be erratic (i.e., increased or decreased) following IM injection, depending largely on blood flow to the specific muscle injection site.

20 Diazepam and temazepam also are metabolized by CYP2C19. Although a relatively minor metabolic pathway for these drugs, it may contribute to significant variance in both therapeutic and undesired effects because of its associated genetic polymorphism. In the U.S., approximately 3% of the people, who are of European continental descent, and 20% of the people, who are of Asian continental descent, have absent or reduced CYP2C19 enzyme activity. Consequently, they are considered to be "poor metabolizers" (Dean, 2016).

cirrhosis of the liver; hepatitis) can slow benzodiazepine metabolism and, consequently, increase toxicity. Some benzodiazepines, including flurazepam (Dalmane®), undergo extensive first-pass hepatic metabolism.[21] Other benzodiazepines, such as lorazepam (Ativan®), oxazepam (Serax®), and temazepam (Restoril®), are metabolized primarily by urinary conjugation to more water-soluble (i.e., polar) glucuronide derivatives that are, subsequently, excreted in the urine.

The benzodiazepines can have slow, intermediate, or rapid elimination profiles. Benzodiazepines that have "slow" elimination profiles are those that produce active metabolites, either as: (1) parent drugs, or compounds; or (2) inactive pro-drugs.

The benzodiazepines that have slow elimination profiles include:

- Active parent drugs, or compounds:
  - Chlordiazepoxide (Librium®);
  - Diazepam (Valium®);
  - Flurazepam (Dalmane®).
- Inactive pro-drugs:
  - Clorazepate (Tranxene®);
  - Halazepam (Paxipam®);
  - Prazepam (Centrax®).

The benzodiazepines that have "intermediate" elimination profiles include:

- Alprazolam (Xanax®);
- Clonazepam (Rivotril®);
- Lorazepam (Ativan®);
- Oxazepam (Serax®);
- Temazepam (Restoril®).

Finally, the benzodiazepines that have "rapid" elimination profiles include:

- Midazolam (Versed®);
- Triazolam (Halcion®).

Benzodiazepine Drug–Drug Interactions

Drug–drug interactions, which involve the benzodiazepines, can be characterized as being either pharmacodynamic or pharmacokinetic in nature (Pagliaro & Pagliaro, 1998).

21 Following ingestion, a drug is transported to the liver by way of the portal venous system before it is released into the general systemic circulation. As it passes through the liver, some, or occasionally most, of the drug is metabolized to a less active or completely inactive form (i.e., the amount metabolized, on this single pass through the liver, is commonly referred to as the "hepatic extraction ratio"). This entire process is called "first pass hepatic metabolism," or the "first-pass effect." The first-pass effect does not occur when drugs or substances of abuse are administered by other common routes that allow them to immediately enter the systemic circulation, such as: buccal placement in the cheek; IM, IV, and SC injection; pulmonary inhalation; rectal insertion (unless insertion is high and near the superior rectal vein); sublingual placement under the tongue; and transdermal and transmucosal delivery.

Pharmacodynamic interactions occur at the receptor sites and generally result in a reduction, or an increase, in the associated effect(s). For example, a reduction in effects (i.e., an amelioration of effects) occur when a psychostimulant (e.g., caffeine; cocaine; nicotine) is used at the same time as a benzodiazepine. Conversely, additive psychodepressant effects occur whenever benzodiazepines are concurrently use with other psychodepressants (e.g., alcohol; opiate analgesics; z-drugs).

Pharmacokinetic interactions occur when the concurrently used drug, or substance of abuse, affects the absorption, distribution, metabolism, or excretion of the benzodiazepines. The majority of these interactions, which can result in a clinically significant effect, involve the metabolism of the benzodiazepines. Because many of the benzodiazepines (e.g., alprazolam; chlordiazepoxide; clonazepam; midazolam; temazepam) are primarily metabolized by the hepatic microsomal enzyme CYP3A4, there is significant risk for the following two types of benzodiazepine metabolic drug–drug interactions:

1. Drugs that strongly "inhibit" CYP3A4 (e.g., clarithromycin; ketoconazole, nefazodone, ritonavir), which may necessitate a decrease in the benzodiazepine dosage;
2. Drugs that moderately "induce" CYP3A4 (e.g., carbamazepine; phenytoin; rifampin), which may necessitate an increase in the benzodiazepine dosage.[22]

Undesired, or Harmful, Effects and Toxicities

As noted earlier in this chapter, the benzodiazepines have a relatively high therapeutic index. Even so, several undesired, or harmful, effects and toxicities have been associated with their use. These effects can generally be classified as "acute" or "chronic" and "other" adverse effects.

ACUTE ADVERSE EFFECTS

Acute adverse effects include: ataxia; blurred vision; diplopia; dizziness; dysarthria; lethargy; muscle weakness; psychomotor impairment; slurred speech; and somnolence. They also include amnesias, particularly anterograde amnesia,[23] and other memory impairments, such as those affecting long-term, explicit (episodic) and implicit (procedural) memory and short-term (active) memory.

These acute harmful effects often occur together (e.g., blurred vision, cognitive impairment, confusion, and dizziness). Consequently, they contribute to a higher risk for: (1) psychomotor impairment and related injury (e.g., falling down a flight of stairs and suffering, for example, a serious head injury); and (2) being involved in a motor vehicle crash (MVC) (e.g., Pagliaro & Pagliaro, 1983; van Strien, Koek, & van Marum, 2013).

Other acute harmful effects include aggression and violent behavior. Often considered to be idiosyncratic personality effects, these effects are, more likely, a consequence of benzodiazepine-induced disinhibition among adolescents and young adults who have preexisting aggressive and hostile tendencies or personalities (Pagliaro & Pagliaro, *Clinical*

22 See also Chapter 5, "Prescription Opiate Analgesic and Heroin," Table 5.3, "Major Inducers and Inhibitors of CYP3A4 and CYP2D6," for a more comprehensive list.

23 This action of the benzodiazepines is used both therapeutically (e.g., to provide amnesia of surgical events for patients requiring surgery) and criminally (e.g., to facilitate crimes including robbery and date rape—see later subsection, "Sexual Assault"). In some contexts of use, the benzodiazepine-related memory impairment resembles alcoholic "blackouts" (see Chapter 1, "Alcohol," for further discussion).

Patient Data Files). (See also the related discussion in the later benzodiazepine subsection, "Physical and Psychological Dependence, Fatalities.")

CHRONIC ADVERSE EFFECTS

Regular, long-term use of the benzodiazepines is associated with: apathy; decreased impulse control; diminished sleep quality;[24] emotional instability; lethargy; memory impairment; mental depression; and rebound anxiety.[25] They also are associated with physical and psychological dependence characterized by tolerance, craving, and the benzodiazepine withdrawal syndrome (see the later benzodiazepine subsection, "Physical and Psychological Dependence").

OTHER ADVERSE EFFECTS

Other effects associated with benzodiazepine abuse, include: fatalities; sexual assault; and, if used during pregnancy, teratogenesis. These and other related effects are discussed in the following sections.

FATALITIES. Potentially fatal harmful effects and toxicities have been associated with the combination of benzodiazepines and other drugs and substances of abuse, particularly, alcohol (see Chapter 1, "Alcohol") and/or opiate analgesics (see Chapter 5, "Prescription Opiate Analgesics and Heroin"). (See also the earlier related subsection, "Benzodiazepine Drug–Drug Interactions.") As noted in the CBHSQ report from SAMHSA:

> Combining benzodiazepines with opioid pain relievers or alcohol significantly increases the risk of serious ED visit outcome for all age groups.
>
> (Day, 2014, p. 1)

The sedative-hypnotic actions of the benzodiazepines are potentiated by the actions of all other psychodepressants (e.g., alcohol; opiate analgesics; z-drugs). In fact, the concomitant use of benzodiazepines and alcohol has resulted in many deaths due to associated respiratory depression (Pagliaro & Pagliaro, 2009; Schmitz, 2016; Tanaka, 2002). (See also the later benzodiazepine subsection, "Overdosage"). Many of these deaths resulted from deliberate, or intentional, suicide attempts that resulted in completed suicides. Mental health professionals should be aware that the risk for suicide attempts among adolescents and young adults, who abuse benzodiazepines, is significantly higher for those, who regularly use higher dosages of the benzodiazepines and concurrently have other mental disorders, including:

- Alcohol dependence or use disorder;
- Borderline Personality Disorder (BPD);
- Major Depressive Disorder (MDD);

24 A decrease in sleep quality appears to be related to the development of the signs and symptoms of mental depression among chronic benzodiazepine abusers (Bourgeois, Elseviers, & Van Bortel, 2014b).

25 Rebound anxiety occurs when the regular, long-term (over 30 days) use of a sedative hypnotic for its anxiolytic effects is abruptly discontinued. In this situation, the anxiety that was initially being treated returns, generally at a much greater intensity.

- Opiate Analgesic dependence or use disorder (Bellivier, Yon, & Luquiens, 2011; Lekka, Paschalis, & Beratis, 2002; Pagliaro & Pagliaro, *Clinical Patient Data Files*; Voaklander, Rowe, & Dryden, 2008).

SEXUAL ASSAULT. Over the last three decades, the benzodiazepines, alone, or in combination with alcohol and other drugs and substances of abuse, frequently have been used to facilitate the perpetration of sexual assaults (i.e., drug-facilitated sexual assaults) (Bechtel & Holstege, 2007; Dowd, Strong, & Janicak, 2002; Gautam, Sharratt, & Cole, 2014; Grela, Gautam, & Cole, 2018; Pagliaro & Pagliaro, 2009).

> The teenager told police she was given a marijuana cigarette laced with Xanax and was then sexually assaulted several times by different people.
>
> (Suarez Sang, 2018, p. 1)

Because they often have been used illicitly in this context, the benzodiazepines, and other sedative-hypnotics—z-drugs, particularly zolpidem (Ambien®), and gamma-hydroxybutyrate (GHB)[26]—have been referred to as:

- Acquaintance rape drugs;
- Drug-assisted rape/sexual assault drugs;
- Date rape drugs (the most commonly used term);
- Intimate partner rape drugs.

(NIDA, 2008; Pagliaro & Pagliaro, 2009, 2012, 2018)

The use of the date rape drugs is estimated to occur in up to 50% of all rapes in the U.S. (Madea & MuBhoff, 2009; Pagliaro & Pagliaro, 2009). Unfortunately, the use of the benzodiazepines, as a means for perpetrating a sexual assault, appears to be increasing. In fact, flunitrazepam (Rohypnol®)—"Forget Me Drug," "Mexican Valium," *Papas*, or "Roofie"—is the benzodiazepine that is most often involved in cases of date rape, being simply slipped into the victim's beverage—without her (or his) knowledge—to induce drowsiness or sleep in order to facilitate the sexual assault. Benzodiazepines also induce anterograde amnesia, which helps the perpetrator to avoid successful prosecution by preventing the victim from:

1. Clearly remembering details of the assault;
2. Identifying the perpetrator;
3. Testifying under oath, in a court of law, that consent was not given for the sexual contact or that other related events did, or did not, occur.

(e.g., Daderman & Edman, 2001; Daderman, Fredriksson, & Kristiansson, 2002; Pagliaro & Pagliaro, *Clinical Patient Data Files*)

26 See also the comprehensive discussions of "Z-Drugs" and "Gamma-Hydroxybutyrate (GHB)," in their specific subsections, later in this chapter.

In addition, it has been increasingly reported, over the new millennium, that adolescent girls and young women commonly ingest flunitrazepam (Rohypnol®)[27] with an alcoholic beverage in a conscious and deliberate attempt to decrease their sexual inhibitions when "clubbing" or attending house parties and raves. In this context, sexual predators often take the opportunity to encourage the use of additional alcohol, benzodiazepines, or other drugs and substances of abuse, including psychodelics (e.g., MDMA), to facilitate the perpetration of the sexual assault (Pagliaro & Pagliaro, *Clinical Patient Data Files*).

PHYSICAL AND PSYCHOLOGICAL DEPENDENCE

The benzodiazepines have a low to moderate potential for physical dependence and a moderate to high potential for psychological dependence (Pagliaro & Pagliaro, 2009; Weaver, 2015). It has long been recognized that psychological dependence can develop with the regular, long-term use of the benzodiazepines at both lower and higher dosages. However, from the time that the benzodiazepines were introduced into medical practice in the 1960s and through the 1980s, it was generally thought that physical dependence, in the strictest sense, did not occur. Available data now indicate that the regular, long-term use of the benzodiazepines, even within therapeutic dosage ranges, can lead to a true, or classic, physical dependence in a significant minority of people (Pagliaro & Pagliaro, 2009), particularly those who have a past personal or family history of alcoholism.

Some general indicators of benzodiazepine physical and psychological dependence, include:

- Regular use of a benzodiazepine extending beyond 30 days;
- An expressed craving for the benzodiazepine;
- A need to increase the dosage of the benzodiazepine to achieve, or maintain, the desired effect(s);[28]
- Characteristic signs and symptoms of the benzodiazepine withdrawal syndrome can occur when the use of the benzodiazepine is abruptly discontinued for any reason, such as:
    - Inability to renew a prescription;
    - Lack of funds to buy more of the drug;
    - Inability to ingest dosages because of illness, including nausea or vomiting.

(Also see the later benzodiazepine subsection, "Benzodiazepine Withdrawal Syndrome.")

As noted by Canham, Gallo, and Simoni-Wastila (2014, p. 873):

> 35% of persons who take benzodiazepines regularly for four weeks or longer will develop dependence; after 4 to 6 months of daily use, the majority of users will develop dependence.

27 Although flunitrazepam is not legally produced in the U.S., it is: (1) widely available for illicit purchase;" (2) legally available in Europe and Mexico under the trade name, Rohypnol®; and (3) easily purchased from vendors over the internet (Pagliaro & Pagliaro, 2009).

28 In this context, a generally related indicator of benzodiazepine dependence or use disorder is a pattern of increasing requests for early refills for benzodiazepine prescriptions (Pagliaro & Pagliaro, *Clinical Patient Data Files*).

BENZODIAZEPINE TOLERANCE. Tolerance to the actions of the benzodiazepines (i.e., the need to use more of the drug more frequently to achieve desired actions) develops within four months of initial, daily use—regardless of the dosage range (i.e., low to high) or if medically prescribed or not. However, the rate of the development of tolerance varies from: (1) individual to individual; (2) benzodiazepine to benzodiazepine; and (3) pharmacological action to pharmacological action (e.g., generally, tolerance develops more quickly to the hypnotic effects of the benzodiazepines than to their anxiolytic effects).

BENZODIAZEPINE WITHDRAWAL SYNDROME. The characteristic signs and symptoms of the benzodiazepine withdrawal syndrome are widely documented in the context of the abrupt discontinuation of regular, long-term benzodiazepine use (e.g., Bateson, 2002; Pagliaro, 1988, 1993).[29] Usually, mild to moderate in intensity, the signs and symptoms of the benzodiazepine withdrawal syndrome may include:

- Anxiety;
- Diaphoresis;
- Irritability;
- Nervousness;
- Rebound Insomnia;
- Seizures;
- Shaking.

These characteristic signs and symptoms, which are essentially the opposite of the desired effects associated with the benzodiazepines, are more likely to occur with:

1. Short-acting benzodiazepines (e.g., alprazolam, Xanax®; lorazepam, Ativan®; triazolam, Halcion®);[30]
2. Higher dosages of benzodiazepines;
3. Regular, daily use of benzodiazepines for four months, or longer;
4. Abrupt discontinuation of benzodiazepines after regular, daily use.

Generally, the benzodiazepine withdrawal syndrome can be avoided, or at least minimized, by gradually decreasing the dosage during the period of drug discontinuation. It is often handled "cold-turkey"—without medical care or adjunctive pharmacotherapy (Bourgeois, Elseviers, & Van Bortel, 2014a). It also can be medically managed with the substitution of an equivalent dose of a long-acting benzodiazepine (e.g., diazepam

29 Interestingly, the signs and symptoms of the benzodiazepine withdrawal syndrome also have been noted with the discontinuation of concurrent pharmacotherapy that inhibits the cytochrome P450 isoenzymes responsible for the metabolism of the benzodiazepines. The discontinuation allows the benzodiazepines to be more quickly metabolized and, consequently, eliminated from the body more rapidly (Ninan, 2001). (See related discussion in the earlier subsection, "Benzodiazepine Drug–Drug Interactions.")

30 Short-acting benzodiazepines are more likely to produce insomnia when they are abruptly discontinued than are long-acting benzodiazepines. Long-acting benzodiazepines are less likely to produce insomnia, or the other signs and symptoms of withdrawal, when they are abruptly discontinued probably because of their longer half-life of elimination. It is generally thought that the longer half-life of elimination may provide a "built-in," tapering-off effect.

[Valium®]) that is gradually reduced over a period of two to three weeks (Pagliaro & Pagliaro, 2009).[31]

Benzodiazepine Overdosage/Unintentional Poisoning

> Benzodiazepine-related overdose mortality has risen dramatically [in the U.S.], from 0.6 per 100,000 adults in 1999 to 4.4 per 100,000 in 2016.
>
> (Agarwal & Landon, 2019, p. 1)

Moreover, during the new millennium, adolescents and young adults in the U.S. have been involved in a significant number of overdosages and ER visits associated with the use of benzodiazepines, particularly the combination of a benzodiazepine (primarily alprazolam [Xanax®]) and/or an opiate analgesic (primarily, oxycodone [Oxycontin®]) (Preidt, 2014; Sharp & Melnik, 2015). Poisonings among adolescents and young adults involving the benzodiazepines increased during the first decade of the new millennium. Among this cohort, intentional poisonings (e.g., involving a deliberate suicide attempts) were highest among adolescent girls and young women between 15 to 24 years-of-age (Cox, Kuo, & Jamieson, 2011).

> The estimated number of ED visits involving nonmedical use of benzodiazepines increased from 143,500 in 2004 to 271,700 in 2008 (i.e., 80%).
>
> (CDC, 2010, p. 706)

Additionally, because of the increasing medical use of z-drugs (see the related discussion in the following subsection) during the second decade of the new millennium, Kaufmann, Spira, and Alexander (2017) analyzed data regarding emergency department (ED) visits involving "benzodiazepine and non-benzodiazepine [e.g., z-drugs] receptor agonists [nBZRAs]" and found that:

> Nineteen percent of visits involving other sedative-hypnotics, 28% involving BZDs-only, 20% involving nBZRAs-only, and 48% involving a combination of BZDs and nBZRAs resulted in a serious disposition. Compared to visits involving other sedative-hypnotics, visits involving BZDs-only had 86% greater odds and visits involving a combination of BZDs and nBZRAs had almost four times increased odds of a serious disposition. Results were similar across age groups.
>
> (p. 1414)

Signs and symptoms of benzodiazepine overdosage, include:

- Blurred vision;
- Coma;

31 Some clinicians and researchers (e.g., Hood, Norman, & Hince, 2014) suggest the use of a low dose "infusion" of the benzodiazepine antagonist, "flumazenil," (Anexate®; Romazicon®) to treat benzodiazepine withdrawal. We have found insufficient data to support the efficacy of this pharmacotherapeutic intervention. Additionally, although a few cases—which were reported in the European literature (e.g., Ramah, Todorovic, & Crnic, 2015)—have suggested efficacy in the treatment of benzodiazepine withdrawal, the approach appears to be counterintuitive. Consequently, we do *not* recommend this suggestion for flumazenil use. It should be noted that others (e.g., Lin, 2014) have advocated the use of acetylcholinesterase inhibitors (e.g., donepezil, rivastigmine)—for the rapid detoxification of benzodiazepine (or z-drug) dependence. As we also noted regarding the suggested use of flumazenil in this context, insufficient supportive data are available for us to recommend this pharmacotherapeutic use of the acetylcholinesterase inhibitors.

- Confusion;
- Diminished reflexes;
- Dizziness;
- Drowsiness;
- Hypotension;
- Hypotonia;
- Incoordination;
- Slurred speech;
- Weakness.

(Gresham, 2018)

Respiratory arrest occurs more commonly with short-acting benzodiazepines (e.g., alprazolam [Xanax®]; midazolam [Versed®]; triazolam [Halcion®]; and when benzodiazepines (e.g., diazepam [Valium®]) are administered by intravenous (IV) injection.[32]

Benzodiazepine overdosage is not usually fatal because the benzodiazepines have a high therapeutic index, or LD_{50}.[33] (See also the related earlier discussion, in the benzodiazepine subsection, "Fatalities.") Alprazolam (Xanax®) has been reported to be the benzodiazepine that is most commonly encountered in ED visits. It also is reported to be "relatively more toxic than others in overdosage" (Gresham, 2018, p. 5).

Regardless of which specific benzodiazepine is involved in the overdosage, benzodiazepine overdosage requires emergency medical support of body systems, with attention to increasing benzodiazepine elimination. The benzodiazepine antagonist, "flumazenil" (Anexate®, Romazicon®), may be required. However, some caution is warranted because flumazenil antagonism may precipitate the benzodiazepine withdrawal syndrome among adolescents and young adults who are physically dependent on the benzodiazepines. Mental health care professionals also should recognize that flumazenil is a relatively short-acting competitive inhibitor of benzodiazepine receptor activity with a half-life of elimination of approximately one hour (Pagliaro & Pagliaro, 1999, 2009). This observation is clinically significant because it explains why overdosages with long-acting benzodiazepines often require management with subsequent additional doses of flumazenil.

In addition, as noted earlier, benzodiazepine overdosage frequently involves the concomitant use of other psychodepressants (e.g., alcohol; barbiturates; opiate analgesics) (Jones, Paulozzi, & Mack, 2014) that are not amenable to the antagonist effects of flumazenil (Pagliaro & Pagliaro, 2009; Sharp & Melnik, 2015). For example, a popular combination of psychodepressants used among young women in Texas since the beginning of the new millennium, consists of: the benzodiazepine, alprazolam (Xanax®)—a miscellaneous sedative-hypnotic from the miscellaneous subgroup, carisoprodol (Soma®)—and the opiate analgesic, hydrocodone (Vicodin®) (Forrester, 2011). As noted by the FDA, overall "overdose deaths that involved both opioid analgesics and

32 Parenteral administration of diazepam (Valium®) or lorazepam (Ativan®) also is accompanied by the risk for propylene glycol poisoning/toxicity. Propylene glycol is used as a diluent and vehicle for injectable solutions of the benzodiazepines—usually in a concentration of 400 mg/ml. Although propylene glycol is "generally recognized as safe" (GRAS) by the FDA, excessively large doses or rapid intravenous injections can rarely cause significant toxicity, including lactic acidosis and coma—particularly among neonates and infants. Treatment of propylene glycol toxicity is primarily supportive and may include the administration of sodium bicarbonate to correct metabolic acidosis and hemodialysis to correct severe hyperosmolality.

33 The LD_{50} is the symbol or abbreviation for the *median* lethal dose, or the dose that would be fatal for one-half of the population. It is more often associated with toxicology testing with population samples of laboratory animals (e.g., Sprague Dawley albino rats).

benzodiazepines [increased significantly] in the U.S. from 2004 to 2011" (Jones & McAninch, 2015, p. 493).

It is important to remember that alcohol is involved in a significant number of opiate analgesic and benzodiazepine related ED visits and drug-related deaths (Jones, Paulozzi, & Mack, 2014, p. 5).

Pregnancy and Lactation

The use of selected benzodiazepines during pregnancy has been associated with teratogenic effects (i.e., birth defects). For example, the use of diazepam (Valium®) during pregnancy, even at usual prescribed dosages, has resulted in cleft lip and cleft palate among some neonates whose mothers were medically prescribed diazepam for the management of their epilepsy. Craniofacial cleft also was reported involving the newborn baby of a mother who ingested 580 mg of diazepam in a single dose on the 43rd day of pregnancy (e.g., Pagliaro & Pagliaro, 2002).

The increased teratogenic risk associated with the use of anticonvulsants/anti-epileptics during pregnancy has long been well documented (Pagliaro & Levin, 1979). However, it has been found to be highest among pregnant women who received benzodiazepine monotherapy for the medical management of epilepsy (Deck, Nadkarni, & Montouris, 2015). Even when teratogenic effects (i.e., major physical abnormalities) have not been documented, the use of the benzodiazepines during pregnancy often has been associated with higher rates of preterm birth, low birth weight, and/or small for gestational age neonates/infants (Okun, Ebert, & Saini, 2015; Wikner, Stiller, & Bergman, 2007).

Only a relatively few and occasional reports of teratogenic effects (e.g., cardiac malformations; facial clefts; intestinal atresia) associated with benzodiazepine use have been reported—usually in the context of high dosages and use during the first trimester of pregnancy. Additionally, longitudinal studies have not identified a "benzodiazepine teratogenic syndrome" and the overall reported incidence of teratogenic effects does not differ from that noted in the general population (e.g., McElhatton, 1994; Ornoy, Arnon, & Shechtman, 1998; Pagliaro & Levin, 1979; Pagliaro & Pagliaro, 2012).[34]

Maternal use of the benzodiazepines during labor may result in neonatal sedation and respiratory depression. The benzodiazepines readily cross the placental barrier and can achieve fetal blood concentrations that are equal to, or higher than, maternal blood concentrations. Regular, long-term abuse of the benzodiazepines by women during pregnancy, or just near term, may result in fetal benzodiazepine physical dependence and, at birth, the expected pharmacological neonatal benzodiazepine effects, including:

- Drowsiness;
- Hypotonia;
- Poor sucking behavior;
- Low Apgar scores;
- Respiratory depression.

In addition, a neonatal benzodiazepine withdrawal syndrome may occur. It is characterized by the following neonatal signs and symptoms:[35]

34 N.B. Additionally, as we have noted on several occasions, the concurrent use of other potential teratogens, including alcohol, during pregnancy significantly confounds interpretation of published data (Pagliaro & Pagliaro, 1997).

35 The noted signs and symptoms, as well their intensity, will vary significantly as a result of the: (1) benzodiazepine; (2) maternal dosage used; (3) duration of maternal use during pregnancy; and (4) timing of maternal use in relation to stage of fetal development during pregnancy.

- Agitation;
- Diarrhea;
- Diaphoresis;
- Hypertension;
- Inconsolable crying;
- Insomnia;
- Seizures;
- Tremor.

Interestingly, but not surprisingly, a large study of the neonatal abstinence syndrome (NAS) (see related discussion in Chapter 5, "Prescription Opiate Analgesics and Heroin") associated with opiate analgesics found that over 40% of the mothers of affected neonates also reported benzodiazepine use during pregnancy (Lind, Petersen, & Lederer, 2015). Thus, health and social care professionals must remain ever vigilant when assessing and diagnosing pregnant women who are likely to have used more than one psychotropic drug or substance of abuse during their pregnancies.

The benzodiazepines also are excreted in breast milk in concentrations that may be sufficient to cause sedation and potential benzodiazepine physical dependence among breastfed neonates and infants. In addition, if regular, long-term maternal benzodiazepine abuse, or breast feeding, is abruptly discontinued, the breastfed neonate or infant is at risk for the benzodiazepine withdrawal syndrome. Maternal benzodiazepine use also has been indirectly associated with such major harmful effects as poor maternal-infant bonding, infant physical abuse and neglect, and infant/toddler failure to thrive.

Trends in New Millennial Benzodiazepine Use

Medical Use of the Benzodiazepines

Currently, the benzodiazepines are approved for several medical conditions, including:

- Anxiety disorders, including panic attacks (e.g., alprazolam, Xanax®);
- Insomnia (e.g., oxazepam, Serax®);
- Lower back pain (e.g., diazepam, Valium®, as a muscle relaxant);
- Management of seizures associated with the alcohol withdrawal syndrome (i.e., long-acting benzodiazepines, such as diazepam, Valium®);
- Pre-medication for medical procedures or surgical adjunct to anesthesia (e.g., lorazepam, Ativan®; midazolam, Versed®);[36]
- Seizure disorders (e.g., clonazepam, Rivotril®; diazepam, Valium®).

(Holbrook, Crowther, & Lotter, 1999; Pagliaro & Pagliaro, 2009)

Since the benzodiazepines were first synthesized, they have been medically used, for their psychodepressant anxiolytic and hypnotic actions. This section presents an overview of the medical use of these prescription sedative-hypnotics.

The first benzodiazepine, "chlordiazepoxide" (Librium®), was synthesized in the early 1950s by Leo Sternbach (1908–2005), a chemist working at a branch of the Swiss pharmaceutical company, Hoffmann-La Roche, in New Jersey. However, its potential

36 Lorazepam (Ativan®) and midazolam (Versed®) are commonly used as surgical/procedural pre-medications to both: (1) decrease anxiety among patients undergoing surgery or procedures (e.g., colonoscopy; endoscopy); and (2) produce anterograde amnesia so that patients do not later recall potentially stressful or distressing surgical/procedural experiences.

use was not immediately recognized, and it sat on a shelf in the laboratory for several years until, by chance, and with the help of a laboratory assistant, Sternbach discovered its efficacy as a sedative-hypnotic. Subsequently, chlordiazepoxide was aggressively marketed as an effective sedative-hypnotic without abuse potential.[37] It was an immediate marketing success. By 1963, a "chemical sister," diazepam (Valium®) joined the market and, over the following decade, more than two dozen additional chemical cousins were synthesized, developed, and marketed in the U.S. (For further related discussion, see Pagliaro & Pagliaro, 2004, 2009).

The use of the benzodiazepines peaked, worldwide, during the late-1970s. Concerns regarding an "over-medicated society" increased and resulted in a re-evaluation of the prescribing practices of physicians. As a result, the use of the benzodiazepines, and the other sedative-hypnotics, generally declined. However, the benzodiazepines continued to be widely prescribed in the U.S.[38] In a serial cross-sectional study of a nationally representative sample of outpatient adults in the U.S., Agarwal and Landon (2019) noted the following changes from January 1, 2003 to December 31, 2015—in regard to "benzodiazepine visits:"

1. ambulatory care "benzodiazepine visit" rates doubled from 3.8% to 7.4%;
2. half of all "benzodiazepine visits" (i.e., 52.3%) were to primary care physicians;
3. "benzodiazepine visit" rate remained stable for psychiatrists (i.e., 29.6% vs 30.2%);
4. "benzodiazepine visit" rate doubled among all non-psychiatric physicians (i.e., 3.6% to 7.5%;
5. "benzodiazepine visit" rate for insomnia remained stable (i.e., 26.9% vs 25.6%);
6. "benzodiazepine visit" rate for back and/or chronic pain more than doubled from 2.6% to 8.5%;
7. co-prescription rate for benzodiazepines and other prescription sedative-hypnotics doubled from 0.7% to 1.5%;
8. co-prescription rate for benzodiazepines and opiate analgesics quadrupled from 0.5% to 2.0%.

Given these observations, it is hardly surprising that several authors have identified the benzodiazepines as being among the most widely over-prescribed and misprescribed drugs in the world (e.g., Sweeney, Laoire, & Linehan, 2015).

Common Misbelief: Drugs and substances of abuse, including the benzodiazepines and z-drugs, do not cause physical dependence when medically prescribed by a physician for an active and appropriate clinical condition.

Not true. The "mis-prescription" and "over-prescription" of benzodiazepines have long been widely associated with a false and dangerous belief that the drugs and substances of abuse are *not* addicting when they are prescribed by a physician—and taken "as directed."

37 Chlordiazepoxide (Librium®) is not unique in this false claim. Throughout the modern history of pharmaceutical synthesis and marketing of various drugs, it seems that, whenever a new psychotropic drug—particularly, one with psychodepressant actions—was developed (e.g., heroin; pentazocine [Talwin®]; zopiclone [Imovane®]), it was aggressively marketed as "non-habit forming." In fact, heroin was specifically marketed during the late 19th century as a cure for "morphinism" (morphine addiction)—see Chapter 5, "Prescription Opiate Analgesics and Heroin."

38 For example, in 2008, according to the CDC, the most prescribed benzodiazepine in the U.S. was alprazolam (Xanax®) (Cai, Crane, & Poneleit, 2010).

As expressed by a psychiatrist, who published a review article on the benzodiazepines:

> It is important to distinguish between addiction to and normal physical dependence on benzodiazepines.... Due to the chronic nature of anxiety, long-term low-dose benzodiazepine treatment may be necessary for some patients; this continuation of treatment should not be considered abuse or addiction.
>
> (O'Brien, 2005, p. 28)[39]

We call attention to this "view" of addiction because it also concerns the prescription of other drugs and substances of abuse (e.g., opiate analgesics, see Chapter 5, "Prescription Opiate Analgesics and Heroin"). Mental health care professionals should both: (1) be aware of this situation that occurs with unacceptable frequency among patients; and (2) utilize this awareness and knowledge in the context of their own practices, particularly when working with adolescents and young adults, whose harmful use of prescription psychotropics may be related, at least initially, to an "iatrogenic" cause.

***Related Professional Reminder:* Mental health care professionals need to be aware of iatrogenic physical and psychological dependence associated with the prescribed sedative-hypnotics, particularly among children, adolescents, and young adults. Hopefully, this awareness will cause prescribers to take the actions required to decrease/eliminate iatrogenic dependence disorders.**

Adolescent and Young Adult Nonmedical or Illicit/Recreational Benzodiazepine Use

Although the overall nonmedical use of the benzodiazepines has significantly decreased from the high levels observed during the end of the last century, their use continues to be significant as indicated by reports from both addiction treatment centers and hospital EDs across the U.S. (e.g., Forrester, 2006; O'Brien, 2008). The benzodiazepines, particularly alprazolam (Xanax®), clonazepam (Rivotril®), diazepam (Valium®), and lorazepam (Ativan®), account for the majority of these reports. In addition, a significant number of adolescents, who seek assistance from addiction counselors for cocaine or opiate analgesic dependence (up to one-third), also have issues with benzodiazepine dependence.

Johnston, O'Malley, and Bachman (2008) found that approximately 6% of U.S. high school students reported benzodiazepine use within the previous 12 months. Esteban McCabe and West (2014) examined the lifetime prevalence of benzodiazepine use, both medical and nonmedical, among a large nationally representative sample of U.S. high school seniors from five

39 This view has become "enshrined" by psychiatrists in the 5th edition of the classification scheme for mental disorders, the *Diagnostic and Statistical Manual for Mental Disorders* (DSM-5):

> According to Charles O'Brien, Chair of the Substance-related Disorders Work Group, the term dependence is misleading because it is often confused with addiction, when in fact the tolerance and withdrawal patients experience are normal responses... So, we're eliminating that bad terminology.
>
> (Cassels, 2010, p. 2)

Perhaps this issue is just a matter of semantics. However, we would like to remind readers of the extremely relevant words of William Shakespeare (1564–1616) in *Romeo and Juliet*, written in 1594: *What's in a name? That which we call a rose by any other name would smell as sweet.* (See additional related discussion in Chapter 5, "Prescription Opiate Analgesics and Heroin.")

independent cohorts from 2007 to 2011. Their major finding was that 10% reported lifetime benzodiazepine exposure. Of these, 75% reported the use in a nonmedical context; 50% reported use in a medical context; and 25% reported both. Later, expanding their analysis to include all "prescription sedatives and anxiolytics," Esteban McCabe, Veliz, and Boyd found that: (1) 20% of adolescents reported lifetime medical or nonmedical use; and (2) of those who reported medical use, 45% also reported nonmedical use.[40]

Adolescents generally obtain benzodiazepines by: (1) "pharming"—stealing prescription benzodiazepines from their parent(s), or other family members, and then sharing them with other children or adolescents or trading them for more desired drugs and substances of abuse; (2) buying available benzodiazepines from illicit dealers, including older siblings and schoolmates; and (3) obtaining specific benzodiazepines by purchase over the internet.[41] As noted by Johnston, O'Malley, and Bachman (2008), in their national study of adolescent drug use in the U.S., for 2007, 20% of the high school students surveyed reported that the benzodiazepines were either fairly easy, or very easy, to obtain.

During the new millennium, the benzodiazepines continued to be used by adolescents and young adults. For example, young women often abuse benzodiazepines to "fully enjoy" the dance and night club scenes (Kurtz, Buttram, & Surratt, 2017; Kurtz, Surratt, & Levi-Minzi, 2011). Adolescents and young adults also use the benzodiazepines for several other reasons, including to:

- Achieve an alcohol-like disinhibitory euphoria, or "high;"
- Facilitate the perpetration of crimes, such as robbery and sexual assault, including "date rape;"
- "Get a good night's sleep" (i.e., manage fatigue related to everyday demands, problems, and worries);
- Prevent, or self-manage, the benzodiazepine withdrawal syndrome.

In addition, during the new millennium, adolescent girls and young women (primarily in their late twenties)—of all continental and other descents and sociocultural norms (e.g., whether living independently or with their parents; whether having dropped out of high school or with some college education)—routinely, concurrently use at least one other drug or substance of abuse (e.g., alcohol; cannabis; cocaine; 3,4-methylenedioxymethamphetamine [MDMA]) with their benzodiazepines. These adolescent girls and young women also share one other major variable, which has not been significantly identified among other cohorts of women—sexual victimization before they were 18 years-of-age.

The exact significance of this pattern of victimization is confounded by the observations made during the new millennium that: (1) sexual victimization is steadily becoming a "norm" in the U.S. (Pagliaro & Pagliaro, 2018); and (2) adolescent girls and young women routinely, and of their own volition, concurrently use benzodiazepines and other drugs and substances of abuse reportedly to decrease their own sexual inhibitions in order to "party" in contexts that may readily place them at higher risk for sexual victimization (Pagliaro & Pagliaro, *Clinical Patient Data Files*).[42]

We now turn to the "Z-drugs."

40 As significant as these findings of benzodiazepine use among adolescents are, it is important to recognize, as noted by Kurtz, Buttram, and Surratt (2017), that: "Young adults ages 18–29 report the highest rates of BZD [benzodiazepine] misuse in the United States" (p 39). Within this age cohort of young adults, benzodiazepine abuse has been noted to be highly correlated with participation in the "club scene" (Pagliaro & Pagliaro, *Clinical Patient Data Files*).

41 By comparison, young adults (26 to 35 years-of-age) primarily obtained benzodiazepines for illicit use through: (1) diversion from pharmacies (e.g., undercounting of capsules/tablets by pharmacy staff; theft by pharmacy staff); and (2) "doctor shopping" (Ibanez, Levi-Minzi, & Rigg, 2013, p. 48).

42 These factors are frequently discussed in the context of public media reviews of high profile cases of sexual assault.

Z-Drugs

The z-drugs are rapidly becoming the most frequently medically prescribed sedative-hypnotics in the U.S. This subgroup of the prescription sedative-hypnotics includes four major drugs: (1) "zaleplon" (Sonata®); (2) "zolpidem" (Ambien®); (3) "zopiclone" (Imovane®); and (4) "eszopiclone" (Lunesta®).[43]

Z-Drug Pharmacology

The z-drugs have a relatively rapid onset (i.e., they reduce sleep latency, or the time it takes to fall asleep after going to bed) and short duration of hypnotic actions. Consequently, they generally are associated with minimal "next day," or "hangover effects." Although their chemical structures are different from the basic benzodiazepine molecular structure, they have a virtually identical spectrum of pharmacological actions—primarily, because they elicit their effects by means of binding to the "benzodiazepine receptors" (i.e., "omega binding sites") (see related discussion in the earlier section, "Benzodiazepines: Pharmacodynamics").

Zaleplon (Sonata®), which is available as an oral capsule, shares many features with the benzodiazepine, triazolam (Halcion®), and another z-drug, zolpidem (Ambien®). However, in comparison to zolpidem, zaleplon appears to produce less sedation and memory impairment (Drover, Lemmens, & Naidu, 2000; Rush, Frey, & Griffiths, 1999). Zaleplon selectively binds to the brain omega-1 site situated on the alpha subunit of the GABA receptor complex.

Zolpidem (Ambien®) is a short-acting z-drug that is available in tablet form for ingestion. It also is the most widely prescribed sedative-hypnotic in the U.S. and, although its pharmacological actions are very similar to the benzodiazepines, it is chemically distinct (Holm & Goa, 2000).

Zopiclone (Imovane®), also a short-acting z-drug, shares a virtually identical spectrum of pharmacological actions with the benzodiazepines. Zopiclone became commercially available in Europe in 1986 and in the United States in 2005. Currently, it is one of the most widely used sedative-hypnotics in the U.S., and throughout the world. Its levorotatory isomer, eszopiclone (Lunesta®) also is available. Eszopiclone was approved in Europe in 1992 and later approved for use in the U.S. in 2004. Zopiclone and eszopiclone have been demonstrated, in young adults, to: reduce sleep latency; decrease the number of nocturnal awakenings; and increase total sleep time (Najib, 2006).

Pharmacodynamics: Mechanism of Action

The z-drugs are not benzodiazepines. However, current data suggest that all of the z-drugs act at the benzodiazepine receptor. Specifically, the z-drugs appear to act at the benzodiazepine recognition site of the $GABA_A$ receptor complex, particularly the omega-1 receptor at its alpha subunit. Working in concert with the inhibitory neurotransmitter GABA, the z-drugs appear to potentiate the GABA-evoked chloride current.[44] A noted placebo-effect also appears to play a significant role in their ability to produce sleep among those who have insomnia or other sleep disorders (Huedo-Medina, Kirsch, & Middlemass, 2012).

43 Eszopiclone is an isomer of zopiclone. An isomer is a closely related chemical that has the exact same molecular formula, but a different physical structure (e.g., one drug may be "dextro," or "right-handed", and the other drug may be "levo," or "left-handed"). Health and social care professionals should be aware that a difference in physical structure may result in a significant difference in actions, particularly when the site of action is a stereospecific drug receptor site.

44 See the related discussion in the earlier Benzodiazepine section, "Pharmacodynamics: Mechanism of Action."

Pharmacokinetics: Absorption, Distribution, Metabolism, and Excretion

The z-drugs are rapidly absorbed following ingestion and achieve peak blood concentrations and related effects within one to two hours. However, absorption is delayed when zolpidem is ingested with food. The half-life of elimination for the Z-drugs usually ranges from one to five hours. Typically, less than 5% of an oral dosage is excreted in unchanged form in the urine. Thus, renal impairment, including that associated with normal aging, does not usually affect their: (1) dosing; (2) half-life of elimination; (3) possible accumulation in the body; or (4) occurrence of undesired, or harmful, effects and toxicities. The Z-drugs are extensively metabolized in the liver by the hepatic microsomal (isoenzyme) system, particularly CYP3A4.[45]

In the following sections, we consider the pharmacokinetics of each of the z-drugs, beginning with zaleplon.

ZALEPLON (SONATA®)

Zaleplon is rapidly absorbed following ingestion and achieves peak blood concentrations within one hour (Dooley & Plosker, 2000). However, because of its extensive first-pass hepatic metabolism, its oral bioavailability is limited (i.e., F = 0.3). A high fat meal may delay oral absorption by up to two hours and reduce the maximum serum concentration by one-third. Approximately 60% of zaleplon is bound to plasma proteins and its apparent volume of distribution is 1.4 L/kg—indicating significant distribution into extravascular tissues. Extensively metabolized to several inactive metabolites by the aldehyde oxidase enzyme and the hepatic microsomal enzyme, CYP3A4, less than 1% of zaleplon is excreted in unchanged form in the urine. The half-life of elimination is approximately one hour (Drover et al., 2000; Gunja, 2013b) and, because of its short half-life of elimination, zaleplon is associated with fewer residual "hang-over" effects when dosed at bedtime (Drover, 2004).

Health care professionals are reminded that, as with other z-drugs, renal impairment does not affect dosing, half-life of elimination, potential accumulation in the body, or associated undesired, or harmful, effects and toxicities. However, hepatic impairment can significantly affect the blood concentration of zaleplon and all the other z-drugs.

ZOLPIDEM (AMBIEN®)

Zolpidem is rapidly and moderately well-absorbed (F = 0.7) following ingestion. It achieves peak blood concentrations within 1.5 hours. However, ingesting zolpidem with food delays and decreases its absorption. Zolpidem is approximately 92% bound to plasma proteins and has an apparent volume of distribution of 0.7 L/kg (Salva & Costa, 1995). It is metabolized extensively in the liver and its metabolites are primarily excreted in the urine. Less than 1% of zolpidem is excreted in unchanged form in the urine.

Metabolism is dependent on the mixed cytochrome P450 isoenzymes, particularly the hepatic isoenzyme, CYP3A4, but also involves CYP2C9 and CYP1A2 (Gunja, 2013b). Total body clearance is ~0.25 ml/kg/min.[46] The mean elimination half-life is two hours (range, one

45 In addition, CYP3A4 is involved in the metabolism of various benzodiazepines (e.g., alprazolam [Xanax®], midazolam [Versed®], and triazolam [Halcion®]). CYP3A4 is significantly inhibited by the selective serotonin reuptake inhibitors (SSRIs)—fluoxetine (Prozac®), fluvoxamine (Luvox®), and sertraline (Zoloft®). It also may be inhibited by the ingestion of grapefruit juice. The consequence of this "inhibition" of CYP3A4 is a significant increase in the blood concentrations of the z-drugs and the benzodiazepines—without any changes in their dosages (see the related discussion in the later subsection, "Drug–Drug Interactions Involving Z-Drugs.")

46 Although zolpidem is not FDA approved for use in children, it should be noted that Salva and Costa (1995) found that "clearance of zolpidem in children is 3 times higher than in young adults" (p. 142).

to three hours) (Drover, Lemmens, & Naidu, 2000). The half-life of elimination may be prolonged in those with hepatic dysfunction (e.g., hepatitis), but is not significantly affected by renal dysfunction.

Vlase, Popa, and Neag have examined potential pharmacokinetic interactions between zolpidem and other drugs, including carbamazepine and ciprofloxacin, following ingestion. In regard to carbamazepine (Tegretol®), they found that the bioavailability of zolpidem is decreased by ~ 60% and that the mean half-life of elimination of zolpidem is reduced from 2.3 hours to 1.6 hours (Vlase, Popa, & Neag, 2011a). In regard to ciprofloxacin (Cipro®), they found that the bioavailability of zolpidem is increased by ~ 50% and that the mean half-life of elimination of zolpidem is increased from 2.4 hours to 3.3 hours (Vlase, Popa, & Neag, 2011b).

ZOPICLONE (IMOVANE®)

Zopiclone is rapidly and moderately well-absorbed following ingestion (F = 0.70) and reaches peak blood concentrations in approximately two hours. However, the ingestion of foods that are high in fat content may delay reaching peak blood concentrations and associated psychodepressant actions. Zopiclone is weakly bound to plasma proteins (i.e., approximately 80%) (Fernandez, Gimenez, & Thuillier, 1999) and is widely distributed in the body with an apparent volume of distribution of approximately 110 L.

Zopiclone is extensively metabolized in the liver, principally by the hepatic isoenzymes CYP3A4 and CYP2E1, to several metabolites, particularly zopiclone-N-oxide (inactive) and N-desmethylzopiclone (active). Total body clearance is 232 ml/min. Only 5% of zopiclone is excreted in unchanged form in the urine. Zopiclone has a mean elimination half-life of approximately five hours (range, four to seven hours). Its longer half-life, in comparison to other z-drugs, may contribute to its greater efficacy in terms of maintaining a full night's sleep with fewer "wake-up" periods (Drover, 2004), but may also contribute to residual "hang-over" effects in the morning upon awakening. Fernandez and colleagues (e.g., Fernandez, Gimenez, & Thuillier, 1999; Fernandez, Maradeix, & Gimenez, 1993; Fernandez, Martin, & Gimenez, 1995) have noted that the pharmacokinetics of zopiclone are stereoselective and that the half-life of elimination differs for the levorotatory enantiomer (i.e., ~ 3.5 hours) versus the dextrorotatory enantiomer (i.e., ~ 6.5 hours).

ESZOPICLONE (LUNESTA®)

Eszopiclone is rapidly and well-absorbed following ingestion and achieves peak plasma levels within one hour. Eszopiclone is weakly bound to plasma proteins (~ 55%). It is extensively metabolized in the liver, primarily by the hepatic microsomal enzymes CYP3A4 and CYP2E1. Less than 10% is excreted as racemic zopiclone in the urine. Eszopiclone has a mean elimination half-life of ~ six hours (Najib, 2006).

Drug–Drug Interactions Involving Z-Drugs

Additive psychodepressant effects occur whenever z-drugs are concurrently used with other psychodepressants (e.g., alcohol; benzodiazepines; opiate analgesics). Also, because the z-drugs are primarily metabolized by the hepatic microsomal enzyme CYP3A4:[47]

1. Z-drugs should not be concurrently used with drugs that strongly "inhibit" CYP3A4 (e.g., clarithromycin, ketoconazole, nefazodone, ritonavir);

47 See also Chapter 5, "Prescription Opiate Analgesics and Heroin," Table 5.3, "Major Inducers and Inhibitors of CYP3A4 and CYP2D6," for a more comprehensive list.

2. Z-drugs may require an increase in dosage if concurrently used with drugs that moderately "induce" CYP3A4 (e.g., carbamazepine; phenytoin; rifampin). (See also the related discussion in the earlier z-drug subsection, "Pharmacokinetics: Zolpidem.")

Undesired, or Harmful, Effects and Toxicities

The spectrum of undesired, or harmful, effects and toxicities associated with the z-drugs appears to be similar to those associated with the benzodiazepines (Gunja, 2013a). In this regard, the z-drugs have been associated with both "acute" and "chronic" toxicities, including physical and psychological dependence. These undesired, or harmful, effects and toxicities are summarized in the following subsections. The noted incidence and severity of these effects and toxicities are significantly increased by the: (1) use of higher dosages; and/or (2) concomitant use of additional sedative-hypnotics (e.g., alcohol; benzodiazepines).

The incidence and nature of these adverse effects, which are associated with the use of the z-drugs—including those related to physical and psychological dependence—are currently incompletely characterized.[48] For example, it was not until April 30, 2019 that the FDA added a boxed warning regarding "serious injuries and deaths resulting from various complex sleep behaviors," such as sleep driving and sleepwalking, associated with the prescription use of the z-drugs (FDA, 2019, p. 1).[49]

ACUTE TOXICITIES

Zaleplon (Sonata®) has been associated with several acute toxicities, such as: anterograde amnesia; ataxia; cognitive impairment; dizziness; falls; hallucinations/illusions (generally, visual and short-lived); headaches; nausea; somnolence; and xerostomia.

Zolpidem (Ambien®) has been associated with several similar acute toxicities, including: anterograde amnesia; asthenia; ataxia; blurred vision; cognitive impairment; confusion; constipation; delirium; diarrhea; dizziness; dyspepsia; falls; hallucinations (i.e., visual, particularly with extremely high dosages); "hangover" effects; headaches; impaired judgment; increased appetite; memory impairment, particularly verbal memory; nausea; nightmares; red eyes; sleep driving (sleep-deprived, or drowsy, driving); somnambulism; somnolence; tinnitus; tremors; and xerostomia.

Zopiclone (Imovane®) also is associated with several acute toxicities. These toxicities include: anterograde amnesia; anxiety; asthenia; ataxia; bitter, metallic taste in the mouth; cognitive impairment; confusion; constipation; daytime fatigue; dizziness; dyspepsia; falls; grogginess and cognitive impairment upon awakening (e.g., "hangover" effects); headache; memory impairment, particularly verbal memory; somnolence; and xerostomia.

CHRONIC TOXICITIES

The major chronic toxicity associated with zaleplon (Sonata®) is mental depression. The major chronic toxicity associated with zopiclone (Imovane®) is mental depression. Eszopiclone (Lunesta®) shares a similar profile of undesired, or harmful, effects and toxicities with its chiral racemic mixture, zopiclone. Both zopiclone and eszopiclone have been associated with increased reports of extended hangover effects lasting over 11 hours and impaired

48 In this regard, the current situation involving the z-drugs is similar to where we were in relation to our knowledge of the benzodiazepines during the 1970s.

49 It should be noted that these same "rare" behaviors have also been noted, generally in forensic contexts, in relation to the use of the benzodiazepdines (Pagliaro & Pagliaro, 1991; Pagliaro & Pagliaro, Clinical Patient Data Files).

driving skills. As a result, in 2014 the FDA recommended the discontinuation of the 3-mg evening dosage for adults and reduction of the starting dosage to one mg (Abramowicz, 2014).

PHYSICAL AND PSYCHOLOGICAL DEPENDENCE

Regular, long-term use of zaleplon (Sonata®) is associated with a low potential for physical dependence and a low to moderate potential for psychological dependence. Based on its similarity to the benzodiazepines (e.g., triazolam), a zaleplon (Sonata®) withdrawal syndrome is expected to occur with regular, long-term use (Rush, Frey, & Griffiths, 1999). Its incidence initially appeared to be low (e.g., Dooley & Plosker, 2000), but has since been confirmed in studies of human case reports to be moderate (Schifano, Chiappini, & Corkery, 2019).

The regular, long-term use of zolpidem (Ambien®) has been associated with the development of low to moderate physical dependence and moderate psychological dependence. In a study evaluating dependence among long-term users of either zolpidem or zopiclone, Yen, Yen, and Ko (2015) found that: (1) zolpidem users reported more severe dependence than did zopiclone users; and (2) severe dependence, which was reported, was significantly correlated with reports of severe mental depression. A zolpidem withdrawal syndrome has been associated with the abrupt discontinuation of its regular, long-term use. Like the benzodiazepine withdrawal syndrome (see earlier benzodiazepine pharmacology subsection—"Benzodiazepine Withdrawal Syndrome"), the zolpidem withdrawal syndrome is characterized, in severe cases, by seizures and drug-induced psychosis (Hypnotic dependence, 2001; Cubala & Landowski, 2007; Mattoo, Gaur, & Das, 2011; Pagliaro & Pagliaro, 2009). The standard seven-day diazepam (Valium®) withdrawal program, which gradually tapers diazepam doses, has been used to successfully manage the zolpidem withdrawal syndrome. (Also see later benzodiazepine subsection, "Pregnancy and Lactation.")

The regular long-term use of zopiclone (Imovane®) has been associated with low potential for physical dependence and low to moderate potential for psychological dependence. However, mental health care professionals are reminded that individual differences in drug response may occur. A zopiclone (Imovane®) withdrawal syndrome, like the alcohol and benzodiazepine withdrawal syndromes, has been observed upon abrupt discontinuation of its regular, long-term medical or nonmedical use (Cimolai, 2007; Pagliaro & Pagliaro, 2009). This withdrawal syndrome is characterized by: agitation; anxiety; confusion; delirium; diaphoresis; flushing; hallucinations; headache; irritability; nightmares; palpitations; rebound anxiety; rebound insomnia; seizures (rare); tachycardia; and tremor. Regular, long-term zopiclone (Imovane®) use should be gradually discontinued in order to avoid the occurrence of this syndrome. Eszopiclone (Lunesta®), the levorotatory isomer (see earlier discussion) of zopiclone, can produce a similar withdrawal syndrome.

***Related Professional Reminder:* Generally, all z-drugs should be considered to have the same abuse potential as the benzodiazepines. Additional clinical data, which are gathered over the next decade, should further clarify individiual differences in the relative potentials for abuse and dependence among the various z-drugs.**

Schifano, Chiappini, and Corkery (2019), in their comprehensive review of related data obtained from the *European Medicines Agency Database*, noted that:

> [analyses] provide firm and large-scale evidence that z-drugs may be abused for recreational purposes.
>
> (p. 270)

In this context of abuse, the tablet forms of the z-drugs are generally orally ingested—often with an alcoholic beverage in order to enhance their euphoric or stress-reducing actions (Pagliaro & Pagliaro, *Clinical Patient Data Files*).

Z-drug Overdosage/Unintentional Poisoning

Overdosages involving the z-drugs alone are generally not life threatening, but may be associated with: ataxia; confusion; dizziness; hypotension; lethargy; respiratory depression; and somnolence. Zolpidem overdosage is also associated with miosis.[50] In cases of severe overdosage, impaired consciousness, ranging from drowsiness to light coma, also can occur. However, being pharmacologically similar to the benzodiazepines (Gunja, 2013a), overdosages involving the z-drugs are rarely fatal—except in the context of overdosages that involve the concurrent use of other drugs and substances of abuse (e.g., alcohol; opiate analgesics). Overdosages involving a deliberate suicide attempt often involve the ingestion of additional drugs and substances of abuse (Forrester, 2007).

Given, both: (1) the significant risk of z-drug overdosages in the context of the concurrent use of other psychodepressants; and (2) the presence of the opiate analgesic epidemic in the U.S. during the new millennium—the FDA added a black box warning, "Warning: Risks from Concomitant Use with Opioids," to the official drug product monographs for the z-drugs.[51]

***Related Professional Reminder:* The concurrent use of a z-drug with other psychodepressants, including alcohol, benzodiazepines, other z-drugs, or opiate analgesics, can significantly increase the risk for fatal overdosage (**Zosel, Osterberg, & Mycyk, 2011**). Fatalities can also be associated with the risky behavior that often accompanies z-drug overdosage (**Pagliaro & Pagliaro, 2009**). For example: (1) driving under the influence (DUI); and (2) sleep driving (**Pressman, 2011**).*

Overdosages involving z-drugs require emergency medical support of body systems, with particular attention to: (1) decreasing zolpidem absorption (e.g., appropriate use of: activated charcoal; syrup of ipecac; or gastric lavage);[52] and (2) maintaining adequate respiratory function (Kurta, Myers, & Krenzelok, 1997). There is no known antidote. The benzodiazepine antagonist, "flumazenil" (Anexate®, Romazicon®), reportedly, may be of some benefit in the management of zolpidem overdosage (Gunja, 2013b). However, caution is required because the use of flumazenil may precipitate a benzodiazepine-like withdrawal syndrome among adolescents and young adults who are physically dependent on zolpidem.

Unintentional poisoning (i.e., accidental poisonings) has usually been reported to occur among young children, under five years-of-age, who, for example, have gained access to their parent's z-drug (or other medications) within their own homes. Most of these cases do not involve any observable signs and symptoms and are conservatively managed at home by the parent or guardian—with the assistance of poison control, call center personnel (Forrester, 2009a, 2009b). Minor and moderate signs and symptoms have been reported and may require more aggressive intervention.

Pregnancy and lactation

Various adverse pregnancy outcomes (e.g., increased rate of preterm births; neonatal low birth weight and/or small for gestational age) have been reported to be higher among women, who received zolpidem (Ambien®) for the management of insomnia during pregnancy, when compared to women, who did not (Wang, Lin, & Lin, 2010). Based on the data of thousands of live births among mothers, who used various z-drugs during pregnancy, it appears, overall,

50 N.B. Miosis is also a common feature of opiate analgesic use and overdosage (see Chapter 5, "Prescription Opiate Analgesics and Heroin," pharmacology subsection, "Undesired, or Harmful, Effects and Toxicities—Prescription Opiate Analgesic and Heroin Overdosage/Unintentional Poisoning").

51 This FDA black box warning was also added to the benzodiazepine drug product monographs.

52 Generally, these approaches are only of benefit when initiated soon after ingestion. Additionally, hemodialysis is not of significant value because of the large volume of distribution of the z-drugs.

that the use of z-drugs by women during pregnancy is not related to teratogenesis (Wikner & Kallen, 2011). However, zolpidem has been demonstrated to cross the placental barrier. Additionally, the maternal use of z-drugs in late pregnancy, particularly near term, has been associated with expected neonatal complications, including: Apgar scores less than seven; hypoglycemia; and respiratory depression. Consequently, cautious use is indicated for adolescent girls and young women who are pregnant (Pagliaro & Pagliaro, 2009).

Data regarding the effects of z-drug use among mothers, who are breastfeeding, is extremely limited. Small amounts (i.e., generally, ~ 1%) of the maternal dose of a z-drugs are excreted in breast milk with peak concentrations occurring ~ 1 hour after maternal use (e.g., Matheson, Sande, & Gaillot, 1990). However, breastfeeding is often listed as a contraindication to the use of the z-drugs and, therefore, caution is recommended if z-drugs are used by mothers who are breastfeeding.

New Millennial Trends in Z-Drug Use

This section presents and discusses the medical and nonmedical use of z-drugs by adolescents and young adults. For an overview of embryo/fetus, neonate/infant, and child exposure to these sedative-hypnotics, see the earlier pharmacology subsections, "Z-Drug Overdosage/ Unintentional Poisoning" and "Pregnancy and Lactation." We begin with the medical use of z-drugs.

Medical Z-Drug Use

The medical use of z-drugs has not been approved by the FDA for children and adolescents. Although their safety and effectiveness—in these population groups—have not been established, they are commonly prescribed, "off-label," for: (1) the short-term adjunctive treatment of insomnia; and (2) comorbid medical, mental, or neurodevelopmental disorders among children and adolescents (e.g., de Zambotti, Goldstone, & Colrain, 2018; Owens, Babcock, & Blumer, 2005; Owens & Moturi, 2009; Owens, Rosen, & Mindell, 2003; Weiss & Garbutt, 2010).

Whenever z-drugs, or other prescription sedative-hypnotic pharmacotherapy are considered or deemed necessary for children and adolescents with sleep disorders, we recommend that it be implemented only after adequate sleep hygiene and appropriate cognitive-behavioral therapy have been implemented.

<u>Related Professional Reminder:</u> Advances in clinical practice frequently outpace formal research and related governmental regulations. Thus, "off-label" use can be rational and justified. In fact, today's "off-label" use quite often becomes tomorrow's "standard of practice." However, because of the limited amount of published research, which is an inherent factor in "off-label" medication use, particular caution and close patient monitoring are essential.

The z-drugs were used for 10 to 25 years in Asia and Europe before being introduced into the U.S. Since the beginning of the new millennium, their medical use increased significantly. Legally produced by pharmaceutical manufacturers in capsule or tablet formulations for ingestion, they are now prescribed more than any other prescription sedative-hypnotic in the U.S.

Zolpidem (Ambien®) was introduced into clinical practice, in the U.S., in 1992 as a sleeping aid that had little risk for physical or psychological dependence. However, its use for the short-term symptomatic medical management of insomnia has now been associated with both physical and psychological dependence—particularly, when prescribed and used in higher dosages or for longer periods of time than recommended. Zolpidem continues to be prescribed for the short-term symptomatic management of sleep disorders, including insomnia.

Unfortunately, since the beginning of the new millennium, prescribers have largely ignored the well-known and well-documented pharmacotherapeutic limitations and precautions associated with the use of zolpidem and other z-drugs. For example, as noted in the review, "Prescrire International:"

> Loss of efficacy can occur after a few weeks of treatment with zolpidem and zopiclone.
> (Hypnotic dependence, 2001, p. 15)

Adolescent and Young Adult Nonmedical or Illicit/Recreational Z-Drug Use

In the U.S., adolescents and young adults use the z-drugs for their psychodepressant actions—to achieve an alcohol-like disinhibitory euphoria, or "high," and to reduce anxiety, or stress. They also use them to prevent or self-manage respective z-drug withdrawal syndromes. Generally obtained by medical prescription, they also are illicitly obtained on-the-street or from internet vendors.

In the following subsection, we consider more specific trends in adolescent and young adult use of the z-drugs. We begin with zaleplon.[53]

ZALEPLON (SONATA®)

During the new millennium in the U.S., adolescent and young adult zaleplon use almost always began with a medical prescription to treat their insomnia. Although generally prescribed for "short-term use only," adolescents and young adults typically continued to use their zaleplon well beyond the prescribed time-frame while often increasing their original daily prescribed dosages by five to 10 times (or more) (see the earlier related discussion in this subsection). Typically, adolescents and young adults, concurrently use their zaleplon with other drugs and substances of abuse, including alcohol. While most ingest their capsules and tablets, many adolescents and young adults—in order to obtain "quick results"—choose to empty their capsules, or pulverize their tablets, and "snort" the resultant fine powder in a manner similar to snorting cocaine, heroin, or other drugs and substances of abuse.

ZOLPIDEM (AMBIEN®)

Known on the street as "A-minus," "No-Go,"[54] "Nappien," or "Tic-Tacs," zolpidem is used to achieve an alcohol-like disinhibitory euphoria, or "high," and optical, or visual, illusions. The tablet is usually crushed and snorted for quick intranasal absorption. Rarely, it is "cooked"—dissolved in a warm liquid and cooled—for IV injection (Pagliaro & Pagliaro, *Clinical Patient Data Files*). In the U.S., most zolpidem users are young adults of European

53 N.B. Because of the paucity of published survey and research studies regarding adolescent and young adult use of the z-drugs in the U.S., many of the references used in the following subsections were obtained from: (1) published European surveys and studies—where clinical experience with the z-drugs is longer and more extensive than that in the U.S.; and (2) our own clinical experience with z-drug use in this population group.

54 Zolpidem is used in the military of the U.S., and other countries, to facilitate sleep and readiness between missions among pilots and special operations personnel. Formal use in the U.S. Air Force is accompanied by a six-hour restriction on subsequent flight operations. Hence, the military argot denoting zolpidem—"no go pills."

continental descent, between 20 and 40 years-of-age. Generally, zolpidem is initially prescribed by their physicians to manage anxiety or sleep disorders. However, because of acquired tolerance, they use higher dosages than prescribed for longer periods of time than recommended (e.g., Madrak & Rosenberg, 2001). As physical dependence develops, adolescents and young adults use zolpidem to prevent, or self-manage, the zolpidem withdrawal syndrome.

Of increasing concern, zolpidem is purposely given to adolescent girls and young women, without their knowledge, to perpetrate drug-facilitated crimes (e.g., robbery; sexual assault, including "date rape") (e.g., Chitale, 2009; Schrotenboer, 2014).

> Ambien has replaced roofies as the rape drug of choice,' said Todd Emanuel, a California attorney who has worked on similar rape cases. "It is very easy to secrete in liquid like wine, and it has a short half-life, so it is usually difficult to detect." …
>
> He [NFL Star Darren Sharper] is out there preying on women between the ages of 20 and 23 years old. He hangs out with them at clubs. He takes them back, and it's the same story every single case … slipping Ambien into women's drinks, rendering them unconscious so he could rape them after a night of partying…
>
> In 2012, a man in Kansas City, Mo., was sentenced to 245 years in federal prison for drugging and molesting 13 children after he admitted to spiking their ice cream and soft drinks with sleeping pills, including zolpidem. Last year, a male nurse in Hawaii was sentenced to two years in prison after being accused of using the drug to spike the beer of a Coast Guard sailor and then sexually assault him.
>
> (Schrotenboer, 2014, pp. 1–5)

Unfortunately, suspected perpetrators are rarely charged and, for those who are charged, convictions are rarely obtained due to a lack of evidence because of the: (1) zolpidem-induced anterograde amnesia experienced by victims; and (2) fact that zolpidem is generally not detected in most routine drug screens (Carter, 2011). Salomone, Gerace, and DiCorcia (2012) have suggested segmental hair analysis of the victim's hair in order to both confirm that zolpidem was ingested and to determine the approximate date of ingestion—as estimated from the distance within the hair sample from the scalp.

***Related Professional Reminder:* Health and social care professionals need to be aware that screening for z-drug abuse is not generally undertaken in drug treatment programs. Thus, z-drugs may be used by adolescents and young adults enrolled in these programs without the knowledge of staff members. The z-drugs also are used in the perpetration of drug-facilitated crimes (e.g., robbery; sexual assault, or "date rape") being given to intended victims without their knowledge.**

ZOPICLONE (IMOVANE®)

Known on the street as "Zim-Zims," zopiclone is used to achieve an alcohol-like euphoria, or "high." It may also be used in an effort to manage the zopiclone withdrawal syndrome or the withdrawal syndrome related to the use of another sedative hypnotic. Although reportedly relatively few in numbers (e.g., Hajak, Muller, & Wittchen, 2003), adolescents and young adults who use zopiclone generally share the following two characteristics:

1. Began use as a medically prescribed drug to facilitate sleep;
2. Are concurrent users of other drugs and substances of abuse.

(e.g., Kuntze, Bullinger, & Mueller-Spahn, 2002; Morinan & Keaney, 2010; Pagliaro & Pagliaro, *Clinical Patient Data Files*; Sikdar, 1998)

Miscellaneous Prescription Sedative-Hypnotics[55]

Suvorexant (Belsomra®), the most recently released miscellaneous prescription sedative-hypnotic, is quite likely nonmedically (i.e., "recreationally" or illicitly) used by adolescents and young adults in the U.S.—but substantiating published research are currently unavailable. Published research is available, however, to substantiate that U.S. adolescents and young adults nonmedically use the much older, miscellaneous prescription sedative-hypnotic, gamma-hydroxybutyrate (GHB), which can be illicitly obtained from peers, dealers on-the-street, or over the internet/darknet. The pharmacology of these prescription sedative-hypnotic drugs is presented and briefly discussed in the following subsections along with trends in their use during the new millennium.

Suvorexant

Suvorexant (Belsomra®) was introduced into clinical practice in 2014 as a prototype for a new subgroup of sedative-hypnotics—"dual orexin receptor antagonists," or "DORAs" (Bennett, Bray, & Neville, 2014; Dubey, Handu, & Mediratta, 2015; Jacobson, Callander, & Hoyer, 2014; Owen, 2016). Suvorexant facilitates both the "onset" and "duration" of sleep and has been found, when compared to a placebo, to be effective for the treatment of insomnia, while improving:

- "Subjective total sleep time;"
- "Wake after sleep onset;"
- "Latency to persistent sleep."

(Patel, Aspesi, & Evoy, 2015, p. 477)

Suvorexant Pharmacology

The pharmacology of suvorexant is unique in comparison to other prescription sedative-hypnotics. Its pharmacology is presented and discussed in the following suvorexant subsections.

PHARMACODYNAMICS: MECHANISM OF ACTION

Orexin (hypocretin) is a neuropeptide that acts in the signaling control of vigilance and sleep/wake states (Reddy, Puvvada, & Kommisetti, 2015; Winrow & Renger, 2014). As such, orexin, as a master regulator of the sleep-wake cycle, displays diurnal variation:

1. During the "wake cycle," orexin displays high activity in the orexin cells found in the lateral hypothalamus (LH).
2. During the "sleep cycle," orexin displays almost no activity.

(Hoyer & Jacobson, 2013)

55 Other miscellaneous prescription sedative-hypnotics—which may be obtained over the internet/darknet for nonmedical, or illicit, use by adolescents and young adults—generally have long histories that can extend back over the past 50 to 150 years. These prescription sedative-hypnotics include the: barbiturates; chloral hydrate; ethchlorvynol; meprobamate; and methaqualone. For detailed information regarding these miscellaneous prescription sedative-hypnotics, readers are referred to Pagliaro and Pagliaro (2004, 2009).

Neurons in the LH produce orexin A and orexin B, which bind to orexin receptors (i.e., OX_1R and OX_2R) producing the desired physiologic response (i.e., wakefulness) (Hopkins, 2012). Acting as an active dual OX_1R and OX_2R antagonist (Yang, 2014), suvorexant blocks the orexin receptors resulting in the promotion of sleep (i.e., suppresses the orexin-mediated wake drive) by reducing arousals and improving sleep consolidation (Lee-Iannotti & Parish, 2016). In addition, suvorexant increases both REM and non-REM sleep (Sutton, 2015).

PHARMACOKINETICS: ABSORPTION, DISTRIBUTION, METABOLISM, AND EXCRETION

Due to the relatively recent introduction of suvorexant for the treatment of insomnia and other sleep disorders, few published research studies are available regarding its pharmacokinetics. However, the following data have been reported:

- Oral bioavailability is high (F = 0.8);
- Onset of action following the ingestion of suvorexant, on an empty stomach, is approximately 30 minutes;
- Absorption and, consequently, latency time from administration to sleep may be delayed when suvorexant is ingested with food or meals;
- Suvorexant is highly bound to plasma proteins (i.e., > 99%);
- Mean volume of distribution is ~ 49 liters;
- Obese adolescents and young adults may have blood suvorexant concentrations 1.5-fold higher than non-obese adolescents and young adults. This effect is particularly prominent among adolescent girls and young women;
- Hepatic metabolism, primarily mediated by CYP3A4, is the major mechanism of elimination;
- Hepatic metabolism, minor route mediated by CYP2C19;
- Renal impairment does not affect blood suvorexant concentrations (i.e., renal excretion of unchanged suvorexant is insignificant);
- The half-life of elimination of suvorexant is ~ 12 hours;
- Hepatic impairment may increase the half-life of elimination for suvorexant by up to 30 hours.

(Cui, Cabalu, & Yee, 2016; Dailey, 2015; Lee-Iannotti & Parish, 2016)

SUVOREXANT DRUG-DRUG INTERACTIONS

Additive psychodepressant effects occur whenever other psychodepressant drugs (e.g., alcohol; benzodiazepines; opiate analgesics; z-drugs) are concurrently used with suvorexant. Additionally, because suvorexant is primarily metabolized by the hepatic microsomal enzyme CYP3A4, it should not be concurrently used with drugs that:

1. Moderately "induce" CYP3A4 (e.g., carbamazepine; phenytoin; rifampin), which may necessitate a significant increase in suvorexant dosage (e.g., increasing a starting dose of five mg to 10 mg);
2. Strongly "inhibit" CYP3A4 (e.g., clarithromycin; ketoconazole; nefazodone; ritonavir), which may necessitate a significant dosage reduction.[56]

56 See also Chapter 5, "Opiate Analgesics and Heroin," Table 5.3, "Major Inducers and Inhibitors of CYP3A4 and CYP2D6," for a more comprehensive list.

UNDESIRED, OR HARMFUL, EFFECTS AND TOXICITIES

Because suvorexant is a relatively new drug from a new drug class of the prescription sedative-hypnotics, available data regarding the undesired, or harmful, effects and toxicities associated with the clinical use of suvorexant are limited. However, it is well-established that the incidence and severity of undesired, or harmful, effects and toxicities, as expected, increase with higher dosages.

The most frequently encountered undesired effects associated with FDA-recommended dosages of suvorexant are: fatigue; headache; impaired driving; somnolence; and xerostomia (Gauld, 2016; Hopkins, 2012; Michelson, Snyder, & Paradis, 2014). Other reported undesired effects include: abnormal dreams; aggressive behavior; amnesia; anxiety; ataxia; confusion; cough; diarrhea; dizziness; dyspepsia; hypnogogic/hypnopompic hallucinations; "hangover" effects; mental depression; muscle weakness; peripheral edema; sleep driving; sleep paralysis; somnambulism; suicide ideation; and a feeling of weakness in the legs (Jacobson, Callander, & Hoyer, 2014; Kishi, Matsunaga, & Iwata, 2015; Michelson, Snyder, & Paradis, 2014).

Overall, because the mechanism of action of suvorexant, which is much more specific than that of other sedative-hypnotics (e.g., alcohol; benzodiazepines; z-drugs), the associated incidence of undesired, or harmful, effects and toxicities (e.g., respiratory depression)—when compared to other sedative-hypnotics—appears to be significantly reduced.

PHYSICAL AND PSYCHOLOGICAL DEPENDENCE

Little published data are available regarding the abuse potential of suvorexant.[57] Preclinical assessment of abuse potential, which was conducted by the pharmaceutical firm Merck & Company® utilizing rat and rhesus monkey models, indicated a probable low abuse potential for suvorexant in humans (Born, Gauvin, & Mukherjee, 2017). The FDA has classified suvorexant as a controlled substance (C-IV). Based on clinical trials, suvorexant also was identified, in a National Drug Monograph, as having human abuse potential similar to that for the z-drug, zolpidem (Dailey, 2015; Schoedel, Sun, & Sellers, 2016).[58] Suvorexant withdrawal signs and symptoms, including rebound insomnia, have been identified, but are reported as generally being nonsignificant (Michelson, Snyder, & Paradis, 2014).

Suvorexant Overdosage/Unintentional Poisoning

The incidence and severity of overdosage increase as the ingested dose increases. Monitoring of vital signs and general symptomatic and supportive measures should be used. Gastric lavage, where appropriate, can be of assistance. However, because suvorexant has significant protein binding, hemodialysis is not expected to significantly increase elimination and, consequently, is not recommended to treat related overdosage and unintentional poisoning. Additional data are *not* currently available.

57 Historically, experience with other prescription sedative-hypnotics suggests that all possess some degree of risk for physical and/or psychological dependence. In addition, data regarding other DORAS, which are not yet on the market (e.g., almorexant), indicate that this pharmacological class of prescription sedative-hypnotics also carry this risk. For example, Cruz, Hoever, and Chakraborty (2014) found that, in a randomized, crossover, placebo-controlled study, subjects reported significant subjective measures of abuse potential (e.g., "drug liking") for almorexant.

58 Based upon the: (1) noted absence of reports of physical dependence; (2) related lack of a demonstrated suvorexant withdrawal syndrome (e.g., Citrome, 2014; Michelson, Snyder, & Paradis, 2014); and (3) the mechanism of suvorexant action, we believe that the probability of physical dependence, if it exists, is low and that the probability of psychological dependence, which likely occurs, is lower than that demonstrated by other currently available prescription sedative-hypnotics.

Pregnancy and Lactation

The effects of the use of suvorexant by adolescent girls and young women, who are pregnant or breastfeeding, is currently unknown. Animal data (i.e., rabbits and rats) failed to demonstrate any teratogenic effects. However, suvorexant was demonstrated to be excreted in rat milk in concentrations that were significantly higher than donor concentrations. Caution is indicated.

New Millennial Trends in Suvorexant Use

In this section, the medical use of suvorexant is presented and discussed with attention to trends in adolescent and young adult use.

Medical Use of Suvorexant

Suvorexant is FDA approved for the treatment of insomnia, characterized by difficulty with sleep onset and/or sleep maintenance in adults. See the related comments, discussion, and recommendations discussion in the earlier z-drug subsection, "Medical Use of Z-Drugs," which also generally apply to suvorexant.

The use of suvorexant has been evaluated for adolescents in a few studies in other countries (e.g., Japan) and, generally, has been found to be safe and effective for the treatment of insomnia (e.g., Kawabe, Horiuchi, & Ochi, 2017). However, currently it is not approved by the FDA for use among children or adolescents.

Gamma-Hydroxybutyrate (GHB)

Gamma-hydroxybutyrate is unique among the prescription miscellaneous sedative-hypnotics because it occurs endogenously in the human body as both a precursor and a metabolite of GABA. As such, it acts as a CNS inhibitory neurotransmitter. GHB is available as an oral solution by its generic, prescription name, "sodium oxybate" (Xyrem®) and is known "on-the-street" by many different names: "Cherry Meth;" "Easy Lay;" "Gamma-Oh;" "Georgia Home Boy;" "Great Hormones at Bedtime;" "Grievous Bodily Harm;" "Liquid G;" "OxySleep;" "Salty Water;" and "Soap."

Illicit GHB, in both oral solutions and powder, is produced,[59] imported,[60] distributed, and sold across the U.S. Adolescents and young adults commonly add GHB oral solution to a bottle of water prior to their attendance at a rave so that they can slowly "swig it" through the night.[61] Colorless, odorless, and virtually tasteless,[62] it also may be mixed into an alcoholic drink at a party or dance club to increase sexual arousal and experiences—or to facilitate date rape (Pagliaro & Pagliaro, *Clinical Patient Data Files*).

59 GHB can be produced from two commonly available chemical precursors: gamma-butyrolactone (GBL); and 1,4-butanediol (BD). GBL and BD can be chemically converted to GHB in vitro by a relatively easy chemical production process—a process that is widely available on several internet sites.

60 GHB is most often produced in Canada, Europe, Mexico, and, to a lesser extent, Israel (National Drug Intelligence Center, 2004).

61 Sold at raves, a single dose of GHB oral solution is often referred to as a "swig."

62 However, when dissolved in water, GHB imparts a distinctly "salty" taste to the water—or other liquid (e.g., alcohol) when sipped).

GHB Pharmacology

Gamma-Hydroxybutyrate has an interesting history. It was synthesized over 140 years ago in 1874 by the Russian chemist, Aleksandr Zaitsev (1841–1910). However, GHB was not used until the 1960s when the French physician, Henri Laborit (1914–1995), began to study its use as an anesthetic and a sedative-hypnotic with human patients. By the 1980s, GHB became widely available in health food stores and was promoted and used as a nutritional supplement, primarily by body builders.

However, by the 1990s, use for its sedative-hypnotic actions grew and became associated with increasing incidents of toxicity and death. As a result, the FDA banned the non-prescription, or over-the-counter, sale of GHB for human consumption. Unfortunately, the effects of GHB had become well-known, and, consequently, through the 1990s, its use as a date rape drug increased significantly (Marinetti & Montgomery, 2010). In response, the *Hillory J. Farias and Samantha Reid Date Rape Drug Prohibition Act* was passed and signed into law in 2000. This Act placed GHB on "Schedule I" of the Controlled Substances Act, prohibiting its prescription or sale in the U.S. (Placement of …, 2000).

Samantha Reid, for whom the act was named, was a victim of one of the first GHB-involved date rape cases that resulted in death:

> Three of the four young men charged in the date-rape-drug death of a 15-year-old girl were found guilty Tuesday of involuntary manslaughter.
>
> Jurors in one of the nation's first trials resulting from a death linked to the date-rape drug GHB also found the three—Joshua Cole, 19, of Southgate, Daniel Brayman, 18, of Trenton and Nicholas Holtschlag, 18, of Wayne County's Brownstown Township—guilty of lesser poisoning charges …
>
> Prosecutors alleged the men gave Samantha a soft drink secretly spiked with GHB, or gamma-hydroxybutyrate, during a January 16, 1999, party at Limmer's Grosse Ile apartment. Samantha died the next day. Her best friend Melanie Sindone, now 16, also ingested the drug and was briefly in a coma, but survived.
>
> (CBS News Staff, 2000, p. 1)

PHARMACODYNAMICS: MECHANISM OF ACTION

The exact mechanism by which GHB produces its sedative-hypnotic actions has not been determined. However, the following five actions have been identified and confirmed:

1. GHB binds to its own endogenous GHB receptors in the CNS, predominantly in the basal ganglia and hippocampus.
2. GHB appears to enhance the inhibitory actions that are modulated by the $GABA_B$ receptors (subunits $GABA_{B1}$ and $GABA_{B2}$).
3. GHB acts both presynaptically and postsynaptically to modulate the activity of other neurotransmitters (e.g., glutamate; norepinephrine; serotonin) in the CNS.
4. GHB presynaptically inhibits the release of dopamine into the synaptic cleft, resulting in an accumulation of dopamine in the presynaptic neuron.
5. GHB activates the $alpha_4$-$GABA_A$ receptor.

(Busardo & Jones, 2015; Carter, Koek, & France, 2009; Okun, Boothby, & Bartfield, 2001; Tunnicliff, 1997)

In addition, GHB appears to affect the cholinergic system, neurosteroidogenesis, and oxytocin release. These collective, proposed mechanisms of GHB action appear to help to account for the observed: (1) therapeutic actions (e.g., euphoria; enhanced sexual experience); (2) undesired, or harmful, effects and toxicities (e.g., cognitive impairment; somnolence); and (3) signs and symptoms of the GHB withdrawal syndrome (e.g., seizures; tachycardia) (Busardo & Jones, 2015; Galloway, Frederick, & Staggers, 1997; Kamal, van Noorden, & Franzek, 2016; Pagliaro & Pagliaro, 2009).

PHARMACOKINETICS: ABSORPTION, DISTRIBUTION, METABOLISM, AND EXCRETION

GHB is rapidly, but incompletely, absorbed from the GI tract. Oral availability is relatively low (F = 0.25) with peak plasma levels obtained approximately 30 minutes after ingestion (Borgen, Okerholm, & Lai, 2004; Schep, Knudsen, & Slaughter, 2012). Onset of action is generally within 10 to 20 minutes following the ingestion of GHB and lasts for approximately five hours. Ingestion with a high-fat content meal significantly delays and reduces absorption. Consequently, in the context of medical use, nocturnal dosing at a consistent time interval—several hours after ingestion of the evening meal—has been recommended (Borgen, Okerholm, & Morrison, 2003). Following absorption into the systemic circulation, GHB is found in equal concentrations in both whole blood and serum—suggesting distribution into erythrocytes (Brailsford, Cowan, & Kieman, 2012).

Metabolism, primarily by GHB dehydrogenase and the Krebs cycle, provides the major elimination pathway for GHB. GHB is metabolized to carbon dioxide and water. Less than 5% is excreted in unchanged form in the urine (Brenneisen, Elsohly, & Murphy, 2004; Busardo & Jones, 2015; Pagliaro & Pagliaro, 2009). The half-life of elimination for GHB is approximately 30 minutes and effects may persist for three to six hours (Busardo & Jones, 2015). Plasma protein binding is less than 1%. The apparent volume of distribution is approximately 50 L and the total body clearance of GHB is approximately one L/min (Brenneisen, Elsohly, & Murphy, 2004; Galloway, Frederick, & Staggers, 1997). GHB appears to follow dose-dependent, or nonlinear, pharmacokinetics (Jones, Eklund, & Kronstrand, 2009; Liechti, Quednow, & Liakoni, 2016; Pagliaro & Pagliaro, 2009).

GHB DRUG–DRUG INTERACTIONS

Adolescents and young adults who use GHB often concurrently use other "club drugs" (e.g., alcohol; MDMA). They also concurrently use methamphetamine and other drugs and substances of abuse (Galloway, Frederick, & Staggers, 1997; Lee & Levounis, 2008; Pagliaro & Pagliaro, 2009). Generally, each of the concurrently used drugs cause expected, associated pharmacologic effects—most often resulting in additive or antagonistic actions. In a few documented cases, these GHB drug–drug interactions have resulted in clinically significant sequelae.

GHB AND ALCOHOL. The concurrent use of alcohol with GHB, as in situations when GHB is added to alcoholic beverages, results in synergistic psychodepressant effects. Additionally, concurrent use of alcohol and GHB may increase the risk of vomiting, aspiration of vomitus, and respiratory depression—particularly during acute GHB intoxication.

GHB AND METHAMPHETAMINE. Concurrent use of GHB and methamphetamine, or other psychostimulants (e.g., cocaine), may increase seizure risk—particularly during GHB withdrawal.

GHB AND OTHER PSYCHODEPRESSANTS. The concurrent use of GHB and other psychodepressants (e.g., alcohol; benzodiazepines; z-drugs) results in additive psychodepression and, consequently, significant increased risk for fatal overdosage (see the related discussion in the later GHB subsection, "GHB Overdosage").

UNDESIRED, OR HARMFUL, EFFECTS AND TOXICITIES

The use of GHB has been associated with several common undesired, or harmful, effects and toxicities, both acute and chronic. These effects—including physical and psychological dependence—are discussed in the following subsections.

ACUTE AND CHRONIC ADVERSE EFFECTS. "Acute" adverse effects include: amnesia; apnea; ataxia; bradycardia; cognitive impairment; coma; confusion; diaphoresis; diarrhea; dizziness; dyspepsia; enuresis; headache; hypotension; hypothermia; nausea; respiratory depression (associated with higher dosages); sleep (deep); slurred speech; somnolence; syncope; vomiting; and weakness.[63]

"Chronic" adverse effects associated with the regular, long-term use of GHB include: mental depression; menstrual cycle irregularities; physical dependence (low); psychological dependence (moderate); somnambulism; tinnitus; and withdrawal syndrome.

PHYSICAL AND PSYCHOLOGICAL DEPENDENCE

The potential for GHB dependence, or use disorder, was first recognized in the 1990s (Galloway, Frederick, & Staggers, 1997). Generally, GHB is associated with a low risk for physical dependence and moderate risk for psychological dependence (Pagliaro & Pagliaro, 2009). However, concern has been raised concerning the possible underreporting of these effects (Brennan & Van Hout, 2014).

GHB WITHDRAWAL SYNDROME. A specific GHB withdrawal syndrome has been reported and likened, in both nature and significance, to the alcohol withdrawal syndrome (see related discussion in Chapter 1, "Alcohol") (Mason & Kerns, 2002; Tarabar & Nelson, 2004). Signs and symptoms of the GHB withdrawal syndrome include:

- Agitation;[64]
- Anxiety;
- Autonomic nervous system excitation, or instability;

63 Interestingly, some researchers (e.g., Zvosec & Smith, 2005) have noted "non-sedative effects" (e.g., agitation; bizarre or self-injurious behavior; combativeness) in association with GHB toxicity. These noted signs and symptoms appear to be quite similar to those occasionally associated with phencyclidine (PCP) (see Chapter 4, "Cannabis and Other Psychodelics"). Upon reflection, we would ascribe the noted "non-sedative" effects to most likely be associated with the:

1. Concurrent use of GHB with another psychotropic, such as a psychostimulant (e.g., methamphetamine, see Chapter 2, "Amphetamines and Cocaine") or psychodelic (e.g., PCP, see Chapter 4, "Cannabis and Other Psychodelics");
2. Exacerbation of an underlying personality-predisposition in association with a GHB-induced decrease in mediated measures of cognitive, and, consequently, social "control."

64 May be quite severe and requires appropriate physical or chemical restraint (or both) to prevent injury to self or others.

- Coma;
- Confusion;
- Delirium;
- Diaphoresis;
- Hallucinations;
- Hypertension;
- Insomnia;
- Nystagmus;
- Paranoid delusions;
- Psychosis;
- Respiratory depression;
- Rhabdomyolysis;
- Seizures;
- Tachycardia;
- Tremor.

(Dyer, Roth, & Hyma, 2001; Pagliaro & Pagliaro, 2009; Wojtowicz, Yarema, & Wax, 2008)

For adolescents and young adults, who are regular, long-term GHB users, the GHB withdrawal syndrome may begin within one hour of the last use of GHB and last for up to 15 days (Galloway, Frederick, & Staggers, 1997). Potentially life-threatening, the GHB withdrawal syndrome is often quite resistant to medical management with benzodiazepines, such as diazepam (Valium®) or lorazepam (Ativan®) (McDonough, Kennedy, & Glasper, 2004). In cases of severe GHB withdrawal, a barbiturate (e.g., pentobarbital [Nembutal®]; phenobarbital [Luminal®]) may be more effective (Ghio, Cervetti, & Respino, 2014; Sivilotti, Burns, & Aaron, 2001).

The GHB withdrawal syndrome, because it is potentially life-threatening, should always be considered a medical emergency that requires prompt and appropriate referral for emergency medical management (Brunt, Van Amsterdam, & van Den Brink, 2014). Severe cases of GHB withdrawal generally require hospitalization (up to five days) for both observation and treatment of associated signs and symptoms (Sivilotti, Burns, & Aaron, 2001; Tarabar & Nelson, 2004; Wojtowicz, Yarema, & Wax, 2008).

GHB Overdosage

Gamma-hydroxybutyrate overdosage is relatively common (Miotto, Darakjian, & Basch, 2001) and may be fatal (Zvosec, Smith, & Porrata, 2011).[65] However, fatalities are rare and are usually associated with the concurrent use of other drugs and substances of abuse (Knudsen, Jonsson, & Abrahamsson, 2010). Alcohol, heroin, and MDMA are most often involved in GHB overdosage (Lee & Levounis, 2008; Pagliaro & Pagliaro, 2009).

Adolescents and young adults, who have overdosed, usually present to the ED in an unconscious state, or coma. Other presenting signs and symptoms of overdosage may include: agitation; ataxia; blurred vision; bradycardia; confusion; delirium; diaphoresis; headache; hypothermia; incontinence; muscle jerks or twitches (myoclonic movements); muscle weakness; respiratory impairment; seizures; and vomiting. Death may occur because of cardiorespiratory depression (Busardo & Jones, 2015).

65 Deaths associated with GHB overdosage, when they do occur, are generally secondary to respiratory failure.

> … responded to a report of a woman that had collapsed after having taken GHB … found the woman passed out in the bathroom. By the time emergency personnel arrived, two more people were in medical distress, after also taking GHB.
>
> (Judd, 2014, p. 1)

> One teenager said three friends were having a bad reaction to the GHB. When officers arrived, they found a 19-year-old man and a 15-year-old girl unresponsive and a 17-year-old girl who was semi-conscious.
>
> (Judd, 2015, p. 1)

GHB overdosage should always be treated as a medical emergency with immediate referral for assistance, as needed. With proper recognition and care, particularly with attention to cardiac and respiratory support,[66] complete recovery within six to eight hours, without any "after effect" associated with the overdosage, generally can be expected (Mason & Kerns, 2002). There is no known antidote for GHB overdosage.

Pregnancy and Lactation

Published data regarding the possible teratogenic effects of GHB in humans are not available. However, because GHB is an endogenous human neurotransmitter (albeit in significantly lower concentrations than when therapeutically administered)—in the absence of contradictory reports of teratogenic effects, the medical use of GHB for pregnant adolescent girls and young women is generally considered to be relatively safe for approved indications.

GHB is excreted in breast milk in concentrations that are 30% to 70% lower than the reported maternal serum concentrations. Breast milk concentrations of GHB generally peak one hour after maternal dosing and remain significantly elevated for at least four hours. In order to minimize the exposure of neonates and infants, who are breastfeeding, to GHB—and associated undesired pharmacological effects—it is recommended that, mothers who are breastfeeding and require GHB (i.e., sodium oxybate) for the treatment of medical conditions (e.g., narcolepsy with associated cataplexy), avoid breastfeeding for at least five hours after their last dose (Barker, Puchowicz, & Letterio, 2017; Busardo, Bertol, & Mannocchi, 2016)—or, as we generally recommend, avoid breastfeeding.

New Millennial Trends in GHB Use

This subsection presents and discusses trends in the medical use of GHB and adolescent and young adult nonmedical or "recreational" use of GHB.

MEDICAL USE OF GHB

In 2002, the FDA approved the prescription use of GHB for the medical management of narcolepsy in patients who experience episodes of cataplexy (National Drug Intelligence Center, 2004). To protect the public, GHB, when used in this medical context, is referred to as, and prescribed by, the alternate generic name and brand/trade name, "sodium oxybate

66 Interestingly, in a three-year retrospective analysis of data from two major inner-city EDs, Dietze, Horyniak, and Agius (2014) found that, in cases of uncomplicated GHB-related coma, conservative airway management—without the use of intubation—was associated with shorter length of stay in the ED.

(Xyrem®)."[67] It is commercially available as an oral solution. Xyrem® has an FDA required black box warning concerning "Central Nervous System Depression, Misuse, and Abuse."[68]

ADOLESCENT AND YOUNG ADULT NONMEDICAL OR ILLICIT/RECREATIONAL GHB USE

During the first two decades of the new millennium, in the U.S., GHB was generally used by adolescents and young adults to achieve such desired effects, as:[69]

1. Alcohol-like disinhibitory euphoria, or "high" (without the "hangover" effect associated with alcohol or other sedative-hypnotic use);[70]
2. Improved body build (i.e., when used as a nutritional/anabolic supplement—often advertised/marketed as a "growth hormone releaser");
3. Enhanced sexual experience;[71]
4. Increased sociability;
5. Means to prevent/self-manage the alcohol withdrawal syndrome;
6. Relaxation;
7. Facilitation of sexual assault[72] (see following discussion).

GHB is also purposely administered to others, without their knowledge, in the context of perpetrating drug-facilitated crimes (e.g., robbery; sexual assault, including

67 GHB also has been used in Europe to treat the alcohol withdrawal syndrome and for the maintenance of abstinence in the treatment of AUD. It is being reviewed for similar clinical use in the U.S. In this clinical context of use, GHB pharmacotherapy has been demonstrated to be equivalent, or superior, to benzodiazepines (e.g., diazepam [Valium®]) or placebo in several studies (e.g., Caputo, Skala, & Mirijello, 2014; Keating, 2014; Leone, Vigna-Taglianti, & Avanzi, 2010; Skala, Caputo, & Mirijello, 2014). However, several researchers (e.g., Keating, 2014) have voiced concern that the use of GHB among those "with alcohol dependence and borderline personality disorder or who are in remission from heroin or cocaine addiction" may be unsuitable because of an increased risk for GHB abuse (p. 63).

68 Because of these identifed risks, the FDA has mandated that Xyrem® only be available in the U.S. through a restricted distribution program referred to as the "Xyrem REMS Program."

69 Because of the relatively short half-life of elimination for GHB (i.e., approximately 30 minutes [see related discussion in the earlier GHB subsection, "Pharmacokinetics"]), GHB is often dosed five or more times daily, particularly for regular, long-term users.

70 As shared by a 20-year-old woman who commonly uses GHB in a social context—similar to that of alcohol:

> I sort of look at it on the same level as having a drink. Often times it affects me for a shorter period of time and I don't have any hangover the next day, it doesn't make me feel crappy … get great sleep.
>
> (Barker, Harris, & Dyer, 2007, p. 123)

71 Kapitany-Foveny, Mervo, and Corazza (2015), in a study of 60 "recreational" GHB users, found their particular "reasons for use" included: (1) increased sexual arousal; (2) more intense attraction toward their partners; and (3) increased openness to having sexual intercourse with strangers. This general use of drugs and substances of abuse to enhance/facilitate sexual experiences is often referred to as "chemsex" (aka "party and play" [PNP]).

Additionally, as noted by Purcell (2017):

> Recreational GHB use has increased due to its popularity in "chemsex" circles. Users claim it has the euphoric effects of alcohol without a hangover, heightening sexual arousal and lowering inhibitions.
>
> (p. 1)

72 GHB, in powder form or solution, may be added to a container of bottled water while attending a rave or mixed into an alcoholic beverage at a circuit party or dance club. It also may be relatively easily, secretly mixed into another person's drink at a bar or mixed into a punch bowl at a social gathering (e.g., frat house party; post game celebration).

"date rape").[73] In this context of use, GHB provides the perpetrator with a means of coercion in an opportunistic situation. For some of these perpetrators, it also satisfies a peculiar paraphilia—a preference for sexual partners who are unconscious (Carey, 2014).

> Mischa Baron, who starred as Marissa Cooper on [the] popular teen drama, The O.C., says she was hospitalized after being drugged with GHB while celebrating her birthday.
>
> (Purcell, 2017, p. 1)

> Abbotsford police are investigating a suspicious case involving two teenage girls who may have ingested GHB (Gamma Hydroxybutyrate), also known as the date rape drug. On Sunday, July 31, a 16-year-old girl had been found wandering alone by some good Samaritans, who then managed to get her to her home. The girl had gone out with her 14-year-old friend earlier in the evening but the two had become separated. One of the 16-year-old's parents found the 14-year-old girl nearby. She also appeared intoxicated and showed symptoms of consuming GHB.
>
> (Judd, 2016, p. 1)

Related Professional Reminder:[74] ***In order to prevent/minimize drug-acquaintance/date rape associated with the use of GHB, we recommend that mental health care professionals, as well as parents and teachers, educate and encourage adolescents and young adults to:***

- ***Avoid going to a bar, party, or rave alone;***
- ***Always carry extra cash for a taxicab;***
- ***Avoid communal drinks (e.g., from a large punchbowl at a "frat" party);***
- ***Avoid the excessive use of alcohol and other drugs and substances of abuse (e.g., don't go out with the deliberate intention to become intoxicated [i.e., drunk; hammered; wasted]).***

And:

- ***Don't take drinks from others, particularly strangers;***
- ***Don't share or exchange drinks;***
- ***Open containers yourself (i.e., don't accept open drinks);***
- ***Watch your drink being poured or mixed at a bar or party;***
- ***Don't leave your drink unattended (if you do, then discard it upon your return);***
- ***If you need to go to the bathroom, take your drink with you (if you can't, then leave it with a trusted friend or simply discard the drink);***
- ***Cover your drink with your hand;***
- ***Don't drink anything that tastes, looks, or smells odd (e.g., don't consume your drink if it tastes salty or appears to have changed color);***
- ***If you feel drunk (e.g., dizzy, lightheaded, nauseous) after consuming only a small amount of alcohol, then seek help right away (e.g., contact a friend, waiter, or bartender and request their assistance getting a taxicab to go home—or to an ED if feeling seriously ill).***

73 Generally used in combination with alcohol for this purpose. Intended victims lose their ability to fend off their assailant and, because of GHB-induced amnesia, become unreliable witnesses if formal, legal charges are brought against the assailant.

74 Drinks in the context of these recommendations apply to all beverages—alcoholic and non-alcoholic (e.g., juices; soda pop).

BISEXUAL AND GAY ADOLESCENT BOYS AND YOUNG MEN. Another population group that is associated with extremely high GHB use is bisexual and gay adolescent boys and young men, regardless of continental descent. In fact, GHB is one of the five main *club drugs* (i.e., cocaine, GHB, ketamine, methamphetamine, and MDMA) commonly socially used by this population group (Pagliaro & Pagliaro, 2012). Bracchi, Stuart, and Castles (2015) noted that over half of a sample of gay adolescent boys and young men, who were HIV-positive, reported frequent concurrent use of three or more "club drugs," including GHB, in the context of "party and play" (see related discussion in Footnote #71). Consequently, GHB use, particularly in this context, has significant implications for the transmission of STDs, including HIV (e.g., Lee & Levounis, 2008; Pollard, Nadarzynski, & Llewellyn, 2017).

> I was lucky. I had fallen into a "G sleep"—a potentially fatal state of unconsciousness triggered by an overdose of the sex drug GHB—and woken up drowsy, naked and in the bed of a stranger. But I was alive, unharmed.
>
> I had met the stranger through the gay dating app, Grindr. The purpose of the hook-up was for more than merely sex, but for a "Party and Play"—a "chemsex"—session.
>
> (Collison, 2017, p. 1)

Because of the relative difficulty associated with obtaining and diverting prescription GHB (i.e., sodium oxybate [Xyrem®]) for personal use,[75] GHB is usually obtained by purchase: (1) over the internet/darknet; or (2) from street dealers, who offer, in addition to GHB, readily available precursors of GHB, y-butyrolactone (GBL) and 1,4-butanediol (BD). Once ingested, both GBL and BD are rapidly converted (T ½ = 1 minute) to GHB (Busardo & Jones, 2015). Regardless of the source, those who use GHB commonly ingest it, multiple times throughout the day until their supply is depleted and they are unable to obtain any additional GHB or GBL or BD (Miotto, Darakjian, & Basch, 2001; Pagliaro & Pagliaro, *Clinical Patient Data Files).*

In their national "Partnership Attitude Tracking Study" (PATS) survey of more than 7,000 students in the 7th through 12th grades, The Partnership for a Drug-Free America (2006) found that 4% of their participants reported use of GHB. Hopfer, Mendelson, and Van Leeuwen (2010), in their study of youth in treatment for substance abuse, found that 7% reported GHB use.

Treatment Approaches for Adolescent and Young Adult GHB Dependence or Use Disorder

Treatment approaches for adolescent and young adults who have been diagnosed with GHB dependence or use disorder require a combination of both appropriate pharmacotherapy and psychotherapy/counseling. For an overview of psychotherapy/counseling approaches, see the related discussion in the "Psychotherapy/Counseling" subsection of Chapter 1, "Alcohol."

Data concerning the pharmacotherapy of GHB use disorder (i.e., GHB detoxification/facilitated withdrawal) are limited, particularly in regard to adolescents and young adults. However, diazepam (Valium®) is generally regarded as the drug of first choice—as per alcohol withdrawal (see the earlier related discussion in the benzodiazepine pharmacology subsection, "Undesired, or Harmful, Effects and Toxicities—Benzodiazepine Withdrawal Syndrome"). Surprisingly, regardless of treatment approach, consensus has not been reached concerning the optimal treatment settings for GHB treatment.

For example, Bell and Collins (2011) suggest the use of a "specialist out-patient clinic and affiliated in-patient detoxification unit" (p. 442). While others (e.g., Zepf, 2011; Zepf,

75 See earlier reference to, and brief discussion of, the "Xyrem REMS Program."

Holtmann, & Duketis, 2009) suggest "in-patient care" (p. 448). Considering the "immaturity" of adolescents and young adults, problems with achieving adequate monitoring and follow-up, and the potential for serious unexpected sequelae (e.g., delirium)—we generally recommend that planned GHB withdrawal, or detoxification for GHB dependence or use disorder, be conducted, for both adolescents and young adults, on an inpatient basis.

References

Abramowicz, M. (2014). Lowering the dose of Lunesta. *The Medical Letter on Drugs and Therapeutics, 56*(1444), 48.

Agarwal, S. D., & Landon, B. E. (2019, January 25). Patterns in outpatient benzodiazepine prescribing in the United States. *JAMA Network Open, 2*(1 e187399) 1–11. doi:10.1001/jamanetworkopen.2018.7399

Atack, J. R. (2005). The benzodiazepine binding site of GABAA receptors as a target for the development of novel anxiolytics. *Expert Opinion on Investigational Drugs, 14*(5), 601–618. doi:10.1517/13543784.14.5.601

Babalonis, S., Lile, J. A., & Martin, C. A. (2011a). Physiological doses of progesterone potentiate the effects of triazolam in healthy, premenopausal women. *Psychopharmacology (Berl), 215*(3), 429–439. doi:10.1007/s00213

Babalonis, S., Lile, J. A., & Martin, C. A. (2011b). Progesterone effects on the discriminative stimulus, subjective and performance effects of triazolam in healthy, premenopausal women. *Behavioural Pharmacology, 22*(5-6), 441–449. doi:10.1097/FBP.0b013e32...

Barker, E. C., Puchowicz, M., & Letterio, J. (2017, August). GHB levels in breast milk of women with narcolepsy with cataplexy treated with sodium oxybate. *Sleep Medicine, 36*, 172–177. doi:10.1016/j.sleep.2017.05.008

Barker, J. C., Harris, S. L., & Dyer, J. E. (2007, June). Experiences of gamma hydroxybutyrate (GHB) ingestion: A focus group study. *Journal of Psychoactive Drugs, 39*(2), 115–129.

Bateson, A. N. (2002). Basic pharmacologic mechanisms involved in benzodiazepine tolerance and withdrawal. *Current Pharmaceutical Design, 8*(1), 5–21.

Bechtel, L. K., & Holstege, C. P. (2007, May). Criminal poisoning: Drug-facilitated sexual assault. *Emergency Medicine Clinics of North America, 25*(2), 499–525.

Belelli, D., & Lambert, J. J. (2005). Neurosteroids: Endogenous regulators of the GABAA receptor. *Nature Reviews in Neuroscience, 6*, 565–575.

Bell, J., & Collins, R. (2011). Gamma-butyrolactone (GBL) dependence and withdrawal. *Addiction, 106*(2), 442–447. doi:10.1111/j.1360-0443.2010.03145.x

Bellivier, F., Yon, L., & Luquiens, A. (2011). Suicidal attempts in bipolar disorder: Results from an observational study (EMBLEM). *Bipolar Disorders, 13*(4), 377–386.

Bennett, R., Bray, D., & Neville, M. W. (2014). Suvorexant, a dual orexin receptor antagonist for the management of insomnia. *Pharmacy and Therapeutics, 39*(4), 264–266.

Bergman, S. A. (1986, September/October). The benzodiazepine receptor. *Anesthesia Progress, 33*(5), 213–219.

Borgen, L. A., Okerholm, R., & Morrison, D. (2003). The influence of gender and food on the pharmacokinetics of sodium oxybate oral solution in healthy subjects. *Journal of Clinical Pharmacology, 43*(1), 59–65.

Borgen, L. A., Okerholm, R. A., & Lai, A. (2004). The pharmacokinetics of sodium oxybate oral solution following acute and chronic administration to narcoleptic patients. *Journal of Clinical Pharmacology, 44*(3), 253–257. doi:10.1177/0091270003262795

Born, S., Gauvin, D. V., & Mukherjee, S. (2017, June). Preclinical assessment of the abuse potential of the orexin receptor antagonist, suvorexant. *Regulatory Toxicology and Pharmacology, 86*, 181–192. doi:10.1016/j.yrtph.2017.03.006

Bourgeois, J., Elseviers, M. M., & Van Bortel, L. (2014a). Feasibility of discontinuing chronic benzodiazepine use in nursing home residents: A pilot study. *European Journal of Pharmacology, 70*(10), 1251–1260. doi:10.1007/s00228-014-1725-7

Bourgeois, J., Elseviers, M. M., & Van Bortel, L. (2014b). One-year evolution of sleep quality in older users of benzodiapines: A longitudinal cohort study in Belgian nursing home residents. *Drugs and Aging, 31*(9), 677–682. doi:10.1007/s40266-014-0203-3

Bracchi, M., Stuart, D., & Castles, R. (2015, August 24). Increasing use of 'party drugs' in people living with HIV on antiretrovirals: A concern for patient safety. *AIDS, 29*(13), 1585–1592. doi:10.1097/QAD.0000000000000786

Brailsford, A. D., Cowan, D. A., & Kieman, A. T. (2012, March). Pharmacokinetc properties of gamma-hydroxybutyrate (GHB) in whole blood, serum, and urine. *Journal of Analytical Toxicology, 36*(2), 88–95. doi:10.1093/jat/bkr023

Brennan, R., & Van Hout, M. C. (2014). Gamma-hydroxybutyrate (GHB): A scoping review of pharmacology, toxicology, motives for use, and user groups. *Journal of Psychoactive Drugs, 46*(3), 243–251. doi:10.1080/02791072.2014.921746

Brenneisen, R., Elsohly, M. A., & Murphy, T. P. (2004, November-December). Pharmacokinetics and excretion of gamma-hydroxybutyrate (GHB) in healthy subjects. *Journal of Analytical Toxicology, 28*(8), 625–630.

Brunt, T. M., Van Amsterdam, J. G., & van Den Brink, W. (2014). GHB, GBL and 1,4-BD addiction. *Current Pharmaceutical Design, 20*(25), 4076–4085.

Busardo, F. P., Bertol, E., & Mannocchi, G. (2016, August). Determination of GHB levels in breast milk and correlation with blood concentrations. *Forensic Science International*, 172–181. doi:10.1016/j.forsclint.2016.02.020

Busardo, F. P., & Jones, A. W. (2015). GHB pharmacology and toxicology: Acute intoxication, concentrations in blood and urine in forensic cases and treatment of the withdrawal syndrome. *Current Neuropharmacology, 13*(1), 47–70. doi:10.2174/1570159X13666141210215423

Cai, R., Crane, E., & Poneleit, K. (2010, June 18). Emergency department visits involving nonmedical use of selected prescription drugs – United States, 2004–2008. *MMWR, Morbidity and Mortality Weekly Report, 59*(23), 705–709.

Canham, S. L., Gallo, J. J., & Simoni-Wastila, L. (2014). Perceptions of benzodiazepine dependence among women age 65 and older. *Journal of Gerontological Social Work, 57*(8), 872–888. doi:10.1080/01634372.2014.901470

Caputo, F., Skala, K., & Mirijello, A. (2014). Sodium oxybate in the treatment of alcohol withdrawal syndrome: A randomized double-blind comparative study versus oxazepam. The GATE 1 trial. *CNS Drugs, 28*(8), 743–752. doi:10.1007/s40263-014-0183-1

Carey, B. (2014, December 8). When a rapist's weapon is a drug. *The New York Times*, 1.

Carter, L. P. (2011). Potential impact of drug effects, availability, pharmacokinetics, and screening on estimates of drugs implicated in cases of assault. *Drug Testing and Analysis, 3*(9), 586–593.

Carter, L. P., Koek, W., & France, C. P. (2009). Behavioral analyses of GHB: Receptor mechanisms. *Pharmacology & Therapeutics, 121*(1), 100–114. doi:10.1016/j.pharmthera.2008.10.003

Cassels, C. (2010, February 10). *APA Releases Proposed Draft of the DSM-5.* Retrieved from Medscape Medical News, pp. 1–4: www.medscape.com/viewarticle/716807?sssdmh=dml.588982&src=nldne&uac=144544HX

CBS News Staff. (2000, March 14). 3 teens guilty in date-rape case. *CBS News*, 1-5.

CDC, Centers for Disease Control and Prevention. (2010). Emergency department visits involving nonmedical use of selected prescription drugs – United States, 2004-2008. *MMWR, Morbidity and Mortality Weekly Report, 59*(23), 705–709.

Chitale, R. (2009, July 24). Did sleeping pills lead to alleged rape? *ABC News*, 1.

Cimolai, N. (2007). Zopiclone: Is it a pharmacologic agent for abuse? *Canadian Family Physician, 53*(12), 2124–2129.

Citrome, L. (2014). Suvorexant for insomnia: A systematic review of the efficacy and safety profile for this newly approved hypnotic - what is the number needed to treat, number needed to harm and likelihood to be helped or harmed? *International Journal of Clinical Practice, 68*(12), 1429–1441. doi:10.1111/ijcp.12568

Collison, C. (2017, July 14). My hazardous journey into the complex world of chemsex. *Mail & Guardian*. Retrieved from htps://mg.co.za/article/2017-07-14-00-my-hazardous-journey-into-the-complex-world-of-chemsex

Cox, S., Kuo, C., & Jamieson, D. J. (2011). Poisoning hospitalisations among reproductive-aged women in the USA, 1998–2006. *Injury Prevention, 17*(5), 332–337. doi:10.1136/ip.2010.029793

Crestani, F., Low, K., & Keist, R. (2001). Molecular targets for the myorelaxant action of diazepam. *Molecular Pharmacology, 59*(3), 442–445.

Cruz, H. G., Hoever, P., & Chakraborty, B. (2014). Assessment of the abuse liability of a dual orexin receptor antagonist: A crossover study of almorexant and zolpidem in recreational drug users. *CNS Drugs, 28*(4), 361–372. doi:10.1007/s40263-014-0150-x

Cubala, W. J., & Landowski, J. (2007, March 30). Seizure following sudden zolpidem withdrawal. *Progress in Neuro-Psychopharmacology and Biological Psychiatry, 31*(2), 539–540. doi:10.1016/j.pnpbp.2006.07.009

Cui, D., Cabalu, T., & Yee, K. L. (2016). In vitro and in vivo characterisation of the metabolism and disposition of suvorexant in humans. *Xenobiotica, 46*(10), 882–895. doi:10.3109/00498254.2015.1129565

Daderman, A. M., & Edman, G. (2001). Flunitrazepam abuse and personality characteristics in male forensic psychiatric patients. *Psychiatry Research, 103*(1), 27–42.

Daderman, A. M., Fredriksson, B., & Kristiansson, M. (2002). Violent behavior, impulsive decision-making, and anterograde amnesia while intoxicated with flunitrazepam and alcohol or other drugs: A case study in forensic psychiatric patients. *The Journal of the American Academy of Psychiatry and the Law, 30*(2), 238–251.

Dailey, J. H. (2015, October). *Suvorexant (Belsomra) National Drug Monograph.* Retrieved June 11, 2016, from VA BPM Services Drug Monographs, pp. 1–14: www.pbm.va.gov

Day, C. (2014, December 18). Benzodiazepines in combination with opioid pain relievers or alcohol: Greater risk of more serious ED visit outcomes. *The CBHSQ Report.*

de Zambotti, M., Goldstone, A., & Colrain, I. M. (2018, June). Insomnia disorder in adolescence: Diagnosis, impact, and treatment. *Sleep Medicine Reviews, 39*, 12–24. doi:10.1016/j.smrv.2017.06.009

Dean, L. (2016, August 25). Diazepam therapy and CYP2C19 genotype. (V. Pratt, H. McLeod, & W. Rubinstein, Eds.), *Medical Genetics Summaries*, 1–3.

Deck, G. M., Nadkarni, N., & Montouris, G. D. (2015). Congenital malformations in infants exposed to antiepileptic medications in utero at Boston Medical Center from 2003 to 2010. *Epilepsy & Behavior, 51*, 166–169. doi:10.1016/j.yebeh.2015.07.001

Dietze, P., Horyniak, D., & Agius, P. (2014). Effect of intubation for gamma-hydroxybutyric acid overdose on emergency department length of stay and hospital admission. *Academic Emergency Medicine, 21*(11), 1226–1231. doi:10.1111/acem.12516

Dooley, M., & Plosker, G. L. (2000, August). A review of its use in the treatment of insomnia. *Drugs, 60*(2), 413–445.

Dowd, S. M., Strong, M. J., & Janicak, P. G. (2002). The behavioral and cognitive effects of two benzodiazepines associated with drug-facilitated sexual assault. *Journal of Forensic Sciences, 47*(5), 1101–1107.

Drover, D., Lemmens, H., & Naidu, S. (2000). Pharmacokinetics, pharmacodynamics, and relative pharmacokinetic/pharmacodynamic profiles of zaleplon and zolpidem. *Clinical Therapeutics, 22*(12), 1443–1461.

Drover, D. R. (2004). Comparative pharmacokinetics and pharmacodynamics of short-acting hypnosedatives: Zaleplon, zolpidem and zopiclone. *Clinical Pharmacokinetics, 43*(4), 227–238. doi:10.2165/00003088-200443040-00002

Dubey, A. K., Handu, S. S., & Mediratta, P. K. (2015, April-June). Suvorexant: The first orexin receptor antagonist to treat insomnia. *Journal of Pharmacology & Therapeutics, 6*(2), 118–121. doi:10.4103/0976-500X.155496

Dyer, J. E., Roth, B., & Hyma, B. A. (2001). Gamma-hydroxybutyrate withdrawal syndrome. *Annals of Emergency Medicine, 37*(2), 147–153. doi:10.1067/mem.2001.112985

Esteban McCabe, S., & West, B. T. (2014). Medical and nonmedical use of prescription benzodiazepine anxiolytics among U.S. high school seniors. *Addictive Behaviors, 39*(5), 959–964. doi:10.1016/j.addbeh.2014.01.009

Farzampour, Z., Reimer, R. J., & Huguenard, J. (2015). Endozepines. *Advances in Pharmacology, 72*, 147–164. doi:10.1016/bs.apha.2014.10.005

FDA, Food and Drug Administration. (2019, April 30). FDA requires stronger warnings about rare but serious incidents related to certain prescription insomnia medications: Updated warnings for eszopiclone, zaleplon and zolpidem, FDA News Alert, 1–2. White Oak, Maryland: FDA.

Fernandez, C., Gimenez, F., & Thuillier, A. (1999, January). Stereoselective binding of zopiclone to human plasma proteins. *Chirality*. doi:10.1002/(SICI)1520-636X(1999)11

Fernandez, C., Maradeix, V., & Gimenez, F. (1993, November-December). Pharmacokinetics of zopiclone and its enantiomers in Caucasian young healthy volunteers. *Drug Metabolism and Disposition, 21*(6), 1125–1128.

Fernandez, C., Martin, C., & Gimenez, F. (1995, December). Clinical pharmacokinetics of zopiclone. *Clinical Pharmacokinetics, 29*(6), 431–441. doi:10.2165/00003088-199529060-00004

Forrester, M. B. (2006). Flunitrazepam abuse and malicious use in Texas, 1998–2003. *Substance Use & Misuse, 41*(3), 427–439.

Forrester, M. B. (2007). Eszopiclone ingestions reported to Texas poison control centers, 2005–2006. *Human & Experimental Toxicology, 26*(10), 795–800.

Forrester, M. B. (2009a). Immediate- and controlled-release zolpidem ingestions reported to Texas poison centers. *Human & Experimental Toxicology, 28*(8), 505–509. doi:10.1177/0960327109106971

Forrester, M. B. (2009b). Pattern of pediatric zolpidem ingestion reported to Texas poison control centers, 2000 to 2006. *Pediatric Emergency Care, 25*(1), 26–30. doi:10.1097/PEC.0b013e318191db3f

Forrester, M. B. (2011). Ingestions of hydrocodone, carisoprodol, and alprazolam in combination reported to Texas poison centers. *Journal of Addictive Diseases, 30*(2), 110–115. doi:10.1080/10550887.2011.554778

Galloway, G. P., Frederick, S. L., & Staggers, F. E. (1997). Gamma-hydroxybutyrate: An emerging drug of abuse that causes physical dependence. *Addiction, 92*(1), 89–96.

Garzone, P. D., & Kroboth, P. D. (1989, June). Pharmacokinetics of the newer benzodiazepines. *Clinical Pharmacokinetics, 16*(6), 337–364.

Gauld, A. R. (2016, June 15). Suvorexant (Belsomra) for insomnia. *American Family Physician, 93*(12), 1016–1020.

Gautam, L., Sharratt, S. D., & Cole, M. D. (2014). Drug facilitated sexual assault: Detection and stability of benzodiazepines in spiked drinks using gas chromatography-mass spectrometry. *PLoS One, 9*(2), e89031. doi:10.1371/journal.pone.0089031

Ghio, L., Cervetti, A., & Respino, M. (2014, July). Management and treatment of gamma butyrolactone withdrawal syndrome: A case report and review. *Journal of Psychiatric Practice, 20*(4), 294–300. doi:10.1097/01.pra.0000452567.84825.07

Grela, A., Gautam, L., & Cole, M. D. (2018, November). A multifactorial critical appraisal of substances found in drug facilitated sexual assault cases. *Forensic Science International, 292*, 50–60. doi:10.1016/j.forsciint.2018.08.034

Gresham, C. (2018, June 13). Benzodiazepine toxicity. *Medscape*, 1–5.

Griffin, C. E., Kaye, A. M., & Rivera Bueno, F. (2013, Summer). Benzodiazepine pharmacology and central nervous system-mediated effects. *The Ochsner Journal, 13*(2), 214–223.

Gunja, N. (2013a). In the Zzz Zone: The effects of Z-drugs on human performance and driving. *Journal of Medicine and Toxicology, 9*, 163–171. doi:10.1007/s13181-013-0294-y

Gunja, N. (2013b, June). The clinical and forensic toxicology of z-drugs. *Journal of Medical Toxicology, 9*(2), 155–162. doi:10.1007/s13181-013-0292-0

Hajak, G., Muller, W. E., & Wittchen, H. U. (2003). Abuse and dependence potential for the non-benzodiazepine hypnotics zolpidem and zopiclone: A review of case reports and epidemiological data. *Addiction, 98*(10), 1371–1378.

Holbrook, A. M., Crowther, R., & Lotter, A. (1999). Meta-Analysis of benzodiazepine use in the treatment of acute alcohol withdrawal. *CMAJ, Canadian Medical Association Journal, 169*(5), 649–655.

Holm, K. J., & Goa, K. L. (2000). Zolpidem: An update of its pharmacology, therapeutic efficacy and tolerability in the treatment of insomnia. *Drugs, 59*(4), 865–889.

Hood, S. D., Norman, A., & Hince, D. A. (2014). Benzodiazepine dependence and its treatment with low dose flumazenil. *British Journal of Clinical Pharmacology*, 77(2), 285–294. doi:10.1111/bcp.12023

Hopfer, C., Mendelson, B., & Van Leeuwen, J. M. (2010). Club drug use among youths in treatment for substance abuse. *The American Journal on Addictions, 15*(1). doi:10.1080/10550490500419144

Hopkins, C. R. (2012). ACS chemical neuroscience molecule spotlight on suvorexant. *ACS Cheimcal Neuroscience, 3*, 647–648. doi:10.1021/cn300086a

Hosie, A. M., Wilkins, M. E., & Da Silva, H. (2006, November 23). Endogenous neurosteroids regulate GABAA receptors through two discrete transmembrane sites. *Nature, 444*, 486–489.

Hoyer, D., & Jacobson, L. H. (2013). Orexin in sleep, addiction and more: Is the perfect insomnia drug at hand? *Neuropeptides*, 47(6), 477–488. doi:10.1016/j.npep.2013.10.009

Huedo-Medina, T. B., Kirsch, I., & Middlemass, J. (2012). Effectiveness of non-benzodiazepine hypnotics in treatment of adult insomnia: Meta-Analysis of data submitted to the Food and Drug Administration. *BMJ, 345*, 1–13. doi:10.1136/bmj.e8343

Hypnotic dependence: Zolpidem and zopiclone too. (2001, February). *Prescrire International, 10*(51), 15.

Ibanez, G. E., Levi-Minzi, M. A., & Rigg, K. K. (2013). Diversion of benzodiazepines through healthcare sources. *Journal of Psychoactive Drugs, 45*(1), 48–56.

Jacobson, L. H., Callander, G. E., & Hoyer, D. (2014). Suvorexant for the treatment of insomnia. *Expert Review of Clinical Pharmacology*, 7(6), 711–730. doi:10.1586/17512433.2014.966813

Johnston, L. D., O'Malley, P. M., & Bachman, J. G. (2008). *Monitoring the Future: National Survey Results on Drug Use, 1975–2008*. Bethesda, MD: National Institute on Drug Abuse.

Jones, A. W., Eklund, A., & Kronstrand, R. (2009, July-August). Concentration-time profiles of gamma-hydroxybutyrate in blood after recreational doses are best described by zero-order rather than first-order kinetics. *Journal of Analytical Toxicology, 33*(6), 332–335.

Jones, C. M., & McAninch, J. K. (2015). Emergency department visits and overdose deaths from combined use of opioids and benzodiazepines. *American Journal of Preventive Medicine, 49*(4), 493–501.

Jones, C. M., Paulozzi, L. J., & Mack, K. A. (2014). Alcohol involvement in opioid pain reliever and benzodiazepine drug abuse–Related emergency department visits and drug-related deaths–United States, 2010. *Morbidity and Mortality Weekly Report (MMWR), 63*(40), 881–885.

Jones, R., Prommer, E., & Backstedt, D. (2016). Naloxegol: A novel therapy in the management of opioid-induced constipation. *American Journal of Hospice Palliative Care, 33*(9), 875–880.

Judd, A. (2014, October 27). 3 people rushed to hospital after intentionally taking 'date rape' drug, GHB. *Global News Online*. Shaw Media. Retrieved November 1, 2016, from http://globalnews.ca/news/1638045/3-people-rushed-to-hospital-after-intentionally-taking-date-rape-drug-ghb/

Judd, A. (2015, June 22). 3 Abbotsford teens in serious condition after overdosing on GHB. *Global News Online*. Shaw Media. Retrieved November 1, 2016, from http://globalnews.ca/news/2068211/3-abbotsford-teens-in-serious-condition-after-overdosing-on-ghb/

Judd, A. (2016, July 31). Two Abbotsford teens allegedly given date rape drug. *Global News*.

Kamal, R. M., van Noorden, M. S., & Franzek, E. (2016). The neurobiological mechanisms of gamma-hydroxybutyrate dependence and withdrawal and their clinical relevance: A review. *Neuropsychobiology, 73*, 65–80. doi:10.1159/000443173

Kapitany-Foveny, M., Mervo, B., & Corazza, O. (2015). Enhancing sexual desire and experience: An investigation of the sexual correlates of gamma-hydroxybutyrate (GHB) use. *Human Psychopharmacology, 30*(4), 276–284. doi:10.1002/hup.2491

Kaufmann, C. N., Spira, A. P., & Alexander, G. C. (2017). Emergency department visits involving benzodiazepines and non-benzodiazepine receptor agonists. *The American Journal of Emergency Medicine, 35*(10), 1414–1419. doi:10.1016/j.ajem.2017.04.023

Kawabe, K., Horiuchi, F., & Ochi, M. (2017). Suvorexant for the treatment of insomnia in adolescents. *Psychopharmacology, 27*(9), 792–795. doi:10.1089/cap.2016.0206

Keating, G. M. (2014). Sodium oxybate: A review of its use in alcohol withdrawal syndrome and in the maintenance of abstinence in alcohol dependence. *Clinical Drug Investigation, 34*(1), 63–80. doi:10.1007/s40261-013-0158-x

Kishi, T., Matsunaga, S., & Iwata, N. (2015). Suvorexant for primary insomnia: A systematic review and meta-analysis of randomized placebo-controlled trials. *PLoS ONE, 10*(8), e0136910. doi:10.1371/journal.pone.0136910

Knudsen, K., Jonsson, U., & Abrahamsson, J. (2010). Twenty-three deaths with gamma-hydroxybutyrate overdose in western Sweden between 2000 and 2007. *Acta Anaesthesiologica Scandinavica, 54*(8), 987–992.

Kuntze, M. F., Bullinger, A. H., & Mueller-Spahn, F. (2002). Excessive use of zopiclone: A case report. *Swiss Medical Weekly, 132*, 523.

Kurta, D. L., Myers, L. B., & Krenzelok, E. P. (1997). Zolpidem (Ambien): A pediatric case series. *Journal of Toxicology. Clinical Toxicology*, *35*(5), 453–457.

Kurtz, S. P., Buttram, M. E., & Surratt, H. L. (2017). Benzodiazepine dependence among young adult participants in the club scene who use drugs. *Journal of Psychoactive Drugs*, *49*(1), 39–46. doi:10.1080/02791072.2016.1269978

Kurtz, S. P., Surratt, H. L., & Levi-Minzi, M. A. (2011). Benzodiazepine dependence among multidrug users in the club scene. *Drug and Alcohol Dependence*, *119*(1-2), 99–105. doi:10.1016/j,drugalcdep.2011.05.036

Lee, S. J., & Levounis, P. (2008, September). Gamma hydroxybutyrate: An ethnographic study of recreational use and abuse. *Journal of Psychoactive Drugs*, *40*(3), 245–253. doi:10.1080/02791072.2008.10400639

Lee-Iannotti, J. K., & Parish, J. M. (2016). Suvorexant: A promising, novel treatment for insomnia. *Neuropsychiatric Disease and Treatment*, *12*, 491–495. doi:10.2147/NDT.S31495

Lekka, N. P., Paschalis, C., & Beratis, S. (2002). Suicide attempts in high-dose benzodiazepine users. *Comprehensive Psychiatry*, *43*(6), 438–442.

Leone, M. A., Vigna-Taglianti, F., & Avanzi, G. (2010, February, 17). Gamma-hydroxybutyrate (GHB) for treatment of alcohol withdrawal and prevention of relapses. *Cochrane Database of Systematic Reviews* (2), CD006266. doi:10.1002/14651858.CD006266.pub2

Liechti, M. E., Quednow, B. B., & Liakoni, E. (2016). Pharmacokinetics and phamacodynamics of gamma-hydroxybutyrate in healthy subjects. *British Journal of Clinical Pharmacology*, *81*(5), 980–988. doi:10.1111/bcp.12863

Lin, S. K. (2014, July). Rapid detoxification of benzodiazepine or Z-drugs dependence using acetylcholinesterase inhibitors. *Medical Hypotheses*, *83*(1), 108–110. doi:10.1016/j.mehy.2014.03.032

Lind, J. N., Petersen, E. E., & Lederer, P. A. (2015). Infant and maternal characteristics in neonatal abstinence syndrome–Selected hospitals in Florida, 2010–2011. *MMWR, Morbidity and Mortality Weekly Report*, *64*(8), 213–216.

Madea, B., & MuBhoff, F. (2009). Knock-out drugs: Their prevalence, modes of action, and means of detection. *Deutsches Azteblatt International*, *106*(20), 341–347.

Madrak, L. N., & Rosenberg, M. (2001, August 1). Zolpidem abuse. *The American Journal of Psychiatry*, 1330. doi:10.1176/appi.ajp.158.8.1330-a

Marinetti, L., & Montgomery, M. A. (2010). The use of GHB to facilitate sexual assault. *Forensic Science Review*, *22*(1), 41–59.

Mason, P. E., & Kerns, W. P. (2002). Gamma hydroxybutyric acid (GHB) intoxication. *Academic Emergency Medicine*, *9* (7), 730–739.

Matheson, I., Sande, H. A., & Gaillot, J. (1990, August). The excretion of zopiclone into breast milk. *British Journal of Clinical Pharmacology*, *30*(2), 267–271.

Mattoo, S. K., Gaur, N., & Das, P. P. (2011, November-December). Zolpidem withdrawal delirium. *Indian Journal of Pharmacology*, *43*(6), 729–730. doi:10.4103/0253-7613.89838

McDonough, M., Kennedy, N., & Glasper, A. (2004, July 15). Clinical features and management of gamma-hydroxybutyrate (GHB) withdrawal: A review. *Drug and Alcohol Dependence*, *75*(1), 3–9. doi:10.1016/j. drugalcdep.2004.01.012

McElhatton, P. R. (1994, November-December). The effects of benzodeiazepdine use during pregnancy and lactation. *Reproductive Toxicology*, *8*(6), 461–475.

Michelson, D., Snyder, E., & Paradis, E. (2014). Safety and efficacy of suvorexant during 1-year treatment of insomnia with subsequent abrupt treatment discontinuation: A phase 3 randomised, double-blind, placebo-controlled trial. *Lancet Neurology*, *13*(5), 461–471. doi:10.1016/S1474-4422(14)70053-5

Miotto, K., Darakjian, J., & Basch, J. (2001). Gamma-hydroxybutyric acid: Patterns of use, effects and withdrawal. *The American Journal on Addictions*, *10*(3), 232–241.

Morinan, A., & Keaney, F. (2010). Long-term misuse of zopiclone in an alcohol dependent woman with a history of anorexia nervosa: A case report. *Journal of Medical Case Reports*, *4*, 403–408.

Najib, J. (2006). Eszopiclone, a nonbenzodiazepine sedative-hypnotic agent for the treatment of transient and chronic insomnia. *Clinical Therapeutics*, *28*(4), 491–516. doi:10.1016/j.clinthera.2006.04.014

National Drug Intelligence Center. (2004, September). GHB trafficking and abuse. *Intelligence Bulletin*. U.S. Department of Justice.

NIDA. (2008, August). *Club Drugs (GHB, Ketamine, and Rohypnol)*. Retrieved from NIDA InfoFacts, pp. 1–3.

Ninan, P. T. (2001). Pharmacokinetically induced benzodiazepine withdrawal. *Psychopharmacology Bulletin*, *35*(4), 94–100.

Nutt, D. J., & Malizia, A. L. (2001). New insights into the role of the GABAA-benzodiazepine receptor in psychiatric disorder. *British Journal of Psychiatry*, *179*, 390–396.

O'Brien, C. P. (2005). Benzodiazepine use, abuse, and dependence. *Journal of Clinical Psychiatry*, *66*(Supplement 2), 28–33.

O'Brien, M. P. (2008, June). Epidemiological trends in drug abuse. *Proceedings of the Community Epidemiology Work Group. Volume 1: Highlights and Executive Summary*. Bethesda, Maryland: National Institute on Drug Abuse, US Department of Health and Human Services.

Okun, M. L., Ebert, R., & Saini, B. (2015). A review of sleep-promoting medications used in pregnancy. *American Journal of Obstetrics and Gynecology*, *212*(4), 428–441. doi:10.1016/j.ajog.2014.10.1106

Okun, M. S., Boothby, L. A., & Bartfield, R. B. (2001). GHB: An important pharmaologic and clinical update. *Journal of Pharmacy and Pharmaceutical Sciences*, *4*(2), 167–175.

Ornoy, A., Arnon, J., & Shechtman, S. (1998, September-October). Is benzodiazepine use during pregnancy really teratogenic? *Reproductive Toxicology*, *12*(5), 511–515.

Owen, R. T. (2016). Suvorexant: Efficacy and safety profile of a dual orexin receptor antagonist in treating insomnia. *Drugs of Today (barcelona, Spain)*, *52*(1), 29–40. doi:10.1358/dot.2016.52.1.2439940

Owens, J. A., Babcock, D., & Blumer, J. (2005). The use of pharmacotherapy in the treatment of pediatric insomnia in primary care: Rational approaches. A consensus meeting summary. *Journal of Clinical Sleep Medicine*, *1*(1), 49–59.

Owens, J. A., & Moturi, S. (2009, October). Pharmacologic treatment of pediatric insomnia. *Child and Adolescent Psychiatric Clinics of North America*, *18*(4), 1001–1016. doi:10.1016/j.chc.2009.04.009

Owens, J. A., Rosen, C. L., & Mindell, J. A. (2003). Medication use in the treatment of pediatric insomnia: Results of a survey of community-based pediatricians. *Pediatrics*, *111*(5), e628-e635.

Pagliaro, A. M., & Pagliaro, L. A. (2018). *Women's Drug and Substance Abuse: A Comprehensive Analysis and Reflective Synthesis*. New York: Routledge.

Pagliaro, L. A., & Levin, R. H. (Eds.). (1979). *Problems in Pediatric Drug Therapy* (1st ed.). Hamilton, Illinois: Drug Intelligence Publications.

Pagliaro, L. A., & Pagliaro, A. M. (1983). *Pharmacologic Aspects of Aging*. St. Louis, MO: C.V. Mosby.

Pagliaro, L. A. (1988). "V" is for valium. *Let's Talk*, *13*(August), 8–9.

Pagliaro, L. A., & Pagliaro, A. M. (1991). Drug induced automatism: Psychological aspects. *Canadian Psychology*, *32*, 204.

Pagliaro, L. A. (1993). The straight dope: Mother's little helper … The benzodiazepines. *Psynopsis*, *15*(1), 8.

Pagliaro, A. M., & Pagliaro, L. A. (1997). Teratogenic effects of in utero exposure to alcohol and other abusable psychotropics. Chapter 2 in P. Budetti & M. Haack (eds.), *Drug-Dependent Mothers and Their Children: Issues in Public Policy and Public Health* (pp. 31–63). New York, NY: Springer.

Pagliaro, L. A., & Pagliaro, A. M. (1998). *The Pharmacological Basis of Psychotherapeutics: An Introduction for Psychologists*. Washington, DC: Brunner/Mazel.

Pagliaro, L. A., & Pagliaro, A. M. (1999). *PPDR: Psychologists' Psychotropic Drug Reference*. Philadelphia, PA: Brunner/ Mazel.

Pagliaro, L. A., & Pagliaro, A. M. (Eds.). (2002). *Problems in Pediatric Drug Therapy* (4th ed.). Washington, DC: American Pharmaceutical Association.

Pagliaro, L. A., & Pagliaro, A. M. (2004). *Pagliaros' Comprehensive Guide to Drugs and Substances of Abuse* (1st ed.). Washington, DC: American Pharmacists Association.

Pagliaro, L. A., & Pagliaro, A. M. (2009). *Pagliaros' Comprehensive Guide to Drugs and Substances of Abuse* (2nd ed.). Washington, DC: American Pharmacists Association.

Pagliaro, L. A., & Pagliaro, A. M. (2012). *Handbook of Child and Adolescent Drug and Substance Abuse: Pharmacological, Developmental, and Clinical Considerations*. Hoboken, NJ: John Wiley & Sons.

Partnership for a Drug-Free America. (2006, May 17). Key findings of: 18th annual Partnership Attitude Tracking Study on Teen Drug Abuse 2005. *Press Release*, 1–2. Partnership for a Drug-Free America.

Patel, K. V., Aspesi, A. V., & Evoy, K. E. (2015). Suvorexant: A dual orexin receptor antagonist for the treatment of sleep onset and sleep maintenance insomnia. *Annals of Pharmacotherapy*, *49*(4), 477–483. doi:10.1177/ 1060028015570467

Placement of gamma-butyrolactone in List I of the Controlled Substances Act (21 U.S.C. 802934). (2000, April 24). Drug Enforcement Administration, Justice. Final rule. *Fed Regist*, *65*(79), 21645–21647.

Pollard, A., Nadarzynski, T., & Llewellyn, C. (2017). Syndemics of stigma, minority-stress, maladaptive coping, risk environments and littoral spaces among men who have sex with men using chemsex. *Culture, Health & Sexuality*, 20(4), 411–427. doi:10.1080/13691058.2017.13507

Preidt, R. (2014, May 22). *Sharp rise in ER visits tied to abuse of sedative, study finds*. Retrieved June 28, 2014, from U.S. News and World Report, pp. 1–2: http://health.usnews.com/health-news/articles/2014/05/22/sharp-rise-in-er-visits-tied-to-ab..

Pressman, M. R. (2011). Sleep driving: Sleepwalking variant or misuse of z-drugs? *Sleep Medicine Review*, *15*(5), 285–292. doi:10.1016/j.smrv.2010.12.004

Purcell, C. (2017, February 2). Everything you need to know about the 'date rape drug' that caused Misca Barton to be hospitalized. *Business Insider*, 1. Mic.

Ramah, A. J., Todorovic, M. M., & Crnic, K. B. (2015). Flumazenil in treatment benzodiazepine withdrawal syndrome: Case report. *Hospital Pharmacology*, *2*(2), 261–265.

Reddy, A., Puvvada, S. C., & Kommisetti, S. (2015). Suvorexant: Something new for sleep? *Acta Neuropsychiatrica*, *27* (1), 53–55. doi:10.1017/neu.2014.31

Rush, C. R., Frey, J. M., & Griffiths, R. R. (1999, August). Zaleplon and triazolam in humans: Acute behavioral effects and abuse potential. *Psychopharmacology*, *145*, 39–51.

Salomone, A., Gerace, E., & DiCorcia, D. (2012). Hair analysis of drugs involved in drug-facilitated sexual assault and detection of zolpidem in a suspected case. *International Journal of Legal Medicine, 126*, 451–459. doi:10.1007/s00414-011-0597-y

Salva, P., & Costa, J. (1995, September). Clinical pharmacokinetics and pharmacodynamics of zolpidem. Therapeutic implications. *Clinical Pharmacokinetics, 29*(3), 142–153. doi:10.2165/00003088-199529030-00002

Schep, L. J., Knudsen, K., & Slaughter, R. J. (2012, July). The clinical toxicology of gamma-hydroxybutyrate, gamma-butyrolactone and 1,4-butanediol. *Clinical Toxicology, 50*(6), 458–470. doi:10.3109/15563650.2012.702218

Schifano, F, Chiappini, S., & Corkery, J. M. (2019, April). An insight into z-drug abuse and dependence: An examination of reports to the European Medicines Agency Database of suspected adverse drug reactions. *International Journal of Neuropsychopharmacology, 22*(4), 270–277.

Schmitz, A. (2016). Benzodiazepine use, misuse, and abuse: A review. *Mental Health Clinician, 6*(3), 120–126. doi:10.9740/mhc.2016.05.120

Schoedel, K. A., Sun, H., & Sellers, D. M. (2016, August). Assessment of the abuse potential of the orexin receptor antagonist, suvorexant, compared with zolpidem in a randomized crossover study. *Journal of Clinical Psychopharmacology, 36*(4), 314–323. doi:10.1097/JCP.0000000000000516

Schrotenboer, B. (2014, March 26). Darren Sharper case spotlights sleep drug's dark side. *USA Today*, 1–5.

Sharp, M. J., & Melnik, T. A. (2015, April 17). Poisoning deaths involving opioid analgesics - New York State, 2003–2013. *MMWR, Morbidity and Mortality Weekly Report, 64*(14), 377–380.

Sieghart, W. (1994). Pharmacology of benzodiazepine receptors: An update. *Journal of Psychiatry & Neuroscience, 19*(1), 24–29.

Sigel, E., & Steinmann, M. E. (2012, November 23). Structure, function, and modulation of GABAA receptors. *Journal of Biological Chemistry, 287*(48), 40224–40231. doi:10.1074/jbc.R112.386664

Sikdar, S. (1998). Physical dependence on zopiclone. *BMJ, 317*, 146. doi:10.1136/bmj.317.7151.146

Sivilotti, M. L., Burns, M. J., & Aaron, C. K. (2001, December). Pentobarbital for severe gamma-butyrolactone withdrawal. *Annals of Emergency Medicine, 38*(6), 660–665. doi:10.1067/mem.2001.119454

Skala, K., Caputo, F., & Mirijello, A. (2014). Sodium oxybate in the treatment of alcohol dependence: From the alcohol withdrawal syndrome to the alcohol relapse prevention. *Expert Opinion on Pharmacotherapy, 15*(2), 245–257. doi:10.1517/14656566.2014.863278

Suarez Sang, L. (2018, January 4). Teenage girl, 16, was held captive, raped and had her head shaved in 'torture chamber', police say. *Fox News*, 1–3. Retrieved from www.foxnews/us/2018/01/04/teenage-girl-16-was-held-captive-raped-and-had-her-head-shaved-in-torture-chamber-police-say.html

Sutton, E. L. (2015). Profile of suvorexant in the management of insomnia. *Drug Design, Development and Therapy, 9*, 6035–6042. doi:10.2147/DDDT.S73224

Sweeney, J., Laoire, F. O., & Linehan, G. (2015). A review of potentially inappropriate prescribing in over 65's in Livinghealth Clinic. *IMJ, Irish Medical Journal, 108*(6), 180–181.

Tanaka, E. (2002). Toxicological interactions between alcohol and benzodiazepines. *Journal of Toxicology. Clinical Toxicology, 40*(1), 69–75.

Tarabar, A. F., & Nelson, L. S. (2004). The gamma-hydroxybutyrate withdrawal syndrome. *Toxicology Reviews, 23*(1), 45–49.

Tunnicliff, G. (1997). Sites of action of gamma-hydroxybutyrate (GHB) – A neuroactive drug with abuse potential. *Journal of Toxicology: Clinical Toxicology, 35*(6), 581–590. doi:10.3109/15563659709001236

van Strien, A. M., Koek, H. L., & van Marum, R. J. (2013). Psychotropic medications, including short acting benzodiazepines, strongly increase the frequency of falls in elderly. *Maturitas, 74*(4), 357–362. doi:10.1016/j.maturitas.2013.01.004

Vlase, L., Popa, A., & Neag, M. (2011a). Pharmacokinetic interaction between zolpidem and carbamazepine in healthy volunteers. *Journal of Clinical Pharmacology, 51*(8), 1233–1236. doi:10.1177/0091270010383690

Vlase, L., Popa, A., & Neag, M. (2011b, January). Pharmacokinetic interaction between zolpidem and ciprofloxacin in healthy volunteers. *European Journal of Drug Metabolism and Pharmacokinetics, 35*(3-4), 83–87. doi:10.1007/s13318-010-0014-9

Voaklander, D. C., Rowe, B. H., & Dryden, D. M. (2008). Medical illness, medication use and suicide in seniors: A population-based case-control study. *Journal of Epidemiology & Community Health, 62*(2), 138–146.

Wang, L. H., Lin, H. C., & Lin, C. C. (2010). Increased risk of adverse pregnancy outcomes in women receiving zolpidem during pregnancy. *Clinical Pharmacology & Therapeutics, 88*(3), 369–374. doi:10.1038/clpt.2010.97

Weaver, M. F. (2015). Prescription sedative misuse and abuse. *Yale Journal of Biology and Medicine, 88*, 247–256.

Weiss, S., & Garbutt, A. (2010, December). Pharmacotherapy in pediatric sleep disorders. *Adolescent Medicine: State of the Art Reviews, 21*(3), 508–521.

Wikner, B. N., & Kallen, B. (2011). Are hypnotic benzodiazepine receptor agonists teratogenic in humans? *Journal of Clinical Psychopharmacology, 31*(3), 356–359. doi:10.1097/JCP.0b013e3182197055

Wikner, B. N., Stiller, C. O., & Bergman, U. (2007). Use of benzodiazepines and benzodiazepine receptor agonists during pregnancy: Neonatal outcome and congenital malformations. *Pharmacoepidemiology and Drug Safety, 16* (11), 1203–1210.

Winrow, C. J., & Renger, J. J. (2014). Discovery and development of orexin receptor antagonists as therapeutics for insomnia. *British Journal of Pharmacology, 171*(2), 283–293. doi:10.1111/bph.12261

Wojtowicz, J. M., Yarema, M. C., & Wax, P. M. (2008). Withdrawl from gamma-hydroxybutyrate, 1,4-butanediol and gamma-butyrolactone: A case report and systematic review. *CJEM, 10*(1), 69–74.

Yang, L. P. (2014). Suvorexant: First global approval. *Drugs, 74*(15), 1817–1822. doi:10.1007/s40265-014-0294-5

Yen, C. F., Yen, C. N., & Ko, C. H. (2015). Correlates of dependence and beliefs about the use of hypnotics among zolpidem and zopiclone users. *Substance Use & Misuse, 50*(3), 350–357. doi:10.3109/10826084.2014.980955

Zepf, F. D. (2011). Commentary on Bell & Collins (2011): Out-patient management of gamma-hydroxybutyric acid (GHB) withdrawal – an alternative strategy for the future? *Addiction, 106*, 448.

Zepf, F. D., Holtmann, M., & Duketis, E. (2009, September). A 16-year-old boy with severe gamma-butyrolactone (GBL) withdrawal delirium. *Pharmacopsychiatry, 42*(5), 202–203. doi:10.1055/s-0029-1224163

Zosel, A., Osterberg, E. C., & Mycyk, M. B. (2011). Zolpidem misuse with other medications or alcohol frequently results in intensive care unit admission. *American Journal of Therapeutics, 18*(4), 305–308. doi:10.1097/MJT.0b013e3181d169ed

Zvosec, D. L., & Smith, S. W. (2005, May). Agitation is common in gamma-hydroxybutyrate toxicity. *The American Journal of Emergency Medicine, 23*(3), 316–320.

Zvosec, D. L., Smith, S. W., & Porrata, T. (2011). Case series of 226 y-hydroxybutyrate-associated deaths: Lethal toxicity and trauma. *The American Journal of Emergency Medicine, 29*(3), 319–332. doi:10.1016/j.ajem.2009.11.008

Index[1, 2, 3, 4, 5, 6]

1 f, followed by the figure number, indicates that the index entry is to be found within the identified figure.
2 fn, followed by the footnote number, indicates that the index entry is to be found within the identified footnote at the bottom of the identified page.
3 t, followed by the table number, indicates that the index entry is to be found within the identified table.
4 Quotation marks around a word indicate that it is a commonly used "street name" for the associated drug or substance of abuse.
5 ® indicates a registered proprietary brand/trade name.
6 Italics signifies a term that is part of the addictions argot.